QUICK LOOK DRUG BOOK

2003

Leonard L. Lance, RPh, BSPharm
Senior Editor
Pharmacist
Lexi-Comp Inc.
Hudson, Ohio

Charles F. Lacy, PharmD, FCSHP
Editor
Facilitative Officer, Clinical Programs and Business Affairs
Nevada College of Pharmacy
Coordinator of Clinical Services
Department of Pharmacy
Cedars-Sinai Health System
Los Angeles, California

Morton P. Goldman, PharmD, BCPS
Associate Editor
Assistant Director, Pharmacotherapy Services
Department of Pharmacy
Cleveland Clinic Foundation
Cleveland, Ohio

Lora L. Armstrong, PharmD, BCPS
Associate Editor
Manager, Clinical Services
Caremark Rx, Inc.
Northbrook, Illinois

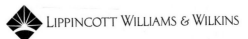

LIPPINCOTT WILLIAMS & WILKINS

Philadelphia • Baltimore • New York • London
Buenos Aires • Hong Kong • Sydney • Tokyo

QUICK LOOK DRUG BOOK

2003

Leonard L. Lance, RPh, BSPharm
Senior Editor
Pharmacist
Lexi-Comp, Inc.
Hudson, Ohio

Charles F. Lacy, PharmD, FCSHP
Editor
Facilitative Officer, Clinical Programs
Professor, Pharmacy Practice
Nevada College of Pharmacy
Las Vegas, Nevada

Morton P. Goldman, PharmD, BCPS
Associate Editor
Assistant Director, Pharmacotherapy Services
Department of Pharmacy
Cleveland Clinic Foundation
Cleveland, Ohio

Lora L. Armstrong, PharmD, BCPS
Associate Editor
Manager, Clinical Services
Caremark Rx, Inc.
Northbrook, Illinois

NOTICE

This handbook is intended to serve the user as a handy quick reference and not as a complete drug information resource. It does not include information on every therapeutic agent available. The publication covers 1578 commonly used drugs and is specifically designed to present certain important aspects of drug data in a more concise format than is generally found in medical literature or product material supplied by manufacturers.

Although great care was taken to ensure the accuracy of the handbook's content when it went to press, the editors, contributors, and publisher cannot be responsible for the continued accuracy of the supplied information due to ongoing research and new developments in the field. Further, the *Quick Look Drug Book* is not offered as a guide to dosing. The reader, herewith, is advised that information shown under the heading **Usual Dosage** is provided only as an indication of the amount of the drug typically given or taken during therapy. Actual dosing amount for any specific drug should be based on an in-depth evaluation of the individual patient's therapy requirement and strong consideration given to such issues as contraindications, warnings, precautions, adverse reactions, along with the interaction of other drugs. The manufacturers' most current product information or other standard recognized references should always be consulted for such detailed information prior to drug use.

The editors and contributors have written this book in their private capacities. No official support or endorsement by any federal agency or pharmaceutical company is intended or inferred.

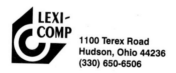

LEXI-COMP

1100 Terex Road
Hudson, Ohio 44236
(330) 650-6506

TABLE OF CONTENTS

ABOUT THE AUTHORS

Leonard L. Lance, RPh, BSPharm

Leonard L. (Bud) Lance has been directly involved in the pharmaceutical industry since receiving his bachelor's degree in pharmacy from Ohio Northern University in 1970. Upon graduation from ONU, Mr Lance spent four years as a navy pharmacist in various military assignments and was instrumental in the development and operation of the first whole hospital I.V. admixture program in a military (Portsmouth Naval Hospital) facility.

After completing his military service, he entered the retail pharmacy field and has managed both an independent and a home I.V. franchise pharmacy operation. Since the late 1970s, Mr Lance has focused much of his interest on using computers to improve pharmacy service. The independent pharmacy he worked for was the first retail pharmacy in the State of Ohio to computerize (1977).

His love for computers and pharmacy led him to Lexi-Comp, Inc. in 1988. He developed Lexi-Comp's first drug database in 1989 and was involved in the editing and publishing of Lexi-Comp's first *Drug Information Handbook* in 1990.

As a result of his strong publishing interest, he serves in the capacity of pharmacy editor and technical advisor as well as pharmacy (information) database coordinator for Lexi-Comp. Along with the *Quick Look Drug Book*, he provides technical support to Lexi-Comp's *Drug Information Handbook for the Allied Health Professional*, and many other titles published by Lexi-Comp, Inc. Mr Lance has also assisted approximately 200 major hospitals in producing their own formulary (pharmacy) publications through Lexi-Comp's custom publishing service.

Mr Lance is a member and past president (1984) of the Summit Pharmaceutical Association (SPA). He is also a member of the Ohio Pharmacists Association (OPA), the American Pharmaceutical Association (APhA), and the American Society of Health-System Pharmacists (ASHP).

Charles F. Lacy, PharmD, FCSHP

Dr Lacy is the Facilitative Officer for Clinical Programs and Professor of Pharmacy Practice at the Nevada College of Pharmacy. In his current capacity, Dr Lacy oversees the clinical curriculum, clinical faculty activities, the computer information systems, student experiential programs, pharmacy residency programs, continuing education programs, entrepreneurial activities, and all of the drug information needs for the college. Prior to coming to the Nevada College of Pharmacy, Dr Lacy was the Clinical Coordinator for the Department of Pharmacy at Cedars-Sinai Medical Center. With over 19 years of clinical experience at one of the nation's largest teaching hospitals, he has developed a reputation as an acknowledged expert in drug information and critical care drug therapy.

Dr Lacy received his doctorate from the University of Southern California School of Pharmacy and still works with the University as a member of their alumni board to advance the curriculum of pharmacy students in the Southern California area.

Presently, Dr Lacy holds teaching affiliations with the Nevada College of Pharmacy, the University of Southern California School of Pharmacy, the University of California at San Francisco School of Pharmacy, the University of the Pacific School of Pharmacy, Western University of Health Sciences School of Pharmacy, and the University of Alberta at Edmonton, School of Pharmacy and Health Sciences.

Dr Lacy is an active member of numerous professional associations including the American Society of Health-System Pharmacists (ASHP), the American College of Clinical Pharmacy (ACCP), the American Society of Consultant Pharmacists (ASCP), the American Association of Colleges of Pharmacy (AACP), American Pharmaceutical Association (APhA), the Nevada Pharmacy Alliance (NPA), and the California Society of Hospital Pharmacists (CSHP), through which he has chaired many committees and subcommittees.

Morton P. Goldman, PharmD, BCPS

Dr Goldman received his bachelor's degree in pharmacy from the University of Pittsburgh, College of Pharmacy and his Doctor of Pharmacy degree from the University of Cincinnati, Division of Graduate Studies and Research. He completed his concurrent 2-year hospital pharmacy residency at the V.A. Medical Center in Cincinnati. Dr Goldman is presently the Assistant Director of Pharmacotherapy Services for the Department of Pharmacy at the Cleveland Clinic Foundation (CCF) after having spent over 4 years at CCF as an Infectious Disease pharmacist and 4 years as Clinical Manager. He holds faculty appointments from Case Western Reserve University, College of Medicine and The University of Toledo. Dr Goldman is a Board-Certified Pharmacotherapy Specialist (BCPS) with added qualifications in infectious diseases.

In his capacity as Assistant Director of Pharmacotherapy Services at CCF, Dr Goldman remains actively involved in patient care and clinical research with the Department of Infectious Disease, as well as the continuing education of the medical and pharmacy staff. He is an editor of CCF's *Guidelines for Antibiotic Use* and participates in their annual Antimicrobial Review retreat. He is a member of the Pharmacy and Therapeutics Committee and many of its subcommittees. Dr Goldman has authored numerous journal articles and lectures locally and nationally on infectious diseases topics and current drug therapies. He is currently a reviewer for the *Annals of Pharmacotherapy* and the *Journal of the American Medical Association*, an editorial board member of the *Journal of Infectious Disease Pharmacotherapy*, and coauthor of the *Infectious Diseases Handbook*, the *Drug Information Handbook*, and the *Drug Information Handbook for the Allied Health Professional* produced by Lexi-Comp, Inc. He also provides technical support to Lexi-Comp's Clinical Reference Library™ publications.

Dr Goldman is an active member of the Ohio College of Clinical Pharmacy, the Society of Infectious Disease Pharmacists, the American College of Clinical Pharmacy, and the American Society of Health-Systems Pharmacists.

Lora L. Armstrong, PharmD, BCPS

Dr Armstrong received her bachelor's degree in pharmacy from Ferris State University and her Doctor of Pharmacy degree from Midwestern University. Dr Armstrong is a Board-Certified Pharmacotherapy Specialist (BCPS).

In her current position, Dr Armstrong serves as the senior manager of the Pharmacy and Therapeutics Committee process at Caremark Rx, Inc, Prescription Services Division. Caremark is a prescription benefit management company (PBM). Dr Armstrong is responsible for coordination of the Caremark National Pharmacy & Therapeutics Committee and she chairs the Caremark Pharmacy & Therapeutics Subcommittee. Dr Armstrong is also responsible for coordinating the Caremark Clinical Practice Committee, monitoring the pharmaceutical product pipeline, monitoring drug surveillance, and communicating Pharmacy & Therapeutics Committee Formulary information to Caremark's internal and external customers.

Prior to joining Caremark Rx, Inc, Dr Armstrong served as the Director of Drug Information Services at the University of Chicago Hospitals. She obtained 17 years of experience in a variety of clinical settings including critical care, hematology, oncology, infectious diseases, and clinical pharmacokinetics. Dr Armstrong played an active role in the education and training of medical, pharmacy, and nursing staff. She coordinated the Drug Information Center, the medical center's Adverse Drug Reaction Monitoring Program, and the continuing Education Program for pharmacists. She also maintained the hospital's strict formulary program and was the editor of the University of Chicago Hospitals' *Formulary of Accepted Drugs* and the drug information center's monthly newsletter *Topics in Drug Therapy*.

Dr Armstrong is an active member of the Academy of Managed Care Pharmacy (AMCP), the American Society of Health-Systems Pharmacists (ASHP), the American Pharmaceutical Association (APhA), and the American College of Clinical Pharmacy (ACCP). Dr Armstrong wrote the chapter entitled "Drugs and Hormones Used in Endocrinology" in the 4th edition of the textbook *Endocrinology*. She also serves on the Editorial Advisory Board of the *Drug INFO Line* Newsletter.

EDITORIAL ADVISORY PANEL

x

PREFACE

Working with clinical pharmacists, hospital pharmacy and therapeutics committees, and hospital drug information centers, the editors of this handbook have directly assisted in the development and production of hospital-specific formulary documentation for several hundred major medical institutions in the United States and Canada. The resultant documentation provides pertinent detail concerning use of medications within the hospital and other clinical settings. The most current information on medications has been extracted, reviewed, coalesced, and cross-referenced by the editors to create this *Quick Look Drug Book*.

Thus, this handbook gives the user quick access to data on 1578 medications with cross referencing to 5679 U.S. and Canadian brand or trade names. Selection of the included medications was based on the analysis of those medications offered in a wide range of hospital formularies. The concise standardized format for data used in this handbook was developed to ensure a consistent presentation of information for all medications.

All generic drug names and synonyms appear in lower case, whereas brand or trade names appear in upper/lower case with the proper trademark information. These three items appear as individual entries in the alphabetical listing of drugs and, thus, there is no requirement for an alphabetical index of drugs.

Mailing and WEB site addresses for Pharmaceutical Manufacturers' and Drug Distributors are provided in the appendix section of this book.

The Indication/Therapeutic Category Index is an expedient mechanism for locating the medication of choice along with its classification. This index will help the user, with knowledge of the disease state, to identify medications which are most commonly used in treatment. All disease states are cross-referenced to a varying number of medications with the most frequently used medication(s) noted.

— L.L. Lance

ACKNOWLEDGMENTS

The *Quick Look Drug Book* exists in its present form as the result of the concerted efforts of the following individuals: Robert D. Kerscher, publisher and president of Lexi-Comp, Inc; Lynn D. Coppinger, managing editor; Barbara F. Kerscher, production manager; Daniel L. Krinsky, director, pharmacotherapy sales and marketing; Ginger S. Stein, project manager; and David C. Marcus, director of information systems.

Special acknowledgment goes to all Lexi-Comp staff for their contributions to this handbook.

USE OF THE HANDBOOK

The *Quick Look Drug Book* is organized into a drug information section, an appendix, and an indication/therapeutic category index.

The drug information section of the handbook, wherein all drugs are listed alphabetically, details information pertinent to each drug. Extensive cross referencing is provided by brand name and synonyms.

Drug information is presented in a consistent format and for quick reference will provide the following:

Generic Name	U.S. Adopted Name (USAN) or International Nonproprietary Name (INN)
	If a drug product is only available in Canada, a *(Canada only)* will be attached to that product and will appear with every occurrence of that drug throughout the book
Pronunciation Guide	Subjective aid for pronouncing drug names
Synonyms	Official names and some slang
Tall-Man	"Tall-Man" lettering revisions recommended by the FDA
U.S./Canadian Brand Names	Common trade names used in the United States and Canada
Therapeutic Category	Lexi-Comp's own system of logical medication classification
Controlled Substance	Drug Enforcement Agency (DEA) classification for federally scheduled controlled substances
Use	Information pertaining to appropriate use of the drug
Usual Dosage	The amount of the drug to be typically given or taken during therapy
Dosage Forms	Information with regard to form, strength and availability of the drug

Appendix

The appendix offers a compilation of tables, guidelines, and conversion information that can often be helpful when considering patient care.

Indication/Therapeutic Category Index

This index provides a listing of accepted drugs for various disease states thus focusing attention on selection of medications most frequently prescribed in relation to a clinical diagnosis. Diseases may have other nonofficial drugs for their treatment and this indication/therapeutic category index should not be used by itself to determine the appropriateness of a particular therapy. The listed indications may encompass varying degrees of severity and, since certain medications may not be appropriate for a given degree of severity, it should not be assumed that the agents listed for specific indications are interchangeable. Also included as a valuable reference is each medication's therapeutic category.

TALL-MAN LETTERS

Confusion between similar drug names is an important cause of medication errors. For years, The Institute for Safe Medication Practices (ISMP), has urged generic manufacturers use a combination of large and small letters as well as bolding (ie, chlorpro**MAZINE** and chlorpro**PAMIDE**) to help distinguish drugs with look-alike names, especially when they share similar strengths. Recently the FDA's Division of Generic Drugs began to issue recommendation letters to manufacturers suggesting this novel way to label their products to help reduce this drug name confusion. Although this project has had marginal success, the method has successfully eliminated problems with products such as diphenhydr**AMINE** and dimenhy**DRINATE**. Hospitals should also follow suit by making similar changes in their own labels, preprinted order forms, computer screens and printouts, and drug storage location labels.

In order for all involved to become more familiar with the FDA's recent suggestion, in this edition of the *Quick Look Drug Book* the "Tall-Man" lettering revisions will be listed in a field called **Tall-Man**.

The following is a list of product names and recommended FDA revisions.

Drug Product	Recommended Revision
acetazolamide	aceta**ZOLAMIDE**
acetohexamide	aceto**HEXAMIDE**
bupropion	bu**PROP**ion
buspirone	bus**PIR**one
chlorpromazine	chlorpro**MAZINE**
chlorpropamide	chlorpro**PAMIDE**
clomiphene	clomi**PHENE**
clomipramine	clomi**PRAMINE**
cycloserine	cyclo**SERINE**
cyclosporine	cyclo**SPORINE**
daunorubicin	**DAUNO**rubicin
dimenhydrinate	dimenhy**DRINATE**
diphenhydramine	diphenhydr**AMINE**
dobutamine	**DOBUT**amine
dopamine	**DOP**amine
doxorubicin	**DOXO**rubicin
glipizide	glipi**ZIDE**
glyburide	gly**BURIDE**
hydralazine	hydr**ALAZINE**
hydroxyzine	hydr**OXY**zine
medroxyprogesterone	medroxy**PROGESTER**one
methylprednisolone	methyl**PREDNIS**olone
methyltestosterone	methyl**TESTOSTER**one

nicardipine	ni**CAR**dipine
nifedipine	**NIFE**dipine
prednisolone	predniso**LONE**
prednisone	predni**SONE**
sulfadiazine	sulfa**DIAZINE**
sulfisoxazole	sulfi**SOXAZOLE**
tolazamide	**TOLAZ**amide
tolbutamide	**TOLBUT**amide
vinblastine	vin**BLAS**tine
vincristine	vin**CRIS**tine

Institute for Safe Medication Practices. "New Tall-Man Lettering Will Reduce Mix-Ups Due to Generic Drug Name Confusion," *ISMP Medication Safety Alert*, September 19, 2001. Available at: http://www.ismp.org.

Institute for Safe Medication Practices. "Prescription Mapping, Can Improve Efficiency While Minimizing Errors With Look-Alike Products," *ISMP Medication Safety Alert*, October 6, 1999. Available at: http://www.ismp.org.

U.S. Pharmacopeia, "USP Quality Review: Use Caution-Avoid Confusion," March 2001, No. 76. Available at: http://www.usp.org.

SAFE WRITING

Health professionals and their support personnel frequently produce handwritten copies of information they see in print; therefore, such information is subjected to even greater possibilities for error or misinterpretation on the part of others. Thus, particular care must be given to how drug names and strengths are expressed when creating written health care documents.

The following are a few examples of safe writing rules suggested by the Institute for Safe Medication Practices, Inc.*

1. There should be a space between a number and its units as it is easier to read. There should be no periods after the abbreviations mg or mL.

Correct	Incorrect
10 mg	10mg
100 mg	100mg

2. Never place a decimal and a zero after a whole number (2 mg is correct and 2.0 mg is incorrect). If the decimal point is not seen because it falls on a line or because individuals are working from copies where the decimal point is not seen, this causes a tenfold overdose.

3. Just the opposite is true for numbers less than one. Always place a zero before a naked decimal (0.5 mL is correct, .5 mL is incorrect).

4. Never abbreviate the word "unit." The handwritten U or u, looks like a 0 (zero), and may cause a tenfold overdose error to be made.

5. IU is not a safe abbreviation for international units. The handwritten IU looks like IV. Write out international units or use int. units.

6. Q.D. is not a safe abbreviation for once daily, as when the Q is followed by a sloppy dot, it looks like QID which means four times daily.

7. O.D. is not a safe abbreviation for once daily, as it is properly interpreted as meaning "right eye" and has caused liquid medications such as saturated solution of potassium iodide and Lugol's solution to be administered incorrectly. There is no safe abbreviation for once daily. It must be written out in full.

8. Do not use chemical names such as 6-mercaptopurine or 6-thioguanine, as 6-fold overdoses have been given when these were not recognized as chemical names. The proper names of these drugs are mercaptopurine or thioguanine.

9. Do not abbreviate drug names (5FC, 6MP, 5-ASA, MTX, HCTZ CPZ, PBZ, etc) as they are misinterpreted and cause error.

10. Do not use the apothecary system or symbols.

11. Do not abbreviate microgram as µg; instead use mcg as there is less likelihood of misinterpretation.

---

*From "Safe Writing" by Davis NM, PharmD and Cohen MR, MS, Lecturers and Consultants for Safe Medication Practices, 1143 Wright Drive, Huntingdon Valley, PA 19006. Phone: (215) 947-7566.

12. When writing an outpatient prescription, write a complete prescription. A complete prescription can prevent the prescriber, the pharmacist, and/or the patient from making a mistake and can eliminate the need for further clarification. The legible prescriptions should contain:

   a.   patient's full name

   b.   for pediatric or geriatric patients: their age (or weight where applicable)

   c.   drug name, dosage form and strength; if a drug is new or rarely prescribed, print this information

   d.   number or amount to be dispensed

   e.   complete instructions for the patient, including the purpose of the medication

   f.   when there are recognized contraindications for a prescribed drug, indicate to the pharmacist that you are aware of this fact (ie, when prescribing a potassium salt for a patient receiving an ACE inhibitor, write "K serum leveling being monitored")

ALPHABETICAL LISTING OF DRUGS

A-200™ Lice [US-OTC] *see* permethrin *on page 505*

A-200™ [US-OTC] *see* pyrethrins *on page 555*

A and D™ Ointment [US-OTC] *see* vitamin A and vitamin D *on page 681*

abacavir (a BAK a veer)
U.S./Canadian Brand Names Ziagen® [US/Can]
Therapeutic Category Nucleoside Reverse Transcriptase Inhibitor (NRTI)
Use Treatment of HIV infections in combination with other antiretroviral agents
Usual Dosage Oral:
Children: 3 months to 16 years: 8 mg/kg body weight twice daily (maximum: 300 mg twice daily) in combination with other antiretroviral agents
Adults: 300 mg twice daily in combination with other antiretroviral agents
Dosage Forms
Solution, oral, as sulfate: 20 mg/mL (240 mL) [strawberry-banana flavor]
Tablet, as sulfate: 300 mg

abacavir, lamivudine, and zidovudine
(a BAK a veer, la MI vyoo deen, & zye DOE vyoo deen)
U.S./Canadian Brand Names Trizivir® [US/Can]
Therapeutic Category Antiretroviral Agent, Nucleoside Reverse Transcriptase Inhibitor (NRTI)
Use Treatment of HIV infection (either alone or in combination with other antiretroviral agents) in patients whose regimen would otherwise contain the components of Trizivir® (based on analyses of surrogate markers in controlled studies with abacavir of up to 24 weeks; there have been no clinical trials conducted with Trizivir®)
Usual Dosage Adolescents and Adults: Oral: 1 tablet twice daily; **Note:** Not recommended for patients <40 kg
Dosage Forms Tablet: Abacavir 300 mg, lamivudine 150 mg, and zidovudine 300 mg

Abbokinase® [US] *see* urokinase *on page 668*

ABCD *see* amphotericin B cholesteryl sulfate complex *on page 39*

abciximab (ab SIK si mab)
Synonyms c7E3
U.S./Canadian Brand Names ReoPro® [US/Can]
Therapeutic Category Platelet Aggregation Inhibitor
Use Adjunct to percutaneous transluminal coronary angioplasty or atherectomy (PTCA) for the prevention of acute cardiac ischemic complications; prevent cardiac ischemic complications in a wider range of percutaneous coronary interventions (PCIs), including balloon angioplasty and stent placement, and without qualification of high risk for abrupt vessel closure; unstable angina that does not respond to conventional therapy when PCI is planned with 24 hours
Usual Dosage I.V.: 0.25 mg/kg bolus followed by an infusion of 10 mcg/minute for 12 hours
Dosage Forms Injection, solution: 2 mg/mL (5 mL)

ABC Pack™ (Avelox®) [US] *see* moxifloxacin *on page 439*

Abelcet® [US/Can] *see* amphotericin B lipid complex *on page 40*

Abenol® [Can] *see* acetaminophen *on next page*

ABLC *see* amphotericin B lipid complex *on page 40*

A/B® Otic [US] *see* antipyrine and benzocaine *on page 47*

Abreva™ [US-OTC] *see* docosanol *on page 208*

absorbable cotton *see* cellulose, oxidized *on page 127*

absorbable gelatin sponge *see* gelatin (absorbable) *on page 294*

Absorbine® Antifungal *(Discontinued)* *see page 814*

Absorbine® Jock Itch *(Discontinued)* *see page 814*

Absorbine Jr.® Antifungal [US-OTC] *see* tolnaftate *on page 644*

acarbose (AY car bose)
U.S./Canadian Brand Names Precose® [US/Can]
Therapeutic Category Antidiabetic Agent, Oral
Use Treatment of noninsulin-dependent diabetes mellitus (NIDDM); as monotherapy or in combination with a sulfonylurea when diet plus acarbose or a sulfonylurea does not result in adequate glycemic control; also used with insulin or metformin in patients with noninsulin-dependent diabetes mellitus (NIDDM)
Usual Dosage Adults: Oral: Dosage must be individualized on the basis of effectiveness and tolerance while not exceeding the maximum recommended dose of 100 mg 3 times/day

Initial dose: 25 mg 3 times/day with the first bite of each main meal
Maintenance dose: Should be adjusted at 4- to 8-week intervals based on 1-hour postprandial glucose levels and tolerance. Dosage may be increased from 25 mg 3 times/day to 50 mg 3 times/day; some patients may benefit from increasing the dose to 100 mg 3 times/day; maintenance dose ranges: 50-100 mg 3 times/day.
Maximum dose:
≤60 kg: 50 mg 3 times/day
>60 kg: 100 mg 3 times/day
Dosage Forms Tablet: 25 mg, 50 mg, 100 mg

A-Caro-25® [US] *see* beta-carotene *on page 82*

Accolate® [US/Can] *see* zafirlukast *on page 688*

AccuNeb™ [US] *see* albuterol *on page 18*

Accupril® [US/Can] *see* quinapril *on page 558*

Accuretic™ [US/Can] *see* quinapril and hydrochlorothiazide *on page 559*

Accutane® [US/Can] *see* isotretinoin *on page 363*

Accuzyme™ [US] *see* papain and urea *on page 492*

acebutolol (a se BYOO toe lole)
U.S./Canadian Brand Names Apo-Acebutolol [Can]; Gen-Acebutolol [Can]; Monitan® [Can]; Novo-Acebutolol [Can]; Nu-Acebutolol [Can]; Rhotral [Can]; Sectral® [US/Can]
Therapeutic Category Antiarrhythmic Agent, Class II; Beta-Adrenergic Blocker
Use Treatment of hypertension; ventricular arrhythmias; angina
Usual Dosage Adults: Oral: 400-800 mg/day in 2 divided doses
Dosage Forms Capsule, as hydrochloride: 200 mg, 400 mg

Aceon® [US] *see* perindopril erbumine *on page 504*

Acephen® [US-OTC] *see* acetaminophen *on this page*

acetaminophen (a seet a MIN oh fen)
Synonyms APAP; n-acetyl-p-aminophenol; paracetamol
U.S./Canadian Brand Names Abenol® [Can]; Acephen® [US-OTC]; Apo®-Acetamino-phen [Can]; Aspirin Free Anacin® Maximum Strength [US-OTC]; Atasol® [Can]; Cetafen Extra® [US-OTC]; Cetafen® [US-OTC]; Feverall® [US-OTC]; Genapap® Children [US-OTC]; Genapap® Extra Strength [US-OTC]; Genapap® Infant [US-OTC]; Genapap® [US-OTC]; Genebs® Extra Strength [US-OTC]; Genebs® [US-OTC]; Infantaire [US-OTC]; Liquiprin® for Children [US-OTC]; Mapap® Children's [US-OTC]; Mapap® Extra Strength [US-OTC]; Mapap® Infants [US-OTC]; Mapap® [US-OTC]; Pediatrix [Can]; Redutemp® [US-OTC]; Silapap® Children's [US-OTC]; Silapap® Infants [US-OTC]; Tempra® [Can]; Tylenol® [US/Can]; Tylenol® Arthritis Pain [US-OTC]; Tylenol® Children's [US-OTC]; Tylenol® Extra Strength [US-OTC]; Tylenol® Infants [US-OTC]; (Continued)

3

acetaminophen *(Continued)*

Tylenol® Junior Strength [US-OTC]; Tylenol® Sore Throat [US-OTC]; Valorin Extra [US-OTC]; Valorin [US-OTC]

Therapeutic Category Analgesic, Non-narcotic; Antipyretic

Use Treatment of mild to moderate pain and fever; does not have antirheumatic or systemic anti-inflammatory effects

Usual Dosage Oral, rectal (if fever not controlled with acetaminophen alone, administer with full doses of aspirin on an every 4- to 6-hour schedule, if aspirin is not otherwise contraindicated):

Children <12 years: 10-15 mg/kg/dose every 4-6 hours as needed; do **not** exceed 5 doses (2.6 g) in 24 hours

Adults: 325-650 mg every 4-6 hours or 1000 mg 3-4 times/day; do **not** exceed 4 g/day

Dosage Forms

Caplet (Genapap® Extra Strength, Genebs® Extra Strength, Tylenol® Extra Strength): 500 mg

Caplet, extended release (Tylenol® Arthritis Pain): 650 mg

Capsule (Mapap® Extra Strength): 500 mg

Elixir: 160 mg/5 mL (5 mL, 10 mL, 20 mL, 120 mL, 240 mL, 500 mL, 3780 mL)

Genapap® Children: 160 mg/5 mL (120 mL) [cherry and grape flavors]

Silapap® Children's: 160 mg/5 mL (120 mL, 240 mL, 480 mL)

Gelcap (Genapap® Extra Strength, Tylenol® Extra Strength): 500 mg

Geltab (Tylenol® Extra Strength): 500 mg

Liquid, oral: 160 mg/5 mL (120 mL, 240 mL, 480 mL, 3870 mL); 500 mg/15 mL (240 mL)

Redutemp®: 500 mg/15 mL (120 mL)

Tylenol® Sore Throat: 500 mg/15 mL (240 mL) [cherry and honey-lemon flavors]

Solution, oral drops: 100 mg/mL (15 mL, 30 mL) [droppers are marked at 0.4 mL (40 mg) and at 0.8 mL (80 mg)]

Genapap® Infant: 80 mg/0.8 mL (15 mL)

Infantaire®, Silapap® Infant's: 80 mg/0.8 mL (15 mL, 30 mL)

Liquiprin® for Children: 80 mg/0.8 mL (30 mL)

Suppository, rectal: 80 mg, 120 mg, 325 mg, 650 mg

Acephen®: 120 mg, 325 mg, 650 mg

Feverall®: 80 mg, 120 mg, 325 mg

Mapap®: 120 mg, 650 mg

Suspension, oral: 160 mg/5 mL (120 mL)

Mapap® Children's: 160 mg/5 mL (120 mL) [cherry, grape, and bubblegum flavors]

Tylenol® Children's: 160 mg/5 mL (120 mL, 240 mL) [cherry, grape, and bubblegum flavors]

Suspension, oral drops: 100 mg/mL (15 mL, 30 mL) [droppers are marked at 0.4 mL (40 mg) and at 0.8 mL (80 mg)]

Mapap® Infants 80 mg/0.8 mL (15 mL, 30 mL) [cherry flavor]

Tylenol® Infants: 80 mg/0.8 mL (15 mL, 30 mL) [cherry and grape flavors]

Syrup, oral: 160 mg/5 mL (120 mL)

Tablet: 160 mg, 325 mg, 500 mg

Aspirin Free Anacin® Maximum Strength, Cetafen® Extra Strength, Genapap® Extra Strength, Genebs® Extra Strength, Mapap® Extra Strength, Redutemp®, Tylenol® Extra Strength, Valorin Extra: 500 mg

Cetafen®, Genapap®, Genebs®, Mapap®, Tylenol®, Valorin: 325 mg

Mapap®: 160 mg

Tablet, chewable: 80 mg, 160 mg

Genapap® Children, Mapap® Children's: 80 mg [contains phenylalanine 3 mg/tablet; fruit and grape flavors]

Tylenol® Children's: 80 mg [fruit and grape flavors contain phenylalanine 3 mg/tablet; bubblegum flavor contains phenylalanine 6 mg/tablet]

Tylenol® Junior Strength: 160 mg [contains phenylalanine 6 mg/tablet; fruit and grape flavors]

acetaminophen and codeine (a seet a MIN oh fen & KOE deen)

Synonyms codeine and acetaminophen

U.S./Canadian Brand Names Capital® and Codeine [US]; Empracet®-30 [Can]; Empracet®-60 [Can]; Emtec-30 [Can]; Lenoltec [Can]; Phenaphen® With Codeine [US]; Triatec-8 [Can]; Triatec-30 [Can]; Triatec-Strong [Can]; Tylenol® with Codeine [US/Can]

Therapeutic Category Analgesic, Narcotic

Controlled Substance C-III; C-V

Use Relief of mild to moderate pain

Usual Dosage Doses should be adjusted according to severity of pain and response of the patient. Adult doses ≥60 mg codeine fail to give commensurate relief of pain but merely prolong analgesia and are associated with an appreciably increased incidence of side effects. Oral:

Children:
Analgesic: 0.5-1 mg codeine/kg/dose every 4-6 hours
Acetaminophen: 10-15 mg/kg/dose every 4 hours up to a maximum of 2.6 g/24 hours for children <12 years
3-6 years: 5 mL 3-4 times/day as needed of elixir
7-12 years: 10 mL 3-4 times/day as needed of elixir
>12 years: 15 mL every 4 hours as needed of elixir
Adults:
Antitussive: Based on codeine (15-30 mg/dose) every 4-6 hours
Analgesic: Based on codeine (30-60 mg/dose) every 4-6 hours
1-2 tablets every 4 hours to a maximum of 12 tablets/24 hours

Dosage Forms
Capsule [C-III]: #3 (Phenaphen® With Codeine): Acetaminophen 325 mg and codeine phosphate 30 mg
Elixir, oral [C-V]: Acetaminophen 120 mg and codeine phosphate 12 mg per 5 mL (5 mL, 10 mL, 12.5 mL, 15 mL, 120 mL, 480 mL, 3840 mL) [contains alcohol 7%]
Tylenol® with Codeine: Acetaminophen 120 mg and codeine phosphate 12 mg per 5 mL (480 mL) [contains alcohol 7%; cherry flavor]
Suspension, oral [C-V] (Capital® and Codeine): Acetaminophen 120 mg and codeine phosphate 12 mg per 5 mL [alcohol free; fruit punch flavor]
Tablet [C-III]:
#2: Acetaminophen 300 mg and codeine phosphate 15 mg
#3 (Tylenol® with Codeine): Acetaminophen 300 mg and codeine phosphate 30 mg [contains sodium metabisulfite]
#4 (Tylenol® with Codeine): Acetaminophen 300 mg and codeine phosphate 60 mg [contains sodium metabisulfite]

acetaminophen and diphenhydramine

(a seet a MIN oh fen & dye fen HYE dra meen)

U.S./Canadian Brand Names Anacin® PM Aspirin Free [US-OTC]; Excedrin® P.M. [US-OTC]; Goody's PM® Powder [US-OTC]; Legatrin PM® [US-OTC]; Tylenol® PM Extra Strength [US-OTC]; Tylenol® Severe Allergy [US-OTC]

Therapeutic Category Analgesic, Non-narcotic

Use Relief of mild to moderate pain or sinus headache

Usual Dosage Oral:
Children <12 years: Not recommended
Adults: 2 caplets or 5 mL of liquid at bedtime or as directed by physician; do not exceed recommended dosage

Dosage Forms
Caplet:
Excedrin® P.M.: Acetaminophen 500 mg and diphenhydramine citrate 38 mg
Legatrin PM®: Acetaminophen 500 mg and diphenhydramine 50 mg
Tylenol® PM Extra Strength: Acetaminophen 500 mg and diphenhydramine 25 mg
Tylenol® Severe Allergy: Acetaminophen 500 mg and diphenhydramine 12.5 mg
Gelcap (Tylenol® PM Extra Strength): Acetaminophen 500 mg and diphenhydramine 25 mg
(Continued)

5

acetaminophen and diphenhydramine *(Continued)*

Geltab:

Excedrin® P.M.: Acetaminophen 500 mg and diphenhydramine citrate 38 mg

Tylenol® PM Extra Strength: Acetaminophen 500 mg and diphenhydramine hydrochloride 25 mg

Powder for oral solution (Goody's PM® Powder): Acetaminophen 500 mg and diphenhydramine citrate 38 mg

Tablet:

Anacin® PM Aspirin-Free, Tylenol® PM Extra Strength: Acetaminophen 500 mg and diphenhydramine hydrochloride 25 mg

Excedrin® P.M.: Acetaminophen 500 mg and diphenhydramine citrate 38 mg

acetaminophen and hydrocodone *see* hydrocodone and acetaminophen *on* page 329

acetaminophen and oxycodone *see* oxycodone and acetaminophen *on* page 485

acetaminophen and phenyltoloxamine

(a seet a MIN oh fen & fen il to LOKS a meen)

U.S./Canadian Brand Names Genesec® [US-OTC]; Percogesic® [US-OTC]; Phenylgesic® [US-OTC]

Therapeutic Category Analgesic, Non-narcotic

Use Relief of mild to moderate pain

Usual Dosage Adults: Oral: 1-2 tablets every 4 hours

Dosage Forms Tablet: Acetaminophen 325 mg and phenyltoloxamine citrate 30 mg

acetaminophen and propoxyphene *see* propoxyphene and acetaminophen *on* page 548

acetaminophen and pseudoephedrine

(a seet a MIN oh fen & soo doe e FED rin)

Synonyms pseudoephedrine and acetaminophen

U.S./Canadian Brand Names Alka-Seltzer Plus® Cold and Sinus [US-OTC]; Children's Tylenol® Sinus [US-OTC]; Dristan® N.D. [Can]; Dristan® N.D., Extra Strength [Can]; Infants Tylenol® Cold [US-OTC]; Medi-Synal [US-OTC]; Ornex® Maximum Strength [US-OTC]; Ornex® [US-OTC]; Sinus-Relief® [US-OTC]; Sinutab® Non Drowsy [Can]; Sinutab® Sinus Maximum Strength Without Drowsiness [US-OTC]; Sudafed® Cold and Sinus [US-OTC]; Sudafed® Head Cold and Sinus Extra Strength [Can]; Sudafed® Sinus Headache [US-OTC]; Tylenol® Decongestant [Can]; Tylenol® Sinus [Can]; Tylenol® Sinus Non-Drowsy [US-OTC]

Therapeutic Category Decongestant/Analgesic

Use Symptomatic relief of congestion, fever, and aches/pain of colds/flu

Usual Dosage Adults: Oral: 2 tablets every 4-6 hours

Dosage Forms

Caplet:

Ornex®: Acetaminophen 325 mg and pseudoephedrine hydrochloride 30 mg

Ornex® Maximum Strength, Sinutab® Sinus Maximum Strength Without Drowsiness, Sudafed® Sinus Headache, Tylenol® Sinus Non-Drowsy: Acetaminophen 500 mg and pseudoephedrine hydrochloride 30 mg

Capsule, liquid (Alka-Seltzer Plus® Cold and Sinus, Sudafed® Cold and Sinus): Acetaminophen 325 mg and pseudoephedrine hydrochloride 30 mg

Gelcap (Tylenol® Sinus Non-Drowsy): Acetaminophen 500 mg and pseudoephedrine hydrochloride 30 mg

Geltab (Tylenol® Sinus Non-Drowsy): Acetaminophen 500 mg and pseudoephedrine hydrochloride 30 mg

Liquid, oral drops (Infants Tylenol® Cold): Acetaminophen 80 mg/0.8 mL and pseudoephedrine 7.5 mg/0.8 mL [bubblegum flavor]

Suspension (Children's Tylenol® Sinus): Acetaminophen 160 mg and pseudoephedrine hydrochloride 15 mg/5 mL [fruit flavor]

Tablet (Sudafed® Sinus Headache): Acetaminophen 500 mg and pseudoephedrine hydrochloride 30 mg

Tablet, chewable (Children's Tylenol® Sinus): Acetaminophen 80 mg and pseudoephedrine hydrochloride 7.5 mg [fruit flavor] [contains phenylalanine 5 mg/tablet]

acetaminophen and tramadol (a seet a MIN oh fen & TRA ma dole)

Synonyms APAP and tramadol

U.S./Canadian Brand Names Ultracet™ [US]

Therapeutic Category Analgesic, Non-narcotic; Analgesic, Miscellaneous

Use Short-term (≤5 days) management of acute pain

Usual Dosage Oral: Adults: Acute pain: Two tablets every 4-6 hours as needed for pain relief (maximum: 8 tablets/day); treatment should not exceed 5 days

Dosage Forms Tablet: Acetaminophen 325 mg and tramadol hydrochloride 37.5 mg

acetaminophen, aspirin, and caffeine

(a seet a MIN oh fen, AS pir in, & KAF een)

U.S./Canadian Brand Names Excedrin® Extra Strength [US-OTC]; Excedrin® Migraine [US-OTC]; Genaced [US-OTC]; Goody's® Extra Strength Headache Powder [US-OTC]; Vanquish® Extra Strength Pain Reliever [US-OTC]

Therapeutic Category Analgesic, Non-narcotic

Use Relief of mild to moderate pain or fever

Usual Dosage Adults: Oral: 1-2 tablets or powders every 2-6 hours as needed for pain

Dosage Forms

Caplet:

Excedrin® Extra Strength: Acetaminophen 250 mg, aspirin 250 mg, and caffeine 65 mg

Vanquish® Extra Strength Pain Reliever: Acetaminophen 194 mg, aspirin 227 mg, and caffeine 33 mg

Geltab (Excedrin® Extra Strength): Acetaminophen 250 mg, aspirin 250 mg, and caffeine 65 mg

Powder (Goody's® Extra Strength Headache Powder): Acetaminophen 260 mg, aspirin 520 mg, and caffeine 32.5 mg

Tablet:

Excedrin® Extra Strength, Excedrin® Migraine, Genaced: Acetaminophen 250 mg, aspirin 250 mg, and caffeine 65 mg

acetaminophen, caffeine, hydrocodone, chlorpheniramine, and phenylephrine *see* hydrocodone, chlorpheniramine, phenylephrine, acetaminophen, and caffeine *on page 332*

acetaminophen, chlorpheniramine, and pseudoephedrine

(a seet a MIN oh fen, klor fen IR a meen, & soo doe e FED rin)

U.S./Canadian Brand Names Alka-Seltzer® Plus Cold Liqui-Gels® [US-OTC]; Children's Tylenol® Cold [US-OTC]; Comtrex® Allergy-Sinus [US-OTC]; Sinutab® Sinus & Allergy [Can]; Sinutab® Sinus Allergy Maximum Strength [US-OTC]; Thera-Flu® Flu and Cold [US]; Tylenol® Allergy Sinus [US/Can]

Therapeutic Category Antihistamine/Decongestant/Analgesic

Use Temporary relief of sinus symptoms

Usual Dosage Adults: Oral: 2 caplets/capsules/tablets every 6 hours

Dosage Forms

Caplet (Sinutab® Sinus Allergy Maximum Strength, Tylenol® Allergy Sinus): Acetaminophen 500 mg, chlorpheniramine maleate 2 mg, and pseudoephedrine hydrochloride 30 mg

Capsule, liquid (Alka-Seltzer® Plus Cold Liqui-Gels®): Acetaminophen 325 mg, chlorpheniramine maleate 2 mg, and pseudoephedrine hydrochloride 30 mg

Gelcap (Tylenol® Allergy Sinus): Acetaminophen 500 mg, chlorpheniramine maleate 2 mg, and pseudoephedrine hydrochloride 30 mg

(Continued)

acetaminophen, chlorpheniramine, and pseudoephedrine
(Continued)

Geltab (Tylenol® Allergy Sinus): Acetaminophen 500 mg, chlorpheniramine maleate 2 mg, and pseudoephedrine hydrochloride 30 mg

Liquid (Children's Tylenol® Cold): Acetaminophen 160 mg, chlorpheniramine maleate 1 mg, and pseudoephedrine hydrochloride 15 mg per 5 mL (120 mL) [grape flavor]

Powder for oral solution [packet] (Thera-Flu® Flu and Cold): Acetaminophen 650 mg, chlorpheniramine maleate 4 mg, and pseudoephedrine hydrochloride 60 mg [lemon flavor]

Tablet (Comtrex® Allergy-Sinus): Acetaminophen 500 mg, chlorpheniramine maleate 2 mg, and pseudoephedrine hydrochloride 30 mg

Tablet, chewable (Children's Tylenol® Cold): Acetaminophen 80 mg, chlorpheniramine maleate 0.5 mg, and pseudoephedrine hydrochloride 7.5 mg [contains phenylalanine 6 mg/tablet; grape flavor]

acetaminophen, dextromethorphan, and pseudoephedrine
(a seet a MIN oh fen, deks troe meth OR fan, & soo doe e FED rin)

Synonyms dextromethorphan, acetaminophen, and pseudoephedrine; pseudoephedrine, acetaminophen, and dextromethorphan; pseudoephedrine, dextromethorphan, and acetaminophen

U.S./Canadian Brand Names Alka-Seltzer® Plus Flu Liqui-Gels® [US-OTC]; Comtrex® Non-Drowsy Cough and Cold [US-OTC]; Contac® Cough, Cold and Flu Day & Night™ [Can]; Contac® Severe Cold and Flu/Non-Drowsy [US-OTC]; Infants' Tylenol® Cold Plus Cough Concentrated Drops [US-OTC]; Sudafed® Cold & Cough Extra Strength [Can]; Sudafed® Severe Cold [US-OTC]; Thera-Flu® Non-Drowsy Flu, Cold and Cough [US-OTC]; Triaminic® Sore Throat Formula [US-OTC]; Tylenol® Cold [Can]; Tylenol® Cold Non-Drowsy [US-OTC]; Tylenol® Flu Non-Drowsy Maximum Strength [US-OTC]; Vicks® DayQuil® Cold and Flu Non-Drowsy [US-OTC]

Therapeutic Category Cold Preparation

Use Symptomatic relief of congestion, fever, cough, and aches/pain of colds/flu

Usual Dosage Oral:

Analgesic: Based on acetaminophen component:

Children: 10-15 mg/kg/dose every 4-6 hours as needed; do **not** exceed 5 doses/24 hours

Adults: 325-650 mg every 4-7 hours as needed; do **not** exceed 4 g/day

Cough suppressant: Based on dextromethorphan component:

Children 6-12 years: 15 mg every 6-8 hours; do **not** exceed 60 mg/24 hours

Children >12 years and Adults: 10-20 mg every 4-8 hours **or** 30 mg every 8 hours; do **not** exceed 120 mg/24 hours

Decongestant: Based on pseudoephedrine component:

Children:

2-6 years: 15 mg every 4 hours (maximum: 90 mg/24 hours)

6-12 years: 30 mg every 4 hours (maximum: 180 mg/24 hours)

Children >12 years and Adults: 60 mg every 4 hours (maximum: 360 mg/24 hours)

Product labeling:

Infants' Tylenol® Cold Plus Cough Concentrated Drops: Children 2-3 years (24-55 lbs): 2 dropperfuls every 4-6 hours (maximum: 4 doses/24 hours)

Sudafed® Severe Cold, Thera-Flu® Non-Drowsy Maximum Strength (gelcap), Tylenol® Flu Non-Drowsy Maximum Strength: Children >12 years and Adults: 2 doses every 6 hours (maximum: 8 doses/24 hours)

Tylenol® Cold Non-Drowsy:

Children 6-11 years: 1 dose every 6 hours (maximum: 4 doses/24 hours)

Children ≥12 years and Adults: 2 doses every 6 hours (maximum: 8 doses/24 hours)

Thera-Flu® Non-Drowsy Maximum Strength: Children >12 years and Adults: 1 packet dissolved in hot water every 6 hours (maximum: 4 packets/24 hours)

Dosage Forms

Caplet:

Contac® Severe Cold and Flu/Non-Drowsy, Sudafed® Severe Cold, Tylenol® Cold Non-Drowsy: Acetaminophen 325 mg, dextromethorphan hydrobromide 15 mg, and pseudoephedrine hydrochloride 30 mg

Comtrex® Non-Drowsy Cough and Cold, Thera-Flu® Non-Drowsy Flu Cold and Cough: Acetaminophen 500 mg, dextromethorphan hydrobromide 15 mg, and pseudoephedrine hydrochloride 30 mg

Capsule, liquid

Alka-Seltzer® Plus Flu Liqui-Gels®: Acetaminophen 325 mg, dextromethorphan hydrobromide 10 mg, and pseudoephedrine hydrochloride 30 mg

Vicks® DayQuil® Cold and Flu Non-Drowsy: Acetaminophen 250 mg, dextromethorphan hydrobromide 10 mg, and pseudoephedrine hydrochloride 30 mg

Gelcap:

Tylenol® Cold Non-Drowsy: Acetaminophen 325 mg dextromethorphan hydrobromide 15 mg, and pseudoephedrine hydrochloride 30 mg

Tylenol® Flu Non-Drowsy Maximum Strength: Acetaminophen 500 mg, dextromethorphan hydrobromide 15 mg, and pseudoephedrine hydrochloride 30 mg

Liquid:

Triaminic® Sore Throat Formula: Acetaminophen 160 mg, dextromethorphan hydrobromide 7.5 mg, and pseudoephedrine hydrochloride 15 mg per 5 mL (120 mL, 240 mL) [grape flavor]

Vicks® DayQuil® Cold and Flu Non-Drowsy: Acetaminophen 325 mg, dextromethorphan hydrobromide 10 mg, and pseudoephedrine hydrochloride 30 mg per 15 mL (175 mL)

Powder for oral solution [packet] (Thera-Flu® Non-Drowsy Flu, Cold and Cough): Acetaminophen 1000 mg, dextromethorphan hydrobromide 30 mg, and pseudoephedrine hydrochloride 60 mg [lemon flavor]

Solution, oral concentrate [drops] (Infants' Tylenol® Cold Plus Cough Concentrated Drops): Acetaminophen 160 mg, dextromethorphan hydrobromide 5 mg, and pseudoephedrine hydrochloride 15 mg per 1.6 mL (15 mL) [1.6 mL = 2 dropperfuls] [cherry flavor]

Tablet (Sudafed® Severe Cold): Acetaminophen 325 mg, dextromethorphan hydrobromide 15 mg, and pseudoephedrine hydrochloride 30 mg

acetaminophen, isometheptene, and dichloralphenazone

(a seet a MIN oh fen, eye soe me THEP teen, & dye KLOR al FEN a zone)

U.S./Canadian Brand Names Midrin® [US]; Migratine® [US]

Therapeutic Category Analgesic, Non-narcotic

Use Relief of migraine and tension headache

Usual Dosage Adults: Oral: 2 capsules at first sign of headache, followed by 1 capsule every 60 minutes until relieved, up to 5 capsules in a 12-hour period

Dosage Forms Capsule: Acetaminophen 325 mg, isometheptene mucate 65 mg, dichloralphenazone 100 mg

Acetasol® HC [US] see acetic acid, propylene glycol diacetate, and hydrocortisone *on next page*

acetazolamide (a set a ZOLE a mide)

Tall-Man aceta**ZOLAMIDE**

U.S./Canadian Brand Names Apo®-Acetazolamide [Can]; Diamox Sequels® [US]; Diamox® [US/Can]

Therapeutic Category Anticonvulsant; Carbonic Anhydrase Inhibitor

Use Reduce elevated intraocular pressure in glaucoma, a diuretic, an adjunct to the treatment of refractory seizures and acute altitude sickness; centrencephalic epilepsies

(Continued)

acetazolamide *(Continued)*

Usual Dosage

Children:

Glaucoma:

Oral: 8-30 mg/kg/day divided every 6-8 hours

I.M., I.V.: 20-40 mg/kg/day divided every 6 hours

Edema: Oral, I.M., I.V.: 5 mg/kg or 150 mg/m^2 once every day or every other day

Epilepsy: Oral: 8-30 mg/kg/day in 2-4 divided doses, not to exceed 1 g/day

Adults:

Glaucoma:

Oral: 250 mg 1-4 times/day or 500 mg sustained release capsule twice daily

I.M., I.V.: 250-500 mg, may repeat in 2-4 hours

Edema: Oral, I.M., I.V.: 250-375 mg once daily

Epilepsy: Oral: 8-30 mg/kg/day in 1-4 divided doses

Altitude sickness: Oral: 250 mg every 8-12 hours

Dosage Forms

Capsule, sustained release (Diamox Sequels®): 500 mg

Injection, powder for reconstitution: 500 mg

Tablet: 125 mg, 250 mg

Diamox®: 250 mg

acetic acid (a SEE tik AS id)

Synonyms ethanoic acid

U.S./Canadian Brand Names Aci-jel® [US]; VōSol® [US]

Therapeutic Category Antibacterial, Otic; Antibacterial, Topical

Use Continuous or intermittent irrigation of the bladder; treatment of superficial bacterial infections of the external auditory canal and vagina

Usual Dosage

Irrigation: For continuous irrigation of the urinary bladder with 0.25% acetic acid irrigation, the rate of administration will approximate the rate of urine flow; usually 500-1500 mL/24 hours; for periodic irrigation of an indwelling urinary catheter to maintain patency, approximately 50 mL of 0.25% acetic acid irrigation is required. (Note: Dosage of an irrigating solution depends on the capacity or surface area of the structure being irrigated.)

Otic: Insert saturated wick, keep moist 24 hours; remove wick and instill 5 drops 3-4 times/day

Vaginal: One applicatorful morning and evening

Dosage Forms

Jelly, vaginal (Aci-jel®): 0.921% [contains oxyquinolone sulfate 0.025%, ricinoleic acid 0.7%, and glycerin 5%] (85 g)

Solution for irrigation: 0.25% (250 mL, 500 mL, 1000 mL)

Solution, otic (VōSol®): 2% [in propylene glycol] (15 mL)

acetic acid and aluminum acetate otic *see* aluminum acetate and acetic acid *on page 27*

acetic acid, propylene glycol diacetate, and hydrocortisone
(a SEE tik AS id, PRO pa leen GLY kole dye AS e tate, & hye droe KOR ti sone)

U.S./Canadian Brand Names Acetasol® HC [US]; VōSol® HC [US/Can]

Therapeutic Category Antibiotic/Corticosteroid, Otic

Use Treatment of superficial infections of the external auditory canal caused by organisms susceptible to the action of the antimicrobial, complicated by inflammation

Usual Dosage Adults: Otic: Instill 4 drops in ear(s) 3-4 times/day

Dosage Forms Solution, otic: Acetic acid 2%, propylene glycol diacetate 3%, and hydrocortisone 1% (10 mL)

acetohexamide (a set oh HEKS a mide)
Tall-Man aceto**HEXAMIDE**
Therapeutic Category Antidiabetic Agent, Oral
Use Adjunct to diet for the management of mild to moderately severe, stable, noninsulin-dependent (type II) diabetes mellitus
Usual Dosage Adults: Oral: 250 mg to 1.5 g/day in 1-2 divided doses
Dosage Forms Tablet: 250 mg, 500 mg

acetohydroxamic acid (a SEE toe hye droks am ik AS id)
Synonyms AHA
U.S./Canadian Brand Names Lithostat® [US]
Therapeutic Category Urinary Tract Product
Use Adjunctive therapy in chronic urea-splitting urinary infection
Usual Dosage Oral:
   Children: Initial: 10 mg/kg/day
   Adults: 250 mg 3-4 times/day for a total daily dose of 10-15 mg/kg/day
Dosage Forms Tablet: 250 mg

Acetoxyl® [Can] *see* benzoyl peroxide *on page 79*

acetoxymethylprogesterone *see* medroxyprogesterone acetate *on page 404*

acetylcholine (a se teel KOE leen)
U.S./Canadian Brand Names Miochol-E® [US/Can]
Therapeutic Category Cholinergic Agent
Use Produces complete miosis in cataract surgery, keratoplasty, iridectomy and other anterior segment surgery where rapid miosis is required
Usual Dosage Adults: Intraocular: 0.5-2 mL of 1% injection (5-20 mg) instilled into anterior chamber before or after securing one or more sutures
Dosage Forms Powder for intraocular suspension, as chloride: 1:100 [10 mg/mL] (2 mL)

acetylcysteine (a se teel SIS teen)
Synonyms mercapturic acid; NAC; *N*-acetylcysteine; *N*-acetyl-L-cysteine
U.S./Canadian Brand Names Acys-5® [US]; Mucomyst® [US/Can]; Parvolex® [Can]
Therapeutic Category Mucolytic Agent
Use Adjunctive therapy in patients with abnormal or viscid mucous secretions in broncho-pulmonary diseases, pulmonary complications of surgery, and cystic fibrosis; diagnostic bronchial studies; antidote for acute acetaminophen toxicity; enema to treat bowel obstruction due to meconium ileus or its equivalent
Usual Dosage
   Acetaminophen poisoning: Children and Adults: Oral: 140 mg/kg; followed by 17 doses of 70 mg/kg every 4 hours; repeat dose if emesis occurs within 1 hour of administration; therapy should continue until all doses are administered even though the acetaminophen plasma level has dropped below the toxic range
   Inhalation: Acetylcysteine 10% and 20% solution (Mucomyst®) (dilute 20% solution with sodium chloride or sterile water for inhalation); 10% solution may be used undiluted
   Infants: 1-2 mL of 20% solution or 2-4 mL 10% solution until nebulized administered 3-4 times/day
   Children: 3-5 mL of 20% solution or 6-10 mL of 10% solution until nebulized administered 3-4 times/day
   Adolescents: 5-10 mL of 10% to 20% solution until nebulized administered 3-4 times/day
   Note: Patients should receive an aerosolized bronchodilator 10-15 minutes prior to acetylcysteine
   Meconium ileus equivalent: Children and Adults: 100-300 mL of 4% to 10% solution by irrigation or orally
Dosage Forms Solution, as sodium: 10% [100 mg/mL] (4 mL, 10 mL, 30 mL); 20% [200 mg/mL] (4 mL, 10 mL, 30 mL, 100 mL)

acetylsalicylic acid *see* aspirin *on page 58*

Aches-N-Pain® *(Discontinued)* *see page 814*

Achromycin® Parenteral *(Discontinued)* *see page 814*

Achromycin® V Capsule *(Discontinued)* *see page 814*

Achromycin® V Oral Suspension *(Discontinued)* *see page 814*

aciclovir *see* acyclovir *on next page*

Acid Reducer 200® **[US-OTC]** *see* cimetidine *on page 146*

Aci-jel® **[US]** *see* acetic acid *on page 10*

Acilac [Can] *see* lactulose *on page 372*

Aciphex™ **[US/Can]** *see* rabeprazole *on page 560*

acitretin (a si TRE tin)

U.S./Canadian Brand Names Soriatane® [US/Can]

Therapeutic Category Retinoid-like Compound

Use Treatment of severe psoriasis (includes erythrodermic and pustular types) and other disorders of keratinization

Usual Dosage Adults: Oral: Individualization of dosage is required to achieve maximum therapeutic response while minimizing side effects

Initial: Therapy should be initiated at 25 mg/day, given as a single dose with the main meal; if by 4 weeks the response is unsatisfactory, and in the absence of toxicity, the daily dose may be gradually increased to a maximum of 75 mg/day; the dose may be reduced if necessary to minimize side effects

Maintenance: Doses of 25 to 50 mg/day may be given after initial response to treatment; the maintenance dose should be based on clinical efficacy and tolerability; it may be necessary in some cases to increase the dose to a maximum of 75 mg/day

Dosage Forms Capsule: 10 mg, 25 mg

Aclovate® **[US]** *see* alclometasone *on page 20*

Acot-Tussin® Allergy [US-OTC] *see* diphenhydramine *on page 202*

acrivastine and pseudoephedrine (AK ri vas teen & soo doe e FED rin)

Synonyms pseudoephedrine and acrivastine

U.S./Canadian Brand Names Semprex®-D [US]

Therapeutic Category Antihistamine/Decongestant Combination

Use Temporary relief of nasal congestion, decongest sinus openings, running nose, itching of nose or throat, and itchy, watery eyes due to hay fever or other upper respiratory allergies

Usual Dosage Adults: 1 capsule 3-4 times/day

Dosage Forms Capsule: Acrivastine 8 mg and pseudoephedrine hydrochloride 60 mg

ACT® *(Discontinued)* *see page 814*

Actagen-C® *(Discontinued)* *see page 814*

Actagen® Syrup *(Discontinued)* *see page 814*

Actagen® Tablet *(Discontinued)* *see page 814*

Act-A-Med® *(Discontinued)* *see page 814*

Actanol® **[US-OTC]** *see* triprolidine and pseudoephedrine *on page 659*

Actedril® **[US-OTC]** *see* triprolidine and pseudoephedrine *on page 659*

ACTH *see* corticotropin *on page 164*

ACTH-40® *(Discontinued)* *see page 814*

Acthar® **[US]** *see* corticotropin *on page 164*

ActHIB® **[US/Can]** *see* Haemophilus B conjugate vaccine *on page 314*

Acticin® **[US]** *see* permethrin *on page 505*

Acticort® **[US]** *see* hydrocortisone (topical) *on page 334*

Actidil® *(Discontinued) see page 814*

Actidose-Aqua® **[US-OTC]** *see* charcoal *on page 131*

Actidose® **[US-OTC]** *see* charcoal *on page 131*

Actifed® **[US/Can]** *see* triprolidine and pseudoephedrine *on page 659*

Actifed® **Allergy Tablet (Night)** *(Discontinued) see page 814*

Actifed® **Syrup** *(Discontinued) see page 814*

Actifed® **With Codeine** *(Discontinued) see page 814*

Actigall™ **[US]** *see* ursodiol *on page 669*

Actimmune® **[US/Can]** *see* interferon gamma-1b *on page 356*

Actinex® *(Discontinued) see page 814*

actinomycin D *see* dactinomycin *on page 173*

Actiq® **[US/Can]** *see* fentanyl *on page 266*

Activase® **[US]** *see* alteplase *on page 26*

Activase® **rt-PA [Can]** *see* alteplase *on page 26*

activated carbon *see* charcoal *on page 131*

activated dimethicone *see* simethicone *on page 591*

activated ergosterol *see* ergocalciferol *on page 232*

activated methylpolysiloxane *see* simethicone *on page 591*

activated protein C, human, recombinant *see* drotrecogin alfa *on page 218*

activated recombinant human blood coagulation factor VII *see* eptacog alfa (activated) *(Canada only) on page 231*

Activella™ **[US]** *see* estradiol and norethindrone *on page 239*

Actonel™ **[US/Can]** *see* risedronate *on page 574*

Actos® **[US/Can]** *see* pioglitazone *on page 516*

Acu-Dyne® **Skin [US-OTC]** *see* povidone-iodine *on page 533*

Acular® **[US/Can]** *see* ketorolac *on page 368*

Acular® **PF [US]** *see* ketorolac *on page 368*

Acutrim® **16 Hours** *(Discontinued) see page 814*

Acutrim® **II, Maximum Strength** *(Discontinued) see page 814*

Acutrim® **Late Day** *(Discontinued) see page 814*

ACV *see* acyclovir *on this page*

acycloguanosine *see* acyclovir *on this page*

acyclovir (ay SYE kloe veer)

Synonyms aciclovir; ACV; acycloguanosine

U.S./Canadian Brand Names Apo®-Acyclovir [Can]; Avirax™ [Can]; Gen-Acyclovir [Can]; Nu-Acyclovir [Can]; Zovirax® [US/Can]

Therapeutic Category Antiviral Agent

Use Treatment of initial and prophylaxis of recurrent mucosal and cutaneous herpes simplex (HSV-1 and HSV-2) infections; herpes simplex encephalitis; herpes zoster infections; varicella-zoster infections in healthy, nonpregnant persons >13 years of age, children >12 months of age who have a chronic skin or lung disorder or are receiving long-term aspirin therapy, and immunocompromised patients

(Continued)

13

acyclovir *(Continued)*

Usual Dosage
Children and Adults: I.V.:
Mucocutaneous HSV infection: 750 mg/m^2/day divided every 8 hours or 15 mg/kg/day divided every 8 hours for 5-10 days
HSV encephalitis: 1500 mg/m^2/day divided every 8 hours or 30 mg/kg/day divided every 8 hours for 10 days
Varicella-zoster virus infection: 1500 mg/m^2/day divided every 8 hours or 30 mg/kg/day divided every 8 hours for 5-10 days
Adults:
Oral: Initial: 200 mg every 4 hours while awake (5 times/day); prophylaxis: 200 mg 3-4 times/day or 400 mg twice daily. Prophylaxis of varicella or herpes zoster in HIV positive patients: 400 mg 5 times/day
Topical: ½" ribbon of ointment every 3 hours (6 times/day)

Herpes zoster in immunocompromised patients:
Children: Oral: 250-600 mg/m^2/dose 4-5 times/day
Adults: Oral: 800 mg every 4 hours (5 times/day) for 7-10 days
Children and Adults: I.V.: 7.5 mg/kg/dose every 8 hours
Varicella-zoster infections: Oral:
Children: 10-20 mg/kg/dose (up to 800 mg) 4 times/day
Adults: 600-800 mg/dose 5 times/day for 7-10 days or 1000 mg every 6 hours for 5 days
Prophylaxis of bone marrow transplant recipients: Children and Adults: I.V.:
Autologous patients who are HSV seropositive: 150 mg/m^2/dose every 12 hours; with clinical symptoms of herpes simplex: 150 mg/m^2/dose every 8 hours
Autologous patients who are CMV seropositive: 500 mg/m^2/dose every 8 hours; for clinically symptomatic CMV infection, ganciclovir should be used in place of acyclovir

Dosage Forms
Capsule: 200 mg
Injection, powder for reconstitution, as sodium: 500 mg, 1000 mg
Injection, solution, as sodium [preservative free]: 50 mg/mL (10 mL, 20 mL)
Ointment, topical: 5% (3 g, 15 g)
Suspension, oral: 200 mg/5 mL (480 mL) [banana flavor]
Tablet: 400 mg, 800 mg

Acys-5® [US] *see* acetylcysteine *on page 11*

Adacel® [Can] *see* diphtheria, tetanus toxoids, and acellular pertussis vaccine *on page 204*

Adagen™ [US/Can] *see* pegademase (bovine) *on page 495*

Adalat® *(Discontinued)* *see page 814*

Adalat® CC [US] *see* nifedipine *on page 459*

Adalat® XL® [Can] *see* nifedipine *on page 459*

adamantanamine *see* amantadine *on page 30*

adapalene *(a DAP a leen)*
U.S./Canadian Brand Names Differin® [US/Can]
Therapeutic Category Acne Products
Use Treatment of acne vulgaris
Usual Dosage Adults: Topical: Apply once daily, before retiring, in a thin film to affected areas after washing; not recommended in children
Dosage Forms
Cream, topical: 0.1% (15 g, 45 g)
Gel, topical: 0.1% (15 g, 45 g) [alcohol free]
Pledget, topical: 0.1% (60s)
Solution, topical: 0.1% (30 mL)

Adderall® **[US]** *see* dextroamphetamine and amphetamine *on page 188*

Adderall XR™ **[US]** *see* dextroamphetamine and amphetamine *on page 188*

Adeflor® **[US]** *see* vitamin (multiple/pediatric) *on page 683*

adefovir (a DEF o veer)
    U.S./Canadian Brand Names Hepsera™ [US]
    Therapeutic Category Antiretroviral Agent, Non-nucleoside Reverse Transcriptase Inhibitor (NNRTI)
    Use Treatment of chronic hepatitis B with evidence of active viral replication (based on persistent elevation of ALT/AST or histologic evidence), including patients with lamivudine-resistant hepatitis B
    Usual Dosage Oral: Adults: 10 mg once daily
    Dosage Forms Tablet, as dipivoxil: 10 mg

ADEKs® **Pediatric Drops [US]** *see* vitamin (multiple/pediatric) *on page 683*

adenine arabinoside *see* vidarabine *on page 677*

Adenocard® **[US/Can]** *see* adenosine *on this page*

Adenoscan® **[US]** *see* adenosine *on this page*

adenosine (a DEN oh seen)
    Synonyms 9-beta-D-ribofuranosyladenine
    U.S./Canadian Brand Names Adenocard® [US/Can]; Adenoscan® [US]
    Therapeutic Category Antiarrhythmic Agent, Miscellaneous
    Use Treatment of paroxysmal supraventricular tachycardia (PSVT)
    Usual Dosage
        Children: Initial: Rapid I.V.: 0.05 mg/kg; if not effective within 2 minutes, increase dose in 0.05 mg/kg increments every 2 minutes to a maximum dose of 0.25 mg/kg or until termination of PSVT; median dose required: 0.15 mg/kg; do not exceed adult doses
        Adults: Rapid I.V. push: 6 mg, if the dose is not effective within 1-2 minutes, a rapid I.V. dose of 12 mg may be administered; may repeat 12 mg bolus if needed
    Dosage Forms Injection, solution [preservative free]:
        Adenocard®: 3 mg/mL (2 mL, 4 mL)
        Adenoscan®: 3 mg/mL (20 mL, 30 mL)

Adipex-P® **[US]** *see* phentermine *on page 509*

Adipost® **(Discontinued)** *see page 814*

Adlone® **Injection (Discontinued)** *see page 814*

Adoxa™ **[US]** *see* doxycycline *on page 215*

Adphen® **(Discontinued)** *see page 814*

ADR *see* doxorubicin *on page 214*

Adrenalin® **Chloride [US/Can]** *see* epinephrine *on page 228*

adrenaline *see* epinephrine *on page 228*

adrenocorticotropic hormone *see* corticotropin *on page 164*

Adriamycin® **[Can]** *see* doxorubicin *on page 214*

Adriamycin PFS® **[US]** *see* doxorubicin *on page 214*

Adriamycin RDF® **[US]** *see* doxorubicin *on page 214*

Adrin® **(Discontinued)** *see page 814*

Adrucil® **[US/Can]** *see* fluorouracil *on page 279*

Adsorbocarpine® **Ophthalmic (Discontinued)** *see page 814*

Adsorbonac® **(Discontinued)** *see page 814*

Adsorbotear® **Ophthalmic Solution (Discontinued)** *see page 814*

Advair™ Diskus® [US/Can] *see* fluticasone and salmeterol *on page 282*

Advanced Formula Oxy® Sensitive Gel *(Discontinued)* *see page 814*

Advantage 24™ [Can] *see* nonoxynol 9 *on page 464*

Advantage-S™ [US-OTC] *see* nonoxynol 9 *on page 464*

Advicor™ [US] *see* niacin and lovastatin *on page 457*

Advil® [US/Can] *see* ibuprofen *on page 342*

Advil® Children's [US-OTC] *see* ibuprofen *on page 342*

Advil® Cold & Sinus Caplets [US-OTC] *see* pseudoephedrine and ibuprofen *on page 553*

Advil® Cold & Sinus Tablet [Can] *see* pseudoephedrine and ibuprofen *on page 553*

Advil® Infants' Concentrated Drops [US-OTC] *see* ibuprofen *on page 342*

Advil® Junior [US-OTC] *see* ibuprofen *on page 342*

Advil® Migraine [US-OTC] *see* ibuprofen *on page 342*

Aeroaid® *(Discontinued)* *see page 814*

AeroBid® [US] *see* flunisolide *on page 276*

AeroBid®-M [US] *see* flunisolide *on page 276*

AeroChamber™ [US] *see* inhalation devices *on page 351*

Aerodine® *(Discontinued)* *see page 814*

Aerolate III® [US] *see* theophylline *on page 630*

Aerolate JR® [US] *see* theophylline *on page 630*

Aerolate® Oral Solution *(Discontinued)* *see page 814*

Aerolate SR® [US] *see* theophylline *on page 630*

Aeroseb-Dex® [US] *see* dexamethasone (topical) *on page 185*

Aeroseb-HC® [US] *see* hydrocortisone (topical) *on page 334*

Aerosporin® Injection *(Discontinued)* *see page 814*

Afrin® Children's Nose Drops *(Discontinued)* *see page 814*

Afrin® Extra Moisturizing [US-OTC] *see* oxymetazoline *on page 486*

Afrinol® *(Discontinued)* *see page 814*

Afrin® Original [US-OTC] *see* oxymetazoline *on page 486*

Afrin® Saline Mist *(Discontinued)* *see page 814*

Afrin® Severe Congestion [US-OTC] *see* oxymetazoline *on page 486*

Afrin® Sinus [US-OTC] *see* oxymetazoline *on page 486*

Afrin® [US-OTC] *see* oxymetazoline *on page 486*

Aftate® for Athlete's Foot [US-OTC] *see* tolnaftate *on page 644*

Aftate® for Jock Itch [US-OTC] *see* tolnaftate *on page 644*

Agenerase® [US/Can] *see* amprenavir *on page 41*

Aggrastat® [US/Can] *see* tirofiban *on page 641*

Aggrenox® [US/Can] *see* dipyridamole and aspirin *on page 206*

AgNO$_3$ *see* silver nitrate *on page 590*

Agoral® Plain *(Discontinued)* *see page 814*

Agrylin® [US/Can] *see* anagrelide *on page 42*

AHA *see* acetohydroxamic acid *on page 11*

AHF *see* antihemophilic factor (human) *on page 45*

A-HydroCort® [US/Can] *see* hydrocortisone (systemic) *on page 333*

AKBeta® *(Discontinued)* see page 814

Ak-Chlor® **Ophthalmic** *(Discontinued)* see page 814

AK-Cide® **[US]** see sulfacetamide and prednisolone on page 611

AK-Con™ **[US]** see naphazoline on page 446

AK-Dex® **[US]** see dexamethasone (ophthalmic) on page 184

AK-Dilate® **Ophthalmic** **[US]** see phenylephrine on page 510

AK-Fluor **[US]** see fluorescein sodium on page 277

Ak-Homatropine® **Ophthalmic** *(Discontinued)* see page 814

Akineton® **[US/Can]** see biperiden on page 86

AK-Mycin® *(Discontinued)* see page 814

AK-Nefrin® **Ophthalmic** **[US]** see phenylephrine on page 510

Akne-Mycin® **[US]** see erythromycin (ophthalmic/topical) on page 235

Akoline® **C.B. Tablet** *(Discontinued)* see page 814

AK-Pentolate® **[US]** see cyclopentolate on page 168

AK-Poly-Bac® **[US]** see bacitracin and polymyxin B on page 68

AK-Pred® **[US]** see prednisolone (ophthalmic) on page 537

AK-Spore® **H.C. Otic** *(Discontinued)* see page 814

AK-Spore® **Ophthalmic Ointment** *(Discontinued)* see page 814

AK-Spore® **Ophthalmic Solution** **[US]** see neomycin, polymyxin B, and gramicidin on page 453

AK-Sulf® **[US]** see sulfacetamide on page 610

AK-Taine® *(Discontinued)* see page 814

AKTob® **[US]** see tobramycin on page 641

AK-Tracin® **[US]** see bacitracin on page 68

AK-Trol® **[US]** see neomycin, polymyxin B, and dexamethasone on page 452

Akwa Tears® **[US-OTC]** see artificial tears on page 56

AK-Zol® *(Discontinued)* see page 814

Ala-Cort® **[US]** see hydrocortisone (topical) on page 334

Alamast™ **[US/Can]** see pemirolast on page 496

Ala-Quin® **[US]** see clioquinol and hydrocortisone on page 152

Ala-Scalp® **[US]** see hydrocortisone (topical) on page 334

Ala-Tet® *(Discontinued)* see page 814

alatrofloxacin see trovafloxacin on page 661

Alazide® *(Discontinued)* see page 814

Albalon® **[US]** see naphazoline on page 446

Albalon®-A Liquifilm **[Can]** see naphazoline and antazoline on page 447

Albalon-A® **Ophthalmic** *(Discontinued)* see page 814

albendazole (al BEN da zole)
   U.S./Canadian Brand Names Albenza® [US]
   Therapeutic Category Anthelmintic
   Use Treatment of parenchymal neurocysticercosis and cystic hydatid disease of the liver, lung, and peritoneum; albendazole may also be useful in the treatment of ascariasis, trichuriasis, enterobiasis, hookworm, strongyloidiasis, giardiasis, and microsporidiosis in AIDS
   (Continued)

albendazole *(Continued)*

Usual Dosage Oral:

Children ≤2 years:

Neurocysticercosis: 15 mg/kg for 8 days; repeat as necessary

Children >2 years and Adults:

Hydatid cyst: 400 mg twice daily with meals for 3 cycles (each cycle consists of 28 days of dosing followed by a 14-day albendazole-free interval)

Neurocysticercosis: 400 mg twice daily for 8-30 days

Roundworm, pinworm, hookworm: 400 mg as a single dose; treatment may be repeated in 3 weeks

Giardiasis: Strongyloidiasis and tapeworm: 400 mg/day for 3 days; treatment may be repeated in 3 weeks (giardiasis is a single course)

Dosage Forms Tablet: 200 mg

Albenza® [US] *see albendazole on previous page*

Albert® Glyburide [Can] *see glyburide on page 301*

Albert® Pentoxifylline [Can] *see pentoxifylline on page 502*

Albert® Tiafen [Can] *see tiaprofenic acid (Canada only) on page 638*

Albumarc® [US] *see albumin on this page*

albumin *(al BYOO min)*

Synonyms albumin (human)

U.S./Canadian Brand Names Albumarc® [US]; Albuminar® [US]; Albutein® [US]; Buminate® [US]; Plasbumin® [US/Can]

Therapeutic Category Blood Product Derivative

Use Treatment of hypovolemia; plasma volume expansion and maintenance of cardiac output in the treatment of certain types of shock or impending shock; hypoproteinemia resulting in generalized edema or decreased intravascular volume (eg, hypoproteinemia associated with acute nephrotic syndrome, premature infants)

Usual Dosage 5% should be used in hypovolemic patients; 25% should be used in patients in whom fluid and sodium intake must be minimized

Children:

Emergency initial dose: 25 g

Nonemergencies: 25% to 50% of the adult dose

Adults: Dosage depends on the condition of patient, usual adult dose is 25 g; no more than 250 g should be administered within 48 hours

Hypoproteinemia: I.V.: 0.5-1 g/kg/dose; repeat every 1-2 days as calculated to replace ongoing losses

Hypovolemia: I.V.: 0.5-1 g/kg/dose; repeat as needed; maximum dose: 6 g/kg/day

Dosage Forms Injection, human: 5% [50 mg/mL] (50 mL, 250 mL, 500 mL, 1000 mL); 25% [250 mg/mL] (20 mL, 50 mL, 100 mL)

Albuminar® [US] *see albumin on this page*

albumin (human) *see albumin on this page*

Albumisol® *(Discontinued)* *see page 814*

Albunex® *(Discontinued)* *see page 814*

Albutein® [US] *see albumin on this page*

albuterol *(al BYOO ter ole)*

Synonyms salbutamol

U.S./Canadian Brand Names AccuNeb™ [US]; Alti-Salbutamol [Can]; Apo®-Salvent [Can]; Novo-Salmol [Can]; Proventil® HFA [US]; Proventil® Repetabs® [US]; Proventil® [US]; Ventolin® HFA [US]; Ventolin® [US]; Volmax® [US]

Therapeutic Category Adrenergic Agonist Agent

Use Bronchodilator in reversible airway obstruction due to asthma or COPD; prevention of exercise-induced bronchospasm

Usual Dosage

Oral:

Children: Bronchospasm (treatment):

2-6 years: 0.1-0.2 mg/kg/dose 3 times/day; maximum dose not to exceed 12 mg/day (divided doses)

6-12 years: 2 mg/dose 3-4 times/day; maximum dose not to exceed 24 mg/day (divided doses)

Extended release: 4 mg every 12 hours; maximum dose not to exceed 24 mg/day (divided doses)

Children >12 years and Adults: Bronchospasm (treatment): 2-4 mg/dose 3-4 times/day; maximum dose not to exceed 32 mg/day (divided doses)

Extended release: 8 mg every 12 hours; maximum dose not to exceed 32 mg/day (divided doses). A 4 mg dose every 12 hours may be sufficient in some patients, such as adults of low body weight.

Elderly: Bronchospasm (treatment): 2 mg 3-4 times/day; maximum: 8 mg 4 times/day

Inhalation: Children ≥4 years and Adults:

Bronchospasm (treatment):

MDI: 90 mcg/spray: 1-2 inhalations every 4-6 hours; maximum: 12 inhalations/day

Capsule: 200-400 mcg every 4-6 hours

Exercise-induced bronchospasm (prophylaxis):

MDI-CFC aerosol: 2 inhalations 15 minutes before exercising

MDI-HFA aerosol: 2 inhalations 15-30 minutes before exercise

Capsule: 200 mcg 15 minutes before exercise

Nebulization:

Children:

Bronchospasm (treatment): 0.01-0.05 mL/kg of 0.5% solution every 4-6 hours

2-12 years: AccuNeb™: 0.63 mg or 1.25 mg 3-4 times/day, as needed, delivered over 5-15 minutes

Children >40 kg, patients with more severe asthma, or children 11-12 years: May respond better with a 1.25 mg dose

Bronchospasm (acute): 0.01-0.05 mL/kg of 0.5% solution every 4-6 hours; intensive care patients may require more frequent administration; minimum dose: 0.1 mL; maximum dose: 1 mL diluted in 1-2 mL normal saline; continuous nebulized albuterol at 0.3 mg/kg/hour has been used safely in the treatment of severe status asthmaticus in children; continuous nebulized doses of 3 mg/kg/hour ± 2.2 mg/kg/hour in children whose mean age was 20.7 months resulted in no cardiac toxicity; the optimal dosage for continuous nebulization remains to be determined.

Adults:

Bronchospasm (treatment): 2.5 mg, diluted to a total of 3 mL, 3-4 times/day over 5-15 minutes

Bronchospasm (acute) in intensive care patients: 2.5-5 mg every 20 minutes for 3 doses, then 2.5-10 mg every 1-4 hours as needed, **or** 10-15 mg/hour continuously

Dosage Forms

Aerosol, oral: 90 mcg/dose (17 g) [200 doses]

Proventil®: 90 mcg/dose (17 g) [200 doses]

Aerosol, oral, as sulfate [chlorofluorocarbon free]:

Proventil® HFA: 90 mcg/dose (6.7 g) [200 doses]

Ventolin® HFA: 90 mcg/dose (18 g) [200 doses]

Solution for oral inhalation, as sulfate: 0.083% (3 mL); 0.5% (20 mL)

AccuNeb™: 0.63 mg/3 mL (5 vials/pouch); 1.25 mg/3 mL (5 vials/pouch)

Proventil®: 0.083% (3 mL); 0.5% (20 mL)

Syrup, as sulfate: 2 mg/5 mL (120 mL, 480 mL)

Tablet, as sulfate: 2 mg, 4 mg

Tablet, extended release, as sulfate:

Proventil® Repetabs®: 4 mg

Volmax®: 4 mg, 8 mg

Alcaine® **[US/Can]** *see* proparacaine *on page 547*

alclometasone (al kloe MET a sone)

U.S./Canadian Brand Names Aclovate® [US]
Therapeutic Category Corticosteroid, Topical
Use Inflammation of corticosteroid-responsive dermatosis
Usual Dosage Topical: Apply a thin film to the affected area 2-3 times/day. Therapy should be discontinued when control is achieved. If no improvement is seen, reassessment of diagnosis may be necessary.
Dosage Forms
  Cream, as dipropionate: 0.05% (15 g, 45 g, 60 g)
  Ointment, topical, as dipropionate: 0.05% (15 g, 45 g, 60 g)

alcohol (ethyl) (AL koe hol ETH il)

Synonyms ethanol
U.S./Canadian Brand Names Biobase™ [Can]; Dilusol® [Can]; Duonalc® [Can]; Duonalc-E® Mild [Can]; Lavacol® [US-OTC]
Therapeutic Category Intravenous Nutritional Therapy; Pharmaceutical Aid
Use Topical anti-infective; pharmaceutical aid; an antidote for ethylene glycol overdose; an antidote for methanol overdose
Usual Dosage
  I.V.: Doses of 100-125 mg/kg/hour to maintain blood levels of 100 mg/dL are recommended after a loading dose of 0.6 g/kg; maximum dose: 400 mL of a 5% solution within 1 hour
  Topical: Use as needed
Dosage Forms
  Infusion [in D_5W]: Alcohol 5% (1000 mL); alcohol 10% (1000 mL)
  Injection, solution [absolute]: 98% (1 mL, 5 mL)
  Injection, solution [dehydrated]: 98% (1 mL, 5 mL)
  Liquid, topical [denatured] (Lavacol®): 70% (473 mL)

Alcomicin® **[Can]** *see* gentamicin *on page 297*

Alconefrin® **Nasal Solution** *(Discontinued)* *see page 814*

Aldactazide® **[US/Can]** *see* hydrochlorothiazide and spironolactone *on page 329*

Aldactone® **[US/Can]** *see* spironolactone *on page 604*

Aldara™ **[US/Can]** *see* imiquimod *on page 346*

aldesleukin (al des LOO kin)

Synonyms interleukin-2
U.S./Canadian Brand Names Proleukin® [US/Can]
Therapeutic Category Biological Response Modulator
Use Primarily investigated in tumors known to have a response to immunotherapy, such as melanoma and renal cell carcinoma; has been used in conjunction with LAK cells, TIL cells, IL-1, and interferon
Usual Dosage All orders should be written in million international units (million int. units) (refer to individual protocols).

Adults: Metastatic renal cell carcinoma:
  Treatment consists of two 5-day treatment cycles separated by a rest period. 600,000 int. units/kg (0.037 mg/kg)/dose administered every 8 hours by a 15-minute I.V. infusion for a total of 14 doses; following 9 days of rest, the schedule is repeated for another 14 doses, for a maximum of 28 doses per course.
Investigational regimen: I.V. continuous infusion: 4.5 million int. units/m²/day in 250-1000 mL of D_5W for 5 days
Dose modification: Hold or interrupt a dose rather than reducing dose; refer to protocol
Retreatment: Patients should be evaluated for response ~4 weeks after completion of a course of therapy and again immediately prior to the scheduled start of the next

treatment course. Additional courses of treatment may be administered to patients only if there is some tumor shrinkage following the last course and retreatment is not contraindicated. Each treatment course should be separated by a rest period of at least 7 weeks from the date of hospital discharge. Tumors have continued to regress up to 12 months following the initiation of therapy.

Dosage Forms Injection, powder for reconstitution: 22 x 10^6 int. units [18 million int. units/mL = 1.1 mg/mL when reconstituted]

Aldoclor® *(Discontinued)* see page 814

Aldomet® **[US/Can]** see methyldopa on page 420

Aldoril® **[US]** see methyldopa and hydrochlorothiazide on page 421

alemtuzumab (ay lem TU zoo mab)

Synonyms campath-1H; DNA-derived humanized monoclonal antibody; humanized IgG1 anti-CD52 monoclonal antibody

U.S./Canadian Brand Names Campath® [US]

Therapeutic Category Antineoplastic Agent, Monoclonal Antibody

Use Treatment of B-cell chronic lymphocytic leukemia (B-CLL) in patients treated with alkylating agents and who have failed fludarabine therapy

Usual Dosage Note: **Dose escalation is required;** usually accomplished in 3-7 days. Do not exceed single doses >30 mg or cumulative doses >90 mg/week. Premedicate with diphenhydramine and acetaminophen 30 minutes before initiation of infusion. Start anti-infective prophylaxis. Discontinue therapy during serious infection, serious hematologic or other serious toxicity until the event resolves. Permanently discontinue if evidence of autoimmune anemia or autoimmune thrombocytopenia occurs.

I.V. infusion: Adults: B-CLL:

Initial: 3 mg/day as a 2-hour infusion; when daily dose is tolerated (eg, infusion-related toxicities at or below Grade 2) increase to 10 mg/day and continue until tolerated; when 10 mg dose tolerated, increase to 30 mg/day

Maintenance: 30 mg/day 3 times/week on alternate days (ie, Monday, Wednesday, Friday) for up to 12 weeks

Dosage Forms Injection, solution: 10 mg/mL (3 mL)

alendronate (a LEN droe nate)

U.S./Canadian Brand Names Fosamax® [US/Can]

Therapeutic Category Bisphosphonate Derivative

Use Treatment of osteoporosis in postmenopausal women, Paget's disease of the bone; treatment of glucocorticoid-induced osteoporosis in males and females with low bone mineral density who are receiving a daily dosage ≥7.5 mg of prednisone (or equivalent)

Usual Dosage Oral:

Adults: Patients with osteoporosis or Paget's disease should receive supplemental calcium and vitamin D if dietary intake is inadequate

Osteoporosis in postmenopausal women: 10 mg once daily. Safety of treatment for >4 years has not been studied (extension studies are ongoing).

Paget's disease of bone: 40 mg once daily for 6 months

Retreatment: Relapses during the 12 months following therapy occurred in 9% of patients who responded to treatment. Specific retreatment data are not available. Retreatment with alendronate may be considered, following a 6-month post-treatment evaluation period, in patients who have relapsed based on increases in serum alkaline phosphatase, which should be measured periodically. Retreatment may also be considered in those who failed to normalize their serum alkaline phosphatase.

Treatment of glucocorticoid-induced osteoporosis: 5 mg once daily. A dose of 10 mg once daily should be used in postmenopausal women who are not receiving estrogen. Patients treated with glucocorticoids should receive adequate amounts of calcium and vitamin D.

Dosage Forms Tablet, as sodium: 5 mg, 10 mg, 35 mg, 40 mg, 70 mg

Alercap® **[US-OTC]** see diphenhydramine on page 202

Aler-Dryl® **[US-OTC]** *see* diphenhydramine *on page 202*

Alertab® **[US-OTC]** *see* diphenhydramine *on page 202*

Alertec® **[Can]** *see* modafinil *on page 434*

Alesse® **[US/Can]** *see* ethinyl estradiol and levonorgestrel *on page 248*

Aleve® **[US-OTC]** *see* naproxen *on page 447*

Alfenta® **[US/Can]** *see* alfentanil *on this page*

alfentanil (al FEN ta nil)

U.S./Canadian Brand Names Alfenta® [US/Can]
Therapeutic Category Analgesic, Narcotic; General Anesthetic
Controlled Substance C-II
Use Analgesia; analgesia adjunct; anesthetic agent
Usual Dosage Doses should be titrated to appropriate effects; wide range of doses is dependent upon desired degree of analgesia/anesthesia

Children <12 years: Dose not established
Adults: Anesthesia of ≤30 minutes: Initial (induction): 8-20 mcg/kg, then 3-5 mcg/kg/ dose or 0.5-1 mcg/kg/minute for maintenance; total dose: 8-40 mcg/kg; higher doses used for longer anesthesia required procedures
Dosage Forms Injection, as hydrochloride [preservative free]: 500 mcg/mL (2 mL, 5 mL, 10 mL, 20 mL)

Alferon® **N [US/Can]** *see* interferon alfa-n3 *on page 356*

alglucerase (al GLOO ser ase)

Synonyms glucocerebrosidase
U.S./Canadian Brand Names Ceredase® [US]
Therapeutic Category Enzyme
Use Long-term enzyme replacement in patients with confirmed Type I Gaucher's disease who exhibit one or more of the following conditions: Moderate to severe anemia; thrombocytopenia and bleeding tendencies; bone disease; hepatomegaly or spleno-megaly
Usual Dosage I.V. infusion: Administer 20-60 units/kg with a frequency ranging from 3 times/week to once every 2 weeks
Dosage Forms Injection, solution: 10 units/mL (5 mL); 80 units/mL (5 mL)

alitretinoin (a li TRET i noyn)

U.S./Canadian Brand Names Panretin™ [US]
Therapeutic Category Antineoplastic Agent, Miscellaneous; Retinoic Acid Derivative
Use Topical treatment of cutaneous lesions in AIDS-related Kaposi's sarcoma; not indicated when systemic therapy for Kaposi's sarcoma is indicated
Usual Dosage Topical: Apply gel twice daily to cutaneous Kaposi's sarcoma lesions
Dosage Forms Gel: 0.1% (60 g)

Alka-Mints® **[US-OTC]** *see* calcium carbonate *on page 104*

Alka-Seltzer Plus® **Cold and Sinus [US-OTC]** *see* acetaminophen and pseudo-ephedrine *on page 6*

Alka-Seltzer® **Plus Cold Liqui-Gels**® **[US-OTC]** *see* acetaminophen, chlorphen-iramine, and pseudoephedrine *on page 7*

Alka-Seltzer® **Plus Flu Liqui-Gels**® **[US-OTC]** *see* acetaminophen, dextrometh-orphan, and pseudoephedrine *on page 8*

Alkeran® **[US/Can]** *see* melphalan *on page 406*

Allbee® **With C [US-OTC]** *see* vitamin B complex with vitamin C *on page 681*

Allegra® **[US/Can]** *see* fexofenadine *on page 270*

Allegra-D® **[US/Can]** *see* fexofenadine and pseudoephedrine *on page 271*

Aller-Chlor® **[US-OTC]** *see* chlorpheniramine *on page 137*

Allercon® **Tablet** *(Discontinued) see page 814*

Allerdryl® **[Can]** *see* diphenhydramine *on page 202*

Allerest® **12 Hour Capsule** *(Discontinued) see page 814*

Allerest® **12 Hour Nasal Solution** *(Discontinued) see page 814*

Allerest® **Eye Drops** *(Discontinued) see page 814*

Allerest® **Maximum Strength [US-OTC]** *see* chlorpheniramine and pseudoephedrine *on page 138*

Allerfed® **[US-OTC]** *see* triprolidine and pseudoephedrine *on page 659*

Allerfrim® **[US-OTC]** *see* triprolidine and pseudoephedrine *on page 659*

Allerfrin® **Syrup** *(Discontinued) see page 814*

Allerfrin® **Tablet** *(Discontinued) see page 814*

Allerfrin® **With Codeine** *(Discontinued) see page 814*

Allergan® **Ear Drops [US]** *see* antipyrine and benzocaine *on page 47*

Allermax® **[US-OTC]** *see* diphenhydramine *on page 202*

Allernix [Can] *see* diphenhydramine *on page 202*

Allerphed® **[US-OTC]** *see* triprolidine and pseudoephedrine *on page 659*

Allersol® **[US]** *see* naphazoline *on page 446*

allopurinol (al oh PURE i nole)

U.S./Canadian Brand Names Aloprim™ [US]; Apo®-Allopurinol [Can]; Zyloprim® [US/Can]

Therapeutic Category Xanthine Oxidase Inhibitor

Use Prevention of attacks of gouty arthritis and nephropathy; also used to treat secondary hyperuricemia which may occur during treatment of tumors or leukemia; prevent recurrent calcium oxalate calculi

Usual Dosage

Oral:

Children: 10 mg/kg/day in 2-3 divided doses or 200-300 mg/m^2/day in 2-4 divided doses, maximum: 600 mg/24 hours

Alternative:

<6 years: 150 mg/day in 3 divided doses

6-10 years: 300 mg/day in 2-3 divided doses

Children >10 years and Adults: Daily doses >300 mg should be administered in divided doses

Myeloproliferative neoplastic disorders: 600-800 mg/day in 2-3 divided doses for prevention of acute uric acid nephropathy for 2-3 days starting 1-2 days before chemotherapy

Gout: 200-300 mg/day (mild); 400-600 mg/day (severe)

Maximum dose: 800 mg/day

I.V.: Intravenous daily dose can be given as a single infusion or in equally divided doses at 6-, 8-, or 12-hour intervals. A fluid intake sufficient to yield a daily urinary output of at least 2 L in adults and the maintenance of a neutral or, preferably, slightly alkaline urine are desirable.

Children: Starting dose: 200 mg/m^2/day

Adults: 200-400 mg/m^2/day (max: 600 mg/day)

Dosage Forms

Injection, powder for reconstitution, as sodium (Aloprim™): 500 mg

Tablet (Zyloprim®): 100 mg, 300 mg

all-*trans*-retinoic acid *see* tretinoin (oral) *on page 649*

almotriptan (al moh TRIP tan)

Synonyms almotriptan malate
U.S./Canadian Brand Names Axert™ [US]
Therapeutic Category Serotonin 5-HT$_{1D}$ Receptor Agonist
Use Acute treatment of migraine with or without aura
Usual Dosage Oral: Adults: Migraine: Initial: 6.25-12.5 mg in a single dose; if the headache returns, repeat the dose after 2 hours; no more than 2 doses in 24-hour period
Note: If the first dose is ineffective, diagnosis needs to be re-evaluated. Safety of treating more than 4 migraines/month has not been established.
Dosage Forms Tablet, as malate: 6.25 mg, 12.5 mg

almotriptan malate see almotriptan on this page

Alocril™ [US/Can] see nedocromil (ophthalmic) on page 450

Aloe Vesta® 2-n-1 Antifungal [US-OTC] see miconazole on page 427

Alomide® [US/Can] see lodoxamide tromethamine on page 389

Alophen® [US-OTC] see bisacodyl on page 87

Aloprim™ [US] see allopurinol on previous page

Alor® 5/500 (Discontinued) see page 814

Alora® [US] see estradiol on page 238

alpha$_1$-PI see alpha$_1$-proteinase inhibitor on this page

alpha$_1$-proteinase inhibitor (al fa won-PRO tee in ase in HI bi tor)

Synonyms alpha$_1$-PI
U.S./Canadian Brand Names Prolastin® [US/Can]
Therapeutic Category Antitrypsin Deficiency Agent
Use Congenital alpha$_1$-antitrypsin deficiency
Usual Dosage Adults: I.V.: 60 mg/kg once weekly
Dosage Forms Injection, human [single-dose vial]: 500 mg alpha$_1$-PI [20 mL diluent]; 1000 mg alpha$_1$-PI [40 mL diluent]

Alphagan® (Discontinued) see page 814

Alphagan® P [US/Can] see brimonidine on page 92

Alphamul® (Discontinued) see page 814

Alphanate® [US] see antihemophilic factor (human) on page 45

AlphaNine® SD [US] see factor IX complex (human) on page 261

Alphatrex® [US] see betamethasone (topical) on page 83

alprazolam (al PRAY zoe lam)

U.S./Canadian Brand Names Alprazolam Intensol® [US]; Alti-Alprazolam [Can]; Apo®-Alpraz [Can]; Gen-Alprazolam [Can]; Novo-Alprazol [Can]; Nu-Alprax [Can]; Xana TS™ [Can]; Xanax® [US/Can]
Therapeutic Category Benzodiazepine
Controlled Substance C-IV
Use Treatment of anxiety; adjunct in the treatment of depression; management of panic attacks
Usual Dosage Oral:
Children <18 years: Dose not established
Adults: 0.25-0.5 mg 2-3 times/day, titrate dose upward; maximum: 4 mg/day (anxiety); 10 mg/day (panic attacks)
Dosage Forms
Solution, oral: 1 mg/mL (30 mL)
Tablet: 0.25 mg, 0.5 mg, 1 mg, 2 mg

Alprazolam Intensol® [US] *see* alprazolam *on previous page*

alprostadil (al PROS ta dill)

Synonyms PGE$_1$; prostaglandin E$_1$

U.S./Canadian Brand Names Caverject® [US/Can]; Edex® [US]; Muse® Pellet [US]; Prostin VR Pediatric® [US/Can]

Therapeutic Category Prostaglandin

Use Temporary maintenance of patency of ductus arteriosus in neonates with ductal-dependent congenital cyanotic or acyanotic heart disease until surgery can be performed; these defects include cyanotic (eg, pulmonary atresia, pulmonary stenosis, tricuspid atresia, Fallot's tetralogy, transposition of the great vessels) and acyanotic (eg, interruption of aortic arch, coarctation of aorta, hypoplastic left ventricle) heart disease. Alprostadil has also been used investigationally for the treatment of pulmonary hypertension in infants and children with congenital heart defects with left-to-right shunts and primary graft nonfunction following liver transplant. Used in penile erectile dysfunction

Usual Dosage

Patent ductus arteriosus (Prostin VR Pediatric®):

I.V. continuous infusion into a large vein, or alternatively through an umbilical artery catheter placed at the ductal opening: 0.05-0.1 mcg/kg/minute with therapeutic response, rate is reduced to lowest effective dosage; with unsatisfactory response, rate is increased gradually; maintenance: 0.01-0.4 mcg/kg/minute

PGE$_1$ is usually given at an infusion rate of 0.1 mcg/kg/minute, but it is often possible to reduce the dosage to $1/2$ or even $1/10$ without losing the therapeutic effect.

Therapeutic response is indicated by increased pH in those with acidosis or by an increase in oxygenation (pO$_2$) usually evident within 30 minutes

Erectile dysfunction:

Caverject®:

Vasculogenic, psychogenic, or mixed etiology: Individualize dose by careful titration; usual dose: 2.5-60 mcg (doses >60 mcg are not recommended); initiate dosage titration at 2.5 mcg, increasing by 2.5 mcg to a dose of 5 mcg and then in increments of 5-10 mcg depending on the erectile response until the dose produces an erection suitable for intercourse, not lasting >1 hour; if there is absolutely no response to initial 2.5 mcg dose, the second dose may increased to 7.5 mcg, followed by increments of 5-10 mcg

Neurogenic etiology (eg, spinal cord injury): Initiate dosage titration at 1.25 mcg, increasing to a doses of 2.5 mcg and then 5 mcg; increase further in increments 5 mcg until the dose is reached that produces an erection suitable for intercourse, not lasting >1 hour

Note: Patient must stay in the physician's office until complete detumescence occurs; if there is no response, then the next higher dose may be given within 1 hour; if there is still no response, a 1-day interval before giving the next dose is recommended; increasing the dose or concentration in the treatment of impotence results in increasing pain and discomfort

Muse® Pellet: Intraurethral: Administer as needed to achieve an erection; duration of action: ~30-60 minutes; use only two systems per 24-hour period

Dosage Forms

Injection:

Caverject®: 5 mcg/mL, 10 mcg/mL, 20 mcg/mL

Edex®: 5 mcg/mL, 10 mcg/mL, 20 mcg/mL, 40 mcg/mL

Prostin VR Pediatric®: 500 mcg/mL (1 mL)

Pellet, urethral (Muse®): 125 mcg, 250 mcg, 500 mcg, 1000 mcg

Alrex™ [US/Can] *see* loteprednol *on page 393*

AL-Rr® Oral (Discontinued) *see page 814*

Altace™ [US/Can] *see* ramipril *on page 564*

Altafed® [US-OTC] *see* triprolidine and pseudoephedrine *on page 659*

Altamist [US-OTC] *see* sodium chloride *on page 595*

Altaryl® **[US-OTC]** *see* diphenhydramine *on page 202*

alteplase (AL te plase)

Synonyms alteplase, recombinant; tissue plasminogen activator, recombinant; t-PA
U.S./Canadian Brand Names Activase® rt-PA [Can]; Activase® [US]; Cathflo™ Activase® [US]
Therapeutic Category Fibrinolytic Agent
Use Management of acute myocardial infarction for the lysis of thrombi in coronary arteries; management of acute massive pulmonary embolism (PE) in adults
Unlabeled use: Peripheral arterial thrombotic obstruction
Usual Dosage
  I.V.:
  Coronary artery thrombi: Front loading dose (weight-based):
  Patients >67 kg: Total dose: 100 mg over 1.5 hours; infuse 15 mg (30 mL) over 1-2 minutes. Infuse 50 mg (100 mL) over 30 minutes. See "Note."
  Patients ≤67 kg: Total dose: 1.25 mg/kg; infuse 15 mg I.V. bolus over 1-2 minutes, then infuse 0.75 mg/kg (not to exceed 50 mg) over next 30 minutes, followed by 0.5 mg/kg over next 60 minutes (not to exceed 35 mg). See "Note."
  Note: Concurrently, begin heparin 60 units/kg bolus (maximum: 4000 units) followed by continuous infusion of 12 units/kg/hour (maximum: 1000 units/hour) and adjust to aPTT target of 1.5-2 times the upper limit of control. Infuse remaining 35 mg (70 mL) of alteplase over the next hour.
  Acute pulmonary embolism: 100 mg over 2 hours.
  Acute ischemic stroke: Doses should be given within the first 3 hours of the onset of symptoms. Load with 0.09 mg/kg as a bolus, followed by 0.81 mg/kg as a continuous infusion over 60 minutes. Maximum total dose should not exceed 90 mg. Heparin should not be started for at least 24 hours after starting alteplase for stroke.
  Intracatheter: Central venous catheter clearance: Cathflo™ Activase®:
  Patients ≥10 to <30 kg: 110% of the internal lumen volume of the catheter (≤2 mg [1 mg/mL]); retain in catheter for ≤2 hours; may instill a second dose if catheter remains occluded
  Patients ≥30 kg: 2 mg (1 mg/mL); retain in catheter for ≤2 hours; may instill a second dose if catheter remains occluded
  Intra-arterial: Peripheral arterial thrombotic obstruction (unlabeled use): 0.02-0.1 mg/kg/hour for 1-8 hours
Dosage Forms Injection, powder for reconstitution, recombinant:
  Activase®: 50 mg [29 million units]; 100 mg [58 million units]
  Cathflo™ Activase®: 2 mg

alteplase, recombinant *see* alteplase *on this page*

ALternaGel® **[US-OTC]** *see* aluminum hydroxide *on page 28*

Alti-Alprazolam [Can] *see* alprazolam *on page 24*

Alti-Amiodarone [Can] *see* amiodarone *on page 34*

Alti-Azathioprine [Can] *see* azathioprine *on page 65*

Alti-Beclomethasone [Can] *see* beclomethasone *on page 73*

Alti-Benzydamine [Can] *see* benzydamine *(Canada only) on page 81*

Alti-Bromazepam [Can] *see* bromazepam *(Canada only) on page 92*

Alti-Captopril [Can] *see* captopril *on page 112*

Alti-Clindamycin [Can] *see* clindamycin *on page 151*

Alti-Clobazam [Can] *see* clobazam *(Canada only) on page 152*

Alti-Clonazepam [Can] *see* clonazepam *on page 154*

Alti-CPA [Can] *see* cyproterone *(Canada only) on page 170*

Alti-Desipramine [Can] *see* desipramine *on page 181*

Alti-Dexamethasone [Can] *see* dexamethasone (systemic) *on page 184*

Alti-Diltiazem [Can] *see* diltiazem *on page 199*

Alti-Diltiazem CD [Can] *see* diltiazem *on page 199*

Alti-Divalproex [Can] *see* valproic acid and derivatives *on page 670*

Alti-Domperidone [Can] *see* domperidone *(Canada only) on page 211*

Alti-Doxepin [Can] *see* doxepin *on page 213*

Alti-Famotidine [Can] *see* famotidine *on page 262*

Alti-Flunisolide [Can] *see* flunisolide *on page 276*

Alti-Fluoxetine [Can] *see* fluoxetine *on page 279*

Alti-Flurbiprofen [Can] *see* flurbiprofen *on page 282*

Alti-Fluvoxamine [Can] *see* fluvoxamine *on page 285*

Alti-Ipratropium [Can] *see* ipratropium *on page 358*

Alti-Minocycline [Can] *see* minocycline *on page 431*

Alti-Moclobemide [Can] *see* moclobemide *(Canada only) on page 434*

Alti-MPA [Can] *see* medroxyprogesterone acetate *on page 404*

Altinac™ [US] *see* tretinoin (topical) *on page 650*

Alti-Nadolol [Can] *see* nadolol *on page 443*

Alti-Nortriptyline [Can] *see* nortriptyline *on page 466*

Alti-Piroxicam [Can] *see* piroxicam *on page 517*

Alti-Prazosin [Can] *see* prazosin *on page 536*

Alti-Ranitidine [Can] *see* ranitidine hydrochloride *on page 564*

Alti-Salbutamol [Can] *see* albuterol *on page 18*

Alti-Sotalol [Can] *see* sotalol *on page 602*

Alti-Sulfasalazine® [Can] *see* sulfasalazine *on page 613*

Alti-Terazosin [Can] *see* terazosin *on page 622*

Alti-Ticlopidine [Can] *see* ticlopidine *on page 639*

Alti-Trazodone [Can] *see* trazodone *on page 649*

Alti-Verapamil [Can] *see* verapamil *on page 675*

Altocor™ [US] *see* lovastatin *on page 393*

altretamine (al TRET a meen)
Synonyms hexamethylmelamine
U.S./Canadian Brand Names Hexalen® [US/Can]
Therapeutic Category Antineoplastic Agent
Use Palliative treatment of persistent or recurrent ovarian cancer
Usual Dosage Adults: Oral (refer to protocol): 4-12 mg/kg/day in 3-4 divided doses for 21-90 days
Alternatively: 240-320 mg/m²/day in 3-4 divided doses for 21 days, repeated every 6 weeks
Alternatively: 260 mg/m²/day for 14-21 days of a 28-day cycle in 4 divided doses
Dosage Forms Capsule: 50 mg

Alu-Cap® [US-OTC] *see* aluminum hydroxide *on next page*

Aludrox® *(Discontinued)* *see* page 814

aluminum acetate and acetic acid
(a LOO mi num AS e tate & a SEE tik AS id)
Synonyms acetic acid and aluminum acetate otic; Burow's otic
U.S./Canadian Brand Names Otic Domeboro® [US]
Therapeutic Category Otic Agent, Anti-infective
(Continued)

aluminum acetate and acetic acid *(Continued)*

Use Treatment of superficial infections of the external auditory canal

Usual Dosage Otic: Instill 4-6 drops in ear(s) every 2-3 hours

Dosage Forms Solution, otic: Aluminum acetate 10% and acetic acid 2% (60 mL)

aluminum chloride hexahydrate

(a LOO mi num KLOR ide heks a HYE drate)

U.S./Canadian Brand Names Drysol™ [US]

Therapeutic Category Topical Skin Product

Use Astringent in the management of hyperhidrosis

Usual Dosage Adults: Topical: Apply at bedtime

Dosage Forms Solution, topical: 20% in SD alcohol 40 (35 mL, 37.5 mL)

aluminum hydroxide (a LOO mi num hye DROKS ide)

U.S./Canadian Brand Names ALternaGel® [US-OTC]; Alu-Cap® [US-OTC]; Amphojel® [Can]; Basaljel® [Can]

Therapeutic Category Antacid

Use Hyperacidity; hyperphosphatemia

Usual Dosage Oral:

Peptic ulcer disease:

Children: 5-15 mL/dose every 3-6 hours or 1 and 3 hours after meals and at bedtime

Adults: 15-45 mL every 3-6 hours or 1 and 3 hours after meals and at bedtime

Prophylaxis against gastrointestinal bleeding:

Infants: 2-5 mL/dose every 1-2 hours

Children: 5-15 mL/dose every 1-2 hours

Adults: 30-60 mL/dose every hour

Titrate to maintain the gastric pH >5

Hyperphosphatemia:

Children: 50 mg to 150 mg/kg/24 hours in divided doses every 4-6 hours, titrate dosage to maintain serum phosphorus within normal range

Adults: 500-1800 mg, 3-6 times/day, between meals and at bedtime

Antacid: Adults: 30 mL 1 and 3 hours postprandial and at bedtime

Dosage Forms

Capsule:

Alu-Cap®: 475 mg

Liquid (ALternaGel®): 600 mg/5 mL

Suspension, oral: 320 mg/5 mL, 450 mg/5 mL, 675 mg/5 mL

aluminum hydroxide and magnesium carbonate

(a LOO mi num hye DROKS ide & mag NEE zhum KAR bun nate)

U.S./Canadian Brand Names Gaviscon® Extra Strength [US-OTC]; Gaviscon® Liquid [US-OTC]

Therapeutic Category Antacid

Use Temporary relief of symptoms associated with gastric acidity

Usual Dosage Adults: Oral: 15-30 mL 4 times/day after meals and at bedtime

Dosage Forms

Liquid:

Gaviscon®: Aluminum hydroxide 31.7 mg and magnesium carbonate 119.3 mg per 5 mL (355 mL) [contains sodium 0.57 mEq/5 mL]

Gaviscon® Extra Strength: Aluminum hydroxide 84.6 mg and magnesium carbonate 79.1 mg per 5 mL (355 mL) [contains sodium 0.9 mEq/5 mL]

Tablet, chewable (Gaviscon® Extra Strength): Aluminum hydroxide 160 mg and magnesium carbonate 105 mg [contains sodium 1.3 mEq/tablet]

aluminum hydroxide and magnesium hydroxide
(a LOO mi num hye DROKS ide & mag NEE zhum hye DROK side)

Synonyms magnesium hydroxide and aluminum hydroxide

U.S./Canadian Brand Names Diovol® [Can]; Diovol® Ex [Can]; Gelusil® [Can]; Gelusil® Extra Strength [Can]; Maalox® TC (Therapeutic Concentrate) [US-OTC]; Maalox® [US-OTC]; Univol® [Can]

Therapeutic Category Antacid

Use Antacid, hyperphosphatemia in renal failure

Usual Dosage Adults: Oral: 5-10 mL or 1-2 tablets 4-6 times/day, between meals and at bedtime; may be used every hour for severe symptoms

Dosage Forms
Suspension (Maalox®): Aluminum hydroxide 225 mg and magnesium hydroxide 200 mg per 5 mL (150 mL, 360 mL, 780 mL)
Suspension, high potency (Maalox® TC): Aluminum hydroxide 600 mg and magnesium hydroxide 300 mg per 5 mL (360 mL)

aluminum hydroxide, magnesium hydroxide, and simethicone
(a LOO mi num hye DROKS ide, mag NEE zhum hye DROKS ide, & sye METH i kone)

U.S./Canadian Brand Names Diovol Plus® [Can]; Maalox® Fast Release Liquid [US-OTC]; Maalox® Max [US-OTC]; Mylanta® [Can]; Mylanta™ Double Strength; Mylanta™ Extra Strength [Can]; Mylanta® Extra Strength Liquid [US-OTC]; Mylanta® Liquid [US-OTC]; Mylanta™ Regular Strength [Can]

Therapeutic Category Antacid; Antiflatulent

Use Temporary relief of hyperacidity associated with gas; may also be used for indications associated with other antacids

Usual Dosage Adults: Oral: 15-30 mL or 2-4 tablets 4-6 times/day between meals and at bedtime; may be used every hour for severe symptoms

Dosage Forms Liquid:
Maalox® Fast Release: Aluminum hydroxide 500 mg, magnesium hydroxide 450 mg, and simethicone 40 mg per 5 mL (360 mL, 780 mL)
Maalox® Max: Aluminum hydroxide 400 mg, magnesium hydroxide 400 mg, and simethicone 40 mg per 5 mL (360 mL)
Mylanta®: Aluminum hydroxide 200 mg, magnesium hydroxide 200 mg, and simethicone 20 mg per 5 mL (180 mL, 360 mL, 720 mL) [original, cherry, mint, and lemon flavors]
Mylanta® Extra Strength: Aluminum hydroxide 400 mg, magnesium hydroxide 400 mg, and simethicone 40 mg per 5 mL (180 mL, 360 mL, 720 mL) [original, cherry, and mint flavors]

aluminum sucrose sulfate, basic *see* sucralfate *on page 609*

aluminum sulfate and calcium acetate
(a LOO mi num SUL fate & KAL see um AS e tate)

U.S./Canadian Brand Names Bluboro® [US-OTC]; Domeboro® [US-OTC]; Pedi-Boro® [US-OTC]

Therapeutic Category Topical Skin Product

Use Astringent wet dressing for relief of inflammatory conditions of the skin and to reduce weeping that may occur in dermatitis

Usual Dosage Topical: Soak affected area in the solution 2-4 times/day for 15-30 minutes or apply wet dressing soaked in the solution 2-4 times/day for 30-minute treatment periods; rewet dressing with solution every few minutes to keep it moist

Dosage Forms Aluminum sulfate and calcium acetate form aluminum acetate when mixed:
Powder, for topical solution (Bluboro®, Domeboro®, Pedi-Boro®): 1 packet/16 ounces of water = 1:40 solution = Modified Burow's Solution
Tablet, effervescent, for topical solution (Domeboro®): 1 tablet/12 ounces of water = 1:40 solution = Modified Burow's Solution

Alupent® **[US]** *see* metaproterenol *on page 413*

Alu-Tab® *(Discontinued) see page 814*

amantadine (a MAN ta deen)

Synonyms adamantanamine
U.S./Canadian Brand Names Endantadine® [Can]; PMS-Amantadine [Can]; Symmetrel® [US/Can]
Therapeutic Category Anti-Parkinson's Agent; Antiviral Agent
Use Prophylaxis and treatment of influenza A viral infection; symptomatic and adjunct treatment of parkinsonism
Usual Dosage Oral:
Children:
1-9 years: 4.4-8.8 mg/kg/day in 1-2 divided doses to a maximum of 150 mg/day
9-12 years: 100-200 mg/day in 1-2 divided doses
After first influenza A virus vaccine dose, amantadine prophylaxis may be administered for up to 6 weeks or until 2 weeks after the second dose of vaccine
Adults:
Parkinson's disease: 100 mg twice daily
Influenza A viral infection: 200 mg/day in 1-2 divided doses
Prophylaxis: Minimum 10-day course of therapy following exposure or continue for 2-3 weeks after influenza A virus vaccine is administered
Dosage Forms
Capsule, as hydrochloride: 100 mg
Syrup, as hydrochloride (Symmetrel®): 50 mg/5 mL (480 mL) [raspberry flavor]
Tablet, as hydrochloride (Symmetrel®): 100 mg

Amaphen® *(Discontinued) see page 814*

Amaryl® **[US/Can]** *see* glimepiride *on page 299*

Amatine® **[Can]** *see* midodrine *on page 430*

ambenonium (am be NOE nee um)

U.S./Canadian Brand Names Mytelase® [US/Can]
Therapeutic Category Cholinergic Agent
Use Treatment of myasthenia gravis
Usual Dosage Adults: Oral: 5-25 mg 3-4 times/day
Dosage Forms Tablet, as chloride: 10 mg

Ambi 10® *(Discontinued) see page 814*

Ambien® **[US/Can]** *see* zolpidem *on page 693*

Ambi® **Skin Tone** *(Discontinued) see page 814*

AmBisome® **[US/Can]** *see* amphotericin B liposomal *on page 40*

amcinonide (am SIN oh nide)

U.S./Canadian Brand Names Cyclocort® [US/Can]
Therapeutic Category Corticosteroid, Topical
Use Relief of the inflammatory and pruritic manifestations of corticosteroid-responsive dermatoses
Usual Dosage Adults: Topical: Apply in a thin film 2-3 times/day. Therapy should be discontinued when control is achieved. If no improvement is seen, reassessment of diagnosis may be necessary.
Dosage Forms
Cream: 0.1% (15 g, 30 g, 60 g) [contains benzyl alcohol]
Lotion: 0.1% (20 mL, 60 mL) [contains benzyl alcohol]
Ointment: 0.1% (15 g, 30 g, 60 g) [contains benzyl alcohol]

Amcort® **Injection** *(Discontinued) see page 814*

Amen® *(Discontinued)* *see page 814*

Amerge® **[US/Can]** *see* naratriptan *on page 448*

Americaine® **Anesthetic Lubricant [US]** *see* benzocaine *on page 77*

Americaine® **[US-OTC]** *see* benzocaine *on page 77*

A-methaPred® **[US]** *see* methylprednisolone *on page 423*

amethocaine *see* tetracaine *on page 627*

amethopterin *see* methotrexate *on page 417*

Ametop™ **[Can]** *see* tetracaine *on page 627*

amfepramone *see* diethylpropion *on page 195*

Amibid LA [US] *see* guaifenesin *on page 307*

Amicar® **[US/Can]** *see* aminocaproic acid *on next page*

Amidate® **[US/Can]** *see* etomidate *on page 259*

amifostine (am i FOS teen)

Synonyms ethiofos; gammaphos
U.S./Canadian Brand Names Ethyol® [US/Can]
Therapeutic Category Antidote
Use Reduce the incidence of moderate to severe xerostomia in patients undergoing postoperative radiation treatment for head and neck cancer, where the radiation port includes a substantial portion of the parotid glands. Protection against cisplatin-induced nephrotoxicity in advanced ovarian cancer patients; it may also provide protection from cisplatin-induced peripheral neuropathy
Usual Dosage I.V.: 910 mg/m^2 beginning 30 minutes before starting chemotherapy; reduction of xerostomia from head and neck radiation: 200 mg/m^2 I.V. (as a 3-minute infusion) once daily, starting 15-30 minutes before standard fraction radiation therapy; dose adjustment is recommended for subsequent doses if the previous dose was interrupted, and not able to be resumed; secondary to hypotension, the recommended dose for subsequent administration is 740 mg/m^2
Dosage Forms Injection, powder for reconstitution: 500 mg

Amigesic® **[US/Can]** *see* salsalate *on page 583*

amikacin (am i KAY sin)

U.S./Canadian Brand Names Amikin® [US/Can]
Therapeutic Category Aminoglycoside (Antibiotic)
Use Treatment of documented gram-negative enteric infection resistant to gentamicin and tobramycin; documented infection of mycobacterial organisms susceptible to amikacin
Usual Dosage I.M., I.V.:
Infants and Children: 15-20 mg/kg/day divided every 8 hours
Adults: 15 mg/kg/day divided every 8-12 hours
Dosage Forms Injection, solution, as sulfate: 50 mg/mL (2 mL, 4 mL); 62.5 mg/mL (8 mL); 250 mg/mL (2 mL, 4 mL) [contains metabisulfite]

Amikin® **[US/Can]** *see* amikacin *on this page*

amiloride (a MIL oh ride)

U.S./Canadian Brand Names Midamor® [US/Can]
Therapeutic Category Diuretic, Potassium Sparing
Use Counteract potassium loss induced by other diuretics in the treatment of hypertension or edematous conditions including CHF, hepatic cirrhosis and hypoaldosteronism; usually used in conjunction with a more potent diuretic such as thiazides or loop diuretics
(Continued)

amiloride *(Continued)*

Usual Dosage Oral:
Children: Although safety and efficacy have not been established by the FDA in children, a dosage of 0.625 mg/kg/day has been used in children weighing 6-20 kg
Adults: 5-10 mg/day (up to 20 mg)
Dosage Forms Tablet, as hydrochloride: 5 mg

amiloride and hydrochlorothiazide
(a MIL oh ride & hye droe klor oh THYE a zide)
Synonyms hydrochlorothiazide and amiloride
U.S./Canadian Brand Names Apo®-Amilzide [Can]; Moduret® [Can]; Moduretic® [US/Can]; Novamilor [Can]; Nu-Amilzide [Can]
Therapeutic Category Diuretic, Combination
Use Antikaliuretic diuretic, antihypertensive
Usual Dosage Adults: Oral: Start with 1 tablet/day, then may be increased to 2 tablets/day if needed; usually administered in a single dose
Dosage Forms Tablet: Amiloride hydrochloride 5 mg and hydrochlorothiazide 50 mg

Amin-Aid® *(Discontinued)* see page 814

2-amino-6-mercaptopurine *see* thioguanine *on page 633*

2-amino-6-trifluoromethoxy-benzothiazole *see* riluzole *on page 573*

aminobenzylpenicillin *see* ampicillin *on page 40*

aminocaproic acid (a mee noe ka PROE ik AS id)
U.S./Canadian Brand Names Amicar® [US/Can]
Therapeutic Category Hemostatic Agent
Use Treatment of excessive bleeding resulting from systemic hyperfibrinolysis and urinary fibrinolysis
Usual Dosage In the management of acute bleeding syndromes, oral dosage regimens are the same as the I.V. dosage regimens in adults and children

Chronic bleeding: Oral, I.V.: 5-30 g/day in divided doses at 3- to 6-hour intervals
Acute bleeding syndrome:
Children: Oral, I.V.: 100 mg/kg or 3 g/m^2 during the first hour, followed by continuous infusion at the rate of 33.3 mg/kg/hour or 1 g/m^2/hour; total dosage should not exceed 18 g/m^2/24 hours
Adults:
Oral: For elevated fibrinolytic activity, administer 5 g during first hour, followed by 1-1.25 g/hour for approximately 8 hours or until bleeding stops
I.V.: Administer 4-5 g in 250 mL of diluent during first hour followed by continuous infusion at the rate of 1-1.25 g/hour in 50 mL of diluent, continue for 8 hours or until bleeding stops
Dosage Forms
Injection, solution: 250 mg/mL (20 mL) [contains benzyl alcohol]
Syrup: 1.25 g/5 mL (480 mL) [raspberry flavor]
Tablet: 500 mg

Amino-Cerv™ [US] *see* urea *on page 666*

aminoglutethimide (a mee noe gloo TETH i mide)
U.S./Canadian Brand Names Cytadren® [US]
Therapeutic Category Antineoplastic Agent
Use Suppression of adrenal function in selected patients with Cushing's syndrome; also used successfully in postmenopausal patients with advanced breast carcinoma and in patients with metastatic prostate carcinoma

Usual Dosage Adults: Oral: 250 mg every 6 hours, may be increased at 1- to 2-week intervals to a total of 2 g/day; administer in divided doses 2-3 times/day to reduce incidence of nausea and vomiting

Dosage Forms Tablet, scored: 250 mg

aminolevulinic acid (a MEE noh lev yoo lin ik AS id)

Synonyms aminolevulinic acid hydrochloride

U.S./Canadian Brand Names Levulan® Kerastick™ [US/Can]

Therapeutic Category Photosensitizing Agent, Topical; Porphyrin Agent, Topical

Use Treatment of non-hyperkeratotic actinic keratoses of the face or scalp; to be used in conjunction with blue light illumination

Usual Dosage Adults: Topical: Apply to actinic keratoses (**not** perilesional skin) followed 14-18 hours later by blue light illumination. Application/treatment may be repeated at a treatment site after 8 weeks.

Dosage Forms Solution, topical: 20% [with applicator]

aminolevulinic acid hydrochloride *see* aminolevulinic acid *on this page*

Amino-Opti-E® [US-OTC] *see* vitamin E *on page 682*

aminophylline (am in OFF i lin)

Synonyms theophylline ethylenediamine

U.S./Canadian Brand Names Phyllocontin®-350 [Can]; Phyllocontin® [Can]

Therapeutic Category Theophylline Derivative

Use Bronchodilator in reversible airway obstruction due to asthma or COPD; increase diaphragmatic contractility; neonatal idiopathic apnea of prematurity

Usual Dosage

Neonates: Apnea of prematurity:

Loading dose: 5 mg/kg for one dose

Maintenance: I.V.:

0-24 days: Begin at 2 mg/kg/day divided every 12 hours and titrate to desired levels and effects

>24 days: 3 mg/kg/day divided every 12 hours; increased dosages may be indicated as liver metabolism matures (usually >30 days of life); monitor serum levels to determine appropriate dosages

Theophylline levels should be initially drawn after 3 days of therapy; repeat levels are indicated 3 days after each increase in dosage or weekly if on a stabilized dosage

Treatment of acute bronchospasm:

Loading dose (in patients not currently receiving aminophylline or theophylline): 6 mg/kg (based on aminophylline) administered I.V. over 20-30 minutes; administration rate should not exceed 25 mg/minute (aminophylline)

Approximate I.V. maintenance dosages are based upon **continuous infusions**; bolus dosing (often used in children <6 months of age) may be determined by multiplying the hourly infusion rate by 24 hours and dividing by the desired number of doses/day

6 weeks to 6 months: 0.5 mg/kg/hour

6 months to 1 year: 0.6-0.7 mg/kg/hour

1-9 years: 1-1.2 mg/kg/hour

9-12 years and young adult smokers: 0.9 mg/kg/hour

12-16 years: 0.7 mg/kg/hour

Adults (healthy, nonsmoking): 0.7 mg/kg/hour

Older patients and patients with cor pulmonale, patients with congestive heart failure or liver failure: 0.25 mg/kg/hour

Dosage should be adjusted according to serum level measurements during the first 12- to 24-hour period; avoid using suppositories due to erratic, unreliable absorption.

Rectal: Adults: 500 mg 3 times/day

Dosage Forms

Injection: 25 mg/mL (10 mL, 20 mL)

Liquid, oral: 105 mg/5 mL (240 mL)

(Continued)

aminophylline *(Continued)*

Suppository, rectal: 250 mg, 500 mg
Tablet: 100 mg, 200 mg

aminosalicylate sodium (a MEE noe sa LIS i late SOW dee um)

Synonyms PAS
U.S./Canadian Brand Names Nemasol® Sodium [Can]
Therapeutic Category Nonsteroidal Anti-inflammatory Drug (NSAID)
Use Treatment of tuberculosis with combination drugs
Usual Dosage Oral:
Children: 150-300 mg/kg/day in 3-4 equally divided doses
Adults: 150 mg/kg/day in 2-3 equally divided doses (usually 12-14 g/day)
Dosage Forms Tablet: 500 mg

5-aminosalicylic acid *see* mesalamine *on page 411*

Aminoxin® [US-OTC] *see* pyridoxine *on page 556*

amiodarone (a MEE oh da rone)

U.S./Canadian Brand Names Alti-Amiodarone [Can]; Cordarone® [US/Can]; Gen-Amiodarone [Can]; Novo-Amiodarone [Can]; Pacerone® [US]
Therapeutic Category Antiarrhythmic Agent, Class III
Use Management of resistant, life-threatening ventricular arrhythmias unresponsive to conventional therapy with less toxic agents; also used for treatment of supraventricular arrhythmias unresponsive to conventional therapy; injectable available from manufacturer via orphan drug status or compassionate use for acute treatment and prophylaxis of life-threatening ventricular tachycardia or ventricular fibrillation (see Dosage Forms)
Usual Dosage Children <1 year should be dosed as calculated by body surface area
Children: Loading dose: 10-15 mg/kg/day or 600-800 mg/1.73 m²/day for 4-14 days or until adequate control of arrhythmia or prominent adverse effects occur (this loading dose may be administered in 1-2 divided doses/day); dosage should then be reduced to 5 mg/kg/day or 200-400 mg/1.73 m²/day administered once daily for several weeks; if arrhythmia does not recur reduce to lowest effective dosage possible; usual daily minimal dose: 2.5 mg/kg; maintenance doses may be administered for 5 of 7 days/week
Adults: Ventricular arrhythmias: 800-1600 mg/day in 1-2 doses for 1-3 weeks, then 600-800 mg/day in 1-2 doses for 1 month; maintenance: 400 mg/day; lower doses are recommended for supraventricular arrhythmias, usually 100-400 mg/day
Dosage Forms
Injection, solution, as hydrochloride: 50 mg/mL (3 mL) [contains benzyl alcohol and polysorbate (Tween®) 80]
Tablet, scored, as hydrochloride: 200 mg
Cordarone®: 200 mg
Pacerone®: 200 mg, 400 mg

Amipaque® [US] *see* radiological/contrast media (non-ionic) *on page 563*

Ami-Tex LA® *(Discontinued)* *see page 814*

Ami-Tex PSE [US] *see* guaifenesin and pseudoephedrine *on page 310*

Amitone® [US-OTC] *see* calcium carbonate *on page 104*

amitriptyline (a mee TRIP ti leen)

U.S./Canadian Brand Names Apo®-Amitriptyline [Can]; Elavil® [US/Can]; Vanatrip® [US]
Therapeutic Category Antidepressant, Tricyclic (Tertiary Amine)
Use Treatment of various forms of depression, often in conjunction with psychotherapy; analgesic for certain chronic and neuropathic pain; migraine prophylaxis

Usual Dosage
Children <12 years: Not recommended
Adolescents: Oral: Initial: 25-50 mg/day; may administer in divided doses; increase gradually to 100 mg/day in divided doses
Adults:
Oral: 30-100 mg/day single dose at bedtime or in divided doses; dose may be gradually increased up to 300 mg/day; once symptoms are controlled, decrease gradually to lowest effective dose
I.M.: 20-30 mg 4 times/day

Dosage Forms
Injection, as hydrochloride: 10 mg/mL (10 mL)
Tablet, as hydrochloride: 10 mg, 25 mg, 50 mg, 75 mg, 100 mg, 150 mg

amitriptyline and chlordiazepoxide
(a mee TRIP ti leen & klor dye az e POKS ide)
Synonyms chlordiazepoxide and amitriptyline
U.S./Canadian Brand Names Limbitrol® DS [US]; Limbitrol® [US/Can]
Therapeutic Category Antidepressant, Tricyclic (Tertiary Amine)
Controlled Substance C-IV
Use Treatment of moderate to severe anxiety and/or agitation and depression
Usual Dosage Oral: Initial: 3-4 tablets in divided doses; this may be increased to 6 tablets/day as required; some patients respond to smaller doses and can be maintained on 2 tablets
Dosage Forms Tablet:
5-12.5: Amitriptyline hydrochloride 12.5 mg and chlordiazepoxide 5 mg
10-25: Amitriptyline hydrochloride 25 mg and chlordiazepoxide 10 mg

amitriptyline and perphenazine (a mee TRIP ti leen & per FEN a zeen)
Synonyms perphenazine and amitriptyline
U.S./Canadian Brand Names Etrafon® [US/Can]; Triavil® [US/Can]
Therapeutic Category Antidepressant/Phenothiazine
Use Treatment of patients with moderate to severe anxiety and depression
Usual Dosage Oral: 1 tablet 2-4 times/day
Dosage Forms Tablet:
2-10: Amitriptyline hydrochloride 10 mg and perphenazine 2 mg
4-10: Amitriptyline hydrochloride 10 mg and perphenazine 4 mg
2-25: Amitriptyline hydrochloride 25 mg and perphenazine 2 mg
4-25: Amitriptyline hydrochloride 25 mg and perphenazine 4 mg
4-50: Amitriptyline hydrochloride 50 mg and perphenazine 4 mg

amlexanox (am LEKS an oks)
U.S./Canadian Brand Names Aphthasol™ [US]
Therapeutic Category Anti-inflammatory Agent, Locally Applied
Use Treating signs and symptoms of canker sores (minor aphthous ulcers)
Usual Dosage Administer directly on ulcers 4 times/day following oral hygiene, after meals, and before going to bed
Dosage Forms Paste: 5% (5 g)

amlodipine (am LOE di peen)
U.S./Canadian Brand Names Norvasc® [US/Can]
Therapeutic Category Calcium Channel Blocker
Use Treatment of hypertension alone or in combination with antihypertensives; chronic stable angina alone or with other antianginal agents; vasospastic angina alone or in combination with other agents
Usual Dosage Oral:
Adults: 2.5-10 mg once daily
Dosage Forms Tablet: 2.5 mg, 5 mg, 10 mg

amlodipine and benazepril (am LOE di peen & ben AY ze pril)
Synonyms benazepril and amlodipine
U.S./Canadian Brand Names Lotrel® [US/Can]
Therapeutic Category Antihypertensive Agent, Combination
Use Treatment of hypertension
Usual Dosage Adults: Oral: 1 capsule daily
Dosage Forms
  Capsule:
    Amlodipine 2.5 mg and benazepril hydrochloride 10 mg
    Amlodipine 5 mg and benazepril hydrochloride 10 mg
    Amlodipine 5 mg and benazepril hydrochloride 20 mg
    Amlodipine 10 mg and benazepril hydrochloride 20 mg

Ammens® Medicated Deodorant [US-OTC] *see* zinc oxide *on page 691*

ammonapse *see* sodium phenylbutyrate *on page 598*

ammonia spirit (aromatic) (a MOE nee ah SPEAR it air oh MAT ik)
Synonyms smelling salts
U.S./Canadian Brand Names Aromatic Ammonia Aspirols® [US]
Therapeutic Category Respiratory Stimulant
Use Respiratory and circulatory stimulant; treatment of fainting
Usual Dosage "Smelling salts" to treat or prevent fainting
Dosage Forms
  Solution: 60 mL, 480 mL
  Vapor for inhalation [ampul]: 0.33 mL

ammonium chloride (a MOE nee um KLOR ide)
Therapeutic Category Electrolyte Supplement, Oral
Use Diuretic or systemic and urinary acidifying agent; treatment of hypochloremic states
Usual Dosage
  Children: Oral, I.V.: 75 mg/kg/day in 4 divided doses for urinary acidification; maximum daily dose: 6 g
  Adults:
    Oral: 2-3 g every 6 hours
    I.V.: 1.5 g/dose every 6 hours
Dosage Forms
  Injection: 26.75% [5 mEq/mL] (20 mL)
  Tablet: 500 mg
  Tablet, enteric coated: 486 mg

ammonium lactate *see* lactic acid with ammonium hydroxide *on page 371*

amobarbital (am oh BAR bi tal)
Synonyms amylobarbitone
U.S./Canadian Brand Names Amytal® [US/Can]
Therapeutic Category Barbiturate
Controlled Substance C-II
Use Used to control status epilepticus or acute seizure episodes; also used in catatonic, negativistic, or manic reactions and in "Amytal® Interviewing" for narcoanalysis
Usual Dosage Hypnotic: Adults:
  I.M.: 65-500 mg, should not exceed 500 mg
  I.V.: 65-500 mg, should not exceed 1000 mg
Dosage Forms Injection, as sodium: 500 mg

amobarbital and secobarbital (am oh BAR bi tal & see koe BAR bi tal)
Synonyms secobarbital and amobarbital
U.S./Canadian Brand Names Tuinal® [US]

Therapeutic Category Barbiturate
Controlled Substance C-II
Use Short-term treatment of insomnia
Usual Dosage Adults: Oral: 1-2 capsules at bedtime
Dosage Forms Capsule: Amobarbital 50 mg and secobarbital 50 mg

Amonidrin® Tablet *(Discontinued)* see page 814

AMO Vitrax® *(Discontinued)* see page 814

amoxapine (a MOKS a peen)

Therapeutic Category Antidepressant, Tricyclic (Secondary Amine)
Use Treatment of neurotic and endogenous depression and mixed symptoms of anxiety and depression
Usual Dosage Oral (once symptoms are controlled, decrease gradually to lowest effective dose):

Children <16 years: Dose not established
Adolescents: Initial: 25-50 mg/day; increase gradually to 100 mg/day; may administer as divided doses or as a single dose at bedtime
Adults: Initial: 25 mg 2-3 times/day, if tolerated, dosage may be increased to 100 mg 2-3 times/day; may be administered in a single bedtime dose when dosage <300 mg/day
Maximum daily dose:
Outpatient: 400 mg
Inpatient: 600 mg
Dosage Forms Tablet: 25 mg, 50 mg, 100 mg, 150 mg

amoxicillin (a moks i SIL in)

Synonyms amoxycillin; *p*-hydroxyampicillin
U.S./Canadian Brand Names Amoxicot® [US]; Amoxil® [US/Can]; Apo®-Amoxi [Can]; Gen-Amoxicillin [Can]; Lin-Amox [Can]; Moxilin® [US]; Novamoxin® [Can]; Nu-Amoxi [Can]; Trimox® [US]; Wymox® [US]
Therapeutic Category Penicillin
Use Treatment of otitis media, sinusitis, and infections involving the respiratory tract, skin, and urinary tract due to susceptible *H. influenzae, N. gonorrhoeae, E. coli, P. mirabilis, E. faecalis*, streptococci, and nonpenicillinase-producing staphylococci; prophylaxis of bacterial endocarditis
Unlabeled use: Postexposure prophylaxis for anthrax exposure with documented susceptible organisms
Usual Dosage Oral:
Children: 25-50 mg/kg/day in divided doses every 8 hours
Uncomplicated gonorrhea: ≥2 years: 50 mg/kg plus probenecid 25 mg/kg in a single dose; do not use this regimen in children <2 years of age, probenecid is contraindicated in this age group
SBE prophylaxis: 50 mg/kg 1 hour before procedure and 25 mg/kg 6 hours later; not to exceed adult dosage
Adults: 250-500 mg every 8 hours or 500-875 mg twice daily; maximum dose: 2-3 g/day
Uncomplicated gonorrhea: 3 g plus probenecid 1 g in a single dose
Endocarditis prophylaxis: 3 g 1 hour before procedure and 1.5 g 6 hours later
Anthrax exposure (unlabeled use): **Note:** Postexposure prophylaxis only with documented susceptible organisms:
<40 kg: 15 mg/kg every 8 hours
≥40 kg: 500 mg every 8 hours
Adults: 250-500 mg every 8 hours or 500-875 mg twice daily; maximum dose: 2-3 g/day
Dosage Forms
Capsule, as trihydrate: 250 mg, 500 mg
Amoxicot®, Amoxil®, Moxilin®, Trimox®: 250 mg, 500 mg
Wymox®: 250 mg
(Continued)

amoxicillin *(Continued)*

Powder for oral suspension, as trihydrate: 125 mg/5 mL (5 mL, 80 mL, 100 mL, 150 mL); 250 mg/5 mL (5 mL, 80 mL, 100 mL, 150 mL)
  Amoxicot®: 125 mg/5 mL (100 mL, 150 mL); 250 mg/5 mL (100 mL, 150 mL)
Powder for oral suspension [drops], as trihydrate (Amoxil®): 50 mg/mL (15 mL, 30 mL) [strawberry flavor]
Tablet, chewable, as trihydrate: 125 mg, 200 mg, 250 mg, 400 mg
  Amoxil® [cherry-banana-peppermint flavor]: 200 mg [contains phenylalanine 1.82 mg/tablet], 400 mg [contains phenylalanine 3.64 mg/tablet]
Tablet, film coated (Amoxil®): 500 mg, 875 mg

amoxicillin and clavulanate potassium

(a moks i SIL in & klav yoo LAN ate poe TASS ee um)
Synonyms amoxicillin and clavulanic acid; clavulanate potassium and amoxicillin
U.S./Canadian Brand Names Augmentin ES-600™ [US]; Augmentin® [US/Can]; Clavulin® [Can]
Therapeutic Category Penicillin
Use Infections caused by susceptible organisms involving the lower respiratory tract, otitis media, sinusitis, skin and skin structure, and urinary tract; spectrum same as amoxicillin in addition to beta-lactamase-producing *B. catarrhalis*, *H. influenzae*, *N. gonorrhoeae*, and *S. aureus* (not MRSA)
Usual Dosage Oral:
Children ≤40 kg: 20-40 mg (amoxicillin)/kg/day in divided doses every 8 hours
Children >40 kg and Adults: 250-500 mg every 8 hours or 875 mg every 12 hours
Dosage Forms
Powder for oral suspension:
  125: Amoxicillin trihydrate 125 mg and clavulanate potassium 31.25 mg per 5 mL (75 mL, 100 mL, 150 mL) [banana flavor]
  200: Amoxicillin 200 mg and clavulanate potassium 28.5 mg per 5 mL (50 mL, 75 mL, 100 mL) [contains phenylalanine 7 mg/5 mL; orange-raspberry flavor]
  250: Amoxicillin trihydrate 250 mg and clavulanate potassium 62.5 mg per 5 mL (75 mL, 100 mL, 150 mL) [orange flavor]
  400: Amoxicillin 400 mg and clavulanate potassium 57 mg per 5 mL (50 mL, 75 mL, 100 mL) [contains phenylalanine 7 mg/5 mL; orange-raspberry flavor]
  600 (ES-600™): Amoxicillin 600 mg and clavulanic potassium 42.9 mg per 5 mL (50 mL, 75 mL, 100 mL, 150 mL) [contains phenylalanine 7 mg/5 mL; orange-raspberry flavor]
Tablet:
  250: Amoxicillin trihydrate 250 mg and clavulanate potassium 125 mg
  500: Amoxicillin trihydrate 500 mg and clavulanate potassium 125 mg
  875: Amoxicillin trihydrate 875 mg and clavulanate potassium 125 mg
Tablet, chewable:
  125: Amoxicillin trihydrate 125 mg and clavulanate potassium 31.25 mg [lemon-lime flavor]
  200: Amoxicillin trihydrate 200 mg and clavulanate potassium 28.5 mg [contains phenylalanine 2.1 mg/tablet; cherry-banana flavor]
  250: Amoxicillin trihydrate 250 mg and clavulanate potassium 62.5 mg [lemon-lime flavor]
  400: Amoxicillin trihydrate 400 mg and clavulanate potassium 57 mg [contains phenylalanine 4.2 mg/tablet; cherry-banana flavor]

amoxicillin and clavulanic acid *see* amoxicillin and clavulanate potassium *on this page*

Amoxicot® [US] *see* amoxicillin *on previous page*

Amoxil® [US/Can] *see* amoxicillin *on previous page*

amoxycillin *see* amoxicillin *on previous page*

amphetamine mixture *see* dextroamphetamine and amphetamine *on page 188*

Amphocin® **[US]** *see* amphotericin B (conventional) *on this page*

Amphojel® *(Discontinued)* *see page 814*

Amphojel® **[Can]** *see* aluminum hydroxide *on page 28*

Amphotec® **[US]** *see* amphotericin B cholesteryl sulfate complex *on this page*

amphotericin B cholesteryl sulfate complex
(am foe TER i sin bee kole LES te ril SUL fate KOM plecks)

Synonyms ABCD; amphotericin B colloidal dispersion

U.S./Canadian Brand Names Amphotec® [US]

Therapeutic Category Antifungal Agent

Use Effective in the treatment of invasive mycoses in patient refractory to or intolerant of conventional amphotericin B

Usual Dosage Children and Adults: 3-4 mg/kg/day I.V. (infusion of 1 mg/kg/hour); maximum: 7.5 mg/kg/day; duration of therapy is often <6 weeks

Dosage Forms Injection, suspension: 50 mg (20 mL); 100 mg (50 mL)

amphotericin B colloidal dispersion *see* amphotericin B cholesteryl sulfate complex *on this page*

amphotericin B (conventional) (am foe TER i sin bee con VEN sha nal)

U.S./Canadian Brand Names Amphocin® [US]; Fungizone® [US/Can]

Therapeutic Category Antifungal Agent

Use Treatment of severe systemic infections and meningitis caused by susceptible fungi such as *Candida* species, *Histoplasma capsulatum*, *Cryptococcus neoformans*, *Aspergillus* species, *Blastomyces dermatitidis*, *Torulopsis glabrata*, and *Coccidioides immitis*; fungal peritonitis; irrigant for bladder fungal infections; and topically for cutaneous and mucocutaneous candidal infections

Usual Dosage

I.V.:

Infants and Children:

Test dose (not required): I.V.: 0.1 mg/kg/dose to a maximum of 1 mg; infuse over 30-60 minutes

Initial therapeutic dose: 0.25 mg/kg gradually increased, usually in 0.25 mg/kg increments on each subsequent day, until the desired daily dose is reached

Maintenance dose: 0.25-1 mg/kg/day given once daily; infuse over 2-6 hours. Once therapy has been established, amphotericin B can be administered on an every other day basis at 1-1.5 mg/kg/dose; cumulative dose: 1.5-2 g over 6-10 weeks

Adults:

Test dose (not required): 1 mg infused over 20-30 minutes

Initial dose: 0.25 mg/kg administered over 2-6 hours, gradually increased on subsequent days to the desired level by 0.25 mg/kg increments per day; in critically ill patients, may initiate with 1-1.5 mg/kg/day with close observation

Maintenance dose: 0.25-1 mg/kg/day or 1.5 mg/kg over 4-6 hours every other day; do not exceed 1.5 mg/kg/day; cumulative dose: 1-4 g over 4-10 weeks

Duration of therapy varies with nature of infection: histoplasmosis, *Cryptococcus*, or blastomycosis may be treated with total dose of 2-4 g

I.T.:

Children.: 25-100 mcg every 48-72 hours; increase to 500 mcg as tolerated

Adults: 25-300 mcg every 48-72 hours; increase to 500 mcg to 1 mg as tolerated

Oral: 1 mL (100 mg) 4 times daily

Topical: Apply to affected areas 2-4 times/day for 1-4 weeks of therapy depending on nature and severity of infection

Administration in dialysate: Children and Adults: 1-2 mg/L of peritoneal dialysis fluid either with or without low-dose I.V. amphotericin B (a total dose of 2-10 mg/kg given over 7-14 days)

Administration via bladder irrigation: Children and Adults: 50 mg/day in 1 L of sterile water irrigation solution instilled over 24 hours for 2-7 days or until cultures are clear

(Continued)

amphotericin B (conventional) *(Continued)*

Dosage Forms
Cream: 3% (20 g)
Lotion: 3% (30 mL)
Injection, powder for reconstitution, as desoxycholate: 50 mg
Suspension, oral: 100 mg/mL (24 mL) [with dropper]

amphotericin B lipid complex (am foe TER i sin bee LIP id KOM pleks)

Synonyms ABLC
U.S./Canadian Brand Names Abelcet® [US/Can]
Therapeutic Category Antifungal Agent
Use Treatment of aspergillosis in patients who are refractory to or intolerant of conventional amphotericin B therapy. This indication is based on results obtained primarily from emergency use studies for the treatment of aspergillosis; orphan drug status for cryptococcal meningitis
Usual Dosage Children and Adults: I.V.: 2.5-5 mg/kg/day as a single infusion **Note:** Significantly higher dose of ABLC are tolerated; it appears that attaining higher doses with ABLC produce more rapid fungicidal activity *in vivo* than standard amphotericin B preparations
Dosage Forms Injection, suspension: 5 mg/mL (10 mL, 20 mL)

amphotericin B liposomal (am foe TER i sin bee lye po SO mal)

Synonyms L-AmB
U.S./Canadian Brand Names AmBisome® [US/Can]
Therapeutic Category Antifungal Agent, Systemic
Use Empirical therapy for presumed fungal infection in febrile, neutropenic patients. Treatment of patients with *Aspergillus* species, *Candida* species and/or *Cryptococcus* species infections refractory to amphotericin B deoxycholate, or in patients where renal impairment or unacceptable toxicity precludes the use of amphotericin B deoxycholate. Treatment of visceral leishmaniasis. In immunocompromised patients with visceral leishmaniasis treated with AmBisome, relapse rates were high following initial clearance of parasites
Usual Dosage Children and Adults: I.V.:
Empirical therapy: Recommended initial dose of 3 mg/kg/day
Systemic fungal infections (*Aspergillus*, *Candida*, *Cryptococcus*): Recommended initial dose of 3-5 mg/kg/day
Treatment of visceral leishmaniasis: AmBisome® achieved high rates of acute parasite clearance in immunocompetent patients when total doses of 12-30 mg/kg were administered. Most of these immunocompetent patients remained relapse-free during follow-up periods of 6 months or longer. While acute parasite clearance was achieved in most of the immunocompromised patients who received total doses of 30-40 mg/kg, the majority of these patients were observed to relapse in the 6 months following the completion of therapy.
Dosage Forms Injection, powder for reconstitution: 50 mg

ampicillin (am pi SIL in)

Synonyms aminobenzylpenicillin
U.S./Canadian Brand Names Apo®-Ampi [Can]; Marcillin® [US]; Novo-Ampicillin [Can]; Nu-Ampi [Can]; Principen® [US]
Therapeutic Category Penicillin
Use Treatment of susceptible bacterial infections caused by streptococci, pneumococci, nonpenicillinase-producing staphylococci, *Listeria*, meningococci; some strains of *H. influenzae*, *Salmonella*, *Shigella*, *E. coli*, *Enterobacter*, and *Klebsiella*
Usual Dosage
Infants and Children:
Oral: 50-100 mg/kg/day divided every 6 hours; maximum dose: 2-3 g/day

I.M., I.V.: 100-200 mg/kg/day in 4-6 divided doses; meningitis: 200-400 mg/kg/day in 4-6 divided doses; maximum dose: 12 g/day

Adults:
Oral: 250-500 mg every 6 hours
I.M., I.V.: 8-12 g/day in 4-6 divided doses

Dosage Forms
Capsule, as anhydrous: 250 mg, 500 mg
Capsule, as trihydrate: 250 mg, 500 mg
Powder for injection, as sodium: 125 mg, 250 mg, 500 mg, 1 g, 2 g, 10 g
Powder for oral suspension, as trihydrate: 125 mg/5 mL (100 mL, 150 mL, 200 mL); 250 mg/5 mL (100 mL, 150 mL, 200 mL)

ampicillin and sulbactam (am pi SIL in & SUL bak tam)

Synonyms sulbactam and ampicillin
U.S./Canadian Brand Names Unasyn® [US/Can]
Therapeutic Category Penicillin
Use Treatment of susceptible bacterial infections involved with skin and skin structure, intra-abdominal infections, gynecological infections; spectrum is that of ampicillin plus organisms producing beta-lactamases such as *S. aureus*, *H. influenzae*, *E. coli*, *Klebsiella*, *Acinetobacter*, *Enterobacter* and anaerobes
Usual Dosage Unasyn® (ampicillin/sulbactam) is a combination product. Each 3 g vial contains 2 g of ampicillin and 1 g of sulbactam. Sulbactam has very little antibacterial activity by itself, but effectively extends the spectrum of ampicillin to include beta-lactamase producing strains that are resistant to ampicillin alone. Therefore, dosage recommendations for Unasyn® are based on the ampicillin component.

I.M., I.V.:
Children: 100-200 mg ampicillin/kg/day (150-300 mg Unasyn®) divided every 6 hours; maximum dose: 8 g ampicillin/day (12 g Unasyn®)
Adults: 1-2 g ampicillin (1.5-3 g Unasyn®) every 6-8 hours; maximum dose: 8 g ampicillin/day (12 g Unasyn®)

Dosage Forms
Injection, powder for reconstitution:
1.5 g [ampicillin sodium 1 g and sulbactam sodium 0.5 g]
3 g [ampicillin sodium 2 g and sulbactam sodium 1 g]
15 g [ampicillin sodium 10 g and sulbactam sodium 5 g] [bulk package]

amprenavir (am PRE na veer)

U.S./Canadian Brand Names Agenerase® [US/Can]
Therapeutic Category Protease Inhibitor
Use Treatment of HIV infections in combination with at least two other antiretroviral agents
Usual Dosage Adults: Oral: 1200 mg twice daily
Dosage Forms
Capsule: 50 mg, 150 mg
Solution, oral: 15 mg/mL (240 mL)

AMPT *see* metyrosine *on page 427* *on page 427*

amrinone *see* inamrinone *on page 348*

Amvisc® *(Discontinued)* *see* *page 814*

Amvisc® Plus *(Discontinued)* *see* *page 814*

amylase, lipase, and protease *see* pancrelipase *on page 489*

amyl nitrite (AM il NYE trite)

Synonyms isoamyl nitrite
Therapeutic Category Vasodilator
(Continued)

amyl nitrite *(Continued)*

Use Coronary vasodilator in angina pectoris; an adjunct in treatment of cyanide poisoning; also used to produce changes in the intensity of heart murmurs

Usual Dosage 1-6 inhalations from 1 capsule are usually sufficient to produce the desired effect

Dosage Forms Vapor for inhalation [crushable glass perles]: 0.3 mL

amylobarbitone *see* amobarbital *on page 36*

Amytal® **[US/Can]** *see* amobarbital *on page 36*

Anabolin® *(Discontinued)* *see page 814*

Anacin-3® **(all products)** *(Discontinued)* *see page 814*

Anacin® **PM Aspirin Free [US-OTC]** *see* acetaminophen and diphenhydramine *on page 5*

Anadrol® **[US]** *see* oxymetholone *on page 486*

Anafranil® **[US/Can]** *see* clomipramine *on page 154*

anagrelide *(an AG gre lide)*

U.S./Canadian Brand Names Agrylin® [US/Can]

Therapeutic Category Platelet Reducing Agent

Use Treatment of thrombocythemia (ET), secondary to myeloproliferative disorders, to reduce the elevated platelet count and the risk of thrombosis, and to ameliorate associated symptoms (including thrombohemorrhagic events)

Usual Dosage Adults: Oral: 0.5 mg 4 times/day or 1 mg twice daily, maintain for ≥1 week, then adjust to the lowest effective dose to reduce and maintain platelet count <600,000 µL ideally to the normal range

Dosage Forms Capsule, as hydrochloride: 0.5 mg, 1 mg

Anaids® **Tablet** *(Discontinued)* *see page 814*

anakinra *(an a KIN ra)*

Synonyms IL-1Ra; interleukin-1 receptor antagonist

U.S./Canadian Brand Names Kineret™ [US]

Therapeutic Category Antirheumatic, Disease Modifying

Use Reduction of signs and symptoms of moderately- to severely-active rheumatoid arthritis in adult patients who have failed one or more disease-modifying antirheumatic drugs (DMARDs); may be used alone or in combination with DMARDs (other than tumor necrosis factor-blocking agents)

Usual Dosage Adults: S.C.: Rheumatoid arthritis: 100 mg once daily (administer at approximately the same time each day)

Dosage Forms Injection [prefilled glass syringe; preservative free]: 100 mg/0.67 mL (1 mL)

Ana-Kit® **[US]** *see* insect sting kit *on page 351*

Analpram-HC® **[US]** *see* pramoxine and hydrocortisone *on page 535*

Anamine® **Syrup** *(Discontinued)* *see page 814*

Anandron® **[Can]** *see* nilutamide *on page 460*

Anaplex® **Liquid** *(Discontinued)* *see page 814*

Anaprox® **[US/Can]** *see* naproxen *on page 447*

Anaprox® **DS [US/Can]** *see* naproxen *on page 447*

Anaspaz® **[US]** *see* hyoscyamine *on page 339*

anastrozole *(an AS troe zole)*

U.S./Canadian Brand Names Arimidex® [US/Can]

Therapeutic Category Antineoplastic Agent

Use Treatment of locally-advanced or metastatic breast cancer (ER-positive or hormone receptor unknown) in postmenopausal women; treatment of advanced breast cancer in postmenopausal women with disease progression following tamoxifen therapy; adjuvant treatment of early ER-positive breast cancer in postmenopausal women

Usual Dosage Breast cancer: Adults: Oral (refer to individual protocols): 1 mg once daily
NOTE: In advanced breast cancer, continue until tumor progression. In early breast cancer, optimal duration of therapy unknown.

Dosage Forms Tablet: 1 mg

Anatrast® **[US]** *see* radiological/contrast media (ionic) *on page 561*

Anatuss® *(Discontinued) see page 814*

Anatuss LA [US] *see* guaifenesin and pseudoephedrine *on page 310*

Anbesol® Baby [US/Can] *see* benzocaine *on page 77*

Anbesol® Maximum Strength [US-OTC] *see* benzocaine *on page 77*

Anbesol® [US-OTC] *see* benzocaine *on page 77*

Ancef® [US/Can] *see* cefazolin *on page 121*

Ancobon® [US/Can] *see* flucytosine *on page 274*

Andehist DM NR Drops [US] *see* carbinoxamine, pseudoephedrine, and dextromethorphan *on page 115*

Andehist NR Drops [US] *see* carbinoxamine and pseudoephedrine *on page 115*

Andehist NR Syrup [US] *see* brompheniramine and pseudoephedrine *on page 94*

Andriol® [Can] *see* testosterone *on page 625*

Androcur® [Can] *see* cyproterone *(Canada only) on page 170*

Androcur® Depot [Can] *see* cyproterone *(Canada only) on page 170*

Androderm® [US] *see* testosterone *on page 625*

Andro/Fem® *(Discontinued) see page 814*

AndroGel® [US] *see* testosterone *on page 625*

Android® [US] *see* methyltestosterone *on page 423*

Andro-L.A.® Injection *(Discontinued) see page 814*

Androlone® *(Discontinued) see page 814*

Androlone®-D *(Discontinued) see page 814*

Andropository® Injection *(Discontinued) see page 814*

Anectine® Chloride [US] *see* succinylcholine *on page 608*

Anectine® Flo-Pack® [US] *see* succinylcholine *on page 608*

Anergan® [US] *see* promethazine *on page 544*

Anergan® 25 Injection *(Discontinued) see page 814*

Anestacon® [US] *see* lidocaine *on page 383*

aneurine *see* thiamine *on page 632*

Anexate® [Can] *see* flumazenil *on page 275*

Anexsia® [US] *see* hydrocodone and acetaminophen *on page 329*

Angio Conray® [US] *see* radiological/contrast media (ionic) *on page 561*

Angiomax™ [US] *see* bivalirudin *on page 89*

Angiovist® [US] *see* radiological/contrast media (ionic) *on page 561*

anisindione (an is in DY one)

U.S./Canadian Brand Names Miradon® [US]

Therapeutic Category Anticoagulant (Other)

Use Prophylaxis and treatment of venous thrombosis, pulmonary embolism, and thromboembolic disorders; atrial fibrillation with risk of embolism; adjunct in the prophylaxis of systemic embolism following myocardial infarction

Usual Dosage Oral: Adults:

Initial: 300 mg on first day, 200 mg on second day, 100 mg on third day

Maintenance dosage: Established by daily PT/INR determinations; range: 25-250 mg/day

Note: When discontinuing therapy, manufacturer recommends tapering dose over 3-4 weeks.

Dosage Forms Tablet: 50 mg

Anodynos-DHC® *(Discontinued)* see page 814

Anolor 300® [US] see butalbital, acetaminophen, and caffeine on page 99

Anoquan® *(Discontinued)* see page 814

Ansaid® Oral [US/Can] see flurbiprofen on page 282

ansamycin see rifabutin on page 571

Antabuse® [US/Can] see disulfiram on page 207

Antagon® *(Discontinued)* see page 814

Antazoline-V® Ophthalmic *(Discontinued)* see page 814

Anthra-Derm® *(Discontinued)* see page 814

Anthraforte® [Can] see anthralin on this page

anthralin (AN thra lin)

Synonyms dithranol

U.S./Canadian Brand Names Anthraforte® [Can]; Anthranol® [Can]; Anthrascalp® [Can]; Drithocreme® [US]; Micanol® [US/Can]

Therapeutic Category Keratolytic Agent

Use Treatment of psoriasis

Usual Dosage Adults: Topical: Generally, apply once daily or as directed. The irritant potential of anthralin is directly related to the strength being used and each patient's individual tolerance. Always commence treatment for at least one week using the lowest strength possible.

Skin application: Apply sparingly only to psoriatic lesions and rub gently and carefully into the skin until absorbed. Avoid applying an excessive quantity which may cause unnecessary soiling and staining of the clothing or bed linen.

Scalp application: Comb hair to remove scalar debris and, after suitably parting, rub cream well into the lesions, taking care to prevent the cream from spreading onto the forehead

Remove by washing or showering; optimal period of contact will vary according to the strength used and the patient's response to treatment. Continue treatment until the skin is entirely clear (ie, when there is nothing to feel with the fingers and the texture is normal)

Dosage Forms Cream: 0.1% (50 g); 0.5% (50 g); 1% (50 g)

Anthranol® [Can] see anthralin on this page

Anthrascalp® [Can] see anthralin on this page

anthrax vaccine, adsorbed (AN thraks vak SEEN, ad SORBED)

U.S./Canadian Brand Names BioThrax™ [US]

Therapeutic Category Vaccine

Use Immunization against *Bacillus anthracis*. Recommended for individuals who may come in contact with animal products which come from anthrax endemic areas and may be contaminated with *Bacillus anthracis* spores; recommended for high-risk persons such as veterinarians and other handling potentially infected animals. Routine immunization for the general population is not recommended.

The Department of Defense is implementing an anthrax vaccination program against the biological warfare agent anthrax, which will be administered to all active duty and reserve personnel.

Usual Dosage
Primary immunization: S.C.: Three injections of 0.5 mL each given 2 weeks apart followed by three additional S.C. injections given at 6, 12, and 18 months
Subsequent booster injections: 0.5 mL at 1-year intervals are recommended for immunity to be maintained

Dosage Forms Injection, suspension: 5 mL [vial stopper contains dry natural rubber]

Antiben® *(Discontinued)* see page 814

AntibiOtic® Ear [US] see neomycin, polymyxin B, and hydrocortisone on page 453

anti-CD20 monoclonal antibodies see rituximab on page 575

antidigoxin Fab fragments see digoxin immune Fab on page 197

antidiuretic hormone (ADH) see vasopressin on page 674

antihemophilic factor (human) (an tee hee moe FIL ik FAK tor HYU man)
Synonyms AHF; factor VIII
U.S./Canadian Brand Names Alphanate® [US]; Hemofil® M [US/Can]; Humate-P® [US/Can]; Koāte®-DVI [US]; Monarc® M [US]; Monoclate-P® [US]
Therapeutic Category Blood Product Derivative
Use Management of hemophilia A in patients whom a deficiency in factor VIII has been demonstrated
Usual Dosage I.V.: Individualize dosage based on coagulation studies performed prior to and during treatment at regular intervals. One AHF unit is the activity present in 1 mL of normal pooled human plasma; dosage should be adjusted to actual vial size currently stocked in the pharmacy.

Hospitalized patients: 20-50 units/kg/dose; may be higher for special circumstances; dose can be administered every 12-24 hours and more frequently in special circumstances
Dosage Forms Injection, human [single-dose vial]: Labeling on cartons and vials indicates number of int. units

antihemophilic factor (porcine) (an tee hee moe FIL ik FAK ter POR seen)
U.S./Canadian Brand Names Hyate®:C [US]
Therapeutic Category Antihemophilic Agent
Use Treatment of congenital hemophiliacs with antibodies to human factor VIII:C and also for previously nonhemophiliac patients with spontaneously acquired inhibitors to human factor VIII:C; patients with inhibitors who are bleeding or who are to undergo surgery
Usual Dosage Clinical response should be used to assess efficacy rather than relying upon a particular laboratory value for recovery of factor VIII:C.

Initial dose:
Antibody level to human factor VIII:C <50 Bethesda units/mL: 100-150 porcine units/kg (body weight) is recommended
Antibody level to human factor VIII:C >50 Bethesda units/mL: Activity of the antibody to porcine factor VIII:C should be determined; **an antiporcine antibody level** >20 Bethesda units/mL indicates that the patient is unlikely to benefit from treatment; for lower titers, a dose of 100-150 porcine units/kg is recommended
(Continued)

45

antihemophilic factor (porcine) *(Continued)*

If a patient has previously been treated with Hyate®:C, this may provide a guide to his likely response and, therefore, assist in estimation of the preliminary dose

Subsequent doses: Following administration of the initial dose, if the recovery of factor VIII:C in the patient's plasma is not sufficient, a further higher dose should be administered; if recovery after the second dose is still insufficient, a third and higher dose may prove effective

Dosage Forms Injection, powder for reconstitution: 400-700 porcine units [to be reconstituted with 20 mL SWFI]

antihemophilic factor (recombinant)

(an tee hee moe FIL ik FAK tor ree KOM be nant)

Synonyms factor VIII recombinant

U.S./Canadian Brand Names Helixate® FS [US]; Kogenate® FS [US/Can]; Recombinate™ [US/Can]

Therapeutic Category Blood Product Derivative

Use Management of hemophilia A in patients whom a deficiency in factor VIII has been demonstrated

Usual Dosage I.V.: Individualize dosage based on coagulation studies performed prior to and during treatment at regular intervals. One AHF unit is the activity present in 1 mL of normal pooled human plasma; dosage should be adjusted to actual vial size currently stocked in the pharmacy.

Hospitalized patients: 20-50 units/kg/dose; may be higher for special circumstances; dose can be administered every 12-24 hours and more frequently in special circumstances

Dosage Forms

Injection, powder for reconstitution, recombinant [preservative free]:

Helixate® FS, Kogenate® FS: 250 int. units/vial, 500 int. units/vial, 1000 int. units/vial [contains sucrose 28 mg/vial]

Recombinate™: 250 int. units/vial, 500 units/vial, 1000 int. units/vial [contains human albumin 12.5 mg/mL]

ReFacto®: 250 int. units/vial, 500 units/vial, 1000 int. units/vial

Antihist-1® *(Discontinued)* see page 814

Antihist-D® *(Discontinued)* see page 814

Anti-Hist® **[US-OTC]** see diphenhydramine on page 202

anti-inhibitor coagulant complex

(an tee-in HI bi tor coe AG yoo lant KOM pleks)

Synonyms coagulant complex inhibitor

U.S./Canadian Brand Names Autoplex® T [US]; Feiba VH Immuno® [US/Can]

Therapeutic Category Hemophilic Agent

Use Patients with factor VIII inhibitors who are to undergo surgery or those who are bleeding

Usual Dosage Dosage range: I.V.: 25-100 factor VIII correctional units per kg depending on the severity of hemorrhage

Dosage Forms

Injection:

Autoplex® T: Each bottle is labeled with correctional units of factor VIII [with heparin 2 units]

Feiba VH Immuno®: Each bottle is labeled with correctional units of factor VIII [heparin free]

Antilirium® *(Discontinued)* see page 814

Antiminth® *(Discontinued)* see page 814

Antinea® **Cream** *(Discontinued)* see page 814

Antiphlogistine Rub A-535 No Odour [Can] *see* triethanolamine salicylate *on page 654*

Antiphogistine Rub A-535 Capsaicin [Can] *see* capsaicin *on page 111*

antipyrine and benzocaine (an tee PYE reen & BEN zoe kane)

Synonyms benzocaine and antipyrine

U.S./Canadian Brand Names A/B® Otic [US]; Allergan® Ear Drops [US]; Auralgan® [US/Can]; Aurodex® [US]; Auroto® [US]; Benzotic® [US]; Dec-Agesic® A.B. [US]; Dolotic® [US]; Rx-Otic® Drops [US]

Therapeutic Category Otic Agent, Analgesic; Otic Agent, Ceruminolytic

Use Temporary relief of pain and reduction of inflammation associated with acute congestive and serous otitis media, swimmer's ear, otitis externa; facilitates ear wax removal

Usual Dosage Otic: Fill ear canal; moisten cotton pledget, place in external ear, repeat every 1-2 hours until pain and congestion is relieved; for ear wax removal instill drops 3-4 times/day for 2-3 days

Dosage Forms Solution, otic: Antipyrine 5.4% and benzocaine 1.4% (10 mL, 15 mL)

Antispas® Injection *(Discontinued)* *see page 814*

antispasmodic compound *see* hyoscyamine, atropine, scopolamine, and phenobarbital *on page 340*

Antispas® Tablet [US] *see* hyoscyamine, atropine, scopolamine, and phenobarbital *on page 340*

antithrombin III (an tee THROM bin three)

Synonyms ATIII; heparin cofactor I

U.S./Canadian Brand Names Thrombate III™ [US/Can]

Therapeutic Category Blood Product Derivative

Use Agent for hereditary antithrombin III deficiency

Usual Dosage After first dose of antithrombin III, level should increase to 120% of normal; thereafter maintain at levels >80%. Generally, achieved by administration of maintenance doses once every 24 hours; initially and until patient is stabilized, measure antithrombin III level at least twice daily, thereafter once daily and always immediately before next infusion.

Initial dosage (units) = [desired AT-III level % - baseline AT-III level %] x body weight (kg) divided by 1%/units/kg

Measure antithrombin III preceding and 30 minutes after dose to calculate *in vivo* recovery rate; maintain level within normal range for 2-8 days depending on type of surgery or procedure

Dosage Forms Injection, powder for reconstitution [with diluent]: 500 int. units, 1000 int. units

antithymocyte globulin (equine) *see* lymphocyte immune globulin *on page 395*

antithymocyte globulin (rabbit) (an te THY moe site GLOB yu lin RAB bit)

U.S./Canadian Brand Names Thymoglobulin® [US]

Therapeutic Category Immunosuppressant Agent

Use Treatment of acute moderate-to-severe renal allograft rejection

Usual Dosage Adults: I.V.: Treatment of acute renal allograft rejection: 1.5 mg/kg/day for 7-14 days.

Dosage Forms Injection [with diluent]: 25 mg vial

Anti-Tuss® Expectorant *(Discontinued)* *see page 814*

antivenin *(Crotalidae)* polyvalent
(an tee VEN in (kroe TAL ih die) pol i VAY lent)

Synonyms crotaline antivenin, polyvalent; North and South American antisnake-bite serum; pit vipers antivenin; snake (pit vipers) antivenin

U.S./Canadian Brand Names Antivenin Polyvalent [Equine] [US]; CroFab™ [Ovine] [US]

Therapeutic Category Antivenin

Use Neutralization of venoms of North and South American crotalids: rattlesnake, copperhead, cottonmouth, tropical moccasins, fer-de-lance, bushmaster

Usual Dosage Initial intradermal sensitivity test. The entire initial dose of antivenin should be administered as soon as possible to be most effective (within 4 hours after the bite).

Children and Adults: I.V.: Minimal envenomation: 20-40 mL; moderate envenomation: 50-90 mL; severe envenomation: 100-150 mL

Additional doses of antivenin is based on clinical response to the initial dose. If swelling continues to progress, symptoms increase in severity, hypotension occurs, or decrease in hematocrit appears, an additional 10-50 mL should be administered.

For I.V. infusion: 1:1-1:10 dilution of reconstituted antivenin in normal saline or D_5W should be prepared. Infuse the initial 5-10 mL of diluted antivenin over 3-5 minutes monitoring closely for signs of sensitivity reactions.

Dosage Forms Injection, powder for reconstitution:
Equine origin [contains phenol and thimerosal] [with 10 mL diluent]
Ovine origin (CroFab™) [contains thimerosal] (2 vials/box)

antivenin *(Latrodectus mactans)* (an tee VEN in lak tro DUK tus MAK tans)
Synonyms black widow spider antivenin (*Latrodectus mactans*); *Latrodectus mactans* antivenin

Therapeutic Category Antivenin

Use Treat patients with symptoms of black widow spider bites

Usual Dosage
Children <12 years (severe or shock): I.V.: 2.5 mL in 10-50 mL over 15 minutes
Children and Adults: I.M.: 2.5 mL

Dosage Forms Powder for injection: 6000 antivenin units (2.5 mL)

antivenin *(Micrurus fulvius)* (an tee VEN in mye KRU rus FUL vee us)
Synonyms North American coral snake antivenin

Therapeutic Category Antivenin

Use Neutralize the venom of Eastern coral snake and Texas coral snake but does not neutralize venom of Arizona or Sonoran coral snake

Usual Dosage I.V.: 3-5 vials by slow injection

Dosage Forms Injection [with diluent]: One vial antivenin

Antivenin Polyvalent [Equine] [US] *see* antivenin *(Crotalidae)* polyvalent *on this page*

Antivert® **[US/Can]** *see* meclizine *on page 403*

Antivert® Chewable Tablet *(Discontinued)* *see page 814*

Antizol® [US] *see* fomepizole *on page 287*

Antrizine® *(Discontinued)* *see page 814*

Antrocol® Capsule & Tablet *(Discontinued)* *see page 814*

Anturane® [US] *see* sulfinpyrazone *on page 614*

Anusol® HC-1 [US-OTC] *see* hydrocortisone (topical) *on page 334*

Anusol® HC-2.5% [US-OTC] *see* hydrocortisone (topical) *on page 334*

Anusol-HC® Suppository [US] *see* hydrocortisone (rectal) *on page 333*

Anusol® [US-OTC] *see* pramoxine *on page 534*

ANX® **[US]** *see* hydroxyzine *on page 339*

Anxanil® Oral *(Discontinued) see page 814*

Anzemet® **[US/Can]** *see* dolasetron *on page 209*

Apacet® *(Discontinued) see page 814*

APAP *see* acetaminophen *on page 3*

APAP and tramadol *see* acetaminophen and tramadol *on page 7*

Apaphen® *(Discontinued) see page 814*

Apatate® **[US-OTC]** *see* vitamin B complex *on page 681*

Aphedrid™ **[US-OTC]** *see* triprolidine and pseudoephedrine *on page 659*

Aphrodyne® **[US]** *see* yohimbine *on page 687*

Aphthasol™ **[US]** *see* amlexanox *on page 35*

A.P.L.® *(Discontinued) see page 814*

Aplicare® **[US-OTC]** *see* povidone-iodine *on page 533*

Aplisol® **[US]** *see* tuberculin tests *on page 662*

Aplitest® *(Discontinued) see page 814*

Apo-Acebutolol [Can] *see* acebutolol *on page 3*

Apo®-Acetaminophen [Can] *see* acetaminophen *on page 3*

Apo®-Acetazolamide [Can] *see* acetazolamide *on page 9*

Apo®-Acyclovir [Can] *see* acyclovir *on page 13*

Apo®-Allopurinol [Can] *see* allopurinol *on page 23*

Apo®-Alpraz [Can] *see* alprazolam *on page 24*

Apo®-Amilzide [Can] *see* amiloride and hydrochlorothiazide *on page 32*

Apo®-Amitriptyline [Can] *see* amitriptyline *on page 34*

Apo®-Amoxi [Can] *see* amoxicillin *on page 37*

Apo®-Ampi [Can] *see* ampicillin *on page 40*

Apo®-ASA [Can] *see* aspirin *on page 58*

Apo®-Atenol [Can] *see* atenolol *on page 60*

Apo®-Baclofen [Can] *see* baclofen *on page 70*

Apo®-Beclomethasone [Can] *see* beclomethasone *on page 73*

Apo®-Benztropine [Can] *see* benztropine *on page 80*

Apo®-Benzydamine [Can] *see* benzydamine *(Canada only) on page 81*

Apo®-Bisacodyl [Can] *see* bisacodyl *on page 87*

Apo®-Bromazepam [Can] *see* bromazepam *(Canada only) on page 92*

Apo® Bromocriptine [Can] *see* bromocriptine *on page 93*

Apo®-Buspirone [Can] *see* buspirone *on page 98*

Apo®-C [Can] *see* ascorbic acid *on page 57*

Apo®-Cal [Can] *see* calcium carbonate *on page 104*

Apo®-Capto [Can] *see* captopril *on page 112*

Apo®-Carbamazepine [Can] *see* carbamazepine *on page 113*

Apo®-Cefaclor [Can] *see* cefaclor *on page 120*

Apo®-Cefadroxil [Can] *see* cefadroxil *on page 121*

Apo®-Cephalex [Can] *see* cephalexin *on page 128*

Apo®-Cetirizine [Can] *see* cetirizine *on page 129*

Apo®-Chlorax [Can] *see* clidinium and chlordiazepoxide *on page 151*

Apo®-Chlordiazepoxide [Can] *see* chlordiazepoxide *on page 134*

Apo®-Chlorpropamide [Can] *see* chlorpropamide *on page 142*

Apo®-Chlorthalidone [Can] *see* chlorthalidone *on page 142*

Apo®-Cimetidine [Can] *see* cimetidine *on page 146*

Apo®-Clomipramine [Can] *see* clomipramine *on page 154*

Apo®-Clonazepam [Can] *see* clonazepam *on page 154*

Apo®-Clonidine [Can] *see* clonidine *on page 155*

Apo®-Clorazepate [Can] *see* clorazepate *on page 156*

Apo®-Cloxi [Can] *see* cloxacillin *on page 157*

Apo®-Cromolyn [Can] *see* cromolyn sodium *on page 166*

Apo®-Cyclobenzaprine [Can] *see* cyclobenzaprine *on page 168*

Apo®-Desipramine [Can] *see* desipramine *on page 181*

Apo®-Diazepam [Can] *see* diazepam *on page 191*

Apo®-Diclo [Can] *see* diclofenac *on page 193*

Apo®-Diclo SR [Can] *see* diclofenac *on page 193*

Apo®-Diflunisal [Can] *see* diflunisal *on page 196*

Apo®-Diltiaz [Can] *see* diltiazem *on page 199*

Apo®-Diltiaz CD [Can] *see* diltiazem *on page 199*

Apo®-Diltiaz SR [Can] *see* diltiazem *on page 199*

Apo®-Dimenhydrinate [Can] *see* dimenhydrinate *on page 200*

Apo®-Dipyridamole FC [Can] *see* dipyridamole *on page 206*

Apo®-Divalproex [Can] *see* valproic acid and derivatives *on page 670*

Apo®-Domperidone [Can] *see* domperidone *(Canada only) on page 211*

Apo®-Doxazosin [Can] *see* doxazosin *on page 213*

Apo®-Doxepin [Can] *see* doxepin *on page 213*

Apo®-Doxy [Can] *see* doxycycline *on page 215*

Apo®-Doxy Tabs [Can] *see* doxycycline *on page 215*

Apo®-Erythro Base [Can] *see* erythromycin (systemic) *on page 235*

Apo®-Erythro E-C [Can] *see* erythromycin (systemic) *on page 235*

Apo®-Erythro-ES [Can] *see* erythromycin (systemic) *on page 235*

Apo®-Erythro-S [Can] *see* erythromycin (systemic) *on page 235*

Apo®-Etodolac [Can] *see* etodolac *on page 258*

Apo®-Famotidine [Can] *see* famotidine *on page 262*

Apo®-Fenofibrate [Can] *see* fenofibrate *on page 265*

Apo®-Feno-Micro [Can] *see* fenofibrate *on page 265*

Apo®-Ferrous Gluconate [Can] *see* ferrous gluconate *on page 268*

Apo®-Ferrous Sulfate [Can] *see* ferrous sulfate *on page 269*

Apo®-Fluconazole [Can] *see* fluconazole *on page 274*

Apo®-Flunisolide [Can] *see* flunisolide *on page 276*

Apo®-Fluoxetine [Can] *see* fluoxetine *on page 279*

Apo®-Fluphenazine [Can] *see* fluphenazine *on page 281*

Apo®-Flurazepam [Can] *see* flurazepam *on page 281*

Apo®-Flurbiprofen [Can] *see* flurbiprofen *on page 282*

Apo-Flutamide [Can] *see* flutamide *on page 282*

Apo®-Fluvoxamine [Can] *see* fluvoxamine *on page 285*

Apo®-Folic [Can] *see* folic acid *on page 285*

Apo®-Furosemide [Can] *see* furosemide *on page 291*

Apo®-Gain [Can] *see* minoxidil *on page 432*

Apo®-Gemfibrozil [Can] *see* gemfibrozil *on page 295*

Apo®-Glyburide [Can] *see* glyburide *on page 301*

Apo®-Haloperidol [Can] *see* haloperidol *on page 316*

Apo®-Hydralazine [Can] *see* hydralazine *on page 327*

Apo®-Hydro [Can] *see* hydrochlorothiazide *on page 328*

Apo®-Hydroxyzine [Can] *see* hydroxyzine *on page 339*

Apo®-Ibuprofen [Can] *see* ibuprofen *on page 342*

Apo®-Imipramine [Can] *see* imipramine *on page 346*

Apo®-Indapamide [Can] *see* indapamide *on page 348*

Apo®-Indomethacin [Can] *see* indomethacin *on page 349*

Apo®-Ipravent [Can] *see* ipratropium *on page 358*

Apo®-ISDN [Can] *see* isosorbide dinitrate *on page 362*

Apo®-K [Can] *see* potassium chloride *on page 530*

Apo®-Keto [Can] *see* ketoprofen *on page 368*

Apo®-Ketoconazole [Can] *see* ketoconazole *on page 367*

Apo®-Keto-E [Can] *see* ketoprofen *on page 368*

Apo®-Ketorolac [Can] *see* ketorolac *on page 368*

Apo®-Keto SR [Can] *see* ketoprofen *on page 368*

Apo®-Ketotifen [Can] *see* ketotifen *on page 368*

Apo®-Levocarb [Can] *see* levodopa and carbidopa *on page 380*

Apo®-Lisinopril [Can] *see* lisinopril *on page 388*

Apo®-Loperamide [Can] *see* loperamide *on page 390*

Apo®-Lorazepam [Can] *see* lorazepam *on page 391*

Apo®-Lovastatin [Can] *see* lovastatin *on page 393*

Apo®-Loxapine [Can] *see* loxapine *on page 394*

Apo®-Mefenamic [Can] *see* mefenamic acid *on page 405*

Apo®-Megestrol [Can] *see* megestrol acetate *on page 405*

Apo®-Meprobamate [Can] *see* meprobamate *on page 409*

Apo®-Metformin [Can] *see* metformin *on page 414*

Apo®-Methazide [Can] *see* methyldopa and hydrochlorothiazide *on page 421*

Apo®-Methoprazine [Can] *see* methotrimeprazine *(Canada only) on page 418*

Apo®-Methyldopa [Can] *see* methyldopa *on page 420*

Apo®-Metoclop [Can] *see* metoclopramide *on page 424*

Apo®-Metoprolol [Can] *see* metoprolol *on page 425*

Apo®-Metronidazole [Can] *see* metronidazole *on page 426*

Apo®-Minocycline [Can] *see* minocycline *on page 431*

Apo®-Moclobemide [Can] *see* moclobemide *(Canada only) on page 434*

apomorphine *(Discontinued)* *see page 814*

Apo®-Nabumetone [Can] *see* nabumetone *on page 443*

Apo®-Nadol [Can] *see* nadolol *on page 443*

Apo®-Napro-Na [Can] *see* naproxen *on page 447*

Apo®-Napro-Na DS [Can] *see* naproxen *on page 447*

Apo®-Naproxen [Can] *see* naproxen *on page 447*

Apo®-Naproxen SR [Can] *see* naproxen *on page 447*

Apo®-Nifed [Can] *see* nifedipine *on page 459*

Apo®-Nifed PA [Can] *see* nifedipine *on page 459*

Apo®-Nitrofurantoin [Can] *see* nitrofurantoin *on page 461*

Apo®-Nizatidine [Can] *see* nizatidine *on page 463*

Apo®-Norflox [Can] *see* norfloxacin *on page 465*

Apo®-Nortriptyline [Can] *see* nortriptyline *on page 466*

Apo®-Oflox [Can] *see* ofloxacin *on page 475*

Apo®-Oxazepam [Can] *see* oxazepam *on page 482*

Apo®-Pentoxifylline SR [Can] *see* pentoxifylline *on page 502*

Apo®-Pen VK [Can] *see* penicillin V potassium *on page 499*

Apo®-Perphenazine [Can] *see* perphenazine *on page 505*

Apo®-Pindol [Can] *see* pindolol *on page 516*

Apo®-Piroxicam [Can] *see* piroxicam *on page 517*

Apo®-Prazo [Can] *see* prazosin *on page 536*

Apo®-Prednisone [Can] *see* prednisone *on page 538*

Apo®-Primidone [Can] *see* primidone *on page 540*

Apo®-Procainamide [Can] *see* procainamide *on page 541*

Apo®-Propranolol [Can] *see* propranolol *on page 549*

Apo®-Quinidine [Can] *see* quinidine *on page 559*

Apo®-Ranitidine [Can] *see* ranitidine hydrochloride *on page 564*

Apo®-Salvent [Can] *see* albuterol *on page 18*

Apo®-Selegiline [Can] *see* selegiline *on page 586*

Apo®-Sertraline [Can] *see* sertraline *on page 589*

Apo®-Sotalol [Can] *see* sotalol *on page 602*

Apo®-Sucralate [Can] *see* sucralfate *on page 609*

Apo®-Sulfatrim [Can] *see* sulfamethoxazole and trimethoprim *on page 612*

Apo®-Sulfinpyrazone [Can] *see* sulfinpyrazone *on page 614*

Apo®-Sulin [Can] *see* sulindac *on page 615*

Apo®-Tamox [Can] *see* tamoxifen *on page 618*

Apo®-Temazepam [Can] *see* temazepam *on page 621*

Apo®-Terazosin [Can] *see* terazosin *on page 622*

Apo®-Tetra [Can] *see* tetracycline *on page 628*

Apo®-Theo LA [Can] *see* theophylline *on page 630*

Apo®-Thioridazine [Can] *see* thioridazine *on page 635*

Apo®-Tiaprofenic [Can] *see* tiaprofenic acid *(Canada only) on page 638*

Apo®-Ticlopidine [Can] *see* ticlopidine *on page 639*

Apo®-Timol [Can] *see* timolol *on page 639*

Apo®-Timop [Can] *see* timolol *on page 639*

Apo®-Tolbutamide [Can] *see* tolbutamide *on page 643*

Apo®-Trazodone [Can] *see* trazodone *on page 649*

Apo®-Trazodone D *see* trazodone *on page 649*

Apo®-Triazide [Can] *see* hydrochlorothiazide and triamterene *on page 329*

Apo®-Triazo [Can] *see* triazolam *on page 653*

Apo®-Trifluoperazine [Can] *see* trifluoperazine *on page 655*

Apo®-Trihex [Can] *see* trihexyphenidyl *on page 655*

Apo®-Trimip [Can] *see* trimipramine *on page 658*

Apo®-Verap [Can] *see* verapamil *on page 675*

Apo®-Zidovudine [Can] *see* zidovudine *on page 689*

Apo®-Zopiclone [Can] *see* zopiclone *(Canada only) on page 693*

APPG *see* penicillin G procaine *on page 499*

apraclonidine (a pra KLOE ni deen)
U.S./Canadian Brand Names Iopidine® [US/Can]
Therapeutic Category Alpha$_2$-Adrenergic Agonist Agent, Ophthalmic
Use 1%: Prevention and treatment of postsurgical intraocular pressure elevation; 0.5%: Short-term adjunctive therapy in patients on maximally tolerated medical therapy who require additional redirection of intraocular pressure
Usual Dosage Adults: Ophthalmic: Instill 1 drop in operative eye 1 hour prior to laser surgery, second drop in eye upon completion of procedure
Dosage Forms Solution, ophthalmic, as hydrochloride: 0.5% (5 mL, 10 mL); 1% (0.1 mL)

Apresazide® *(Discontinued) see page 814*

Apresoline® [US/Can] *see* hydralazine *on page 327*

Apri® [US] *see* ethinyl estradiol and desogestrel *on page 244*

Aprodine® [US-OTC] *see* triprolidine and pseudoephedrine *on page 659*

Aprodine® w/C [US] *see* triprolidine, pseudoephedrine, and codeine *on page 659*

aprotinin (a proe TYE nin)
U.S./Canadian Brand Names Trasylol® [US/Can]
Therapeutic Category Hemostatic Agent
Use Reduction or prevention of blood loss in patients undergoing coronary artery bypass surgery when a high index of suspicion of excessive bleeding potential exists; this includes open heart reoperation, pre-existing coagulopathy, operations on the great vessels, and patients whose religious beliefs prohibit blood transfusions
Usual Dosage Test dose: **All** patients should receive a 1 mL I.V. test dose at least 10 minutes prior to the loading dose to assess the potential for allergic reactions

Regimen A (standard dose):
2 million units (280 mg) loading dose I.V. over 20-30 minutes
2 million units (280 mg) into pump prime volume
500,000 units/hour (70 mg/hour) I.V. during operation
Regimen B (low dose):
1 million units (140 mg) loading dose I.V. over 20-30 minutes
1 million units (140 mg) into pump prime volume
250,000 units/hour (35 mg/hour) I.V. during operation
Dosage Forms Injection: 1.4 mg/mL [10,000 units/mL] (100 mL, 200 mL)

Aquacare® [US-OTC] *see* urea *on page 666*

Aquachloral® Supprettes® [US] *see* chloral hydrate *on page 132*

Aquacort® [Can] *see* hydrocortisone (topical) *on page 334*

Aquacot® [US] *see* trichlormethiazide *on page 653*

Aqua Lube Plus [US-OTC] *see* nonoxynol 9 *on page 464*

AquaMEPHYTON® [US/Can] *see* phytonadione *on page 513*

Aquaphilic® With Carbamide [US-OTC] *see* urea *on page 666*

Aquaphyllin® *(Discontinued) see page 814*

AquaSite® [US-OTC] *see* artificial tears *on page 56*

Aquasol A® [US] *see* vitamin A *on page 680*

Aquasol E® [US-OTC] *see* vitamin E *on page 682*

Aquatab® [US] *see* guaifenesin and pseudoephedrine *on page 310*

Aquatab® C [US] *see* guaifenesin, pseudoephedrine, and dextromethorphan *on page 312*

Aquatab® D Dose Pack [US] *see* guaifenesin and pseudoephedrine *on page 310*

Aquatab® DM [US] *see* guaifenesin and dextromethorphan *on page 308*

AquaTar® *(Discontinued) see page 814*

Aquatensen® [US/Can] *see* methyclothiazide *on page 420*

Aquazide H® [US] *see* hydrochlorothiazide *on page 328*

aqueous procaine penicillin G *see* penicillin G procaine *on page 499*

aqueous testosterone *see* testosterone *on page 625*

Aquest® *(Discontinued) see page 814*

ARA-A *see* vidarabine *on page 677*

arabinofuranosyladenine *see* vidarabine *on page 677*

arabinosylcytosine *see* cytarabine *on page 171*

ARA-C *see* cytarabine *on page 171*

Aralen® Phosphate [US/Can] *see* chloroquine phosphate *on page 136*

Aralen® Phosphate With Primaquine Phosphate *(Discontinued) see page 814*

Aramine® [US/Can] *see* metaraminol *on page 413*

Aranesp™ [US] *see* darbepoetin alfa *on page 175*

Arava™ [US/Can] *see* leflunomide *on page 376*

Arcet® [US] *see* butalbital, acetaminophen, and caffeine *on page 99*

Arcotinic® Tablet *(Discontinued) see page 814*

Arduan® [US/Can] *see* pipecuronium *on page 516*

Aredia® [US/Can] *see* pamidronate *on page 488*

argatroban (ar GA troh ban)

Therapeutic Category Anticoagulant, Thrombin Inhibitor

Use Prophylaxis or treatment of thrombosis in adults with heparin-induced thrombocytopenia

Usual Dosage I.V.: Adults:

Initial dose: 2 mcg/kg/minute

Maintenance dose: Measure aPTT after 2 hours, adjust dose until the steady-state aPTT is 1.5-3.0 times the initial baseline value, not exceeding 100 seconds; dosage should not exceed 10 mcg/kg/minute

Conversion to oral anticoagulant: Because there may be a combined effect on the INR when argatroban is combined with warfarin, loading doses of warfarin should not be used. Warfarin therapy should be started at the expected daily dose.

Patients receiving ≤2 mcg/kg/minute of argatroban: Argatroban therapy can be stopped when the combined INR on warfarin and argatroban is >4; repeat INR measurement in 4-6 hours; if INR is below therapeutic level, argatroban therapy may be restarted. Repeat procedure daily until desired INR on warfarin alone is obtained.

Patients receiving >2 mcg/kg/minute of argatroban: Reduce dose of argatroban to 2 mcg/kg/minute; measure INR for argatroban and warfarin 4-6 hours after dose reduction; argatroban therapy can be stopped when the combined INR on warfarin and argatroban is >4. Repeat INR measurement in 4-6 hours; if INR is below therapeutic level, argatroban therapy may be restarted. Repeat procedure daily until desired INR on warfarin alone is obtained.

Dosage Forms Injection: 100 mg/mL (2.5 mL)

Argesic®-SA [US] *see* salsalate *on page 583*

arginine (AR ji neen)

U.S./Canadian Brand Names R-Gene® [US]

Therapeutic Category Diagnostic Agent

Use Pituitary function test (growth hormone); management of severe, uncompensated, metabolic alkalosis (pH ≥7.55) **after** optimizing therapy with sodium, potassium, or ammonium chloride supplements

Usual Dosage I.V.:

Growth hormone (pituitary function) reserve test:

Children: 500 mg (5 mL) kg/dose administered over 30 minutes

Adults: 30 g (300 mL) administered over 30 minutes

Metabolic alkalosis: Children and Adults: Usual dose: 10 g/hour

Acid required (mEq) =

[1] 0.2 (L/kg) x wt (kg) x [103 - serum chloride] (mEq/L) **or**

[2] 0.3 (L/kg) x wt (kg) x base excess (mEq/L) **or**

[3] 0.5 (L/kg) x wt (kg) x [serum HCO_3 - 24] (mEq/L)

Administer $1/2$ to $2/3$ of calculated dose and re-evaluate

Note: Arginine hydrochloride should never be used as an alternative to chloride supplementation but used in the patient who is unresponsive to sodium chloride or potassium chloride supplementation

Dosage Forms Injection, solution, as hydrochloride: 10% [100 mg/mL = 950 mOsm/L] (300 mL) [contains chloride 0.475 mEq/mL]

8-arginine vasopressin *see* vasopressin *on page 674*

Argyrol® S.S. *(Discontinued)* *see page 814*

Aricept® [US/Can] *see* donepezil *on page 211*

Arimidex® [US/Can] *see* anastrozole *on page 42*

Aristocort® A Topical [US] *see* triamcinolone (topical) *on page 652*

Aristocort® Forte Injection [US] *see* triamcinolone (systemic) *on page 651*

Aristocort® Intralesional Injection [US] *see* triamcinolone (systemic) *on page 651*

Aristocort® Tablet [US/Can] *see* triamcinolone (systemic) *on page 651*

Aristocort® Topical [US/Can] *see* triamcinolone (topical) *on page 652*

Aristospan® Intra-articular Injection [US/Can] *see* triamcinolone (systemic) *on page 651*

Aristospan® Intralesional Injection [US/Can] *see* triamcinolone (systemic) *on page 651*

Arixtra® [US] *see* fondaparinux *on page 287*

Arlex® [US] *see* sorbitol *on page 602*

Arlidin® *(Discontinued)* *see page 814*

Arm-a-Med® Isoetharine *(Discontinued)* *see page 814*

Arm-a-Med® Isoproterenol *(Discontinued)* *see page 814*

Arm-a-Med® Metaproterenol *(Discontinued)* *see page 814*

A.R.M.® Caplet *(Discontinued)* *see page 814*

Armour® Thyroid [US] *see thyroid on page 636*

Aromasin® [US/Can] *see exemestane on page 260*

Aromatic Ammonia Aspirols® [US] *see ammonia spirit (aromatic) on page 36*

Arrestin® (Discontinued) *see page 814*

arsenic trioxide (AR se nik tri OKS id)

U.S./Canadian Brand Names Trisenox™ [US]

Therapeutic Category Antineoplastic Agent, Miscellaneous

Use Induction of remission and consolidation in patients with acute promyelocytic leukemia (APL) which is specifically characterized by t(15;17) translocation or PML/RAR-alpha gene expression. Should be used only in those patients who have relapsed or are refractory to retinoid and anthracycline chemotherapy.

Usual Dosage I.V.: Children >5 years and Adults:

Induction: 0.15 mg/kg/day; administer daily until bone marrow remission; maximum induction: 60 doses

Consolidation: 0.15 mg/kg/day starting 3-6 weeks after completion of induction therapy; maximum consolidation: 25 doses over 5 weeks

Dosage Forms Injection: 1 mg/mL (10 mL)

Artane® [US] *see trihexyphenidyl on page 655*

Artha-G® (Discontinued) *see page 814*

Arth Dr® [US] *see capsaicin on page 111*

Arthricare Hand & Body® [US] *see capsaicin on page 111*

Arthritis Foundation® Ibuprofen (Discontinued) *see page 814*

Arthritis Foundation® Nighttime (Discontinued) *see page 814*

Arthritis Foundation® Pain Reliever, Aspirin Free (Discontinued) *see page 814*

Arthropan® [US-OTC] *see choline salicylate on page 144*

Arthrotec® [US/Can] *see diclofenac and misoprostol on page 194*

Articulose-50® Injection (Discontinued) *see page 814*

artificial tears (ar ti FISH il tears)

Synonyms polyvinyl alcohol

U.S./Canadian Brand Names Akwa Tears® [US-OTC]; AquaSite® [US-OTC]; Bion® Tears [US-OTC]; HypoTears PF [US-OTC]; HypoTears [US-OTC]; Isopto® Tears [US/Can]; Liquifilm® Tears [US-OTC]; Moisture® Eyes PM [US-OTC]; Moisture® Eyes [US-OTC]; Murine® Tears [US-OTC]; Murocel® [US-OTC]; Nature's Tears® [US-OTC]; Nu-Tears® II [US-OTC]; Nu-Tears® [US-OTC]; OcuCoat® [US/Can]; OcuCoat® PF [US-OTC]; Puralube® Tears [US-OTC]; Refresh® Plus [US/Can]; Refresh® Tears [US/Can]; Refresh® [US-OTC]; Teardrops® [Can]; Teargen® II [US-OTC]; Teargen® [US-OTC]; Tearisol® [US-OTC]; Tears Again® [US-OTC]; Tears Naturale® Free [US-OTC]; Tears Naturale® II [US-OTC]; Tears Naturale® [US-OTC]; Tears Plus® [US-OTC]; Tears Renewed® [US-OTC]; Ultra Tears® [US-OTC]; Viva-Drops® [US-OTC]

Therapeutic Category Ophthalmic Agent, Miscellaneous

Use Ophthalmic lubricant; relief of dry eyes and eye irritation

Usual Dosage Ophthalmic: Use as needed to relieve symptoms, 1-2 drops into eye(s) 3-4 times/day

Dosage Forms Solution, ophthalmic: 15 mL and 30 mL with dropper

ASA *see aspirin on page 58*

A.S.A.® (Discontinued) *see page 814*

5-ASA *see mesalamine on page 411*

Asacol® [US/Can] *see mesalamine on page 411*

Asaphen [Can] *see* aspirin *on next page*

Asaphen E.C. [Can] *see* aspirin *on next page*

Asbron-G® Elixir *(Discontinued)* *see page 814*

Asbron-G® Tablet *(Discontinued)* *see page 814*

Ascarel® [US-OTC] *see* pyrantel pamoate *on page 555*

ascorbic acid (a SKOR bik AS id)

Synonyms vitamin C

U.S./Canadian Brand Names Apo®-C [Can]; C-500-GR™ [US-OTC]; Cecon® [US-OTC]; Cevi-Bid® [US-OTC]; C-Gram [US-OTC]; Dull-C® [US-OTC]; Proflavanol C™ [Can]; Revitalose C-1000® [Can]; Vita-C® [US-OTC]

Therapeutic Category Vitamin, Water Soluble

Use Prevention and treatment of scurvy; urinary acidification; dietary supplementation; prevention and reduction in the severity of colds

Usual Dosage Oral, I.M., I.V., S.C.:

Recommended daily allowance (RDA):

<6 months: 30 mg

6 months to 1 year: 35 mg

1-3 years: 40 mg

4-10 years: 45 mg

11-14 years: 50 mg

>14 years and Adults: 60 mg

Children:

Scurvy: 100-300 mg/day in divided doses for at least 2 weeks

Urinary acidification: 500 mg every 6-8 hours

Dietary supplement: 35-100 mg/day

Adults:

Scurvy: 100-250 mg 1-2 times/day for at least 2 weeks

Urinary acidification: 4-12 g/day in 3-4 divided doses

Prevention and treatment of colds: 1-3 g/day

Dietary supplement: 50-200 mg/day

Dosage Forms

Capsule: 500 mg, 1000 mg

C-500-GR™: 500 mg

Capsule, timed release: 500 mg

Crystal (Vita-C®): 4 g/teaspoonful (100 g)

Injection, solution: 250 mg/mL (2 mL, 30 mL); 500 mg/mL (50 mL)

Cenolate®: 500 mg/mL (1 mL, 2 mL) [contains sodium hydrosulfite]

Powder, solution (Dull-C®): 4 g/teaspoonful (100 g, 500 g)

Solution, oral (Cecon®): 90 mg/mL (50 mL)

Tablet: 100 mg, 250 mg, 500 mg, 1000 mg

C-Gram: 1000 mg

Tablet, chewable: 100 mg, 250 mg, 500 mg [some products may contain aspartame]

Tablet, timed release: 500 mg, 1000 mg, 1500 mg

Cevi-Bid®: 500 mg

ascorbic acid and ferrous sulfate *see* ferrous sulfate and ascorbic acid *on page 269*

Ascorbicap® *(Discontinued)* *see page 814*

Ascriptin® Arthritis Pain [US-OTC] *see* aspirin *on next page*

Ascriptin® Enteric [US-OTC] *see* aspirin *on next page*

Ascriptin® Extra Strength [US-OTC] *see* aspirin *on next page*

Ascriptin® [US-OTC] *see* aspirin *on next page*

Asendin® *(Discontinued)* *see page 814*

Asmalix® *(Discontinued)* *see page 814*

asparaginase (a SPIR a ji nase)
Synonyms colaspase
U.S./Canadian Brand Names Elspar® [US/Can]; Kidrolase® [Can]
Therapeutic Category Antineoplastic Agent
Use Treatment of acute lymphocytic leukemia, lymphoma; used for induction therapy
Usual Dosage Refer to individual protocols; the manufacturer recommends performing intradermal sensitivity testing before the initial dose

Children and Adults:
I.M. (preferred route): 6000 units/m² 3 times/week for 3 weeks for combination therapy
I.V.: 1000 units/kg/day for 10 days for combination therapy or 200 units/kg/day for 28 days if combination therapy is inappropriate
Dosage Forms Injection, powder for reconstitution: 10,000 units

A-Spas® S/L [US] *see* hyoscyamine *on page 339*

Aspercin Extra [US-OTC] *see* aspirin *on this page*

Aspercin [US-OTC] *see* aspirin *on this page*

Aspergum® [US-OTC] *see* aspirin *on this page*

aspirin (AS pir in)
Synonyms acetylsalicylic acid; ASA
U.S./Canadian Brand Names Apo®-ASA [Can]; Asaphen [Can]; Asaphen E.C. [Can]; Ascriptin® Arthritis Pain [US-OTC]; Ascriptin® Enteric [US-OTC]; Ascriptin® Extra Strength [US-OTC]; Ascriptin® [US-OTC]; Aspercin Extra [US-OTC]; Aspercin [US-OTC]; Aspergum® [US-OTC]; Bayer® Aspirin Extra Strength [US-OTC]; Bayer® Aspirin Regimen Adult Low Strength [US-OTC]; Bayer® Aspirin Regimen Adult Low Strength with Calcium [US-OTC]; Bayer® Aspirin Regimen Children's [US-OTC]; Bayer® Aspirin Regimen Regular Strength [US-OTC]; Bayer® Aspirin [US-OTC]; Bayer® Plus Extra Strength [US-OTC]; Bufferin® Arthritis Strength [US-OTC]; Bufferin® Extra Strength [US-OTC]; Bufferin® [US-OTC]; Easprin® [US]; Ecotrin® Low Adult Strength [US-OTC]; Ecotrin® Maximum Strength [US-OTC]; Ecotrin® [US-OTC]; Entrophen® [Can]; Halfprin® [US-OTC]; Novasen [Can]; St. Joseph® Pain Reliever [US-OTC]; Sureprin 81™ [US-OTC]; ZORprin® [US]
Therapeutic Category Analgesic, Non-narcotic; Antiplatelet Agent; Antipyretic; Nonsteroidal Anti-inflammatory Drug (NSAID)
Use Treatment of mild to moderate pain, inflammation and fever; adjunctive treatment of Kawasaki disease; may be used for prophylaxis of myocardial infarction and transient ischemic attacks (TIA)
Usual Dosage
Children:
Analgesic and antipyretic: Oral, rectal: 10-15 mg/kg/dose every 4-6 hours
Anti-inflammatory: Oral: Initial: 60-90 mg/kg/day in divided doses; usual maintenance: 80-100 mg/kg/day divided every 6-8 hours; monitor serum concentrations
Kawasaki disease: Oral: 100 mg/kg/day divided every 6 hours; after fever resolves: 8-10 mg/kg/day once daily; monitor serum concentrations
Adults:
Analgesic and antipyretic: Oral, rectal: 325-1000 mg every 4-6 hours up to 4 g/day
Anti-inflammatory: Oral: Initial: 2.4-3.6 g/day in divided doses; usual maintenance: 3.6-5.4 g/day; monitor serum concentrations
Transient ischemic attack: Oral: 1.3 g/day in 2-4 divided doses
Myocardial infarction prophylaxis: 160-325 mg/day
Dosage Forms
Caplet, buffered:
Ascriptin® Arthritis Pain: 325 mg [contains aluminum hydroxide, calcium carbonate, and magnesium hydroxide]
Ascriptin® Extra Strength: 500 mg [contains aluminum hydroxide, calcium carbonate, and magnesium hydroxide]

Gelcap:
 Bayer® Aspirin: 325 mg
 Bayer® Aspirin Extra Strength: 500 mg
Gum (Aspergum®): 227 mg
Suppository, rectal: 60 mg, 120 mg, 125 mg, 200 mg, 300 mg, 325 mg, 600 mg, 650 mg
Tablet: 325 mg, 500 mg
 Aspercin: 325 mg
 Aspercin Extra, Bayer® Aspirin Extra Strength: 500 mg
 Bayer® Aspirin: 325 mg [film coated]
Tablet, buffered:
 Ascriptin®: 325 mg [contains aluminum hydroxide, calcium carbonate, and magnesium hydroxide]
 Bayer® Plus Extra Strength: 500 mg [contains calcium carbonate]
 Bufferin®: 325 mg [contains citric acid]
 Bufferin® Arthritis Strength, Bufferin® Extra Strength: 500 mg [contains citric acid]
Tablet, chewable: 81 mg
 Bayer® Aspirin Regimen Children's Chewable, St. Joseph® Pain Reliever: 81 mg
Tablet, controlled release (ZORprin®): 800 mg
Tablet, enteric coated: 81 mg, 162 mg, 325 mg, 500 mg, 650 mg, 975 mg
 Ascriptin® Enteric, Bayer® Aspirin Regimen Adult Low Strength, Ecotrin® Adult Low Strength, St. Joseph Pain Reliever: 81 mg
 Bayer® Aspirin Regimen Adult Low Strength with Calcium: 81 mg [contains calcium carbonate 250 mg]
 Bayer® Aspirin Regimen Regular Strength, Ecotrin®: 325 mg
 Easprin®: 975 mg
 Ecotrin® Maximum Strength: 500 mg
 Halfprin®: 81 mg, 162 mg
 Sureprin 81™: 81 mg

aspirin and codeine (AS pir in & KOE deen)
Synonyms codeine and aspirin
U.S./Canadian Brand Names Coryphen® Codeine [Can]; Empirin® With Codeine [US]
Therapeutic Category Analgesic, Narcotic
Controlled Substance C-III
Use Relief of mild to moderate pain
Usual Dosage Oral:
 Children:
  Aspirin: 10 mg/kg/dose every 4 hours
  Codeine: 0.5-1 mg/kg/dose every 4 hours
 Adults: 1-2 tablets every 4-6 hours as needed for pain
Dosage Forms Tablet:
 #3: Aspirin 325 mg and codeine phosphate 30 mg
 #4: Aspirin 325 mg and codeine phosphate 60 mg

aspirin and hydrocodone see hydrocodone and aspirin on page 330

aspirin and meprobamate (AS pir in & me proe BA mate)
Synonyms meprobamate and aspirin
U.S./Canadian Brand Names Equagesic® [US]; 292 MEP® [Can]
Therapeutic Category Skeletal Muscle Relaxant
Controlled Substance C-IV
Use Adjunct to treatment of skeletal muscular disease in patients exhibiting tension and/or anxiety
Usual Dosage Oral: 1 tablet 3-4 times/day
Dosage Forms Tablet: Aspirin 325 mg and meprobamate 200 mg

aspirin and methocarbamol see methocarbamol and aspirin on page 417
aspirin and oxycodone see oxycodone and aspirin on page 485

aspirin and propoxyphene *see* propoxyphene and aspirin *on page 549*

Aspirin® Backache [Can] *see* methocarbamol and aspirin *on page 417*

Aspirin Free Anacin® Maximum Strength [US-OTC] *see* acetaminophen *on page 3*

aspirin, orphenadrine, and caffeine *see* orphenadrine, aspirin, and caffeine *on page 480*

Asproject® *(Discontinued) see page 814*

Astelin® [US/Can] *see* azelastine *on page 66*

AsthmaHaler® Mist *(Discontinued) see page 814*

AsthmaNefrin® *(Discontinued) see page 814*

Astramorph™ PF [US] *see* morphine sulfate *on page 437*

Atabrine® Tablet *(Discontinued) see page 814*

Atacand® [US/Can] *see* candesartan *on page 110*

Atacand HCT™ [US] *see* candesartan and hydrochlorothiazide *on page 110*

Atapryl® [US] *see* selegiline *on page 586*

Atarax® [US/Can] *see* hydroxyzine *on page 339*

Atasol® [Can] *see* acetaminophen *on page 3*

atenolol (a TEN oh lole)

U.S./Canadian Brand Names Apo®-Atenol [Can]; Gen-Atenolol [Can]; Novo-Atenol [Can]; Nu-Atenol; PMS-Atenolol [Can]; Rhoxal-atenolol [Can]; Tenolin [Can]; Tenormin® [US/Can]

Therapeutic Category Beta-Adrenergic Blocker

Use Treatment of hypertension, alone or in combination with other agents; management of angina pectoris; antiarrhythmic; postmyocardial infarction patients; acute alcohol withdrawal

Usual Dosage
Oral:
Children: 1-2 mg/kg/dose administered daily
Adults:
Hypertension: 50 mg once daily, may increase to 100 mg/day; doses >100 mg are unlikely to produce any further benefit
Angina pectoris: 50 mg once daily, may increase to 100 mg/day; some patients may require 200 mg/day
Postmyocardial infarction: Follow I.V. dose with 100 mg/day or 50 mg twice daily for 6-9 days postmyocardial infarction
I.V.: Postmyocardial infarction: Early treatment: 5 mg slow I.V. over 5 minutes; may repeat in 10 minutes; if both doses are tolerated, may start oral atenolol 50 mg every 12 hours or 100 mg/day for 6-9 days postmyocardial infarction

Dosage Forms
Injection, solution: 0.5 mg/mL (10 mL)
Tablet: 25 mg, 50 mg, 100 mg

atenolol and chlorthalidone (a TEN oh lole & klor THAL i done)

Synonyms chlorthalidone and atenolol

U.S./Canadian Brand Names Tenoretic® [US/Can]

Therapeutic Category Antihypertensive Agent, Combination

Use Treatment of hypertension with a cardioselective beta-blocker and a diuretic

Usual Dosage Adults: Oral: Initial: 1 tablet (50) once daily, then individualize dose until optimal dose is achieved

Dosage Forms
Tablet:
50: Atenolol 50 mg and chlorthalidone 25 mg
100: Atenolol 100 mg and chlorthalidone 25 mg

ATG *see* lymphocyte immune globulin *on page 395*

Atgam® **[US/Can]** *see* lymphocyte immune globulin *on page 395*

ATIII *see* antithrombin III *on page 47*

Ativan® **[US/Can]** *see* lorazepam *on page 391*

Atolone® **Oral** *(Discontinued)* *see page 814*

atorvastatin (a TORE va sta tin)

U.S./Canadian Brand Names Lipitor® [US/Can]

Therapeutic Category HMG-CoA Reductase Inhibitor

Use Adjunct to diet for the reduction of elevated total and LDL-cholesterol levels in patients with hypercholesterolemia (Type IIa, IIb, and IIc); used in hypercholesterolemic patients without clinically evident heart disease to reduce the risk of myocardial infarction, to reduce the risk for revascularization, and reduce the risk of death due to cardiovascular causes with no increase in death from noncardiovascular diseases

Usual Dosage Adults: Oral: Initial: 10 mg/day, with a range of 10-80 mg/day, administered as a single dose at any time of day, with or without food

Dosage Forms Tablet: 10 mg, 20 mg, 40 mg, 80 mg

atovaquone (a TOE va kwone)

U.S./Canadian Brand Names Mepron™ [US/Can]

Therapeutic Category Antiprotozoal

Use Acute oral treatment of mild to moderate *Pneumocystis carinii* pneumonia (PCP) in patients who are intolerant to co-trimoxazole

Usual Dosage Adults: Oral: 750 mg twice daily with food for 21 days

Dosage Forms Suspension, oral: 750 mg/5 mL (5 mL, 210 mL) [citrus flavor]

atovaquone and proguanil (a TOE va kwone & pro GWA nil)

U.S./Canadian Brand Names Malarone™ [US/Can]

Therapeutic Category Antimalarial Agent

Use Prevention or treatment of acute, uncomplicated *P. falciparum* malaria

Usual Dosage Oral (doses given in mg of atovaquone and proguanil):

Adults:

Prevention of malaria: Atovaquone/proguanil 250 mg/100 mg once daily. Start 1-2 days prior to entering a malaria-endemic area, continue throughout the stay and for 7 days after returning.

Treatment of acute malaria: Atovaquone/proguanil 1 g/400 mg as a single dose, once daily for 3 consecutive days

Children (dosage based on body weight):

Prevention of malaria: Start 1-2 days prior to entering a malaria-endemic area, continue throughout the stay and for 7 days after returning. Take as a single dose, once daily.

11-20 kg: Atovaquone/proguanil 62.5 mg/25 mg

21-30 kg: Atovaquone/proguanil 125 mg/50 mg

31-40 kg: Atovaquone/proguanil 187.5 mg/75 mg

>40 kg: Atovaquone/proguanil 250 mg/100mg

Treatment of acute malaria: Take as a single dose, once daily for 3 consecutive days.

11-20 kg: Atovaquone/proguanil 250 mg/100 mg

21-30 kg: Atovaquone/proguanil 500 mg/200mg

31-40 kg: Atovaquone/proguanil 750 mg/300mg

>40 kg: Atovaquone/proguanil 1 g/400 mg

Dosage Forms

Tablet: Atovaquone 250 mg and proguanil hydrochloride 100 mg

Tablet, pediatric: Atovaquone 62.5 mg and proguanil hydrochloride 25 mg

Atozine® **Oral** *(Discontinued)* *see page 814*

atracurium (a tra KYOO ree um)

U.S./Canadian Brand Names Tracrium® [US]

Therapeutic Category Skeletal Muscle Relaxant

Use Eases endotracheal intubation as an adjunct to general anesthesia and relaxes skeletal muscle during surgery or mechanical ventilation

Usual Dosage I.V.:

Children 1 month to 2 years: Initial: 0.3-0.4 mg/kg followed by maintenance doses of 0.08-0.1 mg/kg as needed to maintain neuromuscular blockade

Children >2 years to Adults: Initial: 0.4-0.5 mg/kg then 0.08-0.1 mg/kg every 20-45 minutes after initial dose to maintain neuromuscular block

Continuous infusion: 0.4-0.8 mg/kg/hour

Dosage Forms

Injection, as besylate: 10 mg/mL (5 mL, 10 mL)

Injection, as besylate [preservative free]: 10 mg/mL (5 mL)

Atrohist® Plus *(Discontinued)* see page 814

Atromid-S® *(Discontinued)* see page 814

Atropair® *(Discontinued)* see page 814

atropine (A troe peen)

U.S./Canadian Brand Names Atropine-Care® [US]; Atropisol® [US/Can]; Isopto® Atropine [US/Can]; Sal-Tropine™ [US]

Therapeutic Category Anticholinergic Agent

Use Preoperative medication to inhibit salivation and secretions; treatment of sinus bradycardia; management of peptic ulcer; treatment of exercise-induced bronchospasm; antidote for organophosphate pesticide poisoning; used to produce mydriasis and cycloplegia for examination of the retina and optic disk and accurate measurement of refractive errors; treatment of uveitis

Usual Dosage Note: Doses <0.1 mg have been associated with paradoxical bradycardia.

Neonates, Infants, and Children:

Preanesthetic: Oral, I.M., I.V., S.C.:

<5 kg: 0.02 mg/kg/dose 30-60 minutes preop then every 4-6 hours as needed. Use of a minimum dosage of 0.1 mg in neonates <5 kg will result in dosages >0.02 mg/kg. There is no documented minimum dosage in this age group.

>5 kg: 0.01-0.02 mg/kg/dose to a maximum 0.4 mg/dose 30-60 minutes preop; minimum dose: 0.1 mg

Bradycardia: I.V., intratracheal: 0.02 mg/kg, minimum dose 0.1 mg, maximum single dose: 0.5 mg in children and 1 mg in adolescents; may repeat in 5-minute intervals to a maximum total dose of 1 mg in children or 2 mg in adolescents. **(Note:** For intratracheal administration, the dosage must be diluted with normal saline to a total volume of 1-2 mL). When treating bradycardia in neonates, reserve use for those patients unresponsive to improved oxygenation and epinephrine.

Children:

Bronchospasm: Inhalation: 0.03-0.05 mg/kg/dose 3-4 times/day

Preprocedure: Ophthalmic: 0.5% solution: Instill 1-2 drops twice daily for 1-3 days before the procedure

Uveitis: Ophthalmic: 0.5% solution: Instill 1-2 drops up to 3 times/day

Adults (doses <0.5 mg have been associated with paradoxical bradycardia):

Asystole: I.V.: 1 mg; may repeat every 3-5 minutes as needed

Preanesthetic: I.M., I.V., S.C.: 0.4-0.6 mg 30-60 minutes preop and repeat every 4-6 hours as needed

Bradycardia: I.V.: 0.5-1 mg every 5 minutes, not to exceed a total of 2 mg or 0.04 mg/kg; may give intratracheal in 1 mg/10 mL dilution only, intratracheal dose should be 2-2.5 times the I.V. dose

Neuromuscular blockade reversal: I.V.: 25-30 mcg/kg 30 seconds before neostigmine or 10 mcg/kg 30 seconds before edrophonium

Organophosphate or carbamate poisoning: I.V.: 1-2 mg/dose every 10-20 minutes until atropine effect (dry flushed skin, tachycardia, mydriasis, fever) is observed, then every 1-4 hours for at least 24 hours; up to 50 mg in first 24 hours and 2 g over several days may be given in cases of severe intoxication

Bronchospasm: Inhalation: 0.025-0.05 mg/kg/dose every 4-6 hours as needed (maximum: 5 mg/dose)

Ophthalmic solution: 1%:

Preprocedure: Instill 1-2 drops 1 hour before the procedure.

Uveitis: Instill 1-2 drops 4 times/day.

Ophthalmic ointment: Apply a small amount in the conjunctival sac up to 3 times/day. Compress the lacrimal sac by digital pressure for 1-3 minutes after instillation.

Dosage Forms

Injection, solution, as sulfate: 0.1 mg/mL (5 mL, 10 mL); 0.4 mg/mL (1 mL, 20 mL); 0.5 mg/mL (1 mL); 1 mg/mL (1 mL)

Ointment, ophthalmic, as sulfate: 1% (3.5 g)

Solution, ophthalmic, as sulfate: 1% (5 mL, 15 mL)

Atropine-Care®: 1% (2 mL)

Atropisol®: 1% (1 mL)

Isopto® Atropine: 1% (5 mL, 15 mL)

Tablet, as sulfate (Sal-Tropine™): 0.4 mg

atropine and difenoxin *see* difenoxin and atropine *on page 196*

atropine and diphenoxylate *see* diphenoxylate and atropine *on page 203*

Atropine-Care® [US] *see* atropine *on previous page*

atropine, hyoscyamine, scopolamine, and phenobarbital *see* hyoscyamine, atropine, scopolamine, and phenobarbital *on page 340*

atropine soluble tablet *(Discontinued) see page 814*

Atropisol® [US/Can] *see* atropine *on previous page*

Atrosept® [US] *see* methenamine, phenyl salicylate, atropine, hyoscyamine, benzoic acid, and methylene blue *on page 416*

Atrovent® [US/Can] *see* ipratropium *on page 358*

A/T/S® [US] *see* erythromycin (ophthalmic/topical) *on page 235*

attapulgite (at a PULL gite)

U.S./Canadian Brand Names Children's Kaopectate® [US-OTC]; Diasorb® [US-OTC]; Kaopectate® Advanced Formula [US-OTC]; Kaopectate® Maximum Strength Caplets [US-OTC]; Kaopectate® [US/Can]; K-Pek® [US-OTC]

Therapeutic Category Antidiarrheal

Use Treatment of uncomplicated diarrhea

Usual Dosage Oral:

Children:

<3 years: Not recommended

3-6 years: 750 mg/dose up to 2250 mg/24 hours

6-12 years: 1200-1500 mg/dose up to 4500 mg/24 hours

Adults: 1200-1500 mg after each loose bowel movement or every 2 hours; 15-30 mL up to 8 times/day, up to 9000 mg/24 hours

Dosage Forms

Caplet (Kaopectate® Maximum Strength): 750 mg

Liquid, oral concentrate: Activated attapulgite 600 mg/15 mL (120 mL, 180 mL, 240 mL); activated attapulgite 750 mg/15 mL (120 mL, 360 mL)

Children's Kaopectate®: Activated attapulgite 300 mg/7.5 mL (180 mL) [cherry flavor]

Diasorb®: Activated attapulgite 750 mg/5 mL (120 mL) [cola flavor; sugar free]

Kaopectate® Advanced Formula: Activated attapulgite 750 mg/15 mL (90 mL, 240 mL, 360 mL) [peppermint flavor]

K-Pek®: Activated attapulgite 750 mg/15 mL (240 mL, 480 mL)

Attenuvax® [US] *see* measles virus vaccine (live) *on page 402*

Augmentin® [US/Can] *see* amoxicillin and clavulanate potassium *on page 38*

Augmentin ES-600™ [US] *see* amoxicillin and clavulanate potassium *on page 38*

Auralgan® [US/Can] *see* antipyrine and benzocaine *on page 47*

auranofin (au RANE oh fin)
U.S./Canadian Brand Names Ridaura® [US/Can]
Therapeutic Category Gold Compound
Use Management of active stage of classic or definite rheumatoid or psoriatic arthritis in patients that do not respond to or tolerate other agents
Usual Dosage Oral:
Children: Initial: 0.1 mg/kg/day divided daily; usual maintenance: 0.15 mg/kg/day in 1-2 divided doses; maximum: 0.2 mg/kg/day in 1-2 divided doses
Adults: 6 mg/day in 1-2 divided doses; after 3 months may be increased to 9 mg/day in 3 divided doses; if still no response after 3 months at 9 mg/day, discontinue drug
Dosage Forms Capsule: 3 mg [gold 29%]

Aureomycin® *(Discontinued)* *see page 814*

Aurodex® [US] *see* antipyrine and benzocaine *on page 47*

Auro® Ear Drops [US-OTC] *see* carbamide peroxide *on page 113*

Aurolate® [US] *see* gold sodium thiomalate *on page 304*

aurothioglucose (aur oh thye oh GLOO kose)
U.S./Canadian Brand Names Solganal® [US/Can]
Therapeutic Category Gold Compound
Use Management of active stage of classic or definite rheumatoid or psoriatic arthritis in patients that do not respond to or tolerate other agents
Usual Dosage I.M. (doses should initially be administered at weekly intervals):
Children 6-12 years: Initial: 0.25 mg/kg/dose first week; increment at 0.25 mg/kg/dose increasing with each weekly dose; maintenance: 0.75-1 mg/kg/dose weekly not to exceed 25 mg/dose to a total of 20 doses, then every 2-4 weeks
Adults: 10 mg first week; 25 mg second and third week; then 50 mg/week until 800 mg to 1 g cumulative dose has been administered - if improvement occurs without adverse reactions, administer 25-50 mg every 2-3 weeks, then every 3-4 weeks
Dosage Forms Injection, suspension: 50 mg/mL [gold 50%] (10 mL)

Auroto® [US] *see* antipyrine and benzocaine *on page 47*

Autoplex® T [US] *see* anti-inhibitor coagulant complex *on page 46*

Avalide® [US/Can] *see* irbesartan and hydrochlorothiazide *on page 359*

Avandia® [US/Can] *see* rosiglitazone *on page 578*

Avapro® [US/Can] *see* irbesartan *on page 359*

Avaxim® [Can] *see* hepatitis A vaccine *on page 319*

AVC™ [US/Can] *see* sulfanilamide *on page 613*

Aveeno® Cleansing Bar [US-OTC] *see* sulfur and salicylic acid *on page 614*

Avelox® [US/Can] *see* moxifloxacin *on page 439*

Aventyl® HCl [US/Can] *see* nortriptyline *on page 466*

Aviane™ [US] *see* ethinyl estradiol and levonorgestrel *on page 248*

Avinza™ [US] *see* morphine sulfate *on page 437*

Avirax™ [Can] *see* acyclovir *on page 13*

Avita® [US] *see* tretinoin (topical) *on page 650*

Avitene® [US] *see* microfibrillar collagen hemostat *on page 428*

Avlosulfon® *(Discontinued)* *see page 814*

Avodart™ **[US]** *see* dutasteride *on page 220*

Avonex® **[US/Can]** *see* interferon beta-1a *on page 356*

Axert™ **[US]** *see* almotriptan *on page 24*

Axid® **[US/Can]** *see* nizatidine *on page 463*

Axid® **AR [US-OTC]** *see* nizatidine *on page 463*

Axocet® **[US]** *see* butalbital, acetaminophen, and caffeine *on page 99*

Axotal® *(Discontinued)* *see page 814*

Aygestin® **[US]** *see* norethindrone *on page 465*

Ayr® **Baby Saline [US-OTC]** *see* sodium chloride *on page 595*

Ayr® **Saline [US-OTC]** *see* sodium chloride *on page 595*

Azactam® **[US/Can]** *see* aztreonam *on page 67*

azatadine (a ZA ta deen)

U.S./Canadian Brand Names Optimine® [US/Can]
Therapeutic Category Antihistamine
Use Treatment of perennial and seasonal allergic rhinitis and chronic urticaria
Usual Dosage Children >12 years and Adults: Oral: 1-2 mg twice daily
Dosage Forms Tablet, as maleate: 1 mg

azatadine and pseudoephedrine (a ZA ta deen & soo doe e FED rin)

Synonyms pseudoephedrine and azatadine
U.S./Canadian Brand Names Rynatan® [US]; Trinalin® Repetabs® [US/Can]
Therapeutic Category Antihistamine/Decongestant Combination
Use Perennial and seasonal allergic rhinitis and other allergic symptoms including urticaria
Usual Dosage Adults: 1 tablet twice daily
Dosage Forms Tablet: Azatadine maleate 1 mg and pseudoephedrine sulfate 120 mg

azathioprine (ay za THYE oh preen)

U.S./Canadian Brand Names Alti-Azathioprine [Can]; Gen-Azathioprine [Can]; Imuran® [US/Can]
Therapeutic Category Immunosuppressant Agent
Use Adjunct with other agents in prevention of transplant rejection; also used as an immunosuppressant in a variety of autoimmune diseases such as systemic lupus erythematosus, severe rheumatoid arthritis unresponsive to other agents, and nephrotic syndrome
Usual Dosage
Children and Adults: Renal transplantation: Oral, I.V.: Initial: 3-5 mg/kg/day; maintenance: 1-3 mg/kg/day
Adults: Rheumatoid arthritis: Oral: 1 mg/kg/day for 6-8 weeks; increase by 0.5 mg/kg every 4 weeks until response or up to 2.5 mg/kg/day I.V. dose is equivalent to oral dose
Dosage Forms
Injection, powder for reconstitution, as sodium: 100 mg
Tablet, scored: 50 mg

Azdone® *(Discontinued)* *see page 814*

azelaic acid (a zeh LAY ik AS id)

U.S./Canadian Brand Names Azelex® [US]; Finevin™ [US]
Therapeutic Category Topical Skin Product
Use Treatment of mild to moderate acne vulgaris
Usual Dosage Adults: Topical: After skin is thoroughly washed and patted dry, gently but thoroughly massage a thin film of azelaic acid cream into the affected areas twice daily,
(Continued)

azelaic acid *(Continued)*

in the morning and evening. The duration of use can vary and depends on the severity of the acne. In the majority of patients with inflammatory lesions, improvement of the condition occurs within 4 weeks.

Dosage Forms
Cream:
Azelex®: 20% (30 g, 50 g)
Finevin™: 20% (30 g)

azelastine (a ZEL as teen)

U.S./Canadian Brand Names Astelin® [US/Can]; Optivar™ [US]
Therapeutic Category Antihistamine; Antihistamine, Ophthalmic
Use
Nasal spray: Treatment of the symptoms of seasonal allergic rhinitis such as rhinorrhea, sneezing, and nasal pruritus in adults and children ≥5 years of age
Ophthalmic: Treatment of itching of the eye associated with seasonal allergic conjunctivitis
Usual Dosage
Nasal spray: Children ≥5 years and Adults: 2 sprays (137 mcg/spray) each nostril twice daily. Before initial use, the delivery system should be primed with 4 sprays or until a fine mist appears. If 3 or more days have elapsed since last use, the delivery system should be reprimed.
Ophthalmic: Instill 1 drop into affected eye(s) twice daily
Dosage Forms
Nasal spray (Astelin®): 1 mg/mL [137 mcg/spray] (17 mL) [contains benzalkonium chloride]
Solution, ophthalmic (Optivar™): 0.05% (6 mL) [contains benzalkonium chloride]

Azelex® [US] *see azelaic acid on previous page*

azidothymidine *see zidovudine* *on page 689*

azithromycin (az ith roe MYE sin)

U.S./Canadian Brand Names Zithromax® [US/Can]; Z-PAK® [US/Can]
Therapeutic Category Macrolide (Antibiotic)
Use
Children: Treatment of acute otitis media due to *H. influenzae*, *M. catarrhalis*, or *S. pneumoniae*; pharyngitis/tonsillitis due to *S. pyogenes*
Adults:
Treatment of mild to moderate upper and lower respiratory tract infections, infections of the skin and skin structure, and sexually transmitted diseases due to susceptible strains of *C. trachomatis*, *M. catarrhalis*, *H. influenzae*, *S. aureus*, *S. pneumoniae*, *Mycoplasma pneumoniae*, and *C. psittaci*; community-acquired pneumonia, pelvic inflammatory disease (PID)
Prevention of (or to delay onset of) infection with *Mycobacterium avium* complex (MAC)
Prevention or (to delay onset of) or treatment of MAC in patients with advanced HIV infection
Prophylaxis of bacterial endocarditis in patients who are allergic to penicillin and undergoing surgical or dental procedures
Usual Dosage Oral:
Children:
Acute otitis media: 10 mg/kg on day 1 (not to exceed 500 mg/day) followed by 5 mg/kg/day once daily on days 2-5 (not to exceed 250 mg/day)
Pharyngitis/tonsillitis: 12 mg/kg/day for 5 days (not to exceed 500 mg/day)
Adolescents ≥16 years and Adults:
Mild to moderate respiratory tract, skin, and soft tissue infections: 500 mg in a single dose on day 1; 250 mg in a single dose on days 2-5
Nongonococcal urethritis and cervicitis: 1 g in a single dose

Chancroid and *Chlamydia*: 1 g in a single dose
I.V.: Adults:
Community-acquired pneumonia: 500 mg as a single dose for at least 2 days, follow I.V. therapy by the oral route with a single daily dose of 500 mg to complete a 7- to 10-day course of therapy
Pelvic inflammatory disease (PID): 500 mg as a single dose for 1-2 days, follow I.V. therapy by the oral route with a single daily dose of 250 mg to complete a 7-day course of therapy

Dosage Forms
Injection, powder for reconstitution, as dihydrate: 500 mg
Powder for oral suspension, as dihydrate: 100 mg/5 mL (15 mL); 200 mg/5 mL (15 mL, 22.5 mL, 30 mL); 1 g [single-dose packet]
Tablet, as dihydrate: 250 mg, 500 mg, 600 mg
Zithromax® TRI-PAK™ [unit-dose pack]: 500 mg (3s)
Zithromax® Z-PAK® [unit-dose pack]: 250 mg (6s)

Azlin® Injection *(Discontinued)* see page 814

Azmacort® [US] see triamcinolone (inhalation, oral) on page 651

Azo-Dine® [US-OTC] see phenazopyridine on page 506

Azo Gantanol® *(Discontinued)* see page 814

Azo Gantrisin® *(Discontinued)* see page 814

Azo-Gesic® [US-OTC] see phenazopyridine on page 506

Azopt® [US/Can] see brinzolamide on page 92

Azo-Standard® [US] see phenazopyridine on page 506

AZT see zidovudine on page 689

AZT™ [Can] see zidovudine on page 689

AZT + 3TC see zidovudine and lamivudine on page 690

azthreonam see aztreonam on this page

aztreonam (AZ tree oh nam)

Synonyms azthreonam
U.S./Canadian Brand Names Azactam® [US/Can]
Therapeutic Category Antibiotic, Miscellaneous
Use Treatment of patients with documented multidrug resistant aerobic gram-negative infection in which beta-lactam therapy is contraindicated; used for urinary tract infection, lower respiratory tract infections, septicemia, skin/skin structure infections, intra-abdominal infections and gynecological infections caused by susceptible Enterobacteriaceae, *H. influenzae*, and *P. aeruginosa*
Usual Dosage
Children >1 month: I.M., I.V.: 90-120 mg/kg/day divided every 6-8 hours
Cystic fibrosis: 50 mg/kg/dose every 6-8 hours (ie, up to 200 mg/kg/day); maximum: 6-8 g/day
Adults:
Urinary tract infection: I.M., I.V.: 500 mg to 1 g every 8-12 hours
Moderately severe systemic infections: 1 g I.V. or I.M. or 2 g I.V. every 8-12 hours
Severe systemic or life-threatening infections (especially caused by *Pseudomonas aeruginosa*): I.V.: 2 g every 6-8 hours; maximum: 8 g/day
Dosage Forms
Injection, powder for reconstitution: 500 mg, 1 g, 2 g
Infusion [premixed]: 1 g (50 mL); 2 g (50 mL)

Azulfidine® EN-tabs® [US] see sulfasalazine on page 613
Azulfidine® Suspension *(Discontinued)* see page 814
Azulfidine® Tablet [US] see sulfasalazine on page 613

Babee® Teething® [US-OTC] *see* benzocaine *on page 77*

BAC *see* benzalkonium chloride *on page 76*

B-A-C® *(Discontinued)* *see page 814*

Bacid® [US/Can] *see* Lactobacillus *on page 372*

Baciguent® [US/Can] *see* bacitracin *on this page*

Baci-IM® [US] *see* bacitracin *on this page*

Bacillus Calmette-Guérin (BCG) Live *see* BCG vaccine *on page 72*

bacitracin (bas i TRAY sin)

U.S./Canadian Brand Names AK-Tracin® [US]; Baciguent® [US/Can]; Baci-IM® [US]

Therapeutic Category Antibiotic, Ophthalmic; Antibiotic, Topical; Antibiotic, Miscellaneous

Use Treatment of pneumonia and emphysema caused by susceptible staphylococci; prevention or treatment of superficial skin infections or infections of the eye caused by susceptible organisms; due to its toxicity, use of bacitracin systemically or as an irrigant should be limited to situations where less toxic alternatives would not be effective; treatment of antibiotic-associated colitis

Usual Dosage I.M. recommended; **do not administer I.V.**:

Infants:

<2.5 kg: 900 units/kg/day in 2-3 divided doses

>2.5 kg: 1000 units/kg/day in 2-3 divided doses

Children: 800-1200 units/kg/day divided every 8 hours

Adults: 10,000-25,000 units/dose every 6 hours; not to exceed 100,000 units/day

Topical: Apply 1-5 times/day

Ophthalmic ointment: $1/4$" to $1/2$" ribbon every 3-4 hours to conjunctival sac for acute infections or 2-3 times/day for mild to moderate infections for 7-10 days

Irrigation, solution: 50-100 units/mL in normal saline, lactated Ringer's, or sterile water for irrigation; soak sponges in solution for topical compresses 1-5 times/day or as needed during surgical procedures

Dosage Forms

Injection, powder for reconstitution (Baci-IM®): 50,000 units

Ointment, ophthalmic (AK-Tracin®): 500 units/g (3.5 g)

Ointment, topical: 500 units/g (0.9 g, 15 g, 30 g, 120 g, 454 g)

Baciguent®: 500 units/g (15 g, 30 g)

bacitracin and polymyxin B (bas i TRAY sin & pol i MIKS in bee)

Synonyms polymyxin B and bacitracin

U.S./Canadian Brand Names AK-Poly-Bac® [US]; LID-Pack® [Can]; Optimyxin® Ophthalmic [Can]; Polycidin® Ophthalmic; Polysporin® Ophthalmic [US]; Polysporin® Topical [US-OTC]

Therapeutic Category Antibiotic, Ophthalmic; Antibiotic, Topical

Use Treatment of superficial infections involving the conjunctiva and/or cornea caused by susceptible organisms; prevent infection in minor cuts, scrapes and burns

Usual Dosage

Ophthalmic: Apply $1/2$" ribbon to the affected eye(s) every 3-4 hours

Topical: Apply to affected area 1-3 times/day; may cover with sterile bandage if needed

Dosage Forms

Ointment, ophthalmic (AK-Poly-Bac®, Polysporin®): Bacitracin 500 units and polymyxin B sulfate 10,000 units per g (3.5 g)

Ointment, topical [OTC]: Bacitracin 500 units and polymyxin B sulfate 10,000 units per g in white petrolatum (15 g, 30 g)

Betadine® First Aid Antibiotics + Moisturizer: Bacitracin 500 units and polymyxin B sulfate 10,000 units per g (14 g)

Polysporin®: Bacitracin 500 units and polymyxin B sulfate 10,000 units per g (15g, 30 g)

Powder, topical (Polysporin®): Bacitracin 500 units and polymyxin B sulfate 10,000 units per g (10 g)

bacitracin, neomycin, and polymyxin B
(bas i TRAY sin, nee oh MYE sin, & pol i MIKS in bee)

Synonyms neomycin, bacitracin, and polymyxin B; polymyxin B, bacitracin, and neomycin

U.S./Canadian Brand Names Mycitracin® [US-OTC]; Neosporin® Ophthalmic Ointment [US/Can]; Neosporin® Topical [US/Can]; Neotopic® [Can]; Triple Antibiotic® [US]

Therapeutic Category Antibiotic, Ophthalmic; Antibiotic, Topical

Use Help prevent infection in minor cuts, scrapes and burns; short-term treatment of superficial external ocular infections caused by susceptible organisms

Usual Dosage Children and Adults:
Ophthalmic ointment: Instill into the conjunctival sac one or more times/day every 3-4 hours for 7-10 days
Topical: Apply 1-3 times/day

Dosage Forms
Ointment, ophthalmic (Neosporin®): Bacitracin 400 units, neomycin sulfate 3.5 mg, and polymyxin B sulfate 10,000 units per g (3.5 g)
Ointment, topical (Triple Antibiotic®): Bacitracin 400 units, neomycin sulfate 3.5 mg, and polymyxin B sulfate 5000 units per g (0.9 g, 15 g, 30 g, 454 g)
Mycitracin®: Bacitracin 400 units, neomycin sulfate 3.5 mg, and polymyxin B sulfate 5000 units per g (14 g)
Neosporin®: Bacitracin 400 units, neomycin sulfate 3.5 mg, and polymyxin B sulfate 5000 units per g (0.9 g, 15 g, 30 g)

bacitracin, neomycin, polymyxin B, and hydrocortisone
(bas i TRAY sin, nee oh MYE sin, pol i MIKS in bee, & hye droe KOR ti sone)

Synonyms hydrocortisone, bacitracin, neomycin, and polymyxin B; neomycin, bacitracin, polymyxin B, and hydrocortisone; polymyxin B, bacitracin, neomycin, and hydrocortisone

U.S./Canadian Brand Names Cortisporin® Ointment [US/Can]

Therapeutic Category Antibiotic/Corticosteroid, Ophthalmic; Antibiotic/Corticosteroid, Topical

Use Prevention and treatment of susceptible superficial topical infections

Usual Dosage
Ophthalmic ointment: Apply ½" ribbon to inside of lower lid every 3-4 hours until improvement occurs
Topical: Apply sparingly 2-4 times/day. Therapy should be discontinued when control is achieved. If no improvement is seen, reassessment of diagnosis may be necessary.

Dosage Forms
Ointment, ophthalmic (Cortisporin®): Bacitracin 400 units, neomycin sulfate 3.5 mg, polymyxin B sulfate 10,000 units, and hydrocortisone 10 mg per g (3.5 g)
Ointment, topical (Cortisporin®): Bacitracin 400 units, neomycin sulfate 3.5 mg, polymyxin B sulfate 10,000 units, and hydrocortisone 10 mg per g (15 g)

bacitracin, neomycin, polymyxin B, and lidocaine
(bas i TRAY sin, nee oh MYE sin, pol i MIKS in bee, & LYE doe kane)

U.S./Canadian Brand Names Spectrocin Plus® [US-OTC]

Therapeutic Category Antibiotic, Topical

Use Prevention and treatment of susceptible superficial topical infections

Usual Dosage Adults: Topical: Apply 1-4 times/day to infected areas; cover with sterile bandage if needed

Dosage Forms Ointment, topical: Bacitracin 500 units, neomycin base 3.5 g, polymyxin B sulfate 5000 units, and lidocaine 40 mg per g (15 g, 30 g)

Backache Pain Relief Extra Strength [US] *see* magnesium salicylate *on page 398*

baclofen (BAK loe fen)

U.S./Canadian Brand Names Apo®-Baclofen [Can]; Gen-Baclofen [Can]; Lioresal® [US/Can]; Liotec [Can]; Nu-Baclo [Can]; PMS-Baclofen [Can]

Therapeutic Category Skeletal Muscle Relaxant

Use Treatment of reversible spasticity associated with multiple sclerosis or spinal cord lesions; intrathecal use for the management of spasticity in patients who are unresponsive to oral baclofen or experience intolerable CNS side effects; treatment of trigeminal neuralgia; adjunctive treatment of tardive dyskinesia

Usual Dosage

Oral:

Children:

2-7 years: Initial: 10-15 mg/24 hours divided every 8 hours; titrate dose every 3 days in increments of 5-15 mg/day to a maximum of 40 mg/day

≥8 years: Maximum: 60 mg/day in 3 divided doses

Adults: 5 mg 3 times/day, may increase 5 mg/dose every 3 days to a maximum of 80 mg/day

Intrathecal:

Test dose: 50-100 mcg, doses >50 mcg should be administered in 25 mcg increments, separated by 24 hours

Maintenance: After positive response to test dose, a maintenance intrathecal infusion can be administered via an implanted intrathecal pump. Initial dose via pump: Infusion at a 24-hourly rate dosed at twice the test dose.

Dosage Forms

Injection, solution, intrathecal [preservative free]: 50 mcg/mL (1 mL); 500 mcg/mL (20 mL); 2000 mcg/mL (5 mL)

Tablet: 10 mg, 20 mg

Bactine® Hydrocortisone [US-OTC] see hydrocortisone (topical) on page 334

Bactocill® (Discontinued) see page 814

BactoShield® (Discontinued) see page 814

Bactrim™ [US] see sulfamethoxazole and trimethoprim on page 612

Bactrim™ DS [US] see sulfamethoxazole and trimethoprim on page 612

Bactroban® [US/Can] see mupirocin on page 440

Bactroban® Nasal [US] see mupirocin on page 440

Baker's P & S [US/Can] see phenol on page 508

baking soda see sodium bicarbonate on page 594

BAL see dimercaprol on page 200

balanced salt solution (BAL anced salt soe LOO shun)

U.S./Canadian Brand Names BSS® Plus [US/Can]; BSS® [US/Can]; Eye-Stream® [US/Can]

Therapeutic Category Ophthalmic Agent, Miscellaneous

Use Intraocular irrigating solution; also used to soothe and cleanse the eye in conjunction with hard contact lenses

Usual Dosage Use as needed for foreign body removal, gonioscopy, and other general ophthalmic office procedures

Dosage Forms Solution, ophthalmic [irrigation]: 15 mL, 30 mL, 250 mL, 500 mL

Baldex® [US] see dexamethasone (ophthalmic) on page 184

BAL in Oil® [US] see dimercaprol on page 200

Balmex® [US-OTC] see zinc oxide on page 691

Balminil® Decongestant [Can] see pseudoephedrine on page 552

Balminil DM D [Can] see pseudoephedrine and dextromethorphan on page 553

Balminil DM + Decongestant + Expectorant [Can] *see* guaifenesin, pseudoe-phedrine, and dextromethorphan *on page 312*

Balminil DM E [Can] *see* guaifenesin and dextromethorphan *on page 308*

Balminil Expectorant [Can] *see* guaifenesin *on page 307*

Balnetar® [US/Can] *see* coal tar, lanolin, and mineral oil *on page 158*

balsalazide (bal SAL a zide)
 Synonyms balsalazide disodium
 U.S./Canadian Brand Names Colazal™ [US]
 Therapeutic Category 5-Aminosalicylic Acid Derivative; Anti-inflammatory Agent
 Use Treatment of mild to moderate active ulcerative colitis
 Usual Dosage Oral: Adults: 2.25 g (three 750 mg capsules) 3 times/day for 8-12 weeks
 Dosage Forms Capsule, as disodium: 750 mg

balsalazide disodium *see* balsalazide *on this page*

Banaril® [US-OTC] *see* diphenhydramine *on page 202*

Bancap® *(Discontinued)* *see page 814*

Bancap HC® [US] *see* hydrocodone and acetaminophen *on page 329*

Banesin® *(Discontinued)* *see page 814*

Banophen® Decongestant Capsule *(Discontinued)* *see page 814*

Banophen® [US-OTC] *see* diphenhydramine *on page 202*

Banthine® *(Discontinued)* *see page 814*

Bantron® *(Discontinued)* *see page 814*

Barbidonna® *(Discontinued)* *see page 814*

Barbita® *(Discontinued)* *see page 814*

Barc™ Liquid *(Discontinued)* *see page 814*

Baricon® [US] *see* radiological/contrast media (ionic) *on page 561*

Baridium® [US] *see* phenazopyridine *on page 506*

Barobag® [US] *see* radiological/contrast media (ionic) *on page 561*

Baro-CAT® [US] *see* radiological/contrast media (ionic) *on page 561*

Baroflave® [US] *see* radiological/contrast media (ionic) *on page 561*

Barosperse® [US] *see* radiological/contrast media (ionic) *on page 561*

Bar-Test® [US] *see* radiological/contrast media (ionic) *on page 561*

Basaljel® *(Discontinued)* *see page 814*

Basaljel® [Can] *see* aluminum hydroxide *on page 28*

basiliximab (ba si LIKS i mab)
 U.S./Canadian Brand Names Simulect® [US/Can]
 Therapeutic Category Immunosuppressant Agent
 Use Prophylaxis of acute organ rejection in renal transplantation
 Usual Dosage I.V.:
  Children: 12 mg/m^2 (maximum: 20 mg) within 2 hours prior to transplant surgery, followed by a second dose of 12 mg/m^2 (maximum: 20 mg) 4 days after transplantation
  Adults: 20 mg within 2 hours prior to transplant surgery, followed by a second 20 mg dose 4 days after transplantation
 Dosage Forms Injection, powder for reconstitution: 20 mg

Bausch & Lomb® Computer Eye Drops [US-OTC] *see* glycerin *on page 302*

Baycol® *(Discontinued)* *see page 814*

Bayer® Aspirin Extra Strength [US-OTC] *see* aspirin *on page 58*

Bayer® Aspirin Regimen Adult Low Strength [US-OTC] *see* aspirin *on page 58*

Bayer® Aspirin Regimen Adult Low Strength with Calcium [US-OTC] *see* aspirin *on page 58*

Bayer® Aspirin Regimen Children's [US-OTC] *see* aspirin *on page 58*

Bayer® Aspirin Regimen Regular Strength [US-OTC] *see* aspirin *on page 58*

Bayer® Aspirin [US-OTC] *see* aspirin *on page 58*

Bayer® Plus Extra Strength [US-OTC] *see* aspirin *on page 58*

BayGam® [US/Can] *see* immune globulin (intramuscular) *on page 346*

BayHep B™ [US/Can] *see* hepatitis B immune globulin *on page 320*

Baypress® *(Discontinued)* *see page 814*

BayRab® [US/Can] *see* rabies immune globulin (human) *on page 561*

BayRho-D® Full-Dose [US] *see* $Rh_o(D)$ immune globulin *on page 569*

BayRho-D® Mini-Dose [US] *see* $Rh_o(D)$ immune globulin *on page 569*

BayTet™ [US/Can] *see* tetanus immune globulin (human) *on page 626*

Baza® Antifungal [US-OTC] *see* miconazole *on page 427*

B-Caro-T™ [US] *see* beta-carotene *on page 82*

BCG vaccine (bee see jee vak SEEN)

Synonyms Bacillus Calmette-Guérin (BCG) Live

U.S./Canadian Brand Names ImmuCyst® [Can]; Oncotice™ [Can]; Pacis™ [Can]; TheraCys® [US]; TICE® BCG [US]

Therapeutic Category Biological Response Modulator

Use BCG vaccine is no longer recommended for adults at high risk for tuberculosis in the United States. BCG vaccination may be considered for infants and children who are skin test-negative to 5 tuberculin units of tuberculin and who cannot be given isoniazid preventive therapy but have close contact with untreated or ineffectively treated active tuberculosis patients or who belong to groups which other control measures have not been successful.

In the United States, tuberculosis control efforts are directed toward early identification, treatment of cases, and preventive therapy with isoniazid.

Usual Dosage Intravesical treatment and prophylaxis for carcinoma *in situ* of the urinary bladder: Begin between 7-14 days after biopsy or transurethral resection. Administer a dose of 3 vials of BCG live intravesically under aseptic conditions once weekly for 6 weeks (induction therapy). Each dose (3 reconstituted vials) is further diluted in an additional 50 mL sterile, preservative free saline for a total of 53 mL. A urethral catheter is inserted into the bladder under aseptic conditions, the bladder is drained, and then the 53 mL suspension is instilled slowly by gravity, following which the catheter is withdrawn. If the bladder catheterization has been traumatic, BCG live should not be administered, and there must be a treatment delay of at least 1 week. Resume subsequent treatment; follow the induction therapy by one treatment administered 3, 6, 12, 18 and 24 months following the initial treatment.

Dosage Forms Injection, powder for reconstitution, intravesical:
TheraCys®: 81 mg [with diluent]
TICE® BCG: 50 mg

BCNU *see* carmustine *on page 118*

B-D™ Glucose [US-OTC] *see* glucose (instant) *on page 300*

becaplermin (be KAP ler min)

U.S./Canadian Brand Names Regranex® [US/Can]

Therapeutic Category Topical Skin Product

Use Treatment of diabetic ulcers that occur on the lower limbs and feet

Usual Dosage Adults: Topical: Apply once daily; applied with a cotton swab or similar tool, as a coating over the ulcer

Dosage Forms Gel, topical: 0.01% (15 g)

beclomethasone (be kloe METH a sone)

U.S./Canadian Brand Names Alti-Beclomethasone [Can]; Apo®-Beclomethasone [Can]; Beconase® AQ [US]; Beconase® [US]; Gen-Beclo [Can]; Nu-Beclomethasone [Can]; Propaderm® [Can]; QVAR™ [US/Can]; Rivanase AQ [Can]; Vancenase® AQ 84 mcg [US]; Vancenase® Pockethaler® [US]; Vanceril® [US/Can]

Therapeutic Category Adrenal Corticosteroid

Use

Oral inhalation: Treatment of bronchial asthma in patients who require chronic administration of corticosteroids

Nasal aerosol: Symptomatic treatment of seasonal or perennial rhinitis and nasal polyposis

Usual Dosage

Inhalation:

Children 6-12 years: 1-2 inhalations 3-4 times/day, not to exceed 10 inhalations/day

Adults: 2-4 inhalations twice daily, not to exceed 20 inhalations/day

Aerosol inhalation (nasal):

Children 6-12 years: 1 spray each nostril 3 times/day

Adults: 2-4 sprays each nostril twice daily

Aqueous inhalation (nasal): 1-2 sprays each nostril twice daily

Dosage Forms

Aerosol for oral inhalation, as dipropionate:

Vanceril®: 42 mcg/inhalation [200 metered doses] (16.8 g)

QVAR™: 40 mcg/inhalation [100 metered doses] (7.3 g); 80 mcg/inhalation [100 metered doses] (7.3 g)

Vanceril® Double Strength: 84 mcg/inhalation [40 metered doses] (5.4 g), 84 mcg/inhalation [120 metered doses] (12.2 g)

Aerosol, intranasal, as dipropionate (Beconase®, Vancenase®): 42 mcg/inhalation: [80 metered doses] (6.7 g); [200 metered doses] (16.8 g)

Suspension, intranasal, aqueous, as dipropionate [spray]:

Beconase® AQ, Vancenase® AQ 0.042%: 42 mcg/inhalation [≥200 metered doses] (25 g)

Vancenase® AQ Double Strength: 84 mcg per inhalation [120 actuations] (19 g)

Becomject-100® *(Discontinued)* see page 814

Beconase® [US] see beclomethasone *on this page*

Beconase® AQ [US] see beclomethasone *on this page*

Becotin® Pulvules® *(Discontinued)* see page 814

Bedoz [Can] see cyanocobalamin *on page 167*

Beepen-VK® *(Discontinued)* see page 814

Beesix® *(Discontinued)* see page 814

Belix® Oral *(Discontinued)* see page 814

belladonna (bel a DON a)

Therapeutic Category Anticholinergic Agent

Use Decrease gastrointestinal activity in functional bowel disorders and to delay gastric emptying as well as decrease gastric secretion

Usual Dosage Tincture: Oral:

Children: 0.03 mL/kg 3 times/day

Adults: 0.6-1 mL 3-4 times/day

Dosage Forms Tincture: Belladonna alkaloids (principally hyoscyamine and atropine) 0.3 mg/mL with alcohol 65% to 70% (120 mL, 480 mL, 3780 mL)

belladonna and opium (bel a DON a & OH pee um)

Synonyms opium and belladonna

U.S./Canadian Brand Names B&O Supprettes® [US]

Therapeutic Category Analgesic, Narcotic

Controlled Substance C-II

Use Relief of moderate to severe pain associated with rectal or bladder tenesmus that may occur in postoperative states and neoplastic situations; pain associated with ureteral spasms not responsive to non-narcotic analgesics and to space intervals between injections of opiates

Usual Dosage Rectal:

Children: Dose not established

Adults: 1 suppository 1-2 times/day, up to 4 doses/day

Dosage Forms Suppository:

#15 A: Belladonna extract 16.2 mg and opium 30 mg

#16 A: Belladonna extract 16.2 mg and opium 60 mg

belladonna, phenobarbital, and ergotamine tartrate
(bel a DON a, fee noe BAR bi tal, & er GOT a meen TAR trate)

Synonyms ergotamine tartrate, belladonna, and phenobarbital; phenobarbital, belladonna, and ergotamine tartrate

U.S./Canadian Brand Names Bellamine S [US]; Bellergal® Spacetabs® [Can]; Bel-Phen-Ergot S® [US]; Bel-Tabs [US]

Therapeutic Category Ergot Alkaloid and Derivative

Use Management and treatment of menopausal disorders, gastrointestinal disorders and recurrent throbbing headache

Usual Dosage Oral: 1 tablet each morning and evening

Dosage Forms Tablet: Belladonna alkaloids 0.2 mg, phenobarbital 40 mg, and ergotamine tartrate 0.6 mg

Bellafoline® *(Discontinued)* see page 814

Bellamine S [US] see belladonna, phenobarbital, and ergotamine tartrate on this page

Bellatal® *(Discontinued)* see page 814

Bellergal-S® *(Discontinued)* see page 814

Bellergal® Spacetabs® [Can] see belladonna, phenobarbital, and ergotamine tartrate on this page

Bel-Phen-Ergot S® [US] see belladonna, phenobarbital, and ergotamine tartrate on this page

Bel-Tabs [US] see belladonna, phenobarbital, and ergotamine tartrate on this page

Bemote® *(Discontinued)* see page 814

Bena-D® *(Discontinued)* see page 814

Benadryl® [US/Can] see diphenhydramine on page 202

Benadryl® 50 mg Capsule *(Discontinued)* see page 814

Benadryl® Cold/Flu *(Discontinued)* see page 814

Benadryl® Decongestant Allergy [US-OTC] see diphenhydramine and pseudoephedrine on page 203

Benahist® Injection *(Discontinued)* see page 814

Ben-Allergin-50® Injection *(Discontinued)* see page 814

Ben-Aqua® *(Discontinued)* see page 814

benazepril (ben AY ze pril)

U.S./Canadian Brand Names Lotensin® [US/Can]

Therapeutic Category Angiotensin-Converting Enzyme (ACE) Inhibitor

Use Treatment of hypertension, either alone or in combination with other antihypertensive agents

Usual Dosage Adults: Oral: 20-40 mg/day as a single dose or 2 divided doses

Dosage Forms Tablet, as hydrochloride: 5 mg, 10 mg, 20 mg, 40 mg

benazepril and amlodipine *see* amlodipine and benazepril *on page 36*

benazepril and hydrochlorothiazide

(ben AY ze pril & hye droe klor oh THYE a zide)

Synonyms hydrochlorothiazide and benazepril

U.S./Canadian Brand Names Lotensin® HCT [US]

Therapeutic Category Antihypertensive Agent, Combination

Use Treatment of hypertension

Usual Dosage Dose is individualized

Dosage Forms Tablet:

Benazepril 5 mg and hydrochlorothiazide 6.25 mg

Benazepril 10 mg and hydrochlorothiazide 12.5 mg

Benazepril 20 mg and hydrochlorothiazide 12.5 mg

Benazepril 20 mg and hydrochlorothiazide 25 mg

bendroflumethiazide (ben droe floo meth EYE a zide)

U.S./Canadian Brand Names Naturetin® [US]

Therapeutic Category Diuretic, Thiazide

Use Management of mild to moderate hypertension, edema associated with congestive heart failure, pregnancy, or nephrotic syndrome; reportedly does not alter serum electrolyte concentrations appreciably at recommended doses

Usual Dosage Oral:

Children: Initial: 0.1-0.4 mg/kg in 1-2 doses; maintenance dose: 0.05-0.1 mg/kg/day in 1-2 doses

Adults: 2.5-20 mg/day or twice daily in divided doses

Dosage Forms Tablet: 5 mg

BeneFix™ [US] *see* factor IX complex (human) *on page 261*

Benemid® *(Discontinued)* *see page 814*

Benicar™ [US] *see* olmesartan *on page 476*

Benoject® *(Discontinued)* *see page 814*

Benoquin® [US] *see* monobenzone *on page 436*

Benoxyl® [Can] *see* benzoyl peroxide *on page 79*

benserazide and levodopa *(Canada only)*

(ben SER a zide & lee voe DOE pa)

U.S./Canadian Brand Names Prolopa® [Can]

Therapeutic Category Anti-Parkinson's Agent

Use Treatment of Parkinson's syndrome with exception of drug-induced parkinsonism

Usual Dosage Adult: Oral: The optimal dose for most patients is usually 4-8 capsules of 100-25 daily (400-800 mg levodopa) divided into 4-6 doses

Dosage Forms Capsule:

50-12.5: Levodopa 50 mg and benserazide 12.5 mg

100-25: Levodopa 100 mg and benserazide 25 mg

200-50: Levodopa 200 mg and benserazide 50 mg

bentoquatam (ben to KWA tam)
U.S./Canadian Brand Names IvyBlock® [US-OTC]
Therapeutic Category Protectant, Topical
Use To protect the skin from rash due to exposure to poison sumac, poison ivy or poison oak
Usual Dosage Topical: Apply to exposed skin at least 15 minutes before potential contact and reapply every 4 hours
Dosage Forms Lotion: 5% (120 mL)

Bentyl® [US] *see* dicyclomine *on page 194*

Bentylol® [Can] *see* dicyclomine *on page 194*

Benuryl™ [Can] *see* probenecid *on page 540*

Benylin® 3.3 mg-D-E [Can] *see* guaifenesin, pseudoephedrine, and codeine *on page 311*

Benylin® Cough Syrup *(Discontinued) see page 814*

Benylin DM® *(Discontinued) see page 814*

Benylin® DM-D [Can] *see* pseudoephedrine and dextromethorphan *on page 553*

Benylin® DM-D-E [Can] *see* guaifenesin, pseudoephedrine, and dextromethorphan *on page 312*

Benylin® DM-E [Can] *see* guaifenesin and dextromethorphan *on page 308*

Benylin® E Extra Strength [Can] *see* guaifenesin *on page 307*

Benylin® Expectorant [US-OTC] *see* guaifenesin and dextromethorphan *on page 308*

Benylin® Pediatric [US-OTC] *see* dextromethorphan *on page 189*

Benzac® [US] *see* benzoyl peroxide *on page 79*

Benzac® AC [US/Can] *see* benzoyl peroxide *on page 79*

Benzac® AC Wash [US] *see* benzoyl peroxide *on page 79*

BenzaClin™ [US] *see* clindamycin and benzoyl peroxide *on page 152*

Benzacot® [US] *see* trimethobenzamide *on page 657*

Benzac® W Gel [US/Can] *see* benzoyl peroxide *on page 79*

Benzac® W Wash [US/Can] *see* benzoyl peroxide *on page 79*

Benzagel® [US] *see* benzoyl peroxide *on page 79*

Benzagel® Wash [US] *see* benzoyl peroxide *on page 79*

benzalkonium chloride (benz al KOE nee um KLOR ide)
Synonyms BAC
U.S./Canadian Brand Names Benza® [US-OTC]; 3M™ Cavilon™ Skin Cleanser [US-OTC]; Ony-Clear [US-OTC]; Zephiran® [US-OTC]
Therapeutic Category Antibacterial, Topical
Use Surface antiseptic and germicidal preservative
Usual Dosage Thoroughly rinse anionic detergents and soaps from the skin or other areas prior to use of solutions because they reduce the antibacterial activity of BAC; to protect metal instruments stored in BAC solution, add crushed Anti-Rust Tablets, 4 tablets per quart, to antiseptic solution, change solution at least once weekly; not to be used for storage of aluminum or zinc instruments, instruments with lenses fastened by cement, lacquered catheters or some synthetic rubber goods
Dosage Forms
Solution, topical:
Benza®: 1:750 (60 mL, 240 mL, 480 mL, 3840 mL)
Ony-Clear: 1% (30 mL)
Zephiran®: 1:750 (240 mL, 3840 mL) [aqueous]
Solution, topical spray (3M™ Cavilon™ Skin Cleanser): 0.11% (240 mL)

benzalkonium chloride, benzocaine, butyl aminobenzoate, tetracaine *see* benzocaine, butyl aminobenzoate, tetracaine, and benzalkonium chloride *on next page*

Benzamycin® [US] *see* erythromycin and benzoyl peroxide *on page 235*

Benzashave® [US] *see* benzoyl peroxide *on page 79*

benzathine benzylpenicillin *see* penicillin G benzathine *on page 498*

benzathine penicillin G *see* penicillin G benzathine *on page 498*

Benza® [US-OTC] *see* benzalkonium chloride *on previous page*

benzazoline *see* tolazoline *on page 643*

Benzedrex® [US-OTC] *see* propylhexedrine *on page 550*

benzene hexachloride *see* lindane *on page 385*

benzhexol *see* trihexyphenidyl *on page 655*

benzocaine (BEN zoe kane)

Synonyms ethyl aminobenzoate

U.S./Canadian Brand Names Americaine® Anesthetic Lubricant [US]; Americaine® [US-OTC]; Anbesol® Baby [US/Can]; Anbesol® Maximum Strength [US-OTC]; Anbesol® [US-OTC]; Babee® Teething® [US-OTC]; Benzodent® [US-OTC]; Chiggerex® [US-OTC]; Chiggertox® [US-OTC]; Cylex® [US-OTC]; Detane® [US-OTC]; Foille® Medicated First Aid [US-OTC]; Foille® Plus [US-OTC]; Foille® [US-OTC]; HDA® Toothache [US-OTC]; Hurricaine® [US]; Mycinettes® [US-OTC]; Orabase®-B [US-OTC]; Orajel® Baby Nighttime [US-OTC]; Orajel® Baby [US-OTC]; Orajel® Maximum Strength [US-OTC]; Orajel® [US-OTC]; Orasol® [US-OTC]; Solarcaine® [US-OTC]; Trocaine® [US-OTC]; Zilactin® Baby [US/Can]; Zilactin®-B [US/Can]

Therapeutic Category Local Anesthetic

Use Temporary relief of pain associated with pruritic dermatosis, pruritus, minor burns, toothache, minor sore throat pain, canker sores, hemorrhoids, rectal fissures; anesthetic lubricant for passage of catheters and endoscopic tubes

Usual Dosage

Children and Adults:

Mucous membranes: Dosage varies depending on area to be anesthetized and vascularity of tissues

Oral mouth/throat preparations: Do not administer for >2 days or in children <2 years of age, unless directed by a physician; refer to specific package labeling

Topical: Apply to affected area as needed

Adults: Nonprescription diet aid: 6-15 mg just prior to food consumption, not to exceed 45 mg/day

Dosage Forms

Aerosol, oral spray (Hurricaine®): 20% (60 mL) [cherry flavor]

Aerosol, topical spray:

Americaine®: 20% (20 mL, 120 mL)

Foille®: 5% (97.5 mL) [contains chloroxylenol 0.63%]

Foille® Plus: 5% (105 mL) [contains chloroxylenol 0.63% and alcohol 57.33%]

Solarcaine®: 20% (90 mL, 120 mL, 135 mL) [contains triclosan, alcohol 0.13%]

Cream, topical: 5% (30 g, 454 g)

Gel, oral:

Anbesol® 6.3% (7.5 g)

Anbesol® Baby, Detane®, Orajel® Baby: 7.5% (7.5 g, 10 g, 15 g)

Anbesol® Maximum Strength, Orajel® Maximum Strength: 20% (6 g, 7.5 g, 10 g)

HDA® Toothache: 6.5% (15 mL) [contains benzyl alcohol]

Hurricaine®: 20% (5 g, 30 g) [mint, pina colada, watermelon, and wild cherry flavors]

Orabase-B®: 20% (7 g)

Orajel®, Orajel® Baby Nighttime, Zilactin®-B, Zilactin® Baby: 10% (6 g, 7.5 g, 10 g)

Gel, topical (Americaine® Anesthetic Lubricant): 20% (2.5 g, 28 g) [contains 0.1% benzethonium chloride

(Continued)

77

benzocaine *(Continued)*

Liquid, oral:
Anbesol®, Orasol®: 6.3% (9 mL, 15 mL, 30 mL)
Anbesol® Maximum Strength: 20% (9 mL, 14 mL)
Hurricaine®: 20% (30 mL) [pina colada and wild cherry flavors]
Orajel®: 10% (13 mL) [contains tartrazine]
Orajel® Baby: 7.5% (13 mL)
Liquid, topical (Chiggertox®): 2% (30 mL)
Lotion, oral (Babee® Teething): 2.5% (15 mL)
Lozenge:
Cylex®, Mycinettes®: 15 mg [Cylex® contains cetylpyridinium chloride 5 mg]
Trocaine®: 10 mg
Ointment, oral (Benzodent®): 20% (30 g)
Ointment, topical:
Chiggerex®: 2% (52 g)
Foille® Medicated First Aid: 5% (3.5 g, 28 g) [contains chloroxylenol 0.1%, benzyl alcohol; corn oil base]
Paste, oral (Orabase®-B): 20% (7 g)

benzocaine and antipyrine *see* antipyrine and benzocaine *on page 47*

benzocaine and cetylpyridinium chloride *see* cetylpyridinium and benzocaine *on page 130*

benzocaine, butyl aminobenzoate, tetracaine, and benzalkonium chloride

(BEN zoe kane, BYOO til a meen oh BENZ oh ate, TET ra kane, & benz al KOE nee um KLOR ide)

Synonyms benzalkonium chloride, benzocaine, butyl aminobenzoate, tetracaine; butyl aminobenzoate, benzocaine, tetracaine, and benzalkonium chloride; tetracaine hydrochloride, benzocaine, butyl aminobenzoate, and benzalkonium chloride

U.S./Canadian Brand Names Cetacaine® [US]

Therapeutic Category Local Anesthetic

Use Topical anesthetic to control pain or gagging

Usual Dosage Topical: Apply to affected area for approximately 1 second or less

Dosage Forms

Aerosol, topical: Benzocaine 14%, butyl aminobenzoate 2%, tetracaine 2%, and benzalkonium chloride 0.5% (56 g)
Gel, topical: Benzocaine 14%, butyl aminobenzoate 2%, tetracaine 2%, and benzalkonium chloride 0.5% (29 g)
Liquid, topical: Benzocaine 14%, butyl aminobenzoate 2%, tetracaine 2%, and benzalkonium chloride 0.5% (56 mL)

benzocaine, gelatin, pectin, and sodium carboxymethylcellulose

(BEN zoe kane, JEL a tin, PEK tin, & SOW dee um kar box ee meth il SEL yoo lose)

U.S./Canadian Brand Names Orabase® With Benzocaine [US-OTC]

Therapeutic Category Local Anesthetic

Use Topical anesthetic and emollient for oral lesions

Usual Dosage Topical: Apply 2-4 times/day

Dosage Forms Paste: Benzocaine 20%, gelatin, pectin, and sodium carboxymethylcellulose (5 g, 15 g)

Benzocol® *(Discontinued)* *see page 814*

Benzodent® [US-OTC] *see* benzocaine *on previous page*

benzoin (BEN zoyn)
Synonyms gum benjamin
U.S./Canadian Brand Names TinBen® [US-OTC]
Therapeutic Category Pharmaceutical Aid; Protectant, Topical
Use Protective application for irritations of the skin; sometimes used in boiling water as steam inhalants for their expectorant and soothing action
Usual Dosage Topical: Apply 1-2 times/day
Dosage Forms
Tincture, USP: (15 mL, 60 mL, 120 mL, 480 mL, 4000 mL)
TinBen®: 120 mL
Tincture, USP [spray]: 120 mL

benzonatate (ben ZOE na tate)
U.S./Canadian Brand Names Tessalon® Perles [US/Can]
Therapeutic Category Antitussive
Use Symptomatic relief of nonproductive cough
Usual Dosage Oral:
Children <10 years: 8 mg/kg in 3-6 divided doses
Children >10 years and Adults: 100 mg 3 times/day up to 600 mg/day
Dosage Forms Capsule: 100 mg, 200 mg

Benzotic® [US] *see* antipyrine and benzocaine *on page 47*

benzoyl peroxide (BEN zoe il peer OKS ide)
U.S./Canadian Brand Names Acetoxyl® [Can]; Benoxyl® [Can]; Benzac® [US]; Benzac® AC [US/Can]; Benzac® AC Wash [US]; Benzac® W Gel [US/Can]; Benzac® W Wash [US/Can]; Benzagel® [US]; Benzagel® Wash [US]; Benzashave® [US]; Brevoxyl® [US]; Brevoxyl® Cleansing [US]; Brevoxyl® Wash [US]; Clinac™ BPO [US]; Del Aqua® [US]; Desquam-E™ [US]; Desquam-X® [US/Can]; Exact® Acne Medication [US-OTC]; Fostex® 10% BPO [US-OTC]; Loroxide® [US-OTC]; Neutrogena® Acne Mask [US-OTC]; Neutrogena® On The Spot® Acne Treatment [US-OTC]; Oxy 10® Balanced Medicated Face Wash [US-OTC]; Oxyderm™ [Can]; Palmer's® Skin Success Acne [US-OTC]; PanOxyl® [US/Can]; PanOxyl®-AQ [US]; PanOxyl® Bar [US-OTC]; Seba-Gel™ [US]; Solugel® [Can]; Triaz® [US]; Triaz® Cleanser [US]; Zapzyt® [US-OTC]
Therapeutic Category Acne Products
Use Adjunctive treatment of mild to moderate acne vulgaris
Usual Dosage Children and Adults:
Cleansers: Wash once or twice daily; control amount of drying or peeling by modifying dose frequency or concentration
Topical: Apply sparingly once daily; gradually increase to 2-3 times/day if needed. If excessive dryness or peeling occurs, reduce dose frequency or concentration; if excessive stinging or burning occurs, remove with mild soap and water; resume use the next day.
Dosage Forms
Cream, topical:
Benzashave®: 5% (120 g); 10% (120 g)
Exact® Acne Medication: 5% (18 g)
Neutrogena® Acne Mask: 5% (60 g)
Neutrogena® On The Spot® Acne Treatment: 2.5% (22.5 g)
Gel, topical: 5% (45 g, 60 g, 90 g); 10% (45 g, 60 g, 90 g)
Benzac® [alcohol based]: 5% (60 g); 10% (60 g) [contains alcohol 12%]
Benzac® AC [water based]: 2.5% (60 g, 90 g); 5% (60 g, 90 g); 10% (60 g, 90 g)
Benzac® W [water based]: 2.5% (60 g, 90 g); 10% (60 g, 90 g)
Benzagel®: 5% (45 g); 10% (45 g)
Benzagel® Wash [water based]: 10% (60 g)
Brevoxyl®: 4% (43 g, 90 g)
Clinac™ BPO: 7% (45 g, 90 g)
Desquam-E™ [water based]: 5% (42.5 g); 10% (42.5 g) [emollient gel]
(Continued)

79

benzoyl peroxide *(Continued)*

Desquam-X®: 5% (42.5 g); 10% (42.5 g)
Fostex® 10% BPO: 10% (45 g)
PanOxyl® [alcohol based]: 5% (57 g, 113 g); 10% (57 g, 113 g)
PanOxyl® AQ [water based]: 2.5% (57 g, 113 g); 5% (57 g, 113 g); 10% (57 g, 113 g)
Seba-Gel™: 5% (60 g, 90 g); 10% (60 g, 90 g)
Triaz®: 3% (42.5 g); 6% (42.5 g); 10% (42.5 g)
Triaz® Cleanser: 3% (170 g, 340 g); 6% (170 g, 340 g); 10% (170 g, 340 g)
Zapzyt®: 10% (30 g)
Liquid, topical: 2.5% (240 mL); 5% (120 mL, 150 mL, 240 mL); 10% (150 mL, 240 mL)
Benzac® AC Wash [water based]: 2.5% (240 mL); 5% (240 mL); 10% (240 mL)
Benzac® W Wash [water based]: 5% (120 mL, 240 mL); 10% (240 mL)
Del-Aqua®: 5% (45 mL); 10% (45 mL)
Oxy-10® Balance Medicated Face Wash: 10% (240 mL)
Lotion, topical: 5% (30 mL); 10% (30 mL)
Brevoxyl® Cleansing: 4% (297 g); 8% (297 g) [in a lathering vehicle]
Brevoxyl® Wash: 4% (170 g); 8% (170 g) [in a lathering vehicle]
Fostex® 10% BPO: 10% (150 mL)
Loroxide®: 5.5% (26 mL)
Palmer's® Skin Success Acne: 10% (30 mL) [contains vitamin E and aloe]
Soap, topical [bar]:
Fostex® 10% BPO: 10% (113 g)
PanOxyl® Bar: 5% (113 g); 10% (113 g)

benzoyl peroxide and clindamycin *see* clindamycin and benzoyl peroxide *on* page 152

benzoyl peroxide and erythromycin *see* erythromycin and benzoyl peroxide *on* page 235

benzoyl peroxide and hydrocortisone

(BEN zoe il peer OKS ide & hye droe KOR ti sone)
Synonyms hydrocortisone and benzoyl peroxide
U.S./Canadian Brand Names Vanoxide-HC® [US/Can]
Therapeutic Category Acne Products
Use Treatment of acne vulgaris and oily skin
Usual Dosage Topical: Shake well; apply thin film 1-3 times/day, gently massage into skin
Dosage Forms Lotion: Benzoyl peroxide 5% and hydrocortisone acetate 0.5% (25 mL)

benzphetamine (benz FET a meen)

U.S./Canadian Brand Names Didrex® [US/Can]
Therapeutic Category Anorexiant
Controlled Substance C-III
Use Short-term adjunct in exogenous obesity
Usual Dosage Adults: Oral: 25-50 mg 2-3 times/day, preferably twice daily, midmorning and midafternoon
Dosage Forms Tablet, as hydrochloride: 50 mg

benztropine (BENZ troe peen)

U.S./Canadian Brand Names Apo®-Benztropine [Can]; Cogentin® [US/Can]
Therapeutic Category Anticholinergic Agent; Anti-Parkinson's Agent
Use Adjunctive treatment of parkinsonism; also used in treatment of drug-induced extra-pyramidal effects (except tardive dyskinesia) and acute dystonic reactions
Usual Dosage Titrate dose in 0.5 mg increments at 5- to 6-day intervals
Extrapyramidal reaction, drug induced: Oral, I.M., I.V.:
Children >3 years: 0.02-0.05 mg/kg/dose 1-2 times/day
Adults: 1-4 mg/dose 1-2 times/day

Parkinsonism: Oral: 0.5-6 mg/day in 1-2 divided doses; if one dose is greater, administer at bedtime

Dosage Forms
Injection, solution, as mesylate: 1 mg/mL (2 mL)
Tablet, as mesylate: 0.5 mg, 1 mg, 2 mg

benzydamine *(Canada only)* (ben ZID a meen)
U.S./Canadian Brand Names Alti-Benzydamine [Can]; Apo®-Benzydamine [Can]; Novo-Benzydamine [Can]; PMS-Benzydamine [Can]; Sun-Benz [Can]; Tantum™ [Can]
Therapeutic Category Analgesic, Topical
Use Local analgesic
Dosage Forms Solution: 0.15% (100 mL, 250 mL)

benzylpenicillin *see* penicillin G (parenteral/aqueous) *on page 499*

benzylpenicillin benzathine *see* penicillin G benzathine *on page 498*

benzylpenicilloyl-polylysine (BEN zil pen i SIL oyl-pol i LIE seen)
Synonyms penicilloyl-polylysine; PPL
U.S./Canadian Brand Names Pre-Pen® [US]
Therapeutic Category Diagnostic Agent
Use As an adjunct in assessing the risk of administering penicillin (penicillin or benzylpenicillin) in patients with a history of clinical penicillin hypersensitivity

Usual Dosage
Use scratch technique with a 20-gauge needle to make 3-5 mm scratch on epidermis, apply a small drop of solution to scratch, rub in gently with applicator or toothpick
A positive reaction consists of a pale wheal surrounding the scratch site which develops within 10 minutes and ranges from 5-15 mm or more in diameter
If the scratch test is negative an intradermal test may be performed
Intradermal test: Use intradermal test with a tuberculin syringe with a 26- to 30-gauge short bevel needle; a dose of 0.01-0.02 mL is injected intradermally. A control of 0.9% sodium chloride should be injected at least 1½" from the PPL test site. Most skin responses to the intradermal test will develop within 5-15 minutes.
(-) = no reaction or increase in size compared to control
(±) = wheal slightly larger with or without erythematous flare and larger than control site
(+) = itching and increase in size of original bleb may exceed 20 mm in diameter
Dosage Forms Injection, solution: 0.25 mL

bepridil (BE pri dil)
U.S./Canadian Brand Names Vascor® [US/Can]
Therapeutic Category Calcium Channel Blocker
Use Treatment of chronic stable angina; only approved indication is hypertension, but may be used for congestive heart failure; doses should not be adjusted for at least 10 days after beginning therapy
Usual Dosage Adults: Oral: Initial: 200 mg/day, then adjust dose until optimal response is achieved; maximum daily dose: 400 mg
Dosage Forms Tablet, as hydrochloride: 200 mg, 300 mg

beractant (ber AKT ant)
Synonyms bovine lung surfactant; natural lung surfactant
U.S./Canadian Brand Names Survanta® [US/Can]
Therapeutic Category Lung Surfactant
Use Prevention and treatment of respiratory distress syndrome (RDS) in premature infants

Prophylactic therapy: Infants with body weight <1250 g who are at risk for developing or with evidence of surfactant deficiency
(Continued)

beractant *(Continued)*

Rescue therapy: Treatment of infants with RDS confirmed by x-ray and requiring mechanical ventilation

Usual Dosage Intratracheal:

Prophylactic treatment: Administer 4 mL/kg as soon as possible; as many as 4 doses may be administered during the first 48 hours of life, no more frequently than 6 hours apart. The need for additional doses is determined by evidence of continuing respiratory distress; if the infant is still intubated and requiring at least 30% inspired oxygen to maintain a PaO$_2$ ≤80 torr.

Rescue treatment: Administer 4 mL/kg as soon as the diagnosis of RDS is made

Dosage Forms Suspension for inhalation: 25 mg/mL (4 mL, 8 mL)

Berocca® **[US]** *see* vitamin B complex with vitamin C and folic acid *on page 681*

Berotec® **[Can]** *see* fenoterol *(Canada only) on page 266*

Berubigen® *(Discontinued) see page 814*

Beta-2® *(Discontinued) see page 814*

beta-carotene (BAY tah-KARE oh teen)

U.S./Canadian Brand Names A-Caro-25® [US]; B-Caro-T™ [US]; Lumitene™ [US]

Therapeutic Category Vitamin, Fat Soluble

Use Reduce the severity of photosensitivity reactions in patients with erythropoietic protoporphyria (EPP)

Usual Dosage Oral:

Children <14 years: 30-150 mg/day

Adults: 30-300 mg/day

Dosage Forms

Capsule: 10,000 int. units (6 mg); 25,000 int. units (15 mg)

A-Caro-25®, B-Caro-T™: 25,000 int. units (15 mg)

Lumitene™: 50,000 int. units (30 mg)

Tablet: 10,000 int. units

Betachron® *(Discontinued) see page 814*

Betaderm® **[Can]** *see* betamethasone (topical) *on next page*

Betadine® **[US/Can]** *see* povidone-iodine *on page 533*

Betadine® **First Aid Antibiotics + Moisturizer** *(Discontinued) see page 814*

9-beta-D-ribofuranosyladenine *see* adenosine *on page 15*

Betagan® **[US/Can]** *see* levobunolol *on page 379*

betahistine *(Canada only)* (bay ta HISS teen)

U.S./Canadian Brand Names Serc® [Can]

Therapeutic Category Antihistamine

Use May be of value in the treatment of Ménière's disease

Usual Dosage Adult: Oral: 4-8 mg 3 times/day

Dosage Forms Tablet, as dihydrochloride: 8 mg, 16 mg

betaine anhydrous (BAY tayne an HY drus)

U.S./Canadian Brand Names Cystadane® [US/Can]

Therapeutic Category Urinary Tract Product

Use Treatment of homocystinuria

Usual Dosage Oral: 6 g/day, usually given in two 3 g doses

Dosage Forms Powder for oral solution: 1 g/scoop (180 g) [1 scoop = 1.7 mL]

Betaject™ **[Can]** *see* betamethasone (systemic) *on next page*

Betalene® **Topical** *(Discontinued) see page 814*

Betalin® **S** *(Discontinued)* see page 814

Betaloc® **[Can]** see metoprolol on page 425

Betaloc® **Durules**® see metoprolol on page 425

Betamethacot® **[US]** see betamethasone (topical) on this page

betamethasone and clotrimazole
(bay ta METH a sone & kloe TRIM a zole)

Synonyms clotrimazole and betamethasone

U.S./Canadian Brand Names Lotrisone® [US/Can]

Therapeutic Category Antifungal/Corticosteroid

Use Topical treatment of various dermal fungal infections (including tinea pedis, cruris, and corpora in patients ≥17 years of age)

Usual Dosage Topical: Apply twice daily

Dosage Forms
Cream: Betamethasone dipropionate 0.05% and clotrimazole 1% (15 g, 45 g)
Lotion: Betamethasone dipropionate 0.05% and clotrimazole 1% (30 mL)

betamethasone (systemic) (bay ta METH a sone sis TEM ik)

U.S./Canadian Brand Names Betaject™ [Can]; Betnesol® [Can]; Celestone® Phosphate [US]; Celestone® Soluspan® [US/Can]; Celestone® [US]; Cel-U-Jec® [US]

Therapeutic Category Adrenal Corticosteroid

Use Anti-inflammatory; immunosuppressant agent; corticosteroid replacement therapy

Usual Dosage Children and Adults:
I.M.: Betamethasone sodium phosphate and betamethasone acetate: 0.5-9 mg/day (¹/₃ to ¹/₂ of oral dose)
Intrabursal, intra-articular: 0.5-2 mL
Oral: 0.6-7.2 mg/day

Dosage Forms
Base (Celestone®), Oral:
Syrup: 0.6 mg/5 mL (118 mL)
Tablet: 0.6 mg
Injection: Sodium phosphate (Celestone® Phosphate, Cel-U-Jec®): 4 mg betamethasone phosphate/mL (equivalent to 3 mg betamethasone/mL) (5 mL)
Injection, suspension: Sodium phosphate and acetate (Celestone® Soluspan®): 6 mg/mL (3 mg of betamethasone sodium phosphate and 3 mg of betamethasone acetate per mL) (5 mL)

betamethasone (topical) (bay ta METH a sone TOP i kal)

Synonyms flubenisolone

U.S./Canadian Brand Names Alphatrex® [US]; Betaderm® [Can]; Betamethacot® [US]; Betatrex® [US]; Beta-Val® [US]; Betnovate® [Can]; Celestoderm®-EV/2 [Can]; Celestoderm®-V [Can]; Del-Beta® [US]; Diprolene® AF [US]; Diprolene® [US/Can]; Diprosone® [US/Can]; Ectosone [Can]; Luxiq™ [US]; Maxivate® [US]; Prevex® [Can]; Qualisone® [US]; Taro-Sone® [Can]; Topilene® [Can]; Topisone®; Valisone® Scalp Lotion [Can]

Therapeutic Category Corticosteroid, Topical

Use Inflammatory dermatoses such as psoriasis, seborrheic or atopic dermatitis, neurodermatitis, inflammatory phase of xerosis, late phase of allergic dermatitis or irritant dermatitis

Usual Dosage Topical: Adults: Apply thin film 2-4 times/day. Therapy should be discontinued when control is achieved. If no improvement is seen, reassessment of diagnosis may be necessary.

Dosage Forms
Dipropionate (Alphatrex®, Diprosone®, Del-Beta®, Maxivate®):
Aerosol: 0.1% (85 g)
Cream: 0.05% (15 g, 45 g)
(Continued)

83

betamethasone (topical) *(Continued)*

Lotion: 0.05% (20 mL, 30 mL, 60 mL)
Ointment: 0.05% (15 g, 45 g)
Dipropionate augmented (Diprolene®, Diprolene® AF):
Cream: 0.05% (15 g, 45 g)
Gel: 0.05% (15 g, 45 g)
Lotion: 0.05% (30 mL, 60 mL)
Ointment, topical: 0.05% (15 g, 45 g)
Valerate (Betamethacot®, Betatrex®, Qualisone®):
Cream: 0.01% (15 g, 60 g); 0.1% (15 g, 45 g, 110 g, 430 g)
Lotion: 0.1% (20 mL, 60 mL)
Ointment: 0.1% (15 g, 45 g)
Valerate (Beta-Val®):
Cream: 0.01% (15 g, 60 g); 0.1% (15 g, 45 g, 110 g, 430 g)
Lotion: 0.1% (20 mL, 60 mL)
Valerate (Luxiq™): Foam: 100 g aluminum can (box of 1)

Betapace® [US] *see* sotalol *on page 602*

Betapace AF™ [US/Can] *see* sotalol *on page 602*

Betapen®-VK *(Discontinued)* *see page 814*

Betasept® [US-OTC] *see* chlorhexidine gluconate *on page 134*

Betaseron® [US/Can] *see* interferon beta-1b *on page 356*

Betatrex® [US] *see* betamethasone (topical) *on previous page*

Beta-Val® [US] *see* betamethasone (topical) *on previous page*

Beta-Val® Ointment (only) *(Discontinued)* *see page 814*

Betaxin® [Can] *see* thiamine *on page 632*

betaxolol (be TAKS oh lol)

U.S./Canadian Brand Names Betoptic® S [US/Can]; Kerlone® [US]
Therapeutic Category Beta-Adrenergic Blocker
Use Treatment of chronic open-angle glaucoma, ocular hypertension; management of hypertension
Usual Dosage Adults:
Ophthalmic: Instill 1 drop twice daily
Oral: 10 mg/day; may increase dose to 20 mg/day after 7-14 days if desired response is not achieved; initial dose in elderly patients: 5 mg/day
Dosage Forms
Solution, ophthalmic, as hydrochloride: 0.5% (5 mL, 10 mL, 15 mL) [contains benzalkonium chloride]
Suspension, ophthalmic, as hydrochloride (Betoptic® S): 0.25% (2.5 mL, 10 mL, 15 mL) [contains benzalkonium chloride]
Tablet, as hydrochloride (Kerlone®): 10 mg, 20 mg

Betaxon® [US/Can] *see* levobetaxolol *on page 379*

bethanechol (be THAN e kole)

U.S./Canadian Brand Names Duvoid® [Can]; Myotonachol™ [Can]; Urecholine® [US]
Therapeutic Category Cholinergic Agent
Use Treatment of nonobstructive urinary retention and retention due to neurogenic bladder; gastroesophageal reflux
Usual Dosage
Children:
Oral:
Abdominal distention or urinary retention: 0.6 mg/kg/day divided 3-4 times/day

Gastroesophageal reflux: 0.1-0.2 mg/kg/dose administered 30 minutes to 1 hour before each meal to a maximum of 4 times/day
Adults:
Oral: 10-50 mg 2-4 times/day
Dosage Forms Tablet, as chloride: 5 mg, 10 mg, 25 mg, 50 mg

Betimol® **[US]** *see* timolol *on page 639*

Betnesol® **[Can]** *see* betamethasone (systemic) *on page 83*

Betnovate® **[Can]** *see* betamethasone (topical) *on page 83*

Betoptic® *(Discontinued) see page 814*

Betoptic® **S [US/Can]** *see* betaxolol *on previous page*

bexarotene (beks AIR oh teen)
U.S./Canadian Brand Names Targretin® [US/Can]
Therapeutic Category Retinoic Acid Derivative; Vitamin A Derivative; Vitamin, Fat Soluble
Use
Oral: Treatment of cutaneous manifestations of cutaneous T-cell lymphoma in patients who are refractory to at least one prior systemic therapy
Topical: Treatment of cutaneous lesions in patients with cutaneous T-cell lymphoma (stage 1A and 1B) who have refractory or persistent disease after other therapies or who have not tolerated other therapies
Usual Dosage
Adults: Oral: 300 mg/m^2/day taken as a single daily dose. If there is no tumor response after 8 weeks and the initial dose was well tolerated, then an increase to 400 mg/m^2/day can be made with careful monitoring. Maintain as long as the patient is deriving benefit.
If the initial dose is not tolerated, then it may be adjusted to 200 mg/m^2/day, then to 100 mg/m^2/day or temporarily suspended if necessary to manage toxicity
Gel: Apply once every other day for first week, then increase on a weekly basis to once daily, 2 times/day, 3 times/day, and finally 4 times/day, according to tolerance
Dosage Forms
Capsule: 75 mg
Gel: 1% (60 g)

Bexophene® *(Discontinued) see page 814*

Bextra™ **[US]** *see* valdecoxib *on page 669*

bezafibrate *(Canada only)* (be za FYE brate)
U.S./Canadian Brand Names Bezalip® [Can]; PMS-Bezafibrate [Can]
Therapeutic Category Antihyperlipidemic Agent, Miscellaneous
Use Adjunct to dietary therapy in the management of hyperlipidemias associated with high triglyceride levels (types III, IV, V); primarily lowers triglycerides and very low density lipoprotein
Usual Dosage Adult: Oral: 200 mg 3 times/day
Dosage Forms
Tablet, immediate release: 200 mg
Tablet, sustained release: 400 mg

Bezalip® **[Can]** *see* bezafibrate *(Canada only) on this page*

Biamine® **Injection** *(Discontinued) see page 814*

Biavax® **II [US]** *see* rubella and mumps vaccines, combined *on page 579*

Biaxin® **[US/Can]** *see* clarithromycin *on page 149*

Biaxin® **XL [US]** *see* clarithromycin *on page 149*

bicalutamide (bye ka LOO ta mide)

U.S./Canadian Brand Names Casodex® [US/Can]

Therapeutic Category Androgen

Use Combination therapy with a luteinizing hormone-releasing hormone (LHRH) analog for the treatment of advanced prostate cancer

Usual Dosage Adults: Oral: 50 mg once daily (morning or evening), with or without food, in combination with a LHRH analog

Dosage Forms Tablet: 50 mg

Bicillin® C-R [US] *see* penicillin G benzathine and procaine combined *on page 498*

Bicillin® C-R 900/300 [US] *see* penicillin G benzathine and procaine combined *on page 498*

Bicillin® L-A [US] *see* penicillin G benzathine *on page 498*

BiCNU® [US/Can] *see* carmustine *on page 118*

Bilezyme® Tablet *(Discontinued)* *see page 814*

Bilopaque® [US] *see* radiological/contrast media (ionic) *on page 561*

Biltricide® [US/Can] *see* praziquantel *on page 535*

bimatoprost (bi MAT oh prost)

U.S./Canadian Brand Names Lumigan™ [US]

Therapeutic Category Ophthalmic Agent, Miscellaneous

Use Reduction of intraocular pressure (IOP) in patients with open-angle glaucoma or ocular hypertension; should be used in patients who are intolerant of other IOP-lowering medications or failed treatment with another IOP-lowering medication

Usual Dosage Ophthalmic: Adult: Open-angle glaucoma or ocular hypertension: Instill 1 drop into affected eye(s) once daily in the evening; do not exceed once-daily dosing (may decrease IOP-lowering effect). If used with other topical ophthalmic agents, separate administration by at least 5 minutes.

Dosage Forms Solution, ophthalmic: 0.03% (2.5 mL, 5 mL) [contains benzalkonium chloride]

Biobase™ [Can] *see* alcohol (ethyl) *on page 20*

Biocef® [US] *see* cephalexin *on page 128*

BioCox® *(Discontinued)* *see page 814*

Biodine® *(Discontinued)* *see page 814*

Biofed-PE® [US-OTC] *see* triprolidine and pseudoephedrine *on page 659*

Biolon® [US/Can] *see* sodium hyaluronate *on page 597*

Biomox® *(Discontinued)* *see page 814*

Bion® Tears [US-OTC] *see* artificial tears *on page 56*

Bio-Statin® [US] *see* nystatin *on page 473*

BioThrax™ [US] *see* anthrax vaccine, adsorbed *on page 44*

Biozyme-C® *(Discontinued)* *see page 814*

biperiden (bye PER i den)

U.S./Canadian Brand Names Akineton® [US/Can]

Therapeutic Category Anticholinergic Agent; Anti-Parkinson's Agent

Use Treatment of all forms of Parkinsonism including drug-induced type (extrapyramidal symptoms)

Usual Dosage Adults:

Parkinsonism: Oral: 2 mg 3-4 times/day

Extrapyramidal: Oral: 2-6 mg 2-3 times/day

Dosage Forms Tablet, as hydrochloride: 2 mg

Biphetamine® *(Discontinued)* *see page 814*

Bisac-Evac™ [US-OTC] *see* bisacodyl *on this page*

bisacodyl (bis a KOE dil)

U.S./Canadian Brand Names Alophen® [US-OTC]; Apo®-Bisacodyl [Can]; Bisac-Evac™ [US-OTC]; Dulcolax® [US/Can]; Feen-A-Mint® [US-OTC]; Femilax™ [US-OTC]; Fleet® Bisacodyl Enema [US-OTC]; Fleet® Stimulant Laxative [US-OTC]; Modane Tablets® [US-OTC]

Therapeutic Category Laxative

Use Treatment of constipation; colonic evacuation prior to procedures or examination

Usual Dosage
Children:
Oral: >6 years: 5-10 mg (0.3 mg/kg) at bedtime or before breakfast
Rectal suppository:
<2 years: 5 mg as a single dose
>2 years: 10 mg
Adults:
Oral: 5-15 mg as single dose (up to 30 mg when complete evacuation of bowel is required)
Rectal suppository: 10 mg as single dose
Tannex:
Enema: 2.5 g in 1000 mL warm water
Barium enema: 2.5-5 g in 1000 mL barium suspension
Do not administer >10 g within a 72-hour period

Dosage Forms
Enema (Fleet® Bisacodyl Enema): 10 mg/30 mL
Suppository, rectal (Bisac-Evac™, Bisacodyl Uniserts®; Dulcolax®): 10 mg
Tablet, enteric coated (Alophen®; Bisac-Evac™, Dulcolax®, Feen-A-Mint®, Femilax™, Fleet® Stimulant Laxative; Modane®): 5 mg

Bisacodyl Uniserts® *(Discontinued)* *see page 814*

bishydroxycoumarin *see* dicumarol *on page 194*

Bismatrol® [US-OTC] *see* bismuth subsalicylate *on this page*

bismuth subgallate (BIZ muth sub GAL ate)

U.S./Canadian Brand Names Devrom® [US-OTC]
Therapeutic Category Gastrointestinal Agent, Miscellaneous
Use Symptomatic treatment of mild, nonspecific diarrhea
Usual Dosage Oral: 1-2 tablets 3 times/day with meals
Dosage Forms Tablet, chewable: 200 mg

bismuth subsalicylate (BIZ muth sub sa LIS i late)

Synonyms pink bismuth
U.S./Canadian Brand Names Bismatrol® [US-OTC]; Diotame® [US-OTC]; Pepto-Bismol® [US-OTC]
Therapeutic Category Gastrointestinal Agent, Miscellaneous
Use Symptomatic treatment of mild, nonspecific diarrhea including traveler's diarrhea; chronic infantile diarrhea
Usual Dosage Oral:
Nonspecific diarrhea:
Children: Up to 8 doses/24 hours:
3-6 years: 1/3 tablet or 5 mL every 30 minutes to 1 hour as needed
6-9 years: 2/3 tablet or 10 mL every 30 minutes to 1 hour as needed
9-12 years: 1 tablet or 15 mL every 30 minutes to 1 hour as needed
Adults: 2 tablets or 30 mL every 30 minutes to 1 hour as needed up to 8 doses/24 hours
(Continued)

bismuth subsalicylate *(Continued)*

Prevention of traveler's diarrhea: 2.1 g/day or 2 tablets 4 times/day before meals and at bedtime

Dosage Forms
Caplet, swallowable: 262 mg
Liquid: 262 mg/15 mL (120 mL, 240 mL, 360 mL, 480 mL); 524 mg/15 mL (120 mL, 240 mL, 360 mL)
Tablet, chewable: 262 mg

bismuth subsalicylate, metronidazole, and tetracycline

(BIZ muth sub sa LIS i late, me troe NI da zole, & tet ra SYE kleen)
U.S./Canadian Brand Names Helidac™ [US]
Therapeutic Category Antidiarrheal
Use In combination with an H_2 antagonist, used to treat and decrease rate of recurrence of active duodenal ulcer associated with *H. pylori* infection
Usual Dosage Adults: Chew 2 bismuth subsalicylate 262.4 mg tablets, swallow 1 metronidazole 250 mg tablet, and swallow 1 tetracycline 500 mg capsule plus an H_2 antagonist 4 times/day at meals and bedtime for 14 days; follow with 8 oz of water
Dosage Forms Each package contains 14 blister cards (2-week supply); each card contains the following:
Capsule: Tetracycline hydrochloride: 500 mg (4)
Tablet:
Bismuth subsalicylate [chewable]: 262.4 mg (8)
Metronidazole: 250 mg (4)

bisoprolol (bis OH proe lol)

U.S./Canadian Brand Names Monocor® [Can]; Zebeta® [US/Can]
Therapeutic Category Beta-Adrenergic Blocker
Use Treatment of hypertension, alone or in combination with other agents
Usual Dosage Adults: Oral: 5 mg once daily, may be increased to 10 mg, and then up to 20 mg once daily, if necessary
Dosage Forms Tablet, as fumarate: 5 mg, 10 mg

bisoprolol and hydrochlorothiazide

(bis OH proe lol & hye droe klor oh THYE a zide)
Synonyms hydrochlorothiazide and bisoprolol
U.S./Canadian Brand Names Ziac® [US/Can]
Therapeutic Category Antihypertensive Agent, Combination
Use Treatment of hypertension
Usual Dosage Adults: Oral: Dose is individualized, administered once daily
Dosage Forms Tablet:
Bisoprolol fumarate 2.5 mg and hydrochlorothiazide 6.25 mg
Bisoprolol fumarate 5 mg and hydrochlorothiazide 6.25 mg
Bisoprolol fumarate 10 mg and hydrochlorothiazide 6.25 mg

bistropamide *see* tropicamide *on page 661*

bitolterol (bye TOLE ter ole)

U.S./Canadian Brand Names Tornalate® [US/Can]
Therapeutic Category Adrenergic Agonist Agent
Use Prevent and treat bronchial asthma and bronchospasm
Usual Dosage Children >12 years and Adults:
Bronchospasm: 2 inhalations at an interval of at least 1-3 minutes, followed by a third inhalation if needed
Prevention of bronchospasm: 2 inhalations every 8 hours

Dosage Forms
Aerosol for oral inhalation, as mesylate: 0.8% [370 mcg/metered spray; 300 inhalations] (15 mL)
Solution for oral inhalation, as mesylate: 0.2% (10 mL, 30 mL, 60 mL)

bivalirudin (bye VAL i roo din)
Synonyms hirulog
U.S./Canadian Brand Names Angiomax™ [US]
Therapeutic Category Anticoagulant (Other)
Use Anticoagulant used in conjunction with aspirin for patients with unstable angina undergoing percutaneous transluminal coronary angioplasty (PTCA)
Usual Dosage Adults: Anticoagulant in patients with unstable angina undergoing PTCA (treatment should be started just prior to PTCA): I.V.: Initial: Bolus: 1 mg/kg, followed by continuous infusion: 2.5 mg/kg/hour over 4 hours; if needed, infusion may be continued at 0.2 mg/kg/hour for up to 20 hours; patients should also receive aspirin 300-325 mg/day
Dosage Forms Injection, powder for reconstitution: 250 mg

Black Draught® [US-OTC] see senna on page 587

black widow spider antivenin (Latrodectus mactans) see antivenin (Latrodectus mactans) on page 48

Blanex® Capsule (Discontinued) see page 814

BlemErase® Lotion (Discontinued) see page 814

Blenoxane® [US/Can] see bleomycin on this page

bleomycin (blee oh MYE sin)
Synonyms BLM
U.S./Canadian Brand Names Blenoxane® [US/Can]
Therapeutic Category Antineoplastic Agent
Use Palliative treatment of squamous cell carcinoma, testicular carcinoma, germ cell tumors, and the following lymphomas: Hodgkin's, lymphosarcoma and reticulum cell sarcoma; sclerosing agent to control malignant effusions
Usual Dosage Refer to individual protocols.
Children and Adults:
Test dose for lymphoma patients: I.M., I.V., S.C.: 1-2 units of bleomycin for the first 2 doses; monitor vital signs every 15 minutes; wait a minimum of 1 hour before administering remainder of dose
I.M., I.V., S.C.: 10-20 units/m² (0.25-0.5 units/kg) 1-2 times/week in combination regimens
I.V. continuous infusion: 15-20 units/m²/day for 4-5 days
Adults: Intracavitary injection for pleural effusion: 15-240 units have been administered
Dosage Forms Injection, powder for reconstitution, as sulfate: 15 units, 30 units [1 unit = 1 mg]

Bleph®-10 [US] see sulfacetamide on page 610

Blephamide® [US/Can] see sulfacetamide and prednisolone on page 611

Blis-To-Sol® [US-OTC] see tolnaftate on page 644

BLM see bleomycin on this page

Blocadren® [US] see timolol on page 639

Bluboro® [US-OTC] see aluminum sulfate and calcium acetate on page 29

Bonamine™ [Can] see meclizine on page 403

Bonefos® [US/Can] see clodronate disodium (Canada only) on page 153

Bonine® [US/Can] see meclizine on page 403

Bontril PDM® [US] see phendimetrazine on page 507

Bontril® **Slow-Release [US]** *see* phendimetrazine *on page 507*

boric acid (BOR ik AS id)
U.S./Canadian Brand Names Borofax® [US-OTC]; Dri-Ear® Otic [US-OTC]; Swim-Ear® Otic [US-OTC]
Therapeutic Category Pharmaceutical Aid
Use
Ophthalmic: Mild antiseptic used for inflamed eyelids
Otic: Prophylaxis of swimmer's ear
Topical ointment: Temporary relief of chapped, chafed, or dry skin, diaper rash, abrasions, minor burns, sunburn, insect bites, and other skin irritations
Usual Dosage
Ophthalmic: Apply to lower eyelid 1-2 times/day
Otic: Place 2-4 drops in ears
Topical: Apply as needed
Dosage Forms
Ointment:
Ophthalmic: 5% (3.5 g); 10% (3.5 g)
Topical: 5% (52.5 g); 10% (28 g)
Topical (Borofax®): 5% boric acid and lanolin (1¾ oz)
Solution, otic: 2.75% with isopropyl alcohol (30 mL)

Born Again Super Pain Relieving® **[US]** *see* capsaicin *on page 111*

Borofax® **[US-OTC]** *see* boric acid *on this page*

bosentan (boe SEN tan)
U.S./Canadian Brand Names Tracleer™ [US]
Therapeutic Category Endothelin Antagonist
Controlled Substance Bosentan (Tracleer™) is available only through a limited distribution program directly from the manufacturer (Actelion Pharmaceuticals 1-866-228-3546). It will not be available through wholesalers or individual pharmacies.
Use Treatment of pulmonary artery hypertension (PAH) in patients with World Health Organization (WHO) Class III or IV symptoms to improve exercise capacity and decrease the rate of clinical deterioration
Usual Dosage Oral: Adults: Initial: 62.5 mg twice daily for 4 weeks; increase to maintenance dose of 125 mg twice daily; adults <40 kg should be maintained at 62.5 mg twice daily
Note: When discontinuing treatment, consider a reduction in dosage to 62.5 mg twice daily for 3-7 days (to avoid clinical deterioration).
Dosage Forms Tablet: 62.5 mg, 125 mg

B&O Supprettes® **[US]** *see* belladonna and opium *on page 74*

Botox® **[US/Can]** *see* botulinum toxin type A *on this page*

Botox® **Cosmetic [US]** *see* botulinum toxin type A *on this page*

botulinum toxin type A (BOT yoo lin num TOKS in type aye)
U.S./Canadian Brand Names Botox® Cosmetic [US]; Botox® [US/Can]
Therapeutic Category Ophthalmic Agent, Toxin
Use Treatment of strabismus and blepharospasm
Usual Dosage
Strabismus: 1.25-5 units (0.05-0.15 mL) injected into any one muscle
Subsequent doses for residual/recurrent strabismus: Re-examine patients 7-14 days after each injection to assess the effect of that dose. Subsequent doses for patients experiencing incomplete paralysis of the target may be increased up to twofold the previously administered dose. Maximum recommended dose as a single injection for any one muscle is 25 units.
Blepharospasm: 1.25-2.5 units (0.05-0.10 mL) injected into the orbicularis oculi muscle

Subsequent doses: Each treatment lasts approximately 3 months. At repeat treatment sessions, the dose may be increased up to twofold if the response from the initial treatment is considered insufficient (usually defined as an effect that does not last >2 months). There appears to be little benefit obtainable from injecting >5 units per site. Some tolerance may be found if treatments are administered any more frequently than every 3 months.

The cumulative dose should not exceed 200 units in a 30-day period

Dosage Forms Injection, powder for reconstitution (Botox®, Botox® Cosmetic): 100 units *Clostridium botulinum* toxin type A

botulinum toxin type B (BOT yoo lin num TOKS in type bee)

U.S./Canadian Brand Names Myobloc® [US]

Therapeutic Category Neuromuscular Blocker Agent, Toxin

Use Treatment of cervical dystonia (spasmodic torticollis)

Usual Dosage

Children: Not established in pediatric patients

Adults: Cervical dystonia: I.M.: Initial: 2500-5000 units divided among the affected muscles in patients **previously treated** with botulinum toxin; initial dose in **previously untreated** patients should be lower. Subsequent dosing should be optimized according to patient's response.

Dosage Forms Injection, solution [single-dose vial]: 5000 units/mL (0.5 mL, 1 mL, 2 mL) [contains albumin 0.05%]

Boudreaux's® Butt Paste [US-OTC] *see* zinc oxide *on page 691*

bovine lung surfactant *see* beractant *on page 81*

Breathe Free® [US-OTC] *see* sodium chloride *on page 595*

Breathe Right® Saline [US-OTC] *see* sodium chloride *on page 595*

Breezee® Mist Antifungal *(Discontinued)* *see page 814*

Breonesin® *(Discontinued)* *see page 814*

Brethaire® *(Discontinued)* *see page 814*

Brethine® [US] *see* terbutaline *on page 623*

bretylium (bre TIL ee um)

Therapeutic Category Antiarrhythmic Agent, Class III

Use Ventricular tachycardia or ventricular fibrillation; other serious ventricular arrhythmias resistant to lidocaine

Usual Dosage

Children:

I.M.: 2-5 mg/kg as a single dose

I.V.: Initial: 5 mg/kg, then attempt electrical defibrillation; repeat with 10 mg/kg if ventricular fibrillation persists

Maintenance dose: I.M., I.V.: 5 mg/kg every 6-8 hours

Adults:

Immediate life-threatening ventricular arrhythmias; ventricular fibrillation; unstable ventricular tachycardia. **Note**: Patients should undergo defibrillation/cardioversion before and after bretylium doses as necessary:

Initial dose: I.V.: 5 mg/kg (undiluted) over 1 minute; if arrhythmia persists, administer 10 mg/kg (undiluted) over 1 minute and repeat as necessary (usually at 15- to 30-minute intervals) up to a total dose of 30 mg/kg

Other life-threatening ventricular arrhythmias:

Initial dose: I.M., I.V.: 5-10 mg/kg, may repeat every 1-2 hours if arrhythmia persist; administer I.V. dose (diluted) over 10-30 minutes

Maintenance dose: I.M.: 5-10 mg/kg every 6-8 hours; I.V. (diluted): 5-10 mg/kg every 6 hours; I.V. infusion (diluted): 1-2 mg/minute (little experience with doses >40 mg/kg/day)

(Continued)

bretylium *(Continued)*

Dosage Forms

Injection, solution, as tosylate: 50 mg/mL (10 mL)

Injection, solution, as tosylate [premixed in D_5W]: 2 mg/mL (250 mL); 4 mg/mL (250 mL)

Bretylol® *(Discontinued)* see page 814

Brevibloc® **[US/Can]** see esmolol on page 237

Brevicon® **[US]** see ethinyl estradiol and norethindrone on page 251

Brevital® **Sodium [US/Can]** see methohexital on page 417

Brevoxyl® **[US]** see benzoyl peroxide on page 79

Brevoxyl® **Cleansing [US]** see benzoyl peroxide on page 79

Brevoxyl® **Wash [US]** see benzoyl peroxide on page 79

Brexidol® **20 [Can]** see piroxicam and cyclodextrin *(Canada only)* on page 518

Bricanyl® *(Discontinued)* see page 814

Bricanyl® **[Can]** see terbutaline on page 623

brimonidine (bri MOE ni deen)

U.S./Canadian Brand Names Alphagan® P [US/Can]

Therapeutic Category Alpha$_2$-Adrenergic Agonist Agent, Ophthalmic

Use Lowering of intraocular pressure in patients with open-angle glaucoma or ocular hypertension

Usual Dosage Adults: Ophthalmic: 1 drop in affected eye(s) 3 times/day (approximately every 8 hours)

Dosage Forms Solution, ophthalmic, as tartrate: 0.15% (5 mL, 10 mL, 15 mL) [contains Purite® 0.005% as preservative]

brinzolamide (brin ZOH la mide)

U.S./Canadian Brand Names Azopt® [US/Can]

Therapeutic Category Carbonic Anhydrase Inhibitor

Use Lowers intraocular pressure to treat glaucoma in patients with ocular hypertension or open-angle glaucoma

Usual Dosage Adults: Ophthalmic: Instill 1 drop in eye(s) 3 times/day

Dosage Forms Suspension, ophthalmic: 1% (5 mL, 10 mL, 15 mL) [contains benzalkonium chloride]

British anti-lewisite see dimercaprol on page 200

Brodspec® **[US]** see tetracycline on page 628

Brofed® **[US]** see brompheniramine and pseudoephedrine on page 94

Bromaline® **Elixir** *(Discontinued)* see page 814

Bromanate® **DC** *(Discontinued)* see page 814

Bromanate® **[US-OTC]** see brompheniramine and pseudoephedrine on page 94

Bromarest® *(Discontinued)* see page 814

Bromatapp® *(Discontinued)* see page 814

bromazepam *(Canada only)* (broe MA ze pam)

U.S./Canadian Brand Names Alti-Bromazepam [Can]; Apo®-Bromazepam [Can]; Gen-Bromazepam [Can]; Lectopam® [Can]; Novo-Bromazepam [Can]; Nu-Bromazepam [Can]

Therapeutic Category Benzodiazepine; Sedative

Use Short-term, symptomatic relief of manifestations of excessive anxiety in patients with anxiety neurosis

Usual Dosage Adults: Oral: 6-18 mg/day in equally divided doses. depending on the severity of symptoms and response of the patient
Dosage Forms Tablet: 1.5 mg, 3 mg, 6 mg

Brombay® *(Discontinued)* see page 814

Bromfed-PD® [US-OTC] *see* brompheniramine and pseudoephedrine *on next page*

Bromfed® [US-OTC] *see* brompheniramine and pseudoephedrine *on next page*

Bromfenex® [US] *see* brompheniramine and pseudoephedrine *on next page*

Bromfenex® PD [US] *see* brompheniramine and pseudoephedrine *on next page*

bromocriptine (broe moe KRIP teen)
U.S./Canadian Brand Names Apo® Bromocriptine [Can]; Parlodel® [US/Can]; PMS-Bromocriptine [Can]
Therapeutic Category Anti-Parkinson's Agent; Ergot Alkaloid and Derivative
Use Treatment of parkinsonism in patients unresponsive or allergic to levodopa; also used in conditions associated with hyperprolactinemia and to suppress lactation
Usual Dosage Oral:
  Parkinsonism: 1.25 mg twice daily, increased by 2.5 mg/day in 2- to 4-week intervals (usual dose range: 30-90 mg/day in 3 divided doses)
  Hyperprolactinemia and postpartum lactation: 2.5 mg 2-3 times/day
Dosage Forms
  Capsule, as mesylate: 5 mg
  Tablet, as mesylate: 2.5 mg

Bromphen® *(Discontinued)* see page 814

Bromphen® DC With Codeine *(Discontinued)* see page 814

brompheniramine (brome fen IR a meen)
Synonyms parabromdylamine
U.S./Canadian Brand Names Colhist® Solution [US-OTC]; Dimetane® Extentabs® [US-OTC]; Dimetapp® Allergy Children's [US-OTC]; Dimetapp® Allergy [US-OTC]; Lodrane® 12 Hour [US-OTC]; ND-Stat® Solution [US-OTC]; Polytapp® Allergy Dye-Free Medication [US-OTC]
Therapeutic Category Antihistamine
Use Perennial and seasonal allergic rhinitis and other allergic symptoms including urticaria
Usual Dosage
  Oral:
  Children:
    <6 years: 0.125 mg/kg/dose administered every 6 hours; maximum: 6-8 mg/day
    6-12 years: 2-4 mg every 6-8 hours; maximum: 12-16 mg/day
    Adults: 4 mg every 4-6 hours or 8 mg of sustained release form every 8-12 hours or 12 mg of sustained release every 12 hours; maximum: 24 mg/day
  I.M., I.V., S.C.:
    Children <12 years: 0.5 mg/kg/24 hours divided every 6-8 hours
    Adults: 5-50 mg every 4-12 hours, maximum: 40 mg/24 hours
Dosage Forms
  Capsule, as maleate: 4 mg
  Elixir, as maleate: 2 mg/5 mL with 3% alcohol (120 mL)
  Liquid, as maleate: 2 mg/5 mL (60 mL, 120 mL, 240 mL)
  Solution, as maleate: 2 mg/5 mL (10 mL)
  Tablet, as maleate: 4 mg
  Tablet, sustained release, as maleate: 6 mg, 12 mg

brompheniramine and pseudoephedrine
(brome fen IR a meen & soo doe e FED rin)

U.S./Canadian Brand Names Andehist NR Syrup [US]; Brofed® [US]; Bromanate® [US-OTC]; Bromfed-PD® [US-OTC]; Bromfed® [US-OTC]; Bromfenex® PD [US]; Bromfenex® [US]; Children's Dimetapp® Elixir Cold & Allergy [US-OTC]; Rondec® Syrup [US]; Touro™ Allergy [US]

Therapeutic Category Antihistamine/Decongestant Combination

Use Temporary relief of symptoms of seasonal and perennial allergic rhinitis, and vasomotor rhinitis, including nasal obstruction

Usual Dosage Oral:
  Capsule, sustained release:
   Based on 60 mg pseudoephedrine:
    Children 6-12 years: 1 capsule every 12 hours
    Children ≥12 years and Adults: 1-2 capsules every 12 hours
   Based on 120 mg pseudoephedrine: Children ≥12 years and Adults: 1 capsule every 12 hours
  Elixir: Children >12 years and Adults:
   Brompheniramine 2 mg/pseudoephedrine 30 mg per 5 mL: 10 mL every 4-6 hours, up to 40 mL/day
   Brompheniramine 4 mg/pseudoephedrine 30 mg per 5 mL: 10 mL 3 times/day
  Tablet: Based on 60 mg pseudoephedrine: Children >12 years and Adults: 1 tablet every 4 hours
   Brompheniramine 4 mg/pseudoephedrine 60 mg per 5 mL: 5 mL 4 times/day
  Syrup:
   Children 2-6 years of age: 2.5 mL 4 times/day
   Children ≥6 years of age and Adults: 5 mL 4 times/day

Dosage Forms
  Capsule, extended release:
   Bromfed®, Bromfenex®: Brompheniramine maleate 12 mg and pseudoephedrine hydrochloride 120 mg
   Bromfed-PD®, Bromfenex® PD: Brompheniramine maleate 6 mg and pseudoephedrine hydrochloride 60 mg
  Capsule, sustained release (Touro™ Allergy): Brompheniramine maleate 5.75 mg and pseudoephedrine hydrochloride 60 mg
  Elixir: Brompheniramine maleate 1 mg and pseudoephedrine hydrochloride 15 mg per 5 mL (120 mL, 480 mL)
   Bromanate®: Brompheniramine maleate 1 mg and pseudoephedrine sulfate 15 mg per 5 mL (120 mL, 240 mL, 480 mL) [alcohol free; grape flavor]
   Children's Dimetapp® Elixir Cold & Allergy: Brompheniramine maleate 1 mg and pseudoephedrine hydrochloride 15 mg per 5 mL (240 mL) [alcohol free; grape flavor]
  Syrup:
   Andehist NR: Brompheniramine maleate 4 mg and pseudoephedrine sulfate 45 mg per 5 mL (473 mL) [raspberry flavor]
   Brofed®: Brompheniramine maleate 4 mg and pseudoephedrine hydrochloride 30 mg per 5 mL (480 mL) [mint flavor]
   Rondec®: Brompheniramine maleate 4 mg and pseudoephedrine hydrochloride 45 mg per 5 mL (120 mL, 480 mL) [cherry flavor]

Brompheril® [US-OTC] see dexbrompheniramine and pseudoephedrine on page 185

Bronchial® (Discontinued) see page 814

Bronchial Mist® [US] see epinephrine on page 228

Broncho Saline® [US] see sodium chloride on page 595

Bronitin® Mist (Discontinued) see page 814

Bronkephrine® (Discontinued) see page 814

Bronkometer® (Discontinued) see page 814

Bronkosol® *(Discontinued)* see page 814

Brontex® **[US]** see guaifenesin and codeine on page 308

Brotane® *(Discontinued)* see page 814

BSS® **[US/Can]** see balanced salt solution on page 70

BSS® **Plus [US/Can]** see balanced salt solution on page 70

B-type natriuretic peptide (human) see nesiritide on page 455

Bucet™ **[US]** see butalbital, acetaminophen, and caffeine on page 99

Bucladin®**-S Softab**® *(Discontinued)* see page 814

budesonide (byoo DES oh nide)

U.S./Canadian Brand Names Entocort™ EC [US/Can]; Gen-Budesonide AQ [Can]; Pulmicort® Nebuamp®; Pulmicort Respules™ [US]; Pulmicort Turbuhaler® [US/Can]; Rhinocort® [US/Can]; Rhinocort® Aqua™ [US/Can]

Therapeutic Category Adrenal Corticosteroid

Use

Intranasal: Children ≥6 years of age and Adults: Management of symptoms of seasonal or perennial rhinitis

Nebulization: Children 12 months to 8 years: Maintenance and prophylactic treatment of asthma

Oral capsule: Treatment of active Crohn's disease (mild to moderate) involving the ileum and/or ascending colon

Oral inhalation: Maintenance and prophylactic treatment of asthma; includes patients who require corticosteroids and those who may benefit from systemic dose reduction/elimination

Usual Dosage

Nasal inhalation: Children ≥6 years and Adults:

Rhinocort®: Initial: 8 sprays (4 sprays/nostril) per day (256 mcg/day), given as either 2 sprays in each nostril in the morning and evening or as 4 sprays in each nostril in the morning; after symptoms decrease (usually by 3-7 days), reduce dose slowly every 2-4 weeks to the smallest amount needed to control symptoms

Rhinocort® Aqua™: 64 mcg/day as a single 32 mcg spray in each nostril. Some patients who do not achieve adequate control may benefit from increased dosage. A reduced dosage may be effective after initial control is achieved.

Maximum dose: Children <12 years: 128 mcg/day; Adults: 256 mcg/day

Nebulization: Children 12 months to 8 years: Pulmicort Respules™: Titrate to lowest effective dose once patient is stable; start at 0.25 mg/day or use as follows:

Previous therapy of bronchodilators alone: 0.5 mg/day administered as a single dose or divided twice daily (maximum daily dose: 0.5 mg)

Previous therapy of inhaled corticosteroids: 0.5 mg/day administered as a single dose or divided twice daily (maximum daily dose: 1 mg)

Previous therapy of oral corticosteroids: 1 mg/day administered as a single dose or divided twice daily (maximum daily dose: 1 mg)

Oral inhalation:

Children ≥6 years:

Previous therapy of bronchodilators alone: 200 mcg twice initially which may be increased up to 400 mcg twice daily

Previous therapy of inhaled corticosteroids: 200 mcg twice initially which may be increased up to 400 mcg twice daily

Previous therapy of oral corticosteroids: The highest recommended dose in children is 400 mcg twice daily

Adults:

Previous therapy of bronchodilators alone: 200-400 mcg twice initially which may be increased up to 400 mcg twice daily

Previous therapy of inhaled corticosteroids: 200-400 mcg twice initially which may be increased up to 800 mcg twice daily

(Continued)

budesonide *(Continued)*

Previous therapy of oral corticosteroids: 400-800 mcg twice daily which may be increased up to 800 mcg twice daily

NIH Guidelines (NIH, 1997) (give in divided doses twice daily):

Children:

"Low" dose: 100-200 mcg/day

"Medium" dose: 200-400 mcg/day (1-2 inhalations/day)

"High" dose: >400 mcg/day (>2 inhalation/day)

Adults:

"Low" dose: 200-400 mcg/day (1-2 inhalations/day)

"Medium" dose: 400-600 mcg/day (2-3 inhalations/day)

"High" dose: >600 mcg/day (>3 inhalation/day)

Oral: Adults: Crohn's disease: 9 mg once daily in the morning; safety and efficacy have not been established for therapy duration >8 weeks; recurring episodes may be treated with a repeat 8-week course of treatment

Note: Treatment may be tapered to 6 mg once daily for 2 weeks prior to complete cessation. Patients receiving CYP3A3/4 inhibitors should be monitored closely for signs and symptoms of hypercorticism; dosage reduction may be required.

Dosage Forms

Capsule, enteric coated (Entocort™ EC): 3 mg

Powder for oral inhalation (Pulmicort Turbuhaler®): 200 mcg/inhalation (104 g) [delivers ~160 mcg/inhalation; 200 metered doses]

Suspension for nasal inhalation (Rhinocort®): 50 mcg/inhalation (7 g) [delivers ~32 mcg/inhalation; 200 metered doses]

Suspension, nasal [spray] (Rhinocort® Aqua™): 32 mcg/inhalation (8.6 g) [120 metered doses]

Suspension for oral inhalation (Pulmicort Respules™): 0.25 mg/2 mL (30s), 0.5 mg/2 mL (30s)

Buffered®, Tri-buffered *(Discontinued)* see page 814

Bufferin® Arthritis Strength [US-OTC] see aspirin on page 58

Bufferin® Extra Strength [US-OTC] see aspirin on page 58

Bufferin® [US-OTC] see aspirin on page 58

Buf-Puf® Acne Cleansing Bar *(Discontinued)* see page 814

bumetanide *(byoo MET a nide)*

U.S./Canadian Brand Names Bumex® [US/Can]; Burinex® [Can]

Therapeutic Category Diuretic, Loop

Use Management of edema secondary to congestive heart failure or hepatic or renal disease including nephrotic syndrome; may also be used alone or in combination with antihypertensives in the treatment of hypertension

Usual Dosage

Children:

<6 months: Dose not established

>6 months:

Oral: Initial: 0.015 mg/kg/dose once daily or every other day; maximum dose: 0.1 mg/kg/day

I.M., I.V.: Dose not established

Adults:

Oral: 0.5-2 mg/dose (maximum: 10 mg/day) 1-2 times/day

I.M., I.V.: 0.5-1 mg/dose (maximum: 10 mg/day)

Dosage Forms

Injection: 0.25 mg/mL (2 mL, 4 mL, 10 mL)

Tablet: 0.5 mg, 1 mg, 2 mg

Bumex® [US/Can] see bumetanide on this page

Buminate® **[US]** *see* albumin *on page 18*

Bupap® **[US]** *see* butalbital, acetaminophen, and caffeine *on page 99*

Buphenyl® **[US]** *see* sodium phenylbutyrate *on page 598*

bupivacaine (byoo PIV a kane)

U.S./Canadian Brand Names Marcaine® Spinal [US]; Marcaine® [US/Can]; Sensor-caine®-MPF [US]; Sensorcaine® [US/Can]

Therapeutic Category Local Anesthetic

Use Local anesthetic (injectable) for peripheral nerve block, infiltration, sympathetic block, caudal or epidural block, retrobulbar block

Usual Dosage Dose varies with procedure, depth of anesthesia, vascularity of tissues, duration of anesthesia and condition of patient

Caudal block (with or without epinephrine):
Children: 1-3.7 mg/kg
Adults: 15-30 mL of 0.25% or 0.5%
Epidural block (other than caudal block):
Children: 1.25 mg/kg/dose
Adults: 10-20 mL of 0.25% or 0.5%
Peripheral nerve block: 5 mL dose of 0.25% or 0.5% (12.5-25 mg); maximum: 2.5 mg/kg (plain); 3 mg/kg (with epinephrine); up to a maximum of 400 mg/day
Sympathetic nerve block: 20-50 mL of 0.25% (no epinephrine) solution

Dosage Forms
Injection, solution, as hydrochloride [preservative free]: 0.25% [2.5 mg/mL] (20 mL, 30 mL, 50 mL); 0.5% [5 mg/mL] (20 mL, 30 mL); 0.75% [7.5 mg/mL] (20 mL, 30 mL)
Marcaine®: 0.25% [2.5 mg/mL] (10 mL, 30 mL, 50 mL); 0.5% [5 mg/mL] (10 mL, 30 mL); 0.75% [7.5 mg/mL] (10 mL, 30 mL)
Marcaine® Spinal: 0.75% [7.5 mg/mL] (2 mL) [in dextrose 8.25%]
Sensorcaine®-MPF: 0.25% [2.5 mg/mL] (10 mL, 30 mL); 0.5% [5 mg/mL] (10 mL, 30 mL); 0.75% [7.5 mg/mL] (10 mL, 30 mL)
Injection, solution, as hydrochloride [with preservative]: 0.25% [2.5 mg/mL] (10 mL, 30 mL, 50 mL); 0.5% [5 mg/mL] (10 mL, 30 mL, 50 mL); 0.75% [7.5 mg/mL] (10 mL, 30 mL)
Marcaine®, Sensorcaine®: 0.25% [2.5 mg/mL] (50 mL); 0.5% [5 mg/mL] (50 mL) [contains methylparaben]
Injection, solution, with epinephrine 1:200,000, as hydrochloride [preservative free]:
Marcaine®: 0.25% [2.5 mg/mL] (10 mL, 30 mL, 50 mL); 0.5% [5 mg/mL] (3 mL, 10 mL, 30 mL); 0.75% [7.5 mg/mL] (30 mL) [contains sodium metabisulfite]
Sensorcaine®-MPF: 0.25% [2.5 mg/mL] (10 mL, 30 mL); 0.5% [5 mg/mL] (5 mL, 10 mL, 30 mL) [contains sodium metabisulfite]
Injection, solution, with epinephrine 1:200,000, as hydrochloride [with preservative] (Marcaine®, Sensorcaine®): 0.25% [2.5 mg/mL] (50 mL); 0.5% [5 mg/mL] (50 mL) [contains methylparaben and sodium metabisulfite]

Buprenex® **[US/Can]** *see* buprenorphine *on this page*

buprenorphine (byoo pre NOR feen)

U.S./Canadian Brand Names Buprenex® [US/Can]

Therapeutic Category Analgesic, Narcotic

Controlled Substance C-V

Use Management of moderate to severe pain

Usual Dosage Adults: I.M., slow I.V.: 0.3-0.6 mg every 6 hours as needed

Dosage Forms Injection, solution, as hydrochloride: 0.3 mg/mL (1 mL)

bupropion (byoo PROE pee on)

Tall-Man buPROPion

U.S./Canadian Brand Names Wellbutrin® [US/Can]; Wellbutrin® SR [US]; Zyban® [US/Can]

(Continued)

bupropion *(Continued)*

Therapeutic Category Antidepressant, Aminoketone

Use Treatment of depression; as an aid to smoking cessation treatment

Usual Dosage Oral:

Adults:

Depression: 100 mg 3 times/day; begin at 100 mg twice daily; may increase to a maximum dose of 450 mg/day

Smoking cessation: Initiate with 150 mg once daily for 3 days; increase to 150 mg twice daily; treatment should continue for 7-12 weeks

Dosage Forms

Tablet (Wellbutrin®): 75 mg, 100 mg

Tablet, sustained release:

Wellbutrin® SR: 100 mg, 150 mg, 200 mg

Zyban®: 150 mg

Burinex® [Can] *see* bumetanide *on page 96*

Burow's otic *see* aluminum acetate and acetic acid *on page 27*

buserelin acetate (BYOO se rel in AS e tate)

Therapeutic Category Luteinizing Hormone-Releasing Hormone Analog

Use For the palliative treatment of patients with hormone-dependent advanced carcinoma of the prostate gland (Stage D). Buserelin is also indicated for the treatment of endometriosis in patients who do not require surgery as primary therapy. The duration of treatment is usually 6 months and should not exceed 9 months. Experience with buserelin for the management of endometriosis has been limited to women 18 years of age and older.

Usual Dosage Buserelin should be administered at approximately equal time intervals to ensure that the desired therapeutic effect is maintained.

Prostatic Cancer: Initial Treatment: For the first 7 days of treatment give buserelin 500 mcg (0.5 mL) every 8 hours by S.C. injection. For patient comfort, vary the injection site.

Maintenance Treatment: Depending upon patient preference, or physician recommendation, maintenance treatment may be by daily S.C. injection or by intranasal administration 3 times daily. During maintenance dosing by the S.C. route, the buserelin dose is 200 mcg (0.2 mL) daily. For patient comfort, vary the site of injection.

During maintenance dosing by the intranasal administration route, the buserelin dose is 400 mcg (200 mcg into each nostril) 3 times daily using the metered-dose pump (nebulizer) provided. Each pump action delivers 100 mcg buserelin acetate or 0.1mL solution.

Endometriosis: The dose of buserelin in patients with endometriosis is 400 mcg (200 mcg into each nostril) 3 times daily using the metered-dose pump (nebulizer) provided. Each pump action delivers 100 mcg or 0.1 mL solution. The treatment duration is usually 6 months and should not exceed 9 months.

Dosage Forms Injection, depot: 6.6 mg [2 month]; 9.9 mg [3 month]

BuSpar® [US/Can] *see* buspirone *on this page*

Buspirex [Can] *see* buspirone *on this page*

buspirone (byoo SPYE rone)

Tall-Man busPIRone

U.S./Canadian Brand Names Apo®-Buspirone [Can]; BuSpar® [US/Can]; Buspirex [Can]; Gen-Buspirone [Can]; Lin-Buspirone [Can]; Novo-Buspirone [Can]; Nu-Buspirone [Can]; PMS-Buspirone [Can]

Therapeutic Category Antianxiety Agent

Use Management of anxiety

Usual Dosage Adults: Oral: 15 mg/day (5 mg 3 times/day); may increase to a maximum of 60 mg/day

Dosage Forms Tablet, as hydrochloride: 5 mg, 7.5 mg, 10 mg, 15 mg, 30 mg
BuSpar®: 5 mg, 10 mg, 15 mg, 30 mg

busulfan (byoo SUL fan)
U.S./Canadian Brand Names Busulfex® [US/Can]; Myleran® [US/Can]
Therapeutic Category Antineoplastic Agent
Use
Injection: Use in combination with cyclophosphamide as a conditioning regimen prior to allogeneic hematopoietic progenitor cell transplantation for chronic myelogenous leukemia
Oral: Chronic myelogenous leukemia and bone marrow disorders, such as polycythemia vera and myeloid metaplasia, conditioning regimens for bone marrow transplantation
Usual Dosage
I.V.: Adult: As a component of a conditioning regimen prior to bone marrow or peripheral blood progenitor cell replacement support is 0.8 mg/kg of ideal body weight or actual body weight, whichever is lower, administered every 6 hours for 4 days (a total of 16 doses)
Oral (**refer to individual protocols**):
Children:
For remission induction of CML: 0.06-0.12 mg/kg/day **or** 1.8-4.6 mg/m^2/day; titrate dosage to maintain leukocyte count above 40,000/mm^3; reduce dosage by 50% if the leukocyte count reaches 30,000-40,000/mm^3; discontinue drug if counts fall to ≤20,000/mm^3
BMT marrow-ablative conditioning regimen: 1 mg/kg/dose (ideal body weight) every 6 hours for 16 doses

Adults:
BMT marrow-ablative conditioning regimen: 1 mg/kg/dose (ideal body weight) every 6 hours for 16 doses
Dosage Forms
Injection, solution (Busulfex®): 6 mg/mL (10 mL)
Tablet (Myleran®): 2 mg

Busulfex® [US/Can] *see busulfan on this page*

butabarbital sodium (byoo ta BAR bi tal SOW dee um)
U.S./Canadian Brand Names Butisol Sodium® [US]
Therapeutic Category Barbiturate
Controlled Substance C-III
Use Sedative, hypnotic
Usual Dosage
Children: Preop: 2-6 mg/kg/dose; maximum: 100 mg
Adults:
Sedative: 15-30 mg 3-4 times/day
Hypnotic: 50-100 mg
Preop: 50-100 mg 1-1½ hours before surgery
Dosage Forms
Elixir, as sodium: 30 mg/5 mL (480 mL) [contains alcohol 7%]
Tablet, as sodium: 30 mg, 50 mg

Butace® (Discontinued) *see page 814*

Butalan® (Discontinued) *see page 814*

butalbital, acetaminophen, and caffeine
(byoo TAL bi tal, a seet a MIN oh fen, & KAF een)
U.S./Canadian Brand Names Anolor 300® [US]; Arcet® [US]; Axocet® [US]; Bucet™ [US]; Bupap® [US]; Butex Forte® [US]; Cephadyn® [US]; Dolgic® [US]; Esgic® [US]; Esgic-Plus™ [US]; Ezol® [US]; Fioricet® [US]; Geone® [US]; Margesic® [US]; Marten-
(Continued)

butalbital, acetaminophen, and caffeine *(Continued)*

Tab® [US]; Medigesic® [US]; Nonbac® [US]; Pacaps® [US]; Phrenilin® [US]; Phrenilin Forte® [US]; Promacet® [US]; Repan® [US]; Repan CF® [US]; Sedapap® [US]; Tenake® [US]; Tencon® [US]; Triad® [US]; Zebutal® [US]

Therapeutic Category Barbiturate/Analgesic

Use Relief of the symptomatic complex of tension or muscle contraction headache

Usual Dosage Adults: Oral: 1-2 tablets or capsules every 4 hours; not to exceed 6/day

Dosage Forms

Capsule:

Anolor 300®; Arcet®, Esgic®, Ezol®, Geone®, Margesic®, Medigesic®, Pacaps®, Tenake®, Triad®: Butalbital 50 mg and acetaminophen 325 mg with caffeine 40 mg

Axocet®, Bucet™, Butex Forte®, Phrenilin Forte®, Tencon®: Butalbital 50 mg and acetaminophen 650 mg

Esgic-Plus™, Zebutal®: Butalbital 50 mg and acetaminophen 500 mg with caffeine 40 mg

Tablet:

Bupap®, Cephadyn®, Dolgic®, Promacet®, Repan CF®, Sedapap®: Butalbital 50 mg and acetaminophen 650 mg

Esgic®, Fioricet®, Marten-Tab®, Nonbac®, Repan®: Butalbital 50 mg and acetaminophen 325 mg with caffeine 40 mg

Phrenilin®: Butalbital 50 mg and acetaminophen 325 mg

butalbital, aspirin, and caffeine (byoo TAL bi tal, AS pir in, & KAF een)

U.S./Canadian Brand Names Butalbital Compound® [US]; Farbital® [US]; Fiorinal® [US/Can]; Fortabs® [US]; Laniroif® [US]; Tecnal® [Can]; Trianal® [Can]

Therapeutic Category Barbiturate/Analgesic

Controlled Substance C-III (Fiorinal®)

Use Relief of the symptomatic complex of tension or muscle contraction headache

Usual Dosage Adults: Oral: 1-2 tablets or capsules every 4 hours; not to exceed 6/day

Dosage Forms

Capsule: (Butalbital Compound®, Fiorinal®, Laniroif®): Butalbital 50 mg, caffeine 40 mg, and aspirin 325 mg

Tablet: (Butalbital Compound®, Farbital®, Fiorinal®, Fortabs®, Laniroif®): Butalbital 50 mg, caffeine 40 mg, and aspirin 325 mg

Butalbital Compound® [US] *see* butalbital, aspirin, and caffeine *on this page*

butalbital compound and codeine

(byoo TAL bi tal KOM pound & KOE deen)

Synonyms codeine and butalbital compound

U.S./Canadian Brand Names Fiorinal®-C 1/2 [Can]; Fiorinal®-C 1/4 [Can]; Fiorinal® With Codeine [US]; Tecnal C 1/2 [Can]; Tecnal C 1/4 [Can]

Therapeutic Category Analgesic, Narcotic; Barbiturate

Controlled Substance C-III

Use Mild to moderate pain when sedation is needed

Usual Dosage Adults: Oral: 1-2 capsules every 4 hours as needed for pain; up to 6/day

Dosage Forms Capsule: Butalbital 50 mg, caffeine 40 mg, aspirin 325 mg, and codeine phosphate 30 mg

butenafine (byoo TEN a fine)

U.S./Canadian Brand Names Lotrimin® Ultra™ [US-OTC]; Mentax® [US]

Therapeutic Category Antifungal Agent

Use Topical treatment of interdigital tinea pedis (athlete's foot) due to *Epidermophyton floccosum*, *Trichophyton mentagrophytes*, or *Trichophyton rubrum*

Usual Dosage Adults: Topical: Apply cream to the affected area and surrounding skin once daily for 4 weeks

Dosage Forms Cream, as hydrochloride:
Mentax®: 1% (15 g, 30 g)
Lotrimin® Ultra™: 1% (12 g, 24 g)

Butex Forte® [US] *see* butalbital, acetaminophen, and caffeine *on page 99*

Buticaps® *(Discontinued) see page 814*

Butisol Sodium® [US] *see* butabarbital sodium *on page 99*

butoconazole (byoo toe KOE na zole)
U.S./Canadian Brand Names Femstat® One [Can]; Gynazole-1™ [US]; Mycelex®-3 [US-OTC]
Therapeutic Category Antifungal Agent
Use Local treatment of vulvovaginal candidiasis
Usual Dosage Adults:
Nonpregnant: Insert 1 applicatorful (~5 g) intravaginally at bedtime for 3 days, may extend for up to 6 days if necessary
Pregnant: **Use only during second or third trimesters**
Dosage Forms
Cream, vaginal, as nitrate:
Mycelex®-3: 2% (20 g) [with disposable applicator]
Gynazole-1™ [prefilled applicator]: 2% (5 g)

butorphanol (byoo TOR fa nole)
U.S./Canadian Brand Names Stadol® NS [US/Can]; Stadol® [US]
Therapeutic Category Analgesic, Narcotic
Controlled Substance C-IV
Use Management of moderate to severe pain
Usual Dosage Adults:
I.M.: 1-4 mg every 3-4 hours as needed
I.V.: 0.5-2 mg every 3-4 hours as needed
Nasal: Initial: 1 mg (1 spray in one nostril), allow 60-90 minutes to elapse before deciding whether a second 1 mg dose is needed; this 2-dose sequence may be repeated in 3-4 hours if needed
Dosage Forms
Injection, solution, as tartrate [preservative free] (Stadol®): 1 mg/mL (1 mL); 2 mg/mL (1 mL, 2 mL)
Injection, solution, as tartrate [with preservative] (Stadol®): 2 mg/mL (10 mL)
Nasal spray, as tartrate (Stadol® NS): 10 mg/mL (2.5 mL) [14-15 doses]

butyl aminobenzoate, benzocaine, tetracaine, and benzalkonium chloride *see* benzocaine, butyl aminobenzoate, tetracaine, and benzalkonium chloride *on page 78*

Byclomine® Injection *(Discontinued) see page 814*

Bydramine® Cough Syrup *(Discontinued) see page 814*

C2B8 monoclonal antibody *see* rituximab *on page 575*

c7E3 *see* abciximab *on page 2*

C8-CCK *see* sincalide *on page 591*

311C90 *see* zolmitriptan *on page 692*

C-500-GR™ [US-OTC] *see* ascorbic acid *on page 57*

cabergoline (ca BER go leen)
U.S./Canadian Brand Names Dostinex® [US]
Therapeutic Category Ergot-like Derivative
Use Treatment of hyperprolactinemia
(Continued)

cabergoline *(Continued)*

Usual Dosage Adults: Oral: 0.25 mg twice weekly; dosage may be increased by 0.25 mg twice weekly to a dose of up to 1 mg twice weekly (according to the patient's prolactin level)

Dosage Forms Tablet: 0.5 mg

Caelyx® [Can] *see* doxorubicin *on page 214*

Cafatine-PB® *(Discontinued) see page 814*

Cafcit® [US/Can] *see* caffeine (citrated) *on this page*

Cafergot® [US/Can] *see* ergotamine *on page 233*

Cafetrate® *(Discontinued) see page 814*

caffeine and sodium benzoate (KAF een & SOW dee um BEN zoe ate)

Synonyms sodium benzoate and caffeine

Therapeutic Category Diuretic, Miscellaneous

Use Emergency stimulant in acute circulatory failure; as a diuretic; and to relieve spinal puncture headache

Usual Dosage

Children: I.M., I.V., S.C.: 8 mg/kg every 4 hours as needed

Adults: I.M., I.V.: 500 mg, maximum single dose: 1 g

Dosage Forms Injection: Caffeine 125 mg and sodium benzoate 125 mg per mL (2 mL)

caffeine (citrated) (KAF een SIT rated)

U.S./Canadian Brand Names Cafcit® [US/Can]

Therapeutic Category Respiratory Stimulant; Stimulant

Use Central nervous system stimulant; used in the treatment of apnea of prematurity (28 to <33 weeks gestational age). Has several advantages over theophylline in the treatment of neonatal apnea, its half-life is about 3 times as long, allowing once daily dosing, drug levels do not need to be drawn at peak and trough; has a wider therapeutic window, allowing more room between an effective concentration and toxicity.

Usual Dosage Apnea of prematurity: Neonates:

Loading dose (usually administered I.V.): 10-20 mg/kg as caffeine citrate (5-10 mg/kg as caffeine base). If theophylline has been administered to the patient within the previous 3 days, a full or modified loading dose (50% to 75% of a loading dose) may be given (caffeine is a significant metabolite of theophylline in the newborn).

Maintenance dose: Oral, I.V.: 5 mg/kg/day as caffeine citrate (2.5 mg/kg/day as caffeine base) once daily starting 24 hours after the loading dose. Maintenance dose is adjusted based on patient's response (efficacy and adverse effects), and serum caffeine concentrations.

Dosage Forms

Injection: 20 mg/mL as caffeine citrate [equivalent to 10 mg/mL caffeine base] (3 mL)

Solution, oral: 20 mg/mL as caffeine citrate [equivalent to 10 mg/mL caffeine base] (3 mL)

caffeine, hydrocodone, chlorpheniramine, phenylephrine, and acetaminophen *see* hydrocodone, chlorpheniramine, phenylephrine, acetaminophen, and caffeine *on page 332*

caffeine, orphenadrine, and aspirin *see* orphenadrine, aspirin, and caffeine *on page 480*

Caladryl® Spray *(Discontinued) see page 814*

Calan® [US/Can] *see* verapamil *on page 675*

Calan® SR [US] *see* verapamil *on page 675*

Calbon® [US] *see* calcium lactate *on page 108*

Cal Carb-HD® [US-OTC] *see* calcium carbonate *on page 104*

Calcibind® [US/Can] *see* cellulose sodium phosphate *on page 127*

Calci-Chew™ [US-OTC] *see* calcium carbonate *on next page*

Calciday-667® *(Discontinued)* *see page 814*

calcifediol (kal si fe DYE ole)
Synonyms 25-D$_3$; 25-hydroxycholecalciferol; 25-hydroxyvitamin D$_3$
U.S./Canadian Brand Names Calderol® [US/Can]
Therapeutic Category Vitamin D Analog
Use Treatment and management of metabolic bone disease associated with chronic renal failure
Usual Dosage Hepatic osteodystrophy: Oral:
Infants: 5-7 mcg/kg/day
Children and Adults: 20-100 mcg/day or every other day; titrate to obtain normal serum calcium/phosphate levels
Dosage Forms Capsule: 20 mcg, 50 mcg

Calciferol™ [US] *see* ergocalciferol *on page 232*

Calcijex™ [US] *see* calcitriol *on next page*

Calcimar® *(Discontinued)* *see page 814*

Calcimar® [Can] *see* calcitonin *on this page*

Calci-Mix™ [US-OTC] *see* calcium carbonate *on next page*

Calcionate® [US-OTC] *see* calcium glubionate *on page 106*

Calciparine® Injection *(Discontinued)* *see page 814*

calcipotriene (kal si POE try een)
U.S./Canadian Brand Names Dovonex® [US]
Therapeutic Category Antipsoriatic Agent
Use Treatment of plaque psoriasis
Usual Dosage Topical: Apply to skin lesions twice daily
Dosage Forms
Cream: 0.005% (30 g, 60 g, 100 g)
Ointment: 0.005% (30 g, 60 g, 100 g)
Solution, topical: 0.005% (60 mL)

Calciquid® [US-OTC] *see* calcium glubionate *on page 106*

calcitonin (kal si TOE nin)
Synonyms calcitonin (salmon)
U.S./Canadian Brand Names Calcimar® [Can]; Caltine® [Can]; Miacalcin® [US/Can]
Therapeutic Category Polypeptide Hormone
Use
Calcitonin (salmon): Treatment of Paget's disease of bone and as adjunctive therapy for hypercalcemia; also used in postmenopausal osteoporosis and osteogenesis imperfecta
Calcitonin (human): Treatment of Paget's disease of bone
Usual Dosage
Children: Dosage not established
Adults:
Paget's disease: Salmon calcitonin:
I.M., S.C.: 100 units/day to start, 50 units/day or 50-100 units every 1-3 days maintenance dose
Human calcitonin: S.C.: Initial: 0.5 mg/day (maximum: 0.5 mg twice daily); maintenance: 0.5 mg 2-3 times/week or 0.25 mg/day
Hypercalcemia: Initial: Salmon calcitonin: I.M., S.C.: 4 units/kg every 12 hours; may increase up to 8 units/kg every 12 hours to a maximum of every 6 hours
(Continued)

calcitonin *(Continued)*

Osteogenesis imperfecta: Salmon calcitonin: I.M., S.C.: 2 units/kg 3 times/week
Postmenopausal osteoporosis: Salmon calcitonin:
I.M., S.C.: 100 units/day
Intranasal: 200 units (1 spray)/day

Dosage Forms
Injection, salmon calcitonin: 200 units/mL (2 mL)
Nasal spray, salmon calcitonin (Miacalcin®): 200 units/activation (0.09 mL/dose) [glass bottle with pump] (2 mL)

calcitonin (salmon) *see* calcitonin *on previous page*

Cal-Citrate® 250 [US-OTC] *see* calcium citrate *on page 106*

calcitriol (kal si TRYE ole)

Synonyms 1,25 dihydroxycholecalciferol
U.S./Canadian Brand Names Calcijex™ [US]; Rocaltrol® [US/Can]
Therapeutic Category Vitamin D Analog
Use Management of hypocalcemia in patients on chronic renal dialysis; reduce elevated parathyroid hormone levels
Unlabeled uses: Decrease severity of psoriatic lesions in psoriatic vulgaris; vitamin D resistant rickets
Usual Dosage Individualize dosage to maintain calcium levels of 9-10 mg/dL
Renal failure: Oral:
Children: Initial: 15 ng/kg/day; maintenance: 30-60 ng/kg/day
Adults: 0.25 mcg/day or every other day (may require 0.5-1 mcg/day)
Unlabeled dose:
Renal failure: I.V.: Adults: 0.5 mcg (0.01 mcg/kg) 3 times/week; most doses in the range of 0.5-3 mcg (0.01-0.05 mcg/kg) 3 times/week
Hypoparathyroidism/pseudohypoparathyroidism: Oral:
Children 1-5 years: 0.25-0.75 mcg/day
Children >6 years and Adults: 0.5-2 mcg/day
Dosage Forms
Capsule: 0.25 mcg, 0.5 mcg
Injection: 1 mcg/mL (1 mL); 2 mcg/mL (1 mL)
Solution, oral: 1 mcg/mL

calcium acetate (KAL see um AS e tate)

U.S./Canadian Brand Names PhosLo® [US]
Therapeutic Category Electrolyte Supplement, Oral
Use Control of hyperphosphatemia in end-stage renal failure and does not promote aluminum absorption
Usual Dosage Adults: Oral: 2 tablets with each meal; dosage may be increased to bring serum phosphate value to <6 mg/dL; most patients require 3-4 tablets with each meal
Dosage Forms Elemental calcium listed in brackets:
Capsule (PhosLo®): 333.5 mg [84.5 mg]; 667 mg [169 mg]
Gelcap (PhosLo®): 667 mg [169 mg]
Injection: 0.5 mEq calcium/mL [calcium acetate/mL 39.55 mg] (10 mL, 50 mL, 100 mL)

calcium carbonate (KAL see um KAR bun ate)

U.S./Canadian Brand Names Alka-Mints® [US-OTC]; Amitone® [US-OTC]; Apo®-Cal [Can]; Cal Carb-HD® [US-OTC]; Calci-Chew™ [US-OTC]; Calci-Mix™ [US-OTC]; Caltrate® 600 [US/Can]; Chooz® [US-OTC]; Florical® [US-OTC]; Mallamint® [US-OTC]; Nephro-Calci® [US-OTC]; Os-Cal® 500 [US/Can]; Oyst-Cal 500 [US-OTC]; Oystercal® 500 [US]; Rolaids® Calcium Rich [US-OTC]; Tums® E-X Extra Strength Tablet [US-OTC]; Tums® Ultra [US-OTC]; Tums® [US-OTC]
Therapeutic Category Antacid; Electrolyte Supplement, Oral
Use Treatment and prevention of calcium depletion; relief of acid indigestion, heartburn

Usual Dosage Dosage is in terms of elemental calcium
Recommended daily allowance (RDA): Oral:
<6 months: 360 mg/day
6-12 months: 540 mg/day
1-10 years: 800 mg/day
10-18 years: 1200 mg/day
Adults: 800 mg/day
Hypocalcemia (dose depends on clinical condition and serum calcium level):
Children: 20-65 mg/kg/day in 4 divided doses
Adults: 1-2 g or more per day
Dosage Forms Elemental calcium listed in brackets:
Capsule: 1500 mg [600 mg]
Calci-Mix™: 1250 mg [500 mg]
Florical®: 364 mg [145.6 mg] with sodium fluoride 8.3 mg
Powder (Cal Carb-HD®): 6.5 g/packet [2.6 g]
Suspension, oral: 1250 mg/5 mL [500 mg]
Tablet: 650 mg [260 mg], 1500 mg [600 mg]
Caltrate® 600, Nephro-Calci®: 1500 mg [600 mg]
Florical®: 364 mg [145.6 mg] with sodium fluoride 8.3 mg
Os-Cal® 500, Oyst-Cal 500, Oystercal® 500: 1250 mg [500 mg]
Tablet, chewable:
Alka-Mints®: 850 mg [340 mg]
Amitone®: 350 mg [140 mg]
Calci-Chew™, Os-Cal® 500: 1.25 g [500 mg]
Chooz®, Dicarbosil®, Tums®: 500 mg [200 mg]
Mallamint®: 420 mg [168 mg]
Rolaids® Calcium Rich: 550 mg [220 mg]
Tums® E-X Extra Strength: 750 mg [300 mg]
Tums® Ultra®: 1000 mg [400 mg]

calcium carbonate and magnesium hydroxide
(KAL see um KAR bun ate & mag NEE zhum hye DROKS ide)
U.S./Canadian Brand Names Mylanta® Gelcaps® [US-OTC]; Mylanta® Tablets [US-OTC]; Mylanta® Ultra Tablet [US-OTC]
Therapeutic Category Antacid
Use Hyperacidity
Usual Dosage Adults: Oral: 2-4 Gelcaps® as needed
Dosage Forms
Gelcap (Mylanta® Gelcaps®): Calcium carbonate 550 mg and magnesium hydroxide 125 mg
Tablet, chewable:
Mylanta®: Calcium carbonate 350 mg and magnesium hydroxide 150 mg
Mylanta® Ultra: Calcium carbonate 700 mg and magnesium hydroxide 300 mg

calcium carbonate and simethicone
(KAL see um KAR bun ate & sye METH i kone)
Synonyms simethicone and calcium carbonate
U.S./Canadian Brand Names Titralac® Plus Liquid [US-OTC]
Therapeutic Category Antacid; Antiflatulent
Use Relief of acid indigestion, heartburn, peptic esophagitis, hiatal hernia, and gas
Usual Dosage Oral: 0.5-2 g 4-6 times/day
Dosage Forms Elemental calcium listed in brackets
Liquid: Calcium carbonate 500 mg [200 mg] and simethicone 20 mg per 5 mL

calcium chloride (KAL see um KLOR ide)

Therapeutic Category Electrolyte Supplement, Oral

Use Emergency treatment of hypocalcemic tetany; treatment of hypermagnesemia; cardiac disturbances of hyperkalemia, hypocalcemia or calcium channel blocking agent toxicity

Usual Dosage I.V.:

Cardiac arrest in the presence of hyperkalemia or hypocalcemia, magnesium toxicity, or calcium antagonist toxicity:

Infants and Children: 10-20 mg/kg; may repeat in 10 minutes if necessary

Adults: 1.5-4 mg/kg/dose or 2.5-5 mL/dose every 10 minutes

Hypocalcemia:

Infants and Children: 10-20 mg/kg/dose, repeat every 4-6 hours if needed

Adults: 500 mg to 1 g at 1- to 3-day intervals

Exchange transfusion: 0.45 mEq after each 100 mL of blood exchanged I.V.

Hypocalcemia secondary to citrated blood transfusion: Administer 0.45 mEq **elemental** calcium for each 100 mL citrated blood infused

Tetany:

Infants and Children: 10 mg/kg over 5-10 minutes; may repeat after 6 hours or follow with an infusion with a maximum dose of 200 mg/kg/day

Adults: 1 g over 10-30 minutes; may repeat after 6 hours

Dosage Forms Elemental calcium listed in brackets:

Injection: 10% = 100 mg/mL [27.2 mg/mL, 1.36 mEq/mL] (10 mL)

calcium citrate (KAL see um SIT rate)

U.S./Canadian Brand Names Cal-Citrate® 250 [US-OTC]; Citracal® [US-OTC]

Therapeutic Category Electrolyte Supplement, Oral

Use Adjunct in prevention of postmenopausal osteoporosis, treatment and prevention of calcium depletion

Usual Dosage Oral (dosage is in terms of elemental calcium): Adults: Oral: 1-2 g/day

Recommended daily allowance (RDA):

<6 months: 360 mg/day

6-12 months: 540 mg/day

1-10 years: 800 mg/day

10-18 years: 1200 mg/day

Adults: 800 mg/day

Dosage Forms Elemental calcium listed in brackets

Tablet: 950 mg [200 mg]

Cal-Citrate®: 250 mg [100% calcium citrate]

Tablet, effervescent: 2376 mg [500 mg]

Calcium Disodium Versenate® [US] *see* edetate calcium disodium *on page 222*

calcium edta *see* edetate calcium disodium *on page 222*

calcium glubionate (KAL see um gloo BYE oh nate)

U.S./Canadian Brand Names Calcionate® [US-OTC]; Calciquid® [US-OTC]

Therapeutic Category Electrolyte Supplement, Oral

Use Treatment and prevention of calcium depletion

Usual Dosage Oral (syrup is a hyperosmolar solution; dosage is in terms of calcium glubionate):

Neonatal hypocalcemia: 1200 mg/kg/day in 4-6 divided doses

Maintenance: Infants and Children: 600-2000 mg/kg/day in 4 divided doses up to a maximum of 9 g/day .

Adults: 6-18 g/day in divided doses

Recommended daily allowance (RDA):

<6 months: 360 mg/day

6-12 months: 540 mg/day

1-10 years: 800 mg/day
10-18 years: 1200 mg/day
Adults: 800 mg/day
Dosage Forms Elemental calcium listed in brackets:
Syrup: 1.8 g/5 mL [115 mg/5 mL] (480 mL)

calcium gluceptate (KAL see um gloo SEP tate)

Therapeutic Category Electrolyte Supplement, Oral
Use Emergency treatment of hypocalcemia; treatment of hypermagnesemia; cardiac disturbances of hyperkalemia, hypocalcemia, or calcium channel blocker toxicity
Usual Dosage I.V.:
Cardiac resuscitation in the presence of hypocalcemia, hyperkalemia, or calcium channel blocker toxicity:
Children: 110 mg/kg/dose or 0.5 mL/kg/dose every 10 minutes
Adults: 5 mL every 10 minutes
Hypocalcemia:
Children: 200-500 mg/kg/day divided every 6 hours
Adults: 500 mg to 1.1 g/dose as needed
Exchange transfusion: 0.45 mEq (0.5 mL) after each 100 mL of blood exchanged
After citrated blood administration: Children and Adults: 0.4 mEq/100 mL blood infused
Dosage Forms Elemental calcium listed in brackets:
Injection: 220 mg/mL [18 mg/mL, 0.9 mEq/mL] (5 mL)

calcium gluconate (KAL see um GLOO koe nate)

U.S./Canadian Brand Names Calfort® [US]; Cal-G® [US]
Therapeutic Category Electrolyte Supplement, Oral
Use Treatment and prevention of hypocalcemia, hypermagnesemia, cardiac disturbances of hyperkalemia, hypocalcemia, or calcium channel blocker toxicity
Usual Dosage Dosage is in terms of elemental calcium
Recommended daily allowance (RDA):
<6 months: 360 mg/day
6-12 months: 540 mg/day
1-10 years: 800 mg/day
10-18 years: 1200 mg/day
Adults: 800 mg/day
Calcium gluconate electrolyte requirement in newborn period:
Premature: 200-1000 mg/kg/24 hours
Term:
0-24 hours: 0-500 mg/kg/24 hours
24-48 hours: 200-500 mg/kg/24 hours
48-72 hours: 200-600 mg/kg/24 hours
>3 days: 200-800 mg/kg/24 hours
Hypocalcemia:
I.V.:
Infants and Children: 200-1000 mg/kg/day as a continuous infusion or in 4 divided doses
Adults: 2-15 g/24 hours as a continuous infusion or in divided doses
Oral:
Children: 200-500 mg/kg/day divided every 6 hours
Adults: 500 mg to 2 g 2-4 times/day
Calcium antagonist toxicity, magnesium intoxication; cardiac arrest in the presence of hyperkalemia or hypocalcemia: I.V.:
Infants and Children: 100 mg/kg/dose
Adults: 1-3 g
Tetany: I.V.: doses or as an infusion
Infants and Children: 100-200 mg/kg/dose over 5-10 minutes; may repeat after 6 hours or follow with an infusion of 500 mg/kg/day
Adults: 1-3 g may be administered until therapeutic response occurs
(Continued)

107

calcium gluconate *(Continued)*

Cardiac resuscitation: I.V.:
Infants and Children: 100 mg/kg/dose (1 mL/kg/dose) every 10 minutes
Adults: 500-800 mg/dose (5-8 mL) every 10 minutes
Hypocalcemia secondary to citrated blood infusion; administer 0.45 mEq **elemental** calcium for each 100 mL citrated blood infused
Exchange transfusion:
Adults: 300 mg/100 mL of citrated blood exchanged
Maintenance electrolyte requirements for total parenteral nutrition: I.V.: Daily requirements: Adults: 10-20 mEq/1000 kcals/24 hours
Dosage Forms Elemental calcium listed in brackets:
Injection: 10% = 100 mg/mL [9 mg/mL] (10 mL, 50 mL, 100 mL, 200 mL)
Tablet: 500 mg [45 mg], 650 mg [58.5 mg], 975 mg [87.75 mg], 1 g [90 mg]

calcium lactate (KAL see um LAK tate)

U.S./Canadian Brand Names Calbon® [US]; Cal-Lac® [US]; Ridactate® [US]
Therapeutic Category Electrolyte Supplement, Oral
Use Treatment and prevention of calcium depletion
Usual Dosage Oral:
Infants: 400-500 mg/kg/day divided every 4-6 hours
Children: 500 mg/kg/day divided every 6-8 hours; maximum daily dose: 9 g
Adults: 1.5-3 g divided every 8 hours
Dosage Forms Elemental calcium listed in brackets
Capsule: 500 mg [90 mg]
Tablet: 325 mg [42.25 mg], 650 mg [84.5 mg]

calcium pantothenate *see* pantothenic acid *on page 491*

calcium phosphate (dibasic) (KAL see um FOS fate dye BAY sik)

Synonyms dicalcium phosphate
U.S./Canadian Brand Names Posture® [US-OTC]
Therapeutic Category Electrolyte Supplement, Oral
Use Adjunct in prevention of postmenopausal osteoporosis, treatment and prevention of calcium depletion
Usual Dosage Oral:
Children: 45-65 mg/kg/day
Adults: 1-2 g/day (doses in g of elemental calcium)
Dosage Forms Elemental calcium listed in brackets
Tablet, sugar free: 1565.2 mg [600 mg]

calcium polycarbophil (KAL see um pol i KAR boe fil)

U.S./Canadian Brand Names Equalactin® Chewable Tablet [US-OTC]; Fiberall® Chewable Tablet [US-OTC]; FiberCon® Tablet [US-OTC]; Fiber-Lax® Tablet [US-OTC]; Mitrolan® Chewable Tablet [US-OTC]
Therapeutic Category Gastrointestinal Agent, Miscellaneous; Laxative
Use Treatment of constipation or diarrhea by restoring a more normal moisture level and providing bulk in the patient's intestinal tract; calcium polycarbophil is supplied as the approved substitute whenever a bulk-forming laxative is ordered in a tablet, capsule, wafer, or other oral solid dosage form
Usual Dosage Oral:
Children:
2-6 years: 500 mg 1-2 times/day, up to 1.5 g/day
6-12 years: 500 mg 1-3 times/day, up to 3 g/day
Adults: 1 g 4 times/day, up to 6 g/day
Dosage Forms
Tablet (FiberCon®, Fiber-Lax®): 625 mg calcium polycarbophil [500 mg polycarbophil] [sodium free]

Tablet, chewable (Equalactin®, Fiberall®, Mitrolan®): 500 mg polycarbophil

CaldeCORT® Anti-Itch Spray [US] *see* hydrocortisone (topical) *on page 334*

CaldeCORT® [US-OTC] *see* hydrocortisone (topical) *on page 334*

Calderol® [US/Can] *see* calcifediol *on page 103*

calfactant (cal FAC tant)
   U.S./Canadian Brand Names Infasurf® [US]
   Therapeutic Category Lung Surfactant
   Use Prevention of respiratory distress syndrome (RDS) in premature infants at high risk for RDS and for the treatment ("rescue") of premature infants who develop RDS; decreases the incidence of RDS, mortality due to RDS, and air leaks associated with RDS
   Usual Dosage Should be administered intratracheally through a side-port adapter into the endotracheal tube; two attendants, one to instill the suspension, the other to monitor the patient and assist in positioning, facilitate the dosing; the dose (3 mL/kg) should be administered in two aliquots of 1.5 mL/kg each; after each aliquot is instilled, the infant should be positioned with either the right or the left side dependent; administration is made while ventilation is continued over 20-30 breaths for each aliquot, with small bursts timed only during the inspiratory cycles; a pause followed by evaluation of the respiratory status and repositioning should separate the two aliquots
   Dosage Forms Suspension, intratracheal: 6 mL (35 mg/mL)

Calfort® [US] *see* calcium gluconate *on page 107*

Cal-G® [US] *see* calcium gluconate *on page 107*

Cal-Lac® [US] *see* calcium lactate *on previous page*

Calm-X® Oral [US-OTC] *see* dimenhydrinate *on page 200*

Calmylin with Codeine [Can] *see* guaifenesin, pseudoephedrine, and codeine *on page 311*

Calphron® *(Discontinued)* *see page 814*

Cal-Plus® *(Discontinued)* *see page 814*

Caltine® [Can] *see* calcitonin *on page 103*

Caltrate® 600 [US/Can] *see* calcium carbonate *on page 104*

Caltrate Jr.® *(Discontinued)* *see page 814*

Camalox® Suspension & Tablet *(Discontinued)* *see page 814*

Campath® [US] *see* alemtuzumab *on page 21*

campath-1H *see* alemtuzumab *on page 21*

Campho-Phenique® [US-OTC] *see* camphor and phenol *on this page*

camphor and phenol (KAM for & FEE nole)
   U.S./Canadian Brand Names Campho-Phenique® [US-OTC]
   Therapeutic Category Topical Skin Product
   Use Relief of pain and for minor infections
   Usual Dosage Topical: Apply as needed
   Dosage Forms Liquid, topical: Camphor 10.8% and phenol 4.7%

camphorated tincture of opium *see* paregoric *on page 493*

camphor, menthol, and phenol (KAM for, MEN thol, & FEE nole)
   U.S./Canadian Brand Names Sarna® [US-OTC]
   Therapeutic Category Topical Skin Product
   Use Relief of dry, itching skin
   Usual Dosage Topical: Apply as needed for dry skin
   (Continued)

camphor, menthol, and phenol *(Continued)*

Dosage Forms Lotion, topical: Camphor 0.5%, menthol 0.5%, and phenol 0.5% in emollient base (240 mL)

Camptosar® **[US/Can]** *see* irinotecan *on page 359*

Canasa™ **[US]** *see* mesalamine *on page 411*

Cancidas® **[US]** *see* caspofungin *on page 119*

candesartan *(kan de SAR tan)*
U.S./Canadian Brand Names Atacand® [US/Can]
Therapeutic Category Angiotensin II Receptor Antagonist
Use Treatment of hypertension; may be used alone or in combination with other antihypertensive agents
Usual Dosage Adults: Oral: Dosage must be individualized; blood pressure response is dose-related over the range of 2-32 mg; the usual recommended starting dose of 16 mg once daily when it is used as monotherapy in patients who are not volume depleted; it can be administered once or twice daily with total daily doses ranging from 8-32 mg; larger doses do not appear to have a greater effect and there is relatively little experience with such doses; most of the antihypertensive effect is present within 2 weeks and maximal blood pressure reduction is generally obtained within 4-6 weeks of treatment
Dosage Forms Tablet, as cilexetil: 4 mg, 8 mg, 16 mg, 32 mg

candesartan and hydrochlorothiazide
(kan de SAR tan & hye droe klor oh THYE a zide)
U.S./Canadian Brand Names Atacand HCT™ [US]
Therapeutic Category Antihypertensive Agent, Combination
Use Treatment of hypertension; combination product should not be used for initial therapy
Usual Dosage Adults: Oral: Replacement therapy: Combination product can be substituted for individual agents; maximum therapeutic effect would be expected within 4 weeks
Usual dosage range:
  Candesartan: 8-32 mg/day, given once daily or twice daily in divided doses
  Hydrochlorothiazide: 12.5-50 mg once daily
Dosage Forms
  Tablet:
    Atacand HCT™ 16-12.5: Candesartan 16 mg and hydrochlorothiazide 12.5 mg
    Atacand HCT™ 32-12.5: Candesartan 32 mg and hydrochlorothiazide 12.5 mg

Candida albicans (Monilia) (KAN dee da AL bi kans mo NIL ya)
Synonyms *Monilia* skin test
U.S./Canadian Brand Names Dermatophytin-O [US]
Therapeutic Category Diagnostic Agent
Use Screen for detection of nonresponsiveness to antigens in immunocompromised individuals
Usual Dosage Intradermal: 0.1 mL, examine reaction site in 24-48 hours; induration of ≥5 mm in diameter is a positive reaction
Dosage Forms
  Injection, intradermal: 1:100 (5 mL)
  Injection, scratch: 1:10 (5 mL)

Candistatin® **[Can]** *see* nystatin *on page 473*

Canesten® **Topical [Can]** *see* clotrimazole *on page 156*

Canesten® **Vaginal [Can]** *see* clotrimazole *on page 156*

Cantharone® *(Discontinued) see page 814*

Cantharone Plus® *(Discontinued) see page 814*

Cantil® **[US/Can]** *see* mepenzolate *on page 408*

Capastat® **Sulfate [US]** *see* capreomycin *on this page*

capecitabine (kap eh SITE a bean)
U.S./Canadian Brand Names Xeloda® [US/Can]
Therapeutic Category Antineoplastic Agent, Antimetabolite
Use Treatment of patients with metastatic colorectal cancer. Treatment of patients with metastatic breast cancer resistant to both paclitaxel and an anthracycline-containing chemotherapy regimen or resistant to paclitaxel and for whom further anthracycline therapy is not indicated (eg, patients who have received cumulative doses of 400 mg/m^2 of doxorubicin or doxorubicin equivalents). Resistance is defined as progressive disease while on treatment, with or without an initial response, or relapse within 6 months of completing treatment with an anthracycline-containing adjuvant regimen.
Usual Dosage Refer to individual protocols.
2510 mg/m^2 days 1-14 every 3 weeks
1657 mg/m^2 days 1-14 every 3 weeks
1331 mg/m^2/day
Dosage Forms Tablet: 150 mg, 500 mg

Capex™ **[US/Can]** *see* fluocinolone *on page 276*

Capital® **and Codeine [US]** *see* acetaminophen and codeine *on page 5*

Capitrol® **[US/Can]** *see* chloroxine *on page 137*

Capoten® **[US/Can]** *see* captopril *on next page*

Capozide® **[US/Can]** *see* captopril and hydrochlorothiazide *on next page*

capreomycin (kap ree oh MYE sin)
U.S./Canadian Brand Names Capastat® Sulfate [US]
Therapeutic Category Antibiotic, Miscellaneous
Use In conjunction with at least one other antituberculosis agent in the treatment of tuberculosis
Usual Dosage Adults: I.M.: 15 mg/kg/day up to 1 g/day for 60-120 days
Dosage Forms Injection, as sulfate: 100 mg/mL (10 mL)

Caprex® **[US]** *see* capsaicin *on this page*

Caprex Plus® **[US]** *see* capsaicin *on this page*

Capsagel® **[US]** *see* capsaicin *on this page*

Capsagel Extra Strength® **[US]** *see* capsaicin *on this page*

Capsagel Maximum Strength® **[US]** *see* capsaicin *on this page*

Capsagesic-HP Arthritis Relief® **[US]** *see* capsaicin *on this page*

capsaicin (kap SAY sin)
U.S./Canadian Brand Names Antiphogistine Rub A-535 Capsaicin [Can]; Arth Dr® [US]; Arthricare Hand & Body® [US]; Born Again Super Pain Relieving® [US]; Caprex® [US]; Caprex Plus® [US]; Capsagel® [US]; Capsagel Extra Strength® [US]; Capsagel Maximum Strength® [US]; Capsagesic-HP Arthritis Relief® [US]; Capsin® [US-OTC]; D-Care Circulation Stimulator® [US]; Double Cap® [US]; Icy Hot Arthritis Therapy® [US]; Pain Enz® [US]; Pharmacist's Capsaicin® [US]; Rid-A-Pain® [US]; Rid-A-Pain-HP® [US]; Sloan's Liniment® [US]; Sportsmed® [US]; Theragen® [US]; Theragen HP® [US]; Therapatch Warm® [US]; Trixaicin® [US]; Trixaicin HP® [US]; Zostrix® [US/Can]; Zostrix High Potency® [US]; Zostrix®-HP [US/Can]; Zostrix Sports® [US]
Therapeutic Category Analgesic, Topical
Use FDA approved for the topical treatment of pain associated with postherpetic neuralgia, rheumatoid arthritis, osteoarthritis, diabetic neuropathy, and postsurgical pain
Unlabeled uses: Treatment of pain associated with psoriasis, chronic neuralgias unresponsive to other forms of therapy, and intractable pruritus
(Continued)

capsaicin *(Continued)*

Usual Dosage Children >2 years and Adults: Topical: Apply to area up to 3-4 times/day only

Dosage Forms
Cream, topical: 0.025% (45 g, 90 g); 0.25% (28 g); 0.075% (30 g, 60 g)
Gel, topical: 0.025% (15 g, 30 g)
Lotion, topical: 0.025% (59 mL); 0.075% (59 mL)
Roll-on, topical: 0.075% (60 mL)

Capsin® [US-OTC] *see* capsaicin *on previous page*

captopril *(KAP toe pril)*

U.S./Canadian Brand Names Alti-Captopril [Can]; Apo®-Capto [Can]; Capoten® [US/Can]; Gen-Captopril [Can]; Novo-Captopril [Can]; Nu-Capto® [Can]; PMS-Captopril® [Can]

Therapeutic Category Angiotensin-Converting Enzyme (ACE) Inhibitor

Use Management of hypertension and treatment of congestive heart failure; in postmyocardial infarction, improves survival in clinically stable patients with left ventricular dysfunction

Usual Dosage Note: Dosage must be titrated according to patient's response; use lowest effective dose. Oral:

Infants: Initial: 0.15-0.3 mg/kg/dose; titrate dose upward to maximum of 6 mg/kg/day in 1-4 divided doses; usual required dose: 2.5-6 mg/kg/day

Children: Initial: 0.5 mg/kg/dose; titrate upward to maximum of 6 mg/kg/day in 2-4 divided doses

Older Children: Initial: 6.25-12.5 mg/dose every 12-24 hours; titrate upward to maximum of 6 mg/kg/day

Adolescents and Adults: Initial: 12.5-25 mg/dose administered every 8-12 hours; increase by 25 mg/dose to maximum of 450 mg/day

Dosage Forms Tablet: 12.5 mg, 25 mg, 50 mg, 100 mg

captopril and hydrochlorothiazide

(KAP toe pril & hye droe klor oh THYE a zide)

Synonyms hydrochlorothiazide and captopril

U.S./Canadian Brand Names Capozide® [US/Can]

Therapeutic Category Antihypertensive Agent, Combination

Use Management of hypertension and treatment of congestive heart failure

Usual Dosage Adults: Oral:
Hypertension: Initial: 25 mg 2-3 times/day; may increase at 1- to 2-week intervals up to 150 mg 3 times/day (captopril dosages)
Congestive heart failure: 6.25-25 mg 3 times/day (maximum: 450 mg/day) (captopril dosages)

Dosage Forms
Tablet:
25/15: Captopril 25 mg and hydrochlorothiazide 15 mg
25/25: Captopril 25 mg and hydrochlorothiazide 25 mg
50/15: Captopril 50 mg and hydrochlorothiazide 15 mg
50/25: Captopril 50 mg and hydrochlorothiazide 25 mg

Capzasin-P® *(Discontinued) see page 814*

Carac™ [US] *see* fluorouracil *on page 279*

Carafate® [US] *see* sucralfate *on page 609*

carbachol *(KAR ba kole)*

Synonyms carbacholine; carbamylcholine chloride

U.S./Canadian Brand Names Carbastat® [US/Can]; Carboptic® [US]; Isopto® Carbachol [US/Can]; Miostat® Intraocular [US/Can]

Therapeutic Category Cholinergic Agent

Use Lower intraocular pressure in the treatment of glaucoma; to cause miosis during surgery

Usual Dosage Adults:

Intraocular: 0.5 mL instilled into anterior chamber before or after securing sutures

Ophthalmic: Instill 1-2 drops up to 4 times/day

Dosage Forms

Solution, intraocular (Carbastat®, Miostat®): 0.01% (1.5 mL)

Solution, ophthalmic:

Carboptic®: 3% (15 mL)

Isopto® Carbachol: 0.75% (15 mL, 30 mL); 1.5% (15 mL, 30 mL); 2.25% (15 mL); 3% (15 mL, 30 mL)

carbacholine *see* carbachol *on previous page*

carbamazepine (kar ba MAZ e peen)

U.S./Canadian Brand Names Apo®-Carbamazepine [Can]; Carbatrol® [US]; Epitol® [US]; Gen-Carbamazepine CR [Can]; Novo-Carbamaz [Can]; Nu-Carbamazepine® [Can]; PMS-Carbamazepine [Can]; Taro-Carbamazepin [Can]; Tegretol® [US/Can]; Tegretol®-XR [US]

Therapeutic Category Anticonvulsant

Use Prophylaxis of generalized tonic-clonic, partial (especially complex partial), and mixed partial or generalized seizure disorder; may be used to relieve pain in trigeminal neuralgia or diabetic neuropathy; has been used to treat bipolar disorders

Usual Dosage Oral (dosage must be adjusted according to patient's response and serum concentrations):

Children:

<6 years: Initial: 5 mg/kg/day; dosage may be increased every 5-7 days to 10 mg/kg/day; then up to 20 mg/kg/day if necessary; administer in 2-4 divided doses/day

6-12 years: Initial: 100 mg twice daily or 10 mg/kg/day in 2 divided doses; increase by 100 mg/day depending upon response; usual maintenance: 15-30 mg/kg/day in 2-4 divided doses/day; maximum: 1000 mg/24 hours

Children >12 years and Adults: 200 mg twice daily to start, increase by 200 mg/day at weekly intervals until therapeutic levels achieved; usual dose: 800-1200 mg/day in 3-4 divided doses; some patients have required up to 1.6-2.4 g/day

Dosage Forms

Capsule, extended release: 200 mg, 300 mg

Suspension, oral: 100 mg/5 mL (450 mL) [citrus-vanilla flavor]

Tablet: 200 mg

Tablet, chewable: 100 mg

Tablet, extended release: 100 mg, 200 mg, 400 mg

carbamide *see* urea *on page 666*

carbamide peroxide (KAR ba mide per OKS ide)

Synonyms urea peroxide

U.S./Canadian Brand Names Auro® Ear Drops [US-OTC]; Debrox® Otic [US-OTC]; E•R•O Ear [US-OTC]; Gly-Oxide® Oral [US-OTC]; Mollifene® Ear Wax Removing Formula [US-OTC]; Murine® Ear Drops [US-OTC]; Orajel® Perioseptic® [US-OTC]; Proxigel® Oral [US-OTC]

Therapeutic Category Anti-infective Agent, Oral; Otic Agent, Ceruminolytic

Use

Oral: Relief of minor inflammation of gums, oral mucosal surfaces and lips including canker sores and dental irritation; adjunct in oral hygiene

Otic: Emulsify and disperse ear wax

Usual Dosage Children >12 years and Adults:

Oral: Apply several drops undiluted to affected area of the mouth 4 times/day and at bedtime for up to 7 days, expectorate after 2-3 minutes; as an adjunct to oral hygiene

(Continued)

113

carbamide peroxide *(Continued)*

after brushing, swish 10 drops for 2-3 minutes, then expectorate; gel: massage on affected area 4 times/day

Otic: Instill 5-10 drops twice daily for up to 4 days; keep drops in ear for several minutes by keeping head tilted or placing cotton in ear

Dosage Forms
Gel, oral (Proxigel®): 10% (34 g)
Solution, oral:
Gly-Oxide®: 10% [in glycerin] (15 mL, 60 mL)
Orajel® Perioseptic®: 15% [in glycerin] (13.3 mL)
Solution, otic (Auro® Ear Drops, Debrox®, E•R•O Ear, Mollifene® Ear Wax Removing, Murine® Ear Drops): 6.5% [in glycerin] (15 mL, 30 mL)

carbamylcholine chloride *see* carbachol *on page 112*

Carbastat® [US/Can] *see* carbachol *on page 112*

Carbatrol® [US] *see* carbamazepine *on previous page*

Carbaxefed DM RF [US] *see* carbinoxamine, pseudoephedrine, and dextromethorphan *on next page*

Carbaxefed RF [US] *see* carbinoxamine and pseudoephedrine *on next page*

carbenicillin (kar ben i SIL in)

Synonyms carindacillin
U.S./Canadian Brand Names Geocillin® [US]
Therapeutic Category Penicillin
Use Treatment of urinary tract infections, asymptomatic bacteriuria, or prostatitis caused by susceptible strains of *Pseudomonas aeruginosa*, *E. coli*, indole-positive *Proteus*, and *Enterobacter*
Usual Dosage Oral:
Children: 30-50 mg/kg/day divided every 6 hours; maximum dose: 2-3 g/day
Adults: 1-2 tablets every 6 hours
Dosage Forms Tablet, film coated, as indanyl sodium ester: 382 mg [base]

carbetocin *(Canada only)* (kar BE toe sin)

U.S./Canadian Brand Names Duratocin™ [Can]
Therapeutic Category Uteronic Agent
Use For the prevention of uterine atony and postpartum hemorrhage following elective cesarean section under epidural or spinal anesthesia.
Usual Dosage A single I.V. dose of 100 mcg (1 mL) is administered by bolus injection, over 1 minute, only when delivery of the infant has been completed by cesarean section under epidural anesthetic. Carbetocin can be administered either before or after delivery of the placenta
Dosage Forms Injection: 1 mcg/mL (1 mL)

carbidopa (kar bi DOE pa)

U.S./Canadian Brand Names Lodosyn® [US]
Therapeutic Category Anti-Parkinson's Agent; Dopaminergic Agent (Anti-Parkinson's)
Use With levodopa in the treatment of parkinsonism to enable a lower dosage of the latter to be used and a more rapid response to be obtained, and to decrease side-effects; for details of administration and dosage
Usual Dosage Adults: Oral: 70-100 mg/day; maximum daily dose: 200 mg
Dosage Forms Tablet: 25 mg

carbidopa and levodopa *see* levodopa and carbidopa *on page 380*

carbinoxamine and pseudoephedrine
(kar bi NOKS a meen & soo doe e FED rin)

Synonyms pseudoephedrine and carbinoxamine

U.S./Canadian Brand Names Andehist NR Drops [US]; Carbaxefed RF [US]; Hydro-Tussin™-CBX [US]; Palgic®-DS [US]; Palgic®-D [US]; Rondec® Drops [US]; Rondec® Tablets [US]; Rondec-TR® [US]

Therapeutic Category Antihistamine/Decongestant Combination

Use Temporary relief of nasal congestion, running nose, sneezing, itching of nose or throat, and itchy, watery eyes due to the common cold, hay fever, or other respiratory allergies

Usual Dosage Oral:
Children:
Drops: 1-18 months: 0.25-1 mL 4 times/day
Syrup:
18 months to 6 years: 2.5 mL 3-4 times/day
>6 years: 5 mL 2-4 times/day
Adults:
Liquid: 5 mL 4 times/day
Tablet: 1 tablet 4 times/day

Dosage Forms
Solution, oral drops:
Andehist NR: Carbinoxamine maleate 1 mg and pseudoephedrine hydrochloride 15 mg per mL (30 mL) [alcohol and sugar free; raspberry flavor]
Carbaxefed RF, Rondec®: Carbinoxamine maleate 1 mg and pseudoephedrine hydrochloride 15 mg per mL (30 mL) [alcohol free; contains sodium benzoate; cherry flavor]
Syrup (Hydro-Tussin™-CBX, Palgic® DS): Carbinoxamine maleate 4 mg and pseudoephedrine hydrochloride 15 mg per 5 mL (480 mL) [alcohol and sugar free; strawberry/pineapple flavor]
Tablet (Rondec®): Carbinoxamine maleate 4 mg and pseudoephedrine hydrochloride 60 mg
Tablet, sustained release:
Palgic®-D: Carbinoxamine maleate 8 mg and pseudoephedrine hydrochloride 90 mg
Rondec-TR®: Carbinoxamine maleate 8 mg and pseudoephedrine hydrochloride 120 mg

carbinoxamine, pseudoephedrine, and dextromethorphan
(kar bi NOKS a meen, soo doe e FED rin, & deks troe meth OR fan)

U.S./Canadian Brand Names Andehist DM NR Drops [US]; Carbaxefed DM RF [US]; Rondec®-DM Drops [US]

Therapeutic Category Antihistamine/Decongestant/Antitussive

Use Relief of coughs and upper respiratory symptoms, including nasal congestion, associated with allergy or the common cold

Usual Dosage
Infants: Drops:
1-3 months: $\frac{1}{4}$ mL 4 times/day
3-6 months: $\frac{1}{2}$ mL 4 times/day
6-9 months: $\frac{3}{4}$ mL 4 times/day
9-18 months: 1 mL 4 times/day
Children $1\frac{1}{2}$ to 6 years: Syrup: 2.5 mL 4 times/day
Children >6 years and Adults: Syrup: 5 mL 4 times/day

Dosage Forms Solution, oral drops:
Andehist DM NR: Carbinoxamine maleate 1 mg, pseudoephedrine hydrochloride 15 mg and dextromethorphan hydrobromide 4 mg per mL (30 mL) [alcohol and sugar free; grape flavor]
Carbaxefed DM RF, Rondec® DM: Carbinoxamine maleate 1 mg, pseudoephedrine hydrochloride 15 mg and dextromethorphan hydrobromide 4 mg per mL (30 mL) [alcohol free; grape flavor]

Carbiset® Tablet *(Discontinued)* see page 814

Carbiset-TR® Tablet *(Discontinued)* see page 814

Carbocaine® [US/Can] see mepivacaine on page 409

Carbodec® Syrup *(Discontinued)* see page 814

Carbodec® Tablet *(Discontinued)* see page 814

Carbodec® TR Tablet *(Discontinued)* see page 814

carbol-fuchsin solution (kar bol-FOOK sin soe LOO shun)
Synonyms Castellani paint
Therapeutic Category Antifungal Agent
Use Treatment of superficial mycotic infections
Usual Dosage Topical: Apply to affected area 2-4 times/day
Dosage Forms
Solution, topical: Basic fuchsin 0.3%, boric acid 1%, phenol 4.5%, resorcinol 10%, acetone 5%, and alcohol 10%
Solution, topical, colorless: Boric acid 1%, phenol 4.5%, resorcinol 10%, acetone 5%, and alcohol 10%

carbolic acid see phenol on page 508

Carbolith™ [Can] see lithium on page 388

carboplatin (KAR boe pla tin)
Synonyms CBDCA
U.S./Canadian Brand Names Paraplatin-AQ [Can]; Paraplatin® [US]
Therapeutic Category Antineoplastic Agent
Use Palliative treatment of ovarian carcinoma; also used in the treatment of small cell lung cancer, squamous cell carcinoma of the esophagus; solid tumors of the bladder, cervix and testes; pediatric brain tumor, neuroblastoma
Usual Dosage I.V. (refer to individual protocols):
Children:
Solid tumor: 560 mg/m^2 once every 4 weeks
Brain tumor: 175 mg/m^2 once weekly for 4 weeks with a 2-week recovery period between courses; dose is then adjusted on platelet count and neutrophil count values
Adults: Single agent: 360 mg/m^2 once every 4 weeks; dose is then adjusted on platelet count and neutrophil count values
Dosage Forms Injection, powder for reconstitution: 50 mg, 150 mg, 450 mg

carbopol 940 *(Canada only)* (KAR boe pol nine forty)
U.S./Canadian Brand Names Lacrinorm [Can]
Therapeutic Category Ophthalmic Agent, Miscellaneous
Use Artificial tear
Dosage Forms Gel, ophthalmic: 20 mg (10 g)

carboprost tromethamine (KAR boe prost tro METH a meen)
U.S./Canadian Brand Names Hemabate™ [US/Can]
Therapeutic Category Prostaglandin
Use Termination of pregnancy
Usual Dosage I.M.: Initial: 250 mcg, then 250 mcg at 1½-hour to 3½-hour intervals depending on uterine response; a 500 mcg dose may be administered if uterine response is not adequate after several 250 mcg doses
Dosage Forms Injection: Carboprost 250 mcg and tromethamine 83 mcg per mL (1 mL)

Carboptic® [US] see carbachol on page 112

carbose d see carboxymethylcellulose on next page

carboxymethylcellulose (kar boks ee meth il SEL yoo lose)
　　Synonyms carbose d; carboxymethylcellulose sodium
　　U.S./Canadian Brand Names Cellufresh® [US-OTC]; Celluvisc® [US/Can]
　　Therapeutic Category Ophthalmic Agent, Miscellaneous
　　Use Preservative-free artificial tear substitute
　　Usual Dosage Adults: Ophthalmic: Instill 1-2 drops into eye(s) 3-4 times/day
　　Dosage Forms Solution, ophthalmic, as sodium [preservative free]: 0.5% (0.3 mL); 1%
　　(0.3 mL)

carboxymethylcellulose sodium *see* carboxymethylcellulose *on this page*

Cardem® *(Discontinued) see page 814*

Cardene® **[US]** *see* nicardipine *on page 457*

Cardene® **I.V. [US]** *see* nicardipine *on page 457*

Cardene® **SR [US]** *see* nicardipine *on page 457*

Cardilate® *(Discontinued) see page 814*

Cardio-Green® *(Discontinued) see page 814*

Cardioquin® *(Discontinued) see page 814*

Cardizem® **[US/Can]** *see* diltiazem *on page 199*

Cardizem® **CD [US/Can]** *see* diltiazem *on page 199*

Cardizem® **SR [US/Can]** *see* diltiazem *on page 199*

Cardura® **[US/Can]** *see* doxazosin *on page 213*

Carimune™ **[US]** *see* immune globulin (intravenous) *on page 347*

carindacillin *see* carbenicillin *on page 114*

carisoprodate *see* carisoprodol *on this page*

carisoprodol (kar i soe PROE dole)
　　Synonyms carisoprodate; isobamate
　　U.S./Canadian Brand Names Soma® [US/Can]
　　Therapeutic Category Skeletal Muscle Relaxant
　　Use Skeletal muscle relaxant
　　Usual Dosage Adults: Oral: 350 mg 3-4 times/day; administer last dose at bedtime;
　　compound: 1-2 tablets 4 times/day
　　Dosage Forms Tablet: 350 mg

carisoprodol and aspirin (kar i soe PROE dole & AS pir in)
　　U.S./Canadian Brand Names Soma® Compound [US]
　　Therapeutic Category Skeletal Muscle Relaxant
　　Use Skeletal muscle relaxant
　　Usual Dosage Adults: Oral: 1-2 tablets 4 times/day
　　Dosage Forms Tablet: Carisoprodol 200 mg and aspirin 325 mg

carisoprodol, aspirin, and codeine
　　(kar i soe PROE dole, AS pir in, and KOE deen)
　　U.S./Canadian Brand Names Soma® Compound w/Codeine [US]
　　Therapeutic Category Skeletal Muscle Relaxant
　　Controlled Substance C-III
　　Use Skeletal muscle relaxant
　　Usual Dosage Adults: Oral: 1-2 tablets 4 times/day
　　Dosage Forms Tablet: Carisoprodol 200 mg, aspirin 325 mg, and codeine phosphate 16
　　mg

Carmol® **10 [US-OTC]** *see* urea *on page 666*

Carmol® 20 [US-OTC] *see* urea *on page 666*

Carmol® 40 [US] *see* urea *on page 666*

Carmol® Deep Cleaning [US] *see* urea *on page 666*

Carmol-HC® [US] *see* urea and hydrocortisone *on page 667*

Carmol® Scalp [US] *see* sulfacetamide *on page 610*

Carmol® Scalp Treatment [US] *see* urea *on page 666*

carmustine (kar MUS teen)
Synonyms BCNU
U.S./Canadian Brand Names BiCNU® [US/Can]; Gliadel® [US]
Therapeutic Category Antineoplastic Agent
Use Treatment of brain tumors (glioblastoma, brainstem glioma, medulloblastoma, astrocytoma, ependymoma, and metastatic brain tumors), multiple myeloma, Hodgkin's disease, non-Hodgkin's lymphomas, melanoma, lung cancer, colon cancer
Gliadel®: Adjunct to surgery in patients with recurrent glioblastoma multiforme
Usual Dosage I.V. (refer to individual protocols):
Children: 200-250 mg/m^2 every 4-6 weeks as a single dose
Adults: Usual dosage (per manufacturer labeling): 150-200 mg/m^2 every 6-8 weeks as a single dose or divided into daily injections on 2 successive days
Next dose is to be determined based on hematologic response to the previous dose. Repeat dose should not be administered until circulating blood elements have returned to acceptable levels (leukocytes >4000, platelets >100,000), usually 6 weeks
Adjunct to surgery in patients with recurrent glioblastoma multiforme (Gliadel®): Implantation: Up to 8 wafers may be placed in the resection cavity (total dose 62.6 mg); should the size and shape not accommodate 8 wafers, the maximum number of wafers allowed should be placed
Dosage Forms
Injection, powder for reconstitution: 100 mg/vial [with 3 mL absolute alcohol as diluent]
Wafer (Gliadel®): Carmustine 7.7 mg

Carnation Instant Breakfast® [US-OTC] *see* nutritional formula, enteral/oral *on page 472*

Carnitor® [US/Can] *see* levocarnitine *on page 379*

Caroid® (Discontinued) *see page 814*

Carrington Antifungal [US-OTC] *see* miconazole *on page 427*

carteolol (KAR tee oh lole)
U.S./Canadian Brand Names Cartrol® Oral [US/Can]; Ocupress® Ophthalmic [US/Can]
Therapeutic Category Beta-Adrenergic Blocker
Use Management of hypertension; treatment of increased intraocular pressure
Usual Dosage Adults:
Oral: 2.5 mg as a single daily dose, maintenance dose: 2.5-5 mg once daily
Ophthalmic: 1 drop in eye(s) twice daily
Dosage Forms
Solution, ophthalmic, as hydrochloride (Ocupress®): 1% (5 mL, 10 mL)
Tablet, as hydrochloride (Cartrol®): 2.5 mg, 5 mg

Carter's Little Pills® (Discontinued) *see page 814*

Cartia® XT [US] *see* diltiazem *on page 199*

Cartrol® Oral [US/Can] *see* carteolol *on this page*

carvedilol (KAR ve dil ole)
U.S./Canadian Brand Names Coreg® [US/Can]
Therapeutic Category Beta-Adrenergic Blocker

Use Management of hypertension, congestive heart failure; can be used alone or in combination with other agents, especially thiazide-type diuretics

Unlabeled use: Angina pectoris

Usual Dosage Adults: Oral:

Hypertension: 6.25 mg twice daily; if tolerated, dose should be maintained for 1-2 weeks, then increased to 12.5 mg twice daily; dosage may be increased to a maximum of 25 mg twice daily after 1-2 weeks; reduce dosage if heart rate drops to <55 beats/minute

Congestive heart failure: 3.125 mg twice daily for 2 weeks; if this dose is tolerated, may increase to 6.25 mg twice daily. Double the dose every 2 weeks to the highest dose tolerated by patient. (Prior to initiating therapy, other heart failure medications should be stabilized.)

Maximum recommended dose:

<85 kg: 25 mg twice daily

>85 kg: 50 mg twice daily

Angina pectoris (unlabeled use): 25-50 mg twice daily

Idiopathic cardiomyopathy (unlabeled use): 6.25-25 mg twice daily

Dosage Forms Tablet: 3.125 mg, 6.25 mg, 12.5 mg, 25 mg

casanthranol and docusate *see* docusate and casanthranol *on page 209*

Casodex® [US/Can] *see* bicalutamide *on page 86*

caspofungin (kas poe FUN jin)

Synonyms caspofungin acetate

U.S./Canadian Brand Names Cancidas® [US]

Therapeutic Category Antifungal Agent, Systemic

Use Treatment of invasive *Aspergillus* infection in patients who do not tolerate or do not respond to other antifungal therapies (including amphotericin B, lipid formulations of amphotericin B, or itraconazole); has not been studied as initial therapy for aspergillosis

Usual Dosage I.V.:

Children: Safety and efficacy in pediatric patients have not been established

Adults: *Aspergillus* infection (invasive):

Initial dose: 70 mg infused slowly (over 1 hour)

Subsequent dosing: 50 mg/day (infused over 1 hour)

Duration of treatment should be determined by patient status and clinical response (limited experience beyond 2 weeks of therapy); efficacy of 70 mg/day dose (in patients not responding to 50 mg/day) has not been adequately studied, although this dose appears to be well tolerated

Patients receiving carbamazepine, dexamethasone, efavirenz, nelfinavir, nevirapine, phenytoin, and rifampin (and possibly other enzyme inducers) may require an increased daily dose of caspofungin (70 mg/day) if response to 50 mg/day is inadequate.

Dosage Forms Injection, powder for reconstitution, as acetate: 50 mg, 70 mg

caspofungin acetate *see* caspofungin *on this page*

Castellani paint *see* carbol-fuchsin solution *on page 116*

castor oil (KAS tor oyl)

Synonyms oleum ricini

U.S./Canadian Brand Names Emulsoil® [US-OTC]; Neoloid® [US-OTC]; Purge® [US-OTC]

Therapeutic Category Laxative

Use Preparation for rectal or bowel examination or surgery; rarely used to relieve constipation; also applied to skin as emollient and protectant

Usual Dosage Oral:

Castor oil:

Infants <2 years: 1-5 mL or 15 mL/m^2/dose as a single dose

Children 2-11 years: 5-15 mL as a single dose

(Continued)

castor oil *(Continued)*

Children ≥12 years and Adults: 15-60 mL as a single dose
Emulsified castor oil:
Infants: 2.5-7.5 mL/dose
Children <2 years: 5-15 mL/dose
Children 2-11 years: 7.5-30 mL/dose
Children ≥12 years and Adults: 30-60 mL/dose

Dosage Forms
Emulsion, oral:
Emulsoil®: 95% (63 mL)
Neoloid®: 36.4% (118 mL)
Liquid, oral: 100% (60 mL, 120 mL, 480 mL)
Purge®: 95% (30 mL, 60 mL)

Cataflam® [US/Can] *see* diclofenac *on page 193*

Catapres® [US/Can] *see* clonidine *on page 155*

Catapres-TTS®-1 [US] *see* clonidine *on page 155*

Catapres-TTS®-2 [US] *see* clonidine *on page 155*

Catapres-TTS®-3 [US] *see* clonidine *on page 155*

Catarase® 1:5000 *(Discontinued)* *see page 814*

Cathflo™ Activase® [US] *see* alteplase *on page 26*

Caverject® [US/Can] *see* alprostadil *on page 25*

CBDCA *see* carboplatin *on page 116*

CCNU *see* lomustine *on page 389*

C-Crystals® *(Discontinued)* *see page 814*

2-CdA *see* cladribine *on page 149*

CDDP *see* cisplatin *on page 148*

Cebid® *(Discontinued)* *see page 814*

Ceclor® [US/Can] *see* cefaclor *on this page*

Ceclor® CD [US] *see* cefaclor *on this page*

Cecon® [US-OTC] *see* ascorbic acid *on page 57*

Cedax® [US] *see* ceftibuten *on page 125*

Cedilanid-D® Injection *(Discontinued)* *see page 814*

Cedocard®-SR [Can] *see* isosorbide dinitrate *on page 362*

CeeNU® [US/Can] *see* lomustine *on page 389*

Ceepryn® *(Discontinued)* *see page 814*

cefaclor (SEF a klor)

U.S./Canadian Brand Names Apo®-Cefaclor [Can]; Ceclor® CD [US]; Ceclor® [US/ Can]; Novo-Cefaclor [Can]; Nu-Cefaclor [Can]; PMS-Cefaclor [Can]
Therapeutic Category Cephalosporin (Second Generation)
Use Infections caused by susceptible organisms including *Staphylococcus aureus, S. pneumoniae,* and *H. influenzae;* treatment of otitis media, sinusitis, and infections involving the respiratory tract, skin and skin structure, bone and joint, and urinary tract
Usual Dosage Oral:
Children >1 month: 20-40 mg/kg/day divided every 8-12 hours; maximum dose: 2 g/day (twice daily option is for treatment of otitis media or pharyngitis)
Adults: 250-500 mg every 8 hours or daily dose can be administered in 2 divided doses
Dosage Forms
Capsule: 250 mg, 500 mg

Powder for oral suspension: 125 mg/5 mL (75 mL, 150 mL); 187 mg/5 mL (50 mL, 100 mL); 250 mg/5 mL (75 mL, 150 mL); 375 mg/5 mL (50 mL, 100 mL) [strawberry flavor]
Tablet, extended release: 375 mg, 500 mg

cefadroxil (sef a DROKS il)

U.S./Canadian Brand Names Apo®-Cefadroxil [Can]; Duricef® [US/Can]; Novo-Cefadroxil [Can]

Therapeutic Category Cephalosporin (First Generation)

Use Treatment of susceptible bacterial infections including group A beta-hemolytic streptococcal pharyngitis or tonsillitis; skin and soft tissue infections caused by streptococci or staphylococci; urinary tract infections caused by *Klebsiella*, *E. coli*, and *Proteus mirabilis*

Usual Dosage Oral:
Children: 30 mg/kg/day divided twice daily up to a maximum of 2 g/day
Adults: 1-2 g/day in 2 divided doses

Dosage Forms
Capsule, as monohydrate: 500 mg
Suspension, oral, as monohydrate: 125 mg/5 mL, 250 mg/5 mL, 500 mg/5 mL (50 mL, 100 mL)
Tablet, as monohydrate: 1 g

Cefadyl® [US/Can] see cephapirin on page 128

cefamandole (sef a MAN dole)

U.S./Canadian Brand Names Mandol® [US]

Therapeutic Category Cephalosporin (Second Generation)

Use Treatment of susceptible bacterial infection; mainly respiratory tract, skin and skin structure, bone and joint, urinary tract and gynecologic as well as septicemia, perioperative prophylaxis

Usual Dosage I.M., I.V.:
Children: 100-150 mg/kg/day in divided doses every 4-6 hours
Adults: 4-12 g/24 hours divided every 4-6 hours 500-1000 mg every 4-8 hours

Dosage Forms Injection, powder for reconstitution, as nafate: 1 g (10 mL, 100 mL); 2 g (20 mL, 100 mL); 10 g (100 mL)

Cefanex® *(Discontinued)* see page 814

cefazolin (sef A zoe lin)

U.S./Canadian Brand Names Ancef® [US/Can]; Kefzol® [US/Can]

Therapeutic Category Cephalosporin (First Generation)

Use Treatment of respiratory tract, skin and skin structure, urinary tract, biliary tract, bone and joint infections and septicemia due to susceptible gram-positive cocci (except enterococcus); some gram-negative bacilli including *E. coli*, *Proteus*, and *Klebsiella* may be susceptible; perioperative prophylaxis

Usual Dosage I.M., I.V.:
Infants and Children: 50-100 mg/kg/day in 3 divided doses; maximum dose: 6 g/day
Adults: 1-2 g every 8 hours

Dosage Forms
Infusion, as sodium [premixed in D_5W, frozen] (Ancef®): 500 mg (50 mL); 1 g (50 mL)
Injection, powder for reconstitution, as sodium (Ancef®, Kefzol®): 500 mg, 1 g, 10 g, 20 g
Injection, powder for reconstitution, as sodium [with 50 mL D_5W in DUPLEX™ container]: 500 mg, 1 g

cefdinir (SEF di ner)

Synonyms CFDN

U.S./Canadian Brand Names Omnicef® [US/Can]

Therapeutic Category Cephalosporin (Third Generation)
(Continued)

cefdinir *(Continued)*

Use Treatment of community-acquired pneumonia, acute exacerbations of chronic bronchitis, acute bacterial otitis media, acute maxillary sinusitis, pharyngitis/tonsillitis, and uncomplicated skin and skin structure infections.

Usual Dosage Oral:

Children (otitis media with effusion): 7 mg/kg orally twice daily or 14 mg/kg orally once daily

Adolescents and Adults: 300 mg orally twice daily; an oral dose of 600 mg once daily has been used in streptococcal pharyngitis

Dosage Forms

Capsule: 300 mg

Suspension, oral: 125 mg/5 mL (60 mL, 100 mL)

cefditoren (sef de TOR en)

Synonyms cefditoren pivoxil

U.S./Canadian Brand Names Spectracef™ [US]

Therapeutic Category Antibiotic, Cephalosporin

Use Treatment of acute bacterial exacerbation of chronic bronchitis or community-acquired pneumonia (due to susceptible organisms including *Haemophilus influenzae, Haemophilus parainfluenzae, Streptococcus pneumoniae*-penicillin susceptible only, *Moraxella catarrhalis*); pharyngitis or tonsillitis (*Streptococcus pyogenes*); and uncomplicated skin and skin-structure infections (*Staphylococcus aureus*-not MRSA, *Streptococcus pyogenes*)

Usual Dosage Oral: Children ≥12 years and Adults:

Acute bacterial exacerbation of chronic bronchitis: 400 mg twice daily for 10 days

Community-acquired pneumonia: 400 mg twice daily for 14 days

Pharyngitis, tonsillitis, uncomplicated skin and skin structure infections: 200 mg twice daily for 10 days

Dosage Forms Tablet, as pivoxil: 200 mg [equivalent to cefditoren] [contains sodium caseinate]

cefditoren pivoxil *see* cefditoren *on this page*

cefepime (SEF e pim)

U.S./Canadian Brand Names Maxipime® [US/Can]

Therapeutic Category Cephalosporin (Fourth Generation)

Use Treatment of respiratory tract infections (including bronchitis and pneumonia), cellulitis and other skin and soft tissue infections, and urinary tract infections; considered a fourth generation cephalosporin because it has good gram-negative coverage similar to third generation cephalosporins, but better gram-positive coverage

Usual Dosage I.V.:

Children: Unlabeled: 50 mg/kg every 8 hours; maximum dose: 2 g

Adults:

Most infections: 1-2 g every 12 hours for 5-10 days; higher doses or more frequent administration may be required in pseudomonal infections

Urinary tract infections, uncomplicated: 500 mg every 12 hours

Dosage Forms

Infusion, as hydrochloride (ADD-Vantage®): 1 g, 2 g

Infusion, piggyback, as hydrochloride: 1 g (100 mL); 2 g (100 mL)

Injection, powder for reconstitution, as hydrochloride: 500 mg, 1 g, 2 g

cefixime (sef IKS eem)

U.S./Canadian Brand Names Suprax® [US/Can]

Therapeutic Category Cephalosporin (Third Generation)

Use Treatment of urinary tract infections, otitis media, respiratory infections due to susceptible organisms including *S. pneumoniae* and *pyogenes, H. influenzae, M. catarrhalis*, and many Enterobacteriaceae; documented poor compliance with other oral antimicrobials; outpatient therapy of serious soft tissue or skeletal infections due to susceptible organisms; single-dose oral treatment of uncomplicated cervical/urethral gonorrhea due to *N. gonorrhoeae*; treatment of shigellosis in areas with a high rate of resistance to TMP-SMX

Usual Dosage Oral:
  Children: 8 mg/kg/day in 1-2 divided doses; maximum dose: 400 mg/day
  Children >50 kg or >12 years and Adults: 400 mg/day in 1-2 divided doses

Dosage Forms
  Powder for oral suspension: 100 mg/5 mL (50 mL, 100 mL) [strawberry flavor]
  Tablet, film coated: 200 mg, 400 mg

Cefizox® [US/Can] *see* ceftizoxime *on page 125*

Cefobid® [US/Can] *see* cefoperazone *on this page*

Cefol® Filmtab® [US] *see* vitamin (multiple/oral) *on page 683*

cefoperazone (sef oh PER a zone)

U.S./Canadian Brand Names Cefobid® [US/Can]

Therapeutic Category Cephalosporin (Third Generation)

Use Treatment of susceptible bacterial infections, mainly respiratory tract, skin and skin structure, urinary tract and sepsis; as a third generation cephalosporin, cefoperazone has activity against gram-negative bacilli (eg, *E. coli*, *Klebsiella*, and *Haemophilus*) but variable activity against *Streptococcus* and *Staphylococcus* species; it has activity against *Pseudomonas aeruginosa*, but less than ceftazidime

Usual Dosage I.M., I.V.:
  Children: 100-150 mg/kg/day divided every 8-12 hours
  Adults: 2-4 g/day in divided doses every 12 hours (up to 12 g/day)

Dosage Forms
  Injection, as sodium [premixed, frozen]: 1 g (50 mL); 2 g (50 mL)
  Injection, powder for reconstitution, as sodium: 1 g, 2 g

Cefotan® [US/Can] *see* cefotetan *on this page*

cefotaxime (sef oh TAKS eem)

U.S./Canadian Brand Names Claforan® [US/Can]

Therapeutic Category Cephalosporin (Third Generation)

Use Treatment of susceptible lower respiratory tract, skin and skin structure, bone and joint, intra-abdominal and genitourinary tract infections; treatment of a documented or suspected meningitis due to susceptible organisms such as *H. influenzae* and *N. meningitidis*; nonpseudomonal gram-negative rod infection in a patient at risk of developing aminoglycoside-induced nephrotoxicity and/or ototoxicity; infection due to an organism whose susceptibilities clearly favor cefotaxime over cefuroxime or an aminoglycoside

Usual Dosage I.M., I.V.:
  Infants and Children 1 month to 12 years:
    <50 kg: 100-200 mg/kg/day in 3-4 divided doses
    Meningitis: 200 mg/kg/day in 4 divided doses
    >50 kg: Moderate to severe infection: 1-2 g every 6-8 hours; life-threatening infection: 2 g/dose every 4 hours; maximum dose: 12 g/day
  Children >12 years and Adults: 1-2 g every 6-8 hours (up to 12 g/day)

Dosage Forms
  Infusion, as sodium [premixed in D_5W, frozen]: 1 g (50 mL); 2 g (50 mL)
  Injection, powder for reconstitution, as sodium: 500 mg, 1 g, 2 g, 10 g

cefotetan (SEF oh tee tan)

U.S./Canadian Brand Names Cefotan® [US/Can]

Therapeutic Category Cephalosporin (Second Generation)

Use Treatment of susceptible lower respiratory tract, skin and skin structure, bone and joint, genitourinary tract, sepsis, gynecologic, and intra-abdominal infections; active
(Continued)

cefotetan *(Continued)*

against anaerobes including *Bacteroides* species of gastrointestinal tract, gram-negative enteric bacilli including *E. coli*, *Klebsiella*, and *Proteus*; active against many strains of *N. gonorrhoeae*; perioperative prophylaxis

Usual Dosage I.M., I.V.:
Children: 40-80 mg/kg/day divided every 12 hours
Adults: 1-6 g/day in divided doses every 12 hours, 1-2 g may be administered every 24 hours for urinary tract infection

Dosage Forms
Infusion, as disodium [premixed, frozen]: 1 g (50 mL); 2 g (50 mL)
Injection, powder for reconstitution, as disodium: 1 g, 2 g, 10 g

cefoxitin *(se FOKS i tin)*

U.S./Canadian Brand Names Mefoxin® [US/Can]
Therapeutic Category Cephalosporin (Second Generation)
Use Treatment of susceptible lower respiratory tract, skin and skin structure, bone and joint, genitourinary tract, sepsis, gynecologic, and intra-abdominal infections; active against anaerobes including *Bacteroides* species of the gastrointestinal tract, gram-negative enteric bacilli including *E. coli*, *Klebsiella*, and *Proteus*; active against many strains of *N. gonorrhoeae*; perioperative prophylaxis

Usual Dosage I.M., I.V.:
Infants >3 months and Children:
Mild-moderate infection: 80-100 mg/kg/day in divided doses every 4-6 hours
Severe infection: 100-160 mg/kg/day in divided doses every 4-6 hours
Maximum dose: 12 g/day
Adults: 1-2 g every 6-8 hours (I.M. injection is painful)

Dosage Forms
Infusion, as sodium [premixed in D_5W, frozen]: 1 g (50 mL); 2 g (50 mL)
Injection, powder for reconstitution, as sodium: 1 g, 2 g, 10 g

cefpodoxime *(sef pode OKS eem)*

U.S./Canadian Brand Names Vantin® [US/Can]
Therapeutic Category Cephalosporin (Second Generation)
Use Treatment of susceptible acute, community-acquired pneumonia caused by *S. pneumoniae* or nonbeta-lactamase producing *H. influenzae*; alternative regimen for acute uncomplicated gonorrhea caused by *N. gonorrhoeae*; uncomplicated skin and skin structure infections caused by *S. aureus* or *S. pyogenes*; acute otitis media caused by *S. pneumoniae*, *H. influenzae*, or *M. catarrhalis*; pharyngitis or tonsillitis; and uncomplicated urinary tract infections caused by *E. coli*, *Klebsiella*, and *Proteus*

Usual Dosage Oral:
Children >6 months to 12 years: 10 mg/kg/day divided every 12 hours for 10 days
Adults: 100-400 mg every 12 hours for 7-14 days

Dosage Forms
Granules for oral suspension, as proxetil: 50 mg/5 mL (100 mL); 100 mg/5 mL (100 mL) [lemon creme flavor]
Tablet, film coated, as proxetil: 100 mg, 200 mg

cefprozil *(sef PROE zil)*

U.S./Canadian Brand Names Cefzil® [US/Can]
Therapeutic Category Cephalosporin (Second Generation)
Use Infections caused by susceptible organisms including *S. pneumoniae*, *H. influenzae*, *M. catarrhalis*, *S. aureus*, *S. pyogenes*; treatment of infections involving the respiratory tract, skin and skin structure, and otitis media

Usual Dosage Oral:
Infants and Children >6 months to 12 years: 15 mg/kg every 12 hours for 10 days
Children >13 years and Adults: 250-500 mg every 12-24 hours for 10 days

Dosage Forms
Powder for oral suspension, as anhydrous: 125 mg/5 mL (50 mL, 75 mL, 100 mL); 250 mg/5 mL (50 mL, 75 mL, 100 mL)
Tablet, as anhydrous: 250 mg, 500 mg

ceftazidime (SEF tay zi deem)

U.S./Canadian Brand Names Ceptaz® [US/Can]; Fortaz® [US/Can]; Tazicef® [US]; Tazidime® [US/Can]

Therapeutic Category Cephalosporin (Third Generation)

Use Treatment of documented susceptible *Pseudomonas aeruginosa* infection and infections due to other susceptible aerobic gram-negative organisms; empiric therapy of a febrile, granulocytopenic patient

Usual Dosage
Infants and Children 1 month to 12 years: 30-50 mg/kg/dose every 8 hours; maximum dose: 6 g/day
Adults: 1-2 g every 8-12 hours (250-500 mg every 12 hours for urinary tract infections)

Dosage Forms
Infusion, as sodium [premixed, frozen] (Fortaz®): 1 g (50 mL); 2 g (50 mL)
Injection, powder for reconstitution:
Ceptaz®: 1 g, 2 g, 10 g [L-arginine formulation]
Fortaz®: 500 mg, 1 g, 2 g, 6 g [contains sodium carbonate]
Tazicef®, Tazidime®: 1 g, 2 g, 6 g [contains sodium carbonate]

ceftibuten (sef TYE byoo ten)

U.S./Canadian Brand Names Cedax® [US]

Therapeutic Category Cephalosporin (Third Generation)

Use Oral cephalosporin for bronchitis, otitis media, and strep throat

Usual Dosage Oral:
Children: 9 mg/kg/day for 10 days; maximum daily dose: 400 mg
Children ≥12 years and Adults: 400 mg once daily for 10 days

Dosage Forms
Capsule: 400 mg
Powder for oral suspension: 90 mg/5 mL (30 mL, 60 mL, 120 mL); 180 mg/5 mL (30 mL, 60 mL, 120 mL) [cherry flavor]

Ceftin® [US/Can] *see* cefuroxime *on next page*

ceftizoxime (sef ti ZOKS eem)

U.S./Canadian Brand Names Cefizox® [US/Can]

Therapeutic Category Cephalosporin (Third Generation)

Use Treatment of susceptible bacterial infections, mainly respiratory tract, skin and skin structure, bone and joint, urinary tract and sepsis; as a third generation cephalosporin, ceftizoxime has activity against gram-negative enteric bacilli (eg, *E. coli*, *Klebsiella*), and cocci (eg, *Neisseria*), and variable activity against gram-positive cocci (*Staphylococcus* and *Streptococcus*); it has some anaerobic coverage but is less active against *B. fragilis* than cefoxitin; also indicated for *Neisseria gonorrhoeae* infections (including uncomplicated cervical and urethral gonorrhea and gonorrhea pelvic inflammatory disease), and *Haemophilus influenzae* meningitis

Usual Dosage I.M., I.V.:
Children ≥6 months: 50 mg/kg every 6-8 hours to 200 mg/kg/day to maximum of 12 g/24 hours
Adults: 1-2 g every 8-12 hours, up to 2 g every 4 hours or 4 g every 8 hours for life-threatening infections

Dosage Forms
Injection, as sodium [in D_5W, frozen]: 1 g (50 mL); 2 g (50 mL)
Injection, powder for reconstitution, as sodium: 500 mg, 1 g, 2 g, 10 g

ceftriaxone (sef trye AKS one)

U.S./Canadian Brand Names Rocephin® [US/Can]

Therapeutic Category Cephalosporin (Third Generation)

Use Treatment of sepsis, meningitis, infections of the lower respiratory tract, skin and skin structure, bone and joint, intra-abdominal and urinary tract due to susceptible organisms as a third generation cephalosporin, ceftriaxone has activity against gram-negative aerobic bacteria (ie, *H. influenzae*, Enterobacteriaceae, *Neisseria*) and variable activity against gram-positive cocci; documented or suspected infection due to susceptible organisms in home care patients and patients without I.V. line access; treatment of documented or suspected gonococcal infection or chancroid; emergency room management of patients at high risk for bacteremia, periorbital or buccal cellulitis, salmonellosis or shigellosis and pneumonia of unestablished etiology (<5 years of age)

Usual Dosage

Gonococcal ophthalmia: 25-50 mg/kg/day administered every 24 hours

Infants and Children: 50-100 mg/kg/day in 1-2 divided doses

Meningitis: 100 mg/kg/day divided every 12 hours; loading dose of 75 mg/kg may be administered at the start of therapy

Chancroid, uncomplicated gonorrhea: I.M.:

<45 kg: 125 mg as a single dose

>45 kg: 250 mg as a single dose

Adults: 1-2 g every 12-24 hours depending on the type and severity of the infection; maximum dose: 4 g/day

Dosage Forms

Infusion, as sodium [premixed, frozen]: 1 g [in $D_{3.8}W$] (50 mL); 2 g [in $D_{2.4}W$] (50 mL)

Injection, powder for reconstitution, as sodium: 250 mg, 500 mg, 1 g, 2 g, 10 g

cefuroxime (se fyoor OKS eem)

U.S./Canadian Brand Names Ceftin® [US/Can]; Kefurox® [US/Can]; Zinacef® [US/Can]

Therapeutic Category Cephalosporin (Second Generation)

Use Second generation cephalosporin useful in infections caused by susceptible staphylococci, group B streptococci, pneumococci, *H. influenzae* (type A and B), *E. coli*, *Enterobacter*, and *Klebsiella*; treatment of susceptible infections of the upper and lower respiratory tract, otitis media, urinary tract, skin and soft tissue, bone and joint, and sepsis

Usual Dosage

Children:

Oral:

<12 years: 125 mg twice daily

>12 years: 250 mg twice daily

I.M., I.V.: 75-150 mg/kg/day divided every 8 hours; maximum dose: 9 g/day

Adults:

Oral: 125-500 mg twice daily, depending on severity of infection

I.M., I.V.: 100-150 mg/kg/day in divided doses every 6-8 hours; maximum: 6 g/24 hours

Dosage Forms

Infusion, as sodium [premixed, frozen] (Zinacef®): 750 mg (50 mL); 1.5 g (50 mL)

Injection, powder for reconstitution, as sodium: 750 mg, 1.5 g, 7.5 g

Kefurox®, Zinacef®: 750 mg, 1.5 g, 7.5 g

Powder for oral suspension, as axetil (Ceftin®): 125 mg/5 mL (50 mL, 100 mL, 200 mL); 250 mg/5 mL (50 mL, 100 mL) [tutti-frutti flavor]

Tablet, as axetil (Ceftin®): 250 mg, 500 mg

Cefzil® [US/Can] *see* cefprozil *on page 124*

Celebrex® [US/Can] *see* celecoxib *on this page*

celecoxib (ce le COX ib)

U.S./Canadian Brand Names Celebrex® [US/Can]

Therapeutic Category Nonsteroidal Anti-inflammatory Drug (NSAID), COX-2 Selective

Use Relief of the signs and symptoms of osteoarthritis; relief of the signs and symptoms of rheumatoid arthritis in adults; decreasing intestinal polyps in familial adenomatous polyposis (FAP); management of acute pain; treatment of primary dysmenorrhea

Usual Dosage Adults: Oral:
Osteoarthritis: 200 mg once/day or 100 mg twice daily
Rheumatoid arthritis: 100-200 mg twice daily

Dosage Forms Capsule: 100 mg, 200 mg, 400 mg

Celectol® *(Discontinued)* *see page 814*

Celestoderm®-EV/2 [Can] *see* betamethasone (topical) *on page 83*

Celestoderm®-V [Can] *see* betamethasone (topical) *on page 83*

Celestone® [US] *see* betamethasone (systemic) *on page 83*

Celestone® Phosphate [US] *see* betamethasone (systemic) *on page 83*

Celestone® Soluspan® [US/Can] *see* betamethasone (systemic) *on page 83*

Celexa™ [US/Can] *see* citalopram *on page 148*

CellCept® [US/Can] *see* mycophenolate *on page 441*

Cellufresh® [US-OTC] *see* carboxymethylcellulose *on page 117*

cellulose, oxidized (SEL yoo lose, OKS i dyzed)
Synonyms absorbable cotton
U.S./Canadian Brand Names Oxycel® [US]; Surgicel® [US]
Therapeutic Category Hemostatic Agent
Use Temporary packing for the control of capillary, venous, or small arterial hemorrhage
Usual Dosage Minimal amounts of an appropriate size are laid on the bleeding site
Dosage Forms
Pad (Oxycel®): 3" x 3" (8 ply)
Pledget (Oxycel®): 2" x 1" x 1"
Strip:
Oxycel®:
5" x ½" (4 ply)
18" x 2" (4 ply)
36" x ½" (4 ply)
Surgicel®:
½" x 2"
2" x 3"
2" x 14"
4" x 8"

cellulose sodium phosphate (sel yoo lose SOW dee um FOS fate)
Synonyms CSP; sodium cellulose phosphate
U.S./Canadian Brand Names Calcibind® [US/Can]
Therapeutic Category Urinary Tract Product
Use Adjunct to dietary restriction to reduce renal calculi formation in absorptive hypercalciuria type I
Usual Dosage Adults: Oral: 5 g 3 times/day with meals; decrease dose to 5 g with main meal and 2.5 g with each of two other meals when urinary calcium declines to <150 mg/day
Dosage Forms Powder: 300 g bulk pack

Celluvisc® [US/Can] *see* carboxymethylcellulose *on page 117*

Celontin® [US/Can] *see* methsuximide *on page 420*

Cel-U-Jec® [US] *see* betamethasone (systemic) *on page 83*

Cenafed® Plus Tablet [US-OTC] *see* triprolidine and pseudoephedrine *on page 659*

Cenafed® [US-OTC] *see* pseudoephedrine *on page 552*

Cena-K® [US] *see* potassium chloride *on page 530*

Cenestin™ [US/Can] *see* estrogens (conjugated A/synthetic) *on page 241*

Cenocort® A-40 *(Discontinued)* *see page 814*

Cenocort® Forte *(Discontinued)* *see page 814*

Cenolate® [US] *see* sodium ascorbate *on page 594*

Centrax® Capsule & Tablet *(Discontinued)* *see page 814*

Cēpacol® Anesthetic Troches [US-OTC] *see* cetylpyridinium and benzocaine *on page 130*

Cēpacol® Mouthwash/Gargle [US-OTC] *see* cetylpyridinium *on page 130*

Cēpastat® [US-OTC] *see* phenol *on page 508*

Cephadyn® [US] *see* butalbital, acetaminophen, and caffeine *on page 99*

cephalexin (sef a LEKS in)
U.S./Canadian Brand Names Apo®-Cephalex [Can]; Biocef® [US]; Keflex® [US]; Keftab® [US/Can]; Novo-Lexin® [Can]; Nu-Cephalex® [Can]
Therapeutic Category Cephalosporin (First Generation)
Use Treatment of susceptible bacterial infections, including those caused by group A beta-hemolytic *Streptococcus*, *Staphylococcus*, *Klebsiella pneumoniae*, *E. coli*, and *Proteus mirabilis*; not active against enterococci; used to treat susceptible infections of the respiratory tract, skin and skin structure, bone, genitourinary tract, and otitis media
Usual Dosage Oral:
Children: 25-50 mg/kg/day every 6 hours; severe infections: 50-100 mg/kg/day in divided doses every 6 hours; maximum: 3 g/24 hours
Adults: 250-1000 mg every 6 hours
Dosage Forms
Capsule, as monohydrate: 250 mg, 500 mg
Tablet, as hydrochloride: 500 mg
Tablet, as monohydrate: 250 mg, 500 mg, 1 g
Powder for oral suspension, as monohydrate: 125 mg/5 mL (5 mL unit dose, 60 mL, 100 mL, 200 mL); 250 mg/5 mL (5 mL unit dose, 100 mL, 200 mL)

cephalothin (sef A loe thin)
U.S./Canadian Brand Names Ceporacin® [Can]
Therapeutic Category Cephalosporin (First Generation)
Use Treatment of respiratory tract, skin and skin structure, urinary tract, bone and joint infections, endocarditis, and septicemia due to susceptible gram-positive cocci (except enterococcus); some gram-negative bacilli including *E. coli*, *Proteus*, and *Klebsiella* may be susceptible; perioperative prophylaxis
Usual Dosage I.M., I.V.:
Children: 75-125 mg/kg/day divided every 4-6 hours; maximum dose: 10 g in a 24-hour period
Adults: 500 mg to 2 g every 4-6 hours
Dosage Forms Injection, powder for reconstitution, as sodium: 1 g, 2 g (50 mL)

cephapirin (sef a PYE rin)
U.S./Canadian Brand Names Cefadyl® [US/Can]
Therapeutic Category Cephalosporin (First Generation)
Use Treatment of respiratory tract, skin and skin structure, urinary tract, bone and joint infections, endocarditis and septicemia due to susceptible gram-positive cocci (except enterococcus); some gram-negative bacilli including *E. coli*, *Proteus*, and *Klebsiella*, may be susceptible; perioperative prophylaxis
Usual Dosage I.M., I.V.:
Children: 10-20 mg/kg every 6 hours up to 4 g/24 hours
Adults: 1 g every 6 hours up to 12 g/day
Dosage Forms Injection, powder for reconstitution, as sodium: 500 mg, 1 g, 2 g, 4 g

cephradine (SEF ra deen)

U.S./Canadian Brand Names Velosef® [US]

Therapeutic Category Cephalosporin (First Generation)

Use Treatment of susceptible bacterial infections, including those caused by group A beta-hemolytic *Streptococcus*

Usual Dosage Oral:

Children ≥9 months: 25-100 mg/kg/day in equally divided doses every 6-12 hours up to 4 g/day

Adults: 2-4 g/day in 4 equally divided doses up to 8 g/day

Dosage Forms

Capsule: 250 mg, 500 mg

Powder for oral suspension: 125 mg/5 mL (5 mL, 100 mL, 200 mL); 250 mg/5 mL (5 mL, 100 mL, 200 mL)

Cephulac® *(Discontinued)* see page 814

Ceporacin® **[Can]** see cephalothin on previous page

Ceptaz® **[US/Can]** see ceftazidime on page 125

Cerebyx® **[US/Can]** see fosphenytoin on page 289

Ceredase® **[US]** see alglucerase on page 22

Cerespan® *(Discontinued)* see page 814

Cerezyme® **[US]** see imiglucerase on page 345

Cerose-DM® **[US-OTC]** see chlorpheniramine, phenylephrine, and dextromethorphan on page 139

Cerubidine® **[US/Can]** see daunorubicin hydrochloride on page 176

Cerumenex® **[US/Can]** see triethanolamine polypeptide oleate-condensate on page 654

Cervidil® **Vaginal Insert [US/Can]** see dinoprostone on page 201

CES see estrogens (conjugated/equine) on page 242

Cesamet® *(Discontinued)* see page 814

Cetacaine® **[US]** see benzocaine, butyl aminobenzoate, tetracaine, and benzalkonium chloride on page 78

Cetacort® see hydrocortisone (topical) on page 334

Cetafen Extra® **[US-OTC]** see acetaminophen on page 3

Cetafen® **[US-OTC]** see acetaminophen on page 3

Cetamide® **[US/Can]** see sulfacetamide on page 610

Cetane® *(Discontinued)* see page 814

Cetapred® **Ophthalmic** *(Discontinued)* see page 814

cetirizine (se TI ra zeen)

Synonyms P-071; UCB-P071

U.S./Canadian Brand Names Apo®-Cetirizine [Can]; Reactine™ [Can]; Zyrtec® [US]

Therapeutic Category Antihistamine

Use Perennial and seasonal allergic rhinitis and other allergic symptoms including urticaria

Usual Dosage Children ≥6 years and Adults: Oral: 5-10 mg once daily, depending upon symptom severity

Dosage Forms

Syrup, as hydrochloride: 5 mg/5 mL (120 mL)

Tablet, as hydrochloride: 5 mg, 10 mg

cetirizine and pseudoephedrine (se TI ra zeen & soo doe e FED rin)
U.S./Canadian Brand Names Zyrtec-D 12 Hour™ [US]
Therapeutic Category Antihistamine/Decongestant Combination
Use Treatment of symptoms of seasonal or perennial allergic rhinitis
Usual Dosage Oral:
   Children ≥12 years and Adults: Seasonal/perennial allergic rhinitis: 1 tablet twice daily
Dosage Forms Tablet, extended release: Cetirizine hydrochloride 5 mg and pseudoephedrine hydrochloride 120 mg

cetrorelix (se troh REE liks)
Synonyms cetrorelix acetate
U.S./Canadian Brand Names Cetrotide™ [US]
Therapeutic Category Antigonadotropic Agent
Use Inhibits premature luteinizing hormone (LH) surges in women undergoing controlled ovarian stimulation
Usual Dosage S.C.: Adults: Female: Used in conjunction with controlled ovarian stimulation therapy using gonadotropins (FSH, HMG):
   Single dose regimen: 3 mg given when serum estradiol levels show appropriate stimulation response, usually stimulation day 7 (range days 5-9). If hCG is not administered within 4 days, continue cetrorelix at 0.25 mg/day until hCG is administered
   Multiple dose regimen: 0.25 mg morning or evening of stimulation day 5, or morning of stimulation day 6; continue until hCG is administered.
Dosage Forms
   Injection [prefilled glass syringe; single-dose vial]:
   0.25 mg with 1 mL SWFI
   3 mg with 3 mL SWFI

cetrorelix acetate see cetrorelix on this page

Cetrotide™ [US] see cetrorelix on this page

cetylpyridinium (SEE til peer i DI nee um)
U.S./Canadian Brand Names Cēpacol® Mouthwash/Gargle [US-OTC]
Therapeutic Category Local Anesthetic
Use Temporary relief of sore throat
Usual Dosage Children >6 years and Adults: Oral: Dissolve 1 lozenge in the mouth every 2 hours as needed
Dosage Forms Mouthwash, as chloride: 0.05% and alcohol 14% (120 mL, 180 mL, 720 mL, 960 mL)

cetylpyridinium and benzocaine
(SEE til peer i DI nee um & BEN zoe kane)
Synonyms benzocaine and cetylpyridinium chloride; cetylpyridinium chloride and benzocaine
U.S./Canadian Brand Names Cēpacol® Anesthetic Troches [US-OTC]
Therapeutic Category Local Anesthetic
Use Symptomatic relief of sore throat
Usual Dosage Oral: Use as needed for sore throat
Dosage Forms Troche: Cetylpyridinium chloride 1:1500 and benzocaine 10 mg (18s)

cetylpyridinium chloride and benzocaine see cetylpyridinium and benzocaine on this page

Cevalin® *(Discontinued)* see page 814

Cevi-Bid® [US-OTC] see ascorbic acid on page 57

cevimeline (se vi ME leen)

Synonyms cevimeline hydrochloride
U.S./Canadian Brand Names Evoxac™ [US/Can]
Therapeutic Category Cholinergic Agent
Use Treatment of symptoms of dry mouth in patients with Sjögren's syndrome
Usual Dosage Adults: Oral: 30 mg 3 times/day
Dosage Forms Capsule: 30 mg

cevimeline hydrochloride *see* cevimeline *on this page*

CFDN *see* cefdinir *on page 121*

CG *see* chorionic gonadotropin (human) *on page 144*

CGP-42446 *see* zoledronic acid *on page 692*

CGP 57148B *see* imatinib *on page 345*

C-Gram [US-OTC] *see* ascorbic acid *on page 57*

Charcadole® [Can] *see* charcoal *on this page*

Charcadole® Aqueous [Can] *see* charcoal *on this page*

Charcadole® TFS [Can] *see* charcoal *on this page*

Charcoaid® *(Discontinued)* *see page 814*

charcoal (CHAR kole)

Synonyms activated carbon; liquid antidote; medicinal carbon
U.S./Canadian Brand Names Actidose-Aqua® [US-OTC]; Actidose® [US-OTC]; Charcadole® Aqueous [Can]; Charcadole® [Can]; Charcadole® TFS [Can]; Liqui-Char® [US/Can]
Therapeutic Category Antidote
Use Emergency treatment in poisoning by drugs and chemicals; repetitive doses for gastrointestinal dialysis in drug overdose to enhance the elimination of certain drugs (eg, theophylline, phenobarbital, and aspirin) and in uremia to adsorb various waste products
Usual Dosage Oral:
  Acute poisoning: Single dose: Charcoal with sorbitol:
    Children 1-12 years: 1-2 g/kg/dose or 15-30 g or approximately 5-10 times the weight of the ingested poison; 1 g adsorbs 100-1000 mg of poison; the use of repeat oral charcoal with sorbitol doses is not recommended. In young children sorbitol should be repeated no more than 1-2 times/day.
    Adults: 30-100 g

  Charcoal in water:
    Single dose:
    Infants <1 year: 1 g/kg
    Children 1-12 years: 15-30 g or 1-2 g/kg
    Adults: 30-100 g or 1-2 g/kg
    Multiple dose:
    Infants <1 year: 1 g/kg every 4-6 hours
    Children 1-12 years: 20-60 g or 1-2 g/kg every 2-6 hours until clinical observations and serum drug concentration have returned to a subtherapeutic range
    Adults: 20-60 g or 1-2 g/kg every 2-6 hours
  Gastric dialysis: Adults: 20-50 g every 6 hours for 1-2 days
Dosage Forms
  Liquid, activated:
    Actidose-Aqua®: 15 g (72 mL); 25 g (120 mL); 50 g (240 mL)
    Liqui-Char®: 15 g (75 mL); 25 g (120 mL); 30 g (120 mL)
  Liquid, activated [with propylene glycol]: 12.5 g (60 mL); 25 g (120 mL)
  Liquid, activated [with sorbitol]:
    Actidose®: 25 g (120 mL); 50 g (240 mL)
    Liqui-Char®: 25 g (120 mL); 50 g (240 mL)
  (Continued)

131

charcoal *(Continued)*

Powder for suspension, activated: 15 g, 30 g, 40 g, 120 g, 240 g

Charcocaps® *(Discontinued)* see page 814

Chealamide® [US] see edetate disodium on page 222

Chemet® [US/Can] see succimer on page 608

Chenix® Tablet *(Discontinued)* see page 814

Cheracol® [US] see guaifenesin and codeine on page 308

Cheracol® D [US-OTC] see guaifenesin and dextromethorphan on page 308

Cheracol® Plus [US-OTC] see guaifenesin and dextromethorphan on page 308

Cheratussin DAC [US] see guaifenesin, pseudoephedrine, and codeine on page 311

chickenpox vaccine see varicella virus vaccine on page 673

Chiggerex® [US-OTC] see benzocaine on page 77

Chiggertox® [US-OTC] see benzocaine on page 77

Children's Dimetapp® Elixir Cold & Allergy [US-OTC] see brompheniramine and pseudoephedrine on page 94

Children's Hold® *(Discontinued)* see page 814

Children's Kaopectate® [US-OTC] see attapulgite on page 63

Children's Nostril® [US] see phenylephrine on page 510

Children's Silfedrine® [US-OTC] see pseudoephedrine on page 552

Children's Sudafed® Cough & Cold [US-OTC] see pseudoephedrine and dextromethorphan on page 553

Children's Sudafed® Nasal Decongestant [US-OTC] see pseudoephedrine on page 552

Children's Tylenol® Cold [US-OTC] see acetaminophen, chlorpheniramine, and pseudoephedrine on page 7

Children's Tylenol® Sinus [US-OTC] see acetaminophen and pseudoephedrine on page 6

children's vitamins see vitamin (multiple/pediatric) on page 683

Chirocaine® [US/Can] see levobupivacaine on page 379

Chlo-Amine® Oral *(Discontinued)* see page 814

Chlorafed® Liquid *(Discontinued)* see page 814

chloral see chloral hydrate on this page

chloral hydrate (KLOR al HYE drate)

Synonyms chloral; trichloroacetaldehyde monohydrate

U.S./Canadian Brand Names Aquachloral® Supprettes® [US]; PMS-Chloral Hydrate [Can]; Somnote® [US]

Therapeutic Category Hypnotic, Nonbarbiturate

Controlled Substance C-IV

Use Short-term sedative and hypnotic (<2 weeks), sedative/hypnotic prior to nonpainful therapeutic or diagnostic procedures (eg, EEG, CT scan, MRI, ophthalmic exam, dental procedure)

Usual Dosage

Children:

Sedation, anxiety: Oral, rectal: 5-15 mg/kg/dose every 8 hours, maximum: 500 mg/dose

Prior to EEG: Oral, rectal: 20-25 mg/kg/dose, 30-60 minutes prior to EEG; may repeat in 30 minutes to maximum of 100 mg/kg or 2 g total

Hypnotic: Oral, rectal: 20-40 mg/kg/dose up to a maximum of 50 mg/kg/24 hours or 1 g/dose or 2 g/24 hours

Sedation, nonpainful procedure: Oral: 50-75 mg/kg/dose 30-60 minutes prior to procedure; may repeat 30 minutes after initial dose if needed, to a total maximum dose of 120 mg/kg or 1 g total

Adults: Oral, rectal:

Sedation, anxiety: 250 mg 3 times/day

Hypnotic: 500-1000 mg at bedtime or 30 minutes prior to procedure, not to exceed 2 g/24 hours

Dosage Forms
Capsule: 500 mg
Suppository, rectal: 324 mg, 500 mg, 648 mg
Syrup: 500 mg/5 mL (5 mL, 10 mL, 480 mL)

chlorambucil (klor AM byoo sil)

U.S./Canadian Brand Names Leukeran® [US/Can]

Therapeutic Category Antineoplastic Agent

Use Management of chronic lymphocytic leukemia (CLL), Hodgkin's and non-Hodgkin's lymphoma; breast and ovarian carcinoma, testicular carcinoma, choriocarcinoma; Waldenström's macroglobulinemia, and nephrotic syndrome unresponsive to conventional therapy

Usual Dosage Children and Adults: Oral (refer to individual protocols):

General short courses: 0.1-0.2 mg/kg/day or 4-8 mg/m^2/day for 2-3 weeks for remission induction, then adjust dose on basis of blood counts; maintenance therapy: 0.03-0.1 mg/kg/day

Nephrotic syndrome: 0.1-0.2 mg/kg/day every day for 5-15 weeks with low-dose prednisone

Chronic lymphocytic leukemia:

Biweekly regimen: Initial: 0.4 mg/kg dose is increased by 0.1 mg/kg every 2 weeks until a response occurs and/or myelosuppression occurs

Monthly regimen: Initial: 0.4 mg/kg, increase dose by 0.2 mg/kg every 4 weeks until a response occurs and/or myelosuppression occurs

Malignant lymphomas:

Non-Hodgkins: 0.1 mg/kg/day

Hodgkins: 0.2 mg/kg/day

Dosage Forms Tablet, sugar-coated: 2 mg

chloramphenicol (klor am FEN i kole)

U.S./Canadian Brand Names Chloromycetin® Parenteral [US/Can]; Chloroptic® Ophthalmic [US]; Diochloram® [Can]; Ocu-Chlor® Ophthalmic [US]; Pentamycetin® [Can]

Therapeutic Category Antibiotic, Ophthalmic; Antibiotic, Otic; Antibiotic, Miscellaneous

Use Treatment of serious infections due to organisms resistant to other less toxic antibiotics or when its penetrability into the site of infection is clinically superior to other antibiotics to which the organism is sensitive; useful in infections caused by *Bacteroides*, *H. influenzae*, *Neisseria meningitidis*, *S. pneumoniae*, *Salmonella*, and *Rickettsia*

Usual Dosage

I.V.:

Infants and Children: 50-75 mg/kg/day divided every 6 hours; maximum daily dose: 4 g/day

Adults: 50 mg/kg/day in divided doses every 6 hours; maximum daily dose: 4 g/day

Ophthalmic: Children and Adults: Instill 1-2 drops or small amount of ointment every 3-6 hours; increase interval between applications after 48 hours

Dosage Forms
Powder for injection, as sodium succinate: 1 g
(Continued)

chloramphenicol (Continued)

Solution:
Ophthalmic: 0.5% [5 mg/mL] (2.5 mL, 7.5 mL, 15 mL)
Otic: 0.5% (15 mL)

Chloraseptic® [US-OTC] *see* phenol *on page 508*

Chlorate® Oral *(Discontinued) see page 814*

chlordiazepoxide (klor dye az e POKS ide)

Synonyms methaminodiazepoxide
U.S./Canadian Brand Names Apo®-Chlordiazepoxide [Can]; Librium® [US]
Therapeutic Category Benzodiazepine
Controlled Substance C-IV
Use Management of anxiety and as a preoperative sedative, symptoms of alcohol withdrawal
Usual Dosage
Children >6 years: Anxiety: Oral, I.M.: 0.5 mg/kg/24 hours divided every 6-8 hours
Adults:
Anxiety: Oral: 15-100 mg divided 3-4 times/day
Severe anxiety: 20-25 mg 3-4 times/day
Preoperative sedation:
Oral: 5-10 mg 3-4 times/day, 1-day preop
I.M.: 50-100 mg 1-hour preop
Alcohol withdrawal symptoms: Oral, I.V.: 50-100 mg to start, dose may be repeated in 2-4 hours as necessary to a maximum of 300 mg/24 hours
Dosage Forms
Capsule, as hydrochloride: 5 mg, 10 mg, 25 mg
Injection, powder for reconstitution, as hydrochloride: 100 mg

chlordiazepoxide and amitriptyline *see* amitriptyline and chlordiazepoxide *on page 35*

chlordiazepoxide and clidinium *see* clidinium and chlordiazepoxide *on page 151*

Chloresium® [US-OTC] *see* chlorophyll *on next page*

Chlorgest-HD® Elixir *(Discontinued) see page 814*

chlorhexidine gluconate (klor HEKS i deen GLOO koe nate)

U.S./Canadian Brand Names Betasept® [US-OTC]; Dyna-Hex® [US-OTC]; Hibiclens® [US-OTC]; Hibistat® [US-OTC]; Peridex® [US]; Periochip® [US]; PerioGard® [US]
Therapeutic Category Antibiotic, Oral Rinse; Antibiotic, Topical
Use
Dental:
Antibacterial dental rinse; chlorhexidine is active against gram-positive and gram-negative organisms, facultative anaerobes, aerobes, and yeast
Chip, for periodontal pocket insertion; indicated as an adjunct to scaling and root planing procedures for reduction of pocket depth in patients with adult periodontitis; may be used as part of a periodontal maintenance program
Medical: Skin cleanser for surgical scrub, cleanser for skin wounds, germicidal hand rinse
Usual Dosage Oral rinse (Peridex®)
Precede use of solution by flossing and brushing teeth, completely rinse toothpaste from mouth; swish 15 mL undiluted oral rinse around in mouth for 30 seconds, then expectorate. Caution patient not to swallow the medicine; avoid eating for 2-3 hours after treatment. (The cap on bottle of oral rinse is a measure for 15 mL.)
When used as a treatment of gingivitis, the regimen begins with oral prophylaxis. Patient treats mouth with 15 mL chlorhexidine; swish for 30 seconds, then expectorate;

this is repeated twice daily (morning and evening). Patient should have a re-evaluation followed by a dental prophylaxis every 6 months.

Dosage Forms
Chip for periodontal pocket insertion (PerioChip®): 2.5 mg
Dressing, with chlorhexidine (Biopatch® [OTC]):
  3/4" (1.9 cm) disk [1.5 mm center hole]
  1" (2.5 cm) disk [4 mm center hole, 7 mm center hole]
Liquid, topical (Stat Touch 2 [OTC]): 2% (118 mL, 946 mL, 3800 mL)
Liquid, topical [with ethyl alcohol 61%]: (3M™ Avagard™): 1% (88 mL, 500 mL) [contains moisturizer]
Liquid, topical [with isopropyl alcohol 2%]:
  Chlorostat®: 2% (360 mL, 3840 mL)
  Dyna-Hex® Skin Cleanser: 2% (120 mL, 240 mL, 480 mL, 960 mL, 4000 mL)
Liquid, topical [with isopropyl alcohol 4%]:
  Betasept®, Hibiclens® Skin Cleanser: 4% (15 mL, 120 mL, 240 mL, 480 mL, 960 mL, 4000 mL)
  Dyna-Hex® Skin Cleanser: 4% (120 mL, 960 mL, 4000 mL)
Rinse, oral [with alcohol 11.6%] (Peridex®, PerioGard®): 0.12% (480 mL) [mint flavor]
Rinse, topical [with isopropyl alcohol 70%] (Hibistat® Hand Rinse): 0.5% (120 mL, 240 mL)
Sponge/Brush [with isopropyl alcohol 4%] (Hibiclens®): 4% (22 mL)
Wipes [with isopropyl alcohol 70%] (Hibistat®): 0.5% (50s)

2-chlorodeoxyadenosine *see* cladribine *on page 149*

chloroethane *see* ethyl chloride *on page 257*

Chlorofon-A® Tablet *(Discontinued)* *see page 814*

Chloromag® [US] *see* magnesium chloride *on page 397*

Chloromycetin® Cream *(Discontinued)* *see page 814*

Chloromycetin® Kapseals® *(Discontinued)* *see page 814*

Chloromycetin® Ophthalmic *(Discontinued)* *see page 814*

Chloromycetin® Otic *(Discontinued)* *see page 814*

Chloromycetin® Palmitate Oral Suspension *(Discontinued)* *see page 814*

Chloromycetin® Parenteral [US/Can] *see* chloramphenicol *on page 133*

chlorophylin *see* chlorophyll *on this page*

chlorophyll (KLOR oh fil)
Synonyms chlorophylin
U.S./Canadian Brand Names Chloresium® [US-OTC]; Derifil® [US-OTC]; Nullo® [US-OTC]; PALS® [US-OTC]
Therapeutic Category Gastrointestinal Agent, Miscellaneous
Use Topically promotes normal healing, relieves pain and inflammation, and reduces malodors in wounds, burns, surface ulcers, abrasions and skin irritations; used orally to control fecal and urinary odors in colostomy, ileostomy, or incontinence
Usual Dosage
Oral: 1-2 tablets/day
Topical: Apply generously and cover with gauze, linen, or other appropriate dressing; do not change dressings more often than every 48-72 hours
Dosage Forms
Ointment, topical (Chloresium®): Chlorophyllin copper complex 0.5% (30 g, 120 g)
Solution, topical, in isotonic saline (Chloresium®): Chlorophyllin copper complex 0.2% (240 mL, 946 mL)
Tablet: 20 mg [sodium free, sugar free]
  Chloresium®: Chlorophyllin copper complex 14 mg
  Derifil®: Water soluble chlorophyll: 100 mg
  Nullo®: Chlorophyllin copper complex 33.3 mg
(Continued)

chlorophyll *(Continued)*

PALS®: Chlorophyllin copper complex 100 mg

chloroprocaine (klor oh PROE kane)

U.S./Canadian Brand Names Nesacaine®-CE [Can]; Nesacaine®-MPF [US]; Nesacaine® [US]

Therapeutic Category Local Anesthetic

Use For infiltration anesthesia and for peripheral and epidural anesthesia

Usual Dosage Dosage varies with anesthetic procedure, the area to be anesthetized, the vascularity of the tissues, depth of anesthesia required, degree of muscle relaxation required, and duration of anesthesia

Dosage Forms

Injection, as hydrochloride (Nesacaine®) [with preservative]: 1% (30 mL); 2% (30 mL)

Injection, as hydrochloride (Nesacaine®-MPF) [preservative free]: 2% (20 mL); 3% (20 mL)

Chloroptic® Ophthalmic [US] *see* chloramphenicol *on page 133*

Chloroptic-P® Ophthalmic *(Discontinued)* *see page 814*

chloroquine phosphate (KLOR oh kwin FOS fate)

U.S./Canadian Brand Names Aralen® Phosphate [US/Can]

Therapeutic Category Aminoquinoline (Antimalarial)

Use Suppression or chemoprophylaxis of malaria; treatment of uncomplicated or mild-moderate malaria; extraintestinal amebiasis; rheumatoid arthritis; discoid lupus erythematosus, scleroderma, pemphigus

Usual Dosage Oral:

Malaria (excluding resistant *P. falciparum*):

Suppression or prophylaxis in endemic areas (begin 1-2 weeks prior to, and continue for 6-8 weeks after the period of potential exposure):

Children: 5 mg base/kg/dose weekly, up to a maximum of 300 mg/dose

Adults: 300 mg/dose weekly

Treatment:

Children: 10 mg base/kg/dose, up to a maximum of 600 mg base/dose one time, followed by 5 mg base/kg/dose one time after 6 hours, and then daily for 2 days (total dose of 25 mg base/kg)

Adults: 600 mg base/dose one time, followed by 300 mg base/dose one time after 6 hours, and then daily for 2 days

Extraintestinal amebiasis: Dosage expressed in mg base:

Children: 10 mg/kg once daily for 2-3 weeks (up to 300 mg base/day)

Adults: 600 mg base/day for 2 days followed by 300 mg base/day for at least 2-3 weeks

Rheumatoid arthritis: Adults: 150 mg base once daily

Melanoma treatment: Children: 10 mg/kg base/dose (maximum: 600 mg) as a single dose followed by 5 mg/kg base one time after 6 hours, then daily for 2 days

Dosage Forms

Injection, as hydrochloride: 50 mg/mL [equivalent to 40 mg base/mL] (5 mL)

Tablet, as phosphate: 250 mg [equivalent to 150 mg base]; 500 mg [equivalent to 300 mg base]

Chloroserpine® *(Discontinued)* *see page 814*

chlorothiazide (klor oh THYE a zide)

U.S./Canadian Brand Names Diuril® [US/Can]

Therapeutic Category Diuretic, Thiazide

Use Management of mild to moderate hypertension; edema associated with congestive heart failure, pregnancy, or nephrotic syndrome

Usual Dosage I.V. has been limited in infants and children and is generally not recommended

Infants <6 months and patients with pulmonary interstitial edema:
Oral: 20-40 mg/kg/day in 2 divided doses
I.V.: 2-8 mg/kg/day in 2 divided doses
Infants >6 months and Children:
Oral: 20 mg/kg/day in 2 divided doses
I.V.: 4 mg/kg/day
Adults:
Oral: 500 mg to 2 g/day divided in 1-2 doses
I.V.: 100-500 mg/day

Dosage Forms
Injection, powder for reconstitution, as sodium: 500 mg
Suspension, oral: 250 mg/5 mL (237 mL)
Tablet: 250 mg, 500 mg

chloroxine (klor OKS een)

U.S./Canadian Brand Names Capitrol® [US/Can]

Therapeutic Category Antiseborrheic Agent, Topical

Use Treatment of dandruff or seborrheic dermatitis of the scalp

Usual Dosage Topical: Use twice weekly, massage into wet scalp, lather should remain on the scalp for approximately 3 minutes, then rinsed; application should be repeated and scalp rinsed thoroughly

Dosage Forms Shampoo, topical: 2% (120 mL)

Chlorphed® *(Discontinued)* *see page 814*

Chlorphed®-LA Nasal Solution *(Discontinued)* *see page 814*

chlorpheniramine (klor fen IR a meen)

U.S./Canadian Brand Names Aller-Chlor® [US-OTC]; Chlor-Trimeton® [US-OTC]; Chlor-Tripolon® [Can]

Therapeutic Category Antihistamine

Use Perennial and seasonal allergic rhinitis and other allergic symptoms including urticaria

Usual Dosage
Children: Oral: 0.35 mg/kg/day in divided doses every 4-6 hours
2-6 years: 1 mg every 4-6 hours, not to exceed 6 mg in 24 hours
6-12 years: 2 mg every 4-6 hours, not to exceed 12 mg/day or sustained release 8 mg at bedtime
Children >12 years and Adults: Oral: 4 mg every 4-6 hours, not to exceed 24 mg/day or sustained release 8-12 mg every 8-12 hours, not to exceed 24 mg/day
Adults: Allergic reactions: I.M., I.V., S.C.: 10-20 mg as a single dose; maximum recommended dose: 40 mg/24 hours

Dosage Forms
Injection, as maleate: 10 mg/mL (30 mL)
Syrup, as maleate: 2 mg/5 mL (120 mL)
Tablet, as maleate: 4 mg
Tablet, chewable, as maleate: 2 mg
Tablet, timed release, as maleate: 8 mg, 12 mg

chlorpheniramine and acetaminophen

(klor fen IR a meen & a seet a MIN oh fen)

U.S./Canadian Brand Names Coricidin® [US-OTC]

Therapeutic Category Antihistamine/Analgesic

Use Symptomatic relief of congestion, headache, aches, and pains of colds and flu

Usual Dosage Adults: Oral: 2 tablets every 4 hours, up to 20 tablets/day

Dosage Forms Tablet: Chlorpheniramine maleate 2 mg and acetaminophen 325 mg

chlorpheniramine and hydrocodone *see* hydrocodone and chlorpheniramine *on page 330*

chlorpheniramine and phenylephrine (klor fen IR a meen & fen il EF rin)

Synonyms phenylephrine and chlorpheniramine

U.S./Canadian Brand Names Ed A-Hist® [US]; Histatab® Plus [US-OTC]

Therapeutic Category Antihistamine/Decongestant Combination

Use Temporary relief of nasal congestion and eustachian tube congestion as well as runny nose, sneezing, itching of nose or throat, itchy and watery eyes

Usual Dosage Oral:

Children:

2-5 years: 2.5 mL every 4 hours

6-12 years: 5 mL every 4 hours

Adults: 10 mL every 4 hours or 1-2 regular tablets 3-4 times daily or 1 sustained release capsule every 12 hours

Dosage Forms

Liquid:

Ed A-Hist® Liquid: Chlorpheniramine maleate 4 mg and phenylephrine hydrochloride 10 mg per 5 mL

Tablet (Histatab® Plus): Chlorpheniramine maleate 2 mg and phenylephrine hydrochloride 5 mg

chlorpheniramine and pseudoephedrine
(klor fen IR a meen & soo doe e FED rin)

Synonyms pseudoephedrine and chlorpheniramine

U.S./Canadian Brand Names Allerest® Maximum Strength [US-OTC]; Chlor-Trimeton® Allergy/Decongestant [US-OTC]; Codimal-LA® Half [US-OTC]; Codimal-LA® [US-OTC]; Deconamine® SR [US-OTC]; Deconamine® [US-OTC]; Hayfebrol® [US-OTC]; Histalet® [US-OTC]; Rhinosyn-PD® [US-OTC]; Rhinosyn® [US-OTC]; Ryna® [US-OTC]; Sudafed® Cold & Allergy [US-OTC]

Therapeutic Category Antihistamine/Decongestant Combination

Use Relief of nasal congestion associated with the common cold, hay fever, and other allergies, sinusitis, eustachian tube blockage, and vasomotor and allergic rhinitis

Usual Dosage Oral:

Capsule: 1 capsule every 12 hours

Liquid: 5 mL 3-4 times/day

Tablet: 1 tablet 3-4 times/day

Dosage Forms

Capsule, sustained release:

Codimal-LA® Half: Chlorpheniramine maleate 4 mg and pseudoephedrine hydrochloride 60 mg

Deconamine® SR: Chlorpheniramine maleate 8 mg and pseudoephedrine hydrochloride 120 mg

Liquid:

Anamine®, Deconamine®, Hayfebrol®, Rhinosyn-PD®, Ryna®: Chlorpheniramine maleate 2 mg and pseudoephedrine sulfate 30 mg per 5 mL

Histalet®: Chlorpheniramine maleate 3 mg and pseudoephedrine sulfate 45 mg per 5 mL

Rhinosyn®: Chlorpheniramine maleate 2 mg and pseudoephedrine sulfate 60 mg per 5 mL

Tablet:

Allerest® Maximum Strength: Chlorpheniramine maleate 2 mg and pseudoephedrine hydrochloride 30 mg

Chlor-Trimeton® 4-Hour, Deconamine®, Fedahist®, Sudafed® Cold & Allergy: Chlorpheniramine maleate 4 mg and pseudoephedrine hydrochloride 60 mg

Chlor-Trimeton® 12-Hour: Chlorpheniramine maleate 8 mg and pseudoephedrine hydrochloride 120 mg

chlorpheniramine, ephedrine, phenylephrine, and carbetapentane

(klor fen IR a meen, e FED rin, fen il EF rin, & kar bay ta PEN tane)

U.S./Canadian Brand Names Rentamine® [US-OTC]; Rynatuss® Pediatric Suspension [US-OTC]; Rynatuss® [US-OTC]

Therapeutic Category Antihistamine/Decongestant/Antitussive

Use Symptomatic relief of cough

Usual Dosage Children: Oral:

<2 years: Titrate dose individually

2-6 years: 2.5-5 mL every 12 hours

>6 years: 5-10 mL every 12 hours

Dosage Forms

Liquid: Carbetapentane tannate 30 mg, ephedrine tannate 5 mg, phenylephrine tannate 5 mg, and chlorpheniramine tannate 4 mg per 5 mL

Tablet: Carbetapentane tannate 60 mg, ephedrine tannate 10 mg, phenylephrine tannate 10 mg, and chlorpheniramine tannate 5 mg per 5 mL

chlorpheniramine, hydrocodone, phenylephrine, acetaminophen, and caffeine *see* hydrocodone, chlorpheniramine, phenylephrine, acetaminophen, and caffeine *on page 332*

chlorpheniramine, phenylephrine, and codeine

(klor fen IR a meen, fen il EF rin, & KOE deen)

U.S./Canadian Brand Names Pediacof® [US]; Pedituss® [US]

Therapeutic Category Antihistamine/Decongestant/Antitussive

Controlled Substance C-IV

Use Symptomatic relief of rhinitis, nasal congestion, and cough due to colds or allergy

Usual Dosage Children 6 months to 12 years: Oral: 1.25-10 mL every 4-6 hours

Dosage Forms

Liquid:

Pediacof®: Chlorpheniramine maleate 0.75 mg, phenylephrine hydrochloride 2.5 mg, and codeine phosphate 5 mg with potassium iodide 75 mg per 5 mL [contains alcohol 5%]

Pedituss®: Chlorpheniramine maleate 0.75 mg, phenylephrine hydrochloride 2.5 mg, and codeine phosphate 5 mg with potassium iodide 75 mg per 5 mL

chlorpheniramine, phenylephrine, and dextromethorphan

(klor fen IR a meen, fen il EF rin, & deks troe meth OR fan)

U.S./Canadian Brand Names Cerose-DM® [US-OTC]

Therapeutic Category Antihistamine/Decongestant/Antitussive

Use Temporary relief of cough due to minor throat and bronchial irritation; relief of nasal congestion, runny nose, and sneezing

Usual Dosage Adults: Oral: 5-10 mL 4 times/day

Dosage Forms Liquid: Chlorpheniramine maleate 4 mg, phenylephrine hydrochloride 10 mg, and dextromethorphan hydrobromide 15 mg per 5 mL

chlorpheniramine, phenylephrine, and methscopolamine

(klor fen IR a meen, fen il EF rin, & meth skoe POL a meen)

U.S./Canadian Brand Names D.A.II™ [US]; Dallergy® [US]; Dura-Vent®/DA [US]; Extendryl JR [US]; Extendryl SR [US]; Extendryl [US]

Therapeutic Category Antihistamine/Decongestant/Anticholinergic

Use Relief of nasal congestion, runny nose, and sneezing

Usual Dosage Adults: Oral: 1 capsule or caplet every 12 hours or 5 mL every 4-6 hours

Dosage Forms

Caplet, sustained release (Dallergy®): Chlorpheniramine maleate 8 mg, phenylephrine hydrochloride 20 mg, and methscopolamine nitrate 2.5 mg

(Continued)

chlorpheniramine, phenylephrine, and methscopolamine
(Continued)

Capsule:
Extendryl JR: Chlorpheniramine maleate 4 mg, phenylephrine hydrochloride 10 mg, and methscopolamine nitrate 1.25 mg
Extendryl SR: Chlorpheniramine maleate 8 mg, phenylephrine hydrochloride 20 mg, and methscopolamine nitrate 2.5 mg
Syrup (Extendryl): Chlorpheniramine maleate 2 mg, phenylephrine hydrochloride 10 mg, and methscopolamine nitrate 1.25 mg per 5 mL [root beer flavor]
Tablet:
D.A.II™: Chlorpheniramine maleate 4 mg, phenylephrine hydrochloride 10 mg, and methscopolamine nitrate 1.25 mg
Dura-Vent®/DA: Chlorpheniramine maleate 8 mg, phenylephrine hydrochloride 20 mg, and methscopolamine nitrate 2.5 mg
Tablet, chewable:
D.A. Chewable®: Chlorpheniramine maleate 2 mg, phenylephrine hydrochloride 10 mg, and methscopolamine nitrate 1.25 mg [orange flavor, phenylalanine 7.5 mg/tablet]
Extendryl: Chlorpheniramine maleate 2 mg, phenylephrine hydrochloride 10 mg, and methscopolamine nitrate 1.25 mg [root beer flavor]

chlorpheniramine, phenylephrine, and phenyltoloxamine
(klor fen IR a meen, fen il EF rin, & fen il tole LOKS a meen)
U.S./Canadian Brand Names Comhist® LA [US]; Comhist® [US]
Therapeutic Category Antihistamine/Decongestant Combination
Use Symptomatic relief of rhinitis and nasal congestion due to colds or allergy
Usual Dosage Oral: 1 capsule every 8-12 hours or 1-2 tablets 3 times/day
Dosage Forms
Capsule, sustained release (Comhist® LA): Chlorpheniramine maleate 4 mg, phenylephrine hydrochloride 20 mg, and phenyltoloxamine citrate 50 mg
Tablet (Comhist®): Chlorpheniramine maleate 2 mg, phenylephrine hydrochloride 10 mg, and phenyltoloxamine citrate 25 mg

chlorpheniramine, pseudoephedrine, and codeine
(klor fen IR a meen, soo doe e FED rin, & KOE deen)
U.S./Canadian Brand Names Decohistine® DH [US]; Dihistine® DH [US]; Ryna-C® [US]
Therapeutic Category Antihistamine/Decongestant/Antitussive
Controlled Substance C-V
Use Temporary relief of cough associated with minor throat or bronchial irritation; relief of nasal congestion due to common cold, allergic rhinitis, or sinusitis
Usual Dosage Oral:
Children:
25-50 lb: 1.25-2.50 mL every 4-6 hours, up to 4 doses in a 24-hour period
50-90 lb: 2.5-5 mL every 4-6 hours, up to 4 doses in a 24-hour period
Adults: 10 mL every 4-6 hours, up to 4 doses in a 24-hour period
Dosage Forms Liquid: Chlorpheniramine maleate 2 mg, pseudoephedrine hydrochloride 30 mg, and codeine phosphate 10 mg (120 mL, 480 mL)

chlorpheniramine, pseudoephedrine, and methscopolamine
(klor fen IR a meen, soo doe e FED rin, & meth skoe POL a meen)
U.S./Canadian Brand Names Xiral® [US]
Therapeutic Category Antihistamine/Decongestant/Anticholinergic
Use Treatment of upper respiratory symptoms such as respiratory congestion, allergic rhinitis, vasomotor rhinitis, sinusitis, and allergic skin reactions of urticaria and angioedema
Usual Dosage Oral:
Children 6-12 years: 1/2 tablet every 12 hours up to 1 tablet daily

Children ≥12 years and Adults: 1 tablet every 12 hours up to 2 tablets daily

Dosage Forms Tablet, sustained release: Chlorpheniramine maleate 8 mg, pseudoephedrine hydrochloride 120 mg, and methscopolamine nitrate 2.5 mg

chlorpheniramine, pyrilamine, and phenylephrine
(klor fen IR a meen, pye RIL a meen, & fen il EF rin)

U.S./Canadian Brand Names Rhinatate® [US]; R-Tannamine® [US]; R-Tannate® [US]; Rynatan® Pediatric Suspension [US]; Triotann® [US]; Tri-Tannate® [US]

Therapeutic Category Antihistamine/Decongestant Combination

Use Symptomatic relief of nasal congestion associated with upper respiratory tract condition

Usual Dosage Oral:

Children:

<2 years: Titrate dose individually

2-6 years: 2.5-5 mL every 12 hours

Children >6 years and Adults: 5-10 mL every 12 hours

Dosage Forms

Suspension, pediatric: Chlorpheniramine tannate 2 mg, pyrilamine tannate 12.5 mg, and phenylephrine tannate 5 mg per 5 mL

Tablet: Chlorpheniramine tannate 8 mg, pyrilamine maleate 25 mg, and phenylephrine tannate 25 mg

Chlor-Pro® Injection *(Discontinued)* see page 814

Chlorpromanyl® [Can] see chlorpromazine on this page

chlorpromazine (klor PROE ma zeen)

Tall-Man chlorproMAZINE

U.S./Canadian Brand Names Chlorpromanyl® [Can]; Largactil® [Can]; Thorazine® [US]

Therapeutic Category Phenothiazine Derivative

Use Treatment of nausea and vomiting; psychoses; Tourette's syndrome; mania; intractable hiccups (adults); behavioral problems (children)

Usual Dosage

Children >6 months:

Psychosis:

Oral: 0.5-1 mg/kg/dose every 4-6 hours; older children may require 200 mg/day or higher

I.M., I.V.: 0.5-1 mg/kg/dose every 6-8 hours; maximum I.M./I.V. dose for <5 years (22.7 kg): 40 mg/day; maximum I.M./I.V. for 5-12 years (22.7-45.5 kg): 75 mg/day

Nausea and vomiting:

Oral: 0.5-1 mg/kg/dose every 4-6 hours as needed

I.M., I.V.: 0.5-1 mg/kg/dose every 6-8 hours; maximum dose: Same as psychoses

Rectal: 1 mg/kg/dose every 6-8 hours as needed

Adults:

Psychosis:

Oral: Range: 30-800 mg/day in 1-4 divided doses, initiate at lower doses and titrate as needed; usual dose is 200 mg/day; some patients may require 1-2 g/day

I.M., I.V.: Initial: 25 mg, may repeat (25-50 mg) in 1-4 hours, gradually increase to a maximum of 400 mg/dose every 4-6 hours until patient controlled; usual dose: 300-800 mg/day

Nausea and vomiting:

Oral: 10-25 mg every 4-6 hours

I.M., I.V.: 25-50 mg every 4-6 hours

Rectal: 50-100 mg every 6-8 hours

Intractable hiccups: Oral, I.M.: 25-50 mg 3-4 times/day

Dosage Forms

Capsule, sustained action, as hydrochloride: 30 mg, 75 mg, 150 mg, 200 mg, 300 mg

Injection, as hydrochloride: 25 mg/mL (1 mL, 2 mL, 10 mL)

(Continued)

chlorpromazine *(Continued)*

Solution, oral concentrate, as hydrochloride: 30 mg/mL (120 mL); 100 mg/mL (60 mL, 240 mL)
Suppository, rectal, as base: 25 mg, 100 mg
Syrup, as hydrochloride: 10 mg/5 mL (120 mL)
Tablet, as hydrochloride: 10 mg, 25 mg, 50 mg, 100 mg, 200 mg

chlorpropamide (klor PROE pa mide)

Tall-Man chlorpro**PAMIDE**
U.S./Canadian Brand Names Apo®-Chlorpropamide [Can]; Diabinese® [US]
Therapeutic Category Antidiabetic Agent, Oral
Use Control blood sugar in adult onset, noninsulin-dependent diabetes (type II)
Usual Dosage The dosage of chlorpropamide is variable and should be individualized based upon the patient's response

Adults: Oral: 250 mg once daily; initial dose in elderly patients: 100 mg once daily; subsequent dosages may be increased or decreased by 50-125 mg/day at 3- to 5-day intervals; maximum daily dose: 750 mg
Dosage Forms Tablet: 100 mg, 250 mg

Chlor-Rest® Tablet *(Discontinued)* see page 814

Chlortab® *(Discontinued)* see page 814

chlorthalidone (klor THAL i done)

U.S./Canadian Brand Names Apo®-Chlorthalidone [Can]; Thalitone® [US]
Therapeutic Category Diuretic, Miscellaneous
Use Management of mild to moderate hypertension, used alone or in combination with other agents; treatment of edema associated with congestive heart failure, nephrotic syndrome, or pregnancy
Usual Dosage Oral:
Children: 2 mg/kg 3 times/week
Adults: 25-100 mg/day or 100 mg 3 times/week
Dosage Forms
Tablet: 25 mg, 50 mg, 100 mg
Thalitone®: 15 mg

chlorthalidone and atenolol see atenolol and chlorthalidone on page 60

chlorthalidone and clonidine see clonidine and chlorthalidone on page 155

Chlor-Trimeton® Allergy/Decongestant [US-OTC] see chlorpheniramine and pseudoephedrine on page 138

Chlor-Trimeton® [US-OTC] see chlorpheniramine on page 137

Chlor-Tripolon® [Can] see chlorpheniramine on page 137

Chlor-Tripolon ND® [Can] see loratadine and pseudoephedrine on page 391

chlorzoxazone (klor ZOKS a zone)

U.S./Canadian Brand Names Parafon Forte® [Can]; Parafon Forte™ DSC [US]; Strifon Forte® [Can]
Therapeutic Category Skeletal Muscle Relaxant
Use Symptomatic treatment of muscle spasm and pain associated with acute musculoskeletal conditions
Usual Dosage Oral:
Children: 20 mg/kg/day or 600 mg/m^2/day in 3-4 divided doses
Adults: 250-500 mg 3-4 times/day up to 750 mg 3-4 times/day
Dosage Forms
Caplet (Parafon Forte® DSC): 500 mg
Tablet: 250 mg

Cholac® [US] *see* lactulose *on page 372*

Cholan-HMB® [US-OTC] *see* dehydrocholic acid *on page 178*

Cholebrine® [US] *see* radiological/contrast media (ionic) *on page 561*

cholecalciferol (kole e kal SI fer ole)
Synonyms D_3
U.S./Canadian Brand Names Delta-D® [US]; D-Vi-Sol® [Can]
Therapeutic Category Vitamin D Analog
Use Dietary supplement, treatment of vitamin D deficiency or prophylaxis of deficiency
Usual Dosage Adults: Oral: 400-1000 units/day
Dosage Forms Tablet: 400 int. units; 1000 int. units

Choledyl® *(Discontinued) see page 814*

Choledyl SA® [US] *see* oxtriphylline *on page 484*

cholera vaccine (KOL er a vak SEEN)
U.S./Canadian Brand Names Mutacol Berna® [Can]
Therapeutic Category Vaccine, Inactivated Bacteria
Use Primary immunization for cholera prophylaxis
Usual Dosage I.M., S.C.:
  Children:
    6 months to 4 years: 0.2 mL with same dosage schedule
    5-10 years: 0.3 mL with same dosage schedule
    Children >10 years and Adults: 0.5 mL in 2 doses 1 week to 1 month or more apart
Dosage Forms Injection: Suspension of killed *Vibrio cholerae* (Inaba and Ogawa types)
  8 units of each serotype per mL (1.5 mL, 20 mL)

cholestyramine resin (koe LES tir a meen REZ in)
U.S./Canadian Brand Names LoCHOLEST® [US]; LoCHOLEST® Light [US]; Novo-Cholamine [Can]; Novo-Cholamine Light [Can]; PMS-Cholestyramine [Can]; Prevalite® [US]; Questran® Light [US/Can]; Questran® Powder [US/Can]
Therapeutic Category Bile Acid Sequestrant
Use Adjunct in the management of primary hypercholesterolemia; pruritus associated with elevated levels of bile acids; diarrhea associated with excess fecal bile acids; pseudomembranous colitis
Usual Dosage Dosages are expressed in terms of anhydrous resin. Oral:
  Children: 240 mg/kg/day in 3 divided doses; need to titrate dose depending on indication
  Adults: 3-4 g 3-4 times/day to a maximum of 16-32 g/day in 2-4 divided doses
Dosage Forms
  Powder: 4 g of resin/9 g of powder (9 g, 378 g)
  Powder for oral suspension:
    With aspartame: 4 g of resin/5 g of powder (5 g, 210 g)
    With phenylalanine: 4 g of resin/5.5 g of powder (60s)

choline magnesium trisalicylate
(KOE leen mag NEE zhum trye sa LIS i late)
U.S./Canadian Brand Names Tricosal® [US]; Trilisate® [US/Can]
Therapeutic Category Analgesic, Non-narcotic; Nonsteroidal Anti-inflammatory Drug (NSAID)
Use Management of osteoarthritis, rheumatoid arthritis, and other arthritides
Usual Dosage Oral (based on total salicylate content):
  Children: 30-60 mg/kg/day administered in 3-4 divided doses
  Adults: 500 mg to 1.5 g 1-3 times/day
  (Continued)

choline magnesium trisalicylate *(Continued)*

Dosage Forms
Liquid: 500 mg/5 mL total salicylate (293 mg/5 mL choline salicylate and 362 mg/5 mL magnesium salicylate)
Tablet:
500 mg total salicylate (293 mg choline salicylate and 362 mg magnesium salicylate)
750 mg total salicylate (440 mg choline salicylate and 544 mg magnesium salicylate)
1000 mg total salicylate (587 mg choline salicylate and 725 mg magnesium salicylate)

choline salicylate (KOE leen sa LIS i late)

U.S./Canadian Brand Names Arthropan® [US-OTC]; Teejel® [Can]

Therapeutic Category Analgesic, Non-narcotic; Nonsteroidal Anti-inflammatory Drug (NSAID)

Use Temporary relief of pain of rheumatoid arthritis, rheumatic fever, osteoarthritis, and other conditions for which oral salicylates are recommended; useful in patients in which there is difficulty in administering doses in a tablet or capsule dosage form, because of the liquid dosage form

Usual Dosage Adults: Oral: 5 mL every 3-4 hours, if necessary, but not more than 6 doses in 24 hours

Dosage Forms Liquid: 870 mg/5 mL (240 mL, 480 mL) [mint flavor]

choline theophyllinate *see* oxtriphylline *on page 484*

Cholografin® Meglumine [US] *see* radiological/contrast media (ionic) *on page 561*

Choloxin® *(Discontinued)* *see page 814*

chondroitin sulfate-sodium hyaluronate

(kon DROY tin SUL fate-SOW de um hye a loo ROE nate)

Synonyms sodium hyaluronate-chrondroitin sulfate

U.S./Canadian Brand Names Viscoat® [US]

Therapeutic Category Ophthalmic Agent, Viscoelastic

Use Surgical aid in anterior segment procedures, protects corneal endothelium and coats intraocular lens thus protecting it

Usual Dosage Ophthalmic: Carefully introduce into anterior chamber after thoroughly cleaning the chamber with a balanced salt solution

Dosage Forms Solution, ophthalmic: Sodium chondroitin 40 mg and sodium hyaluronate 30 mg (0.25 mL, 0.5 mL)

Chooz® [US-OTC] *see* calcium carbonate *on page 104*

Chorex® [US] *see* chorionic gonadotropin (human) *on this page*

choriogonadotropin alfa *see* chorionic gonadotropin (recombinant) *on next page*

chorionic gonadotropin (human)

(kor ee ON ik goe NAD oh troe pin HYU man)

Synonyms CG; HCG

U.S./Canadian Brand Names Chorex® [US]; Novarel™ [US]; Pregnyl® [US/Can]; Profasi® HP [Can]; Profasi® [US]

Therapeutic Category Gonadotropin

Use Treatment of hypogonadotropic hypogonadism, prepubertal cryptorchidism; induce ovulation

Usual Dosage Children: I.M.:
Prepubertal cryptorchidism: 1000-2000 units/m^2/dose 3 times/week for 3 weeks
Hypogonadotropic hypogonadism: 500-1000 USP units 3 times/week for 3 weeks, followed by the same dose twice weekly for 3 weeks

Dosage Forms Powder for injection: 5000 units, 10,000 units

chorionic gonadotropin (recombinant)
(kor ee ON ik goe NAD oh troe pin ree KOM be nant)
Synonyms choriogonadotropin alfa; r-hCG
U.S./Canadian Brand Names Ovidrel® [US]
Therapeutic Category Gonadotropin; Ovulation Stimulator
Use As part of an assisted reproductive technology (ART) program, induces ovulation in infertile females who have been pretreated with follicle stimulating hormones (FSH); induces ovulation and pregnancy in infertile females when the cause of infertility is functional
Usual Dosage S.C.:
Adults: Female:
Assisted reproductive technologies (ART) and ovulation induction: 250 mcg given 1 day following the last dose of follicle stimulating agent. Use only after adequate follicular development has been determined. Hold treatment when there is an excessive ovarian response.
Dosage Forms Injection [single-dose vial]: 285 mcg r-hCG per vial with 1 mL SWFI [delivers 250 mcg r-hCG following reconstitution]

Choron® *(Discontinued)* see page 814

Chromagen® OB [US-OTC] see vitamin (multiple/prenatal) on page 683

Chroma-Pak® [US] see trace metals on page 646

chromium injection see trace metals on page 646

Chronovera® [Can] see verapamil on page 675

Chronulac® *(Discontinued)* see page 814

Chymex® *(Discontinued)* see page 814

Cibacalcin® *(Discontinued)* see page 814

ciclopirox (sye kloe PEER oks)
U.S./Canadian Brand Names Loprox® [US/Can]; Penlac™ [US/Can]
Therapeutic Category Antifungal Agent
Use Treatment of tinea pedis, tinea cruris, tinea corporis, cutaneous candidiasis, tinea versicolor
Usual Dosage Children >10 years and Adults: Topical: Apply twice daily, gently massage into affected areas; safety and efficacy in children <10 years have not been established
Dosage Forms
Cream, as olamine: 1% (15 g, 30 g, 90 g)
Lotion, as olamine: 1% (30 mL, 60 mL)
Solution, topical nail lacquer: 8% (3.3 mL)

cidofovir (si DOF o veer)
U.S./Canadian Brand Names Vistide® [US]
Therapeutic Category Antiviral Agent
Use Treatment of CMV retinitis in patients with acquired immunodeficiency syndrome (AIDS)
Usual Dosage
Induction treatment: 5 mg/kg once weekly for 2 consecutive weeks
Maintenance treatment: 5 mg/kg administered once every 2 weeks
Probenecid must be administered orally with each dose of cidofovir
Probenecid dose: 2 g 3 hours prior to cidofovir dose, 1 g 2 hours and 8 hours after completion of the infusion; patients should also receive 1 L of normal saline intravenously prior to each infusion of cidofovir; saline should be infused over 1-2 hours
Dosage Forms Injection: 75 mg/mL (5 mL)

cilastatin and imipenem see imipenem and cilastatin on page 345

cilazapril *(Canada only)* (sye LAY za pril)
U.S./Canadian Brand Names Inhibace® [Can]
Therapeutic Category Angiotensin-Converting Enzyme (ACE) Inhibitor
Use Management of hypertension and treatment of congestive heart failure
Usual Dosage Adults: Oral:
  Congestive heart failure: Recommended starting dose is 0.5 mg once daily, usual maintenance dose: 1-2.5 mg/day
  Hypertension: 2.5-5 mg once daily
Dosage Forms Tablet: 1 mg, 2.5 mg, 5 mg

cilostazol (sil OH sta zol)
U.S./Canadian Brand Names Pletal® [US/Can]
Therapeutic Category Platelet Aggregation Inhibitor
Use Symptomatic management of peripheral vascular disease, primarily intermittent claudication
Usual Dosage Adults: Oral: 100 mg twice daily taken at least 30 minutes before or 2 hours after breakfast and dinner; dosage should be reduced to 50 mg twice daily during concurrent therapy with inhibitors of CYP3A4 or CYP2C19
Dosage Forms Tablet: 50 mg, 100 mg

Ciloxan™ [US/Can] *see* ciprofloxacin *on next page*

cimetidine (sye MET i deen)
U.S./Canadian Brand Names Acid Reducer 200® [US-OTC]; Apo®-Cimetidine [Can]; Gen-Cimetidine [Can]; Heartburn 200® [US-OTC]; Heartburn Relief 200® [US-OTC]; Novo-Cimetidine [Can]; Nu-Cimet® [Can]; PMS-Cimetidine [Can]; Tagamet® HB [US/Can]; Tagamet® [US/Can]
Therapeutic Category Histamine H_2 Antagonist
Use Short-term treatment of active duodenal ulcers and benign gastric ulcers; long-term prophylaxis of duodenal ulcer; gastric hypersecretory states; gastroesophageal reflux
Usual Dosage Oral, I.M., I.V.:
  Infants: 10-20 mg/kg/day divided every 6-12 hours
  Children: 20-30 mg/kg/day in divided doses every 6 hours

  Patients with an active bleed: Administer cimetidine as a continuous infusion
  Adults:
    Short-term treatment of active ulcers:
      Oral: 300 mg 4 times/day or 800 mg at bedtime or 400 mg twice daily for up to 8 weeks
      I.M., I.V.: 300 mg every 6 hours or 37.5 mg/hour by continuous infusion; I.V. dosage should be adjusted to maintain an intragastric pH of 5 or greater
    Duodenal ulcer prophylaxis: Oral: 400-800 mg at bedtime
    Gastric hypersecretory conditions: Oral, I.M., I.V.: 300-600 mg every 6 hours; dosage not to exceed 2.4 g/day
Dosage Forms
  Infusion, as hydrochloride, in NS: 300 mg (50 mL)
  Injection, as hydrochloride: 150 mg/mL (2 mL, 8 mL)
  Liquid, oral, as hydrochloride: 200 mg/20 mL; 300 mg/5 mL [with alcohol 2.8%] (5 mL, 240 mL) [mint-peach flavor]
  Tablet: 100 mg, 200 mg, 300 mg, 400 mg, 800 mg

Cinobac® [US/Can] *see* cinoxacin *on this page*

cinoxacin (sin OKS a sin)
U.S./Canadian Brand Names Cinobac® [US/Can]
Therapeutic Category Quinolone
Use Urinary tract infections
Usual Dosage Children >12 years and Adults: Oral: 1 g/day in 2-4 doses

Dosage Forms Capsule: 250 mg, 500 mg

Cipralan® *(Discontinued)* see page 814

Cipro® [US/Can] see ciprofloxacin on this page

ciprofloxacin (sip roe FLOKS a sin)

U.S./Canadian Brand Names Ciloxan™ [US/Can]; Cipro® [US/Can]

Therapeutic Category Antibiotic, Ophthalmic; Quinolone

Use Treatment of documented or suspected infections of the lower respiratory tract, sinuses, skin and skin structure, bone/joints, and urinary tract (including prostatitis) due to susceptible bacterial strains; especially indicated for pseudomonal infections and those due to multidrug-resistant gram-negative organisms, chronic bacterial prostatitis, infectious diarrhea, complicated gram-negative and anaerobic intra-abdominal infections (with metronidazole) due to *E. coli* (enteropathic strains), *B. fragilis*, *P. mirabilis*, *K. pneumoniae*, *P. aeruginosa*, *Campylobacter jejuni* or *Shigella*; approved for acute sinusitis caused by *H. influenzae* or *M. catarrhalis*; also used in treatment of typhoid fever due to *Salmonella typhi* (although eradication of the chronic typhoid carrier state has not been proven), osteomyelitis when parenteral therapy is not feasible, acute uncomplicated cystitis in females, to reduce incidence or progression of disease following exposure to aerolized *Bacillus anthracis*, and sexually-transmitted diseases such as uncomplicated cervical and urethral gonorrhea due to *Neisseria gonorrhoeae*; used ophthalmologically for superficial ocular infections (corneal ulcers, conjunctivitis) due to susceptible strains

Usual Dosage

Children: Oral: 20-30 mg/kg/day in 2 divided doses; maximum dose: 1.5 g/day

Adults:

Oral: 250-750 mg every 12 hours, depending on severity of infection and susceptibility

Ophthalmic: Instill 1-2 drops in eye(s) every 2 hours while awake for 2 days and 1-2 drops every 4 hours while awake for the next 5 days

I.V.: 200-400 mg every 12 hours depending on severity of infection

Dosage Forms

Infusion, as hydrochloride [in D_5W]: 400 mg (200 mL)

Infusion, as hydrochloride [in NS or D_5W]: 200 mg (100 mL) [latex-free PVC]

Injection, as hydrochloride: 200 mg (20 mL); 400 mg (40 mL)

Ointment, ophthalmic, as hydrochloride: 3.33 mg/g [0.3% base] (3.5 g)

Solution, ophthalmic, as hydrochloride: 3.33 mg/g [0.3% base] (2.5 mL, 5 mL. 10 mL)

Suspension, oral: 250 mg/5 mL (100 mL); 500 mg/5 mL (100 mL)

Tablet, as hydrochloride: 100 mg, 250 mg, 500 mg, 750 mg

ciprofloxacin and hydrocortisone

(sip roe FLOKS a sin & hye droe KOR ti sone)

U.S./Canadian Brand Names Cipro® HC Otic [US/Can]

Therapeutic Category Antibiotic/Corticosteroid, Otic

Use Treatment of acute otitis externa, sometimes known as "swimmer's ear"

Usual Dosage Children >1 year of age and Adults: Otic: The recommended dosage for all patients is three drops of the suspension in the affected ear twice daily for seven day; twice-daily dosing schedule is more convenient for patients than that of existing treatments with hydrocortisone, which are typically administered three or four times a day; a twice-daily dosage schedule may be especially helpful for parents and caregivers of young children

Dosage Forms Suspension, otic: Ciprofloxacin hydrochloride 0.2% and hydrocortisone 1% (10 mL)

Cipro® HC Otic [US/Can] see ciprofloxacin and hydrocortisone on this page

cisapride (SIS a pride)

U.S./Canadian Brand Names Propulsid® [US]

Therapeutic Category Gastrointestinal Agent, Prokinetic

(Continued)

cisapride (Continued)

Use Treatment of nocturnal symptoms of gastroesophageal reflux disease (GERD), also demonstrated effectiveness for gastroparesis, refractory constipation, and nonulcer dyspepsia

Usual Dosage Adults: Oral: 10 mg 4 times/day at least 15 minutes before meals and at bedtime; in some patients the dosage will need to be increased to 20 mg to obtain a satisfactory result

Dosage Forms
Suspension, oral: 1 mg/mL (450 mL) [cherry cream flavor]
Tablet, scored: 10 mg, 20 mg

cisatracurium (sis a tra KYOO ree um)

U.S./Canadian Brand Names Nimbex® [US/Can]

Therapeutic Category Skeletal Muscle Relaxant

Use As an adjunct to general anesthesia to facilitate endotracheal intubation and to relax skeletal muscles during surgery; to facilitate mechanical ventilation in ICU patients; does not relieve pain or produce sedation

Usual Dosage I.V.: Dose to effect; doses will vary due to interpatient variability; use ideal body weight for obese patients

Surgery:
Children 2-12 years: 0.1 mg/kg, produces clinically effective block for 28 minutes
Adults: 0.15-0.2 mg/kg, then 0.03 mg/kg 40-60 minutes after initial dose to maintain neuromuscular block, followed by repeat doses of 0.03 mg/kg at 20-minute intervals; initial dose after succinylcholine for intubation: 0.1 mg/kg
Continuous infusion: At initial signs of recovery from bolus dose, begin at 3 mcg/kg/minute, block usually maintained by a rate of 1-2 mcg/kg/minute
Pretreatment/priming: 10% of intubating dose given 3-5 minutes before initial dose
ICU: Adults: 0.1 mg/kg bolus; at initial signs of recovery begin at rate of 3 mcg/kg/minute and adjust accordingly (rates of 0.5-10 mcg/kg/minute reported)

Dosage Forms Injection, as besylate: 2 mg/mL (5 mL, 10 mL); 10 mg/mL (20 mL)

cisplatin (SIS pla tin)

Synonyms CDDP

U.S./Canadian Brand Names Platinol®-AQ [US]; Platinol® [US]

Therapeutic Category Antineoplastic Agent

Use Management of metastatic testicular or ovarian carcinoma, advanced bladder cancer, osteosarcoma, Hodgkin's and non-Hodgkin's lymphoma, head or neck cancer, cervical cancer, lung cancer, brain tumors, neuroblastoma; used alone or in combination with other agents

Usual Dosage Children and Adults (refer to individual protocols): I.V.:
Intermittent dosing schedule: 37-75 mg/m^2 once every 2-3 weeks or 50-120 mg/m^2 once every 3-4 weeks
Daily dosing schedule: 15-20 mg/m^2/day for 5 days every 3-4 weeks

Dosage Forms
Injection, aqueous: 1 mg/mL (50 mL, 100 mL, 200 mL)
Injection, powder for reconstitution: 10 mg, 50 mg

13-*cis*-retinoic acid *see* isotretinoin *on page 363*

citalopram (sye TAL oh pram)

Synonyms citalopram hydrobromide; nitalapram

U.S./Canadian Brand Names Celexa™ [US/Can]

Therapeutic Category Antidepressant

Use Depression

Usual Dosage Oral: 20-60 mg/day

Dosage Forms
Solution, oral: 10 mg/5 mL [alcohol free; peppermint flavor; sugar free]

Tablet, as hydrobromide: 10 mg, 20 mg, 40 mg

citalopram hydrobromide *see* citalopram *on previous page*

Citanest® Forte [Can] *see* prilocaine *on page 539*

Citanest® Plain [US/Can] *see* prilocaine *on page 539*

Cithalith-S® Syrup *(Discontinued)* *see page 814*

Citracal® [US-OTC] *see* calcium citrate *on page 106*

citrate of magnesia *see* magnesium citrate *on page 397*

citric acid and d-gluconic acid irrigant *see* citric acid bladder mixture *on this page*

citric acid and potassium citrate *see* potassium citrate and citric acid *on page 531*

citric acid bladder mixture (SI trik AS id BLAD dur MIKS chur)

Synonyms citric acid and d-gluconic acid irrigant; hemiacidrin

U.S./Canadian Brand Names Renacidin® [US]

Therapeutic Category Irrigating Solution

Use Preparing solutions for irrigating indwelling urethral catheters; to dissolve or prevent formation of calcifications

Usual Dosage 30-60 mL of 10% (sterile) solution 2-3 times/day by means of a rubber syringe

Dosage Forms

Powder for solution: Citric acid 156-171 g, magnesium hydroxycarbonate 75-87 g, D-gluconic acid 21-30 g, magnesium acid citrate 9-15 g, calcium carbonate 2-6 g (150 g, 300 g)

Solution, irrigation: Citric acid 6.602 g, magnesium hydroxycarbonate 3.177 g, glucono-delta-lactone 0.198 g, and benzoic acid 0.023 g per 100 mL (500 mL)

Citro-Mag® [Can] *see* magnesium citrate *on page 397*

Citro-Nesia™ Solution *(Discontinued)* *see page 814*

Citrotein® [US-OTC] *see* nutritional formula, enteral/oral *on page 472*

citrovorum factor *see* leucovorin *on page 377*

Citrucel® [US-OTC] *see* methylcellulose *on page 420*

CI-719 *see* gemfibrozil *on page 295*

CLA *see* clarithromycin *on this page*

cladribine (KLA dri been)

Synonyms 2-CdA; 2-chlorodeoxyadenosine

U.S./Canadian Brand Names Leustatin™ [US/Can]

Therapeutic Category Antineoplastic Agent

Use Hairy cell and chronic lymphocytic leukemias

Usual Dosage Adults: I.V. continuous infusion: 0.09 mg/kg/day

Dosage Forms Injection [preservative free]: 1 mg/mL (10 mL)

Claforan® [US/Can] *see* cefotaxime *on page 123*

Clarinex® [US] *see* desloratadine *on page 182*

clarithromycin (kla RITH roe mye sin)

Synonyms CLA

U.S./Canadian Brand Names Biaxin® [US/Can]; Biaxin® XL [US]

Therapeutic Category Macrolide (Antibiotic)

Use Treatment of upper and lower respiratory tract infections, acute otitis media, and infections of the skin and skin structure due to susceptible strains of *S. aureus, S. pyogenes, S. pneumoniae, H. influenzae, M. catarrhalis, Mycoplasma pneumoniae, C.* (Continued)

clarithromycin *(Continued)*

trachomatis, *Legionella* sp, and *M. avium*; prophylaxis of disseminated *M. avium* complex (MAC) infections in HIV-infected patients

Usual Dosage Oral: 250-500 mg every 12 hours for 7-14 days; Biaxin® XL: 2 x 500 mg once daily for 7-14 days

Upper respiratory tract: 250-500 mg every 12 hours for 10-14 days

Pharyngitis/tonsillitis: 250 mg every 12 hours for 10 days

Acute maxillary sinusitis: 500 mg every 12 hours for 14 days

Lower respiratory tract: 250-500 mg every 12 hours for 7-14 days

Acute exacerbation of chronic bronchitis due to:

S. *pneumoniae*: 250 mg every 12 hours for 7-14 days

M. *catarrhalis*: 250 mg every 12 hours for 7-14 days

H. *influenzae*: 500 mg every 12 hours for 7-14 days

Pneumonia due to:

S. *pneumoniae*: 250 mg every 12 hours for 7-14 days

M. *pneumoniae*: 250 mg every 12 hours for 7-14 days

Uncomplicated skin and skin structure: 250 mg every 12 hours for 7-14 days

Dosage Forms

Granules for oral suspension: 125 mg/5 mL (50 mL, 100 mL); 187.5 mg/5 mL (100 mL); 250 mg/5 mL (50 mL, 100 mL)

Tablet, film coated: 250 mg, 500 mg

Tablet, film coated, extended release: 500 mg

Claritin® **[US/Can]** *see* loratadine *on page 391*

Claritin-D® **12-Hour [US]** *see* loratadine and pseudoephedrine *on page 391*

Claritin-D® **24-Hour [US]** *see* loratadine and pseudoephedrine *on page 391*

Claritin® **Extra [Can]** *see* loratadine and pseudoephedrine *on page 391*

Claritin® **RediTabs®** **[US]** *see* loratadine *on page 391*

clavulanate potassium and amoxicillin *see* amoxicillin and clavulanate potassium *on page 38*

clavulanic acid and ticarcillin *see* ticarcillin and clavulanate potassium *on page 638*

Clavulin® **[Can]** *see* amoxicillin and clavulanate potassium *on page 38*

Clear Away® **Disc** *(Discontinued) see page 814*

Clear By Design® **Gel** *(Discontinued) see page 814*

Clear Eyes® **ACR [US-OTC]** *see* naphazoline *on page 446*

Clear Eyes® **[US-OTC]** *see* naphazoline *on page 446*

Clearsil® **Maximum Strength** *(Discontinued) see page 814*

Clear Tussin® **30** *(Discontinued) see page 814*

clemastine *(KLEM as teen)*

U.S./Canadian Brand Names Tavist® [US]; Tavist®-1 [US-OTC]

Therapeutic Category Antihistamine

Use Perennial and seasonal allergic rhinitis and other allergic symptoms including urticaria

Usual Dosage Oral:

Children:

<12 years: 0.67-1.34 mg every 8-12 hours as needed

>12 years: 1.34 mg twice daily to 2.68 mg 3 times/day; do not exceed 8.04 mg/day

Adults: 1.34 mg twice daily to 2.68 mg 3 times/day; do not exceed 8.04 mg/day

Dosage Forms

Syrup, as fumarate: 0.67 mg/5 mL [with alcohol 5.5%] (120 mL) [citrus flavor]

Tablet, as fumarate: 1.34 mg, 2.68 mg

Cleocin® **[US]** *see* clindamycin *on this page*

Cleocin HCl® **[US]** *see* clindamycin *on this page*

Cleocin Pediatric® **[US]** *see* clindamycin *on this page*

Cleocin Phosphate® **[US]** *see* clindamycin *on this page*

Cleocin T® **[US]** *see* clindamycin *on this page*

clidinium and chlordiazepoxide (kli DI nee um & klor dye az e POKS ide)

Synonyms chlordiazepoxide and clidinium

U.S./Canadian Brand Names Apo®-Chlorax [Can]; Librax® [US/Can]

Therapeutic Category Anticholinergic Agent

Use Adjunct treatment of peptic ulcer, treatment of irritable bowel syndrome

Usual Dosage Oral: 1-2 capsules 3-4 times/day, before meals or food and at bedtime

Dosage Forms Capsule: Clidinium bromide 2.5 mg and chlordiazepoxide hydrochloride 5 mg

Climacteron® **[Can]** *see* estradiol and testosterone *on page 240*

Climara® **[US/Can]** *see* estradiol *on page 238*

Clinac™ **BPO [US]** *see* benzoyl peroxide *on page 79*

Clindagel™ **[US]** *see* clindamycin *on this page*

clindamycin (klin da MYE sin)

U.S./Canadian Brand Names Alti-Clindamycin [Can]; Cleocin HCl® [US]; Cleocin Pediatric® [US]; Cleocin Phosphate® [US]; Cleocin T® [US]; Cleocin® [US]; Clindagel™ [US]; Clindets® [US]; Dalacin® C [Can]

Therapeutic Category Acne Products; Antibiotic, Miscellaneous

Use Useful agent against most aerobic gram-positive staphylococci and streptococci (except enterococci); also useful against *Fusobacterium*, *Bacteroides* sp. and *Actinomyces* for treatment of respiratory tract infections, skin and soft tissue infections, sepsis, intra-abdominal infections, and infections of the female pelvis and genital tract; used topically in treatment of severe acne

Usual Dosage Avoid in neonates (contains benzyl alcohol)

Infants and Children:
Oral: 10-30 mg/kg/day in 3-4 divided doses
I.M., I.V.: 25-40 mg/kg/day in 3-4 divided doses
Children and Adults: Topical: Apply twice daily
Adults:
Oral: 150-450 mg/dose every 6-8 hours; maximum dose: 1.8 g/day
I.M., I.V.: 1.2-1.8 g/day in 2-4 divided doses; maximum dose: 4.8 g/day
Vaginal: 1 full applicator (100 mg) inserted intravaginally once daily before bedtime for 7 consecutive days

Dosage Forms

Capsule, as hydrochloride (Cleocin HCl®): 75 mg [contains tartrazine], 150 mg [contains tartrazine], 300 mg

Cream, vaginal, as phosphate (Cleocin®): 2% (40 g) [packaged with 7 disposable applicators]

Gel, topical, as phosphate: 1% [10 mg/g] (30 g, 60 g)
Cleocin T®: 1% [10 mg/g] (30 g, 60 g)
Clindagel™: 1% [10 mg/g] (42 g, 77 g)

Granules for oral solution, as palmitate (Cleocin Pediatric®): 75 mg/5 mL (100 mL) [cherry flavor]

Infusion, as phosphate [premixed in D_5W] (Cleocin Phosphate®): 300 mg (50 mL); 600 mg (50 mL); 900 mg (50 mL)

Injection, solution, as phosphate (Cleocin Phosphate®): 150 mg/mL (2 mL, 4 mL, 6 mL, 60 mL) [contains benzyl alcohol]

Lotion, as phosphate (Cleocin T®): 1% [10 mg/mL] (60 mL)

Pledgets, topical: 1% (60s)

(Continued)

clindamycin *(Continued)*

Clindets®: 1% (69s)
Cleocin T®: 1% (60s)
Solution, topical, as phosphate (Cleocin T®): 1% [10 mg/mL] (30 mL, 60 mL)
Suppository, vaginal, as phosphate (Cleocin®): 100 mg (3s)

clindamycin and benzoyl peroxide

(klin da MYE sin & BEN zoe il peer OKS ide)
Synonyms benzoyl peroxide and clindamycin
U.S./Canadian Brand Names BenzaClin™ [US]
Therapeutic Category Topical Skin Product; Topical Skin Product, Acne
Use Topical treatment of acne vulgaris
Usual Dosage Topical: Children ≥12 years and Adults: Acne: Apply twice daily (morning and evening) to affected areas after skin has been cleansed and dried
Dosage Forms Gel, topical: Clindamycin 1% and benzol peroxide 5% (25 g, 50 g)

Clindets® **[US]** *see* clindamycin *on previous page*

Clindex® *(Discontinued) see page 814*

Clinoril® **[US]** *see* sulindac *on page 615*

clioquinol (klye oh KWIN ole)

Therapeutic Category Antifungal Agent
Use Treatment of tinea pedis, tinea cruris, and skin infections caused by dermatophytic fungi (ring worm)
Usual Dosage Children and Adults: Topical: Apply 2-4 times/day; do not use for >7 days
Dosage Forms
Cream: 3% (30 g)
Ointment, topical: 3% (30 g)

clioquinol and hydrocortisone (klye oh KWIN ole & hye droe KOR ti sone)

Synonyms hydrocortisone and clioquinol; iodochlorhydroxyquin and hydrocortisone
U.S./Canadian Brand Names Ala-Quin® [US]; Dek-Quin® [US]
Therapeutic Category Antifungal/Corticosteroid
Use Contact or atopic dermatitis; eczema; neurodermatitis; anogenital pruritus; mycotic dermatoses; moniliasis
Usual Dosage Topical: Apply in a thin film 3-4 times/day
Dosage Forms Cream: Clioquinol 3% and hydrocortisone 0.5% (15 g, 30 g); clioquinol 3% and hydrocortisone 1% (20 g, 30 g, 454 g)

Clistin® **Tablet** *(Discontinued) see page 814*

clobazam *(Canada only)* (KLOE ba zam)

U.S./Canadian Brand Names Alti-Clobazam [Can]; Frisium® [Can]; Novo-Clobazam [Can]
Therapeutic Category Anticonvulsant; Antidepressant
Use Antianxiety, anticonvulsant, and sedative agent
Usual Dosage Adults: 20-30 mg/day in divided doses or at night; maximum daily dose: 60 mg
Dosage Forms Tablet: 10 mg

clobetasol (kloe BAY ta sol)

U.S./Canadian Brand Names Cormax® [US]; Dermovate® [Can]; Gen-Clobetasol [Can]; Novo-Clobetasol [Can]; Olux™ [US]; Temovate® [US]
Therapeutic Category Corticosteroid, Topical
Use Short-term relief of inflammation of moderate to severe corticosteroid-responsive dermatosis

Usual Dosage Topical: Apply twice daily for up to 2 weeks with no more than 50 g/week. Therapy should be discontinued when control is achieved. If no improvement is seen, reassessment of diagnosis may be necessary.

Dosage Forms
Cream, as propionate: 0.05% (15 g, 30 g, 45 g)
Cream, as propionate [in emollient base]: 0.05% (15 g, 30 g, 60 g)
Foam, scalp, as propionate (Olux™): 0.05% (100 g)
Gel, as propionate: 0.05% (15 g, 30 g, 45 g)
Ointment, as propionate: 0.05% (15 g, 30 g, 45 g)
Solution, scalp, as propionate: 0.05% (25 mL, 50 mL)

Clocort® Maximum Strength [US-OTC] see hydrocortisone (topical) on page 334

clocortolone (kloe KOR toe lone)
U.S./Canadian Brand Names Cloderm® [US/Can]
Therapeutic Category Corticosteroid, Topical
Use Inflammation of corticosteroid-responsive dermatoses
Usual Dosage Topical: Apply sparingly and gently rub into affected area 1-4 times/day. Therapy should be discontinued when control is achieved. If no improvement is seen, reassessment of diagnosis may be necessary.
Dosage Forms Cream, as pivalate: 0.1% (15 g, 45 g)

Cloderm® [US/Can] see clocortolone on this page

clodronate disodium *(Canada only)* (KLOE droh nate dy SOW de um)
U.S./Canadian Brand Names Bonefos® [US/Can]; Ostac® [US/Can]
Therapeutic Category Bisphosphonate Derivative
Use For the management of hypercalcemia of malignancy. Prior to treatment with clodronate renal excretion of excess calcium should be promoted by restoration and maintenance of adequate fluid balance and urine output. In responsive patients I.V. infusion of clodronate decreases the flux of calcium from the bones by inhibiting the osteoclastic activity and bone resorption, thus reducing the calcium level in blood. Treatment with oral clodronate following I.V. infusion has been found to prolong the duration of action.
Usual Dosage
I.V. Infusion: The recommended adult dose is 300 mg/day (one 5 mL ampul). The contents of the ampul must be diluted in 500 mL of sodium chloride 0.9% injection or dextrose 5% injection and administered by infusion lasting at least 2 hours. Treatment should be continued until plasma calcium returns to normal, this generally being achieved after 2 to 5 days of treatment. Treatment should not be prolonged beyond 7 days.
Capsule: The oral recommended daily maintenance dose following I.V. therapy is in the range of 1600 mg (4 capsules) to 2400 mg (6 capsules) given in single or 2 divided doses. Maximal recommended daily dose is 3200 mg (8 capsules). The drug should be taken at least 2 hours before or after food, because food may decrease the amount of clodronate absorbed by the body.
Dosage Forms
Injection, as disodium: 30 mg/mL (10 mL); 60 mg/mL (5 mL)
Capsule, as disodium: 400 mg

clofazimine (kloe FA zi meen)
U.S./Canadian Brand Names Lamprene® [US/Can]
Therapeutic Category Leprostatic Agent
Use Treatment of dapsone-resistant lepromatous leprosy (*Mycobacterium leprae*); multibacillary dapsone-sensitive leprosy; erythema nodosum leprosum; *Mycobacterium avium-intracellulare* (MAI) infections
(Continued)

clofazimine *(Continued)*

Usual Dosage Oral:

Children: Leprosy: 1 mg/kg/day every 24 hours in combination with dapsone and rifampin

Adults:

Dapsone-resistant leprosy: 50-100 mg/day in combination with one or more antileprosy drugs for 2 years; then alone 50-100 mg/day

Dapsone-sensitive multibacillary leprosy: 50-100 mg/day in combination with two or more antileprosy drugs for at least 2 years and continue until negative skin smears are obtained, then institute single drug therapy with appropriate agent

Erythema nodosum leprosum: 100-200 mg/day for up to 3 months or longer then taper dose to 100 mg/day when possible

MAI: Combination therapy using clofazimine 100 mg 1 or 3 times/day in combination with other antimycobacterial agents

Dosage Forms Capsule, as palmitate: 50 mg

Clomid® **[US/Can]** *see* clomiphene *on this page*

clomiphene (KLOE mi feen)

Tall-Man clomi**PHENE**

U.S./Canadian Brand Names Clomid® [US/Can]; Serophene® [US/Can]

Therapeutic Category Ovulation Stimulator

Use Treatment of ovulatory failure in patients desiring pregnancy

Usual Dosage Oral: 50 mg/day for 5 days (first course); start the regimen on or about the fifth day of cycle; if ovulation occurs do not increase dosage; if not, increase next course to 100 mg/day for 5 days

Dosage Forms Tablet, as citrate: 50 mg

clomipramine (kloe MI pra meen)

Tall-Man clomi**PRAMINE**

U.S./Canadian Brand Names Anafranil® [US/Can]; Apo®-Clomipramine [Can]; Gen-Clomipramine [Can]; Novo-Clopramine [Can]

Therapeutic Category Antidepressant, Tricyclic (Tertiary Amine)

Use Treatment of obsessive-compulsive disorder (OCD)

Usual Dosage Oral:

Children: Initial: 25 mg/day and gradually increase, as tolerated to a maximum of 3 mg/kg or 100 mg, whichever is smaller

Adults: Initial: 25 mg/day and gradually increase, as tolerated to 100 mg/day the first 2 weeks, may then be increased to a total of 250 mg/day

Dosage Forms Capsule, as hydrochloride: 25 mg, 50 mg, 75 mg

Clonapam [Can] *see* clonazepam *on this page*

clonazepam (kloe NA ze pam)

U.S./Canadian Brand Names Alti-Clonazepam [Can]; Apo®-Clonazepam [Can]; Clonapam [Can]; Gen-Clonazepam [Can]; Klonopin™ [US/Can]; Novo-Clonazepam [Can]; Nu-Clonazepam [Can]; PMS-Clonazepam [Can]; Rho-Clonazepam [Can]; Rivotril® [Can]

Therapeutic Category Benzodiazepine

Controlled Substance C-IV

Use Prophylaxis of absence (petit mal), petit mal variant (Lennox-Gastaut), akinetic, and myoclonic seizures

Usual Dosage Oral:

Children <10 years or 30 kg:

Initial daily dose: 0.01-0.03 mg/kg/day (maximum: 0.05 mg/kg/day) administered in 2-3 divided doses; increase by no more than 0.5 mg every third day until seizures are controlled or adverse effects are seen

Maintenance dose: 0.1-0.2 mg/kg/day divided 3 times/day; not to exceed 0.2 mg/kg/day

Adults:

Initial daily dose not to exceed 1.5 mg administered in 3 divided doses; may increase by 0.5-1 mg every third day until seizures are controlled or adverse effects seen

Maintenance dose: 0.05-0.2 mg/kg; do not exceed 20 mg/day

Dosage Forms Tablet: 0.5 mg, 1 mg, 2 mg

clonidine (KLOE ni deen)

U.S./Canadian Brand Names Apo®-Clonidine [Can]; Catapres-TTS®-1 [US]; Catapres-TTS®-2 [US]; Catapres-TTS®-3 [US]; Catapres® [US/Can]; Dixarit® [Can]; Duraclon™ [US]; Novo-Clonidine [Can]; Nu-Clonidine® [Can]

Therapeutic Category Alpha-Adrenergic Agonist

Use Management of mild to moderate hypertension; either used alone or in combination with other antihypertensives

Orphan drug: Duraclon™: For continuous epidural administration as adjunctive therapy with intraspinal opiates for treatment of cancer pain in patients tolerant to or unresponsive to intraspinal opiates

Usual Dosage

Epidural infusion (continuous): 30 mcg/hour, titrated up or down depending on pain relief

Oral:

Children: Initial: 5-10 mcg/kg/day in divided doses every 8-12 hours; increase gradually at 5- to 7-day intervals to 25 mcg/kg/day in divided doses every 6 hours; maximum: 0.9 mg/day

Clonidine tolerance test (test of growth hormone release from pituitary): 0.15 mg/m^2 or 4 mcg/kg as single dose

Adults: Initial dose: 0.1 mg twice daily, usual maintenance dose: 0.2-1.2 mg/day in 2-4 divided doses; maximum recommended dose: 2.4 mg/day

Nicotine withdrawal symptoms: 0.1 mg twice daily to maximum of 0.4 mg/day for 3-4 weeks

Transdermal: Apply once every 7 days; for initial therapy start with 0.1 mg and increase by 0.1 mg at 1- to 2-week intervals; dosages >0.6 mg do not improve efficacy

Dosage Forms

Injection, as hydrochloride [preservative free]: 100 mcg/mL (10 mL); 500 mcg/mL (10 mL)

Patch, transdermal, as hydrochloride [7-day duration]:

Catapres-TTS®-1: 0.1 mg/day (4s)

Catapres-TTS®-2: 0.2 mg/day (4s)

Catapres-TTS®-3: 0.3 mg/day (4s)

Tablet, as hydrochloride: 0.1 mg, 0.2 mg, 0.3 mg

clonidine and chlorthalidone (KLOE ni deen & klor THAL i done)

Synonyms chlorthalidone and clonidine

U.S./Canadian Brand Names Combipres® [US]

Therapeutic Category Antihypertensive Agent, Combination

Use Management of mild to moderate hypertension

Usual Dosage Oral: 1 tablet 1-2 times/day

Dosage Forms

Tablet:

0.1: Clonidine 0.1 mg and chlorthalidone 15 mg

0.2: Clonidine 0.2 mg and chlorthalidone 15 mg

0.3: Clonidine 0.3 mg and chlorthalidone 15 mg

clopidogrel (kloh PID oh grel)

U.S./Canadian Brand Names Plavix® [US/Can]

Therapeutic Category Antiplatelet Agent

(Continued)

clopidogrel *(Continued)*

Use The reduction of atherosclerotic events (myocardial infarction, stroke, vascular deaths) in patients with atherosclerosis documented by recent myocardial infarctions, recent stroke or established peripheral arterial disease

Usual Dosage Adults: Oral: 75 mg once daily

Dosage Forms Tablet, as bisulfate: 75 mg

Clopixol® [Can] *see* zuclopenthixol *(Canada only)* on page 693

Clopixol-Acuphase® [Can] *see* zuclopenthixol *(Canada only)* on page 693

Clopixol® Depot [Can] *see* zuclopenthixol *(Canada only)* on page 693

Clopra® *(Discontinued)* see page 814

clorazepate (klor AZ e pate)

U.S./Canadian Brand Names Apo®-Clorazepate [Can]; Novo-Clopate [Can]; Tranxene® [US/Can]

Therapeutic Category Anticonvulsant; Benzodiazepine

Controlled Substance C-IV

Use Treatment of generalized anxiety and panic disorders; management of alcohol withdrawal; adjunct anticonvulsant in management of partial seizures

Usual Dosage Oral:

Anticonvulsant:

Children:

<9 years: Dose not established

9-12 years: Initial: 3.75-7.5 mg/dose twice daily; increase dose by 3.75 mg at weekly intervals, not to exceed 60 mg/day in 2-3 divided doses

Children >12 years and Adults: Initial: Up to 7.5 mg/dose 2-3 times/day; increase dose by 7.5 mg at weekly intervals; usual dose: 0.5-1 mg/kg/day; not to exceed 90 mg/day (up to 3 mg/kg/day has been used)

Anxiety: Adults: 7.5-15 mg 2-4 times/day, or administered as single dose of 15-22.5 mg at bedtime

Alcohol withdrawal: Adults: Initial: 30 mg, then 15 mg 2-4 times/day on first day; maximum daily dose: 90 mg; gradually decrease dose over subsequent days

Dosage Forms Tablet, as dipotassium:

Tranxene®-SD™: 22.5 mg [once daily]

Tranxene®-SD™ Half Strength: 11.25 mg [once daily]

Tranxene® T-Tab®: 3.75 mg, 7.5 mg, 15 mg

Clorpactin® WCS-90 [US-OTC] *see* oxychlorosene on page 484

Clorpactin® XCB Powder *(Discontinued)* see page 814

Clotrimaderm [Can] *see* clotrimazole on this page

clotrimazole (kloe TRIM a zole)

U.S./Canadian Brand Names Canesten® Topical [Can]; Canesten® Vaginal [Can]; Clotrimaderm [Can]; Cruex® [US-OTC]; Gyne-Lotrimin® 3 [US-OTC]; Gyne-Lotrimin® [US-OTC]; Gynix® [US-OTC]; Lotrimin® [US]; Mycelex® [US]; Mycelex®-7 [US-OTC]; Mycelex® Twin Pack [US-OTC]

Therapeutic Category Antifungal Agent

Use Treatment of susceptible fungal infections, including oropharyngeal candidiasis, dermatophytoses, superficial mycoses, cutaneous candidiasis, as well as vulvovaginal candidiasis; limited data suggests that the use of clotrimazole troches may be effective for prophylaxis against oropharyngeal candidiasis in neutropenic patients

Usual Dosage

Children >3 years and Adults:

Oral:

Prophylaxis: 10 mg troche dissolved 3 times/day for the duration of chemotherapy or until steroids are reduced to maintenance levels

Treatment: 10 mg troche dissolved slowly 5 times/day for 14 consecutive days

Topical: Apply twice daily; if no improvement occurs after 4 weeks of therapy, re-evaluate diagnosis

Children >12 years and Adults:

Vaginal:

Cream:

1%: Insert 1 applicatorful vaginal cream daily (preferably at bedtime) for 7 consecutive days

2%: Insert 1 applicatorful vaginal cream daily (preferably at bedtime) for 3 consecutive days

Tablet: Insert 100 mg/day for 7 days or 500 mg single dose

Topical: Apply to affected area twice daily (morning and evening) for 7 consecutive days

Dosage Forms

Combination pack:

Gyne-Lotrimin®, Mycelex®-7: Vaginal tablet 100 mg (7s) and vaginal cream 1% (7 g)

Gyne-Lotrimin® 3: Vaginal tablet 200 mg (3s) and vaginal cream 1%

Mycelex® Twin Pack: Vaginal tablet 500 mg (1s) and vaginal cream 1% (7 g)

Cream, topical (Lotrimin®, Mycelex®, Mycelex® OTC): 1% (15 g, 30 g, 45 g, 90 g)

Cream, vaginal:

Gyne-Lotrimin®, Mycelex®-7: 1% (45 g, 90 g)

Gyne-Lotrimin® 3: 2% (25 g)

Lotion (Lotrimin®): 1% (30 mL)

Solution, topical (Lotrimin®, Mycelex®, Mycelex® OTC): 1% (10 mL, 30 mL)

Tablet, vaginal:

Gyne-Lotrimin®, Mycelex®-7: 100 mg (7s)

Troche (Mycelex®): 10 mg

clotrimazole and betamethasone *see* betamethasone and clotrimazole *on page 83*

cloxacillin (kloks a SIL in)

U.S./Canadian Brand Names Apo®-Cloxi [Can]; Novo-Cloxin [Can]; Nu-Cloxi® [Can]

Therapeutic Category Penicillin

Use Treatment of susceptible bacterial infections of the respiratory tract, skin and skin structure, bone and joint caused by penicillinase-producing staphylococci

Usual Dosage Oral:

Children >1 month: 50-100 mg/kg/day in divided doses every 6 hours; up to a maximum of 4 g/day

Adults: 250-500 mg every 6 hours

Dosage Forms

Capsule, as sodium: 250 mg, 500 mg

Powder for oral suspension, as sodium: 125 mg/5 mL (100 mL, 200 mL)

Cloxapen® *(Discontinued)* *see page 814*

clozapine (KLOE za peen)

U.S./Canadian Brand Names Clozaril® [US/Can]

Therapeutic Category Antipsychotic Agent, Dibenzodiazepine

Use Management of schizophrenic patients

Usual Dosage Adults: Oral: Initial: 25 mg once or twice daily, increase as tolerated to a target dose of 300-450 mg/day, may require doses as high as 600-900 mg/day

Dosage Forms Tablet: 25 mg, 100 mg

Clozaril® [US/Can] *see* clozapine *on this page*

Clysodrast® *(Discontinued)* *see page 814*

CMV-IGIV *see* cytomegalovirus immune globulin (intravenous-human) *on page 172*

CoActifed® **[Can]** *see* triprolidine, pseudoephedrine, and codeine *on page 659*

coagulant complex inhibitor *see* anti-inhibitor coagulant complex *on page 46*

coagulation factor VIIa *see* factor VIIa (recombinant) *on page 262*

coal tar (KOLE tar)

Synonyms crude coal tar; LCD; pix carbonis

U.S./Canadian Brand Names Denorex® [US-OTC]; DHS® Tar [US-OTC]; Duplex® T [US-OTC]; Estar® [US/Can]; Fototar® [US-OTC]; Neutrogena® T/Derm [US]; Oxipor® VHC [US-OTC]; Pentrax® [US-OTC]; Polytar® [US-OTC]; psoriGel® [US-OTC]; Targel® [Can]; Tegrin® Dandruff Shampoo [US-OTC]; T/Gel® [US-OTC]; Zetar® [US/Can]

Therapeutic Category Antipsoriatic Agent; Antiseborrheic Agent, Topical

Use Topically for controlling dandruff, seborrheic dermatitis, or psoriasis

Usual Dosage
Bath: Add appropriate amount to bath water, for adults usually 60-90 mL of a 5% to 20% solution or 15-25 mL of 30% lotion; soak 5-20 minutes, then pat dry; use once daily for 3 days

Shampoo: Rub shampoo onto wet hair and scalp, rinse thoroughly; repeat; leave on 5 minutes; rinse thoroughly; apply twice weekly for the first 2 weeks then once weekly or more often if needed

Skin: Apply to the affected area 1-4 times/day; decrease frequency to 2-3 times/week once condition has been controlled

Scalp psoriasis: Tar oil bath or coal tar solution may be painted sparingly to the lesions 3-12 hours before each shampoo

Psoriasis of the body, arms, legs: Apply at bedtime; if thick scales are present, use product with salicylic acid and apply several times during the day

Dosage Forms
Cream, topical: 2% to 5%
Gel, topical: Coal tar extract: 2.5% to 8%
Lotion, topical: 5%, 25%
Oil, topical: Coal tar extract: 5%
Shampoo, topical: Coal tar: 0.5% to 12.5%
Soap, topical: Coal tar 1% and coal tar 5% solution combination
Solution, topical: Coal tar: 20%

coal tar and salicylic acid (KOLE tar & sal i SIL ik AS id)

U.S./Canadian Brand Names Neutrogena® T/Sal [US-OTC]; P & S Plus® [US-OTC]; Sebcur/T® [Can]; X-Seb™ T [US-OTC]

Therapeutic Category Antipsoriatic Agent; Antiseborrheic Agent, Topical

Use Treatment of seborrheal dermatitis, dandruff

Usual Dosage Topical: Shampoo twice weekly

Dosage Forms
Gel, topical (P & S Plus®): Coal tar solution 8% and salicylic acid 2%
Shampoo, topical:
Neutrogena® T/Sal: Coal tar extract 2% with salicylic acid 2% (60 mL)
X-Seb™ T: Coal tar solution 10% and salicylic acid 4% (120 mL)

coal tar, lanolin, and mineral oil (KOLE tar, LAN oh lin, & MIN er al oyl)

U.S./Canadian Brand Names Balnetar® [US/Can]

Therapeutic Category Antipsoriatic Agent; Antiseborrheic Agent, Topical

Use Treatment of psoriasis, seborrheal dermatitis, atopic dermatitis, eczematoid dermatitis

Usual Dosage Add to bath water, soak for 5-20 minutes then pat dry

Dosage Forms Oil, bath: Water-dispersible emollient tar 2.5%, lanolin fraction, and mineral oil (225 mL)

Cobal® **[US]** *see* cyanocobalamin *on page 167*

Cobalasine® **Injection** *(Discontinued)* *see page 814*

Cobex® *(Discontinued)* *see page 814*

Cobolin-M® [US] *see* cyanocobalamin *on page 167*

cocaine (koe KANE)
Therapeutic Category Local Anesthetic
Controlled Substance C-II
Use Topical anesthesia for mucous membranes
Usual Dosage Topical: Use lowest effective dose; do not exceed 1 mg/kg; patient tolerance, anesthetic technique, vascularity of tissue and area to be anesthetized will determine dose needed
Dosage Forms
Powder, as hydrochloride: 5 g, 25 g
Solution, topical, as hydrochloride: 4% [40 mg/mL] (4 mL, 10 mL); 10% [100 mg/mL] (4 mL, 10 mL)
Solution, viscous, topical, as hydrochloride: 4% [40 mg/mL] (4 mL, 10 mL); 10% [100 mg/mL] (4 mL, 10 mL)

Codafed® Expectorant [US] *see* guaifenesin, pseudoephedrine, and codeine *on page 311*

Codafed® Pediatric Expectorant [US] *see* guaifenesin, pseudoephedrine, and codeine *on page 311*

Codamine® *(Discontinued)* *see page 814*

Codamine® Pediatric *(Discontinued)* *see page 814*

Codehist® DH *(Discontinued)* *see page 814*

codeine (KOE deen)
Synonyms methylmorphine
Therapeutic Category Analgesic, Narcotic; Antitussive
Controlled Substance C-II
Use Treatment of mild to moderate pain; antitussive in lower doses
Usual Dosage Doses should be titrated to appropriate analgesic effect; when changing routes of administration, note that oral dose is $2/3$ as effective as parenteral dose

Analgesic: Oral, I.M., S.C.:
  Children: 0.5-1 mg/kg/dose every 4-6 hours as needed; maximum: 60 mg/dose
  Adults: 30 mg/dose; range: 15-60 mg every 4-6 hours as needed
Antitussive: Oral (for nonproductive cough):
  Children: 1-1.5 mg/kg/day in divided doses every 4-6 hours as needed: Alternatively dose according to age:
  2-6 years: 2.5-5 mg every 4-6 hours as needed; maximum: 30 mg/day
  6-12 years: 5-10 mg every 4-6 hours as needed; maximum: 60 mg/day
  Adults: 10-20 mg/dose every 4-6 hours as needed; maximum: 120 mg/day
Dosage Forms
Injection, as phosphate: 30 mg (1 mL, 2 mL); 60 mg (1 mL, 2 mL)
Solution, oral, as phosphate: 15 mg/5 mL
Tablet, as sulfate: 15 mg, 30 mg, 60 mg
Tablet, soluble, as phosphate: 30 mg, 60 mg
Tablet, soluble, as sulfate: 15 mg, 30 mg, 60 mg

codeine and acetaminophen *see* acetaminophen and codeine *on page 5*

codeine and aspirin *see* aspirin and codeine *on page 59*

codeine and butalbital compound *see* butalbital compound and codeine *on page 100*

codeine and guaifenesin *see* guaifenesin and codeine *on page 308*

codeine and promethazine *see* promethazine and codeine *on page 545*

codeine, guaifenesin, and pseudoephedrine *see* guaifenesin, pseudoephedrine, and codeine *on page 311*

codeine, promethazine, and phenylephrine *see* promethazine, phenylephrine, and codeine *on page 546*

Codiclear® DH [US] *see* hydrocodone and guaifenesin *on page 331*

Codimal-A® Injection *(Discontinued)* *see page 814*

Codimal® Expectorant *(Discontinued)* *see page 814*

Codimal-LA® Half [US-OTC] *see* chlorpheniramine and pseudoephedrine *on page 138*

Codimal-LA® [US-OTC] *see* chlorpheniramine and pseudoephedrine *on page 138*

cod liver oil *see* vitamin A and vitamin D *on page 681*

Cogentin® [US/Can] *see* benztropine *on page 80*

Co-Gesic® [US] *see* hydrocodone and acetaminophen *on page 329*

Cognex® [US] *see* tacrine *on page 617*

Colace® [US/Can] *see* docusate *on page 208*

colaspase *see* asparaginase *on page 58*

Colax-C® [Can] *see* docusate *on page 208*

Colazal™ [US] *see* balsalazide *on page 71*

ColBenemid® *(Discontinued)* *see page 814*

colchicine (KOL chi seen)

Therapeutic Category Antigout Agent
Use Treat acute gouty arthritis attacks and to prevent recurrences of such attacks; management of familial Mediterranean fever
Usual Dosage
Acute gouty arthritis:
Oral: Initial: 0.5-1.2 mg, then 0.5-0.6 mg every 1-2 hours or 1-1.2 mg every 2 hours until relief or GI side effects occur to a maximum total dose of 8 mg, wait 3 days before initiating a second course
I.V.: Initial: 1-3 mg, then 0.5 mg every 6 hours until response, not to exceed 4 mg/day; following a full course of colchicine (4 mg), wait 7 days before initiating another course of colchicine (by any route)
Prophylaxis of recurrent attacks: Oral:
<1 attack/year: 0.5 or 0.6 mg/day/dose for 3-4 days/week
>1 attack/year: 0.5 or 0.6 mg/day/dose
Severe cases: 1-1.8 mg/day
Dosage Forms
Injection: 0.5 mg/mL (2 mL)
Tablet: 0.5 mg, 0.6 mg

colchicine and probenecid (KOL chi seen & proe BEN e sid)

Synonyms probenecid and colchicine
Therapeutic Category Antigout Agent
Use Treatment of chronic gouty arthritis when complicated by frequent, recurrent acute attacks of gout
Usual Dosage Adults: Oral: 1 tablet daily for 1 week, then 1 tablet twice daily thereafter
Dosage Forms Tablet: Colchicine 0.5 mg and probenecid 0.5 g

Cold & Allergy® Elixir *(Discontinued)* *see page 814*

Coldlac-LA® *(Discontinued)* *see page 814*

Coldloc® *(Discontinued)* *see page 814*

colesevelam (koh le SEV a lam)

U.S./Canadian Brand Names WelChol™ [US/Can]

Therapeutic Category Antihyperlipidemic Agent, Miscellaneous; Bile Acid Sequestrant

Use Adjunctive therapy to diet and exercise in the management of elevated LDL in primary hypercholesterolemia (Fredrickson Type IIa) when used alone or in combination with an HMG-CoA reductase inhibitor.

Usual Dosage

Adults: Oral: Monotherapy: 3 tablets twice daily with meals or 6 tablets once daily with a meal; maximum dose: 7 tablets/day

Combination therapy with an HMG-CoA reductase inhibitor: 4-6 tablets daily; maximum dose: 6 tablets/day

Dosage Forms Tablet: 625 mg

Colestid® [US/Can] *see* colestipol *on this page*

colestipol (koe LES ti pole)

U.S./Canadian Brand Names Colestid® [US/Can]

Therapeutic Category Antihyperlipidemic Agent, Miscellaneous

Use Adjunct in the management of primary hypercholesterolemia; to relieve pruritus associated with elevated levels of bile acids, possibly used to decrease plasma half-life of digoxin as an adjunct in the treatment of toxicity

Usual Dosage Oral: 15-30 g/day in divided doses 2-4 times/day

Dosage Forms

Granules, as hydrochloride: 5 g packet, 300 g, 500 g

Tablet, as hydrochloride: 1 g

colfosceril palmitate (kole FOS er il PALM i tate)

Synonyms dipalmitoylphosphatidylcholine; DPPC; synthetic lung surfactant

U.S./Canadian Brand Names Exosurf® Neonatal™ [US/Can]

Therapeutic Category Lung Surfactant

Use Neonatal respiratory distress syndrome (RDS):

Prophylactic therapy: Infants at risk for developing RDS with body weight <1350 g; infants with evidence of pulmonary immaturity with body weight >1350 g

Rescue therapy: Treatment of infants with RDS based on respiratory distress not attributable to any other causes and chest radiographic findings consistent with RDS

Usual Dosage

Prophylactic treatment: Administer 5 mL/kg as soon as possible; the second and third doses should be administered at 12 and 24 hours later to those infants remaining on ventilators

Rescue treatment: Administer 5 mL/kg as soon as the diagnosis of RDS is made; the second 5 mL/kg dose should be administered 12 hours later

Dosage Forms Injection, powder for reconstitution: 108 mg (10 mL)

Colhist® Solution [US-OTC] *see* brompheniramine *on page 93*

colistimethate (koe lis ti METH ate)

U.S./Canadian Brand Names Coly-Mycin® M [US/Can]

Therapeutic Category Antibiotic, Miscellaneous

Use Treatment of infections due to sensitive strains of certain gram-negative bacilli

Usual Dosage Children and Adults: I.M., I.V.: 2.5-5 mg/kg/day in 2-4 divided doses

Dosage Forms Injection, powder for reconstitution: 150 mg

collagenase (KOL la je nase)

U.S./Canadian Brand Names Plaquase® [US]; Santyl® [US/Can]

Therapeutic Category Enzyme

Use Promote debridement of necrotic tissue in dermal ulcers and severe burns

(Continued)

collagenase *(Continued)*

Usual Dosage Topical: Apply once daily (or more frequently if the dressing becomes soiled)

Dosage Forms

Injection, powder for reconstitution (Plaquase®): 10,000 units/vial

Ointment (Santyl®): 250 units/g (15 g, 30 g)

collagen implants (KOL a jen im PLANTS)

Therapeutic Category Ophthalmic Agent, Miscellaneous

Use Relief of dry eyes; enhance the effect of ocular medications

Usual Dosage Implants inserted by physician

Dosage Forms Implant, ophthalmic: 0.2 mm, 0.3 mm, 0.4 mm, 0.5 mm, 0.6 mm

Collyrium Fresh® [US-OTC] *see* tetrahydrozoline *on page 629*

Colocort™ [US] *see* hydrocortisone (rectal) *on page 333*

Coly-Mycin® M [US/Can] *see* colistimethate *on previous page*

Coly-Mycin® S Oral *(Discontinued)* *see page 814*

Coly-Mycin® S Otic [US] *see* neomycin, colistin, hydrocortisone, and thonzonium *on page 452*

Colyte® [US/Can] *see* polyethylene glycol-electrolyte solution *on page 525*

Combantrin™ [Can] *see* pyrantel pamoate *on page 555*

CombiPatch™ [US] *see* estradiol and norethindrone *on page 239*

Combipres® [US] *see* clonidine and chlorthalidone *on page 155*

Combivent® [US/Can] *see* ipratropium and albuterol *on page 359*

Combivir® [US/Can] *see* zidovudine and lamivudine *on page 690*

Comfort® Ophthalmic *(Discontinued)* *see page 814*

Comfort® Tears Solution *(Discontinued)* *see page 814*

Comhist® [US] *see* chlorpheniramine, phenylephrine, and phenyltoloxamine *on page 140*

Comhist® LA [US] *see* chlorpheniramine, phenylephrine, and phenyltoloxamine *on page 140*

Compazine® [US/Can] *see* prochlorperazine *on page 542*

compound E *see* cortisone acetate *on page 164*

compound F *see* hydrocortisone (systemic) *on page 333*

compound S *see* zidovudine *on page 689*

Compound W® [US-OTC] *see* salicylic acid *on page 581*

Compoz® Nighttime Sleep Aid [US-OTC] *see* diphenhydramine *on page 202*

Compro™ [US] *see* prochlorperazine *on page 542*

Comtan® [US/Can] *see* entacapone *on page 227*

Comtrex® Allergy-Sinus [US-OTC] *see* acetaminophen, chlorpheniramine, and pseudoephedrine *on page 7*

Comtrex® Non-Drowsy Cough and Cold [US-OTC] *see* acetaminophen, dextromethorphan, and pseudoephedrine *on page 8*

Comvax® [US] *see* Haemophilus B conjugate and hepatitis B vaccine *on page 314*

Conceptrol® [US-OTC] *see* nonoxynol 9 *on page 464*

Concerta™ [US] *see* methylphenidate *on page 422*

Condyline™ [Can] *see* podofilox *on page 523*

Condylox® [US] *see* podofilox *on page 523*

Conex® *(Discontinued)* see page 814

Congess® **Jr** *(Discontinued)* see page 814

Congess® **Sr** *(Discontinued)* see page 814

Congest [Can] see estrogens (conjugated/equine) on page 242

Congestac® **[US]** see guaifenesin and pseudoephedrine on page 310

Congestant D® *(Discontinued)* see page 814

conjugated estrogen and methyltestosterone see estrogens and methyltestosterone on page 241

conjugated estrogens see estrogens (conjugated/equine) on page 242

Conray® **[US]** see radiological/contrast media (ionic) on page 561

Constant-T® **Tablet** *(Discontinued)* see page 814

Constilac® **[US]** see lactulose on page 372

Constulose® **[US]** see lactulose on page 372

Contac® **Cold 12 Hour Relief Non Drowsy** see pseudoephedrine on page 552

Contac® **Cough, Cold and Flu Day & Night**™ **[Can]** see acetaminophen, dextromethorphan, and pseudoephedrine on page 8

Contac® **Cough Formula Liquid** *(Discontinued)* see page 814

Contac® **Severe Cold and Flu/Non-Drowsy [US-OTC]** see acetaminophen, dextromethorphan, and pseudoephedrine on page 8

Control® *(Discontinued)* see page 814

Control-L® *(Discontinued)* see page 814

Contuss® *(Discontinued)* see page 814

Contuss® **XT** *(Discontinued)* see page 814

Copaxone® **[US/Can]** see glatiramer acetate on page 299

Cophene-B® *(Discontinued)* see page 814

Cophene XP® *(Discontinued)* see page 814

copolymer-1 see glatiramer acetate on page 299

copper injection see trace metals on page 646

Co-Pyronil® **2 Pulvules**® *(Discontinued)* see page 814

Cordarone® **[US/Can]** see amiodarone on page 34

Cordran® **[US/Can]** see flurandrenolide on page 281

Cordran® **SP [US]** see flurandrenolide on page 281

Coreg® **[US/Can]** see carvedilol on page 118

Corgard® **[US/Can]** see nadolol on page 443

Corgonject® *(Discontinued)* see page 814

Coricidin® **[US-OTC]** see chlorpheniramine and acetaminophen on page 137

Corliprol® *(Discontinued)* see page 814

Corlopam® **[US/Can]** see fenoldopam on page 265

Cormax® **[US]** see clobetasol on page 152

CortaGel® **[US-OTC]** see hydrocortisone (topical) on page 334

Cortaid® **Maximum Strength [US-OTC]** see hydrocortisone (topical) on page 334

Cortaid® **Ointment** *(Discontinued)* see page 814

Cortaid® **with Aloe [US-OTC]** see hydrocortisone (topical) on page 334

Cortatrigen® **Otic** *(Discontinued)* see page 814

Cort-Dome® [US] *see* hydrocortisone (topical) *on page 334*

Cortef® [US/Can] *see* hydrocortisone (systemic) *on page 333*

Cortenema® [US/Can] *see* hydrocortisone (rectal) *on page 333*

Corticaine® [US] *see* dibucaine and hydrocortisone *on page 193*

corticotropin (kor ti koe TROE pin)

Synonyms ACTH; adrenocorticotropic hormone
U.S./Canadian Brand Names Acthar® [US]; H.P. Acthar® Gel [US]
Therapeutic Category Adrenal Corticosteroid
Use Infantile spasms; diagnostic aid in adrenocortical insufficiency; acute exacerbations of multiple sclerosis; severe muscle weakness in myasthenia gravis
Usual Dosage
  Acute exacerbation of multiple sclerosis: I.M.: 80-120 units/day for 2-3 weeks
  Diagnostic purposes:
   I.M., S.C.: 20 units 4 times/day
   I.V.: 10-25 units in 500 mL 5% dextrose in water over 8 hours
Dosage Forms
  Injection, repository (H.P. Acthar® Gel): 40 units/mL (1 mL, 5 mL); 80 units/mL (1 mL, 5 mL)
  Powder for injection (Acthar®): 25 units, 40 units

Cortifoam® [US/Can] *see* hydrocortisone (rectal) *on page 333*

Cortimyxin® [Can] *see* neomycin, polymyxin B, and hydrocortisone *on page 453*

cortisone acetate (KOR ti sone AS e tate)

Synonyms compound E
U.S./Canadian Brand Names Cortone® [Can]
Therapeutic Category Adrenal Corticosteroid
Use Management of adrenocortical insufficiency
Usual Dosage Depends upon the condition being treated and the response of the patient
  Children:
   Anti-inflammatory or immunosuppressive:
    Oral: 2.5-10 mg/kg/day or 20-300 mg/m^2/day in divided doses every 6-8 hours
   Physiologic replacement:
    Oral: 0.5-0.75 mg/kg/day in divided doses every 8 hours
  Adults: Oral: 20-300 mg/day
Dosage Forms Tablet: 5 mg, 10 mg, 25 mg

Cortisporin® Cream [US] *see* neomycin, polymyxin B, and hydrocortisone *on page 453*

Cortisporin® Ointment [US/Can] *see* bacitracin, neomycin, polymyxin B, and hydrocortisone *on page 69*

Cortisporin® Ophthalmic [US/Can] *see* neomycin, polymyxin B, and hydrocortisone *on page 453*

Cortisporin® Otic [US/Can] *see* neomycin, polymyxin B, and hydrocortisone *on page 453*

Cortisporin®-TC Otic [US] *see* neomycin, colistin, hydrocortisone, and thonzonium *on page 452*

Cortisporin® Topical Cream *(Discontinued)* *see page 814*

Cortizone®-5 [US-OTC] *see* hydrocortisone (topical) *on page 334*

Cortizone®-10 [US-OTC] *see* hydrocortisone (topical) *on page 334*

Cortoderm [Can] *see* hydrocortisone (topical) *on page 334*

Cortone® [Can] *see* cortisone acetate *on this page*

Cortone® **Acetate** *(Discontinued)* *see page 814*

Cortrophin-Zinc® *(Discontinued)* *see page 814*

Cortrosyn® **[US/Can]** *see cosyntropin on this page*

Corvert® **[US]** *see ibutilide on page 344*

Coryphen® **Codeine [Can]** *see aspirin and codeine on page 59*

Cosmegen® **[US/Can]** *see dactinomycin on page 173*

Cosopt® **[US/Can]** *see dorzolamide and timolol on page 212*

cosyntropin (koe sin TROE pin)
  Synonyms synacthen; tetracosactide
  U.S./Canadian Brand Names Cortrosyn® [US/Can]
  Therapeutic Category Diagnostic Agent
  Use Diagnostic test to differentiate primary adrenal from secondary (pituitary) adrenocortical insufficiency
  Usual Dosage
    Adrenocortical insufficiency: I.M., I.V.:
      Children <2 years: 0.125 mg injected over 2 minutes
      Children >2 years and Adults: 0.25 mg injected over 2 minutes
      When greater cortisol stimulation is needed, an I.V. infusion may be used: I.V. infusion: 0.25 mg administered over 4-8 hours

      Congenital adrenal hyperplasia evaluation: 1 mg/m^2/dose up to a maximum of 1 mg
  Dosage Forms Injection, powder for reconstitution: 0.25 mg

Cotazym® **[US/Can]** *see pancrelipase on page 489*

Cotazym-S® **[US]** *see pancrelipase on page 489*

Cotrim® *(Discontinued) see page 814*

Cotrim® **DS** *(Discontinued) see page 814*

co-trimoxazole *see sulfamethoxazole and trimethoprim on page 612*

Coumadin® **[US/Can]** *see warfarin on page 685*

Covera® **[Can]** *see verapamil on page 675*

Covera-HS® **[US]** *see verapamil on page 675*

Coversyl® **[Can]** *see perindopril erbumine on page 504*

Cozaar® **[US/Can]** *see losartan on page 392*

CP-99,219-27 *see trovafloxacin on page 661*

CPM *see cyclophosphamide on page 169*

Creon® *(Discontinued) see page 814*

Creon® **5 [US/Can]** *see pancrelipase on page 489*

Creon® **10 [US/Can]** *see pancrelipase on page 489*

Creon® **20 [US/Can]** *see pancrelipase on page 489*

Creon® **25 [Can]** *see pancrelipase on page 489*

Creo-Terpin® **[US-OTC]** *see dextromethorphan on page 189*

Cresylate® **[US]** *see m-cresyl acetate on page 402*

Crinone® **[US/Can]** *see progesterone on page 543*

Critic-Aid Skin Care® **[US-OTC]** *see zinc oxide on page 691*

Criticare HN® **[US-OTC]** *see nutritional formula, enteral/oral on page 472*

Crixivan® **[US/Can]** *see indinavir on page 348*

CroFab™ **[Ovine] [US]** *see antivenin (Crotalidae) polyvalent on page 48*

Crolom® **[US]** *see cromolyn sodium on next page*

cromoglicic acid *see* cromolyn sodium *on this page*

cromolyn sodium (KROE moe lin SOW dee um)

Synonyms cromoglicic acid; disodium cromoglycate; DSCG
U.S./Canadian Brand Names Apo®-Cromolyn [Can]; Crolom® [US]; Gastrocrom® [US]; Intal® [US/Can]; Nalcrom® [Can]; Nasalcrom® [US-OTC]; Nu-Cromolyn [Can]; Opticrom® [US/Can]
Therapeutic Category Mast Cell Stabilizer
Use Adjunct in the prophylaxis of allergic disorders, including rhinitis, conjunctivitis, and asthma; inhalation product may be used for prevention of exercise-induced bronchospasm

Ophthalmologic: Vernal conjunctivitis, vernal keratoconjunctivitis, and vernal keratitis
Systemic: Mastocytosis, food allergy, and treatment of inflammatory bowel disease
Usual Dosage
Children:
Inhalation: >2 years: 20 mg 4 times/day
Nebulization solution: >5 years: 2 inhalations 4 times/day by metered spray, or 20 mg 4 times/day (Spinhaler®); taper frequency to the lowest effective level
For prevention of exercise-induced bronchospasm: Single dose of 2 inhalations (aerosol) just prior to exercise
Nasal: >6 years: 1 spray in each nostril 3-4 times/day
Adults: Nasal: 1 spray in each nostril 3-4 times/day

Systemic mastocytosis: Oral:
Infants ≤2 years: 20 mg/kg/day in 4 divided doses, not to exceed 30 mg/kg/day
Children 2-12 years: 100 mg 4 times/day; not to exceed 40 mg/kg/day
Adults: 200 mg 4 times/day
Food allergy and inflammatory bowel disease: Oral:
Children: 100 mg 4 times/day 15-20 minutes before meals, not to exceed 40 mg/kg/day
Adults: 200 mg 4 times/day 15-20 minutes before meal, up to 400 mg 4 times/day
Dosage Forms
Solution, oral spray, as sodium (Intal®): 800 mcg/inhalation (8.1 g) [112 metered inhalations; 56 doses], (14.2 g) [200 metered inhalations; 100 doses]
Solution for nebulization, as sodium (Intal®): 20 mg/2 mL (60s, 120s)
Nasal spray, as sodium (Nasalcrom®): 40 mg/mL (13 mL, 26 mL) [5.2 mg/inhalation]
Solution, ophthalmic, as sodium (Crolom®, Opticrom®): 4% (2.5 mL, 10 mL) [contains benzalkonium chloride]
Solution, oral, as sodium (Gastrocrom®): 100 mg/5 mL (96s)

crotaline antivenin, polyvalent *see* antivenin *(Crotalidae)* polyvalent *on page 48*

crotamiton (kroe TAM i tonn)

U.S./Canadian Brand Names Eurax® Topical [US]
Therapeutic Category Scabicides/Pediculicides
Use Treatment of scabies (*Sarcoptes scabiei*) in infants and children
Usual Dosage Scabicide: Children and Adults: Topical: Wash thoroughly and scrub away loose scales, then towel dry; apply a thin layer and massage drug onto skin of the entire body from the neck to the toes (with special attention to skin folds, creases, and interdigital spaces). Repeat application in 24 hours; patient should take a cleansing bath 48 hours after the final application.
Dosage Forms
Cream: 10% (60 g)
Lotion: 10% (60 mL, 454 mL)

crude coal tar *see* coal tar *on page 158*
Cruex® [US-OTC] *see* clotrimazole *on page 156*
Cryselle™ [US] *see* ethinyl estradiol and norgestrel *on page 255*

crystalline penicillin *see* penicillin G (parenteral/aqueous) *on page 499*

Crystamine® *(Discontinued) see page 814*

Crysticillin® A.S. *(Discontinued) see page 814*

Crystodigin® *(Discontinued) see page 814*

CSP *see* cellulose sodium phosphate *on page 127*

CTX *see* cyclophosphamide *on page 169*

Cuprimine® [US/Can] *see* penicillamine *on page 497*

Curosurf® [US/Can] *see* poractant alfa *on page 527*

Cutivate™ [US] *see* fluticasone (topical) *on page 284*

CYA *see* cyclosporine *on page 169*

cyanide antidote kit (SYE a nide AN tee dote kit)

Therapeutic Category Antidote

Use Treatment of cyanide poisoning

Usual Dosage Cyanide poisoning: 0.3 mL ampul of amyl nitrite is crushed every minute and vapor is inhaled for 15-30 seconds until an I.V. sodium nitrite infusion is available. Following administration of 300 mg I.V. sodium nitrite, inject 12.5 g sodium thiosulfate I.V. (over ~10 minutes), if needed; injection of both may be repeated at $\frac{1}{2}$ the original dose.

Dosage Forms Kit: Sodium nitrite 300 mg/10 mL (#2); sodium thiosulfate 12.5 g/50 mL (#2); amyl nitrite 0.3 mL (#12); also disposable syringes, stomach tube, tourniquet, and instructions

cyanocobalamin (sye an oh koe BAL a min)

Synonyms vitamin B_{12}

U.S./Canadian Brand Names Bedoz [Can]; Cobal® [US]; Cobolin-M® [US]; LA-12® [US]; Nascobal® [US]; Neuroforte-R® [US]; Twelve Resin-K® [US]; Vita® #12 [US]; Vitabee® 12 [US]

Therapeutic Category Vitamin, Water Soluble

Use Pernicious anemia; vitamin B_{12} deficiency; increased B_{12} requirements due to pregnancy, thyrotoxicosis, hemorrhage, malignancy, liver or kidney disease

Usual Dosage

Congenital pernicious anemia (if evidence of neurologic involvement): I.M.: 1000 mcg/day for at least 2 weeks; maintenance: 50 mcg/month

Vitamin B_{12} deficiency: I.M., S.C. (oral is not recommended due to poor absorption):

Children: 100 mcg/day for 10-15 days (total dose of 1-1.5 mg), then once or twice weekly for several months; may taper to 250-1000 mcg every month

Adults: 100 mcg/day for 6-7 days

Hematologic signs only:

Children: 10-50 mcg/day for 5-10 days, then maintenance: 100-250 mcg/dose every 2-4 weeks

Adults: 30 mcg/day for 5-10 days, followed by 100-200 mcg/month

Methylmalonic aciduria: I.M.: 1 mg/day

Dosage Forms

Gel, intranasal (Nascobal®): 500 mcg/0.1 mL (5 mL)

Injection: 100 mcg/mL (1 mL, 10 mL, 30 mL); 1000 mcg/mL (1 mL, 10 mL, 30 mL)

Tablet [OTC]: 50 mcg, 100 mcg, 250 mcg, 500 mcg, 1000 mcg

cyanocobalamin, folic acid, and pyridoxine *see* folic acid, cyanocobalamin, and pyridoxine *on page 286*

Cyanoject® *(Discontinued) see page 814*

cyclandelate (sye KLAN de late)

Therapeutic Category Vasodilator, Peripheral

Use Considered as "possibly effective" for adjunctive therapy in peripheral vascular disease and possibly senility due to cerebrovascular disease or multi-infarct dementia; migraine prophylaxis, vertigo, tinnitus, and visual disturbances secondary to cerebrovascular insufficiency and diabetic peripheral polyneuropathy

Usual Dosage Adults: Oral: Initial: 1.2-1.6 g/day in divided doses before meals and at bedtime until response; maintenance therapy: 400-800 mg/day in 2-4 divided doses; start with lowest dose in elderly due to hypotensive potential; decrease dose by 200 mg decrements to achieve minimal maintenance dose; improvement can usually be seen over weeks of therapy and prolonged use; short courses of therapy are usually ineffective and not recommended

Dosage Forms Capsule: 200 mg, 400 mg

Cyclessa® [US] *see* ethinyl estradiol and desogestrel *on page 244*

cyclobenzaprine (sye kloe BEN za preen)

U.S./Canadian Brand Names Apo®-Cyclobenzaprine [Can]; Flexeril® [US/Can]; Flexitec [Can]; Gen-Cyclobenzaprine [Can]; Novo-Cycloprine [Can]; Nu-Cyclobenzaprine [Can]

Therapeutic Category Skeletal Muscle Relaxant

Use Treatment of muscle spasm associated with acute painful musculoskeletal conditions; supportive therapy in tetanus

Usual Dosage Oral:
Children: Dosage has not been established
Adults: 20-40 mg/day in 2-4 divided doses; maximum dose: 60 mg/day

Dosage Forms Tablet, as hydrochloride: 10 mg

Cyclocort® [US/Can] *see* amcinonide *on page 30*

Cyclogyl® [US/Can] *see* cyclopentolate *on this page*

Cyclomen® [Can] *see* danazol *on page 174*

Cyclomydril® Ophthalmic [US] *see* cyclopentolate and phenylephrine *on this page*

cyclopentolate (sye kloe PEN toe late)

U.S./Canadian Brand Names AK-Pentolate® [US]; Cyclogyl® [US/Can]; Diopentolate® [Can]

Therapeutic Category Anticholinergic Agent

Use Diagnostic procedures requiring mydriasis and cycloplegia

Usual Dosage Ophthalmic:
Infants: Instill 1 drop of 0.5% into each eye 5-10 minutes before examination
Children: Instill 1 drop of 0.5%, 1%, or 2% in eye followed by 1 drop of 0.5% or 1% in 5 minutes, if necessary
Adults: Instill 1 drop of 1% followed by another drop in 5 minutes; 2% solution in heavily pigmented iris

Dosage Forms Solution, ophthalmic, as hydrochloride: 0.5% (2 mL, 5 mL, 15 mL); 1% (2 mL, 5 mL, 15 mL); 2% (2 mL, 5 mL, 15 mL)

cyclopentolate and phenylephrine (sye kloe PEN toe late & fen il EF rin)

Synonyms phenylephrine and cyclopentolate

U.S./Canadian Brand Names Cyclomydril® Ophthalmic [US]

Therapeutic Category Anticholinergic/Adrenergic Agonist

Use Induce mydriasis greater than that produced with cyclopentolate HCl alone

Usual Dosage Ophthalmic: Instill 1 drop every 5-10 minutes, not to exceed 3 instillations

Dosage Forms Solution, ophthalmic: Cyclopentolate hydrochloride 0.2% and phenylephrine hydrochloride 1% (2 mL, 5 mL)

cyclophosphamide (sye kloe FOS fa mide)

Synonyms CPM; CTX; CYT

U.S./Canadian Brand Names Cytoxan® [US/Can]; Neosar® [US]; Procytox® [Can]

Therapeutic Category Antineoplastic Agent

Use Management of Hodgkin's disease, malignant lymphomas, multiple myeloma, leukemias, sarcomas, mycosis fungoides, neuroblastoma, ovarian carcinoma, breast carcinoma, a variety of other tumors; nephrotic syndrome, lupus erythematosus, severe rheumatoid arthritis, and rheumatoid vasculitis

Usual Dosage
Patients with compromised bone marrow function may require a 33% to 50% reduction in initial loading dose
Children:
SLE: I.V.: 500-750 mg/m^2 every month; maximum dose: 1 g/m^2
JRA/vasculitis: I.V.: 10 mg/kg every 2 weeks
Children and Adults:
Oral: 50-100 mg/m^2/day as continuous therapy or 400-1000 mg/m^2 in divided doses over 4-5 days as intermittent therapy
I.V.:
Single Doses: 400-1800 mg/m^2 (30-50 mg/kg) per treatment course (1-5 days) which can be repeated at 2-4 week intervals
MAXIMUM SINGLE DOSE WITHOUT BMT is 7 g/m^2 (190 mg/kg) SINGLE AGENT THERAPY
Continuous daily doses: 60-120 mg/m^2 (1-2.5 mg/kg) per day
Autologous BMT: IVPB: 50 mg/kg/dose x 4 days or 60 mg/kg/dose for 2 days; total dose is usually divided over 2-4 days
Nephrotic syndrome: Oral: 2-3 mg/kg/day every day for up to 12 weeks when corticosteroids are unsuccessful

Dosage Forms
Injection, powder for reconstitution: 100 mg, 200 mg, 500 mg, 1 g, 2 g
Tablet: 25 mg, 50 mg

cycloserine (sye kloe SER een)

Tall-Man cycloSERINE

U.S./Canadian Brand Names Seromycin® Pulvules® [US]

Therapeutic Category Antibiotic, Miscellaneous

Use Adjunctive treatment in pulmonary or extrapulmonary tuberculosis; treatment of acute urinary tract infections caused by *E. coli* or *Enterobacter* sp. when less toxic conventional therapy has failed or is contraindicated

Usual Dosage Oral:
Tuberculosis:
Children: 10-20 mg/kg/day in 2 divided doses up to 1000 mg/day
Adults: Initial: 250 mg every 12 hours for 14 days, then administer 500 mg to 1 g/day in 2 divided doses
Urinary tract infection: Adults: 250 mg every 12 hours for 14 days

Dosage Forms Capsule: 250 mg

Cyclospasmol® *(Discontinued)* see page 814

cyclosporin A see cyclosporine *on this page*

cyclosporine (SYE kloe spor een)

Synonyms CYA; cyclosporin A

Tall-Man cycloSPORINE

U.S./Canadian Brand Names Gengraf™ [US]; Neoral® [US/Can]; Sandimmune® [US/Can]

Therapeutic Category Immunosuppressant Agent

Use Immunosuppressant used with corticosteroids to prevent graft vs host disease in patients with kidney, liver, heart, and bone marrow transplants; has been used in the
(Continued)

cyclosporine *(Continued)*

treatment of nephrotic syndrome in patients with documented focal glomerulosclerosis when corticosteroids and cyclophosphamide were unsuccessful; monotherapy or in combination with methotrexate for treatment of severe active rheumatoid arthritis where the disease has not adequately responded to methotrexate

Usual Dosage Children and Adults:

Oral: Initial: 14-18 mg/kg/dose daily, beginning 4-12 hours prior to organ transplantation; maintenance: 5-10 mg/kg/day

I.V.: Initial: 5-6 mg/kg/day in divided doses every 12-24 hours; patients should be switched to oral cyclosporine as soon as possible

Dosage Forms

Capsule, soft gel, modified: 25 mg, 100 mg [contains castor oil, ethanol]

Gengraf™: 25 mg, 100 mg [contains ethanol, castor oil, propylene glycol]

Neoral®: 25 mg, 100 mg [contains dehydrated ethanol, corn oil, castor oil, propylene glycol]

Capsule, soft gel, non-modified (Sandimmune®): 25 mg, 100 mg [contains dehydrated ethanol, corn oil]

Injection, solution, non-modified (Sandimmune®): 50 mg/mL (5 mL) [contains Cremophor® EL (polyoxyethylated castor oil), ethanol]

Solution, oral, modified (Neoral®): 100 mg/mL (50 mL) [contains dehydrated ethanol, corn oil, castor oil, propylene glycol]

Solution, oral, non-modified (Sandimmune®): 100 mg/mL (50 mL) [contains olive oil, ethanol]

Cycofed® Pediatric *(Discontinued)* see page 814

Cycrin® 10 mg Tablet *(Discontinued)* see page 814

Cyklokapron® [US/Can] see tranexamic acid on page 647

Cylert® [US] see pemoline on page 496

Cylex® [US-OTC] see benzocaine on page 77

Cyomin® *(Discontinued)* see page 814

cyproheptadine (si proe HEP ta deen)

U.S./Canadian Brand Names Periactin® [US/Can]

Therapeutic Category Antihistamine

Use Perennial and seasonal allergic rhinitis and other allergic symptoms including urticaria

Usual Dosage Oral:

Children: 0.25 mg/kg/day in 2-3 divided doses **or**

2-6 years: 2 mg every 8-12 hours (not to exceed 12 mg/day)

7-14 years: 4 mg every 8-12 hours (not to exceed 16 mg/day)

Adults: 12-16 mg/day every 8 hours (not to exceed 0.5 mg/kg/day)

Dosage Forms

Syrup, as hydrochloride: 2 mg/5 mL [with alcohol 5%] (473 mL)

Tablet, as hydrochloride: 4 mg

cyproterone *(Canada only)* (sye PROE ter one)

U.S./Canadian Brand Names Alti-CPA [Can]; Androcur® [Can]; Androcur® Depot [Can]; Gen-Cyproterone [Can]; Novo-Cyproterone [Can]

Therapeutic Category Antiandrogen; Progestin

Use Palliative treatment of patients with advanced prostatic carcinoma

Usual Dosage Adults:

I.M.: 300 mg (3 mL) once a week

Oral: 200-300 mg divided into 2-3 doses and taken after meals

Dosage Forms

Injection, as acetate: 100 mg/mL (3 mL)

Tablet, as acetate: 50 mg

Cystadane® **[US/Can]** *see* betaine anhydrous *on page 82*

Cystagon® **[US]** *see* cysteamine *on this page*

cysteamine (sis TEE a meen)
U.S./Canadian Brand Names Cystagon® [US]
Therapeutic Category Urinary Tract Product
Use Nephropathic cystinosis in children and adults
Usual Dosage Initiate therapy with $1/4$ to $1/8$ of maintenance dose; titrate slowly upward over 4-6 weeks
Children <12 years: Oral: Maintenance: 1.3 g/m²/day divided into 4 doses
Children >12 years and Adults (>110 lbs): Oral: 2 g/day in 4 divided doses; dosage may in increased to 1.95 g/m²/day if cystine levels are <1 nmol/$1/2$ cystine/mg protein, although intolerance and incidence of adverse events may be increased
Dosage Forms Capsule, as bitartrate: 50 mg, 150 mg

cysteine (SIS teen)
Therapeutic Category Nutritional Supplement
Use Total parenteral nutrition of infants as an additive to meet the I.V. amino acid requirements
Usual Dosage Combine 500 mg of cysteine with 12.5 g of amino acid, then dilute with 50% dextrose
Dosage Forms Injection, as hydrochloride: 50 mg/mL [~0.285 mmol/mL] (10 mL)

Cystistat® **[Can]** *see* sodium hyaluronate *on page 597*

Cystografin® **[US]** *see* radiological/contrast media (ionic) *on page 561*

Cystospaz® **[US/Can]** *see* hyoscyamine *on page 339*

Cystospaz-M® **[US]** *see* hyoscyamine *on page 339*

CYT *see* cyclophosphamide *on page 169*

Cytadren® **[US]** *see* aminoglutethimide *on page 32*

cytarabine (sye TARE a been)
Synonyms arabinosylcytosine; ARA-C; cytosine arabinosine
U.S./Canadian Brand Names Cytosar® [Can]; Cytosar-U® [US]
Therapeutic Category Antineoplastic Agent
Use In combination regimens for the treatment of leukemias and non-Hodgkin's lymphomas
Usual Dosage Children and Adults (refer to individual protocols):
Induction remission:
I.T.: 5-75 mg/m² once daily for 4 days or 1 every 4 days until CNS
I.V.: 200 mg/m²/day for 5 days at 2-week intervals; 100-200 mg/m²/day for 5- to 10-day therapy course or every day until remission administered I.V. continuous drip, or in 2-3 divided doses findings normalize
Maintenance remission:
I.M., S.C.: 1-1.5 mg/kg single dose for maintenance at 1- to 4-week intervals
I.V.: 70-200 mg/m²/day for 2-5 days at monthly intervals
High-dose therapies: Doses as high as 1-3 g/m² have been used for refractory or secondary leukemias or refractory non-Hodgkins lymphoma; dosages of 3 g/m² every 12 hours for up to 12 doses have been used
Dosage Forms
Injection, powder for reconstitution: 100 mg, 500 mg, 1 g, 2 g
Cytosar-U®: 100 mg, 500 mg, 1 g, 2 g

cytarabine (liposomal) (sye TARE a been lip po SOE mal)
U.S./Canadian Brand Names DepoCyt™ [US/Can]
Therapeutic Category Antineoplastic Agent, Antimetabolite (Purine)
(Continued)

171

cytarabine (liposomal) *(Continued)*

Use Intrathecal treatment of lymphomatous meningitis
Usual Dosage Adults:
Induction: 50 mg intrathecally every 14 days for a total of 2 doses (weeks 1 and 3)
Consolidation: 50 mg intrathecally every 14 days for 3 doses (weeks 5, 7, and 9), followed by an additional dose at week 13
Maintenance: 50 mg intrathecally every 28 days for 4 doses (weeks 17, 21, 25, and 29)
If drug-related neurotoxicity develops, the dose should be reduced to 25 mg; if toxicity persists, treatment with liposomal cytarabine should be discontinued

Note: Patients should be started on dexamethasone 4 mg twice daily (oral or I.V.) for 5 days, beginning on the day of liposomal cytarabine injection
Dosage Forms Injection: 10 mg/mL (5 mL)

CytoGam® [US] *see* cytomegalovirus immune globulin (intravenous-human) *on this page*

cytomegalovirus immune globulin (intravenous-human)

(sye toe meg a low VYE rus i MYUN GLOB yoo lin in tra VEE nus-HYU man)
Synonyms CMV-IGIV
U.S./Canadian Brand Names CytoGam® [US]
Therapeutic Category Immune Globulin
Use Attenuation of primary CMV disease associated with kidney transplantation
Usual Dosage I.V.: Adults:
Kidney transplant:
Initial dose (within 72 hours of transplant): 150 mg/kg/dose
2-, 4-, 6-, and 8 weeks after transplant: 100 mg/kg/dose
12 and 16 weeks after transplant: 50 mg/kg/dose
Liver, lung, pancreas, or heart transplant:
Initial dose (within 72 hours of transplant): 150 mg/kg/dose
2-, 4-, 6-, and 8 weeks after transplant: 150 mg/kg/dose
12 and 16 weeks after transplant: 100 mg/kg/dose
Severe CMV pneumonia: Various regimens have been used, including 400 mg/kg CMV-IGIV in combination with ganciclovir on days 1, 2, 7, or 8, followed by 200 mg/kg CMV-IGIV on days 14 and 21
Dosage Forms Injection, powder for reconstitution, detergent-treated: 2500 mg ± 500 mg (50 mL); 1000 mg ± 200 mg (20 mL)

Cytomel® [US/Can] *see* liothyronine *on page 386*

Cytosar® [Can] *see* cytarabine *on previous page*

Cytosar-U® [US] *see* cytarabine *on previous page*

cytosine arabinosine *see* cytarabine *on previous page*

Cytotec® [US/Can] *see* misoprostol *on page 432*

Cytovene® [US/Can] *see* ganciclovir *on page 293*

Cytoxan® [US/Can] *see* cyclophosphamide *on page 169*

D₃ *see* cholecalciferol *on page 143*

25-D₃ *see* calcifediol *on page 103*

d-3-mercaptovaline *see* penicillamine *on page 497*

d4T *see* stavudine *on page 605*

dacarbazine (da KAR ba zeen)

Synonyms DIC; imidazole carboxamide
U.S./Canadian Brand Names DTIC® [Can]; DTIC-Dome® [US]
Therapeutic Category Antineoplastic Agent

Use Singly or in various combination therapy to treat malignant melanoma, Hodgkin's disease, soft-tissue sarcomas (fibrosarcomas, rhabdomyosarcoma), islet cell carcinoma, medullary carcinoma of the thyroid, and neuroblastoma

Usual Dosage Refer to individual protocols. I.V.:

Children:

Solid tumors: 200-470 mg/m^2/day over 5 days every 21-28 days

Neuroblastoma: 800-900 mg/m^2 as a single dose every 3-4 weeks in combination therapy

Adults:

Malignant melanoma: 2-4.5 mg/kg/day for 10 days, repeat in 4 weeks or may use 250 mg/m^2/day for 5 days, repeat in 3 weeks

Hodgkin's disease: 150 mg/m^2/day for 5 days, repeat every 4 weeks or 375 mg/m^2 on day 1, repeat in 15 days of each 28-day cycle in combination with other agents

Dosage Forms Injection: 100 mg (10 mL, 20 mL); 200 mg (20 mL, 30 mL); 500 mg (50 mL)

daclizumab (da KLIK si mab)

U.S./Canadian Brand Names Zenapax® [US/Can]

Therapeutic Category Immunosuppressant Agent

Use Part of an immunosuppressive regimen (including cyclosporine and corticosteroids) for the prophylaxis of acute organ rejection in patients receiving renal transplant

Usual Dosage Children and Adults: IVPB: 1 mg/kg, used as part of an immunosuppressive regimen that includes cyclosporine and corticosteroids for a total of 5 doses; give the first dose ≤24 hours before transplantation. The 4 remaining doses should be administered at intervals of 14 days.

Dosage Forms Injection: 5 mg/mL (5 mL)

Dacodyl® *(Discontinued)* see page 814

dactinomycin (dak ti noe MYE sin)

Synonyms actinomycin D

U.S./Canadian Brand Names Cosmegen® [US/Can]

Therapeutic Category Antineoplastic Agent

Use Management, either alone or in combination with other treatment modalities of Wilms' tumor, rhabdomyosarcoma, neuroblastoma, retinoblastoma, Ewing's sarcoma, trophoblastic neoplasms, testicular carcinoma, and other malignancies

Usual Dosage Refer to individual protocols; dosage should be based on body surface area in obese or edematous patients

Children >6 months and Adults: I.V.: 15 mcg/kg/day or 400-600 mcg/m^2/day for 5 days, may repeat every 3-6 weeks; or 2.5 mg/m^2 administered in divided doses over 1 week; 0.75-2 mg/m^2 as a single dose administered at intervals of 1-4 weeks have been used

Dosage Forms Injection, powder for reconstitution: Dactinomycin 0.5 mg and mannitol 20 mg

D.A.II™ [US] *see* chlorpheniramine, phenylephrine, and methscopolamine *on page 139*

Dairyaid® [Can] *see* lactase *on page 371*

Dairy Ease® [US-OTC] *see* lactase *on page 371*

Dakin's solution *see* sodium hypochlorite solution *on page 597*

Dakrina® Ophthalmic Solution *(Discontinued)* see page 814

Dalacin® C [Can] *see* clindamycin *on page 151*

Dalgan® *(Discontinued)* see page 814

Dallergy® [US] *see* chlorpheniramine, phenylephrine, and methscopolamine *on page 139*

Dallergy-D® Syrup *(Discontinued)* see page 814

Dalmane® **[US/Can]** *see* flurazepam *on page 281*

***d*-alpha tocopherol** *see* vitamin E *on page 682*

dalteparin (dal TE pa rin)

U.S./Canadian Brand Names Fragmin® [US/Can]
Therapeutic Category Anticoagulant (Other)
Use Prevent deep vein thrombosis following abdominal surgery
Usual Dosage Adults: S.C.: 2500 units 1-2 hours prior to surgery, then once daily for 5-10 days postoperatively
Dosage Forms
Injection, solution [multidose vial]: Antifactor Xa 10,000 int. units per 1 mL (9.5 mL) [contains benzyl alcohol]
Injection, solution [preservative free; prefilled syringe]: Antifactor Xa 2500 int. units per 0.2 mL (0.2 mL); antifactor Xa 5000 int. units per 0.2 mL (0.2 mL); antifactor Xa 7500 int. units per 0.3 mL (0.3 mL); antifactor Xa 10,000 int. units per 1 mL (1 mL)

D-Amp® *(Discontinued)* *see page 814*

danaparoid (da NAP a roid)

U.S./Canadian Brand Names Orgaran® [US/Can]
Therapeutic Category Anticoagulant (Other)
Use Prophylaxis of postoperative deep vein thrombosis (DVT)
Usual Dosage Adults: S.C.: 750 anti-Xa units twice daily beginning 1-4 hours preoperatively, and then not sooner than 2 hours hours after surgery
Dosage Forms Injection, as sodium: 750 anti-Xa units/0.6 mL

danazol (DA na zole)

U.S./Canadian Brand Names Cyclomen® [Can]; Danocrine® [US/Can]
Therapeutic Category Androgen
Use Treatment of endometriosis, fibrocystic breast disease, and hereditary angioedema
Usual Dosage Adults: Oral:
Endometriosis: 200-400 mg twice daily
Fibrocystic breast disease: 100-400 mg twice daily for 3-6 months (may extend to 9 months)
Hereditary angioedema: 400-600 mg/day in 2-3 divided doses
Dosage Forms Capsule: 50 mg, 100 mg, 200 mg

Danex® **Shampoo** *(Discontinued)* *see page 814*

Danocrine® **[US/Can]** *see* danazol *on this page*

Dantrium® **[US/Can]** *see* dantrolene *on this page*

dantrolene (DAN troe leen)

U.S./Canadian Brand Names Dantrium® [US/Can]
Therapeutic Category Skeletal Muscle Relaxant
Use Treatment of spasticity associated with upper motor neuron disorders such as spinal cord injury, stroke, cerebral palsy, or multiple sclerosis; also used as treatment of malignant hyperthermia
Usual Dosage
Spasticity: Oral:
Children: Initial: 0.5 mg/kg/dose twice daily, increase frequency to 3-4 times/day at 4- to 7-day intervals, then increase dose by 0.5 mg/kg to a maximum of 3 mg/kg/dose 2-4 times/day up to 400 mg/day
Adults: 25 mg/day to start, increase frequency to 3-4 times/day, then increase dose by 25 mg every 4-7 days to a maximum of 100 mg 2-4 times/day or 400 mg/day
Hyperthermia: Children and Adults:
Oral: 4-8 mg/kg/day in 4 divided doses

I.V.: 1 mg/kg; may repeat dose up to cumulative dose of 10 mg/kg (mean effective dose: 2.5 mg/kg), then switch to oral dosage

Dosage Forms
Capsule, as sodium: 25 mg, 50 mg, 100 mg
Injection, powder for reconstitution, as sodium: 20 mg

Dapacin® Cold Capsule (Discontinued) see page 814

dapiprazole (DA pi pray zole)

U.S./Canadian Brand Names Rēv-Eyes™ [US]

Therapeutic Category Alpha-Adrenergic Blocking Agent

Use Treatment of iatrogenically induced mydriasis produced by adrenergic or parasympatholytic agents

Usual Dosage Ophthalmic: Instill 2 drops followed 5 minutes later by an additional 2 drops applied to the conjunctiva

Dosage Forms Powder, ophthalmic, as hydrochloride: 25 mg [0.5% solution when mixed with supplied diluent]

dapsone (DAP sone)

Synonyms DDS; diaminodiphenylsulfone

Therapeutic Category Sulfone

Use Treatment of leprosy due to susceptible strains of *M. leprae*; treatment of dermatitis herpetiformis; prophylaxis against *Pneumocystis carinii* in children who cannot tolerate sulfamethoxazole/trimethoprim or aerosolized pentamidine

Usual Dosage Oral:
Leprosy:
Children: 1-2 mg/kg/24 hours, up to a maximum of 100 mg/day
Adults: 50-100 mg/day for 3-10 years
Dermatitis herpetiformis: Adults: Start at 50 mg/day, increase to 300 mg/day, or higher to achieve full control, reduce dosage to minimum level as soon as possible
Pneumocystis carinii pneumonia:
Prophylaxis:
Children >1 month: 2 mg/kg/day once daily (maximum dose: 100 mg/day) or 4 mg/kg/dose once weekly (maximum dose: 200 mg)
Adults: 100 mg/day
Treatment: Adults: 100 mg/day in combination with trimethoprim (15-20 mg/kg/day) for 21 days

Dosage Forms Tablet: 25 mg, 100 mg

Daptacel™ [US] see diphtheria, tetanus toxoids, and acellular pertussis vaccine on page 204

Daranide® [US/Can] see dichlorphenamide on page 193

Daraprim® [US/Can] see pyrimethamine on page 557

darbepoetin alfa (dar be POE e tin AL fa)

Synonyms erythropoiesis stimulating protein

U.S./Canadian Brand Names Aranesp™ [US]

Therapeutic Category Colony-Stimulating Factor; Growth Factor; Recombinant Human Erythropoietin

Use Treatment of anemia associated with chronic renal failure (CRF), including patients on dialysis (ESRD) and patients not on dialysis; anemia associated with chemotherapy for non-myeloid malignancies

Usual Dosage I.V., S.C.:
Correction of anemia:
Initial: 0.45 mcg/kg once weekly; dosage should be titrated to limit increases in hemoglobin to <1 g/dL over any 2-week interval, with a target concentration of <12 g/dL. (Continued)

darbepoetin alfa *(Continued)*

Maintenance: Titrated to hematologic response. Some patients may require doses <0.45 mcg/kg once weekly. Selected patients may be managed by administering S.C. doses every 2 weeks.

Dosage Forms Injection, solution, with human albumin 2.5 mg/mL [preservative free, single-dose vial]: 25 mcg/mL (1 mL); 40 mcg/mL (1 mL); 60 mcg/mL (1 mL); 100 mcg/mL (1 mL); 150 mcg/0.75 mL (0.75 mL); 200 mcg/mL (1 mL); 300 mcg/mL (1 mL); 500 mcg/mL (1 mL)

Darbid® Tablet *(Discontinued)* see page 814

Daricon® *(Discontinued)* see page 814

Darvocet-N® 50 [US/Can] see propoxyphene and acetaminophen on page 548

Darvocet-N® 100 [US/Can] see propoxyphene and acetaminophen on page 548

Darvon® [US] see propoxyphene on page 548

Darvon® 32 mg Capsule *(Discontinued)* see page 814

Darvon® Compound-65 [US] see propoxyphene and aspirin on page 549

Darvon-N® Oral Suspension *(Discontinued)* see page 814

Darvon-N® Tablet [US/Can] see propoxyphene on page 548

Datril® Extra Strength *(Discontinued)* see page 814

daunomycin see daunorubicin hydrochloride on this page

daunorubicin citrate (liposomal)

(daw noe ROO bi sin SI trate lip po SOE mal)

Tall-Man **DAUNO**rubicin citrate (liposomal)

U.S./Canadian Brand Names DaunoXome® [US]

Therapeutic Category Antineoplastic Agent

Use Advanced HIV-associated Kaposi's sarcoma

Usual Dosage I.V. (refer to individual protocols):

Children:

ALL combination therapy: Remission induction: 25-45 mg/m² on day 1 every week for 4 cycles **or** 30-45 mg/m²/day for 3 days

In children <2 years or <0.5 m², daunorubicin should be based on weight (mg/kg): 1 mg/kg per protocol with frequency dependent on regimen employed

Cumulative dose should not exceed 300 mg/m² in children >2 years or 10 mg/kg in children <2 years

Adults: 30-60 mg/m²/day for 3-5 days, repeat dose in 3-4 weeks

Single agent induction for AML: 60 mg/m²/day for 3 days; repeat every 3-4 weeks

Combination therapy induction for AML: 45 mg/m²/day for 3 days of the first course of induction therapy; subsequent courses: Every day for 2 days

ALL combination therapy: 45 mg/m²/day for 3 days

Cumulative dose should not exceed 400-600 mg/m²

Dosage Forms Injection: 2 mg/mL [equivalent to 50 mg daunorubicin base] (1 mL, 4 mL, 10 mL unit packs)

daunorubicin hydrochloride (daw noe ROO bi sin hye droe KLOR ide)

Synonyms daunomycin; DNR; rubidomycin

Tall-Man **DAUNO**rubicin hydrochloride

U.S./Canadian Brand Names Cerubidine® [US/Can]

Therapeutic Category Antineoplastic Agent

Use In combination with other agents in the treatment of leukemias (ALL, AML)

Usual Dosage I.V.:

Children:

Combination therapy: Remission induction for ALL: 25-45 mg/m² on day 1 every week for 4 cycles

<2 years or <0.5 m^2: Manufacturer recommends that the dose is based on body weight rather than body surface area

Adults: 30-60 mg/m^2/day for 3-5 days, repeat dose in 3-4 weeks; total cumulative dose should not exceed 400-600 mg/m^2

Single agent induction for AML: 60 mg/m^2/day for 3 days; repeat every 3-4 weeks

Combination therapy induction for AML: 45 mg/m^2/day for 3 days; Subsequent courses: Every day for 2 days

Combination therapy: Remission induction for ALL: 45 mg/m^2 on days 1, 2, and 3

Dosage Forms Injection, powder for reconstitution: 5 mg/mL (4 mL, 10 mL)

DaunoXome® **[US]** *see* daunorubicin citrate (liposomal) *on previous page*

Daypro™ **[US/Can]** *see* oxaprozin *on page 482*

Dayto Himbin® *(Discontinued)* *see page 814*

1-Day™ **[US-OTC]** *see* tioconazole *on page 640*

DC 240® **Softgel®** *(Discontinued)* *see page 814*

D-Care Circulation Stimulator® **[US]** *see* capsaicin *on page 111*

DCF *see* pentostatin *on page 502*

DDAVP® **[US/Can]** *see* desmopressin acetate *on page 182*

ddC *see* zalcitabine *on page 688*

ddl *see* didanosine *on page 195*

DDS *see* dapsone *on page 175*

1-deamino-8-d-arginine vasopressin *see* desmopressin acetate *on page 182*

Debrisan® **[US-OTC]** *see* dextranomer *on page 188*

Debrox® **Otic [US-OTC]** *see* carbamide peroxide *on page 113*

Decadron® **[US/Can]** *see* dexamethasone (systemic) *on page 184*

Decadron® **0.25 mg & 6 mg Tablets** *(Discontinued)* *see page 814*

Decadron®-LA [US] *see* dexamethasone (systemic) *on page 184*

Decadron® **Ocumeter®** **[US]** *see* dexamethasone (ophthalmic) *on page 184*

Decadron® **Phosphate Ophthalmic Ointment** *(Discontinued)* *see page 814*

Deca-Durabolin® **[US/Can]** *see* nandrolone *on page 446*

Dec-Agesic® **A.B. [US]** *see* antipyrine and benzocaine *on page 47*

Decaject® **[US]** *see* dexamethasone (systemic) *on page 184*

Decaject-LA® **[US]** *see* dexamethasone (systemic) *on page 184*

Decaspray® *(Discontinued)* *see page 814*

Decholin® *(Discontinued)* *see page 814*

Declomycin® **[US/Can]** *see* demeclocycline *on page 179*

Decofed® **[US-OTC]** *see* pseudoephedrine *on page 552*

Decohistine® **DH [US]** *see* chlorpheniramine, pseudoephedrine, and codeine *on page 140*

Deconamine® **SR [US-OTC]** *see* chlorpheniramine and pseudoephedrine *on page 138*

Deconamine® **[US-OTC]** *see* chlorpheniramine and pseudoephedrine *on page 138*

Decongest [Can] *see* xylometazoline *on page 687*

Deconsal® **II [US]** *see* guaifenesin and pseudoephedrine *on page 310*

Defen-LA® **[US]** *see* guaifenesin and pseudoephedrine *on page 310*

deferoxamine (de fer OKS a meen)
U.S./Canadian Brand Names Desferal® [US/Can]
Therapeutic Category Antidote
Use Acute iron intoxication; chronic iron overload secondary to multiple transfusions; diagnostic test for iron overload

Investigational use: Treatment of aluminum accumulation in renal failure
Usual Dosage
Children and Adults: Acute iron toxicity: I.V. route is used when severe toxicity is evidenced by systemic symptoms (coma, shock, metabolic acidosis, or severe gastrointestinal bleeding) or potentially severe intoxications (serum iron level >500 mcg/dL). When severe symptoms are not present, the I.M. route may be preferred; however, the use of deferoxamine in situations where the serum iron concentration is <500 mcg/dL or when severe toxicity is not evident is a subject of some clinical debate.
Dose: 15 mg/kg/hour (although rates up to 40-50 mg/kg/hour have been given in patients with massive iron intoxication); maximum recommended dose: 6 g/day (however, doses as high as 16-37 g have been administered)
Children:
Chronic iron overload:
I.V.: 15 mg/kg/hour
S.C.: 20-40 mg/kg/day over 8-12 hours
Aluminum-induced bone disease: 20-40 mg/kg every hemodialysis treatment, frequency dependent on clinical status of the patient
Adults:
Chronic iron overload:
I.M.: 0.5-1 g every day
S.C.: 1-2 g every day over 8-24 hours
Dosage Forms Injection, powder for reconstitution, as mesylate: 500 mg, 2 g

Deficol® *(Discontinued)* see page 814

Definity® [US] see perflutren lipid microspheres on page 503

Degest® 2 Ophthalmic *(Discontinued)* see page 814

Dehist® *(Discontinued)* see page 814

Dehydral® [Can] see methenamine on page 416

dehydrocholic acid (dee hye droe KOE lik AS id)
U.S./Canadian Brand Names Cholan-HMB® [US-OTC]
Therapeutic Category Laxative
Use Relief of constipation; adjunct to various biliary tract conditions
Usual Dosage Children >12 years and Adults: Oral: 250-500 mg 2-3 times/day after meals up to 1.5 g/day
Dosage Forms Tablet: 250 mg

Dek-Quin® [US] see clioquinol and hydrocortisone on page 152

Deladumone® *(Discontinued)* see page 814

Del Aqua® [US] see benzoyl peroxide on page 79

Delatest® Injection *(Discontinued)* see page 814

Delatestryl® [US/Can] see testosterone on page 625

delavirdine (de la VIR deen)
Synonyms U-90152S
U.S./Canadian Brand Names Rescriptor® [US/Can]
Therapeutic Category Antiviral Agent
Use Treatment of HIV-1 infection in combination with appropriate antiretrovirals
Usual Dosage Adults: Oral: 400 mg 3 times/day
Dosage Forms Tablet: 100 mg, 200 mg

Del-Beta® [US] *see* betamethasone (topical) *on page 83*

Delcort® [US] *see* hydrocortisone (topical) *on page 334*

Delestrogen® [US/Can] *see* estradiol *on page 238*

Delfen® [US-OTC] *see* nonoxynol 9 *on page 464*

Del-Mycin® Topical *(Discontinued) see page 814*

Delsym® [US-OTC] *see* dextromethorphan *on page 189*

Delta-Cortef® [US] *see* prednisolone (systemic) *on page 537*

deltacortisone *see* prednisone *on page 538*

Delta-D® [US] *see* cholecalciferol *on page 143*

deltadehydrocortisone *see* prednisone *on page 538*

deltahydrocortisone *see* prednisolone (systemic) *on page 537*

Deltalin® Capsule *(Discontinued) see page 814*

Deltasone® [US] *see* prednisone *on page 538*

Delta-Tritex® Topical *(Discontinued) see page 814*

Del-Vi-A® *(Discontinued) see page 814*

Demadex® [US] *see* torsemide *on page 646*

Demazin® Syrup *(Discontinued) see page 814*

demeclocycline (dem e kloe SYE kleen)
 Synonyms demethylchlortetracycline
 U.S./Canadian Brand Names Declomycin® [US/Can]
 Therapeutic Category Tetracycline Derivative
 Use Treatment of susceptible bacterial infections (acne, gonorrhea, pertussis, chronic bronchitis, and urinary tract infections) caused by both gram-negative and gram-positive organisms; treatment of chronic syndrome of inappropriate antidiuretic hormone (SIADH) secretion
 Usual Dosage Oral:
  Children ≥8 years: 8-12 mg/kg/day divided every 6-12 hours
  Adults: 150 mg 4 times/day or 300 mg twice daily
   Uncomplicated gonorrhea: 600 mg stat, 300 mg every 12 hours for 4 days (3 g total)
   SIADH: Initial: 900-1200 mg/day or 13-15 mg/kg/day divided every 6-8 hours, then decrease to 0.6-0.9 g/day
 Dosage Forms Tablet, as hydrochloride: 150 mg, 300 mg

Demerol® [US/Can] *see* meperidine *on page 408*

4-demethoxydaunorubicin *see* idarubicin *on page 344*

demethylchlortetracycline *see* demeclocycline *on this page*

Demser® [US/Can] *see* metyrosine *on page 427*

Demulen® [US] *see* ethinyl estradiol and ethynodiol diacetate *on page 246*

Demulen® 30 [Can] *see* ethinyl estradiol and ethynodiol diacetate *on page 246*

Denavir™ [US] *see* penciclovir *on page 497*

denileukin diftitox (de ne LU kin DIFT e tox)
 U.S./Canadian Brand Names ONTAK® [US]
 Therapeutic Category Antineoplastic Agent, Miscellaneous
 Use Treatment of patients with persistent or recurrent cutaneous T-cell lymphoma whose malignant cells express the CD25 component of the IL-2 receptor
 Usual Dosage Adults: I.V.: A treatment cycle consists of 9 or 18 mcg/kg/day for 5 consecutive days administered every 21 days. The optimal duration of therapy has not been determined. Only 2% of patients who failed to demonstrate a response (at least a
 (Continued)

denileukin diftitox *(Continued)*

25% decrease in tumor burden) prior to the fourth cycle responded to subsequent treatment.

Dosage Forms Injection: 150 mcg/mL (2 mL)

Denorex® [US-OTC] *see* coal tar *on page 158*

deodorized opium tincture *see* opium tincture *on page 478*

2′-deoxycoformycin *see* pentostatin *on page 502*

Depacon® [US] *see* valproic acid and derivatives *on page 670*

Depakene® [US/Can] *see* valproic acid and derivatives *on page 670*

Depakote® Delayed Release [US] *see* valproic acid and derivatives *on page 670*

Depakote® ER [US] *see* valproic acid and derivatives *on page 670*

Depakote® Sprinkle® [US] *see* valproic acid and derivatives *on page 670*

depAndrogyn® *(Discontinued)* *see page 814*

depAndro® Injection *(Discontinued)* *see page 814*

Depen® [US/Can] *see* penicillamine *on page 497*

depGynogen® Injection *(Discontinued)* *see page 814*

depMedalone® Injection *(Discontinued)* *see page 814*

DepoCyt™ [US/Can] *see* cytarabine (liposomal) *on page 171*

Depo®-Estradiol [US/Can] *see* estradiol *on page 238*

Depoject® Injection *(Discontinued)* *see page 814*

Depo-Medrol® [US/Can] *see* methylprednisolone *on page 423*

Deponit® Patch *(Discontinued)* *see page 814*

Depopred® [US] *see* methylprednisolone *on page 423*

Depo-Provera® [US/Can] *see* medroxyprogesterone acetate *on page 404*

Depo-Provera® 100 mg/mL *(Discontinued)* *see page 814*

Depo-Testadiol® [US] *see* estradiol and testosterone *on page 240*

Depotest® Injection *(Discontinued)* *see page 814*

Depotestogen® *(Discontinued)* *see page 814*

Depo®-Testosterone [US] *see* testosterone *on page 625*

deprenyl *see* selegiline *on page 586*

Deprol® *(Discontinued)* *see page 814*

Dequadin® [Can] *see* dequalinium *(Canada only)* *on this page*

dequalinium *(Canada only)* (de kwal LI ne um)

U.S./Canadian Brand Names Dequadin® [Can]

Therapeutic Category Antibacterial, Topical; Antifungal Agent, Topical

Use Treatment of mouth and throat infections

Usual Dosage Adults:

Lozenge: One lozenge sucked slowly every 2-3 hours

Oral paint: Apply freely to infected area, every 2-3 hours, or as directed by physician

Dosage Forms

Lozenge, as chloride: 0.25 mg (20s)

Oral paint, as chloride: 0.5% (25 mL)

Derifil® [US-OTC] *see* chlorophyll *on page 135*

Dermacort® [US] *see* hydrocortisone (topical) *on page 334*

Dermaflex® Gel [US] *see* lidocaine *on page 383*

Dermamycin® [US-OTC] *see* diphenhydramine *on page 202*

Derma-Pax® [US-OTC] *see* diphenhydramine *on page 202*

Dermarest Dricort® [US] *see* hydrocortisone (topical) *on page 334*

Derma-Smoothe/FS® [US/Can] *see* fluocinolone *on page 276*

Dermatop® [US] *see* prednicarbate *on page 536*

Dermatophytin® [US] *see* Trichophyton skin test *on page 654*

Dermatophytin-O [US] *see* Candida albicans (Monilia) *on page 110*

Dermazene® [US] *see* iodoquinol and hydrocortisone *on page 358*

Dermazin™ [Can] *see* silver sulfadiazine *on page 590*

Dermolate® [US-OTC] *see* hydrocortisone (topical) *on page 334*

Dermovate® [Can] *see* clobetasol *on page 152*

Dermoxyl® Gel *(Discontinued)* *see page 814*

Dermtex® HC with Aloe [US-OTC] *see* hydrocortisone (topical) *on page 334*

DES *see* diethylstilbestrol *on page 196*

deserpidine and methyclothiazide *see* methyclothiazide and deserpidine *on page 420*

Desferal® [US/Can] *see* deferoxamine *on page 178*

desflurane (des FLOO rane)

U.S./Canadian Brand Names Suprane® [US/Can]

Therapeutic Category General Anesthetic

Use Induction or maintenance of anesthesia for adults in outpatient and inpatient surgery

Usual Dosage

Children: Maintenance: Surgical levels of anesthesia may be maintained with concentrations of 5.2% to 10% desflurane, with or without nitrous oxide

Adults: Titrate dose based on individual response; see table in the product packaging for specific details; minimum alveolar concentration (MAC) should be reduced in elderly patients

Induction: Frequent starting concentration 3%; increased in 0.5% to 1% increments every 2-3 breaths; end tidal concentrations of 4% to 11% desflurane with and without nitrous oxide produce anesthesia within 2-4 minutes

Maintenance: Surgical levels of anesthesia in adults may be maintained with concentrations of 2.5% to 8.5% desflurane, with or without nitrous oxide

Note: Because of the higher vapor pressure and higher MAC of desflurane, special vaporizer canisters must be used. Equipment is **not** interchangeable with that for isoflurane.

Dosage Forms Liquid: 240 mL

desiccated thyroid *see* thyroid *on page 636*

desipramine (des IP ra meen)

Synonyms desmethylimipramine

U.S./Canadian Brand Names Alti-Desipramine [Can]; Apo®-Desipramine [Can]; Norpramin® [US/Can]; Novo-Desipramine [Can]; Nu-Desipramine [Can]; PMS-Desipramine

Therapeutic Category Antidepressant, Tricyclic (Secondary Amine)

Use Treatment of various forms of depression, often in conjunction with psychotherapy; analgesic in chronic pain, peripheral neuropathies

Usual Dosage Oral (not recommended for use in children <12 years):

Adolescents: Initial: 25-50 mg/day; gradually increase to 100 mg/day in single or divided doses; maximum: 150 mg/day

Adults: Initial: 75 mg/day in divided doses; increase gradually to 150-200 mg/day in divided or single dose; maximum: 300 mg/day

(Continued)

desipramine *(Continued)*

Dosage Forms Tablet, as hydrochloride: 10 mg, 25 mg, 50 mg, 75 mg, 100 mg, 150 mg

Desitin® Creamy [US-OTC] *see* zinc oxide *on page 691*

Desitin® [US-OTC] *see* zinc oxide, cod liver oil, and talc *on page 691*

desloratadine (des lor AT a deen)

U.S./Canadian Brand Names Clarinex® [US]
Therapeutic Category Antihistamine, Nonsedating
Use Relief of nasal and non-nasal symptoms of seasonal allergic rhinitis
Usual Dosage Oral: Adults and Children ≥12 years: 5 mg once daily
Dosage Forms
Tablet: 5 mg
Tablet, orally-disintegrating (RediTabs®): 5 mg [contains phenylalanine 1.75 mg/tablet; tutti-frutti flavor]

desmethylimipramine *see* desipramine *on previous page*

desmopressin acetate (des moe PRES in AS e tate)

Synonyms 1-deamino-8-d-arginine vasopressin
U.S./Canadian Brand Names DDAVP® [US/Can]; Octostim® [Can]; Stimate™ [US]
Therapeutic Category Vasopressin Analog, Synthetic
Use Treatment of diabetes insipidus and controlling bleeding in certain types of hemophilia
Usual Dosage
Children:
Diabetes insipidus: 3 months to 12 years: Intranasal: Initial: 5 mcg/day divided 1-2 times/day; range: 5-30 mcg/day divided 1-2 times/day
Hemophilia: >3 months: I.V.: 0.3 mcg/kg by slow infusion; may repeat dose if needed
Nocturnal enuresis: ≥6 years: Intranasal: Initial: 20 mcg at bedtime; range: 10-40 mcg
Adults:
Diabetes insipidus: I.V., S.C.: 2-4 mcg/day in 2 divided doses or $\frac{1}{10}$ of the maintenance intranasal dose; intranasal: 5-40 mcg/day 1-3 times/day
Hemophilia: I.V.: 0.3 mcg/kg by slow infusion
Dosage Forms
Injection, solution, as acetate (DDAVP®): 4 mcg/mL (1 mL, 10 mL)
Solution, intranasal, as acetate, (DDAVP®): 100 mcg/mL (2.5 mL) [with rhinal tube]
Nasal spray, as acetate:
DDAVP®: 100 mcg/mL (5 mL) [delivers 10 mcg/spray]
Stimate™: 1.5 mg/mL (2.5 mL)
Tablet, as acetate (DDAVP®): 0.1 mg, 0.2 mg

Desocort® [Can] *see* desonide *on this page*

Desogen® [US] *see* ethinyl estradiol and desogestrel *on page 244*

desogestrel and ethinyl estradiol *see* ethinyl estradiol and desogestrel *on page 244*

desonide (DES oh nide)

U.S./Canadian Brand Names Desocort® [Can]; DesOwen® [US]; Tridesilon® [US]
Therapeutic Category Corticosteroid, Topical
Use Adjunctive therapy for inflammation in acute and chronic corticosteroid responsive dermatosis
Usual Dosage Topical: Apply 2-4 times/day. Therapy should be discontinued when control is achieved. If no improvement is seen, reassessment of diagnosis may be necessary.
Dosage Forms
Cream: 0.05% (15 g, 60 g)

Lotion: 0.05% (60 mL, 120 mL)
Ointment: 0.05% (15 g, 60 g)

DesOwen® [US] *see* desonide *on previous page*

desoximetasone (des oks i MET a sone)

U.S./Canadian Brand Names Taro-Desoximetasone [Can]; Topicort®-LP [US]; Topicort® [US/Can]

Therapeutic Category Corticosteroid, Topical

Use Relief of inflammation and pruritic symptoms of corticosteroid-responsive dermatosis

Usual Dosage Topical:

Children: Apply sparingly in a very thin film to affected area 1-2 times/day

Adults: Apply sparingly in a thin film twice daily

Note: Therapy should be discontinued when control is achieved. If no improvement is seen, reassessment of diagnosis may be necessary.

Dosage Forms

Cream:

Topicort®: 0.25% (15 g, 60 g, 120 g)

Topicort®-LP: 0.05% (15 g, 60 g)

Gel (Topicort®): 0.05% (15 g, 60 g)

Ointment (Topicort®): 0.25% (15 g, 60 g)

desoxyephedrine *see* methamphetamine *on page 415*

Desoxyn® [US/Can] *see* methamphetamine *on page 415*

Desoxyn® Gradumet® [US] *see* methamphetamine *on page 415*

desoxyphenobarbital *see* primidone *on page 540*

Despec® Liquid *(Discontinued)* *see page 814*

Desquam-E™ [US] *see* benzoyl peroxide *on page 79*

Desquam-X® [US/Can] *see* benzoyl peroxide *on page 79*

Desquam-X® Wash *(Discontinued)* *see page 814*

Desyrel® [US/Can] *see* trazodone *on page 649*

Detane® [US-OTC] *see* benzocaine *on page 77*

Detrol® [US/Can] *see* tolterodine *on page 644*

Detrol® LA [US] *see* tolterodine *on page 644*

Detussin® Expectorant *(Discontinued)* *see page 814*

Detussin® Liquid [US] *see* hydrocodone and pseudoephedrine *on page 331*

Devrom® [US-OTC] *see* bismuth subgallate *on page 87*

Dex4 Glucose [US-OTC] *see* glucose (instant) *on page 300*

Dexacen-4® *(Discontinued)* *see page 814*

Dexacen® LA-8 *(Discontinued)* *see page 814*

Dexacidin® [US] *see* neomycin, polymyxin B, and dexamethasone *on page 452*

Dexacine™ [US] *see* neomycin, polymyxin B, and dexamethasone *on page 452*

Dexacort® Phosphate in Respihaler® [US] *see* dexamethasone (oral inhalation) *on next page*

Dexacort® Phosphate Turbinaire® [US] *see* dexamethasone (nasal) *on next page*

dexamethasone and neomycin *see* neomycin and dexamethasone *on page 451*

dexamethasone and tobramycin *see* tobramycin and dexamethasone *on page 642*

dexamethasone (nasal) (deks a METH a sone NAY sal)
U.S./Canadian Brand Names Dexacort® Phosphate Turbinaire® [US]
Therapeutic Category Adrenal Corticosteroid
Use Chronic inflammation and/or allergic conditions
Dosage Forms Dexamethasone sodium phosphate: Aerosol, nasal 84 mcg/activation [170 metered doses] (12.6 g)

dexamethasone, neomycin, and polymyxin B *see* neomycin, polymyxin B, and dexamethasone *on page 452*

dexamethasone (ophthalmic) (deks a METH a sone op THAL mik)
U.S./Canadian Brand Names AK-Dex® [US]; Baldex® [US]; Decadron® Ocumeter® [US]; Diodex® [Can]; Maxidex® [US/Can]
Therapeutic Category Adrenal Corticosteroid
Use Inflammatory or allergic conjunctivitis
Usual Dosage Ophthalmic: Instill 3-4 times/day
Dosage Forms Dexamethasone base:
Solution, ophthalmic: 0.1% (5 mL)
Suspension, ophthalmic: 0.1% (5 mL, 15 mL)

dexamethasone (oral inhalation)
(deks a METH a sone OR al in hil LA shun)
U.S./Canadian Brand Names Dexacort® Phosphate in Respihaler® [US]
Therapeutic Category Adrenal Corticosteroid
Use Chronic inflammation or allergic conditions
Dosage Forms Aerosol, oral: 84 mcg/activation [170 metered doses] (12.6 g)

dexamethasone (systemic) (deks a METH a sone sis TEM ik)
U.S./Canadian Brand Names Alti-Dexamethasone [Can]; Decadron®-LA [US]; Decadron® [US/Can]; Decaject-LA® [US]; Decaject® [US]; Dexasone® L.A. [US]; Dexasone® [US/Can]; Dexone® LA [US]; Dexone® [US]; Hexadrol® [US/Can]; PMS-Dexamethasone [Can]; Solurex L.A.® [US]
Therapeutic Category Adrenal Corticosteroid
Use Systemically for chronic inflammation, allergic, hematologic, neoplastic, and autoimmune diseases; may be used in management of cerebral edema, septic shock, and as a diagnostic agent
Usual Dosage
Children:
Antiemetic (prior to chemotherapy): 10 mg/m^2/dose for first dose then 5 mg/m^2/dose every 6 hours as needed
Physiologic replacement: Oral, I.M., I.V.: 0.03-0.15 mg/kg/day or 0.6-0.75 mg/m^2/day in divided doses every 6-12 hours
Extubation or airway edema: Oral, I.M., I.V.: 0.5-1 mg/kg/day in divided doses every 6 hours beginning 24 hours prior to extubation and continuing for 4-6 doses afterwards
Anti-inflammatory: Oral, I.M., I.V.: 0.75-9 mg/day in divided doses every 6-12 hours
Cerebral edema: I.V. 10 mg stat, 4 mg I.M./I.V. every 6 hours until response is maximized, then switch to oral regimen, then taper off if appropriate
Diagnosis for Cushing's syndrome: Oral: 1 mg at 11 PM, draw blood at 8 AM
ANLL protocol: I.V.: 2 mg/m^2/dose every 8 hours for 12 doses
Dosage Forms
Dexamethasone acetate:
Injection:
Decadron®-LA, Decaject-LA®, Dexasone® L.A., Dexone® LA, Solurex L.A.®: 8 mg/mL (1 mL, 5 mL)
Dexamethasone base:
Elixir (Decadron®, Hexadrol®): 0.5 mg/5 mL (5 mL, 20 mL, 100 mL, 120 mL, 240 mL, 500 mL)

Injection:
Decadron® Phosphate, Decaject®, Dexasone®, Hexadrol® Phosphate: 4 mg/mL (1 mL, 2 mL, 2.5 mL, 5 mL, 10 mL, 30 mL)
Decadron® Phosphate: 24 mg/mL (5 mL, 10 mL)
Hexadrol® Phosphate: 10 mg/mL (1 mL, 10 mL); 20 mg/mL (5 mL)
Solution, oral: 0.5 mg/5 mL (5 mL, 20 mL, 500 mL)
Solution, oral concentrate: 0.5 mg/0.5 mL (30 mL)
Tablet (Decadron®, Dexone®, Hexadrol®): 0.25 mg, 0.5 mg, 0.75 mg, 1 mg, 1.5 mg, 2 mg, 4 mg, 6 mg
Therapeutic pack: Six 1.5 mg tablets and eight 0.75 mg tablets

dexamethasone (topical) (deks a METH a sone TOP i kal)
U.S./Canadian Brand Names Aeroseb-Dex® [US]
Therapeutic Category Adrenal Corticosteroid
Use For chronic inflammation and/or allergic conditions
Usual Dosage Topical: Apply 2-4 times daily. Therapy should be discontinued when control is achieved. If no improvement is seen, reassessment of diagnosis may be necessary.
Dosage Forms Dexamethasone base:
Aerosol, topical: 0.01% (58 g)
Cream: 0.1% (15 g, 30 g)

Dexasone® [US/Can] *see* dexamethasone (systemic) *on previous page*
Dexasone® L.A. [US] *see* dexamethasone (systemic) *on previous page*
Dexatrim® Pre-Meal *(Discontinued)* *see page 814*

dexbrompheniramine and pseudoephedrine
(deks brom fen EER a meen & soo doe e FED rin)
Synonyms pseudoephedrine and dexbrompheniramine
U.S./Canadian Brand Names B10mpheril® [US-OTC]; Disobrom® [US-OTC]; Disophrol® Chronotabs® [US-OTC]; Drixomed® [US]; Drixoral® [Can]; Drixoral® Cold & Allergy [US-OTC]; Histrodrix® [US]; Resporal® [US]
Therapeutic Category Antihistamine/Decongestant Combination
Use Relief of symptoms of upper respiratory mucosal congestion in seasonal and perennial nasal allergies, acute rhinitis, rhinosinusitis and eustachian tube blockage
Usual Dosage Children >12 years and Adults: Oral: 1 tablet every 12 hours, may require 1 tablet every 8 hours
Dosage Forms Tablet, timed release (Disobrom®, Drixomed®, Drixoral® Cold & Allergy, Histrodrix®, Resporal®): Dexbrompheniramine maleate 6 mg and pseudoephedrine sulfate 120 mg

Dexchlor® *(Discontinued)* *see page 814*

dexchlorpheniramine (deks klor fen EER a meen)
U.S./Canadian Brand Names Polaramine® [US]
Therapeutic Category Antihistamine
Use Perennial and seasonal allergic rhinitis and other allergic symptoms including urticaria
Usual Dosage Oral:
Children:
2-5 years: 0.5 mg every 4-6 hours
6-11 years: 1 mg every 4-6 hours or 4 mg timed release at bedtime
Adults: 2 mg every 4-6 hours or 4-6 mg timed release at bedtime or 8-10 hours
Dosage Forms
Syrup, as maleate: 2 mg/5 mL (480 mL) [contains alcohol 6%; orange flavor]
Tablet, as maleate: 2 mg
Tablet, sustained action, as maleate: 4 mg, 6 mg

Dexedrine® Elixir *(Discontinued)* see page 814

Dexedrine® Spansule® [US/Can] see dextroamphetamine on page 188

Dexedrine® Tablet [US/Can] see dextroamphetamine on page 188

Dexferrum® [US] see iron dextran complex on page 360

Dexiron™ [Can] see iron dextran complex on page 360

dexmedetomidine (deks MED e toe mi deen)

Synonyms dexmedetomidine hydrochloride

U.S./Canadian Brand Names Precedex™ [US/Can]

Therapeutic Category Alpha-Adrenergic Agonist - Central-Acting (Alpha$_2$-Agonists); Sedative

Use Sedation of initially intubated and mechanically ventilated patients during treatment in an intensive care setting; duration of infusion should not exceed 24 hours.

Usual Dosage Adults: I.V.: Solution must be diluted prior to administration. Initial: Loading infusion 1 mcg/kg over 10 minutes, followed by a maintenance infusion of 0.2-0.7 mcg/kg/hour. Maintenance: Dosing should be individualized and titrated to the desired level of sedation. Not indicated for infusions lasting longer than 24 hours.

Dosage Forms Injection: 100 mcg/mL (2 mL vial, 2 mL ampul)

dexmedetomidine hydrochloride see dexmedetomidine on this page

dexmethylphenidate (dex meth il FEN i date)

U.S./Canadian Brand Names Focalin™ [US]

Therapeutic Category Central Nervous System Stimulant, Nonamphetamine

Controlled Substance C-II

Use Treatment of attention-deficit/hyperactivity disorder (ADHD)

Usual Dosage Oral: Children ≥6 years and Adults: Treatment of ADHD: Initial: 2.5 mg twice daily in patients not currently taking methylphenidate; dosage may be adjusted in 2.5-5 mg increments at weekly intervals (maximum dose: 20 mg/day); doses should be taken at least 4 hours apart

When switching from methylphenidate to dexmethylphenidate, the starting dose of dexmethylphenidate should be half that of methylphenidate (maximum dose: 20 mg/day)

Safety and efficacy for long-term use of dexmethylphenidate have not yet been established. Patients should be re-evaluated at appropriate intervals to assess continued need of the medication.

Dose reductions and discontinuation: Reduce dose or discontinue in patients with paradoxical aggravation. Discontinue if no improvement is seen after one month of treatment.

Dosage Forms Tablet, as hydrochloride: 2.5 mg, 5 mg, 10 mg

Dexone® [US] see dexamethasone (systemic) on page 184

Dexone® LA [US] see dexamethasone (systemic) on page 184

dexpanthenol (deks PAN the nole)

Synonyms pantothenyl alcohol

U.S./Canadian Brand Names D-Pan® Plus [US-OTC]; D-Pan® [US]; Panthoderm® Cream [US-OTC]

Therapeutic Category Gastrointestinal Agent, Stimulant

Use Prophylactic use to minimize paralytic ileus, treatment of postoperative distention

Usual Dosage

Children and Adults: Relief of itching and aid in skin healing: Topical: Apply to affected area 1-2 times/day

Adults:

Relief of gas retention: Oral: 2-3 tablets 3 times/day

Prevention of postoperative ileus: I.M.: 250-500 mg stat, repeat in 2 hours, followed by doses every 6 hours until danger passes

Paralyzed ileus: I.M.: 500 mg stat, repeat in 2 hours, followed by doses every 6 hours, if needed

Dosage Forms
Cream: 2% (30 g, 60 g)
Injection: 250 mg/mL (2 mL, 10 mL, 30 mL)
Tablet: 50 mg with choline bitartrate 25 mg

dexrazoxane (deks ray ZOKS ane)

Synonyms ICRF-187

U.S./Canadian Brand Names Zinecard® [US/Can]

Therapeutic Category Cardiovascular Agent, Other

Use Prevention of cardiomyopathy associated with doxorubicin administration

Usual Dosage I.V.: 1000 mg/m^2 30 minutes before administration of doxorubicin; maximal doses in patients with and without prior treatment with nitrosoureas, respectively = 750 mg/m^2 and 120 mg/m^2; 3500 mg/m^2/day for 3 days has been maximally used in pediatric patients. The recommended dosage ratio of dexrazoxane:doxorubicin is 10:1.

Dosage Forms Injection, powder for reconstitution: 250 mg, 500 mg (10 mg/mL when reconstituted)

dextran (DEKS tran)

Synonyms dextran, high molecular weight; dextran, low molecular weight

U.S./Canadian Brand Names Gentran® [US/Can]; LMD® [US]; Macrodex® [US]; Rheomacrodex® [US]

Therapeutic Category Plasma Volume Expander

Use Fluid replacement and blood volume expander used in the treatment of hypovolemia, shock, or near shock states

Usual Dosage I.V.:
Children: Total dose should not be >20 mL/kg during first 24 hours
Adults: 500-1000 mL at rate of 20-40 mL/minute

Dosage Forms
Injection, high molecular weight:
Dextran: 6% dextran 75 [in sodium chloride 0.9%] (500 mL)
Gentran®, Macrodex®: 6% dextran 70 [in sodium chloride 0.9%] (500 mL)
Macrodex®: 6% dextran 70 [in dextrose 5%] (500 mL)
Macrodex®: 6% dextran 75 [in dextrose 5%] (500 mL)
Injection, low molecular weight (Gentran®, LMD®, Rheomacrodex®):
10% dextran 40 [in dextrose 5%] (500 mL)
10% dextran 40 [in sodium chloride 0.9%] (500 mL)

dextran 1 (DEKS tran won)

U.S./Canadian Brand Names Promit® [US]

Therapeutic Category Plasma Volume Expander

Use Prophylaxis of serious anaphylactic reactions to I.V. infusion of dextran

Usual Dosage I.V. (time between dextran 1 and dextran solution should not exceed 15 minutes):
Children: 0.3 mL/kg 1-2 minutes before I.V. infusion of dextran
Adults: 20 mL 1-2 minutes before I.V. infusion of dextran

Dosage Forms Injection: 150 mg/mL (20 mL)

dextran, high molecular weight *see* dextran *on this page*

dextran, low molecular weight *see* dextran *on this page*

dextranomer (deks TRAN oh mer)

U.S./Canadian Brand Names Debrisan® [US-OTC]

Therapeutic Category Topical Skin Product

Use Clean exudative wounds; no controlled studies have found dextranomer to be more effective than conventional therapy

Usual Dosage Topical: Apply to affected area once or twice daily

Dosage Forms

Beads, topical: 4 g, 25 g, 60 g, 120 g

Paste, topical [foil pack]: 10 g

dextroamphetamine (deks troe am FET a meen)

U.S./Canadian Brand Names Dexedrine® Spansule® [US/Can]; Dexedrine® Tablet [US/Can]; Dextrostat® [US]

Therapeutic Category Amphetamine

Controlled Substance C-II

Use Adjunct in treatment of attention-deficit/hyperactivity disorder (ADHD) in children, narcolepsy, exogenous obesity

Usual Dosage Oral:

Children:

Narcolepsy: 6-12 years: Initial: 5 mg/day, may increase at 5 mg increments in weekly intervals until side effects appear; maximum dose: 60 mg/day

Attention deficit disorder:

3-5 years: Initial: 2.5 mg/day administered every morning; increase by 2.5 mg/day in weekly intervals until optimal response is obtained, usual range is 0.1-0.5 mg/kg/dose every morning with maximum of 40 mg/day

≥6 years: 5 mg once or twice daily; increase in increments of 5 mg/day at weekly intervals until optimal response is reached, usual range is 0.1-0.5 mg/kg/dose every morning (5-20 mg/day) with maximum of 40 mg/day

Adults:

Narcolepsy: Initial: 10 mg/day, may increase at 10 mg increments in weekly intervals until side effects appear; maximum: 60 mg/day

Exogenous obesity: 5-30 mg/day in divided doses of 5-10 mg 30-60 minutes before meals

Dosage Forms

Capsule, sustained release, as sulfate: 5 mg, 10 mg, 15 mg

Tablet, as sulfate: 5 mg [contains tartrazine], 10 mg

dextroamphetamine and amphetamine

(deks troe am FET a meen & am FET a meen)

Synonyms amphetamine mixture; dextroamphetamine sulfate, dextroamphetamine saccharate, amphetamine aspartate, and amphetamine sulfate

U.S./Canadian Brand Names Adderall® [US]; Adderall XR™ [US]

Therapeutic Category Amphetamine

Controlled Substance C-II

Use Attention-deficit/hyperactivity disorder (ADHD); narcolepsy

Usual Dosage Oral: **Note:** Use lowest effective individualized dose; administer first dose as soon as awake

ADHD:

Children: <3 years: Not recommended

Children: 3-5 years (Adderall®): Initial 2.5 mg/day given every morning; increase daily dose in 2.5 mg increments at weekly intervals until optimal response is obtained (maximum dose: 40 mg/day given in 1-3 divided doses); use intervals of 4-6 hours between additional doses

Children: ≥6 years:

Adderall®: Initial: 5 mg 1-2 times/day; increase daily dose in 5 mg increments at weekly intervals until optimal response is obtained (usual maximum dose: 40 mg/day given in 1-3 divided doses); use intervals of 4-6 hours between additional doses

Adderall XR™: 10 mg once daily in the morning; if needed, may increase daily dose in 10 mg increments at weekly intervals (maximum dose: 30 mg/day)

Narcolepsy: Adderall®

Children: 6-12 years: Initial: 5 mg/day; increase daily dose in 5 mg at weekly intervals until optimal response is obtained (maximum dose: 60 mg/day given in 1-3 divided doses)

Children >12 years and Adults: Initial: 10 mg/day; increase daily dose in 10 mg increments at weekly intervals until optimal response is obtained (maximum dose: 60 mg/day given in 1-3 divided doses)

Dosage Forms

Capsule (Adderall XR™):

5 mg [dextroamphetamine sulfate 1.25 mg, dextroamphetamine saccharate 1.25 mg, amphetamine aspartate monohydrate 1.25 mg, amphetamine sulfate 1.25 mg] (equivalent to amphetamine base 3.1 mg)

10 mg [dextroamphetamine sulfate 2.5 mg, dextroamphetamine saccharate 2.5 mg, amphetamine aspartate monohydrate 2.5 mg, amphetamine sulfate 2.5 mg] (equivalent to amphetamine base 6.3 mg)

15 mg [dextroamphetamine sulfate 3.75 mg, dextroamphetamine saccharate 3.75 mg, amphetamine aspartate monohydrate 3.75 mg, amphetamine sulfate 3.75 mg] (equivalent to amphetamine base 9.4 mg)

20 mg [dextroamphetamine sulfate 5 mg, dextroamphetamine saccharate 5 mg, amphetamine aspartate monohydrate 5 mg, amphetamine sulfate 5 mg] (equivalent to amphetamine base 12.5 mg)

25 mg [dextroamphetamine sulfate 6.25 mg, dextroamphetamine saccharate 6.25 mg, amphetamine aspartate monohydrate 6.25 mg, amphetamine sulfate 6.25 mg] (equivalent to amphetamine base 15.6 mg)

30 mg [dextroamphetamine sulfate 7.5 mg, dextroamphetamine saccharate 7.5 mg, amphetamine aspartate monohydrate 7.5 mg, amphetamine sulfate 7.5 mg] (equivalent to amphetamine base 18.8 mg)

Tablet (Adderall®):

5 mg [dextroamphetamine sulfate 1.25 mg, dextroamphetamine saccharate 1.25 mg, amphetamine aspartate 1.25 mg, amphetamine sulfate 1.25 mg] (equivalent to amphetamine base 3.13 mg)

7.5 mg [dextroamphetamine 1.875 mg, dextroamphetamine saccharate 1.875 mg, amphetamine aspartate 1.875 mg, amphetamine sulfate 1.875 mg] (equivalent to amphetamine base 4.7 mg)

10 mg [dextroamphetamine sulfate 2.5 mg, dextroamphetamine saccharate 2.5 mg, amphetamine aspartate 2.5 mg, amphetamine sulfate 2.5 mg] (equivalent to amphetamine base 6.3 mg)

12.5 mg [dextroamphetamine sulfate 3.125 mg, dextroamphetamine saccharate 3.125 mg, amphetamine aspartate 3.125 mg, amphetamine sulfate 3.125 mg] (equivalent to amphetamine base 7.8 mg)

15 mg [dextroamphetamine sulfate 3.75 mg, dextroamphetamine saccharate 3.75 mg, amphetamine aspartate 3.75 mg, amphetamine sulfate 3.75 mg] (equivalent to amphetamine base 9.4 mg)

20 mg [dextroamphetamine sulfate 5 mg, dextroamphetamine saccharate 5 mg, amphetamine aspartate 5 mg, amphetamine sulfate 5 mg] (equivalent to amphetamine base 12.6 mg)

30 mg [dextroamphetamine sulfate 7.5 mg, dextroamphetamine saccharate 7.5 mg, amphetamine aspartate 7.5 mg, amphetamine sulfate 7.5 mg] (equivalent to amphetamine base 18.8 mg)

dextroamphetamine sulfate, dextroamphetamine saccharate, amphetamine aspartate, and amphetamine sulfate *see* dextroamphetamine and amphetamine *on previous page*

dextromethorphan (deks troe meth OR fan)

U.S./Canadian Brand Names Benylin® Pediatric [US-OTC]; Creo-Terpin® [US-OTC]; Delsym® [US-OTC]; Hold® DM [US-OTC]; Pertussin® CS [US-OTC]; Pertussin® ES [US-(Continued)

dextromethorphan *(Continued)*

OTC]; Robitussin® Cough Calmers [US-OTC]; Robitussin® Pediatric [US-OTC]; Scot-Tussin DM® Cough Chasers [US-OTC]; Silphen DM® [US-OTC]; St. Joseph® Cough Suppressant [US-OTC]; Trocal® [US-OTC]; Vicks Formula 44® Pediatric Formula [US-OTC]; Vicks Formula 44® [US-OTC]

Therapeutic Category Antitussive

Use Symptomatic relief of coughs caused by minor viral upper respiratory tract infections or inhaled irritants; most effective for a chronic nonproductive cough

Usual Dosage Oral:

Children:

2-5 years: 2.5-5 mg every 4 hours or 7.5 mg every 6-8 hours; extended release is 50 mg twice daily

6-11 years: 5-10 mg every 4 hours or 15 mg every 6-8 hours; extended release is 30 mg twice daily

Adults: 10-20 mg every 4 hours or 30 mg every 6-8 hours; extended release is 60 mg twice daily

Dosage Forms

Liquid:

Creo-Terpin®: 10 mg/15 mL (120 mL)

Pertussin® CS: 3.5 mg/5 mL (120 mL)

Pertussin® ES: 15 mg/5 mL (120 mL, 240 mL)

Robitussin® Pediatric, St. Joseph® Cough Suppressant: 7.5 mg/5 mL (60 mL, 120 mL, 240 mL)

Liquid, sustained release, as polistirex (Delsym®): 30 mg/5 mL (89 mL) [alcohol 0.26%]

Lozenge:

Hold® DM, Robitussin® Cough Calmers: 5 mg

Scot-Tussin DM® Cough Chasers: 2.5 mg

Trocal®: 7.5 mg

Syrup:

Benylin® Pediatric: 7.5 mg/mL (118 mL)

Silphen DM®: 10 mg/5 mL (120 mL, 3780 mL)

Vicks Formula 44® Pediatric Formula: 15 mg/15 mL (120 mL)

dextromethorphan, acetaminophen, and pseudoephedrine *see* acetaminophen, dextromethorphan, and pseudoephedrine *on page 8*

dextromethorphan and guaifenesin *see* guaifenesin and dextromethorphan *on page 308*

dextromethorphan and promethazine *see* promethazine and dextromethorphan *on page 545*

dextromethorphan, guaifenesin, and pseudoephedrine *see* guaifenesin, pseudoephedrine, and dextromethorphan *on page 312*

dextropropoxyphene *see* propoxyphene *on page 548*

dextrose, levulose and phosphoric acid *see* phosphorated carbohydrate solution *on page 512*

Dextrostat® [US] *see* dextroamphetamine *on page 188*

Dey-Dose® Isoproterenol *(Discontinued)* *see page 814*

Dey-Dose® Metaproterenol *(Discontinued)* *see page 814*

Dey-Lute® Isoetharine *(Discontinued)* *see page 814*

DFMO *see* eflornithine *on page 224*

DHAD *see* mitoxantrone *on page 433*

DHC® [US] *see* hydrocodone and acetaminophen *on page 329*

DHC Plus® [US] *see* dihydrocodeine compound *on page 198*

D.H.E. 45® [US] *see* dihydroergotamine *on page 198*

DHPG sodium *see* ganciclovir *on page 293*

DHS® Tar [US-OTC] *see* coal tar *on page 158*

DHS Zinc® [US-OTC] *see* pyrithione zinc *on page 557*

DHT™ [US] *see* dihydrotachysterol *on page 198*

DiaBeta® [US/Can] *see* glyburide *on page 301*

Diabetic Tussin® DM Maximum Strength [US-OTC] *see* guaifenesin and dextromethorphan *on page 308*

Diabetic Tussin® DM [US-OTC] *see* guaifenesin and dextromethorphan *on page 308*

Diabetic Tussin® EX [US-OTC] *see* guaifenesin *on page 307*

Diabinese® [US] *see* chlorpropamide *on page 142*

Dialose® Capsule *(Discontinued)* *see page 814*

Dialose® Plus Capsule *(Discontinued)* *see page 814*

Dialose® Tablet *(Discontinued)* *see page 814*

Dialume® *(Discontinued)* *see page 814*

Diamicron® [Can] *see* gliclazide *(Canada only) on page 299*

Diamine T.D.® *(Discontinued)* *see page 814*

diaminodiphenylsulfone *see* dapsone *on page 175*

Diamode® [US-OTC] *see* loperamide *on page 390*

Diamox® [US/Can] *see* acetazolamide *on page 9*

Diamox Sequels® [US] *see* acetazolamide *on page 9*

Diaparene® Cradol® *(Discontinued)* *see page 814*

Diapid® Nasal Spray *(Discontinued)* *see page 814*

Diar-aid® *(Discontinued)* *see page 814*

Diarr-Eze [Can] *see* loperamide *on page 390*

Diasorb® [US-OTC] *see* attapulgite *on page 63*

Diastat® [US/Can] *see* diazepam *on this page*

Diazemuls® [Can] *see* diazepam *on this page*

Diazemuls® Injection *(Discontinued)* *see page 814*

diazepam (dye AZ e pam)

U.S./Canadian Brand Names Apo®-Diazepam [Can]; Diastat® [US/Can]; Diazemuls® [Can]; Diazepam Intensol® [US]; Valium® [US/Can]

Therapeutic Category Benzodiazepine

Controlled Substance C-IV

Use Management of general anxiety disorders, panic disorders; to provide preoperative sedation, light anesthesia, and amnesia; treatment of status epilepticus, alcohol withdrawal symptoms; used as a skeletal muscle relaxant

Usual Dosage

Children:

Sedation or muscle relaxation or anxiety:

Oral: 0.12-0.8 mg/kg/day in divided doses every 6-8 hours

I.M., I.V.: 0.04-0.3 mg/kg/dose every 2-4 hours to a maximum of 0.6 mg/kg within an 8-hour period if needed

Status epilepticus: I.V.:

Infants 30 days to 5 years: 0.05-0.3 mg/kg/dose administered over 2-3 minutes, every 15-30 minutes to a maximum total dose of 5 mg; repeat in 2-4 hours as needed or 0.2-0.5 mg/dose every 2-5 minutes to a maximum total dose of 5 mg

>5 years: 0.05-0.3 mg/kg/dose administered over 2-3 minutes, every 15-30 minutes to a maximum total dose of 10 mg; repeat in 2-4 hours as needed or 1 mg/dose every 2-5 minutes to a maximum of 10 mg;

(Continued)

diazepam *(Continued)*

Adults:
Anxiety:
Oral: 2-10 mg 2-4 times/day
I.M., I.V.: 2-10 mg, may repeat in 3-4 hours if needed
Skeletal muscle relaxation:
Oral: 2-10 mg 2-4 times/day
I.M., I.V.: 5-10 mg, may repeat in 2-4 hours
Status epilepticus: I.V.: 0.2-0.5 mg/kg/dose every 15-30 minutes for 2-3 doses; maximum dose: 30 mg

Dosage Forms
Gel, rectal [delivery system; twin pack] (Diastat®):
Adult rectal tip (6 cm): 5 mg/mL (10 mg, 15 mg, 20 mg)
Pediatric rectal tip (4.4 cm): 5 mg/mL (2.5 mg, 5 mg, 10 mg)
Injection: 5 mg/mL (1 mL, 2 mL, 5 mL, 10 mL)
Solution, oral: 5 mg/5 mL (5 mL, 10 mL, 500 mL) [wintergreen-spice flavor]
Solution, oral concentrate (Diazepam Intensol®): 5 mg/mL (30 mL)
Tablet: 2 mg, 5 mg, 10 mg

Diazepam Intensol® [US] *see* diazepam *on previous page*

diazoxide (dye az OKS ide)

U.S./Canadian Brand Names Hyperstat® I.V. [US/Can]; Proglycem® [US/Can]
Therapeutic Category Antihypertensive Agent; Antihypoglycemic Agent
Use I.V.: Emergency lowering of blood pressure; Oral: Hypoglycemia related to hyperinsulinism secondary to islet cell adenoma, carcinoma, or hyperplasia; adenomatosis; nesidioblastosis (persistent hyperinsulinemic hypoglycemia of infancy); leucine sensitivity, or extrapancreatic malignancy
Usual Dosage
Hyperinsulinemic hypoglycemia: Oral:
Newborns and Infants: 8-15 mg/kg/day in divided doses every 8-12 hours
Children and Adults: 3-8 mg/kg/day in divided doses every 8-12 hours
Hypertension: Children and Adults: I.V.: 1-3 mg/kg (maximum: 150 mg in a single injection); repeat dose in 5-15 minutes until blood pressure adequately reduced; repeat administration every 4-24 hours; monitor blood pressure closely
Dosage Forms
Capsule (Proglycem®): 50 mg
Injection (Hyperstat®): 15 mg/mL (1 mL, 20 mL)
Suspension, oral (Proglycem®): 50 mg/mL (30 mL) [chocolate-mint flavor]

Dibent® Injection *(Discontinued)* see page 814
Dibenzyline® [US/Can] *see* phenoxybenzamine *on page 509*

dibucaine (DYE byoo kane)

U.S./Canadian Brand Names Nupercainal® [US-OTC]
Therapeutic Category Local Anesthetic
Use Fast, temporary relief of pain and itching due to hemorrhoids, minor burns, other minor skin conditions
Usual Dosage Children and Adults:
Rectal: Hemorrhoids: Insert ointment into rectum using a rectal applicator; administer each morning,evening, and after each bowel movement
Topical: Apply gently to the affected areas; no more than 30 g for adults or 7.5 g for children should be used in any 24-hour period
Dosage Forms
Cream: 0.5% (45 g)
Ointment, topical: 1% (30 g, 60 g)

dibucaine and hydrocortisone (DYE byoo kane & hye droe KOR ti sone)
Synonyms hydrocortisone and dibucaine
U.S./Canadian Brand Names Corticaine® [US]
Therapeutic Category Anesthetic/Corticosteroid
Use Relief of the inflammatory and pruritic manifestations of corticosteroid-responsive dermatoses and for external anal itching
Usual Dosage Topical: Apply to affected areas 2-4 times/day
Dosage Forms Cream: Dibucaine 5% and hydrocortisone 5%

DIC *see* dacarbazine *on page 172*

dicalcium phosphate *see* calcium phosphate (dibasic) *on page 108*

Dicarbosil® *(Discontinued)* *see page 814*

Dicetel® [Can] *see* pinaverium *(Canada only)* *on page 515*

dichlorodifluoromethane and trichloromonofluoromethane
(dye klor oh dye flor oh METH ane & tri klor oh mon oh flor oh METH ane)
U.S./Canadian Brand Names Fluori-Methane® [US]
Therapeutic Category Analgesic, Topical
Use Management of myofascial pain, restricted motion, muscle pain; control of pain associated with injections
Usual Dosage Topical: Apply to area from approximately 12" away
Dosage Forms Aerosol, topical: Dichlorodifluoromethane 15% and trichloromonofluoromethane 85% (103 mL)

dichlorotetrafluoroethane and ethyl chloride *see* ethyl chloride and dichlorotetrafluoroethane *on page 257*

dichlorphenamide (dye klor FEN a mide)
Synonyms diclofenamide
U.S./Canadian Brand Names Daranide® [US/Can]
Therapeutic Category Carbonic Anhydrase Inhibitor
Use Adjunct in treatment of open-angle glaucoma and perioperative treatment for angle-closure glaucoma
Usual Dosage Adults: Oral: 100-200 mg to start followed by 100 mg every 12 hours until desired response is obtained; maintenance dose: 25-50 mg 1-3 times/day
Dosage Forms Tablet: 50 mg

dichysterol *see* dihydrotachysterol *on page 198*

diclofenac (dye KLOE fen ak)
U.S./Canadian Brand Names Apo®-Diclo [Can]; Apo®-Diclo SR [Can]; Cataflam® [US/Can]; Diclotec [Can]; Novo-Difenac® [Can]; Novo-Difenac-K [Can]; Novo-Difenac® SR [Can]; Nu-Diclo [Can]; Nu-Diclo-SR [Can]; PMS-Diclofenac [Can]; PMS-Diclofenac SR [Can]; Riva-Diclofenac [Can]; Riva-Diclofenac-K [Can]; Solaraze™ [US]; Voltaren Rapide® [Can]; Voltaren® [US/Can]; Voltaren®-XR [US]; Voltare Ophtha® [Can]
Therapeutic Category Analgesic, Non-narcotic; Nonsteroidal Anti-inflammatory Drug (NSAID)
Use Acute treatment of mild to moderate pain; acute and chronic treatment of rheumatoid arthritis, ankylosing spondylitis, and osteoarthritis; used for juvenile rheumatoid arthritis, gout, dysmenorrhea; ophthalmic solution for postoperative inflammation after cataract extraction; temporary relief of pain and photophobia in patients undergoing corneal refractive surgery
Usual Dosage Adults:
  Oral:
   Rheumatoid arthritis: 150-200 mg/day in 2-4 divided doses
   Osteoarthritis: 100-150 mg/day in 2-3 divided doses
   Ankylosing spondylitis: 100-125 mg/day in 4-5 divided doses
  (Continued)

diclofenac *(Continued)*

Ophthalmic: Instill 1 drop into affected eye 4 times/day beginning 24 hours after cataract surgery and continuing for 2 weeks

Dosage Forms

Gel, as sodium (Solaraze™): 30 mg/g (25 g, 50 g)

Solution, ophthalmic, as sodium (Voltaren®): 0.1% (2.5 mL, 5 mL)

Tablet, as potassium (Cataflam®): 50 mg

Tablet, delayed release: 25 mg, 50 mg, 75 mg

Tablet, enteric coated, as sodium: 25 mg, 50 mg, 75 mg

Voltaren®: 25 mg, 50 mg, 75 mg

Tablet, extended release, as sodium (Voltaren®-XR): 100 mg

diclofenac and misoprostol (dye KLOE fen ak & mye soe PROST ole)

Synonyms misoprostol and diclofenac

U.S./Canadian Brand Names Arthrotec® [US/Can]

Therapeutic Category Analgesic, Non-narcotic; Prostaglandin

Use The diclofenac component is indicated for the treatment of osteoarthritis and rheumatoid arthritis; the misoprostol component is indicated for the prophylaxis of NSAID-induced gastric and duodenal ulceration

Usual Dosage Adults: Oral: 1 tablet 2-3 times/day with food; tablets should be swallowed whole, not chewed

Dosage Forms Tablet: Diclofenac 50 mg and misoprostol 200 mcg; diclofenac 75 mg and misoprostol 200 mcg

diclofenamide *see dichlorphenamide on previous page*

Diclotec [Can] *see diclofenac on previous page*

dicloxacillin (dye kloks a SIL in)

U.S./Canadian Brand Names Dynapen® [US]

Therapeutic Category Penicillin

Use Treatment of skin and soft tissue infections, pneumonia and follow-up therapy of osteomyelitis caused by susceptible penicillinase-producing staphylococci

Usual Dosage Oral:

Children <40 kg: 12.5-50 mg/kg/day divided every 6 hours; doses of 50-100 mg/kg/day in divided doses every 6 hours have been used for follow-up therapy of osteomyelitis

Children >40 kg and Adults: 125-500 mg every 6 hours

Dosage Forms

Capsule, as sodium: 125 mg, 250 mg, 500 mg

Powder for oral suspension, as sodium: 62.5 mg/5 mL (80 mL, 100 mL, 200 mL)

dicumarol (dye KOO ma role)

Synonyms bishydroxycoumarin

Therapeutic Category Anticoagulant (Other)

Use Prophylaxis and treatment of thromboembolic disorders

Usual Dosage Adults: Oral: 25-200 mg/day based on prothrombin time (PT) determinations

Dosage Forms Tablet: 25 mg

Dicyclocot® [US] *see dicyclomine on this page*

dicyclomine (dye SYE kloe meen)

Synonyms dicycloverine

U.S./Canadian Brand Names Bentylol® [Can]; Bentyl® [US]; Dicyclocot® [US]; Formulex® [Can]; Lomine [Can]

Therapeutic Category Anticholinergic Agent

Use Treatment of functional disturbances of GI motility such as irritable bowel syndrome

Usual Dosage
Oral:
Infants >6 months: 5 mg/dose 3-4 times/day
Children: 10 mg/dose 3-4 times/day
Adults: Begin with 80 mg/day in 4 equally divided doses, then increase up to 160 mg/day
I.M. **(should not be used I.V.)**: 80 mg/day in 4 divided doses (20 mg/dose)
Dosage Forms
Capsule, as hydrochloride: 10 mg
Injection, as hydrochloride: 10 mg/mL (2 mL, 10 mL)
Syrup, as hydrochloride: 10 mg/5 mL (118 mL, 473 mL, 946 mL)
Tablet, as hydrochloride: 20 mg

dicycloverine *see* dicyclomine *on previous page*

didanosine (dye DAN oh seen)

Synonyms ddl
U.S./Canadian Brand Names Videx® EC [US]; Videx® [US/Can]
Therapeutic Category Antiviral Agent
Use Treatment of patients with advanced HIV infection which is resistant to zidovudine therapy or in those patients with zidovudine intolerance; has been used in asymptomatic patients with very low CD4$^+$ lymphocyte counts (<200 cells/mm^3) with or without AIDS-related complex
Usual Dosage Administer on an empty stomach: Oral:
Children (dosing is based on body surface area (m^2)):
<0.4: 25 mg tablets twice daily or 31 mg powder twice daily
0.5-0.7: 50 mg tablets twice daily or 62 mg powder twice daily
0.8-1: 75 mg tablets twice daily or 94 mg powder twice daily
1.1-1.4: 100 mg tablets twice daily or 125 mg powder twice daily
Adults: Dosing is based on patient weight:
35-49 kg: 125 mg tablets twice daily or 167 mg buffered powder twice daily
50-74 kg: 200 mg tablets twice daily or 250 mg buffered powder twice daily
≥75 mg: 300 mg tablets twice daily or 375 mg buffered powder twice daily

Note: Children >1 year and Adults should receive 2 tablets per dose and children <1 year should receive 1 tablet per dose for adequate buffering and absorption; tablets should be chewed
Dosage Forms
Capsule, sustained release: 125 mg, 200 mg, 250 mg, 400 mg
Powder, oral solution, buffered [single-dose packet]: 100 mg, 167 mg, 250 mg
Powder, oral solution, pediatric: 2 g, 4 g
Tablet, buffered, chewable/dispersible: 25 mg, 50 mg, 100 mg, 150 mg, 200 mg [mint flavor]

dideoxycytidine *see* zalcitabine *on page 688*

Didrex® [US/Can] *see* benzphetamine *on page 80*

Didronel® [US/Can] *see* etidronate disodium *on page 258*

dietary supplements *see* nutritional formula, enteral/oral *on page 472*

diethylpropion (dye eth il PROE pee on)

Synonyms amfepramone
U.S./Canadian Brand Names Tenuate® Dospan® [US/Can]; Tenuate® [US/Can]
Therapeutic Category Anorexiant
Controlled Substance C-IV
Use Short-term adjunct in exogenous obesity
Usual Dosage Adults: Oral: 25 mg 3 times/day before meals or food or 75 mg controlled release tablet at midmorning
(Continued)

diethylpropion *(Continued)*

Dosage Forms
Tablet, as hydrochloride: 25 mg
Tablet, controlled release, as hydrochloride: 75 mg

diethylstilbestrol (dye eth il stil BES trole)

Synonyms DES; stilbestrol
U.S./Canadian Brand Names Honvol® [Can]; Stilphostrol® [US]
Therapeutic Category Estrogen Derivative
Use Management of severe vasomotor symptoms of menopause, for estrogen replacement, and for palliative treatment of inoperable metastatic prostatic carcinoma
Usual Dosage Adults:
Hypogonadism and ovarian failure: Oral: 0.2-0.5 mg/day
Menopausal symptoms: Oral: 0.1-2 mg/day for 3 weeks and then off 1 week
Postmenopausal breast carcinoma: Oral: 15 mg/day
Prostate carcinoma: Oral: 1-3 mg/day
Prostatic cancer: I.V.: 0.5 g to start, then 1 g every 2-5 days followed by 0.25-0.5 g 1-2 times/week as maintenance
Diphosphate:
Oral: 50 mg 3 times/day; increase up to 200 mg or more 3 times/day
I.V.: Administer 0.5 g, dissolved in 250 mL of saline or D_5W, administer slowly the first 10-15 minutes then adjust rate so that the entire amount is administered in 1 hour
Dosage Forms
Injection, as diphosphate sodium: 0.25 g (5 mL)
Tablet: 50 mg

difenoxin and atropine (dye fen OKS in & A troe peen)

Synonyms atropine and difenoxin
U.S./Canadian Brand Names Motofen® [US]
Therapeutic Category Antidiarrheal
Controlled Substance C-IV
Use Treatment of diarrhea
Usual Dosage Adults: Oral: Initial: 2 tablets, then 1 tablet after each loose stool; 1 tablet every 3-4 hours, up to 8 tablets in a 24-hour period; if no improvement after 48 hours, continued administration is not indicated
Dosage Forms Tablet: Difenoxin hydrochloride 1 mg and atropine sulfate 0.025 mg

Differin® [US/Can] *see* adapalene *on page 14*

diflorasone (dye FLOR a sone)

U.S./Canadian Brand Names Maxiflor® [US]; Psorcon™ [US/Can]; Psorcon™ E [US]
Therapeutic Category Corticosteroid, Topical
Use Relief of inflammation and pruritic symptoms of corticosteroid-responsive dermatosis
Usual Dosage Topical:
Cream: Apply 2-4 times/day
Ointment: Apply sparingly 1-3 times/day
Note: Therapy should be discontinued when control is achieved. If no improvement is seen, reassessment of diagnosis may be necessary.
Dosage Forms
Cream, as diacetate: 0.05% (15 g, 30 g, 60 g)
Ointment, as diacetate: 0.05% (15 g, 30 g, 60 g)

Diflucan® [US/Can] *see* fluconazole *on page 274*

diflunisal (dye FLOO ni sal)

U.S./Canadian Brand Names Apo®-Diflunisal [Can]; Dolobid® [US]; Novo-Diflunisal [Can]; Nu-Diflunisal [Can]

Therapeutic Category Analgesic, Non-narcotic; Nonsteroidal Anti-inflammatory Drug (NSAID)

Use Management of inflammatory disorders usually including rheumatoid arthritis and osteoarthritis; can be used as an analgesic for treatment of mild to moderate pain

Usual Dosage Adults: Oral:
Pain: Initial: 500-1000 mg followed by 250-500 mg every 8-12 hours
Inflammatory condition: 500-1000 mg/day in 2 divided doses

Dosage Forms Tablet: 250 mg, 500 mg

Digepepsin® *(Discontinued)* *see page 814*

Digibind® **[US/Can]** *see* digoxin immune Fab *on this page*

DigiFab™ **[US]** *see* digoxin immune Fab *on this page*

Digitek® **[US]** *see* digoxin *on this page*

digoxin (di JOKS in)

U.S./Canadian Brand Names Digitek® [US]; Lanoxicaps® [US/Can]; Lanoxin® Pediatric [US]; Lanoxin® [US/Can]

Therapeutic Category Antiarrhythmic Agent, Miscellaneous; Cardiac Glycoside

Use Treatment of congestive heart failure; slows the ventricular rate in tachyarrhythmias such as atrial fibrillation, atrial flutter, supraventricular tachycardia

Usual Dosage Adults (based on lean body weight and normal renal function for age. Decrease dose in patients with decreased renal function)

Total digitalizing dose: Administer $\frac{1}{2}$ as initial dose, then administer $\frac{1}{4}$ of the total digitalizing dose (TDD) in each of 2 subsequent doses at 8- to 12-hour intervals; obtain EKG 6 hours after each dose to assess potential toxicity
Oral: 0.75-1.5 mg
I.M., I.V.: 0.5-1 mg
Daily maintenance dose:
Oral: 0.125-0.5 mg
I.M., I.V.: 0.1-0.4 mg

Dosage Forms
Capsule: 50 mcg, 100 mcg, 200 mcg
Elixir, pediatric: 50 mcg/mL (60 mL) [contains alcohol 10%; lime flavor]
Injection: 250 mcg/mL (1 mL, 2 mL)
Injection, pediatric: 100 mcg/mL (1 mL)
Tablet: 125 mcg, 250 mcg, 500 mcg

digoxin immune Fab (di JOKS in i MYUN fab)

Synonyms antidigoxin Fab fragments

U.S./Canadian Brand Names Digibind® [US/Can]; DigiFab™ [US]

Therapeutic Category Antidote

Use Treatment of potentially life-threatening digoxin or digitoxin intoxication in carefully selected patients

Usual Dosage Each vial of Digibind® will bind approximately 0.5 mg of digoxin or digitoxin

I.V.: To determine the dose of digoxin immune Fab, first determine the total body load of digoxin (TBL using either an approximation of the amount ingested or a postdistribution serum digoxin concentration). If neither ingestion amount or serum level is known: Adult dosage is 20 vials (760 mg) I.V. infusion.

Dosage Forms Injection, powder for reconstitution:
Digibind®: 38 mg
DigiFab™: 40 mg

Dihistine® **DH [US]** *see* chlorpheniramine, pseudoephedrine, and codeine *on page 140*

Dihistine® **Expectorant [US]** *see* guaifenesin, pseudoephedrine, and codeine *on page 311*

dihydrocodeine compound (dye hye droe KOE deen KOM pound)

U.S./Canadian Brand Names DHC Plus® [US]; Synalgos®-DC [US]

Therapeutic Category Analgesic, Narcotic

Controlled Substance C-III

Use Management of mild to moderate pain that requires relaxation

Usual Dosage Adults: Oral: 1-2 capsules every 4-6 hours as needed for pain

Dosage Forms Capsule:

DHC Plus®: Dihydrocodeine bitartrate 16 mg, acetaminophen 356.4 mg, and caffeine 30 mg

Synalgos®-DC: Dihydrocodeine bitartrate 16 mg, aspirin 356.4 mg, and caffeine 30 mg

dihydroergotamine (dye hye droe er GOT a meen)

U.S./Canadian Brand Names D.H.E. 45® [US]; Migranal® [US/Can]

Therapeutic Category Ergot Alkaloid and Derivative

Use Abort or prevent vascular headaches

Usual Dosage Adults:

I.M.: 1 mg at first sign of headache; repeat hourly to a maximum dose of 3 mg total

I.V.: Up to 2 mg maximum dose for faster effects; maximum dose: 6 mg/week

Intranasal: One spray (0.5 mg) of nasal spray should be administered into each nostril; if the condition has not sufficiently improved approximately fifteen minutes later, an additional spray should be administered to each nostril. The usual dosage required to obtain optimal efficacy is a total dosage of 4 sprays (2 mg); nasal spray is exclusively indicated for the symptomatic treatment of migraine attacks; no more than 4 sprays (2 mg) should be administered for any single migraine attack; an interval of at least 6-8 hours should be observed before treating another migraine attack with the nasal spray or any drug containing dihydroergotamine or ergotamine; no more than 8 sprays (4 mg) (corresponding to the use of 2 ampuls) should be administered during any 24-hour period; the maximum weekly dosage is 24 sprays (12 mg)

Dosage Forms

Injection, solution, as mesylate (D.H.E. 45®): 1 mg/mL (1 mL) [contains ethanol 94%]

Nasal spray, as mesylate (Migranal®): 4 mg/mL [0.5 mg/spray] (1 mL) [contains caffeine 10 mg/mL]

dihydroergotoxine *see* ergoloid mesylates *on page 233*

dihydrohydroxycodeinone *see* oxycodone *on page 484*

dihydromorphinone *see* hydromorphone *on page 335*

dihydrotachysterol (dye hye droe tak IS ter ole)

Synonyms dichysterol

U.S./Canadian Brand Names DHT™ [US]; Hytakerol® [US/Can]

Therapeutic Category Vitamin D Analog

Use Treatment of hypocalcemia associated with hypoparathyroidism; prophylaxis of hypocalcemic tetany following thyroid surgery; suppress hyperparathyroidism and treat renal osteodystrophy in patients with chronic renal failure

Usual Dosage Oral:

Hypoparathyroidism:

Infants and young Children: 0.1-0.5 mg/day

Older Children and Adults: 0.5-1 mg/day

Nutritional rickets: 0.5 mg as a single dose or 13-50 mcg/day until healing occurs

Renal osteodystrophy: 0.6-6 mg/24 hours; maintenance: 0.25-0.6 mg/24 hours adjusted as necessary to achieve normal serum calcium levels and promote bone healing

Dosage Forms

Capsule (Hytakerol®): 0.125 mg

Solution, oral concentrate (DHT™): 0.2 mg/mL (30 mL)

Tablet (DHT™): 0.125 mg, 0.2 mg, 0.4 mg

1,25 dihydroxycholecalciferol *see* calcitriol *on page 104*

dihydroxypropyl theophylline *see* dyphylline *on page 221*
Dihyrex® Injection *(Discontinued)* *see page 814*
diiodohydroxyquin *see* iodoquinol *on page 357*
Dilacor® XR [US] *see* diltiazem *on this page*
Dilantin® [US/Can] *see* phenytoin *on page 511*
Dilantin-30® Pediatric Suspension *(Discontinued)* *see page 814*
Dilantin® With Phenobarbital *(Discontinued)* *see page 814*
Dilatrate®-SR [US] *see* isosorbide dinitrate *on page 362*
Dilaudid® [US/Can] *see* hydromorphone *on page 335*
Dilaudid® 1 mg & 3 mg Tablet *(Discontinued)* *see page 814*
Dilaudid-5® [US] *see* hydromorphone *on page 335*
Dilaudid® Cough Syrup *(Discontinued)* *see page 814*
Dilaudid-HP® [US/Can] *see* hydromorphone *on page 335*
Dilaudid-HP-Plus® [Can] *see* hydromorphone *on page 335*
Dilaudid-XP® [Can] *see* hydromorphone *on page 335*
Dilocaine® Injection *(Discontinued)* *see page 814*
Dilomine® Injection *(Discontinued)* *see page 814*
Dilor® [US/Can] *see* dyphylline *on page 221*
Diltia® XT [US] *see* diltiazem *on this page*

diltiazem (dil TYE a zem)

U.S./Canadian Brand Names Alti-Diltiazem [Can]; Alti-Diltiazem CD [Can]; Apo®-Diltiaz [Can]; Apo®-Diltiaz CD [Can]; Apo®-Diltiaz SR [Can]; Cardizem® [US/Can]; Cardizem® CD [US/Can]; Cardizem® SR [US/Can]; Cartia® XT [US]; Dilacor® XR [US]; Diltia® XT [US]; Gen-Diltiazem [Can]; Novo-Diltazem [Can]; Novo-Diltazem SR [Can]; Nu-Diltiaz [Can]; Nu-Diltiaz-CD [Can]; Rhoxal-diltiazem SR [Can]; Syn-Diltiazem® [Can]; Tiazac® [US/Can]

Therapeutic Category Calcium Channel Blocker

Use

Oral: Hypertension; chronic stable angina or angina from coronary artery spasm

Injection: Atrial fibrillation or atrial flutter; paroxysmal supraventricular tachycardias (PSVT)

Usual Dosage Adults:

Oral: 30-120 mg 3-4 times/day; dosage should be increased gradually, at 1- to 2-day intervals until optimum response is obtained; usual maintenance dose: 240-360 mg/day

Sustained-release capsules (SR): Initial dose of 60-120 mg twice daily

Sustained-release capsules (CD, XR): 180-300 mg once daily

I.V.: Initial: 0.25 mg/kg as a bolus over 2 minutes, then continuous infusion of 5-15 mg/hour for up to 24 hours

Dosage Forms

Capsule, sustained release, as hydrochloride: 60 mg, 90 mg, 120 mg, 180 mg, 240 mg, 300 mg

Cardizem® CD, Cartia® XT: 120 mg, 180 mg, 240 mg, 300 mg

Cardizem® SR: 60 mg, 90 mg, 120 mg

Dilacor® XR: 180 mg, 240 mg

Diltia XT®: 120 mg, 180 mg, 240 mg

Tiazac®: 120 mg, 180 mg, 240 mg, 300 mg, 360 mg, 420 mg

Injection, as hydrochloride: 5 mg/mL (5 mL, 10 mL)

Cardizem®: 5 mg/mL (5 mL, 10 mL)

Cardizem® Lyo-Ject®: 5 mg/mL (5 mL)

Injection for infusion, as hydrochloride (Cardizem® Monovial®): 100 mg

(Continued)

diltiazem *(Continued)*
Tablet, as hydrochloride (Cardizem®): 30 mg, 60 mg, 90 mg, 120 mg

Dilusol® **[Can]** *see* alcohol (ethyl) *on page 20*

Dimaphen® **Elixir** *(Discontinued)* *see page 814*

Dimaphen® **Tablets** *(Discontinued)* *see page 814*

dimenhydrinate (dye men HYE dri nate)
Tall-Man dimenhy**DRINATE**
U.S./Canadian Brand Names Apo®-Dimenhydrinate [Can]; Calm-X® Oral [US-OTC]; Dramamine® Oral [US-OTC]; Gravol® [Can]; Hydrate® [US]; TripTone® Caplets® [US-OTC]
Therapeutic Category Antihistamine
Use Treatment and prevention of nausea, vertigo, and vomiting associated with motion sickness
Usual Dosage Oral:
Children:
2-5 years: 12.5-25 mg every 6-8 hours, maximum: 75 mg/day
6-12 years: 25-50 mg every 6-8 hours, maximum: 75 mg/day
or
Alternately: 5 mg/kg/day in 4 divided doses, not to exceed 300 mg/day
Adults: 50-100 mg every 4-6 hours, not to exceed 400 mg/day
Dosage Forms
Injection: 50 mg/mL (1 mL, 5 mL, 10 mL)
Liquid: 12.5 mg/4 mL (90 mL, 473 mL); 12.5 mg/5 mL (120 mL); 16.62 mg/5 mL (480 mL)
Tablet: 50 mg
Tablet, chewable: 50 mg

dimercaprol (dye mer KAP role)
Synonyms BAL; British anti-lewisite; dithioglycerol
U.S./Canadian Brand Names BAL in Oil® [US]
Therapeutic Category Chelating Agent
Use Antidote to gold, arsenic, and mercury poisoning; adjunct to edetate calcium disodium in lead poisoning
Usual Dosage Children and Adults: I.M.:
Mild arsenic and gold poisoning: 2.5 mg/kg/dose every 6 hours for 2 days, then every 12 hours on the third day, and once daily thereafter for 10 days
Severe arsenic and gold poisoning: 3 mg/kg/dose every 4 hours for 2 days then every 6 hours on the third day, then every 12 hours thereafter for 10 days
Mercury poisoning: Initial: 5 mg/kg followed by 2.5 mg/kg/dose 1-2 times/day for 10 days
Lead poisoning (use with edetate calcium disodium):
Mild: 3 mg/kg/dose every 4 hours for 5-7 days
Severe: 4 mg/kg/dose every 4 hours for 5-7 days
Acute encephalopathy: Initial: 4 mg/kg/dose, then every 4 hours
Dosage Forms Injection: 100 mg/mL (3 mL)

Dimetabs® **Oral** *(Discontinued)* *see page 814*

Dimetane® *(Discontinued)* *see page 814*

Dimetane®-DC *(Discontinued)* *see page 814*

Dimetane® **Decongestant Elixir** *(Discontinued)* *see page 814*

Dimetane® **Extentabs®** **[US-OTC]** *see* brompheniramine *on page 93*

Dimetapp® **4-Hour Liqui-Gel Capsule** *(Discontinued)* *see page 814*

Dimetapp® **Allergy Children's** **[US-OTC]** *see* brompheniramine *on page 93*

Dimetapp® Allergy [US-OTC] *see* brompheniramine *on page 93*

Dimetapp® Decongestant Liqui-Gels® [US-OTC] *see* pseudoephedrine *on page 552*

Dimetapp® Elixir *(Discontinued)* *see page 814*

Dimetapp® Extentabs® *(Discontinued)* *see page 814*

Dimetapp® Sinus Caplets *(Discontinued)* *see page 814*

Dimetapp® Tablet *(Discontinued)* *see page 814*

β,β-dimethylcysteine *see* penicillamine *on page 497*

dimethyl sulfoxide (dye meth il sul FOKS ide)

Synonyms DMSO
U.S./Canadian Brand Names Kemsol® [Can]; Rimso®-50 [US/Can]
Therapeutic Category Urinary Tract Product
Use Symptomatic relief of interstitial cystitis
Usual Dosage Instill 50 mL directly into bladder and allow to remain for 15 minutes; repeat every 2 weeks until maximum symptomatic relief is obtained
Dosage Forms Solution: 50% [500 mg/mL] (50 mL)

Dinate® Injection *(Discontinued)* *see page 814*

dinoprostone (dye noe PROST one)

Synonyms PGE_2; prostaglandin E_2
U.S./Canadian Brand Names Cervidil® Vaginal Insert [US/Can]; Prepidil® Vaginal Gel [US/Can]; Prostin E_2® Vaginal Suppository [US/Can]
Therapeutic Category Prostaglandin
Use Terminate pregnancy from 12th through 28th week of gestation; evacuate uterus in cases of missed abortion or intrauterine fetal death; manage benign hydatidiform mole
Usual Dosage Vaginal: Insert 1 suppository high in vagina, repeat at 3- to 5-hour intervals until abortion occurs up to 240 mg (maximum dose)
Dosage Forms
Gel, endocervical: 0.5 mg in 3 g syringes [each package contains a 10 mm and 20 mm shielded catheter]
Insert, vaginal (Cervidil®): 10 mg
Suppository, vaginal: 20 mg

Diocaine® [Can] *see* proparacaine *on page 547*

Diocarpine [Can] *see* pilocarpine *on page 514*

Diochloram® [Can] *see* chloramphenicol *on page 133*

Diocto C® [US-OTC] *see* docusate and casanthranol *on page 209*

Diocto-K® *(Discontinued)* *see page 814*

Diocto-K Plus® *(Discontinued)* *see page 814*

Dioctolose Plus® *(Discontinued)* *see page 814*

Diocto® [US-OTC] *see* docusate *on page 208*

dioctyl calcium sulfosuccinate *see* docusate *on page 208*

dioctyl sodium sulfosuccinate *see* docusate *on page 208*

Diodex® [Can] *see* dexamethasone (ophthalmic) *on page 184*

Diodoquin® [Can] *see* iodoquinol *on page 357*

Diofluor™ [Can] *see* fluorescein sodium *on page 277*

Diogent® [Can] *see* gentamicin *on page 297*

Diomycin® [Can] *see* erythromycin (systemic) *on page 235*

Dionephrine® [Can] *see* phenylephrine *on page 510*

Dionosil Oily® [US] *see* radiological/contrast media (ionic) *on page 561*

Diopentolate® [Can] *see* cyclopentolate *on page 168*

Diopred® [Can] *see* prednisolone (ophthalmic) *on page 537*

Dioptimyd® [Can] *see* sulfacetamide and prednisolone *on page 611*

Dioptrol® [Can] *see* neomycin, polymyxin B, and dexamethasone *on page 452*

Diosulf™ [Can] *see* sulfacetamide *on page 610*

Diotame® [US-OTC] *see* bismuth subsalicylate *on page 87*

Diotrope® [Can] *see* tropicamide *on page 661*

Dioval® Injection *(Discontinued)* *see page 814*

Diovan™ [US/Can] *see* valsartan *on page 671*

Diovan HCT™ [US/Can] *see* valsartan and hydrochlorothiazide *on page 671*

Diovol® [Can] *see* aluminum hydroxide and magnesium hydroxide *on page 29*

Diovol® Ex [Can] *see* aluminum hydroxide and magnesium hydroxide *on page 29*

Diovol Plus® [Can] *see* aluminum hydroxide, magnesium hydroxide, and simethicone *on page 29*

dipalmitoylphosphatidylcholine *see* colfosceril palmitate *on page 161*

Dipentum® [US/Can] *see* olsalazine *on page 476*

Diphenacen 50® Injection *(Discontinued)* *see page 814*

Diphenatol® [US] *see* diphenoxylate and atropine *on next page*

Diphendryl® [US-OTC] *see* diphenhydramine *on this page*

Diphenhist® [US-OTC] *see* diphenhydramine *on this page*

diphenhydramine (dye fen HYE dra meen)

Tall-Man diphenhydrAMINE

U.S./Canadian Brand Names Acot-Tussin® Allergy [US-OTC]; Alercap® [US-OTC]; Aler-Dryl® [US-OTC]; Alertab® [US-OTC]; Allerdryl® [Can]; Allermax® [US-OTC]; Allernix [Can]; Altaryl® [US-OTC]; Anti-Hist® [US-OTC]; Banaril® [US-OTC]; Banophen® [US-OTC]; Benadryl® [US/Can]; Compoz® Nighttime Sleep Aid [US-OTC]; Dermamycin® [US-OTC]; Derma-Pax® [US-OTC]; Diphendryl® [US-OTC]; Diphenhist® [US-OTC]; Diphen® [US-OTC]; Diphenyl® [US-OTC]; Dormin® Sleep Aid [US-OTC]; Dytuss® [US-OTC]; Genahist® [US-OTC]; Geridryl® [US-OTC]; Hydramine® [US-OTC]; Hyrexin® [US-OTC]; Mediphedryl® [US-OTC]; Miles® Nervine [US-OTC]; Nytol™ [Can]; Nytol™ Extra Strength [Can]; Nytol® Quickcaps® [US-OTC]; PMS-Diphenhydramine [Can]; Polydryl® [US-OTC]; Q-Dryl® [US-OTC]; Quenalin® [US-OTC]; Siladryl® Allerfy® [US-OTC]; Silphen® [US-OTC]; Simply Sleep® [US-OTC]; Sleepinal® [US-OTC]; Sleep® Tabs [US-OTC]; Sominex® [US-OTC]; Truxadryl® [US-OTC]; Tusstat® [US-OTC]; Twilite® [US-OTC]; Unison® Sleepgels® Maximum Strength [US-OTC]

Therapeutic Category Antihistamine

Use Symptomatic relief of allergic symptoms caused by histamine release which include nasal allergies and allergic dermatosis; mild nighttime sedation, prevention of motion sickness, as an antitussive; treatment of phenothiazine-induced dystonic reactions

Usual Dosage

Children: Oral, I.M., I.V.: 5 mg/kg/day or 150 mg/m^2/day in divided doses every 6-8 hours, not to exceed 300 mg/day

Adults:

Oral: 25-50 mg every 4-6 hours

I.M., I.V.: 10-50 mg in a single dose every 2-4 hours, not to exceed 400 mg/day

Topical: For external application, not longer than 7 days

Dosage Forms

Capsule, as hydrochloride: 25 mg, 50 mg

Cream, as hydrochloride: 1%, 2%

Elixir, as hydrochloride: 12.5 mg/5 mL (5 mL, 10 mL, 20 mL, 120 mL, 480 mL, 3780 mL)
Injection, as hydrochloride: 10 mg/mL (10 mL, 30 mL); 50 mg/mL (1 mL, 10 mL)
Liquid, as hydrochloride: 6.25/5 mL
Lotion, as hydrochloride: 1% (75 mL)
Solution, topical spray, as hydrochloride: 1% (60 mL), 2%
Syrup, as hydrochloride: 12.5 mg/5 mL (5 mL, 120 mL, 240 mL, 480 mL, 3780 mL)
Tablet, as hydrochloride: 25 mg, 50 mg
Tablet, chewable, as hydrochloride: 12.5 mg

diphenhydramine and pseudoephedrine
(dye fen HYE dra meen & soo doe e FED rin)
U.S./Canadian Brand Names Benadryl® Decongestant Allergy [US-OTC]
Therapeutic Category Antihistamine/Decongestant Combination
Use Relief of symptoms of upper respiratory mucosal congestion in seasonal and perennial nasal allergies, acute rhinitis, rhinosinusitis, and eustachian tube blockage
Usual Dosage Adults: Oral: 1 capsule or tablet every 4-6 hours, up to 4/day
Dosage Forms Tablet: Diphenhydramine hydrochloride 25 mg and pseudoephedrine hydrochloride 60 mg

diphenoxylate and atropine (dye fen OKS i late & A troe peen)
Synonyms atropine and diphenoxylate
U.S./Canadian Brand Names Diphenatol® [US]; Lomocot® [US]; Lomotil® [US/Can]; Lonox® [US]
Therapeutic Category Antidiarrheal
Controlled Substance C-V
Use Treatment of diarrhea
Usual Dosage Oral (as diphenoxylate): Initial dose:
Children: 0.3-0.4 mg/kg/day in 2-4 divided doses
<2 years: Not recommended
2-5 years: 2 mg 3 times/day
5-8 years: 2 mg 4 times/day
8-12 years: 2 mg 5 times/day
Adults: 15-20 mg/day in 3-4 divided doses
Reduce dosage as soon as initial control of symptoms is achieved
Dosage Forms
Solution, oral: Diphenoxylate hydrochloride 2.5 mg and atropine sulfate 0.025 mg per 5 mL (4 mL, 10 mL, 60 mL)
Tablet: Diphenoxylate hydrochloride 2.5 mg and atropine sulfate 0.025 mg

Diphen® [US-OTC] *see* diphenhydramine *on previous page*

Diphenylan Sodium® (Discontinued) *see page 814*

diphenylhydantoin *see* phenytoin *on page 511*

Diphenyl® [US-OTC] *see* diphenhydramine *on previous page*

diphtheria and tetanus toxoid (dif THEER ee a & TET a nus TOKS oyd)
Synonyms DT; Td; tetanus and diphtheria toxoid
Therapeutic Category Toxoid
Use Active immunity against diphtheria and tetanus
Usual Dosage I.M.:
Infants and Children:
6 weeks to 1 year: Three 0.5 mL doses at least 4 weeks apart; administer a reinforcing dose 6-12 months after the third injection
1-6 years: Administer two 0.5 mL doses at least 4 weeks apart; reinforcing dose 6-12 months after second injection; if final dose is administered after seventh birthday, use adult preparation
(Continued)

diphtheria and tetanus toxoid *(Continued)*

4-6 years (booster immunization): 0.5 mL; not necessary if all 4 doses were administered after fourth birthday - routinely administer booster doses at 10-year intervals with the adult preparation

Children >7 years and Adults: 2 primary doses of 0.5 mL each, administered at an interval of 4-6 weeks; third (reinforcing) dose of 0.5 mL 6-12 months later; boosters every 10 years

Dosage Forms

Injection, adult:

Diphtheria 2 Lf units and tetanus 2 Lf units per 0.5 mL (5 mL) [Massachusetts Biological Laboratories]

Diphtheria 2 Lf units and tetanus 5 Lf units per 0.5 mL (0.5 mL, 5 mL) [Wyeth]

Diphtheria 2 Lf units and tetanus 5 Lf units per 0.5 mL (5 mL) [Lederle, Aventis/Pasteur]

Injection, pediatric:

Diphtheria 6.7 Lf units and tetanus 5 Lf units per 0.5 mL (5 mL) [Aventis/Pasteur]

Diphtheria 7.5 Lf units and tetanus 7.5 Lf units per 0.5 mL (5 mL) [Massachusetts Biological Laboratories]

Diphtheria 10 Lf units and tetanus 5 Lf units per 0.5 mL (0.5 mL, 5 mL) [Wyeth-Ayerst]

Diphtheria 12.5 Lf units and tetanus 5 Lf units per 0.5 mL (5 mL) [Lederle]

diphtheria antitoxin (dif THEER ee a an tee TOKS in)

Therapeutic Category Antitoxin

Use Passive prevention and treatment of diphtheria

Usual Dosage I.M. or slow I.V. infusion: Dosage varies; range: 20,000-120,000 units

Dosage Forms Injection: ≥500 units/mL (40 mL) [20,000 units/vial]

diphtheria CRM$_{197}$ protein *see* pneumococcal conjugate vaccine (7-valent) *on* page 521

diphtheria, tetanus toxoids, and acellular pertussis vaccine

(dif THEER ee a, TET a nus TOKS oyds, & ay CEL yoo lar per TUS sis vak SEEN)

Synonyms DTAP

U.S./Canadian Brand Names Adacel® [Can]; Daptacel™ [US]; Infanrix® [US]; Tripedia® [US]

Therapeutic Category Toxoid

Use Fourth or fifth immunization of children 15 months to 7 years of age (prior to seventh birthday) who have been previously immunized with 3 or 4 doses of whole-cell pertussis DTP vaccine

Usual Dosage I.M.: After at least 3 doses of whole-cell DTP, administer 0.5 mL at ~18 months (at least 6 months after third DTWP dose), then another dose at 4-5 years of age

Dosage Forms

Injection, suspension:

Daptacel™: Diphtheria 15 Lf units, tetanus 5 Lf units, and acellular pertussis vaccine 10 mcg per 0.5 mL (0.5 mL)

Infanrix®: Diphtheria 25 Lf units, tetanus 10 Lf units, and acellular pertussis vaccine 25 mcg per 0.5 mL (0.5 mL)

Tripedia®: Diphtheria 6.7 Lf units, tetanus 5 Lf units, and acellular pertussis vaccine 46.8 mcg per 0.5 mL (7.5 mL) [contains thimerosal]

Note: Tripedia® vaccine is also used to reconstitute ActHIB® to prepare TriHIBit® vaccine (diphtheria, tetanus toxoids, and acellular pertussis vaccine and *Haemophilus influenzae* b conjugate vaccine combination)

diphtheria, tetanus toxoids, and acellular pertussis vaccine and *Haemophilus* b conjugate vaccine

(dif THEER ee a, TET a nus TOKS oyds, & ay CEL yoo lar per TUS sis vak SEEN, & hem OF fi lus bee KON joo gate vak SEEN)

U.S./Canadian Brand Names TriHIBit® [US]

Therapeutic Category Toxoid; Vaccine, Inactivated Bacteria

Use Active immunization of children 15-18 months of age for prevention of diphtheria, tetanus, pertussis, and invasive disease caused by *H. influenzae* type b.

Usual Dosage Children >15 months of age: I.M.: 0.5 mL; vaccine should be used within 30 minutes of reconstitution.

Dosage Forms Injection: 5 Lf units tetanus toxoid, 6.7 Lf units diphtheria toxoid, 46.8 mcg pertussis antigens, and 10 mcg *H. influenzae* type b purified capsular polysaccharide [Tripedia® vaccine is used to reconstitute ActHIB®] (0.5 mL)

diphtheria, tetanus toxoids, and whole-cell pertussis vaccine

(dif THEER ee a, TET a nus TOKS oyds, & hole-sel per TUS sis vak SEEN)

Synonyms DPT

U.S./Canadian Brand Names Pentacel™ [Can]

Therapeutic Category Toxoid

Use Active immunization of infants and children through 6 years of age (between 2 months and the seventh birthday) against diphtheria, tetanus, and pertussis; recommended for both primary immunization and routine recall; start immunization at once if whooping cough or diphtheria is present in the community

Usual Dosage The primary immunization for children 2 months to 6 years of age, ideally beginning at the age of 2-3 months or at 6-week check-up. Administer 0.5 mL I.M. on 3 occasions at 4- to 8-week intervals with a re-enforcing dose administered 1 year after the third injection. The booster doses (0.5 mL I.M.) are administered when the child is 4-6 years of age.

Dosage Forms Injection: 0.5 mL

diphtheria, tetanus toxoids, whole-cell pertussis, and *Haemophilus* B conjugate vaccine

(dif THEER ee a, TET a nus TOKS oyds, hole-sel per TUS sis, & hem OF fil us bee KON joo gate vak SEEN)

Synonyms DTwP-HIB

Therapeutic Category Toxoid

Use Active immunization of infants and children through 5 years of age (between 2 months and the sixth birthday) against diphtheria, tetanus, and pertussis and *Haemophilus* B disease when indications for immunization with DTP vaccine and HIB vaccine coincide

Usual Dosage The primary immunization for children 2 months to 5 years of age, ideally beginning at the age of 2-3 months or at 6-week check-up; administer 0.5 mL I.M. on 3 occasions at ~2 month intervals, followed by a fourth 0.5 mL dose at ~15 months of age

Dosage Forms Injection: Diphtheria toxoid 12.5 Lf units, tetanus toxoid 5 Lf units, and whole-cell pertussis vaccine 4 units, and *Haemophilus influenzae* type b oligosaccharide 10 mcg per 0.5 mL (5 mL)

dipivalyl epinephrine *see* dipivefrin *on this page*

dipivefrin (dye PI ve frin)

Synonyms dipivalyl epinephrine; DPE

U.S./Canadian Brand Names Ophtho-Dipivefrin™ [Can]; PMS-Dipivefrin [Can]; Propine® [US/Can]

Therapeutic Category Adrenergic Agonist Agent

Use Reduces elevated intraocular pressure in chronic open-angle glaucoma; treatment of ocular hypertension

(Continued)

dipivefrin (Continued)

Usual Dosage Adults: Ophthalmic: Initial: 1 drop every 12 hours
Dosage Forms Solution, ophthalmic, as hydrochloride: 0.1% (5 mL, 10 mL, 15 mL)

Diprivan® **[US/Can]** see propofol on page 548

Diprolene® **[US/Can]** see betamethasone (topical) on page 83

Diprolene® **AF [US]** see betamethasone (topical) on page 83

dipropylacetic acid see valproic acid and derivatives on page 670

Diprosone® **[US/Can]** see betamethasone (topical) on page 83

dipyridamole (dye peer ID a mole)

U.S./Canadian Brand Names Apo®-Dipyridamole FC [Can]; Novo-Dipiradol [Can]; Persantine® [US/Can]
Therapeutic Category Antiplatelet Agent; Vasodilator
Use Maintain patency after surgical grafting procedures including coronary artery bypass; with warfarin to decrease thrombosis in patients after artificial heart valve replacement; for chronic management of angina pectoris; with aspirin to prevent coronary artery thrombosis; in combination with aspirin or warfarin to prevent other thromboembolic disorders; dipyridamole may also be administered 2 days prior to open heart surgery to prevent platelet activation by extracorporeal bypass pump; diagnostic agent I.V. (dipyridamole stress test) for coronary artery disease
Usual Dosage
Children: Oral: 3-6 mg/kg/day in 3 divided doses
Dipyridamole stress test (for evaluation of myocardial perfusion): I.V.: 0.14 mg/kg/minute for a total of 4 minutes
Adults: Oral: 75-400 mg/day in 3-4 divided doses
Dosage Forms
Injection: 5 mg/mL (2 mL, 10 mL)
Tablet: 25 mg, 50 mg, 75 mg

dipyridamole and aspirin (dye peer ID a mole & AS pir in)

U.S./Canadian Brand Names Aggrenox® [US/Can]
Therapeutic Category Antiplatelet Agent
Use Combined therapy with dipyridamole and aspirin is indicated in patients who are recovering from a myocardial infarction; the rate of reinfarction is significantly reduced by such therapy; combined treatment is also indicated for the prevention of occlusion of saphenous vein coronary artery bypass grafts
Usual Dosage Adults: Oral: 1 capsule (dipyridamole 200 mg, aspirin 25 mg) twice daily.
Dosage Forms Capsule: Dipyridamole (extended release) 200 mg and aspirin 25 mg

Diquinol® **[US]** see iodoquinol on page 357

dirithromycin (dye RITH roe mye sin)

U.S./Canadian Brand Names Dynabac® [US]
Therapeutic Category Macrolide (Antibiotic)
Use Treatment of mild to moderate upper and lower respiratory tract infections, infections of the skin and skin structure, and sexually transmitted diseases due to susceptible strains
Usual Dosage Adults: Oral: 500 mg once daily for 7-14 days
Dosage Forms Tablet, enteric coated: 250 mg

Disalcid® **[US]** see salsalate on page 583

disalicylic acid see salsalate on page 583

Disanthrol® **(Discontinued)** see page 814

Disobrom® **[US-OTC]** see dexbrompheniramine and pseudoephedrine on page 185

disodium cromoglycate *see* cromolyn sodium *on page 166*

***d*-isoephedrine** *see* pseudoephedrine *on page 552*

Disonate® *(Discontinued)* *see page 814*

Disophrol® Chronotabs® [US-OTC] *see* dexbrompheniramine and pseudoephedrine *on page 185*

disopyramide (dye soe PEER a mide)

U.S./Canadian Brand Names Norpace® CR [US]; Norpace® [US/Can]; Rythmodan® [Can]; Rythmodan®-LA [Can]

Therapeutic Category Antiarrhythmic Agent, Class I-A

Use Suppression and prevention of unifocal and multifocal ventricular premature complexes, coupled ventricular premature complexes, and/or paroxysmal ventricular tachycardia; also effective in the conversion and prevention of recurrence of atrial fibrillation, atrial flutter, and paroxysmal atrial tachycardia

Usual Dosage Oral:

Children:

<1 year: 10-30 mg/kg/24 hours in 4 divided doses

1-4 years: 10-20 mg/kg/24 hours in 4 divided doses

4-12 years: 10-15 mg/kg/24 hours in 4 divided doses

12-18 years: 6-15 mg/kg/24 hours in 4 divided doses

Adults:

<50 kg: 100 mg every 6 hours or 200 mg every 12 hours (controlled release)

>50 kg: 150 mg every 6 hours or 300 mg every 12 hours (controlled release); if no response, may increase to 200 mg every 6 hours; maximum dose required for patients with severe refractory ventricular tachycardia is 400 mg every 6 hours

Dosage Forms

Capsule, as phosphate: 100 mg, 150 mg

Capsule, sustained action, as phosphate: 100 mg, 150 mg

Disotate® [US] *see* edetate disodium *on page 222*

Di-Spaz® Injection *(Discontinued)* *see page 814*

Di-Spaz® Oral *(Discontinued)* *see page 814*

Dispos-a-Med® Isoproterenol *(Discontinued)* *see page 814*

disulfiram (dye SUL fi ram)

U.S./Canadian Brand Names Antabuse® [US/Can]

Therapeutic Category Aldehyde Dehydrogenase Inhibitor Agent

Use Management of chronic alcoholics

Usual Dosage Oral:

Maximum daily dose: 500 mg/day in a single dose for 1-2 weeks

Average maintenance dose: 250 mg/day; range: 125-500 mg; duration of therapy is to continue until the patient is fully recovered socially and a basis for permanent self control has been established; maintenance therapy may be required for months or even years

Dosage Forms Tablet: 250 mg, 500 mg

Dital® *(Discontinued)* *see page 814*

dithioglycerol *see* dimercaprol *on page 200*

dithranol *see* anthralin *on page 44*

Ditropan® [US/Can] *see* oxybutynin *on page 484*

Ditropan® XL [US] *see* oxybutynin *on page 484*

Diucardin® *(Discontinued)* *see page 814*

Diupress® *(Discontinued)* *see page 814*

Diurigen® *(Discontinued)* *see page 814*

Diuril® **[US/Can]** *see* chlorothiazide *on page 136*

Dixarit® **[Can]** *see* clonidine *on page 155*

Dizac® Injectable Emulsion *(Discontinued)* *see page 814*

Dizmiss® *(Discontinued)* *see page 814*

Dizymes® Tablet *(Discontinued)* *see page 814*

dl-alpha tocopherol *see* vitamin E *on page 682*

d-mannitol *see* mannitol *on page 400*

4-dmdr *see* idarubicin *on page 344*

D-Med® Injection *(Discontinued)* *see page 814*

DMSO *see* dimethyl sulfoxide *on page 201*

DNA-derived humanized monoclonal antibody *see* alemtuzumab *on page 21*

DNASE *see* dornase alfa *on page 212*

DNR *see* daunorubicin hydrochloride *on page 176*

Doan's®, Original [US-OTC] *see* magnesium salicylate *on page 398*

dobutamine (doe BYOO ta meen)
Tall-Man **DOBUT**amine
U.S./Canadian Brand Names Dobutrex® [US/Can]
Therapeutic Category Adrenergic Agonist Agent
Use Short-term management of patients with cardiac decompensation
Usual Dosage I.V. infusion:
  Children: 2.5-15 mcg/kg/minute, titrate to desired response
  Adults: 2.5-15 mcg/kg/minute; maximum: 40 mcg/kg/minute, titrate to desired response
Dosage Forms Infusion, as hydrochloride: 12.5 mg/mL (20 mL)

Dobutrex® **[US/Can]** *see* dobutamine *on this page*

docetaxel (doe se TAKS el)
U.S./Canadian Brand Names Taxotere® [US/Can]
Therapeutic Category Antineoplastic Agent
Use Treatment of breast cancer; advanced or metastatic nonsmall-cell lung cancer in patients whose disease has progressed after platinum-based chemotherapy
Usual Dosage Adults: I.V.: 60-100 mg/m^2 administered over 1 hour every 3 weeks
Dosage Forms Injection, solution: 20 mg/0.5 mL (0.5 mL); 80 mg/2 mL (2 mL) [diluent contains ethanol 13%]

docosanol (doe KOE san ole)
U.S./Canadian Brand Names Abreva™ [US-OTC]
Therapeutic Category Antiviral Agent, Topical
Use Treatment of herpes simplex of the face or lips
Usual Dosage Children ≥12 years and Adults: Topical: Apply 5 times/day to affected area of face or lips. Start at first sign of cold sore or fever blister and continue until healed.
Dosage Forms Cream: 10% (2 g)

docusate (DOK yoo sate)
Synonyms dioctyl calcium sulfosuccinate; dioctyl sodium sulfosuccinate; DOSS; DSS
U.S./Canadian Brand Names Colace® [US/Can]; Colax-C® [Can]; Diocto® [US-OTC]; DOS® Softgel® [US-OTC]; D-S-S® [US-OTC]; Ex-Lax® Stool Softener [US-OTC]; PMS-Docusate Calcium [Can]; PMS-Docusate Sodium [Can]; Regulex® [Can]; Selax® [Can]; Soflax™ [Can]; Surfak® [US-OTC]
Therapeutic Category Stool Softener

Use Stool softener in patients who should avoid straining during defecation and constipation associated with hard, dry stools

Usual Dosage Docusate salts are interchangeable; the amount of sodium, calcium, or potassium per dosage unit is clinically insignificant

Infants and Children <3 years: Oral: 10-40 mg/day in 1-4 divided doses

Children: Oral:

3-6 years: 20-60 mg/day in 1-4 divided doses

6-12 years: 40-150 mg/day in 1-4 divided doses

Adolescents and Adults: Oral: 50-500 mg/day in 1-4 divided doses

Older Children and Adults: Rectal: Add 50-100 mg of docusate liquid to enema fluid (saline or water); administer as retention or flushing enema

Dosage Forms

Capsule, as calcium (Surfak® Liquigel): 240 mg

Capsule, as sodium:

Colace®: 50 mg, 100 mg

DOS® Softgel®: 100 mg, 250 mg

D-S-S®: 100 mg

Modane® Soft: 100 mg

Liquid, as sodium (Colace®, Diocto®): 150 mg/15 mL (480 mL)

Syrup, as sodium: 50 mg/15 mL (15 mL, 30 mL)

Colace®, Diocto®: 60 mg/15 mL (480 mL)

Tablet, as sodium (Ex-Lax® Stool Softener): 100 mg

docusate and casanthranol (DOK yoo sate & ka SAN thra nole)

Synonyms casanthranol and docusate; DSS with casanthranol

U.S./Canadian Brand Names Diocto C® [US-OTC]; Doxidan® [US-OTC]; Genasoft® Plus [US-OTC]; Peri-Colace® [US/Can]; Silace-C® [US-OTC]

Therapeutic Category Laxative/Stool Softener

Use Treatment of constipation generally associated with dry, hard stools and decreased intestinal motility

Usual Dosage Oral:

Children: 5-15 mL of syrup at bedtime or 1 capsule at bedtime

Adults: 1-2 capsules or 15-30 mL syrup at bedtime, may be increased to 2 capsules or 30 mL twice daily or 3 capsules at bedtime

Dosage Forms

Capsule (Doxidan®, Genasoft® Plus, Peri-Colace®): Docusate sodium 100 mg and casanthranol 30 mg

Syrup (Diocto C®, Peri-Colace®, Silace-C®): Docusate sodium 60 mg and casanthranol 30 mg per 15 mL (240 mL, 480 mL, 4000 mL) [with alcohol 10%]

dofetilide (doe FET il ide)

Synonyms UK-68-798

U.S./Canadian Brand Names Tikosyn™ [US/Can]

Therapeutic Category Antiarrhythmic Agent, Class III

Use Prevention and treatment of fibrillation (atrial), flutter (atrial), paroxysmal tachycardia (ventricular), tachycardia (ventricular), fibrillation (ventricular); used in conjunction of implantable defibrillator

Usual Dosage Adults: Oral: Initial: 500 mcg orally twice daily.

Dosage Forms Capsule: 125 mcg, 250 mcg, 500 mcg

Doktors® Nasal Solution *(Discontinued)* see page 814

Dolacet® [US] *see* hydrocodone and acetaminophen on page 329

Dolacet® Forte *(Discontinued)* see page 814

dolasetron (dol A se tron)

U.S./Canadian Brand Names Anzemet® [US/Can]

Therapeutic Category Selective 5-HT₃ Receptor Antagonist

(Continued)

dolasetron *(Continued)*

Use The prevention of nausea and vomiting associated with moderately emetogenic cancer chemotherapy, including initial and repeat courses; the prevention of postoperative nausea and vomiting.

Usual Dosage

Oral:

Prevention of cancer chemotherapy-induced nausea and vomiting:

Children 2-16 years: 1.8 mg/kg given within 1 hour before chemotherapy, up to a maximum of 100 mg; safety and effectiveness in pediatric patients <2 years of age have not been established

Adults: 100 mg given within 1 hour before chemotherapy

Use in the elderly, renal failure patients, or hepatically impaired patients: No dosage adjustment is recommended

Prevention of postoperative nausea and vomiting:

Children 2-16 years: 1.2 mg/kg given within 2 hours before surgery, up to a maximum of 100 mg; safety and effectiveness in pediatric patients <2 years of age have not been established

Adults: 100 mg within 2 hours before surgery

Parenteral (injection):

Prevention of cancer chemotherapy-induced nausea and vomiting:

Children 2-16 years: 1.8 mg/kg given as a single dose approximately 30 minutes before chemotherapy, up to a maximum of 100 mg; safety and effectiveness in pediatric patients <2 years of age have not been established. Injection mixed in apple or apple-grape juice may be used for oral dosing of pediatric patients. When injection is administered orally, the recommended dosage in pediatric patients 2-16 years of age is 1.8 mg/kg up to a maximum 100 mg dose given within 1 hour before chemotherapy. The diluted product may be kept up to 2 hours at room temperature before use.

Adults: From clinical trials, the dose is 1.8 mg/kg given as a single dose approximately 30 minutes before chemotherapy; alternatively, for most patients, a fixed dose of 100 mg can be administered over 30 seconds

Prevention of postoperative nausea and/or vomiting:

Children 2-16 years: 0.35 mg/kg, with a maximum dose of 12.5 mg, given as a single dose approximately 15 minutes before the cessation of anesthesia or as soon as nausea or vomiting presents. Safety and effectiveness in pediatric patients <2 years of age have not been established. Injection mixed in apple or apple-grape juice may be used for oral dosing of pediatric patients; dosage in pediatric patients 2-16 years is 1.2 mg/kg up to a maximum 100 mg dose given before surgery.

Adults: 12.5 mg given as a single dose approximately 15 minutes before the cessation of anesthesia (prevention) or as soon as nausea or vomiting presents (treatment)

Dosage Forms

Injection, as mesylate: 20 mg/mL (0.625 mL, 5 mL)

Tablet, as mesylate: 50 mg, 100 mg

Dolene® *(Discontinued)* see page 814

Dolgic® **[US]** see butalbital, acetaminophen, and caffeine on page 99

Dolobid® **[US]** see diflunisal on page 196

Dolophine® **[US/Can]** see methadone on page 415

Dolorac™ *(Discontinued)* see page 814

Dolorex® *(Discontinued)* see page 814

Dolotic® **[US]** see antipyrine and benzocaine on page 47

Dolsed® **[US]** see methenamine, phenyl salicylate, atropine, hyoscyamine, benzoic acid, and methylene blue on page 416

Domeboro® **[US-OTC]** see aluminum sulfate and calcium acetate on page 29

Dommanate® **Injection** *(Discontinued)* see page 814

domperidone *(Canada only)* (dom PE ri done)

U.S./Canadian Brand Names Alti-Domperidone [Can]; Apo®-Domperidone [Can]; Motilium® [Can]; Novo-Domperidone [Can]; Nu-Domperidone [Can]; PMS-Domperidone [Can]

Therapeutic Category Dopamine Antagonist

Use Symptomatic management of upper gastrointestinal motility disorders associated with chronic and subacute gastritis and diabetic gastroparesis; may also be used to prevent gastrointestinal symptoms associated with the use of dopamine agonist antiparkinsonian agents

Usual Dosage Adults: Oral:

Upper gastrointestinal motility disorders: Usual dosage in adults: 10 mg 3-4 times/day, 15-30 minutes before meals and at bedtime if required. In severe or resistant cases the dose may be increased to a maximum of 20 mg 3-4 times/day.

Nausea and vomiting associated with dopamine agonist antiparkinsonian agents: Usual dosage in adults: 20 mg 3-4 times/day. Higher doses may be required to achieve symptom control while titration of the antiparkinsonian medication is occurring.

Dosage Forms Tablet: 10 mg [domperidone maleate 12.72 mg]

donepezil (don EH pa zil)

Synonyms E2020

U.S./Canadian Brand Names Aricept® [US/Can]

Therapeutic Category Acetylcholinesterase Inhibitor; Cholinergic Agent

Use Treatment of mild to moderate dementia of the Alzheimer's type

Usual Dosage Adults: Oral: Initial: 5 mg at bedtime; may be increased to 10 mg at bedtime after 4-6 weeks; a 10 mg dose may provide additional benefit for some patients

Dosage Forms Tablet: 5 mg, 10 mg

Donnamar® *(Discontinued)* see page 814

Donnapectolin-PG® [US] see hyoscyamine, atropine, scopolamine, kaolin, pectin, and opium on page 341

Donnapine® [US] see hyoscyamine, atropine, scopolamine, and phenobarbital on page 340

Donnatal® [US] see hyoscyamine, atropine, scopolamine, and phenobarbital on page 340

Donnazyme® *(Discontinued)* see page 814

Donphen® Tablet *(Discontinued)* see page 814

dopamine (DOE pa meen)

Tall-Man DOPamine

U.S./Canadian Brand Names Intropin® [Can]

Therapeutic Category Adrenergic Agonist Agent

Use Adjunct in the treatment of shock which persists after adequate fluid volume replacement

Usual Dosage I.V. infusion:

Children: 1-20 mcg/kg/minute, maximum: 50 mcg/kg/minute continuous infusion, titrate to desired response

Adults: 1 mcg/kg/minute up to 50 mcg/kg/minute, titrate to desired response

If dosages >20-30 mcg/kg/minute are needed, a more direct acting pressor may be more beneficial (ie, epinephrine, norepinephrine)

Hemodynamic effects of dopamine are dose-dependent:

Low-dose: 1-5 mcg/kg/minute, increased renal blood flow and urine output

Intermediate-dose: 5-15 mcg/kg/minute, increased renal blood flow, heart rate, cardiac contractility, and cardiac output

High-dose: >15 mcg/kg/minute, alpha-adrenergic effects begin to predominate, vasoconstriction, increased blood pressure

(Continued)

dopamine *(Continued)*

Dosage Forms
Infusion, as hydrochloride [in D₅W]: 0.8 mg/mL (250 mL, 500 mL); 1.6 mg/mL (250 mL, 500 mL); 3.2 mg/mL (250 mL, 500 mL)
Injection, as hydrochloride: 40 mg/mL (5 mL, 10 mL, 20 mL); 80 mg/mL (5 mL, 20 mL); 160 mg/mL (5 mL)

Dopar® *(Discontinued)* *see page 814*

Dopastat® Injection *(Discontinued)* *see page 814*

Dopram® [US] *see* doxapram *on next page*

Doral® [US/Can] *see* quazepam *on page 558*

Doriden® Tablet *(Discontinued)* *see page 814*

Dormarex® 2 Oral *(Discontinued)* *see page 814*

Dormin® Sleep Aid [US-OTC] *see* diphenhydramine *on page 202*

dornase alfa (DOOR nase AL fa)

Synonyms DNASE; recombinant human deoxyribonuclease
U.S./Canadian Brand Names Pulmozyme® [US/Can]
Therapeutic Category Enzyme
Use Management of cystic fibrosis patients to reduce the frequency of respiratory infections and to improve pulmonary function
Usual Dosage Children >5 years and Adults: Inhalation: 2.5 mg once daily through selected nebulizers in conjunction with a Pulmo-Aide® or a Pari-Proneb® compressor
Dosage Forms Solution for nebulization: 1 mg/mL (2.5 mL)

Doryx® [US] *see* doxycycline *on page 215*

dorzolamide (dor ZOLE a mide)

U.S./Canadian Brand Names Trusopt® [US/Can]
Therapeutic Category Carbonic Anhydrase Inhibitor
Use Lower intraocular pressure to treat glaucoma
Usual Dosage Adults: Ophthalmic: 1 drop in eye(s) 3 times/day
Dosage Forms Solution, ophthalmic, as hydrochloride: 2%

dorzolamide and timolol (dor ZOLE a mide & TYE moe lole)

U.S./Canadian Brand Names Cosopt® [US/Can]
Therapeutic Category Beta-Adrenergic Blocker; Carbonic Anhydrase Inhibitor
Use Lowers intraocular pressure to treat glaucoma in patients with ocular hypertension or open-angle glaucoma
Usual Dosage Adults: ophthalmic: One drop in eye(s) twice daily
Dosage Forms Solution, ophthalmic: Dorzolamide 2% and timolol 0.5% (5 mL, 10 mL)

DOSS *see* docusate *on page 208*

DOS® Softgel® [US-OTC] *see* docusate *on page 208*

Dostinex® [US] *see* cabergoline *on page 101*

Double Cap® [US] *see* capsaicin *on page 111*

Dovonex® [US] *see* calcipotriene *on page 103*

doxacurium (doks a KYOO ri um)

U.S./Canadian Brand Names Nuromax® [US/Can]
Therapeutic Category Skeletal Muscle Relaxant
Use Doxacurium is indicated for use as an adjunct to general anesthesia. It provides skeletal muscle relaxation during surgery or endotracheal intubation; increases pulmonary compliance during mechanical ventilation

Usual Dosage I.V. (in obese patients, use ideal body weight to calculate dosage):

Children >2 years: Initial: 0.03-0.05 mg/kg followed by maintenance doses of 0.005-0.01 mg/kg after 30-45 minutes

Adults: Surgery: 0.05 mg/kg with thiopental/narcotic or 0.025 mg/kg with succinylcholine; maintenance dose: 0.005-0.01 mg/kg after 60-100 minutes

Dosage Forms Injection, as chloride: 1 mg/mL (5 mL)

doxapram (DOKS a pram)

U.S./Canadian Brand Names Dopram® [US]

Therapeutic Category Respiratory Stimulant

Use Respiratory and CNS stimulant; idiopathic apnea of prematurity refractory to xanthines

Usual Dosage I.V.:

Neonatal apnea (apnea of prematurity):

Initial: 0.5 mg/kg/hour

Maintenance: 0.5-2.5 mg/kg/hour, titrated to the lowest rate at which apnea is controlled

Adults: Respiratory depression following anesthesia:

Initial: 0.5-1 mg/kg; may repeat at 5-minute intervals; maximum total dose: 2 mg/kg; single doses should not exceed 1.5 mg/kg

I.V. infusion: Initial: 5 mg/minute until adequate response or adverse effects seen; decrease to 1-3 mg/minute; usual total dose: 0.5-4 mg/kg; maximum: 300 mg

Dosage Forms Injection, as hydrochloride: 20 mg/mL (20 mL)

doxazosin (doks AYE zoe sin)

U.S./Canadian Brand Names Apo®-Doxazosin [Can]; Cardura® [US/Can]; Gen-Doxazosin [Can]; Novo-Doxazosin [Can]

Therapeutic Category Alpha-Adrenergic Blocking Agent

Use Alpha-adrenergic blocking agent for treatment of hypertension

Usual Dosage Adults: Oral: 1 mg once daily, may be increased to 2 mg once daily thereafter up to 16 mg if needed

Dosage Forms Tablet: 1 mg, 2 mg, 4 mg, 8 mg

doxepin (DOKS e pin)

U.S./Canadian Brand Names Alti-Doxepin [Can]; Apo®-Doxepin [Can]; Novo-Doxepin [Can]; Sinequan® [US/Can]; Zonalon® Cream [US/Can]

Therapeutic Category Antidepressant, Tricyclic (Tertiary Amine); Topical Skin Product

Use

Oral: Treatment of various forms of depression, usually in conjunction with psychotherapy; treatment of anxiety disorders; analgesic for certain chronic and neuropathic pain

Topical: Adults: Short-term (<8 days) therapy of moderate pruritus due to atopic dermatitis or lichen simplex chronicus

Usual Dosage

Oral:

Adolescents: Initial: 25-50 mg/day in single or divided doses; gradually increase to 100 mg/day

Adults: Initial: 30-150 mg/day at bedtime or in 2-3 divided doses; may increase up to 300 mg/day; single dose should not exceed 150 mg; select patients may respond to 25-50 mg/day

Topical: Apply in a thin film 4 times/day

Dosage Forms

Capsule, as hydrochloride (Sinequan®): 10 mg, 25 mg, 50 mg, 75 mg, 100 mg, 150 mg

Cream (Zonalon®): 5% (30 g, 45 g)

Solution, oral concentrate, as hydrochloride (Sinequan®): 10 mg/mL (120 mL)

doxercalciferol (dox er kal si fe FEER ole)

U.S./Canadian Brand Names Hectorol® [US/Can]

Therapeutic Category Vitamin D Analog

Use Reduction of elevated intact parathyroid hormone (iPTH) in the management of secondary hyperparathyroidism in patients on chronic hemodialysis.

Usual Dosage

Oral:

If the iPTH >400 pg/mL, then the initial dose is 10 mcg 3 times/week at dialysis. The dose is adjusted at 8-week intervals based upon the iPTH levels.

If the iPTH level is decreased by 50% and >300 pg/mL, then the dose can be increased to 12.5 mcg 3 times/week for 8 more weeks. This titration process can continue at 8-week intervals up to a maximum dose of 20 mcg 3 times/week. Each increase should be by 2.5 mcg/dose.

If the iPTH is between 150-300 pg/mL, maintain the current dose.

If the iPTH is <100 pg/mL, then suspend the drug for 1 week; resume doxercalciferol at a reduced dose. Decrease each dose (not weekly dose) by at least 2.5 mcg.

I.V.:

If the iPTH >400 pg/mL, then the initial dose is 4 mcg 3 times/week after dialysis, administered as a bolus dose

If the iPTH level is decreased by 50% and >300 pg/mL, then the dose can be increased by 1-2 mcg at 8-week intervals as necessary

If the iPTH is between 150-300 pg/mL, maintain the current dose.

If the iPTH is <100 pg/mL, then suspend the drug for 1 week; resume doxercalciferol at a reduced dose (at least 1 mcg lower)

Dosage Forms

Capsule: 2.5 mcg

Injection: 2 mcg/mL

Doxidan® [US-OTC] see docusate and casanthranol *on page 209*

Doxil® [US/Can] see doxorubicin (liposomal) *on next page*

Doxinate® Capsule (Discontinued) see page 814

doxorubicin (doks oh ROO bi sin)

Synonyms ADR; hydroxydaunomycin

Tall-Man DOXOrubicin

U.S./Canadian Brand Names Adriamycin® [Can]; Adriamycin PFS® [US]; Adriamycin RDF® [US]; Caelyx® [Can]; Rubex® [US]

Therapeutic Category Antineoplastic Agent

Use Treatment of various solid tumors including ovarian, breast, and bladder tumors; various lymphomas and leukemias (ANL, ALL), soft tissue sarcomas, neuroblastoma, osteosarcoma

Usual Dosage I.V. (refer to individual protocols; patient's ideal weight should be used to calculate body surface area):

Children: 35-75 mg/m^2 as a single dose, repeat every 21 days; or 20 mg/m^2 once weekly

Adults: 60-75 mg/m^2 as a single dose, repeat every 21 days or other dosage regimens like 20-30 mg/m^2/day for 2-3 days, repeat in 4 weeks or 20 mg/m^2 once weekly

The lower dose regimen should be administered to patients with decreased bone marrow reserve, prior therapy or marrow infiltration with malignant cells

Dosage Forms

Injection, as hydrochloride [preservative free]: 2 mg/mL (5 mL, 10 mL, 25 mL, 37.5 mL)

Injection, aqueous, as hydrochloride: 2 mg/mL (5 mL, 10 mL, 25 mL, 100 mL)

Injection, powder for reconstitution, as hydrochloride: 10 mg, 20 mg, 50 mg, 100 mg

Injection, powder for reconstitution, rapid dissolution formula, as hydrochloride: 10 mg, 20 mg, 50 mg, 150 mg

doxorubicin (liposomal) (doks oh ROO bi sin lip pah SOW mal)

Tall-Man DOXOrubicin (liposomal)

U.S./Canadian Brand Names Doxil® [US/Can]

Therapeutic Category Antineoplastic Agent

Use Treatment of AIDS-related Kaposi's sarcoma in patients with disease that has progressed on prior combination chemotherapy or in patients who are intolerant to such therapy; treatment of metastatic carcinoma of the ovary in patients with disease that is refractory to both paclitaxel and platinum-based regimens

Usual Dosage Refer to individual protocols.

I.V. (patient's ideal weight should be used to calculate body surface area): 20 mg/m^2 over 30 minutes, once every 3 weeks, for as long as patients respond satisfactorily and tolerate treatment.

AIDS-KS patients: I.V.: 20 mg/m^2/dose over 30 minutes once every 3 weeks for as long as patients respond satisfactorily and tolerate treatment

Breast cancer: I.V.: 20-80 mg/m^2/dose has been studied in a limited number of phase I/II trials

Ovarian cancer: I.V.: 50 mg/m^2/dose repeated every 4 weeks (minimum of 4 courses is recommended)

Solid tumors: I.V.: 50-60 mg/m^2/dose repeated every 3-4 weeks has been studied in a limited number of phase I/II trials

Dosage Forms Injection, as hydrochloride: 2 mg/mL (10 mL)

Doxy-100™ [US] *see* doxycycline *on this page*

Doxycin [Can] *see* doxycycline *on this page*

doxycycline (doks i SYE kleen)

U.S./Canadian Brand Names Adoxa™ [US]; Apo®-Doxy [Can]; Apo®-Doxy Tabs [Can]; Doryx® [US]; Doxy-100™ [US]; Doxycin [Can]; Doxytec [Can]; Monodox® [US]; Novo-Doxylin [Can]; Nu-Doxycycline [Can]; Periostat® [US]; Vibramycin® [US]; Vibra-Tabs® [US/Can]

Therapeutic Category Tetracycline Derivative

Use

Children, Adolescents, and Adults: Treatment of Rocky Mountain spotted fever caused by susceptible *Rickettsia* or brucellosis

Older Children, Adolescents, and Adults: Treatment of Lyme disease, mycoplasmal disease, or *Legionella*; management of malignant pleural effusions when intrapleural therapy is indicated

Adolescents and Adults: Treatment of nongonococcal pelvic inflammatory disease and urethritis due to *Chlamydia*; treatment for victims of sexual assault

Adults: Periostat® (20 mg capsule) is used as an adjunct to scaling and root planing to promote attachment level gain and to reduce pocket depth in patients with adult periodontitis

Unapproved use: Treatment for syphilis in penicillin-allergic patients; sclerosing agent for pleural effusions

Usual Dosage Oral, I.V.:

Children ≥8 years (<45 kg): 2-5 mg/kg/day in 1-2 divided doses, not to exceed 200 mg/day

Children >8 years (>45 kg) and Adults: 100-200 mg/day in 1-2 divided doses

Sclerosing agent for pleural effusion injection: 500 mg as a single dose in 30-50 mL of NS or SWI

Adults: Periodontitis: 20 mg twice/day for up to 9 months; safety beyond 12 months and efficacy beyond 9 months have not been established

Dosage Forms

Capsule, as hyclate (Vibramycin®): 50 mg, 100 mg

Capsule, as monohydrate (Monodox®): 50 mg, 100 mg

Capsule, coated pellets, as hyclate (Doryx®): 100 mg

Injection, powder for reconstitution, as hyclate (Doxy-100™): 100 mg

(Continued)

doxycycline *(Continued)*

Powder for oral suspension, as monohydrate (Vibramycin®): 25 mg/5 mL (60 mL) [raspberry flavor]

Syrup, as calcium (Vibramycin®): 50 mg/5 mL (480 mL) [raspberry-apple flavor]

Tablet, as hyclate:

Periostat®: 20 mg

Vibra-Tabs®: 100 mg

Tablet, as monohydrate (Adoxa™): 50 mg, 100 mg

doxylamine (dox IL a meen)

U.S./Canadian Brand Names Medi-Sleep® [US-OTC]; Night-Time Sleep Aid [US-OTC]; Sleep-Aid® [US-OTC]; Unisom® [US-OTC]

Therapeutic Category Antihistamine

Use Sleep aid; antihistamine for hypersensitivity reactions and antiemetic

Usual Dosage Oral: Children >12 years and adults: 25 mg at bedtime

Dosage Forms Tablet, as succinate: 25 mg

Doxytec [Can] *see* doxycycline *on previous page*

DPA *see* valproic acid and derivatives *on page 670*

D-Pan® [US] *see* dexpanthenol *on page 186*

D-Pan® Plus [US-OTC] *see* dexpanthenol *on page 186*

DPE *see* dipivefrin *on page 205*

d-penicillamine *see* penicillamine *on page 497*

DPH *see* phenytoin *on page 511*

DPPC *see* colfosceril palmitate *on page 161*

DPT *see* diphtheria, tetanus toxoids, and whole-cell pertussis vaccine *on page 205*

Dramamine® II [US-OTC] *see* meclizine *on page 403*

Dramamine® Injection *(Discontinued)* *see page 814*

Dramamine® Oral [US-OTC] *see* dimenhydrinate *on page 200*

Dramilin® Injection *(Discontinued)* *see page 814*

Dramocen® *(Discontinued)* *see page 814*

Dramoject® *(Discontinued)* *see page 814*

Dri-Ear® Otic [US-OTC] *see* boric acid *on page 90*

Drinex® *(Discontinued)* *see page 814*

Drisdol® [US/Can] *see* ergocalciferol *on page 232*

Dristan® Long Lasting Nasal [Can] *see* oxymetazoline *on page 486*

Dristan® Long Lasting Nasal Solution *(Discontinued)* *see page 814*

Dristan® N.D. [Can] *see* acetaminophen and pseudoephedrine *on page 6*

Dristan® N.D., Extra Strength [Can] *see* acetaminophen and pseudoephedrine *on page 6*

Dristan® Saline Spray *(Discontinued)* *see page 814*

Dristan® Sinus Caplets [US] *see* pseudoephedrine and ibuprofen *on page 553*

Dristan® Sinus Tablet [Can] *see* pseudoephedrine and ibuprofen *on page 553*

Drithocreme® [US] *see* anthralin *on page 44*

Dritho-Scalp® *(Discontinued)* *see page 814*

Drixomed® [US] *see* dexbrompheniramine and pseudoephedrine *on page 185*

Drixoral® [Can] *see* dexbrompheniramine and pseudoephedrine *on page 185*

Drixoral® Cold & Allergy [US-OTC] *see* dexbrompheniramine and pseudoephedrine *on page 185*

Drixoral® Cough & Congestion Liquid Caps *(Discontinued) see page 814*

Drixoral® Cough Liquid Caps *(Discontinued) see page 814*

Drixoral® Nasal [Can] *see* oxymetazoline *on page 486*

Drixoral® Non-Drowsy *(Discontinued) see page 814*

dronabinol (droe NAB i nol)

Synonyms tetrahydrocannabinol; THC
U.S./Canadian Brand Names Marinol® [US/Can]
Therapeutic Category Antiemetic
Controlled Substance C-III
Use Treatment of nausea and vomiting secondary to cancer chemotherapy in patients who have not responded to conventional antiemetics; treatment of anorexia associated with weight loss in AIDS patients
Usual Dosage Oral:
  Children: NCI protocol recommends 5 mg/m^2 starting 6-8 hours before chemotherapy and every 4-6 hours after to be continued for 12 hours after chemotherapy is discontinued
  Adults: 5 mg/m^2 1-3 hours before chemotherapy, then administer 5 mg/m^2/dose every 2-4 hours after chemotherapy for a total of 4-6 doses/day; dose may be increased up to a maximum of 15 mg/m^2/dose if needed (dosage may be increased by 2.5 mg/m^2 increments)
Dosage Forms Capsule: 2.5 mg, 5 mg, 10 mg

droperidol (droe PER i dole)

U.S./Canadian Brand Names Inapsine® [US]
Therapeutic Category Antiemetic; Antipsychotic Agent, Butyrophenone
Use Tranquilizer and antiemetic in surgical and diagnostic procedures; antiemetic for cancer chemotherapy; preoperative medication
Usual Dosage Titrate carefully to desired effect
  Children 2-12 years:
  Premedication: I.M.: 0.088-0.165 mg/kg; smaller doses may be sufficient for control of nausea or vomiting
  Adjunct to general anesthesia: I.V. induction: 0.088-0.165 mg/kg
  Nausea and vomiting: I.M., I.V.: 0.05-0.06 mg/kg/dose every 4-6 hours as needed
  Adults:
  Premedication: I.M., I.V.: 2.5-10 mg 30 minutes to 1 hour preoperatively
  Adjunct to general anesthesia: I.V. induction: 0.22-0.275 mg/kg; maintenance: 1.25-2.5 mg/dose
  Alone in diagnostic procedures: I.M.: Initial: 2.5-10 mg 30 minutes to 1 hour before; then 1.25-2.5 mg if needed
  Nausea and vomiting: I.M., I.V.: 2.5-5 mg/dose every 3-4 hours as needed
Dosage Forms Solution for injection: 2.5 mg/mL (1 mL, 2 mL)

droperidol and fentanyl (droe PER i dole & FEN ta nil)

Synonyms fentanyl and droperidol
U.S./Canadian Brand Names Innovar® [US]
Therapeutic Category Analgesic, Narcotic
Use Produce and maintain analgesia and sedation during diagnostic or surgical procedures (neuroleptanalgesia and neuroleptanesthesia); adjunct to general anesthesia
Usual Dosage
  Children:
  Premedication: I.M.: 0.03 mL/kg 30-60 minutes prior to surgery
  Adjunct to general anesthesia: I.V.: Total dose: 0.05 mL/kg as slow infusion (1 mL/1-2 minutes) until sleep occurs
  (Continued)

droperidol and fentanyl *(Continued)*

Adults:

Premedication: I.M.: 0.5-2 mL 30-60 minutes prior to surgery

Adjunct to general anesthesia: I.V.: 0.09-0.11 mL/kg as slow infusion (1 mL/1-2 minutes) until sleep occurs

Dosage Forms Injection: Droperidol 2.5 mg and fentanyl 50 mcg per mL (2 mL, 5 mL)

drospirenone and ethinyl estradiol *see* ethinyl estradiol and drospirenone *on page 245*

drotrecogin alfa *(droe tre KOE jin AL fa)*

Synonyms activated protein C, human, recombinant; drotrecogin alfa, activated; protein C (activated), human, recombinant

U.S./Canadian Brand Names Xigris™ [US]

Therapeutic Category Protein C (Activated)

Use Reduction of mortality from severe sepsis (associated with organ dysfunction) in adults at high risk of death (based on APACHE II score ≥25)

Usual Dosage I.V.: Adults: 24 mcg/kg/hour for a total of 96 hours; stop infusion **immediately** if clinically-important bleeding is identified

Dosage Forms Injection, powder for reconstitution [preservative free]: 5 mg, 20 mg

drotrecogin alfa, activated *see* drotrecogin alfa *on this page*

Droxia™ [US] *see* hydroxyurea *on page 338*

Dr Scholl's Athlete's Foot [US-OTC] *see* tolnaftate *on page 644*

Dr Scholl's® Disk [US-OTC] *see* salicylic acid *on page 581*

Dr Scholl's Maximum Strength Tritin [US-OTC] *see* tolnaftate *on page 644*

Dr Scholl's® Wart Remover [US-OTC] *see* salicylic acid *on page 581*

Drug Products No Longer Available in the U.S. *see page 814*

Dry Eye® Therapy Solution *(Discontinued)* *see page 814*

Dryox® Gel *(Discontinued)* *see page 814*

Dryox® Wash *(Discontinued)* *see page 814*

Drysol™ [US] *see* aluminum chloride hexahydrate *on page 28*

DSCG *see* cromolyn sodium *on page 166*

DSMC Plus® *(Discontinued)* *see page 814*

DSS *see* docusate *on page 208*

D-S-S Plus® *(Discontinued)* *see page 814*

D-S-S® [US-OTC] *see* docusate *on page 208*

DSS with casanthranol *see* docusate and casanthranol *on page 209*

DT *see* diphtheria and tetanus toxoid *on page 203*

DTAP *see* diphtheria, tetanus toxoids, and acellular pertussis vaccine *on page 204*

DTIC® [Can] *see* dacarbazine *on page 172*

DTIC-Dome® [US] *see* dacarbazine *on page 172*

DTO *see* opium tincture *on page 478*

***d*-tubocurarine** *see* tubocurarine *on page 662*

DTwP-HIB *see* diphtheria, tetanus toxoids, whole-cell pertussis, and *Haemophilus* B conjugate vaccine *on page 205*

Duadacin® Capsule *(Discontinued)* *see page 814*

Dulcolax® [US/Can] *see* bisacodyl *on page 87*

Dull-C® [US-OTC] *see* ascorbic acid *on page 57*

DuoCet™ *(Discontinued)* see page 814

Duo-Cyp® *(Discontinued)* see page 814

Duofilm® Solution [US] see salicylic acid and lactic acid on page 581

DuoFilm® [US-OTC] see salicylic acid on page 581

Duoforte® 27 [Can] see salicylic acid on page 581

Duo-Medihaler® *(Discontinued)* see page 814

Duonalc® [Can] see alcohol (ethyl) on page 20

Duonalc-E® Mild [Can] see alcohol (ethyl) on page 20

DuoNeb™ [US] see ipratropium and albuterol on page 359

DuoPlant® [US-OTC] see salicylic acid on page 581

Duo-Trach® Injection *(Discontinued)* see page 814

Duotrate® *(Discontinued)* see page 814

DuP 753 see losartan on page 392

Duphalac® *(Discontinued)* see page 814

Duplex® T [US-OTC] see coal tar on page 158

Durabolin® [Can] see nandrolone on page 446

Duracid® *(Discontinued)* see page 814

Duraclon™ [US] see clonidine on page 155

Duract® *(Discontinued)* see page 814

Duradyne DHC® *(Discontinued)* see page 814

Duragesic® [US/Can] see fentanyl on page 266

Dura-Gest® *(Discontinued)* see page 814

Duralith® [Can] see lithium on page 388

Duralone® Injection *(Discontinued)* see page 814

Duramist® Plus [US-OTC] see oxymetazoline on page 486

Duramorph® [US] see morphine sulfate on page 437

Duranest® [US/Can] see etidocaine on page 258

Duratest® Injection *(Discontinued)* see page 814

Duratestrin® *(Discontinued)* see page 814

Durathate® Injection *(Discontinued)* see page 814

Duration® [US-OTC] see oxymetazoline on page 486

Duratocin™ [Can] see carbetocin *(Canada only)* on page 114

Duratuss™ [US] see guaifenesin and pseudoephedrine on page 310

Duratuss® DM [US] see guaifenesin and dextromethorphan on page 308

Duratuss-G® [US] see guaifenesin on page 307

Duratuss™ GP [US] see guaifenesin and pseudoephedrine on page 310

Duratuss® HD [US] see hydrocodone, pseudoephedrine, and guaifenesin on page 332

Dura-Vent® *(Discontinued)* see page 814

Dura-Vent®/DA [US] see chlorpheniramine, phenylephrine, and methscopolamine on page 139

Duricef® [US/Can] see cefadroxil on page 121

Durrax® Oral *(Discontinued)* see page 814

dutasteride (doo TAS teer ide)
U.S./Canadian Brand Names Avodart™ [US]
Therapeutic Category Antineoplastic Agent, Anthracenedione
Use Treatment of symptomatic benign prostatic hyperplasia (BPH)
Usual Dosage Oral: Adults: Male: 0.5 mg once daily
Dosage Forms Capsule: 0.5 mg

Duvoid® *(Discontinued)* see page 814

Duvoid® [Can] see bethanechol on page 84

D-Vi-Sol® [Can] see cholecalciferol on page 143

DV® Vaginal Cream *(Discontinued)* see page 814

Dwelle® Ophthalmic Solution *(Discontinued)* see page 814

d-xylose (dee ZYE lose)
Synonyms wood sugar
U.S./Canadian Brand Names Xylo-Pfan® [US-OTC]
Therapeutic Category Diagnostic Agent
Use Evaluating intestinal absorption and diagnosing malabsorptive states
Usual Dosage Oral:
Infants and young Children: 500 mg/kg as a 5% to 10% aqueous solution
Children: 5 g is dissolved in 250 mL water; additional fluids are permitted and are encouraged for children
Adults: 25 g dissolved in 200-300 mL water followed with an additional 200-400 mL water **or** 5 g dissolved in 200-300 mL water followed by an additional 200-400 mL water
Dosage Forms Powder for oral solution: 25 g

Dyazide® [US] see hydrochlorothiazide and triamterene on page 329

Dycill® *(Discontinued)* see page 814

Dyclone® [US] see dyclonine on this page

dyclonine (DYE kloe neen)
U.S./Canadian Brand Names Dyclone® [US]; Sucrets® [US-OTC]
Therapeutic Category Local Anesthetic
Use Local anesthetic prior to laryngoscopy, bronchoscopy, or endotracheal intubation; used topically for temporary relief of pain associated with oral mucosa, skin, episiotomy, or anogenital lesions; the 0.5% topical solution may be used to block the gag reflex, and to relieve the pain of oral ulcers or stomatitis
Usual Dosage
Children and Adults: Topical solution:
Mouth sores: 5-10 mL of 0.5% or 1% to oral mucosa (swab or swish and then spit) 3-4 times/day as needed; maximum single dose: 200 mg (40 mL of 0.5% solution or 20 mL of 1% solution)
Bronchoscopy: Use 2 mL of the 1% solution or 4 mL of the 0.5% solution sprayed onto the larynx and trachea every 5 minutes until the reflex has been abolished
Children >3 years and Adults: Lozenge: Dissolve 1 in mouth slowly every 2 hours
Dosage Forms
Lozenge, as hydrochloride: 1.2 mg, 2 mg, 3 mg
Solution, topical, as hydrochloride: 0.5% (30 mL); 1% (30 mL)

Dyflex-400® Tablet *(Discontinued)* see page 814

Dymelor® *(Discontinued)* see page 814

Dymenate® Injection *(Discontinued)* see page 814

Dynabac® [US] see dirithromycin on page 206

Dynacin® [US] see minocycline on page 431

DynaCirc® **[US/Can]** *see* isradipine *on page 363*
DynaCirc® **CR [US]** *see* isradipine *on page 363*
Dyna-Hex® **[US-OTC]** *see* chlorhexidine gluconate *on page 134*
Dynapen® **[US]** *see* dicloxacillin *on page 194*

dyphylline (DYE fi lin)
  Synonyms dihydroxypropyl theophylline
  U.S./Canadian Brand Names Dilor® [US/Can]; Lufyllin® [US/Can]
  Therapeutic Category Theophylline Derivative
  Use Bronchodilator in reversible airway obstruction due to asthma or COPD
  Usual Dosage
    Children: I.M.: 4.4-6.6 mg/kg/day in divided doses
    Adults:
     Oral: Up to 15 mg/kg 4 times/day, individualize dosage
     I.M.: 250-500 mg, do not exceed total dosage of 15 mg/kg every 6 hours
  Dosage Forms
    Elixir:
     Dilor®: 160 mg/15 mL (473 mL) [contains alcohol 18%]
     Lufyllin®: 100 mg/15 mL (473 mL, 3780 mL) [contains alcohol 20%]
    Injection (Dilor®, Lufyllin®): 250 mg/mL (2 mL)
    Tablet: 200 mg, 400 mg
    Dilor®, Lufyllin®: 200 mg, 400 mg

Dyrenium® **[US/Can]** *see* triamterene *on page 653*
Dyrexan-OD® *(Discontinued)* *see page 814*
Dytuss® **[US-OTC]** *see* diphenhydramine *on page 202*
E2020 *see* donepezil *on page 211*
Easprin® **[US]** *see* aspirin *on page 58*

echothiophate iodide (ek oh THYE oh fate EYE oh dide)
  Synonyms ecostigmine iodide
  U.S./Canadian Brand Names Phospholine Iodide® [US]
  Therapeutic Category Cholinesterase Inhibitor
  Use Reverse toxic CNS effects caused by anticholinergic drugs; used as miotic in treatment of glaucoma
  Usual Dosage Adults: Ophthalmic: Glaucoma: Instill 1 drop twice daily into eyes with one dose just prior to bedtime; some patients have been treated with 1 dose/day or every other day. Use lowest concentration and frequency which gives satisfactory response, with a maximum dose of 0.125% once daily, although more intensive therapy may be used for short periods of time
  Dosage Forms Powder, ophthalmic: 1.5 mg [0.03%] (5 mL); 3 mg [0.06%] (5 mL); 6.25 mg [0.125%] (5 mL); 12.5 mg [0.25%] (5 mL)

EC-Naprosyn® **[US]** *see* naproxen *on page 447*
E-Complex-600® **[US-OTC]** *see* vitamin E *on page 682*

econazole (e KONE a zole)
  U.S./Canadian Brand Names Ecostatin® [Can]; Spectazole™ [US/Can]
  Therapeutic Category Antifungal Agent
  Use Topical treatment of tinea pedis, tinea cruris, tinea corporis, tinea versicolor, and cutaneous candidiasis
  Usual Dosage Children and Adults: Topical: Apply a sufficient amount to cover affected areas once daily; for cutaneous candidiasis: apply twice daily; candidal infections and tinea cruris, versicolor, and corporis should be treated for 2 weeks and tinea pedis for 1 month; occasionally, longer treatment periods may be required
  (Continued)

econazole *(Continued)*

Dosage Forms Cream, as nitrate: 1% (15 g, 30 g, 85 g)

Econopred® **[US]** *see* prednisolone (ophthalmic) *on page 537*

Econopred® **Plus [US]** *see* prednisolone (ophthalmic) *on page 537*

Ecostatin® **[Can]** *see* econazole *on previous page*

ecostigmine iodide *see* echothiophate iodide *on previous page*

Ecotrin® Low Adult Strength [US-OTC] *see* aspirin *on page 58*

Ecotrin® Maximum Strength [US-OTC] *see* aspirin *on page 58*

Ecotrin® [US-OTC] *see* aspirin *on page 58*

Ectosone [Can] *see* betamethasone (topical) *on page 83*

Ed A-Hist® **[US]** *see* chlorpheniramine and phenylephrine *on page 138*

edathamil disodium *see* edetate disodium *on this page*

Edecrin® **[US/Can]** *see* ethacrynic acid *on page 243*

edetate calcium disodium (ED e tate KAL see um dye SOW dee um)

Synonyms calcium edta

U.S./Canadian Brand Names Calcium Disodium Versenate® [US]

Therapeutic Category Chelating Agent

Use Treatment of acute and chronic lead poisoning; also used as an aid in the diagnosis of lead poisoning

Usual Dosage

Children:

Diagnosis of lead poisoning: Mobilization test: (Asymptomatic patients or lead levels <55 mcg/dL: (**Note:** Urine is collected for 24 hours after first EDTA dose and analyzed for lead content; if the ratio of mcg of lead in urine to mg calcium EDTA given is >1, then test is considered positive): Children: 500 mg/m^2 (maximum: 1 g/dose) I.M. or I.V. over 1 hour **or** 2 doses of 500 mg/m^2 at 12-hour intervals

Asymptomatic lead poisoning: (Blood lead concentration >55 mcg/dL or blood lead concentrations of 25-55 mcg/dL with blood erythrocyte protoporphyrin concentrations of ≥35 mcg/dL and positive mobilization test) or symptomatic lead poisoning without encephalopathy with lead level <100 mcg/dL: 1 g/m^2/day I.M./I.V. in divided doses every 8-12 hours for 3-5 days (usually 5 days); maximum: 1 g/24 hours or 50 mg/kg/day

Symptomatic lead poisoning with encephalopathy with lead level >100 mcg/dL (treatment with calcium EDTA and dimercaprol is preferred): 250 mg/m^2 I.M. or intermittent I.V. infusion 4 hours after dimercaprol, then at 4-hour intervals thereafter for 5 days (1.5 g/m^2/day); dose (1.5 g/m^2/day) can also be administered as a single I.V. continuous infusion over 12-24 hours/day for 5 days; maximum: 1 g/24 hours or 75 mg/kg/day

Note: Course of therapy may be repeated in 2-3 weeks until blood lead level is normal

Adults: I.M., I.V.:

Diagnosis of lead poisoning: 500 mg/m^2 (maximum: 1 g/dose) over 1 hour

Treatment: 2 g/day or 1.5 g/m^2/day in divided doses every 12-24 hours for 5 days; may repeat course one time after at least 2 days (usually after 2 weeks)

Dosage Forms Injection: 200 mg/mL (5 mL)

edetate disodium (ED e tate dye SOW dee um)

Synonyms edathamil disodium; EDTA; sodium edetate

U.S./Canadian Brand Names Chealamide® [US]; Disotate® [US]; Endrate® [US]

Therapeutic Category Chelating Agent

Use Emergency treatment of hypercalcemia; control digitalis-induced cardiac dysrhythmias (ventricular arrhythmias)

Usual Dosage I.V.:
Hypercalcemia:
Children: 40-70 mg/kg slow infusion over 3-4 hours
Adults: 50 mg/kg/day over 3 or more hours
Dysrhythmias: Children and Adults: 15 mg/kg/hour up to 60 mg/kg/day
Dosage Forms Injection: 150 mg/mL (20 mL)

Edex® **[US]** *see* alprostadil *on page 25*

edrophonium (ed roe FOE nee um)
U.S./Canadian Brand Names Enlon® [US/Can]; Reversol® [US]; Tensilon® [US]
Therapeutic Category Cholinergic Agent
Use Diagnosis of myasthenia gravis; differentiation of cholinergic crises from myasthenia crises; reversal of nondepolarizing neuromuscular blockers; treatment of paroxysmal atrial tachycardia
Usual Dosage
Infants: I.V.: Initial: 0.1 mg, followed by 0.4 mg if no response; total dose: 0.5 mg
Children:
Diagnosis: Initial: 0.04 mg/kg followed by 0.16 mg/kg if no response, to a maximum total dose of 5 mg for children ≤34 kg, or 10 mg for children >34 kg
Titration of oral anticholinesterase therapy: 0.04 mg/kg once; if strength improves, an increase in neostigmine or pyridostigmine dose is indicated
Adults:
Diagnosis: I.V.: 2 mg test dose administered over 15-30 seconds; 8 mg administered 45 seconds later if no response is seen. Test dose may be repeated after 30 minutes.
Titration of oral anticholinesterase therapy: 1-2 mg administered 1 hour after oral dose of anticholinesterase; if strength improves, an increase in neostigmine or pyridostigmine dose is indicated
Differentiation of cholinergic from myasthenic crisis: I.V.: 1 mg, may repeat after 1 minute (**Note:** Intubation and controlled ventilation may be required if patient has cholinergic crises.)
Reversal of nondepolarizing neuromuscular blocking agents (neostigmine with atropine usually preferred): I.V.: 10 mg, may repeat every 5-10 minutes up to 40 mg
Termination of paroxysmal atrial tachycardia: I.V.: 5-10 mg
Dosage Forms Injection, as chloride: 10 mg/mL (1 mL, 10 mL, 15 mL)

ED-SPAZ® *(Discontinued) see page 814*

EDTA *see* edetate disodium *on previous page*

E.E.S.® **[US/Can]** *see* erythromycin (systemic) *on page 235*

efavirenz (e FAV e renz)
U.S./Canadian Brand Names Sustiva® [US/Can]
Therapeutic Category Non-nucleoside Reverse Transcriptase Inhibitor (NNRTI)
Use Treatment of HIV-1 infections in combination with at least 2 other antiretroviral agents. Also has some activity against hepatitis B virus and herpes viruses.
Usual Dosage Dosing at bedtime is recommended to limit central nervous system effects; should not be used as single-agent therapy
Oral:
Adults: 600 mg once daily
Children: Dosage is based on body weight
10 to <15 kg: 200 mg
15 to <20 kg: 250 mg
20 to <25 kg: 300 mg
25 to <32.5 kg: 350 mg
32.5 to <40 kg: 400 mg
≥40 kg: 600 mg
Dosage Forms
Capsule: 50 mg, 100 mg, 200 mg
(Continued)

efavirenz *(Continued)*
Tablet: 600 mg

Effer-K™ [US] *see* potassium bicarbonate and potassium citrate, effervescent *on page 529*

Effer-Syllium® *(Discontinued) see page 814*

Effexor® [US/Can] *see* venlafaxine *on page 675*

Effexor® XR [US/Can] *see* venlafaxine *on page 675*

Efidac/24® [US-OTC] *see* pseudoephedrine *on page 552*

eflornithine (ee FLOR ni theen)
Synonyms DFMO; eflornithine hydrochloride
U.S./Canadian Brand Names Vaniqa™ [US]
Therapeutic Category Antiprotozoal; Topical Skin Product
Use Cream: Females ≥12 years: Reduce unwanted hair from face and adjacent areas under the chin
Orphan status: Injection: Treatment of meningoencephalitic stage of *Trypanosoma brucei gambiense* infection (sleeping sickness)
Dosage Forms
Cream, as hydrochloride: 13.9% (30 g)
Injection, as hydrochloride: 200 mg/mL (100 mL) [orphan drug status]

eflornithine hydrochloride *see* eflornithine *on this page*

Efodine® *(Discontinued) see page 814*

Efudex® [US/Can] *see* fluorouracil *on page 279*

EHDP *see* etidronate disodium *on page 258*

ELA-Max® [US-OTC] *see* lidocaine *on page 383*

Elase® [US] *see* fibrinolysin and desoxyribonuclease *on page 271*

Elase®-Chloromycetin® Ointment *(Discontinued) see page 814*

Elavil® [US/Can] *see* amitriptyline *on page 34*

Eldecort® [US] *see* hydrocortisone (topical) *on page 334*

Eldepryl® [US/Can] *see* selegiline *on page 586*

Eldepryl® Tablet (only) *(Discontinued) see page 814*

Eldercaps® [US-OTC] *see* vitamin (multiple/oral) *on page 683*

Eldopaque Forte® [US] *see* hydroquinone *on page 336*

Eldopaque® [US-OTC] *see* hydroquinone *on page 336*

Eldoquin® [US/Can] *see* hydroquinone *on page 336*

Eldoquin® Forte® [US] *see* hydroquinone *on page 336*

Eldoquin® Lotion *(Discontinued) see page 814*

electrolyte lavage solution *see* polyethylene glycol-electrolyte solution *on page 525*

Elidel® [US] *see* pimecrolimus *on page 515*

Eligard™ [US] *see* leuprolide acetate *on page 377*

Elimite® [US] *see* permethrin *on page 505*

Elitek™ [US] *see* rasburicase *on page 565*

Elixomin® *(Discontinued) see page 814*

Elixophyllin® [US] *see* theophylline *on page 630*

Elixophyllin® GG [US] *see* theophylline and guaifenesin *on page 631*

Elixophyllin SR® *(Discontinued) see page 814*

Ellence™ [US/Can] *see* epirubicin *on page 230*

Elmiron® [US/Can] *see* pentosan polysulfate sodium *on page 502*

Elocon® [US/Can] *see* mometasone furoate *on page 435*

E-Lor® Tablet *(Discontinued)* *see page 814*

Elspar® [US/Can] *see* asparaginase *on page 58*

Eltor® [Can] *see* pseudoephedrine *on page 552*

Eltroxin® [Can] *see* levothyroxine *on page 382*

Emadine® [US] *see* emedastine *on this page*

Emcyt® [US/Can] *see* estramustine *on page 240*

Emecheck® *(Discontinued)* *see page 814*

emedastine (em e DAS teen)
   U.S./Canadian Brand Names Emadine® [US]
   Therapeutic Category Antihistamine, H_1 Blocker, Ophthalmic
   Use Treatment of allergic conjunctivitis
   Usual Dosage Ophthalmic: Children ≥3 years and Adults: Instill 1 drop in affected eye up to 4 times/day
   Dosage Forms Solution, ophthalmic, as difumarate: 0.05% (5 mL) [contains benzalkonium chloride]

Emete-Con® Injection *(Discontinued)* *see page 814*

emetine hydrochloride *(Discontinued)* *see page 814*

Emetrol® [US-OTC] *see* phosphorated carbohydrate solution *on page 512*

Emgel® [US] *see* erythromycin (ophthalmic/topical) *on page 235*

Emitrip® *(Discontinued)* *see page 814*

Emko® [US-OTC] *see* nonoxynol 9 *on page 464*

EMLA® [US/Can] *see* lidocaine and prilocaine *on page 384*

Emo-Cort® [Can] *see* hydrocortisone (rectal) *on page 333*

Empirin® With Codeine [US] *see* aspirin and codeine *on page 59*

Empracet®-30 [Can] *see* acetaminophen and codeine *on page 5*

Empracet®-60 [Can] *see* acetaminophen and codeine *on page 5*

Emtec-30 [Can] *see* acetaminophen and codeine *on page 5*

EmTet® [US] *see* tetracycline *on page 628*

Emulsoil® [US-OTC] *see* castor oil *on page 119*

E-Mycin® *(Discontinued)* *see page 814*

E-Mycin-E® *(Discontinued)* *see page 814*

ENA 713 *see* rivastigmine *on page 575*

enalapril (e NAL a pril)
   U.S./Canadian Brand Names Vasotec® I.V. [US/Can]; Vasotec® [US/Can]
   Therapeutic Category Angiotensin-Converting Enzyme (ACE) Inhibitor
   Use Management of mild to severe hypertension, congestive heart failure, and asymptomatic left ventricular dysfunction
   Usual Dosage Use lower listed initial dose in patients with hyponatremia, hypovolemia, severe congestive heart failure, decreased renal function, or in those receiving diuretics
   Children:
      Investigational initial oral doses of enalapril of 0.1 mg/kg/day increasing over 2 weeks to 0.12-0.43 mg/kg/day have been used to treat severe congestive heart failure in infants (n=8)
   (Continued)

enalapril *(Continued)*

Investigational I.V. doses of enalaprilat of 5-10 mcg/kg/dose administered every 8-24 hours (as determined by blood pressure readings) have been used for the treatment of neonatal hypertension (n=10); monitor patients carefully; select patients may require higher doses

Adults:

Oral: **Enalapril**: 2.5-5 mg/day then increase as required, usually 10-40 mg/day in 1-2 divided doses

I.V.: **Enalaprilat**: 0.625-1.25 mg/dose, administered over 5 minutes every 6 hours

Dosage Forms

Injection, as enalaprilat: 1.25 mg/mL (1 mL, 2 mL)

Tablet, as maleate: 2.5 mg, 5 mg, 10 mg, 20 mg

enalapril and diltiazem (e NAL a pril & dil TYE a zem)

U.S./Canadian Brand Names Teczem® [US/Can]

Therapeutic Category Antihypertensive Agent, Combination

Use Combination drug for treatment of hypertension

Usual Dosage Adults: Oral: One tablet daily, if further blood pressure control is required, increase dosage to two tablets daily

Dosage Forms Tablet, extended release: Enalapril maleate 5 mg and diltiazem maleate 180 mg

enalapril and felodipine (e NAL a pril & fe LOE di peen)

U.S./Canadian Brand Names Lexxel™ [US/Can]

Therapeutic Category Antihypertensive Agent, Combination

Use Treatment of hypertension

Usual Dosage Adults: Oral: The dose of this combination when given as a replacement to patients taking both components separately should be equal to the component doses previously used. Patients whose blood pressure is not sufficiently controlled on either component may be switched to one combination tablet (5 mg enalapril and 5 mg extended-release felodipine) daily. If control remains inadequate after 1 or 2 weeks, the dosage may be increased to two tablets daily, and if lack of control persists, a thiazide diuretic may be added

Dosage Forms

Tablet, extended release:

Enalapril maleate 5 mg and felodipine 2.5 mg

Enalapril maleate 5 mg and felodipine 5 mg

enalapril and hydrochlorothiazide

(e NAL a pril & hye droe klor oh THYE a zide)

Synonyms hydrochlorothiazide and enalapril

U.S./Canadian Brand Names Vaseretic® [US/Can]

Therapeutic Category Antihypertensive Agent, Combination

Use Treatment of hypertension

Usual Dosage Oral: Dose is individualized

Dosage Forms

Tablet:

Enalapril maleate 5 mg and hydrochlorothiazide 12.5 mg

Enalapril maleate 10 mg and hydrochlorothiazide 25 mg

Enbrel® [US] *see* etanercept *on page 243*

Encare® [US-OTC] *see* nonoxynol 9 *on page 464*

Endal® [US] *see* guaifenesin and phenylephrine *on page 310*

Endantadine® [Can] *see* amantadine *on page 30*

Endep® 25 mg, 50 mg, 100 mg *(Discontinued)* *see page 814*

End Lice® [US-OTC] *see* pyrethrins *on page 555*

Endocet® **[US/Can]** see oxycodone and acetaminophen on page 485

Endodan® **[US/Can]** see oxycodone and aspirin on page 485

Endo®**-Levodopa/Carbidopa [Can]** see levodopa and carbidopa on page 380

Endolor® **(Discontinued)** see page 814

Endrate® **[US]** see edetate disodium on page 222

Enduron® **[US/Can]** see methyclothiazide on page 420

Enduron® **2.5 mg Tablet (Discontinued)** see page 814

Enduronyl® **[US/Can]** see methyclothiazide and deserpidine on page 420

Enduronyl® **Forte [US/Can]** see methyclothiazide and deserpidine on page 420

Enecat® **[US]** see radiological/contrast media (ionic) on page 561

Ener-B® **(Discontinued)** see page 814

enflurane (EN floo rane)
  U.S./Canadian Brand Names Ethrane® [US]
  Therapeutic Category General Anesthetic
  Use General induction and maintenance of anesthesia (inhalation)
  Usual Dosage Inhalation: 0.5% to 3%
  Dosage Forms Liquid: 125 mL, 250 mL

Engerix-B® **[US/Can]** see hepatitis B vaccine on page 320

Enisyl® **(Discontinued)** see page 814

Enkaid® **(Discontinued)** see page 814

Enlon® **[US/Can]** see edrophonium on page 223

Enomine® **(Discontinued)** see page 814

Enovid® **(Discontinued)** see page 814

Enovil® **(Discontinued)** see page 814

enoxaparin (ee noks a PA rin)
  U.S./Canadian Brand Names Lovenox® [US/Can]
  Therapeutic Category Anticoagulant (Other)
  Use Prophylaxis and treatment of thromboembolic disorders (deep vein thrombosis)
  Usual Dosage Adults: S.C.: 30 mg twice daily
  Dosage Forms
    Injection, as sodium [ampul; preservative free]: 30 mg/0.3 mL
    Injection, as sodium [graduated prefilled syringe; preservative free]: 60 mg/0.6 mL, 80 mg/0.8 mL, 90 mg/0.6 mL, 100 mg/mL, 120 mg/0.8 mL, 150 mg/mL
    Injection, as sodium [prefilled syringe; preservative free]: 30 mg/0.3 mL, 40 mg/0.4 mL

Enpresse™ **[US]** see ethinyl estradiol and levonorgestrel on page 248

Ensure Plus® **[US-OTC]** see nutritional formula, enteral/oral on page 472

Ensure® **[US-OTC]** see nutritional formula, enteral/oral on page 472

E.N.T.® **(Discontinued)** see page 814

entacapone (en TA ka pone)
  U.S./Canadian Brand Names Comtan® [US/Can]
  Therapeutic Category Anti-Parkinson's Agent; Reverse COMT Inhibitor
  Use Adjunct to levodopa/carbidopa therapy in patients with idiopathic Parkinson's disease who experience "wearing-off" symptoms at the end of a dosing interval
  Usual Dosage Adults: Oral: 200 mg dose, up to a maximum of 8 times/day; maximum daily dose: 1600 mg/day. Always administer with levodopa/carbidopa. To optimize therapy the levodopa/carbidopa dosage must be reduced, usually by 25%. This reduction is usually necessary when the patient is taking more than 800 mg of levodopa daily. (Continued)

entacapone *(Continued)*
Dosage Forms Tablet: 200 mg

Entertainer's Secret® **[US-OTC]** *see* saliva substitute *on page 582*

Entex® *(Discontinued)* *see page 814*

Entex® LA [US] *see* guaifenesin and phenylephrine *on page 310*

Entex® PSE [US] *see* guaifenesin and pseudoephedrine *on page 310*

Entocort™ EC [US/Can] *see* budesonide *on page 95*

Entozyme® *(Discontinued)* *see page 814*

Entrobar® [US] *see* radiological/contrast media (ionic) *on page 561*

Entrophen® [Can] *see* aspirin *on page 58*

Entsol® Mist [US-OTC] *see* sodium chloride *on page 595*

Entsol® Single Use [US-OTC] *see* sodium chloride *on page 595*

Entsol® [US-OTC] *see* sodium chloride *on page 595*

Entuss-D® Liquid *(Discontinued)* *see page 814*

Enulose® [US] *see* lactulose *on page 372*

Enzone® [US] *see* pramoxine and hydrocortisone *on page 535*

Epaxal Berna® [Can] *see* hepatitis A vaccine *on page 319*

EPEG *see* etoposide *on page 259*

ephedrine (e FED rin)
U.S./Canadian Brand Names Pretz-D® [US-OTC]
Therapeutic Category Adrenergic Agonist Agent
Use Bronchial asthma; nasal congestion; acute bronchospasm; acute hypotensive states
Usual Dosage
Children:
Oral, S.C.: 3 mg/kg/day or 25-100 mg/m^2/day in 4-6 divided doses every 4-6 hours
I.M., slow I.V. push: 0.2-0.3 mg/kg/dose every 4-6 hours
Adults:
Oral: 25-50 mg every 3-4 hours as needed
I.M., S.C.: 25-50 mg, parenteral adult dose should not exceed 150 mg in 24 hours
I.V.: 5-25 mg/dose slow I.V. push repeated after 5-10 minutes as needed, then every 3-4 hours not to exceed 150 mg/24 hours
Dosage Forms
Capsule, as sulfate: 25 mg, 50 mg
Injection, as sulfate: 50 mg/mL (1 mL)
Nasal spray, as sulfate (Pretz-D®): 0.25% (50 mL)

Epi-C® [US] *see* radiological/contrast media (ionic) *on page 561*

Epifoam® [US] *see* pramoxine and hydrocortisone *on page 535*

Epifrin® [US] *see* epinephrine *on this page*

E-Pilo-x® Ophthalmic *(Discontinued)* *see page 814*

Epinal® [US] *see* epinephryl borate *on page 230*

epinephrine (ep i NEF rin)
Synonyms adrenaline
U.S./Canadian Brand Names Adrenalin® Chloride [US/Can]; Bronchial Mist® [US];
Epifrin® [US]; EpiPen® Jr [US/Can]; EpiPen® [US/Can]; Primatene® Mist [US-OTC];
Vaponefrin® [Can]
Therapeutic Category Adrenergic Agonist Agent
Use Treatment of bronchospasm, anaphylactic reactions, cardiac arrest, and management of open-angle (chronic simple) glaucoma

Usual Dosage

Bronchodilator:

Children: S.C.: 10 mcg/kg (0.01 mL/kg of 1:1000) (single doses not to exceed 0.5 mg); injection suspension (1:200): 0.005 mL/kg/dose (0.025 mg/kg/dose) to a maximum of 0.15 mL (0.75 mg for single dose) every 8-12 hours

Adults:

I.M., S.C. (1:1000): 0.1-0.5 mg every 10-15 minutes to 4 hours

Suspension (1:200) S.C.: 0.1-0.3 mL (0.5-1.5 mg)

I.V.: 0.1-0.25 mg (single dose maximum: 1 mg)

Cardiac arrest:

Neonates: I.V. or intratracheal: 0.01-0.03 mg/kg (0.1-0.3 mL/kg of 1:10,000 solution) every 3-5 minutes as needed; dilute intratracheal doses in 1-2 mL of normal saline

Infants and Children: Asystole or pulseless arrest:

I.V., intraosseous: First dose: 0.01 mg/kg (0.1 mL/kg of a 1:10,000 solution); subsequent doses: 0.1 mg/kg (0.1 mL/kg of a 1:1000 solution); doses as high as 0.2 mg/kg may be effective; repeat every 3-5 minutes

Intratracheal: 0.1 mg/kg (0.1 mL/kg of a 1:1000 solution); doses as high as 0.2 mg/kg may be effective

Adults: Asystole:

I.V.: 1 mg every 3-5 minutes; if this approach fails, alternative regimens include: Intermediate: 2-5 mg every 3-5 minutes; Escalating: 1 mg, 3 mg, 5 mg at 3-minute intervals; High: 0.1 mg/kg every 3-5 minutes

Intratracheal: Although optimal dose is unknown, doses of 2-2.5 times the I.V. dose may be needed

Bradycardia: Children:

I.V.: 0.01 mg/kg (0.1 mL/kg of 1:10,000 solution) every 3-5 minutes as needed (maximum: 1 mg/10 mL)

Intratracheal: 0.1 mg/kg (0.1 mL/kg of 1:1000 solution every 3-5 minutes); doses as high as 0.2 mg/kg may be effective

Refractory hypotension (refractory to dopamine/dobutamine): I.V. infusion administration requires the use of an infusion pump:

Children: Infusion rate 0.1-4 mcg/kg/minute

Adults: I.V. infusion: 1 mg in 250 mL NS/D_5W at 0.1-1 mcg/kg/minute; titrate to desired effect

Hypersensitivity reaction:

Children: S.C.: 0.01 mg/kg every 15 minutes for 2 doses then every 4 hours as needed (single doses not to exceed 0.5 mg)

Adults: I.M., S.C.: 0.2-0.5 mg every 20 minutes to 4 hours (single dose maximum: 1 mg)

Nebulization:

Children <2 years: 0.25 mL of 1:1000 diluted in 3 mL NS with treatments ordered individually

Children >2 years and Adolescents: 0.5 mL of 1:1000 concentration diluted in 3 mL NS

Children >2 years and Adults (racemic epinephrine):

<10 kg: 2 mL of 1:8 dilution over 15 minutes every 1-4 hours

10-15 kg: 2 mL of 1:6 dilution over 15 minutes every 1-4 hours

15-20 kg: 2 mL of 1:4 dilution over 15 minutes every 1-4 hours

>20 kg: 2 mL of 1:3 dilution over 15 minutes every 1-4 hours

Adults: Instill 8-15 drops into nebulizer reservoirs; administer 1-3 inhalations 4-6 times/day

Ophthalmic: Instill 1-2 drops in eye(s) once or twice daily

Intranasal: Children ≥6 years and Adults: Apply locally as drops or spray or with sterile swab

Dosage Forms

Aerosol for oral inhalation (Primatene®): 0.2 mg/spray (15 mL, 22.5 mL)

Aerosol for oral inhalation, as bitartrate (AsthmaHaler®, Bronitin®, Primatene® Suspension): 0.3 mg/spray [epinephrine base 0.16 mg/spray] (10 mL, 15 mL, 22.5 mL)

(Continued)

epinephrine *(Continued)*

Auto-injector:
  EpiPen®: Delivers 0.3 mg I.M. of epinephrine 1:1000 (2 mL)
  EpiPen® Jr.: Delivers 0.15 mg I.M. of epinephrine 1:2000 (2 mL)
Injection (Adrenalin®): 1 mg/mL [1:1000] (2 mL)
Injection for solution: 0.1 mg/mL [1:10,000] (10 mL)
Injection for solution, pediatric: 0.1 mg/mL [1:10,000] (5 mL)
Injection for suspension (Sus-Phrine®): 5 mg/mL [1:200] (0.3 mL, 5 mL)
Solution for oral inhalation:
  Adrenalin®: 1% [10 mg/mL, 1:100] (7.5 mL)
  AsthmaNefrin®, microNefrin®: Racepinephrine 2% [epinephrine base 1.125%] (7.5 mL, 15 mL, 30 mL)
Nasal spray: 0.1% [1 mg/mL, 1:1000] (30 mL)
Solution, ophthalmic, as borate (Epinal®): 0.5% (7.5 mL); 1% (7.5 mL)
Solution, ophthalmic, as hydrochloride (Epifrin®, Glaucon®): 0.1% (1 mL); 0.5% (15 mL); 1% (10 mL, 15 mL); 2% (10 mL, 15 mL)

epinephrine and lidocaine *see* lidocaine and epinephrine *on page 384*

epinephrine and pilocarpine *see* pilocarpine and epinephrine *on page 515*

epinephryl borate (ep i NEF ril BOR ate)

U.S./Canadian Brand Names Epinal® [US]
Therapeutic Category Adrenergic Agonist Agent
Use Reduces elevated intraocular pressure in chronic open-angle glaucoma
Usual Dosage Adults: Ophthalmic: Instill 1 drop into the eyes once or twice daily
Dosage Forms Solution, ophthalmic: 0.5% (7.5 mL); 1% (7.5 mL)

EpiPen® [US/Can] *see* epinephrine *on page 228*

EpiPen® Jr [US/Can] *see* epinephrine *on page 228*

epirubicin (ep i ROO bi sin)

U.S./Canadian Brand Names Ellence™ [US/Can]; Pharmorubicin® [Can]
Therapeutic Category Antineoplastic Agent, Anthracycline; Antineoplastic Agent, Antibiotic
Use As a component of adjuvant therapy following primary resection of primary breast cancer in patients with evidence of axillary node tumor involvement
Usual Dosage Adults: I.V. (refer to individual protocols): 100-120 mg/m^2, repeated in 3- to 4-week cycles. The total dose of epirubicin may be given on Day 1 of each cycle or the dose may be divided equally and given on Day 1 and Day 8 of each cycle.
Dosage Forms Injection: 2 mg/mL (25 mL, 100 mL)

Epitol® [US] *see* carbamazepine *on page 113*

Epival® I.V. [Can] *see* valproic acid and derivatives *on page 670*

Epivir® [US] *see* lamivudine *on page 373*

Epivir®-HBV™ [US] *see* lamivudine *on page 373*

E.P. Mycin® Capsule *(Discontinued)* *see page 814*

EPO *see* epoetin alfa *on this page*

epoetin alfa (e POE e tin AL fa)

Synonyms EPO; erythropoietin; RHUEPO-α
U.S./Canadian Brand Names Epogen® [US]; Eprex® [Can]; Procrit® [US]
Therapeutic Category Colony-Stimulating Factor
Use Anemia associated with end-stage renal disease; anemia related to therapy with AZT-treated HIV-infected patients; anemia in cancer patients receiving chemotherapy; anemia of prematurity

Usual Dosage

In patients on dialysis, epoetin alfa usually has been administered as an I.V. bolus 3 times/week; while the administration is independent of the dialysis procedure, it may be administered into the venous line at the end of the dialysis procedure to obviate the need for additional venous access. In patients with CRF not on dialysis, epoetin alfa may be administered either as an I.V. or S.C. injection.

AZT-treated HIV-infected patients: I.V., S.C.: Initial: 100 units/kg/dose 3 times/week for 8 weeks; after 8 weeks of therapy the dose can be adjusted by 50-100 units/kg increments 3 times/week to a maximum dose of 300 units/kg 3 times/week; if the hematocrit exceeds 40%, the dose should be discontinued until the hematocrit drops to 36%

Anemia of prematurity: S.C.: 25-100 units/kg/dose 3 times/week

Dosage Forms

Solution [multidose vial; with preservative]: 20,000 units/mL (1 mL)
Solution [single-dose vial; preservative free]: 2000 units/mL (1 mL); 3000 units/mL (1 mL); 4000 units/mL (1 mL); 10,000 units/mL (1 mL); 40,000 units/mL (1 mL)
Solution [multidose vial; with preservative]: 10,000 units/mL (2 mL)

Epogen® [US] *see* epoetin alfa *on previous page*

epoprostenol (e poe PROST en ole)

U.S./Canadian Brand Names Flolan® [US/Can]
Therapeutic Category Platelet Inhibitor
Use Long-term intravenous treatment of primary pulmonary hypertension (PPH)
Usual Dosage I.V. continuous infusion: 2 ng/kg/minute
Dosage Forms Injection, as sodium [with 50 mL sterile diluent]: 0.5 mg/vial, 1.5 mg/vial

Eprex® [Can] *see* epoetin alfa *on previous page*

eprosartan (ep roe SAR tan)

U.S./Canadian Brand Names Teveten® [US]
Therapeutic Category Angiotensin II Receptor Antagonist
Use Treatment of hypertension; may be used alone or in combination with other antihypertensives
Usual Dosage Adults: Oral: Dosage must be individualized; can administer once or twice daily with total daily doses of 400-800 mg. Usual starting dose is 600 mg once daily as monotherapy in patients who are euvolemic. Limited clinical experience with doses >800 mg.
Dosage Forms
Tablet: 600 mg
Tablet, scored: 400 mg

epsom salts *see* magnesium sulfate *on page 398*

EPT *see* teniposide *on page 622*

eptacog alfa (activated) *(Canada only)* (EP ta cog AL fa AK ti vay ted)

Synonyms activated recombinant human blood coagulation factor VII
U.S./Canadian Brand Names NiaStase® [Can]
Therapeutic Category Coagulation Factor
Use In hemophilia A/B patients with inhibitors to FVIII or FIX, respectively, for the treatment of bleeding episodes (including treatment and prevention of those occurring during and after surgery). Based on the data obtained so far with eptacog alfa (activated) in the treatment of hemophilia patients with inhibitors, the apparent lack of anamnestic response during and after exposure to eptacog alfa (activated) makes it suitable for use in all inhibitor patients.
Usual Dosage Eptacog alfa (activated) is intended for I.V. bolus administration only. The recommended dose range, dose, frequency, and duration of eptacog alfa (activated) administration as a single agent. Evaluation of hemostasis should be used to determine
(Continued)

eptacog alfa (activated) *(Canada only)* *(Continued)*

the effectiveness of eptacog alfa (activated) and to provide a basis for modification of the eptacog alfa (activated) treatment schedule. Coagulation parameters should not be used to evaluate eptacog alfa (activated) effectiveness.

Dosage Forms Injection: Each vial of sterile, white lyophilized powder for reconstitution, contains: Eptacog alfa (activated) 1.2 mg, 2.4 mg, 4.8 mg

eptifibatide (ep TIF i ba tide)

U.S./Canadian Brand Names Integrilin® [US/Can]

Therapeutic Category Antiplatelet Agent

Use Treatment of patients with acute coronary syndrome (UA/NQMI), including patients who are to be managed medically and those undergoing percutaneous coronary intervention (PCI); it has been shown to decrease the rate of a combined endpoint of death or new myocardial infarction. For the treatment of patients undergoing PCI, it has been shown to decrease the rate of a combined endpoint of death, new myocardial infarction, or need for urgent intervention.

Usual Dosage Adults: I.V.:

Acute coronary syndrome: Bolus of 180 mcg/kg as soon as possible following diagnosis, followed by a continuous infusion of 2 mcg/kg/minute until hospital discharge or initiation of CABG surgery, up to 72 hours. If a patient is to undergo a percutaneous coronary intervention (PCI) while receiving eptifibatide, consideration can be given to decreasing the infusion rate to 0.5 mcg/kg/minute (the infusion rate in IMPACT II) at the time of the procedure. Infusion should be continued for an additional 20-24 hours after the procedure, allowing for up to 96 hours of therapy.

Percutaneous coronary intervention (PCI) in patients not presenting with an acute coronary syndrome: Bolus of 135 mcg/kg administered immediately before the initiation of PCI followed by a continuous infusion of 0.5 mcg/kg/minute for 20-24 hours. In the IMPACT II Study, there was little experience in patients weighing more than 143 kg.

Dosage Forms Injection: 0.75 mg/mL (100 mL); 2 mg/mL (10 mL, 100 mL)

Equagesic® [US] *see* aspirin and meprobamate *on page 59*

Equalactin® Chewable Tablet [US-OTC] *see* calcium polycarbophil *on page 108*

Equanil® *(Discontinued)* *see page 814*

Equilet® *(Discontinued)* *see page 814*

Ercaf® *(Discontinued)* *see page 814*

Ergamisol® [US/Can] *see* levamisole *on page 378*

ergocalciferol (er goe kal SIF e role)

Synonyms activated ergosterol; viosterol; vitamin D_2

U.S./Canadian Brand Names Calciferol™ [US]; Drisdol® [US/Can]; Ostoforte® [Can]

Therapeutic Category Vitamin D Analog

Use Refractory rickets; hypophosphatemia; hypoparathyroidism

Usual Dosage

Dietary supplementation: Oral:
Premature infants: 10-20 mcg/day (400-800 units), up to 750 mcg/day (30,000 units)
Infants and healthy Children: 10 mcg/day (400 units)
Renal failure: Oral:
Children: 0.1-1 mg/day (4000-40,000 units)
Adults: 0.5 mg/day (20,000 units)
Hypoparathyroidism: Oral:
Children: 1.25-5 mg/day (50,000-200,000 units) and calcium supplements
Adults: 625 mcg to 5 mg/day (25,000-200,000 units) and calcium supplements
Vitamin D-dependent rickets: Oral:
Children: 75-125 mcg/day (3000-5000 units)
Adults: 250 mcg to 1.5 mg/day (10,000-60,000 units)

Nutritional rickets and osteomalacia:
Oral:
 Children and Adults (with normal absorption): 25 mcg/day (1000 units)
 Children with malabsorption: 250-625 mcg/day (10,000-25,000 units)
 I.M.: Adults: 250 mcg/day
Dosage Forms
 Capsule (Drisdol®): 50,000 units [1.25 mg]
 Injection (Calciferol™): 500,000 units/mL [12.5 mg/mL] (1 mL)
 Liquid (Calciferol™, Drisdol®): 8000 units/mL [200 mcg/mL] (60 mL)

ergoloid mesylates (ER goe loid MES i lates)

Synonyms dihydroergotoxine; hydrogenated ergot alkaloids
U.S./Canadian Brand Names Germinal® [US]; Hydergine® LC [US]; Hydergine® [US/Can]
Therapeutic Category Ergot Alkaloid and Derivative
Use Treatment of cerebrovascular insufficiency in primary progressive dementia, Alzheimer's dementia, and senile onset
Usual Dosage Adults: Oral: 1 mg 3 times/day up to 4.5-12 mg/day; up to 6 months of therapy may be necessary
Dosage Forms
 Capsule, liquid (Hydergine® LC): 1 mg
 Liquid (Hydergine®): 1 mg/mL (100 mL)
 Tablet (Hydergine®): 1 mg
 Tablet, sublingual (Gerimal®, Hydergine®): 0.5 mg, 1 mg

Ergomar® *(Discontinued)* see page 814

ergonovine (er goe NOE veen)

U.S./Canadian Brand Names Ergotrate® Maleate Injection [US]
Therapeutic Category Ergot Alkaloid and Derivative
Use Prevention and treatment of postpartum and postabortion hemorrhage caused by uterine atony or subinvolution
Usual Dosage Adults:
 Oral: 1-2 tablets (0.2-0.4 mg) every 6-12 hours for up to 48 hours
 I.M., I.V. (I.V. should be reserved for emergency use only): 0.2 mg, repeat dose in 2-4 hours as needed
Dosage Forms
 Injection, as maleate: 0.2 mg/mL (1 mL)
 Tablet, as maleate: 0.2 mg

Ergostat® *(Discontinued)* see page 814

ergotamine (er GOT a meen)

Synonyms ergotamine tartrate; ergotamine tartrate and caffeine; ergotamine tartrate with belladonna alkaloids, and phenobarbital
U.S./Canadian Brand Names Cafergot® [US/Can]; Wigraine® [US]
Therapeutic Category Ergot Alkaloid and Derivative
Use Prevent or abort vascular headaches, such as migraine or cluster
Usual Dosage
 Older Children and Adolescents: Oral: 1 tablet at onset of attack; then 1 tablet every 30 minutes as needed, up to a maximum of 3 tablets per attack
 Adults:
 Oral (Cafergot®): 2 tablets at onset of attack; then 1 tablet every 30 minutes as needed; maximum: 6 tablets per attack; do not exceed 10 tablets/week
 Oral (Ergostat®): 1 tablet under tongue at first sign, then 1 tablet every 30 minutes, 3 tablets/24 hours, 5 tablets/week
(Continued)

ergotamine *(Continued)*

Rectal (Cafergot® suppositories, Wigraine® suppositories, Cafatine-PB® suppositories): 1 at first sign of an attack; follow with second dose after 1 hour, if needed; maximum dose: 2 per attack; do not exceed 5/week

Dosage Forms

Suppository, rectal (Cafergot®): Ergotamine tartrate 2 mg and caffeine 100 mg (12s)

Tablet (Cafergot®, Wigraine®): Ergotamine tartrate 1 mg and caffeine 100 mg

Tablet, sublingual (Ergomar®): Ergotamine tartrate 2 mg

ergotamine tartrate *see* ergotamine *on previous page*

ergotamine tartrate and caffeine *see* ergotamine *on previous page*

Ergotamine Tartrate and Caffeine Cafatine® *(Discontinued)* *see page 814*

ergotamine tartrate, belladonna, and phenobarbital *see* belladonna, phenobarbital, and ergotamine tartrate *on page 74*

ergotamine tartrate with belladonna alkaloids, and phenobarbital *see* ergotamine *on previous page*

Ergotrate® Maleate Injection [US] *see* ergonovine *on previous page*

Eridium® *(Discontinued)* *see page 814*

E•R•O Ear [US-OTC] *see* carbamide peroxide *on page 113*

ertapenem (er ta PEN em)

Synonyms ertapenem sodium; L-749,345; MK-0826

U.S./Canadian Brand Names Invanz™ [US]

Therapeutic Category Antibiotic, Carbapenem

Use Treatment of moderate-severe, complicated intra-abdominal infections, skin and skin structure infections, pyelonephritis, acute pelvic infections, and community-acquired pneumonia. Antibacterial coverage includes aerobic gram-positive organisms, aerobic gram-negative organisms, anaerobic organisms.

Methicillin-resistant *Staphylococcus*, *Enterococcus* spp, penicillin-resistant strains of *Streptococcus pneumoniae,* beta-lactamase-positive strains of *Haemophilus influenzae* are **resistant** to ertapenem, as are most *Pseudomonas aeruginosa*.

Usual Dosage Adults: I.V., I.M.: **Note:** I.V. therapy may be administered for up to 14 days; I.M. for up to 7 days

Intra-abdominal infection: 1 g/day for 5-14 days

Skin and skin structure infections: 1 g/day for 7-14 days

Community-acquired pneumonia: 1 g/day; duration of total antibiotic treatment: 10-14 days

Urinary tract infections/pyelonephritis: 1 g/day; duration of total antibiotic treatment: 10-14 days

Acute pelvic infections: 1 g/day for 3-10 days

Dosage Forms Injection, powder for reconstitution, as sodium: 1 g

ertapenem sodium *see* ertapenem *on this page*

Erybid™ [Can] *see* erythromycin (systemic) *on next page*

Eryc® [US/Can] *see* erythromycin (systemic) *on next page*

Erycette® [US] *see* erythromycin (ophthalmic/topical) *on next page*

EryDerm® [US] *see* erythromycin (ophthalmic/topical) *on next page*

Erygel® [US] *see* erythromycin (ophthalmic/topical) *on next page*

EryPed® [US] *see* erythromycin (systemic) *on next page*

Ery-Sol® Topical Solution *(Discontinued)* *see page 814*

Ery-Tab® [US] *see* erythromycin (systemic) *on next page*

Erythra-Derm™ [US] *see* erythromycin (ophthalmic/topical) *on next page*

Erythrocin® **[US/Can]** *see* erythromycin (systemic) *on this page*

erythromycin and benzoyl peroxide
(er ith roe MYE sin & BEN zoe il per OKS ide)
Synonyms benzoyl peroxide and erythromycin
U.S./Canadian Brand Names Benzamycin® [US]
Therapeutic Category Acne Products
Use Topical control of acne vulgaris
Usual Dosage Topical: Apply twice daily (morning and evening)
Dosage Forms Gel: Erythromycin 30 mg and benzoyl peroxide 50 mg per g (23 g, 47 g)

erythromycin and sulfisoxazole (er ith roe MYE sin & sul fi SOKS a zole)
Synonyms sulfisoxazole and erythromycin
U.S./Canadian Brand Names Eryzole® [US]; Pediazole® [US/Can]
Therapeutic Category Macrolide (Antibiotic); Sulfonamide
Use Treatment of susceptible bacterial infections of the upper and lower respiratory tract; otitis media in children caused by susceptible strains of *Haemophilus influenzae*; other infections in patients allergic to penicillin
Usual Dosage Dosage recommendation is based on the product's erythromycin content; Oral:
Children ≥2 months: 40-50 mg/kg/day of erythromycin in divided doses every 6-8 hours; not to exceed 2 g erythromycin or 6 g sulfisoxazole/day or approximately 1.25 mL/kg/day divided every 6-8 hours
Adults: 400 mg erythromycin and 1200 mg sulfisoxazole every 6 hours
Dosage Forms Suspension, oral: Erythromycin ethylsuccinate 200 mg and sulfisoxazole acetyl 600 mg per 5 mL (100 mL, 150 mL, 200 mL, 250 mL)

erythromycin (ophthalmic/topical)
(er ith roe MYE sin op THAL mik/TOP i kal)
U.S./Canadian Brand Names Akne-Mycin® [US]; A/T/S® [US]; Emgel® [US]; Erycette® [US]; EryDerm® [US]; Erygel® [US]; Erythra-Derm™ [US]; Romycin® [US]; Staticin® [US]; Theramycin Z® [US]; T-Stat® [US]
Therapeutic Category Acne Products; Antibiotic, Ophthalmic; Antibiotic, Topical
Use Topical treatment of acne vulgaris
Usual Dosage Children and Adults:
Ophthalmic: Instill one or more times daily depending on the severity of the infection
Topical: Apply 2% solution over the affected area twice daily after the skin has been thoroughly washed and patted dry
Dosage Forms
Gel, topical: 2% (30 g, 60 g)
A/T/S®: 2% (30 g)
Emgel®: 2% (27 g, 50 g)
Erygel®: 2% (30 g, 60 g)
Ointment, ophthalmic: 0.5% [5 mg/g] (1 g, 3.5 g)
Romycin®: 0.5% [5 mg/g] (3.5 g)
Ointment, topical (Akne-Mycin®): 2% (25 g)
Solution, topical: 1.5% (60 mL); 2% (60 mL)
Staticin®: 1.5% (60 mL)
A/T/S/®, EryDerm®, Erythra-Derm™, T-Stat®, Theramycin™ Z: 2% (60 mL)
Swab (Erycette®, T-Stat®): 2% (60s)

erythromycin (systemic) (er ith roe MYE sin sis TEM ik)
U.S./Canadian Brand Names Apo®-Erythro Base [Can]; Apo®-Erythro E-C [Can]; Apo®-Erythro-ES [Can]; Apo®-Erythro-S [Can]; Diomycin® [Can]; E.E.S.® [US/Can]; Erybid™ [Can]; Eryc® [US/Can]; EryPed® [US]; Ery-Tab® [US]; Erythrocin® [US/Can]; Nu-Erythromycin-S [Can]; PCE® [US/Can]; PMS-Erythromycin [Can]
Therapeutic Category Macrolide (Antibiotic)
(Continued)

erythromycin (systemic) *(Continued)*

Use Treatment of mild to moderately severe infections of the upper and lower respiratory tract, pharyngitis and skin infections due to susceptible streptococci and staphylococci; other susceptible bacterial infections including *Mycoplasma* pneumonia, *Legionella* pneumonia, diphtheria, pertussis, chancroid, *Chlamydia*, and *Campylobacter* gastroenteritis; used in conjunction with neomycin for decontaminating the bowel for surgery; dental procedure prophylaxis in penicillin allergic patients

Usual Dosage

Infants and Children:

Oral: Do not exceed 2 g/day

Base and ethylsuccinate: 30-50 mg/kg/day divided every 6-8 hours

Estolate: 30-50 mg/kg/day divided every 8-12 hours

Stearate: 20-40 mg/kg/day divided every 6 hours

Pre-op bowel preparation: 20 mg/kg erythromycin base at 1, 2, and 11 PM on the day before surgery combined with mechanical cleansing of the large intestine and oral neomycin

I.V.: Lactobionate: 20-40 mg/kg/day divided every 6 hours, not to exceed 4 g/day

Adults:

Oral:

Base: 333 mg every 8 hours

Estolate, stearate or base: 250-500 mg every 6-12 hours

Ethylsuccinate: 400-800 mg every 6-12 hours

Pre-op bowel preparation: 1 g erythromycin base at 1, 2, and 11 PM on the day before surgery combined with mechanical cleansing of the large intestine and oral neomycin

I.V.: 15-20 mg/kg/day divided every 6 hours or administered as a continuous infusion over 24 hours

Dosage Forms

Capsule, delayed release, enteric-coated pellets, as base (Eryc®): 250 mg

Granules for oral suspension, as ethylsuccinate (E.E.S.®): 200 mg/5 mL (100 mL, 200 mL) [cherry flavor]

Injection, powder for reconstitution, as lactobionate (Erythrocin®): 500 mg, 1 g

Powder for oral suspension, as ethylsuccinate (Ery-Ped®): 200 mg/5 mL (5 mL, 100 mL, 200 mL) [fruit flavor]; 400 mg/5 mL (5 mL, 60 mL, 100 mL, 200 mL) [banana flavor]

Powder for oral suspension, as ethylsuccinate [drops] (Ery-Ped®): 100 mg/2.5 mL (50 mL) [fruit flavor]

Suspension, oral, as estolate: 125 mg/5 mL (480 mL); 250 mg/5 mL (480 mL) [orange flavor]

Suspension, oral, as ethylsuccinate: 200 mg/5 mL (480 mL); 400 mg/5 mL (480 mL)

E.E.S.®: 200 mg/5 mL (100 mL, 480 mL) [fruit flavor]; 400 mg/5 mL (100 mL, 480 mL) [orange flavor]

Tablet, chewable, as ethylsuccinate (EryPed®): 200 mg [fruit flavor]

Tablet, delayed release, enteric coated, as base (Ery-Tab®): 250 mg, 333 mg, 500 mg

Tablet, film coated, as base: 250 mg, 500 mg

Tablet, film coated, as ethylsuccinate (E.E.S.®): 400 mg

Tablet, film coated, as stearate (Erythrocin®): 250 mg, 500 mg

Tablet, polymer-coated particles, as base (PCE®): 333 mg, 500 mg

erythropoiesis stimulating protein *see* darbepoetin alfa *on page 175*

erythropoietin *see* epoetin alfa *on page 230*

Eryzole® [US] *see* erythromycin and sulfisoxazole *on previous page*

escitalopram (es sye TAL oh pram)

Synonyms Lu-26-054; S-Citalopram

U.S./Canadian Brand Names Lexapro™ [US]

Therapeutic Category Antidepressant, Selective Serotonin Reuptake Inhibitor

Use Treatment of major depressive disorder

Usual Dosage Oral:
  Adults: Depression: Initial: 10 mg/day; dose may be increased to 20 mg/day after at least 1 week
Dosage Forms Tablet: 5 mg, 10 mg, 20 mg

Esclim® **[US]** *see* estradiol *on next page*

Esgic® **[US]** *see* butalbital, acetaminophen, and caffeine *on page 99*

Esgic-Plus™ **[US]** *see* butalbital, acetaminophen, and caffeine *on page 99*

Esidrix® *(Discontinued) see page 814*

Eskalith® **[US]** *see* lithium *on page 388*

Eskalith CR® **[US]** *see* lithium *on page 388*

esmolol (ES moe lol)

U.S./Canadian Brand Names Brevibloc® [US/Can]
Therapeutic Category Antiarrhythmic Agent, Class II; Beta-Adrenergic Blocker
Use Supraventricular tachycardia (primarily to control ventricular rate) and hypertension (especially perioperatively)
Usual Dosage Must be adjusted to individual response and tolerance
  Children: An extremely limited amount of information regarding esmolol use in pediatric patients is currently available. Some centers have utilized doses of 100-500 mcg/kg administered over 1 minute for control of supraventricular tachycardias. Loading doses of 500 mcg/kg/minute over 1 minute with maximal doses of 50-250 mcg/kg/minute (mean 173) have been used in addition to nitroprusside in a small number of patients (7 patients; 7-19 years of age; median 13 years) to treat postoperative hypertension after coarctation of aorta repair.
  Adults: I.V.: Loading dose: 500 mcg/kg over 1 minute; follow with a 50 mcg/kg/minute infusion for 4 minutes; if response is inadequate, rebolus with another 500 mcg/kg loading dose over 1 minute, and increase the maintenance infusion to 100 mcg/kg/minute. Repeat this process until a therapeutic effect has been achieved or to a maximum recommended maintenance dose of 200 mcg/kg/minute. Usual dosage range: 50-200 mcg/kg/minute with average dose = 100 mcg/kg/minute.
Dosage Forms Injection, as hydrochloride: 10 mg/mL (10 mL); 250 mg/mL (10 mL)

E-Solve-2® **Topical** *(Discontinued) see page 814*

esomeprazole (es oh ME pray zol)

Synonyms esomeprazole magnesium
U.S./Canadian Brand Names Nexium™ [US]
Therapeutic Category Proton Pump Inhibitor
Use Short-term (4-8 weeks) treatment of erosive esophagitis; maintaining symptom resolution and healing of erosive esophagitis; treatment of symptomatic gastroesophageal reflux disease; as part of a multidrug regimen for *Helicobacter pylori* eradication in patients with duodenal ulcer disease (active or history of within the past 5 years)
Usual Dosage Note: Delayed-release capsules should be swallowed whole and taken at least 1 hour before eating
  Children: Safety and efficacy have not been established in pediatric patients
  Adults: Oral:
    Erosive esophagitis (healing): 20-40 mg once daily for 4-8 weeks; maintenance: 20 mg once daily
    Symptomatic GERD: 20 mg once daily for 4 weeks
    H. pylori eradication: 40 mg once daily **with** amoxicillin 1000 mg twice daily **and** clarithromycin 500 mg twice daily for a total of 10 days
Dosage Forms Capsule, delayed release: 20 mg, 40 mg

esomeprazole magnesium *see* esomeprazole *on this page*

Esoterica® **Facial [US-OTC]** *see* hydroquinone *on page 336*

Esoterica® Regular [US-OTC] *see* hydroquinone *on page 336*

Esoterica® Sensitive Skin Formula [US-OTC] *see* hydroquinone *on page 336*

Esoterica® Sunscreen [US-OTC] *see* hydroquinone *on page 336*

Estar® [US/Can] *see* coal tar *on page 158*

estazolam (es TA zoe lam)

U.S./Canadian Brand Names ProSom™ [US]
Therapeutic Category Benzodiazepine
Controlled Substance C-IV
Use Short-term management of insomnia
Usual Dosage Adults: Oral: 1 mg at bedtime, some patients may require 2 mg
Dosage Forms Tablet: 1 mg, 2 mg

esterified estrogen and methyltestosterone *see* estrogens and methyltestosterone *on page 241*

esterified estrogens *see* estrogens (esterified) *on page 242*

Estinyl® [US] *see* ethinyl estradiol *on page 244*

Estivin® II Ophthalmic *(Discontinued)* *see page 814*

Estrace® [US/Can] *see* estradiol *on this page*

Estraderm® [US/Can] *see* estradiol *on this page*

estradiol (es tra DYE ole)

Synonyms estradiol hemihydrate
U.S./Canadian Brand Names Alora® [US]; Climara® [US/Can]; Delestrogen® [US/Can]; Depo®-Estradiol [US/Can]; Esclim® [US]; Estrace® [US/Can]; Estraderm® [US/Can]; Estring® [US/Can]; Estrogel® [Can]; Gynodiol™ [US]; Oesclim® [Can]; Vagifem® [US/Can]; Vivelle-Dot® [US]; Vivelle® [US/Can]
Therapeutic Category Estrogen Derivative
Use Atrophic vaginitis, atrophic dystrophy of vulva, menopausal symptoms, female hypogonadism
Usual Dosage Adults (all dosage needs to be adjusted based upon the patient's response):

Male: Prostate cancer: Valerate:
I.M.: ≥30 mg or more every 1-2 weeks
Oral: 1-2 mg 3 times/day
Female:
Hypogonadism:
Oral: 1-2 mg/day in a cyclic regimen for 3 weeks on drug, then 1 week off drug
I.M.: Cypionate: 1.5-2 mg/month; valerate: 10-20 mg/month
Transdermal: 0.05 mg patch initially (titrate dosage to response) applied twice weekly in a cyclic regimen, for 3 weeks on drug and 1 week off drug
Atrophic vaginitis, kraurosis vulvae: Vaginal: Insert 2-4 g/day for 2 weeks then gradually reduce to ½ the initial dose for 2 weeks followed by a maintenance dose of 1 g 1-3 times/week
Moderate to severe vasomotor symptoms: I.M.:
Cypionate: 1-5 mg every 3-4 weeks
Valerate: 10-20 mg every 4 weeks
Postpartum breast engorgement: I.M.: Valerate: 10-25 mg at end of first stage of labor
Dosage Forms
Cream, vaginal (Estrace®): 0.1 mg/g (42.5 g)
Injection, as cypionate (Depo®-Estradiol): 5 mg/mL (5 mL) [chlorobutanol as preservative; in cottonseed oil]
Injection, as valerate: 20 mg/mL (10 mL); 40 mg/mL (10 mL) [may contain benzyl alcohol; may be in castor oil]

Delestrogen®:
  10 mg/mL (5 mL) [chlorobutanol as preservative; in sesame oil]
  20 mg/mL (5 mL) [contains benzyl alcohol; in castor oil]
  40 mg/mL (5 mL) [contains benzyl alcohol; in castor oil]
Ring, vaginal (Estring®): 2 mg [gradually released over 90 days]
Tablet, micronized:
  Estrace®: 0.5 mg, 1 mg, 2 mg
  Gynodiol™: 0.5 mg, 1 mg, 1.5 mg, 2 mg
Tablet, vaginal (Vagifem®): 25.8 mcg of estradiol hemihydrate [equivalent to 25 mcg estradiol]
Transdermal system:
  Alora®:
    0.025 mg/24 hours [9 cm^2] [total estradiol 0.75 mg]
    0.05 mg/24 hours [18 cm^2] [total estradiol 1.5 mg]
    0.075 mg/24 hours [27 cm^2] [total estradiol 2.3 mg]
    0.1 mg/24 hours [36 cm^2] [total estradiol 3 mg]
  Climara®:
    0.025 mg/24 hours [6.5 cm^2] [total estradiol 2.04 mg]
    0.05 mg/24 hours [12.5 cm^2] [total estradiol 3.9 mg]
    0.075 mg/24 hours [18.75 cm^2] [total estradiol 5.85 mg]
    0.1 mg/24 hours [25 cm^2] [total estradiol 7.8 mg]
  Esclim®, Vivelle®:
    0.025 mg/day
    0.0375 mg/day
    0.05 mg/day
    0.075 mg/day
    0.1 mg/day
  Estraderm®:
    0.05 mg/24 hours [10 cm^2] [total estradiol 4 mg]
    0.1 mg/24 hours [20 cm^2] [total estradiol 8 mg]
  Vivelle-Dot®:
    0.025 mg/day
    0.0375 mg/day
    0.05 mg/day
    0.075 mg/day
    0.1 mg/day

estradiol and NGM *see* estradiol and norgestimate *on this page*

estradiol and norethindrone (es tra DYE ole & nor eth IN drone)
U.S./Canadian Brand Names Activella™ [US]; CombiPatch™ [US]
Therapeutic Category Estrogen and Progestin Combination
Use Treatment of moderate to severe vasomotor symptoms associated with menopause; treatment of vulvar and vaginal atrophy
Usual Dosage Adults: Oral: Take one tablet daily
Dosage Forms
  Tablet (Activella™): Estradiol 1 mg and norethindrone acetate 0.5 mg (28s)
  Transdermal system (CombiPatch™):
  9 sq cm: Estradiol 0.05 mg and norethindrone acetate 0.14 mg per day
  16 sq cm: Estradiol 0.05 mg and norethindrone acetate 0.25 mg per day

estradiol and norgestimate (es tra DYE ole & nor JES ti mate)
Synonyms estradiol and NGM; norgestimate and estradiol
U.S./Canadian Brand Names Ortho-Prefest® [US]
Therapeutic Category Estrogen and Progestin Combination
Use Women with an intact uterus: Treatment of moderate to severe vasomotor symptoms associated with menopause; treatment of atrophic vaginitis; prevention of osteoporosis
Usual Dosage Oral: Adults: Females with an intact uterus:
  (Continued)

estradiol and norgestimate *(Continued)*

Treatment of menopausal symptoms, atrophic vaginitis: Treatment is cyclical and consists of the following: One tablet of estradiol 1 mg (pink tablet) once daily for 3 days, followed by 1 tablet of estradiol 1 mg and norgestimate 0.09 mg (white tablet) once daily for 3 days; repeat sequence continuously. **Note:** This dose may not be the lowest effective combination for these indications. In case of a missed tablet, restart therapy with next available tablet in sequence (taking only 1 tablet each day).

Prevention of osteoporosis: See "Treatment of menopausal symptoms"

Dosage Forms Tablet: Estradiol 1 mg [15 pink tablets] and estradiol 1 mg and norgestimate 0.09 mg [15 white tablets] (supplied in blister card of 30)

estradiol and testosterone (es tra DYE ole & tes TOS ter one)

U.S./Canadian Brand Names Climacteron® [Can]; Depo-Testadiol® [US]; Valertest No.1® [US]

Therapeutic Category Estrogen and Androgen Combination

Use Vasomotor symptoms associated with menopause; postpartum breast engorgement

Usual Dosage Adults (all dosage needs to be adjusted based upon the patient's response)

Dosage Forms

Injection [in oil]:

Depo-Testadiol®, Depotestogen®: Estradiol cypionate 2 mg and testosterone cypionate 50 mg per mL (10 mL) [in cottonseed oil]

Valertest No.1®: Estradiol valerate 4 mg and testosterone enanthate 90 mg per mL (10 mL) [in sesame oil]

estradiol cypionate and medroxyprogesterone acetate

(es tra DYE ole sip pe OH nate & me DROKS ee proe JES te rone AS e tate)

U.S./Canadian Brand Names Lunelle™ [US]

Therapeutic Category Contraceptive

Use Prevention of pregnancy

Usual Dosage Adults: Female: I.M.: 0.5 mL

First dose: Within first 5 days of menstrual period or within 5 days of a complete first trimester abortion; do not administer <4 weeks postpartum **if not breast-feeding** or <6 weeks postpartum **if breast-feeding**

Maintenance dose: Monthly, every 28-30 days following previous injection; do not exceed 33 days; pregnancy must be ruled out if >33 days have past between injections; bleeding episodes cannot be used to guide injection schedule; shortening schedule may lead to menstrual pattern changes

Switching from other forms of contraception: First injection should be given within 7 days of last active oral contraceptive pill; when switching from other methods, timing of injection should ensure continuous contraceptive coverage

Dosage Forms Injection, suspension: Estradiol cypionate 5 mg and medroxyprogesterone acetate 25 mg per 0.5 mL

estradiol hemihydrate *see* estradiol *on page 238*

Estradurin® Injection *(Discontinued)* *see page 814*

Estra-L® Injection *(Discontinued)* *see page 814*

estramustine (es tra MUS teen)

U.S./Canadian Brand Names Emcyt® [US/Can]

Therapeutic Category Antineoplastic Agent

Use Palliative treatment of prostatic carcinoma

Usual Dosage Oral: 1 capsule for each 22 lb/day, in 3-4 divided doses

Dosage Forms Capsule, as phosphate sodium: 140 mg

Estratab® [US] *see* estrogens (esterified) *on page 242*

Estratest® [US] *see* estrogens and methyltestosterone *on next page*

Estratest® H.S. [US] *see* estrogens and methyltestosterone *on this page*

Estring® [US/Can] *see* estradiol *on page 238*

Estro-Cyp® Injection *(Discontinued)* *see page 814*

Estrogel® [Can] *see* estradiol *on page 238*

estrogenic substance aqueous *see* estrone *on next page*

estrogens and medroxyprogesterone
(ES troe jenz & me DROKS ee proe JES te rone)

Synonyms medroxyprogesterone and estrogens

U.S./Canadian Brand Names Premphase® [US/Can]; Prempro™ [US/Can]

Therapeutic Category Estrogen and Progestin Combination

Use Women with an intact uterus for the treatment of moderate to severe vasomotor symptoms associated with the menopause; treatment of atrophic vaginitis; primary ovarian failure; osteoporosis prophylactic

Usual Dosage Adults: Oral:

Premphase®: Conjugated estrogen 0.625 mg [Premarin®] and taken orally for 28 days and medroxyprogesterone acetate [Cycrin®] 5 mg (14s) which are taken orally with a Premarin® tablet on days 15 through 28

Prempro™: Conjugated estrogen 0.625 mg [Premarin®] and medroxyprogesterone acetate [Cycrin®] 2.5 mg are taken continuously one each day

Dosage Forms

Tablet:

Premphase® [therapy pack contains 2 separate tablets]: Conjugated estrogens 0.625 mg (14s) and conjugated estrogen 0.625 mg/medroxyprogesterone acetate 5 mg (14s)

Prempro™:

Conjugated estrogens 0.625 mg and medroxyprogesterone acetate 2.5 mg (28s)

Conjugated estrogens 0.625 mg and medroxyprogesterone acetate 5 mg (28s)

estrogens and methyltestosterone
(ES troe jenz & meth il tes TOS te rone)

Synonyms conjugated estrogen and methyltestosterone; esterified estrogen and methyltestosterone

U.S./Canadian Brand Names Estratest® H.S. [US]; Estratest® [US]

Therapeutic Category Estrogen and Androgen Combination

Use Atrophic vaginitis; hypogonadism; primary ovarian failure; vasomotor symptoms of menopause; prostatic carcinoma; osteoporosis prophylactic

Usual Dosage Oral: Lowest dose that will control symptoms should be chosen, normally administered 3 weeks on and 1 week off

Dosage Forms

Tablet:

Estratest®: Esterified estrogen 1.25 mg and methyltestosterone 2.5 mg

Estratest® H.S.: Esterified estrogen 0.625 mg and methyltestosterone 1.25 mg

estrogens (conjugated A/synthetic)
(ES troe jenz KON joo gate ed aye/sin THET ik)

U.S./Canadian Brand Names Cenestin™ [US/Can]

Therapeutic Category Estrogen Derivative

Use Treatment of moderate to severe vasomotor symptoms of menopause

Usual Dosage Moderate to severe vasomotor symptoms: Oral: 0.625 mg/day; may be titrated up to 1.25 mg daily. Attempts to discontinue medication should be made at 3-6 month intervals.

Dosage Forms Tablet: 0.3 mg, 0.625 mg, 0.9 mg, 1.25 mg

estrogens (conjugated/equine) (ES troe jenz KON joo gate ed/EE kwine)

Synonyms CES; conjugated estrogens

U.S./Canadian Brand Names Congest [Can]; PMS-Conjugated Estrogens [Can]; Premarin® [US/Can]

Therapeutic Category Estrogen Derivative

Use Dysfunctional uterine bleeding, atrophic vaginitis, hypogonadism, vasomotor symptoms of menopause

Usual Dosage Adults:

Male: Prostate cancer: Oral: 1.25-2.5 mg 3 times/day

Female:

Hypogonadism: Oral: 2.5-7.5 mg/day for 20 days, off 10 days and repeat until menses occur

Abnormal uterine bleeding:

Oral: 2.5-5 mg/day for 7-10 days; then decrease to 1.25 mg/day for 2 weeks

I.V.: 25 mg every 6-12 hours until bleeding stops

Moderate to severe vasomotor symptoms: Oral: 0.625-1.25 mg/day

Postpartum breast engorgement: Oral: 3.75 mg every 4 hours for 5 doses, then 1.25 mg every 4 hours for 5 days

Dosage Forms

Cream, vaginal: 0.625 mg/g (42.5 g)

Injection: 25 mg (5 mL)

Tablet: 0.3 mg, 0.625 mg, 0.9 mg, 1.25 mg, 2.5 mg

estrogens (esterified) (ES troe jenz es TER i fied)

Synonyms esterified estrogens

U.S./Canadian Brand Names Estratab® [US]; Menest® [US]

Therapeutic Category Estrogen Derivative

Use Atrophic vaginitis; hypogonadism; primary ovarian failure; vasomotor symptoms of menopause; prostatic carcinoma; osteoporosis prophylactic

Usual Dosage Adults: Oral:

Male: Prostate cancer: 1.25-2.5 mg 3 times/day

Female:

Hypogonadism: 2.5-7.5 mg/day for 20 days, off 10 days and repeat until menses occur

Moderate to severe vasomotor symptoms: 0.3-1.25 mg/day

Dosage Forms Tablet: 0.3 mg, 0.625 mg, 1.25 mg, 2.5 mg

Estroject-2® Injection *(Discontinued)* see page 814

Estroject-L.A.® Injection *(Discontinued)* see page 814

estrone (ES trone)

Synonyms estrogenic substance aqueous

U.S./Canadian Brand Names Kestrone® [US/Can]; Oestrilin [Can]

Therapeutic Category Estrogen Derivative

Use Atrophic vaginitis; hypogonadism; primary ovarian failure; vasomotor symptoms of menopause; prostatic carcinoma; osteoporosis prophylactic

Usual Dosage Adults: I.M.:

Vasomotor symptoms, atrophic vaginitis: 0.1-0.5 mg 2-3 times/week

Primary ovarian failure, hypogonadism: 0.1-1 mg/week, up to 2 mg/week

Prostatic carcinoma: 2-4 mg 2-3 times/week

Dosage Forms Injection: 2 mg/mL (10 mL); 5 mg/mL (10 mL)

Estronol® Injection *(Discontinued)* see page 814

estropipate (ES troe pih pate)

Synonyms piperazine estrone sulfate

U.S./Canadian Brand Names Ogen® [US/Can]; Ortho-Est® [US]

Therapeutic Category Estrogen Derivative

Use Atrophic vaginitis; hypogonadism; primary ovarian failure; vasomotor symptoms of menopause; prostatic carcinoma; osteoporosis prophylactic

Usual Dosage Adults: Female:

Moderate to severe vasomotor symptoms: Oral: 0.625-5 mg/day

Hypogonadism: Oral: 1.25-7.5 mg/day for 3 weeks followed by an 8- to 10-day rest period

Atrophic vaginitis or kraurosis vulvae: Vaginal: Instill 2-4 g/day 3 weeks on and 1 week off

Dosage Forms

Cream, vaginal (Ogen®): 0.15% [estropipate 1.5 mg/g] (42.5 g tube)

Tablet (Ogen®, Ortho-Est®): 0.625 mg [estropipate 0.75 mg]; 1.25 mg [estropipate 1.5 mg]; 2.5 mg [estropipate 3 mg]

Estrostep® 21 *(Discontinued)* see page 814

Estrostep® Fe [US] see ethinyl estradiol and norethindrone on page 251

Estrovis® *(Discontinued)* see page 814

etanercept (et a NER cept)

U.S./Canadian Brand Names Enbrel® [US]

Therapeutic Category Antirheumatic, Disease Modifying

Use Reduction in signs and symptoms of moderately to severely active rheumatoid arthritis, moderately to severely active polyarticular juvenile arthritis, or psoriatic arthritis in patients who have had an inadequate response to one or more disease-modifying antirheumatic drugs (DMARDs)

Usual Dosage S.C.:

Children: 0.4 mg/kg (maximum: 25 mg dose)

Adult: 25 mg given twice weekly; if the physician determines that it is appropriate, patients may self-inject after proper training in injection technique

Dosage Forms Injection, powder for reconstitution: 25 mg

ethacrynic acid (eth a KRIN ik AS id)

Synonyms sodium ethacrynate

U.S./Canadian Brand Names Edecrin® [US/Can]

Therapeutic Category Diuretic, Loop

Use Management of edema secondary to congestive heart failure; hepatic or renal disease, hypertension

Usual Dosage

Children:

Oral: 25 mg/day to start, increase by 25 mg/day at intervals of 2-3 days as needed, to a maximum of 3 mg/kg/day

I.V.: 1 mg/kg/dose, (maximum: 50 mg/dose); repeat doses not recommended

Adults:

Oral: 50-100 mg/day increased in increments of 25-50 mg at intervals of several days to a maximum of 400 mg/24 hours

I.V.: 0.5-1 mg/kg/dose (maximum: 50 mg/dose); repeat doses not recommended

Dosage Forms

Injection, powder for reconstitution, as ethacrynate sodium: 50 mg (50 mL)

Tablet: 25 mg, 50 mg

ethambutol (e THAM byoo tole)

U.S./Canadian Brand Names Etibi® [Can]; Myambutol® [US]

Therapeutic Category Antimycobacterial Agent

Use Treatment of tuberculosis and other mycobacterial diseases in conjunction with other antimycobacterial agents

Usual Dosage Oral (not recommended in children <12 years of age):

Children >12 years: 15 mg/kg/day once daily

Adolescents and Adults: 15-25 mg/kg/day once daily, not to exceed 2.5 g/day

(Continued)

ethambutol *(Continued)*
Dosage Forms Tablet, as hydrochloride: 100 mg, 400 mg

Ethamolin® **[US]** *see* ethanolamine oleate *on this page*

ethanoic acid *see* acetic acid *on page 10*

ethanol *see* alcohol (ethyl) *on page 20*

ethanolamine oleate (ETH a nol a meen OH lee ate)
U.S./Canadian Brand Names Ethamolin® [US]
Therapeutic Category Sclerosing Agent
Use Mild sclerosing agent used for bleeding esophageal varices
Usual Dosage Adults: 1.5-5 mL per varix, up to 20 mL total or 0.4 mL/kg; patients with severe hepatic dysfunction should receive less than recommended maximum dose
Dosage Forms Injection: 5% [50 mg/mL] (2 mL)

Ethaquin® *(Discontinued)* *see page 814*
Ethatab® *(Discontinued)* *see page 814*

ethaverine (eth AV er een)
U.S./Canadian Brand Names Ethavex-100® [US]
Therapeutic Category Vasodilator
Use Peripheral and cerebral vascular insufficiency associated with arterial spasm
Usual Dosage Adults: Oral: 100 mg 3 times/day
Dosage Forms Tablet, as hydrochloride: 100 mg

Ethavex-100® **[US]** *see* ethaverine *on this page*

ethchlorvynol (eth klor VI nole)
U.S./Canadian Brand Names Placidyl® [US]
Therapeutic Category Hypnotic, Nonbarbiturate
Controlled Substance C-IV
Use Short-term management of insomnia
Usual Dosage Oral: 500-1000 mg at bedtime
Dosage Forms Capsule: 200 mg, 500 mg, 750 mg

ethinyl estradiol (ETH in il es tra DYE ole)
U.S./Canadian Brand Names Estinyl® [US]
Therapeutic Category Estrogen Derivative
Use Atrophic vaginitis; hypogonadism; primary ovarian failure; vasomotor symptoms of menopause; prostatic carcinoma; osteoporosis prophylactic
Usual Dosage Adults: Oral:
  Hypogonadism: 0.05 mg 1-3 times/day for 2 weeks
  Prostatic carcinoma: 0.15-2 mg/day
  Vasomotor symptoms: 0.02-0.05 mg for 21 days, off 7 days and repeat
Dosage Forms Tablet: 0.02 mg [contains tartrazine], 0.05 mg

ethinyl estradiol and desogestrel
(ETH in il es tra DYE ole & des oh JES trel)
Synonyms desogestrel and ethinyl estradiol
U.S./Canadian Brand Names Apri® [US]; Cyclessa® [US]; Desogen® [US]; Kariva™ [US]; Marvelon® [Can]; Mircette® [US]; Ortho-Cept® [US/Can]
Therapeutic Category Contraceptive, Oral
Use Prevention of pregnancy
Usual Dosage Oral: Adults: Female: Contraception:
  Schedule 1 (Sunday starter): Dose begins on first Sunday after onset of menstruation; if the menstrual period starts on Sunday, take first tablet that very same day. **With a**

Sunday start, an additional method of contraception should be used until after the first 7 days of consecutive administration.

For 21-tablet package: Dosage is 1 tablet daily for 21 consecutive days, followed by 7 days off of the medication; a new course begins on the 8th day after the last tablet is taken.

For 28-tablet package: Dosage is 1 tablet daily without interruption.

Schedule 2 (Day 1 starter): Dose starts on first day of menstrual cycle taking 1 tablet daily.

For 21-tablet package: Dosage is 1 tablet daily for 21 consecutive days, followed by 7 days off of the medication; a new course begins on the 8th day after the last tablet is taken.

For 28-tablet package: Dosage is 1 tablet daily without interruption.

If all doses have been taken on schedule and one menstrual period is missed, continue dosing cycle. If two consecutive menstrual periods are missed, pregnancy test is required before new dosing cycle is started.

Missed doses monophasic formulations (refer to package insert for complete information):

One dose missed: Take as soon as remembered or take 2 tablets next day

Two consecutive doses missed in the first 2 weeks: Take 2 tablets as soon as remembered or 2 tablets next 2 days. **An additional method of contraception should be used for 7 days after missed dose.**

Two consecutive doses missed in week 3 or three consecutive doses missed at any time: Schedule 1 (Sunday starter): Continue to take 1 tablet daily until Sunday, then discard the rest of the pack, and a new pack is started that same day. Schedule 2 (Day 1 starter): Current pack should be discarded, and a new pack started that same day. **An additional method of contraception should be used for 7 days after missed dose.**

Dosage Forms Tablet:

Low-dose formulation:

Kariva™:

Day 1-21: Ethinyl estradiol 0.02 mg and desogestrel 0.15 mg [21 white tablets]

Day 22-23: 2 inactive light green tablets

Day 24-28: Ethinyl estradiol 0.01 mg [5 light blue tablets] (28s)

Mircette®:

Day 1-21: Ethinyl estradiol 0.02 mg and desogestrel 0.15 mg [21 white tablets]

Day 22-23: 2 inactive green tablets

Day 24-28: Ethinyl estradiol 0.01 mg [5 yellow tablets] (28s)

Monophasic formulations:

Apri® 28: Ethinyl estradiol 0.03 mg and desogestrel 0.15 mg [21 rose tablets and 7 white inactive tablets] (28s)

Desogen®: Ethinyl estradiol 0.03 mg and desogestrel 0.15 mg [21 white tablets and 7 green inactive tablets] (28s)

Ortho-Cept® 28: Ethinyl estradiol 0.03 mg and desogestrel 0.15 mg [21 orange tablets and 7 green inactive tablets] (28s)

Triphasic formulation: Cyclessa®:

Day 1-7:Ethinyl estradiol 0.025 mg and desogestrel 0.1 mg [7 light yellow tablets]

Day 8-14: Ethinyl estradiol 0.025 mg and desogestrel 0.125 mg [7 orange tablets]

Day 14-21: Ethinyl estradiol 0.025 mg and desogestrel 0.15 mg [7 red tablets]

Day 21-28: 7 green inactive tablets (28s)

ethinyl estradiol and drospirenone

(ETH in il es tra DYE ole & droh SPYE re none)

Synonyms drospirenone and ethinyl estradiol

U.S./Canadian Brand Names Yasmin® [US]

Therapeutic Category Contraceptive

Use Prevention of pregnancy

Usual Dosage Oral: Adults: Female: Contraception: Dosage is 1 tablet daily for 28 consecutive days. Dose should be taken at the same time each day, either after the evening meal or at bedtime. Dosing may be started on the first day of menstrual period (Continued)

ethinyl estradiol and drospirenone *(Continued)*

(Day 1 starter) or on the first Sunday after the onset of the menstrual period (Sunday starter).

Day 1 starter: Dose starts on first day of menstrual cycle taking 1 tablet daily.

Sunday starter: Dose begins on first Sunday after onset of menstruation; if the menstrual period starts on Sunday, take first tablet that very same day. **With a Sunday start, an additional method of contraception should be used until after the first 7 days of consecutive administration.**

If all doses have been taken on schedule and one menstrual period is missed, continue dosing cycle. If two consecutive menstrual periods are missed, pregnancy test is required before new dosing cycle is started.

If doses have been missed during the first 3 weeks and the menstrual period is missed, pregnancy should be ruled out prior to continuing treatment.

Missed doses (monophasic formulations) (refer to package insert for complete information):

One dose missed: Take as soon as remembered or take 2 tablets next day

Two consecutive doses missed in the first 2 weeks: Take 2 tablets as soon as remembered or 2 tablets next 2 days. **An additional method of contraception should be used for 7 days after missed dose.**

Two consecutive doses missed in week 3 or three consecutive doses missed at any time: **An additional method of contraception must be used for 7 days after a missed dose.**

Day 1 starter: Current pack should be discarded, and a new pack should be started that same day.

Sunday starter: Continue dose of 1 tablet daily until Sunday, then discard the rest of the pack, and a new pack should be started that same day.

Any number of doses missed in week 4: Continue taking one pill each day until pack is empty; no back-up method of contraception is needed

Dosage Forms Tablet: Ethinyl estradiol 0.03 mg and drospirenone 3 mg [21 yellow round active tablets and 7 white inert round tablets] (28s)

ethinyl estradiol and ethynodiol diacetate

(ETH in il es tra DYE ole & e thye noe DYE ole dye AS e tate)

Synonyms ethynodiol diacetate and ethinyl estradiol

U.S./Canadian Brand Names Demulen® 30 [Can]; Demulen® [US]; Zovia™ [US]

Therapeutic Category Contraceptive, Oral

Use Prevention of pregnancy; treatment of hypermenorrhea, endometriosis, female hypogonadism

Usual Dosage Oral: Adults: Female: Contraception:

Schedule 1 (Sunday starter): Dose begins on first Sunday after onset of menstruation; if the menstrual period starts on Sunday, take first tablet that very same day. **With a Sunday start, an additional method of contraception should be used until after the first 7 days of consecutive administration.**

For 21-tablet package: Dosage is 1 tablet daily for 21 consecutive days, followed by 7 days off of the medication; a new course begins on the 8th day after the last tablet is taken.

For 28-tablet package: Dosage is 1 tablet daily without interruption.

Schedule 2 (Day 1 starter): Dose starts on first day of menstrual cycle taking 1 tablet daily.

For 21-tablet package: Dosage is 1 tablet daily for 21 consecutive days, followed by 7 days off of the medication; a new course begins on the 8th day after the last tablet is taken.

For 28-tablet package: Dosage is 1 tablet daily without interruption.

If all doses have been taken on schedule and one menstrual period is missed, continue dosing cycle. If two consecutive menstrual periods are missed, pregnancy test is required before new dosing cycle is started.

Missed doses monophasic formulations (refer to package insert for complete information):

One dose missed: Take as soon as remembered or take 2 tablets next day

Two consecutive doses missed in the first 2 weeks: Take 2 tablets as soon as remembered or 2 tablets next 2 days. **An additional method of contraception should be used for 7 days after missed dose,**

Two consecutive doses missed in week 3 or three consecutive doses missed at any time: Schedule 1 (Sunday starter): Continue dose of 1 tablet daily until Sunday, then discard the rest of the pack, and a new pack should be started that same day. Schedule 2 (Day 1 starter): Current package should be discarded, and a new pack should be started that same day. **An additional method of contraception should be used for 7 days after missed doses.**

Dosage Forms Tablet, monophasic formulations:

Demulin® 1/35-21: Ethinyl estradiol 0.035 mg and ethynodiol diacetate 1 mg [white tablets] (21s)

Demulin® 1/35-28: Ethinyl estradiol 0.035 mg and ethynodiol diacetate 1 mg [21 white tablets and 7 blue inactive tablets] (28s)

Demulin® 1/50-21: Ethinyl estradiol 0.05 mg and ethynodiol diacetate 1 mg [white tablets] (21s)

Demulin® 1/50-28: Ethinyl estradiol 0.05 mg and ethynodiol diacetate 1 mg [21 white tablets and 7 pink inactive tablets] (28s)

Zovia™ 1/35-21: Ethinyl estradiol 0.035 mg and ethynodiol diacetate 1 mg [light pink tablets] (21s)

Zovia™ 1/35-28: Ethinyl estradiol 0.035 mg and ethynodiol diacetate 1 mg [21 light pink tablets and 7 white inactive tablets] (28s)

Zovia™ 1/50-21: Ethinyl estradiol 0.05 mg and ethynodiol diacetate 1 mg [pink tablets] (21s)

Zovia™ 1/50-28: Ethinyl estradiol 0.05 mg and ethynodiol diacetate 1 mg [21 pink tablets and 7 white inactive tablets] (28s)

ethinyl estradiol and etonogestrel

(ETH in il es tra DYE ole & et oh noe JES trel)

Synonyms etonogestrel and ethinyl estradiol

U.S./Canadian Brand Names NuvaRing® [US]

Therapeutic Category Contraceptive; Estrogen and Progestin Combination

Use Prevention of pregnancy

Usual Dosage Vaginal: Adults: Female: Contraception: One ring, inserted vaginally and left in place for 3 consecutive weeks, then removed for 1 week. A new ring is inserted 7 days after the last was removed (even if bleeding is not complete) and should be inserted at approximately the same time of day the ring was removed the previous week.

Initial treatment should begin as follows (pregnancy should always be ruled out first):

No hormonal contraceptive use in the past month: Using the first day of menstruation as "Day 1," insert the ring on or prior to "Day 5," even if bleeding is not complete. An additional form of contraception should be used for the following 7 days.*

Switching from combination oral contraceptive: Ring should be inserted within 7 days after the last active tablet was taken and no later than the first day a new cycle of tablets would begin. Additional forms of contraception are not needed.

Switching from progestin-only contraceptive: An additional form of contraception should be used for the following 7 days with any of the following.*

If previously using a progestin-only mini-pill, insert the ring on any day of the month; do not skip days between the last pill and insertion of the ring.

If previously using an implant, insert the ring on the same day of implant removal.

If previously using a progestin-containing IUD, insert the ring on day of IUD removal.

If previously using a progestin injection, insert the ring on the day the next injection would be given.

Following complete 1st trimester abortion: Insert ring within the first five days of abortion. If not inserted within five days, follow instructions for "No hormonal contraceptive

(Continued)

ethinyl estradiol and etonogestrel *(Continued)*

use within the past month" and instruct patient to use a nonhormonal contraceptive in the interim.

Following delivery or 2nd trimester abortion: Insert ring 4 weeks postpartum (in women who are not breast-feeding) or following 2nd trimester abortion. An additional form of contraception should be used for the following 7 days.*

If the ring is accidentally removed from the vagina at anytime during the 3-week period of use, it may be rinsed with cool or luke-warm water (not hot) and reinserted as soon as possible. If the ring is not reinserted within three hours, contraceptive effectiveness will be decreased. An additional form of contraception should be used until the ring has been inserted for 7 continuous days.*

If the ring has been removed for longer than 1 week, pregnancy must be ruled out prior to restarting therapy. An additional form of contraception should be used for the following 7 days.*

If the ring has been left in place for >3 weeks, a new ring should be inserted following a 1-week (ring-free) interval. Pregnancy must be ruled out prior to insertion and an additional form of contraception should be used for the following 7 days.*

Note: Diaphragms may interfere with proper ring placement, and therefore, are not recommended for use as an additional form of contraception.

Dosage Forms Ring, intravaginal [3-week duration]: Ethinyl estradiol 0.015 mg/day and etonogestrel 0.12 mg/day (1s, 3s)

ethinyl estradiol and levonorgestrel

(ETH in il es tra DYE ole & LEE voe nor jes trel)

Synonyms levonorgestrel and ethinyl estradiol

U.S./Canadian Brand Names Alesse® [US/Can]; Aviane™ [US]; Enpresse™ [US]; Lessina™ [US]; Levlen® [US]; Levlite™ [US]; Levora® [US]; Min-Ovral® [Can]; Nordette® [US]; Portia™ [US]; PREVEN™ [US]; Tri-Levlen® [US]; Triphasil® [US/Can]; Triquilar® [Can]; Trivora® [US]

Therapeutic Category Contraceptive, Oral

Use Prevention of pregnancy; treatment of hypermenorrhea, endometriosis, female hypogonadism

Usual Dosage Oral: Adults: Female: Contraception:

Schedule 1 (Sunday starter): Dose begins on first Sunday after onset of menstruation; if the menstrual period starts on Sunday, take first tablet that very same day. **With a Sunday start, an additional method of contraception should be used until after the first 7 days of consecutive administration.**

For 21-tablet package: Dosage is 1 tablet daily for 21 consecutive days, followed by 7 days off of the medication; a new course begins on the 8th day after the last tablet is taken.

For 28-tablet package: Dosage is 1 tablet daily without interruption.

Schedule 2 (Day 1 starter): Dose starts on first day of menstrual cycle taking 1 tablet daily.

For 21-tablet package: Dosage is 1 tablet daily for 21 consecutive days, followed by 7 days off of the medication; a new course begins on the 8th day after the last tablet is taken.

For 28-tablet package: Dosage is 1 tablet daily without interruption.

If all doses have been taken on schedule and one menstrual period is missed, continue dosing cycle. If two consecutive menstrual periods are missed, pregnancy test is required before new dosing cycle is started.

Missed doses monophasic formulations (refer to package insert for complete information):

One dose missed: Take as soon as remembered or take 2 tablets next day

Two consecutive doses missed in the first 2 weeks: Take 2 tablets as soon as remembered or 2 tablets next 2 days. **An additional method of contraception should be used for 7 days after missed dose.**

Two consecutive doses missed in week 3 or three consecutive doses missed at any time: **An additional method of contraception must be used for 7 days after a missed dose:**

Schedule 1 (Sunday starter): Continue dose of 1 tablet daily until Sunday, then discard the rest of the pack, and a new pack should be started that same day.

Schedule 2 (Day 1 starter): Current pack should be discarded, and a new pack should be started that same day.

Missed doses biphasic/triphasic formulations (refer to package insert for complete information):

One dose missed: Take as soon as remembered or take 2 tablets next day.

Two consecutive doses missed in week 1 or week 2 of the pack: Take 2 tablets as soon as remembered and 2 tablets the next day. Resume taking 1 tablet daily until the pack is empty. **An additional method of contraception should be used for 7 days after a missed dose.**

Two consecutive doses missed in week 3 of the pack; **An additional method of contraception must be used for 7 days after a missed dose.**

Schedule 1 (Sunday Starter): Take 1 tablet every day until Sunday. Discard the remaining pack and start a new pack of pills on the same day.

Schedule 2 (Day 1 starter): Discard the remaining pack and start a new pack the same day.

Three or more consecutive doses missed; **An additional method of contraception must be used for 7 days after a missed dose.**

Schedule 1 (Sunday Starter): Take 1 tablet every day until Sunday; on Sunday, discard the pack and start a new pack.

Schedule 2 (Day 1 Starter): Discard the remaining pack and begin new pack of tablets starting on the same day.

Dosage Forms Tablet:

PREVEN™: Ethinyl estradiol 0.05 mg and levonorgestrel 0.25 mg (4s) [also available as a kit containing 4 tablets and a pregnancy test]

Low-dose formulations:

Alesse® 21: Ethinyl estradiol 0.02 mg and levonorgestrel 0.1 mg [pink tablets] (21s)

Alesse® 28: Ethinyl estradiol 0.02 mg and levonorgestrel 0.1 mg [21 pink tablets and 7 light green inactive tablets] (28s)

Aviane™ 28: Ethinyl estradiol 0.02 mg and levonorgestrel 0.1 mg [21 orange tablets and 7 light green inactive tablets] (28s)

Lessina™ 21, Levlite™ 21: Ethinyl estradiol 0.02 mg and levonorgestrel 0.1 mg [pink tablets] (21s)

Lessina™ 28, Levlite™ 28: Ethinyl estradiol 0.02 mg and levonorgestrel 0.1 mg [21 pink tablets and 7 white inactive tablets] (28s)

Monophasic formulations:

Levlen® 21: Ethinyl estradiol 0.03 mg and levonorgestrel 0.15 mg [light orange tablets] (21s)

Levlen® 28: Ethinyl estradiol 0.03 mg and levonorgestrel 0.15 mg [21 light orange tablets and 7 pink inactive tablets] (28s)

Levora® 21: Ethinyl estradiol 0.03 mg and levonorgestrel 0.15 mg [white tablets] (21s)

Levora® 28: Ethinyl estradiol 0.03 mg and levonorgestrel 0.15 mg [21 white tablets and 7 peach inactive tablets] (28s)

Nordette® 21: Ethinyl estradiol 0.03 mg and levonorgestrel 0.15 mg [light orange tablets] (21s)

Nordette® 28: Ethinyl estradiol 0.03 mg and levonorgestrel 0.15 mg [21 light orange tablets and 7 pink inactive tablets] (28s)

Portia™ 21: Ethinyl estradiol 0.03 mg and levonorgestrel 0.15 mg [pink tablets] (21s)

Portia™ 28: Ethinyl estradiol 0.03 mg and levonorgestrel 0.15 mg [21 pink tablets and 7 white inactive tablets] (28s)

Triphasic formulations:

Enpresse™:

Day 1-6: Ethinyl estradiol 0.03 mg and levonorgestrel 0.05 mg [6 pink tablets]

Day 7-11: Ethinyl estradiol 0.04 mg and levonorgestrel 0.075 mg [5 white tablets]

(Continued)

ethinyl estradiol and levonorgestrel *(Continued)*

Day 12-21: Ethinyl estradiol 0.03 mg and levonorgestrel 0.125 mg [10 orange tablets]
Day 22-28: 7 light green inactive tablets (28s)
Tri-Levlen® 21, Triphasil® 21:
Day 1-6: Ethinyl estradiol 0.03 mg and levonorgestrel 0.05 mg [6 brown tablets]
Day 7-11: Ethinyl estradiol 0.04 mg and levonorgestrel 0.075 mg [5 white tablets]
Day 12-21: Ethinyl estradiol 0.03 mg and levonorgestrel 0.125 mg [10 light yellow tablets] (21s)
Trivora® 21:
Day 1-6: Ethinyl estradiol 0.03 mg and levonorgestrel 0.05 mg [6 blue tablets]
Day 7-11: Ethinyl estradiol 0.04 mg and levonorgestrel 0.075 mg [5 white tablets]
Day 12-21: Ethinyl estradiol 0.03 mg and levonorgestrel 0.125 mg [10 pink tablets] (21s)
Tri-Levlen® 28, Triphasil® 28:
Day 1-6: Ethinyl estradiol 0.03 mg and levonorgestrel 0.05 mg [6 brown tablets]
Day 7-11: Ethinyl estradiol 0.04 mg and levonorgestrel 0.075 mg [5 white tablets]
Day 12-21: Ethinyl estradiol 0.03 mg and levonorgestrel 0.125 mg [10 light yellow tablets]
Day 22-28: 7 light green inactive tablets (28s)
Trivora® 28:
Day 1-6: Ethinyl estradiol 0.03 mg and levonorgestrel 0.05 mg [6 blue tablets]
Day 7-11: Ethinyl estradiol 0.04 mg and levonorgestrel 0.075 mg [5 white tablets]
Day 12-21: Ethinyl estradiol 0.03 mg and levonorgestrel 0.125 mg [10 pink tablets]
Day 22-28: 7 peach inactive tablets (28s)

ethinyl estradiol and norelgestromin

(ETH in il es tra DYE ole & nor el JES troe min)
Synonyms norelgestromin and ethinyl estradiol
U.S./Canadian Brand Names Ortho Evra™ [US]
Therapeutic Category Contraceptive; Estrogen and Progestin Combination
Use Prevention of pregnancy
Usual Dosage Topical: Adults: Female:
Contraception: Apply one patch each week for 3 weeks (21 total days); followed by one week that is patch-free. Each patch should be applied on the same day each week ("patch change day") and only one patch should be worn at a time. No more than 7 days should pass during the patch-free interval.
Schedule 1 (Sunday starter): Dose begins on first Sunday after onset of menstruation; if the menstrual period starts on Sunday, apply one patch that very same day. With a Sunday start, an additional method of contraception (nonhormonal) should be used until after the first 7 days of consecutive administration. Each patch change will then occur on Sunday.
Schedule 2 (Day 1 starter): Dose starts on first day of menstrual cycle, applying one patch during the first 24 hours of menstrual cycle. No back-up method of contraception is needed as long as the patch is applied on the first day of cycle. Each patch change will then occur on that same day of the week.

Additional dosing considerations:
No bleeding during patch-free week/missed menstrual period: If patch has been applied as directed, continue treatment on usual "patch change day". If used correctly, no bleeding during patch-free week does not necessarily indicate pregnancy. However, if no withdrawal bleeding occurs for 2 consecutive cycles, pregnancy should be ruled out. If patch has not been applied as directed, and one menstrual period is missed, pregnancy should be ruled out prior to continuing treatment.
If a patch becomes partially or completely detached for <24 hours: Try to reapply to same place, or replace with a new patch immediately. Do not reapply if patch is no longer sticky, if it is sticking to itself or another surface, or if it has material sticking to it.
If a patch becomes partially or completely detached for >24 hours (or time period is unknown): Apply a new patch and use this day of the week as the new "patch change

day" from this point on. An additional method of contraception (nonhormonal) should be used until after the first 7 days of consecutive administration.

Switching from oral contraceptives: Apply first patch on the first day of withdrawal bleeding. If there is no bleeding within 5 days of taking the last active tablet, pregnancy must first be ruled out. If patch is applied later than the first day of bleeding, **an additional method of contraception (nonhormonal) should be used until after the first 7 days of consecutive administration**

Use after childbirth: Therapy should not be started <4 weeks after childbirth. Pregnancy should be ruled out prior to treatment if menstrual periods have not restarted. **An additional method of contraception (nonhormonal) should be used until after the first 7 days of consecutive administration.**

Use after abortion or miscarriage: Therapy may be started immediately if abortion/ miscarriage occur within the first trimester. If therapy is not started within 5 days, follow instructions for first time use. If abortion/miscarriage occur during the second trimester, therapy should not be started for at least 4 weeks. Follow directions for use after childbirth.

Dosage Forms Patch, transdermal: Ethinyl estradiol 0.75 mg and norelgestromin 6 mg [releases ethinyl estradiol 20 mcg and norelgestromin 150 mcg per day] (1s, 3s)

ethinyl estradiol and norethindrone

(ETH in il es tra DYE ole & nor eth IN drone)

Synonyms norethindrone acetate and ethinyl estradiol

U.S./Canadian Brand Names Brevicon® [US]; Estrostep® Fe [US]; femhrt® [US/Can]; Jenest™-28 [US]; Loestrin® Fe [US]; Loestrin® [US/Can]; Microgestin™ Fe [US]; Minestrin™ 1/20 [Can]; Modicon® [US]; Necon® 0.5/35 [US]; Necon® 1/35 [US]; Necon® 10/11 [US]; Norinyl® 1+35 [US]; Nortrel™ [US]; Ortho-Novum® [US]; Ovcon® [US]; Select™ 1/ 35 [Can]; Synphasic® [Can]; Tri-Norinyl® [US]

Therapeutic Category Contraceptive, Oral

Use Prevention of pregnancy; treatment of hypermenorrhea, endometriosis, female hypogonadism

Usual Dosage Adults: Female:

Moderate to severe vasomotor symptoms associated with menopause: 1 tablet daily (ethinyl estradiol 5 mcg and norethindrone 1 mg) and patients should be re-evaluated at 3- to 6-month intervals to determine if treatment is still necessary

Prevention of osteoporosis: 1 tablet daily (ethinyl estradiol 5 mcg and norethindrone 1 mg)

Contraception: Oral:

Schedule 1 (Sunday starter): Dose begins on first Sunday after onset of menstruation; if the menstrual period starts on Sunday, take first tablet that very same day. **With a Sunday start, an additional method of contraception should be used until after the first 7 days of consecutive administration.**

For 21-tablet package: Dosage is 1 tablet daily for 21 consecutive days, followed by 7 days off of the medication; a new course begins on the 8th day after the last tablet is taken.

For 28-tablet package: Dosage is 1 tablet daily without interruption.

Schedule 2 (Day 1 starter): Dose starts on first day of menstrual cycle taking 1 tablet daily.

For 21-tablet package: Dosage is 1 tablet daily for 21 consecutive days, followed by 7 days off of the medication; a new course begins on the 8th day after the last tablet is taken.

For 28-tablet package: Dosage is 1 tablet daily without interruption.

If all doses have been taken on schedule and one menstrual period is missed, continue dosing cycle. If two consecutive menstrual periods are missed, pregnancy test is required before new dosing cycle is started.

Missed doses monophasic formulations (refer to package insert for complete information):

One dose missed: Take as soon as remembered or take 2 tablets next day

(Continued)

ethinyl estradiol and norethindrone *(Continued)*

Two consecutive doses missed in the first 2 weeks: Take 2 tablets as soon as remembered or 2 tablets next 2 days. **An additional method of contraception should be used for 7 days after missed dose.**

Two consecutive doses missed in week 3 or three consecutive doses missed at any time: **An additional method of contraception must be used for 7 days after a missed dose.**

Schedule 1 (Sunday starter): Continue dose of 1 tablet daily until Sunday, then discard the rest of the pack, and a new pack should be started that same day.

Schedule 2 (Day 1 starter): Current pack should be discarded, and a new pack should be started that same day.

Missed doses biphasic/triphasic formulations (refer to package insert for complete information):

One dose missed: Take as soon as remembered or take 2 tablets next day.

Two consecutive doses missed in week 1 or week 2 of the pack: Take 2 tablets as soon as remembered and 2 tablets the next day. Resume taking 1 tablet daily until the pack is empty. **An additional method of contraception should be used for 7 days after a missed dose.**

Two consecutive doses missed in week 3 of the pack; **An additional method of contraception must be used for 7 days after a missed dose.**

Schedule 1 (Sunday Starter): Take 1 tablet every day until Sunday. Discard the remaining pack and start a new pack of pills on the same day.

Schedule 2 (Day 1 starter): Discard the remaining pack and start a new pack the same day.

Three or more consecutive doses missed; **An additional method of contraception must be used for 7 days after a missed dose.**

Schedule 1 (Sunday Starter): Take 1 tablet every day until Sunday; on Sunday, discard the pack and start a new pack.

Schedule 2 (Day 1 Starter): Discard the remaining pack and begin new pack of tablets starting on the same day.

Dosage Forms Tablet:

femhrt® 1/5: Ethinyl estradiol 0.005 mg and norethindrone acetate 1 mg [white tablets]

Monophasic formulations:

Brevicon®: Ethinyl estradiol 0.035 mg and norethindrone 0.5 mg [21 blue tablets and 7 orange inactive tablets] (28s)

Loestrin® 21 1/20: Ethinyl estradiol 0.02 mg and norethindrone acetate 1 mg [white tablets] (21s)

Loestrin® 21 1.5/30: Ethinyl estradiol 0.03 mg and norethindrone acetate 1.5 mg [green tablets] (21s)

Loestrin® Fe 1/20, Microgestin™ Fe 1/20: Ethinyl estradiol 0.02 mg and norethindrone acetate 1mg [21 white tablets] and ferrous fumarate 75 mg [7 brown tablets] (28s)

Loestrin® Fe 1.5/30, Microgestin™ Fe 1.5/30: Ethinyl estradiol 0.03 mg and norethindrone acetate 1.5 mg [21 green tablets] and ferrous fumarate 75 mg [7 brown tablets] (28s)

Modicon® 21: Ethinyl estradiol 0.035 mg and norethindrone 0.5 mg [white tablets] (21s)

Modicon® 28: Ethinyl estradiol 0.035 mg and norethindrone 0.5 mg [21 white tablets and 7 green inactive tablets] (28s)

Necon® 0.5/35-21: Ethinyl estradiol 0.035 mg and norethindrone 0.5 mg [light yellow tablets] (21s)

Necon® 0.5/35-28: Ethinyl estradiol 0.035 mg and norethindrone 0.5 mg [21 light yellow tablets and 7 white inactive tablets] (28s)

Necon® 1/35-21: Ethinyl estradiol 0.035 mg and norethindrone 1 mg [dark yellow tablets] (21s)

Necon® 1/35-28: Ethinyl estradiol 0.035 mg and norethindrone 1 mg [21 dark yellow tablets and 7 white inactive tablets] (28s)

Norinyl® 1+35: Ethinyl estradiol 0.035 mg and norethindrone 1 mg [21 yellow-green tablets and 7 orange inactive tablets] (28s)

Nortrel™ 0.5/35 mg:
   Ethinyl estradiol 0.035 mg and norethindrone 0.5 mg [light yellow tablets] (21s)
   Ethinyl estradiol 0.035 mg and norethindrone 0.5 mg [21 light yellow tablets and 7 white inactive tablets] (28s)
Nortrel™ 1/35 mg:
   Ethinyl estradiol 0.035 mg and norethindrone 1 mg [yellow tablets] (21s)
   Ethinyl estradiol 0.035 mg and norethindrone 1 mg [21 yellow tablets and 7 white inactive tablets] (28s)
Ortho-Novum® 1/35 21: Ethinyl estradiol 0.035 mg and norethindrone 1 mg [peach tablets] (21s)
Ortho-Novum® 1/35 28: Ethinyl estradiol 0.035 mg and norethindrone 1 mg [21 peach tablets and 7 green inactive tablets] (28s)
Ovcon® 35 21-day: Ethinyl estradiol 0.035 mg and norethindrone 0.4 mg [peach tablets] (21s)
Ovcon® 35 28-day: Ethinyl estradiol 0.035 mg and norethindrone 0.4 mg [21 peach tablets and 7 green inactive tablets] (28s)
Ovcon® 50: Ethinyl estradiol 0.05 mg and norethindrone 1 mg [21 yellow tablets and 7 green inactive tablets] (28s)

Biphasic formulations:
Jenest™-28:
   Day 1-7: Ethinyl estradiol 0.035 mg and norethindrone 0.5 mg [7 white tablets]
   Day 8-21: Ethinyl estradiol 0.035 mg and norethindrone 1 mg [14 peach tablets]
   Day 22-28: 7 green inactive tablets (28s)
Necon® 10/11-21:
   Day 1-10: Ethinyl estradiol 0.035 mg and norethindrone 0.5 mg [10 light yellow tablets]
   Day 11-21: Ethinyl estradiol 0.035 mg and norethindrone 1 mg [11 dark yellow tablets] (21s)
Necon® 10/11-28:
   Day 1-10: Ethinyl estradiol 0.035 mg and norethindrone 0.5 mg [10 light yellow tablets]
   Day 11-21: Ethinyl estradiol 0.035 mg and norethindrone 1 mg [11 dark yellow tablets]
   Day 22-28: 7 white inactive tablets (28s)
Ortho-Novum® 10/11-21:
   Day 1-10: Ethinyl estradiol 0.035 mg and norethindrone 0.5 mg [10 white tablets]
   Day 11-21: Ethinyl estradiol 0.035 mg and norethindrone 1 mg [11 peach tablet] (21s)
Ortho-Novum® 10/11-28:
   Day 1-10: Ethinyl estradiol 0.035 mg and norethindrone 0.5 mg [10 white tablets]
   Day 11-21: Ethinyl estradiol 0.035 mg and norethindrone 1 mg [11 peach tablet]
   Day 22-28: 7 green inactive tablets (28s)

Triphasic formulations:
Estrostep® 21:
   Day 1-5: Ethinyl estradiol 0.02 mg and norethindrone acetate 1mg [5 white triangular tablets]
   Day 6-12: Ethinyl estradiol 0.03 mg and norethindrone acetate 1 mg [7 white square tablets]
   Day 13-21: Ethinyl estradiol 0.035 mg and norethindrone acetate 1 mg [9 white round tablets] (21s)
Estrostep® Fe:
   Day 1-5: Ethinyl estradiol 0.02 mg and norethindrone acetate 1 mg [5 white triangular tablets]
   Day 6-12: Ethinyl estradiol 0.03 mg and norethindrone acetate 1 mg [7 white square tablets]
   Day 13-21: Ethinyl estradiol 0.035 mg and norethindrone acetate 1 mg [9 white round tablets]
   Day 22-28: Ferrous fumarate 75 mg [7 brown tablets] (28s)
Ortho-Novum® 7/7/7 21:
   Day 1-7: Ethinyl estradiol 0.035 mg and norethindrone 0.5 mg [7 white tablets]
   Day 8-14: Ethinyl estradiol 0.035 mg and norethindrone 0.75 mg [7 light peach tablets]
   Day 15-21: Ethinyl estradiol 0.035 mg and norethindrone 1 mg [7 peach tablet] (21s)
(Continued)

ethinyl estradiol and norethindrone *(Continued)*

Ortho-Novum® 7/7/7 28:
Day 1-7: Ethinyl estradiol 0.035 mg and norethindrone 0.5 mg [7 white tablets]
Day 8-14: Ethinyl estradiol 0.035 mg and norethindrone 0.75 mg [7 light peach tablets]
Day 15-21: Ethinyl estradiol 0.035 mg and norethindrone 1 mg [7 peach tablet]
Day 22-28: 7 green inactive tablets (28s)

Tri-Norinyl® 28:
Day 1-7: Ethinyl estradiol 0.035 mg and norethindrone 0.5 mg [7 blue tablets]
Day 8-16: Ethinyl estradiol 0.035 mg and norethindrone 1 mg [9 yellow-green tablets]
Day 17-21: Ethinyl estradiol 0.035 mg and norethindrone 0.5 mg [5 blue tablets]
Day 22-28: 7 orange inactive tablets (28s)

ethinyl estradiol and norgestimate

(ETH in il es tra DYE ole & nor JES ti mate)

Synonyms norgestimate and ethinyl estradiol

U.S./Canadian Brand Names Ortho-Cyclen® [US/Can]; Ortho-Tri-Cyclen® Lo [US]; Ortho Tri-Cyclen® [US/Can]

Therapeutic Category Contraceptive, Oral

Use Prevention of pregnancy

Usual Dosage Oral: Adults: Female: Contraception:

Schedule 1 (Sunday starter): Dose begins on first Sunday after onset of menstruation; if the menstrual period starts on Sunday, take first tablet that very same day. **With a Sunday start, an additional method of contraception should be used until after the first 7 days of consecutive administration.**

For 21-tablet package: Dosage is 1 tablet daily for 21 consecutive days, followed by 7 days off of the medication; a new course begins on the 8th day after the last tablet is taken.

For 28-tablet package: Dosage is 1 tablet daily without interruption.

Schedule 2 (Day 1 starter): Dose starts on first day of menstrual cycle taking 1 tablet daily.

For 21-tablet package: Dosage is 1 tablet daily for 21 consecutive days, followed by 7 days off of the medication; a new course begins on the 8th day after the last tablet is taken.

For 28-tablet package: Dosage is 1 tablet daily without interruption.

If all doses have been taken on schedule and one menstrual period is missed, continue dosing cycle. If two consecutive menstrual periods are missed, pregnancy test is required before new dosing cycle is started.

Missed doses monophasic formulations (refer to package insert for complete information):

One dose missed: Take as soon as remembered or take 2 tablets next day

Two consecutive doses missed in the first 2 weeks: Take 2 tablets as soon as remembered or 2 tablets next 2 days. **An additional method of contraception should be used for 7 days after missed dose.**

Two consecutive doses missed in week 3 or three consecutive doses missed at any time: **An additional method of contraception must be used for 7 days after a missed dose:**

Schedule 1 (Sunday starter): Continue dose of 1 tablet daily until Sunday, then discard the rest of the pack, and a new pack should be started that same day.

Schedule 2 (Day 1 starter): Current pack should be discarded, and a new pack should be started that same day.

Missed doses biphasic/triphasic formulations (refer to package insert for complete information):

One dose missed: Take as soon as remembered or take 2 tablets next day.

Two consecutive doses missed in week 1 or week 2 of the pack: Take 2 tablets as soon as remembered and 2 tablets the next day. Resume taking 1 tablet daily until the pack is empty. **An additional method of contraception should be used for 7 days after a missed dose.**

Two consecutive doses missed in week 3 of the pack; **An additional method of contraception must be used for 7 days after a missed dose.**

Schedule 1 (Sunday Starter): Take 1 tablet every day until Sunday. Discard the remaining pack and start a new pack of pills on the same day.

Schedule 2 (Day 1 starter): Discard the remaining pack and start a new pack the same day.

Three or more consecutive doses missed; **An additional method of contraception must be used for 7 days after a missed dose.**

Schedule 1 (Sunday Starter): Take 1 tablet every day until Sunday; on Sunday, discard the pack and start a new pack.

Schedule 2 (Day 1 Starter): Discard the remaining pack and begin new pack of tablets starting on the same day.

Dosage Forms Tablet:

Monophasic formulation (Ortho-Cyclen®): Ethinyl estradiol 0.035 mg and norgestimate 0.25 mg [21 blue tablets and 7 green inactive tablets] (28s)

Triphasic formulations:

Ortho Tri-Cyclen®:

Day 1-7: Ethinyl estradiol 0.035 mg and norgestimate 0.18 mg [7 white tablets]

Day 8-14: Ethinyl estradiol 0.035 mg and norgestimate 0.215 mg [7 light blue tablets]

Day 15-21: Ethinyl estradiol 0.035 mg and norgestimate 0.25 mg [7 blue tablets]

Day 22-28: 7 green inactive tablets (28s)

Ortho Tri-Cyclen® Lo:

Day 1-7: Ethinyl estradiol 0.025 mg and norgestimate 0.18 mg [7 white tablets]

Day 8-14: Ethinyl estradiol 0.025 mg and norgestimate 0.215 mg [7 light blue tablets]

Day 15-21: Ethinyl estradiol 0.025 mg and norgestimate 0.25 mg [7 dark blue tablets]

Day 22-28: 7 green inactive tablets (28s)

ethinyl estradiol and norgestrel (ETH in il es tra DYE ole & nor JES trel)

Synonyms norgestrel and ethinyl estradiol

U.S./Canadian Brand Names Cryselle™ [US]; Lo/Ovral® [US]; Low-Ogestrel® [US]; Ogestrel®; Ovral® [US/Can]

Therapeutic Category Contraceptive, Oral

Use Prevention of pregnancy; treatment of hypermenorrhea, endometriosis, female hypogonadism

Usual Dosage Oral: Adults: Female: Contraception: Some products recommend starting with one schedule over the other (refer to product information for more details):

Schedule 1 (Sunday starter): Dose begins on first Sunday after onset of menstruation; if the menstrual period starts on Sunday, take first tablet that very same day. **With a Sunday start, an additional method of contraception should be used until after the first 7 days of consecutive administration.**

For 21-tablet package: Dosage is 1 tablet daily for 21 consecutive days, followed by 7 days off of the medication; a new course begins on the 8th day after the last tablet is taken.

For 28-tablet package: Dosage is 1 tablet daily without interruption.

Schedule 2 (Day 1 starter): Dose starts on first day of menstrual cycle taking 1 tablet daily.

For 21-tablet package: Dosage is 1 tablet daily for 21 consecutive days, followed by 7 days off of the medication; a new course begins on the 8th day after the last tablet is taken.

For 28-tablet package: Dosage is 1 tablet daily without interruption.

If all doses have been taken on schedule and one menstrual period is missed, continue dosing cycle. If two consecutive menstrual periods are missed, pregnancy test is required before new dosing cycle is started.

Missed doses monophasic formulations (refer to package insert for complete information):

One dose missed: Take as soon as remembered or take 2 tablets next day

Two consecutive doses missed in the first 2 weeks: Take 2 tablets as soon as remembered or 2 tablets next 2 days. **An additional method of contraception should be used for 7 days after missed dose.**

(Continued)

ethinyl estradiol and norgestrel *(Continued)*

Two consecutive doses missed in week 3 or three consecutive doses missed at any time: Schedule 1 (Sunday starter): Continue to take 1 tablet daily until Sunday, then discard the rest of the pack, and a new pack is started that same day. Schedule 2 (Day 1 starter): Current pack should be discarded, and a new pack started that same day. **An additional method of contraception should be used for 7 days after missed dose.**

Postcoital contraception or "morning after" pill: Oral (50 mcg ethinyl estradiol and 0.5 mg norgestrel): 2 tablets at initial visit and 2 tablets 12 hours later

Dosage Forms Tablet, monophasic formulations:

Cryselle™: Ethinyl estradiol 0.03 mg and norgestrel 0.3 mg [21 white tablets and 7 light green inactive tablets] (28s)

Lo/Ovral®, Low-Ogestrel® 21: Ethinyl estradiol 0.03 mg and norgestrel 0.3 mg [white tablets] (21s)

Low-Ogestrel® 28: Ethinyl estradiol 0.03 mg and norgestrel 0.3 mg [21 white tablets and 7 peach inactive tablets] (28s)

Lo/Ovral® 28: Ethinyl estradiol 0.03 mg and norgestrel 0.3 mg [21 white tablets and 7 pink inactive tablets] (28s)

Ogestrel® 21, Ovral® 21: Ethinyl estradiol 0.05 mg and norgestrel 0.5 mg [white tablets] (21s)

Ogestrel® 28: Ethinyl estradiol 0.05 mg and norgestrel 0.5 mg [21 white tablets and 7 peach inactive tablets] (28s)

Ovral® 28: Ethinyl estradiol 0.05 mg and norgestrel 0.5 mg [21 white tablets and 7 pink inactive tablets] (28s)

Ethiodol® [US] *see* radiological/contrast media (ionic) *on page 561*

ethiofos *see* amifostine *on page 31*

ethionamide (e thye on AM ide)

U.S./Canadian Brand Names Trecator®-SC [US/Can]

Therapeutic Category Antimycobacterial Agent

Use In conjunction with other antituberculosis agents in the treatment of tuberculosis and other mycobacterial diseases

Usual Dosage Oral:

Children: 15-20 mg/kg/day in 2 divided doses, not to exceed 1 g/day

Adults: 500-1000 mg/day in 1-3 divided doses

Dosage Forms Tablet, sugar coated: 250 mg

Ethmozine® [US/Can] *see* moricizine *on page 437*

ethopropazine *(Canada only)* (eth oh PROE pa zeen)

U.S./Canadian Brand Names Parsitan® [Can]

Therapeutic Category Anti-Parkinson's Agent

Use Symptomatic treatment of drug induced extrapyramidal manifestations and of Parkinson's disease of postencephalitic, arteriosclerotic or idiopathic etiology.

Usual Dosage Must be adapted to each individual. In drug induced extrapyramidal reactions 100 mg twice daily usually brings about good control of symptoms. In post encephalitic, arteriosclerotic or idiopathic parkinsonism, initiate treatment at a low dose of 50 mg 3 times a day and increase from 50 to 100 mg daily every 2 to 3 days until the optimum effect is obtained or the limit of tolerance is attained. Drowsiness and anticholinergic effects which may appear at the beginning of treatment generally subside after a few days. The normal daily dose usually ranges between 100 and 500 mg but it may reach 1 g or more per day in certain patients.

Dosage Forms Tablet, as hydrochloride: 50 mg

ethosuximide (eth oh SUKS i mide)

U.S./Canadian Brand Names Zarontin® [US/Can]

Therapeutic Category Anticonvulsant

Use Management of absence (petit mal) seizures, myoclonic seizures, and akinetic epilepsy

Usual Dosage Oral:

Children 3-6 years:

Initial: 250 mg

Increment: 250 mg/day at 4- to 7-day intervals

Maintenance: 20-40 mg/kg/day

Maximum: 1500 mg/day in 2 divided doses

Children >6 years and Adults:

Initial: 500 mg/day

Increment: 250 mg/day at 4- to 7-day intervals

Maintenance: 20-40 mg/kg/day

Maximum: 1500 mg/day in 2 divided doses

Dosage Forms

Capsule: 250 mg

Syrup: 250 mg/5 mL (473 mL) [raspberry flavor]

ethotoin (ETH oh toyn)

Synonyms ethylphenylhydantoin

U.S./Canadian Brand Names Peganone® [US/Can]

Therapeutic Category Hydantoin

Use Generalized tonic-clonic or complex-partial seizures

Usual Dosage Oral:

Children: 250 mg twice daily, up to 250 mg 4 times/day

Adults: 250 mg 4 times/day after meals, may be increased up to 3 g/day in divided doses 4 times/day

Dosage Forms Tablet: 250 mg, 500 mg

ethoxynaphthamido penicillin sodium *see* nafcillin *on page 444*

Ethrane® [US] *see* enflurane *on page 227*

ethyl aminobenzoate *see* benzocaine *on page 77*

ethyl chloride (ETH il KLOR ide)

Synonyms chloroethane

Therapeutic Category Local Anesthetic

Use Local anesthetic in minor operative procedures and to relieve pain caused by insect stings and burns, and irritation caused by myofascial and visceral pain syndromes

Usual Dosage Topical: Dosage varies with use

Dosage Forms Aerosol: 100 mL, 120 mL

ethyl chloride and dichlorotetrafluoroethane

(ETH il KLOR ide & dye klor oh te tra floo or oh ETH ane)

Synonyms dichlorotetrafluoroethane and ethyl chloride

U.S./Canadian Brand Names Fluro-Ethyl® Aerosol [US]

Therapeutic Category Local Anesthetic

Use Topical refrigerant anesthetic to control pain associated with minor surgical procedures, dermabrasion, injections, contusions, and minor strains

Usual Dosage Topical: Press gently on side of spray valve allowing the liquid to emerge as a fine mist approximately 2" to 4" from site of application

Dosage Forms Aerosol: Ethyl chloride 25% and dichlorotetrafluoroethane 75% (225 g)

ethylphenylhydantoin *see* ethotoin *on this page*

ethynodiol diacetate and ethinyl estradiol *see* ethinyl estradiol and ethynodiol diacetate *on page 246*

Ethyol® [US/Can] *see* amifostine *on page 31*

Etibi® [Can] *see* ethambutol *on page 243*

etidocaine (e TI doe kane)

U.S./Canadian Brand Names Duranest® [US/Can]

Therapeutic Category Local Anesthetic

Use Infiltration anesthesia; peripheral nerve blocks; central neural blocks

Usual Dosage Varies with procedure; use 1% for peripheral nerve block, central nerve block, lumbar peridural caudal; use 1.5% for maxillary infiltration or inferior alveolar nerve block; use 1% or 1.5% for intra-abdominal or pelvic surgery, lower limb surgery, or caesarean section

Dosage Forms
Injection, as hydrochloride: 1% [10 mg/mL] (30 mL)
Injection, with epinephrine 1:200,000, as hydrochloride: 1% [10 mg/mL] (30 mL); 1.5% [15 mg/mL] (20 mL)

etidronate disodium (e ti DROE nate dye SOW dee um)

Synonyms EHDP; sodium etidronate

U.S./Canadian Brand Names Didronel® [US/Can]

Therapeutic Category Bisphosphonate Derivative

Use Symptomatic treatment of Paget's disease and heterotopic ossification due to spinal cord injury; hypercalcemia associated with malignancy

Usual Dosage Adults: Oral:
Paget's disease: 5 mg/kg/day administered every day for no more than 6 months; may administer 10 mg/kg/day for up to 3 months. Daily dose may be divided if adverse GI effects occur.
Heterotopic ossification with spinal cord injury: 20 mg/kg/day for 2 weeks, then 10 mg/kg/day for 10 weeks (this dosage has been used in children, however, treatment >1 year has been associated with a rachitic syndrome)
Hypercalcemia associated with malignancy: I.V.: 7.5 mg/kg/day for 3 days

Dosage Forms
Injection: 50 mg/mL (6 mL)
Tablet: 200 mg, 400 mg

etodolac (ee toe DOE lak)

Synonyms etodolic acid

U.S./Canadian Brand Names Apo®-Etodolac [Can]; Gen-Etodolac [Can]; Lodine® [US/Can]; Lodine® XL [US]; Utradol™ [Can]

Therapeutic Category Analgesic, Non-narcotic; Nonsteroidal Anti-inflammatory Drug (NSAID)

Use Acute and long-term use in the management of signs and symptoms of osteoarthritis and management of pain

Usual Dosage Adults: Oral:
Acute pain: 200-400 mg every 6-8 hours, as needed, not to exceed total daily doses of 1200 mg
Osteoarthritis: Initial: 800-1200 mg/day administered in divided doses: 400 mg 2 or 3 times/day; 300 mg 2, 3 or 4 times/day; 200 mg 3 or 4 times/day; total daily dose should not exceed 1200 mg; for patients weighing <60 kg, total daily dose should not exceed 20 mg/kg; extended release dose: one tablet daily

Dosage Forms
Capsule (Lodine®): 200 mg, 300 mg
Tablet (Lodine®): 400 mg, 500 mg
Tablet, extended release (Lodine® XL): 400 mg, 500 mg, 600 mg

etodolic acid *see* etodolac *on this page*

etomidate (e TOM i date)
U.S./Canadian Brand Names Amidate® [US/Can]
Therapeutic Category General Anesthetic
Use Induction of general anesthesia
Usual Dosage Children >10 years and Adults: I.V.: 0.2-0.6 mg/kg over period of 30-60 seconds
Dosage Forms Injection: 2 mg/mL (10 mL, 20 mL)

etonogestrel and ethinyl estradiol *see* ethinyl estradiol and etonogestrel *on page 247*

Etopophos® [US] *see* etoposide phosphate *on this page*

etoposide (e toe POE side)
Synonyms EPEG; VP-16
U.S./Canadian Brand Names Toposar® [US]; VePesid® [US/Can]
Therapeutic Category Antineoplastic Agent
Use Treatment of testicular and lung carcinomas, malignant lymphoma, Hodgkin's disease, leukemias (ALL, AML), neuroblastoma; also used in the treatment of Ewing's sarcoma, rhabdomyosarcoma, Wilms' tumor, brain tumors, and as a conditioning regimen for bone marrow transplantation in patients with advanced hematologic malignancies
Usual Dosage Refer to individual protocols.
Pediatric solid tumors: I.V.: 60-120 mg/m^2/day for 3-5 days every 3-6 weeks
Leukemia in children: I.V.: 100-200 mg/m^2/day for 5 days
Testicular cancer: I.V.: 50-100 mg/m^2/day on days 1-5 or 100 mg/m^2/day on days 1, 3 and 5 every 3-4 weeks for 3-4 courses
Small cell lung cancer:
Oral: Twice the I.V. dose rounded to the nearest 50 mg administered once daily if total dose ≤400 mg or in divided doses if >400 mg
I.V.: 35 mg/m^2/day for 4 days or 50 mg/m^2/day for 5 days every 3-4 weeks
Dosage Forms
Capsule (VePesid®): 50 mg
Injection (Toposar®, VePesid®): 20 mg/mL (5 mL, 7.5 mL, 25 mL, 50 mL)

etoposide phosphate (e toe POE side FOS fate)
U.S./Canadian Brand Names Etopophos® [US]
Therapeutic Category Antineoplastic Agent
Use Treatment of refractory testicular tumors and small cell lung cancer
Usual Dosage Refer to individual protocols. Adults:
Small cell lung cancer:
I.V. (in combination with other approved chemotherapeutic drugs): **Equivalent doses of etoposide phosphate to an etoposide dosage** range of 35 mg/m^2/day for 4 days to 50 mg/m^2/day for 5 days. Courses are repeated at 3- to 4-week intervals after adequate recovery from any toxicity.
Testicular cancer:
I.V. (in combination with other approved chemotherapeutic agents): **Equivalent dose of etoposide phosphate to etoposide dosage** range of 50-100 mg/m^2/day on days 1-5 to 100 mg/m^2/day on days 1, 3, and 5. Courses are repeated at 3- to 4-week intervals after adequate recovery from any toxicity.
Dosage Forms Injection, powder for reconstitution: 119.3 mg (100 mg base, 500 mg base)

Etrafon® [US/Can] *see* amitriptyline and perphenazine *on page 35*

etretinate (e TRET i nate)
U.S./Canadian Brand Names Tegison® [US]
Therapeutic Category Antipsoriatic Agent
(Continued)

etretinate *(Continued)*

Use Treatment of severe recalcitrant psoriasis in patients intolerant of or unresponsive to standard therapies

Usual Dosage Adults: Oral (individualized): Initial: 0.75-1 mg/kg/day in divided doses up to 1.5 mg/kg/day; maintenance dose established after 8-10 weeks of therapy 0.5-0.75 mg/kg/day

Dosage Forms Capsule: 10 mg, 25 mg

ETS-2%® **Topical** *(Discontinued)* see page 814

Eudal®**-SR [US]** see guaifenesin and pseudoephedrine on page 310

Euflex® **[Can]** see flutamide on page 282

Euglucon® **[Can]** see glyburide on page 301

Eulexin® **[US/Can]** see flutamide on page 282

Eurax® **Topical [US]** see crotamiton on page 166

Euthroid® **Tablet** *(Discontinued)* see page 814

Eutron® *(Discontinued)* see page 814

Evac-Q-Mag® *(Discontinued)* see page 814

Evalose® *(Discontinued)* see page 814

Everone® **Injection** *(Discontinued)* see page 814

Evista® **[US/Can]** see raloxifene on page 563

E-Vitamin® **[US-OTC]** see vitamin E on page 682

Evoxac™ **[US/Can]** see cevimeline on page 131

Exact® **Acne Medication [US-OTC]** see benzoyl peroxide on page 79

Excedrin® **Extra Strength [US-OTC]** see acetaminophen, aspirin, and caffeine on page 7

Excedrin® **IB** *(Discontinued)* see page 814

Excedrin® **Migraine [US-OTC]** see acetaminophen, aspirin, and caffeine on page 7

Excedrin® **P.M. [US-OTC]** see acetaminophen and diphenhydramine on page 5

Exelderm® **[US/Can]** see sulconazole on page 610

Exelon® **[US/Can]** see rivastigmine on page 575

exemestane (ex e MES tane)
U.S./Canadian Brand Names Aromasin® [US/Can]
Therapeutic Category Antineoplastic Agent, Miscellaneous
Controlled Substance [EX196]cancer
Use Treatment of advanced breast cancer in postmenopausal women whose disease has progressed following tamoxifen therapy
Dosage Forms Tablet: 25 mg

Exidine® **Scrub** *(Discontinued)* see page 814

Ex-Lax® **[US]** see senna on page 587

Ex-Lax® **Maximum Relief [US]** see senna on page 587

Ex-Lax® **Stool Softener [US-OTC]** see docusate on page 208

Exna® *(Discontinued)* see page 814

Exosurf® **Neonatal**™ **[US/Can]** see colfosceril palmitate on page 161

Exsel® **[US]** see selenium sulfide on page 587

Extendryl [US] see chlorpheniramine, phenylephrine, and methscopolamine on page 139

Extendryl JR [US] *see* chlorpheniramine, phenylephrine, and methscopolamine *on page 139*

Extendryl SR [US] *see* chlorpheniramine, phenylephrine, and methscopolamine *on page 139*

Extra Action Cough Syrup *(Discontinued)* *see page 814*

Extra Strength Doan's® [US-OTC] *see* magnesium salicylate *on page 398*

Eye-Lube-A® Solution *(Discontinued)* *see page 814*

Eye-Sed® Ophthalmic *(Discontinued)* *see page 814*

Eyesine® [US-OTC] *see* tetrahydrozoline *on page 629*

Eyestil [Can] *see* sodium hyaluronate *on page 597*

Eye-Stream® [US/Can] *see* balanced salt solution *on page 70*

Ezide® [US] *see* hydrochlorothiazide *on page 328*

Ezol® [US] *see* butalbital, acetaminophen, and caffeine *on page 99*

f₃t *see* trifluridine *on page 655*

factor IX complex (human) (FAK ter nyne KOM pleks HYU man)

U.S./Canadian Brand Names AlphaNine® SD [US]; BeneFix™ [US]; Hemonyne® [US]; Konȳne® 80 [US]; Profilnine® SD [US]; Proplex® T [US]

Therapeutic Category Antihemophilic Agent

Use

Control bleeding in patients with factor IX deficiency (hemophilia B or Christmas disease). **Note:** Factor IX concentrate containing ONLY factor IX is also available and preferable for this indication.

Prevention/control of bleeding in hemophilia A patients with inhibitors to factor VIII

Prevention/control of bleeding in patients with factor VII deficiency

Emergency correction of the coagulopathy of warfarin excess in critical situations

Usual Dosage Factor IX deficiency (1 unit/kg raises IX levels 1%)

Children and Adults: I.V.:

Hospitalized patients: 20-50 units/kg/dose; may be higher in special cases; may be administered every 24 hours or more often in special cases

Inhibitor patients: 75-100 units/kg/dose; may be administered every 6-12 hours

Dosage Forms

Injection:

AlphaNine® SD [single-dose vial]: Factors II, VII, IX, X

BeneFix™: 250 units, 500 units, 1000 units [purified factor IX recombinant]

Hemonyne®: 20 mL, 40 mL [factors II, VIII, IX, X]

Konȳne® 80: 20 mL, 40 mL [factors II, VII, I, X]

Profilnine® SD [single-dose vial]: Factors II, VII, IX, X

Proplex® T: 30 mL [factors II, VII, IX, X]

factor IX purified *see* factor IX (purified/human) *on this page*

factor IX (purified/human) (FAK ter nyne PURE eh fide/HYU man)

Synonyms factor IX purified; monoclonal antibody purified

U.S./Canadian Brand Names Immunine® VH [Can]; Mononine® [US]

Therapeutic Category Antihemophilic Agent

Use

Control bleeding in patients with factor IX deficiency (hemophilia B or Christmas disease)

Mononine® contains **nondetectable levels of factors II, VII, and X** (<0.0025 units per factor IX unit using standard coagulation assays) and is, therefore, **NOT INDICATED** for replacement therapy of any of these clotting factors

Mononine® is also **NOT INDICATED** in the treatment or reversal of coumarin-induced anticoagulation or in a hemorrhagic state caused by hepatitis-induced lack of production of liver dependent coagulation factors.

(Continued)

factor IX (purified/human) *(Continued)*

Usual Dosage Children and Adults: Dosage is expressed in units of factor IX activity and must be individualized. I.V. only:

Formula for units required to raise blood level %:

Number of factor IX Units Required = body weight (in kg) x desired factor IX level increase (% normal) x 1 unit/kg

For example, for a 100% level a patient who has an actual level of 20%: Number of factor IX Units needed = 70 kg x 80% x 1 Unit/kg = 5,600 Units

Dosage Forms Factor IX units listed per vial and per lot to lot variation of factor IX. Injection: 250 units, 500 units, 1000 units

factor VIIa (recombinant) (factor seven ay ree KOM be nant)

Synonyms coagulation factor VIIa; rFVIIa

U.S./Canadian Brand Names Novo-Seven® [US]

Therapeutic Category Antihemophilic Agent; Blood Product Derivative

Use Treatment of bleeding episodes in patients with hemophilia A or B when inhibitors to factor VIII or factor IX are present

Usual Dosage Children and Adults: I.V. administration only: 90 mcg/kg every 2 hours until hemostasis is achieved or until the treatment is judged ineffective. The dose and interval may be adjusted based upon the severity of bleeding and the degree of hemostasis achieved. The duration of therapy following hemostasis has not been fully established; for patients experiencing severe bleeds, dosing should be continued at 3- to 6-hour intervals after hemostasis has been achieved and the duration of dosing should be minimized.

In clinical trials, dosages have ranged from 35-120 mcg/kg and a decision on the final therapeutic dosages was reached within 8 hours in the majority of patients

Dosage Forms Injection, powder for reconstitution: 1.2 mg, 2.4 mg, 4.8 mg

factor VIII *see* antihemophilic factor (human) *on page 45*

factor VIII recombinant *see* antihemophilic factor (recombinant) *on page 46*

Factrel® [US] *see* gonadorelin *on page 304*

famciclovir (fam SYE kloe veer)

U.S./Canadian Brand Names Famvir™ [US/Can]

Therapeutic Category Antiviral Agent

Use Management of acute herpes zoster (shingles); treatment of recurrent herpes simplex in immunocompetent patients; treatment of recurrent mucocutaneous herpes simplex infections in HIV-infected patients

Usual Dosage Adults: Oral:

Acute herpes zoster: 500 mg every 8 hours for 7 days

Recurrent herpes simplex in immunocompetent patients: 125 mg twice daily for 5 days

Herpes simplex infections in HIV-infected patients: 500 mg twice daily

Dosage Forms Tablet: 125 mg, 250 mg, 500 mg

famotidine (fa MOE ti deen)

U.S./Canadian Brand Names Alti-Famotidine [Can]; Apo®-Famotidine [Can]; Gen-Famotidine [Can]; Novo-Famotidine [Can]; Nu-Famotidine [Can]; Pepcid® [US/Can]; Pepcid® AC [US/Can]; Rhoxal-famotidine [Can]; Ulcidine® [Can]

Therapeutic Category Histamine H_2 Antagonist

Use Therapy and treatment of duodenal ulcer, gastric ulcer, control gastric pH in critically ill patients, symptomatic relief in gastritis, gastroesophageal reflux, active benign ulcer, and pathological hypersecretory conditions

Usual Dosage

Children: Oral, I.V.: Doses of 1-2 mg/kg/day have been used; maximum dose: 40 mg

Adults:
 Oral:
  Duodenal ulcer, gastric ulcer: 40 mg/day at bedtime for 4-8 weeks
  Hypersecretory conditions: Initial: 20 mg every 6 hours, may increase up to 160 mg every 6 hours
  GERD: 20 mg twice daily for 6 weeks
 I.V.: 20 mg every 12 hours
Dosage Forms
 Gelcap (Pepcid® AC): 10 mg
 Infusion [premixed in NS]: 20 mg (50 mL)
 Injection [single-dose vial]: 10 mg/mL (2 mL, 4 mL)
 Powder for oral suspension (Pepcid®): 40 mg/5 mL (50 mL) [cherry-banana-mint flavor]
 Tablet (Pepcid® AC): 10 mg
 Tablet, chewable (Pepcid® AC): 10 mg [contains 1.4 mg phenylalanine/tablet]
 Tablet, film coated (Pepcid®): 20 mg, 40 mg

famotidine, calcium carbonate, and magnesium hydroxide
(fa MOE ti deen, KAL see um KAR bun ate, & mag NEE zhum hye DROKS ide)
U.S./Canadian Brand Names Pepcid® Complete [US-OTC]
Therapeutic Category Antacid; Histamine H$_2$ Antagonist
Use Relief of heartburn due to acid indigestion
Usual Dosage Children ≥12 years and Adults: Relief of heartburn due to acid indigestion: Oral: Pepcid® Complete: 1 tablet as needed; no more than 2 tablets in 24 hours; do **not** swallow whole, chew tablet completely before swallowing; do not use for longer than 14 days
Dosage Forms Tablet, chewable (Pepcid® Complete): Famotidine 10 mg, calcium carbonate 800 mg, and magnesium hydroxide 165 mg

Famvir™ [US/Can] *see* famciclovir *on previous page*

Fansidar® [US] *see* sulfadoxine and pyrimethamine *on page 612*

Farbital® [US] *see* butalbital, aspirin, and caffeine *on page 100*

Fareston® [US/Can] *see* toremifene *on page 646*

Faslodex® [US] *see* fulvestrant *on page 290*

Fastin® *(Discontinued)* *see page 814*

fat emulsion (fat e MUL shun)
Synonyms intravenous fat emulsion
U.S./Canadian Brand Names Intralipid® [US/Can]; Liposyn® [US]; Nutrilipid® [US]; Soyacal® [US]
Therapeutic Category Intravenous Nutritional Therapy
Use Source of calories and essential fatty acids for patients requiring parenteral nutrition of extended duration
Usual Dosage Fat emulsion should not exceed 60% of the total daily calories
 Initial dose:
  Infants, premature: 0.25-0.5 g/kg/day, increase by 0.25-0.5 g/kg/day to a maximum of 3-4 g/kg/day; maximum rate of infusion: 0.15 g/kg/hour (0.75 mL/kg/hour of 20% solution)
  Infants and Children: 0.5-1 g/kg/day, increase by 0.5 g/kg/day to a maximum of 3-4 g/kg/day; maximum rate of infusion: 0.25 g/kg/hour (1.25 mL/kg/hour of 20% solution)
  Adolescents and Adults: 1 g/kg/day, increase by 0.5-1 g/kg/day to a maximum of 2.5 g/kg/day; maximum rate of infusion: 0.25 g/kg/hour (1.25 mL/kg/hour of 20% solution); do not exceed 50 mL/hour (20%) or 100 mL/hour (10%)
 Fatty acid deficiency: Children and Adults: 8% to 10% of total caloric intake; infuse once or twice weekly

Note: At the onset of therapy, the patient should be observed for any immediate allergic reactions such as dyspnea, cyanosis, and fever. Slower initial rates of infusion may be
(Continued)

fat emulsion *(Continued)*

used for the first 10-15 minutes of the infusion (eg, 0.1 mL/minute of 10% or 0.05 mL/minute of 20% solution).

Dosage Forms Injection: 10% [100 mg/mL] (100 mL, 250 mL, 500 mL); 20% [200 mg/mL] (100 mL, 250 mL, 500 mL); 30% (500 mL)

5-FC *see* flucytosine *on page 274*

FC1157a *see* toremifene *on page 646*

Fe-40® [US-OTC] *see* ferrous gluconate *on page 268*

Fedahist® Expectorant *(Discontinued)* *see page 814*

Fedahist® Expectorant Pediatric *(Discontinued)* *see page 814*

Fedahist® Tablet *(Discontinued)* *see page 814*

Feen-A-Mint® [US-OTC] *see* bisacodyl *on page 87*

Feiba VH Immuno® [US/Can] *see* anti-inhibitor coagulant complex *on page 46*

felbamate (FEL ba mate)

U.S./Canadian Brand Names Felbatol® [US]

Therapeutic Category Anticonvulsant

Use Not a first-line agent; reserved for patients who do not adequately respond to alternative agents and whose epilepsy is so severe that benefit outweighs risk of liver failure or aplastic anemia; used as monotherapy and adjunctive therapy in patients ≥14 years of age with partial seizures with and without secondary generalization; adjunctive therapy in children ≥2 years of age who have partial and generalized seizures associated with Lennox-Gastaut syndrome

Usual Dosage Oral:

Monotherapy: 1200 mg/day in divided doses 3 or 4 times/day; titrate previously untreated patients under close clinical supervision, increasing the dosage in 600 mg increments every 2 weeks to 2400 mg/day based on clinical response and thereafter to 3600 mg/day in clinically indicated

Conversion to monotherapy: Initiate at 1200 mg/day in divided doses 3 or 4 times/day, reduce the dosage of the concomitant anticonvulsant(s) by 33% at the initiation of felbamate therapy; at week 2, increase the felbamate dosage to 2400 mg/day while reducing the dosage of the other anticonvulsant(s) up to an additional 33% of their original dosage; at week 3, increase the felbamate dosage up to 3600 mg/day and continue to reduce the dosage of the other anticonvulsant(s) as clinically indicated

Adjunctive therapy:

Week 1:

Felbamate: 1200 mg/day initial dose

Concomitant anticonvulsant(s): Reduce original dosage by 20% to 33%

Week 2:

Felbamate: 2400 mg/day (Therapeutic range)

Concomitant anticonvulsant(s): Reduce original dosage by up to an additional 33%

Week 3:

Felbamate: 3600 mg/day (Therapeutic range)

Concomitant anticonvulsant(s): Reduce original dosage as clinically indicated

Dosage Forms

Suspension, oral: 600 mg/5 mL (240 mL, 960 mL)

Tablet: 400 mg, 600 mg

Felbatol® [US] *see* felbamate *on this page*

Feldene® [US/Can] *see* piroxicam *on page 517*

felodipine (fe LOE di peen)

U.S./Canadian Brand Names Plendil® [US/Can]; Renedil® [Can]

Therapeutic Category Calcium Channel Blocker

Use Management of angina pectoris due to coronary insufficiency, hypertension
Usual Dosage Oral:
    Adults: Initial: 5 mg once daily; dosage range: 2.5-10 mg once daily; may increase dose up to a maximum of 10 mg
Dosage Forms Tablet, extended release: 2.5 mg, 5 mg, 10 mg

Femara® [US/Can] *see* letrozole *on page 377*

FemCare® *(Discontinued) see page 814*

Femcet® *(Discontinued) see page 814*

Femguard® *(Discontinued) see page 814*

femhrt® [US/Can] *see* ethinyl estradiol and norethindrone *on page 251*

Femilax™ [US-OTC] *see* bisacodyl *on page 87*

Femiron® [US-OTC] *see* ferrous fumarate *on page 268*

Femstat® *(Discontinued) see page 814*

Femstat® One [Can] *see* butoconazole *on page 101*

Fenesin™ [US] *see* guaifenesin *on page 307*

Fenesin™ DM [US] *see* guaifenesin and dextromethorphan *on page 308*

fenofibrate (fen oh FYE brate)
Synonyms procetofene; proctofene
U.S./Canadian Brand Names Apo®-Fenofibrate [Can]; Apo®-Feno-Micro [Can]; Gen-Fenofibrat Micro [Can]; Lipidil Micro® [Can]; Lipidil Supra® [Can]; Nu-Fenofibrate [Can]; PMS-Fenofibrate Micro [Can]; TriCor® [US/Can]
Therapeutic Category Antihyperlipidemic Agent, Miscellaneous
Use Adjunct to dietary therapy for the treatment of adults with very high elevations of serum triglyceride levels (types IV and V hyperlipidemia) who are at risk of pancreatitis and who do not respond adequately to a determined dietary effort; its efficacy can be enhanced by combination with other hypolipidemic agents that have a different mechanism of action; safety and efficacy may be greater than that of clofibrate
Usual Dosage
    Adults:
    Hypertriglyceridemia: Initial: 54 mg/day with meals, up to 160 mg/day
    Hypercholesterolemia or mixed hyperlipidemia: Initial: 160 mg/day with meals
Dosage Forms Tablet: 54 mg, 160 mg

fenoldopam (fe NOL doe pam)
U.S./Canadian Brand Names Corlopam® [US/Can]
Therapeutic Category Antihypertensive Agent
Use Patients presenting with emergency hypertension and those requiring blood pressure control during hospitalization pose a challenge due to the associated risk of renal failure and end-organ compromise
Usual Dosage
    Oral: 100 mg 2-4 times/day
    I.V.: Severe hypertension: Initial: 0.1 mcg/kg/minute; may be increased in increments of 0.05-0.2 mcg/kg/minute; maximal infusion rate: 1.6 mcg/kg/minute
Dosage Forms Injection: 10 mg/mL (5 mL)

fenoprofen (fen oh PROE fen)
U.S./Canadian Brand Names Nalfon® [US/Can]
Therapeutic Category Analgesic, Non-narcotic; Nonsteroidal Anti-inflammatory Drug (NSAID)
Use Symptomatic treatment of acute and chronic rheumatoid arthritis and osteoarthritis; relief of mild to moderate pain
(Continued)

fenoprofen *(Continued)*

Usual Dosage Oral:
Children: Juvenile arthritis: 900 mg/m^2/day, then increase over 4 weeks to 1.8 g/m^2/day
Adults:
Arthritis: 300-600 mg 3-4 times/day up to 3.2 g/day
Pain: 200 mg every 4-6 hours as needed

Dosage Forms
Capsule, as calcium: 200 mg, 300 mg
Tablet, as calcium: 600 mg

fenoterol *(Canada only)* (fen oh TER ole)

U.S./Canadian Brand Names Berotec® [Can]

Therapeutic Category Beta$_2$-Adrenergic Agonist Agent

Use For the symptomatic relief and acute prophylaxis of bronchial obstruction in asthma and other conditions in which reversible bronchospasm is a complicating factor, such as chronic bronchitis or emphysema.

Usual Dosage Adults:
MDI: Acute symptoms: One puff will usually be adequate to relieve bronchospasm in the majority of patients, however, if required, a second puff may be taken preferably after waiting 5 minutes for the effect of the first puff to be obtained. This delay allows better assessment of the effectiveness of 1 puff and deeper penetration of the second puff. If an attack has not been relieved by 2 puffs, further puffs may be required. In these cases, patients should immediately consult the physician or the nearest hospital. If, despite other adequate maintenance therapy, regular use of beta-agonists remains necessary for the control of bronchospasm, the recommended dose is 1-2 puffs of the 100 mcg inhaler 3-4 times/day. A maximum of 8 puffs/day should not be exceeded.
Solution: Dosage should be individualized, and patient response should be monitored by the prescribing physician on an ongoing basis. Should be used only under medical supervision.
Motorized, compressed air or ultrasonic nebulizers: These nebulizers generate low pressure, low velocity aerosols. The average single dose is 0.5 to 1 mg of fenoterol. In more refractory cases, up to 2.5 mg of fenoterol may be given. Fenoterol solution should be diluted to 5 mL with preservative-free sterile sodium chloride inhalation solution, USP 0.9% (normal saline) and the total volume should be nebulized over a period of 10 to 15 minutes. Optimal deposition in the lungs is achieved with the patient breathing quietly and slowly. Treatment may be repeated every 6 hours if necessary.
Intermittent positive pressure ventilation: Fenoterol solution may be used in conjunction with Intermittent Positive Pressure Ventilation (IPPV) when such therapy is indicated. The average single dose is 0.5 to 1 mg of fenoterol. In more refractory cases, up to 2.5 mg of fenoterol may be given. Fenoterol solution should be diluted to 5 mL with preservative-free sterile sodium chloride inhalation solution, USP 0.9% and the total volume should be nebulized over a period of 10-15 minutes. The inspiratory pressure is usually 10 to 20 cm H$_2$O and optimal deposition of the drug in the lungs is achieved with the patient breathing quietly and slowly. Treatment may be repeated every 6 hours if necessary. If a previous effective dosage regimen fails to provide the usual relief, or the effects of a dose last for less than 3 hours, medical advice should be sought immediately; this is a sign of seriously worsening asthma that requires reassessment of therapy. In accordance with the present practice for asthma treatment, concomitant anti-inflammatory therapy should be part of the regimen if fenoterol inhalation solution needs to be used on a regular daily basis.

Dosage Forms
Aerosol for inhalation, as hydrobromide: MDI: 100 mcg/dose [200 doses]
Solution for inhalation, as hydrobromide: 0.625 mg/mL (2 mL); 0.25 mg/mL (2 mL)

fentanyl (FEN ta nil)

U.S./Canadian Brand Names Actiq® [US/Can]; Duragesic® [US/Can]; Sublimaze® [US]

Therapeutic Category Analgesic, Narcotic; General Anesthetic

Controlled Substance C-II

Use Sedation; relief of pain; preoperative medication; adjunct to general or regional anesthesia; management of chronic pain (transdermal product)

Oral transmucosal: Hospital setting use only as preoperative anesthetic agent or to induce conscious sedation before procedures

Usual Dosage Doses should be titrated to appropriate effects; wide range of doses, dependent upon desired degree of analgesia/anesthesia

Children:

Sedation for minor procedures/analgesia: I.M., I.V.:

1-3 years: 2-3 mcg/kg/dose; may repeat after 30-60 minutes as required

3-12 years: 1-2 mcg/kg/dose; may repeat at 30- to 60-minute intervals as required. **Note:** Children 18-36 months of age may require 2-3 mcg/kg/dose

Continuous sedation/analgesia: Initial I.V. bolus: 1-2 mcg/kg then 1 mcg/kg/hour; titrate upward; usual: 1-3 mcg/kg/hour

Transdermal: Not recommended

Children <12 years and Adults:

Sedation for minor procedures/analgesia: 0.5-1 mcg/kg/dose; higher doses are used for major procedures

Preoperative sedation, adjunct to regional anesthesia, postoperative pain: I.M., I.V.: 50-100 mcg/dose

Adjunct to general anesthesia: I.M., I.V.: 2-50 mcg/kg

General anesthesia without additional anesthetic agents: I.V. 50-100 mcg/kg with O_2 and skeletal muscle relaxant

Transdermal: Initial: 25 mcg/hour system; if currently receiving opiates, convert to fentanyl equivalent and administer equianalgesic dosage (see package insert for further information)

Dosage Forms

Injection, as citrate [preservative free]: 0.05 mg/mL (2 mL, 5 mL, 10 mL, 20 mL, 30 mL, 50 mL)

Lozenge, oral transmucosal, as citrate [mounted on a plastic radiopaque handle] (Actiq®): 200 mcg, 400 mcg, 600 mcg, 800 mcg, 1200 mcg, 1600 mcg [raspberry flavor]

Transdermal system: 25 mcg/hour [10 cm^2]; 50 mcg/hour [20 cm^2]; 75 mcg/hour [30 cm^2]; 100 mcg/hour [40 cm^2] (5s)

fentanyl and droperidol *see* droperidol and fentanyl *on page 217*

Fentanyl Oralet® *(Discontinued)* *see page 814*

Feosol® [US-OTC] *see* ferrous sulfate *on page 269*

Feostat® [US-OTC] *see* ferrous fumarate *on next page*

Feracid® [US] *see* glutamic acid *on page 301*

Ferancee® *(Discontinued)* *see page 814*

Feratab® [US-OTC] *see* ferrous sulfate *on page 269*

Fergon Plus® *(Discontinued)* *see page 814*

Fergon® [US-OTC] *see* ferrous gluconate *on next page*

Feridex I.V.® [US] *see* ferumoxides *on page 270*

Fer-in-Sol® Capsule (only) *(Discontinued)* *see page 814*

Fer-In-Sol® Drops [US/Can] *see* ferrous sulfate *on page 269*

Fer-Iron® [US-OTC] *see* ferrous sulfate *on page 269*

Fermalac [Can] *see* Lactobacillus *on page 372*

Fermalox® *(Discontinued)* *see page 814*

Ferndex® *(Discontinued)* *see page 814*

Ferodan™ [Can] *see* ferrous sulfate *on page 269*

Fero-Grad 500® [US-OTC] *see* ferrous sulfate and ascorbic acid *on page 269*

Fero-Gradumet® *(Discontinued)* *see page 814*

Feronate® **[US-OTC]** *see* ferrous gluconate *on this page*

Ferospace® *(Discontinued)* *see page 814*

Ferralet® *(Discontinued)* *see page 814*

Ferralyn® **Lanacaps**® *(Discontinued)* *see page 814*

Ferra-TD® *(Discontinued)* *see page 814*

ferric gluconate (FER ik GLOO koe nate)

U.S./Canadian Brand Names Ferrlecit® [US]

Therapeutic Category Iron Salt

Use Repletion of total body iron content in patients with iron deficiency anemia who are undergoing hemodialysis in conjunction with erythropoietin therapy

Usual Dosage Adults:

Test dose (recommended): 2 mL diluted in 50 mL 0.9% sodium chloride over 60 minutes

Repletion of iron in hemodialysis patients: I.V.: 125 mg (10 mL) in 100 mL 0.9% sodium chloride over 1 hour during hemodialysis. Most patients will require a cumulative dose of 1 g elemental iron over approximately 8 sequential dialysis treatments to achieve a favorable response.

Dosage Forms Injection: 12.5 mg elemental iron/mL (5 mL) [contains benzyl alcohol 9 mg/mL]

Ferrlecit® **[US]** *see* ferric gluconate *on this page*

Ferro-Sequels® **[US-OTC]** *see* ferrous fumarate *on this page*

ferrous fumarate (FER us FYOO ma rate)

U.S./Canadian Brand Names Femiron® [US-OTC]; Feostat® [US-OTC]; Ferro-Sequels® [US-OTC]; Hemocyte® [US-OTC]; Ircon® [US-OTC]; Nephro-Fer™ [US-OTC]; Palafer® [Can]

Therapeutic Category Electrolyte Supplement, Oral

Use Prevention and treatment of iron deficiency anemias

Usual Dosage Oral:

Children: 3 mg/kg 3 times/day

Adults: 200 mg 3-4 times/day

Dosage Forms Elemental iron listed in brackets:

Capsule, controlled release (Span-FF®): 325 mg [106 mg]

Solution, oral drops (Feostat®): 45 mg/0.6 mL [15 mg/0.6 mL] (60 mL)

Suspension, oral (Feostat®): 100 mg/5 mL [33 mg/5 mL] (240 mL)

Tablet: 325 mg [106 mg]

Femiron®: 63 mg [20 mg]

Hemocyte®: 324 mg [106 mg]

Nephro-Fer™: 350 mg [115 mg]

Tablet, chewable (Feostat®): 100 mg [33 mg] [chocolate flavor]

Tablet, timed release (Ferro-Sequels®): Ferrous fumarate 150 mg [50 mg]

ferrous gluconate (FER us GLOO koe nate)

U.S./Canadian Brand Names Apo®-Ferrous Gluconate [Can]; Fe-40® [US-OTC]; Fergon® [US-OTC]; Feronate® [US-OTC]

Therapeutic Category Electrolyte Supplement, Oral

Use Prevention and treatment of iron deficiency anemias

Usual Dosage Oral (dose expressed in terms of elemental iron):

Iron deficiency anemia: 3-6 Fe mg/kg/day in 3 divided doses

Maintenance:

Preterm infants:

Birthweight <1000 g: 4 Fe mg/kg/day

Birthweight 1000-1500 g: 3 Fe mg/kg/day

Birthweight 1500-2500 g: 2 Fe mg/kg/day

Term Infants and Children: 1-2 Fe mg/kg/day in 3 divided doses, up to a maximum of 18 Fe mg/day

Adults: 60-100 Fe mg/day in 3 divided doses

Dosage Forms Elemental iron listed in brackets:

Tablet: 300 mg [34 mg]; 325 mg [36 mg]

Fergon®: 240 mg [27 mg]

ferrous sulfate (FER us SUL fate)

Synonyms FeSO₄

U.S./Canadian Brand Names Apo®-Ferrous Sulfate [Can]; Feosol® [US-OTC]; Feratab® [US-OTC]; Fer-In-Sol® Drops [US/Can]; Fer-Iron® [US-OTC]; Ferodan™ [Can]; Slow FE® [US-OTC]

Therapeutic Category Electrolyte Supplement, Oral

Use Prevention and treatment of iron deficiency anemias

Usual Dosage Oral (dose expressed in terms of elemental iron):

Children:

Severe iron deficiency anemia: 4-6 mg Fe/kg/day in 3 divided doses

Mild to moderate iron deficiency anemia: 3 mg Fe/kg/day in 1-2 divided doses

Prophylaxis: 1-2 mg Fe/kg/day up to a maximum of 15 mg/day

Adults: Iron deficiency: 60-100 Fe/kg/day in divided doses

Dosage Forms Elemental iron listed in brackets:

Elixir (Feosol®): 220 mg/5 mL [44 mg/5 mL] (473 mL, 4000 mL) [contains alcohol 5%]

Solution, oral drops (Fer-In-Sol®, Fer-Iron®): 75 mg/0.6 mL [15 mg/0.6 mL] (50 mL)

Syrup (Fer-In-Sol®): 90 mg/5 mL [18 mg/5 mL] (480 mL) [contains alcohol 5%]

Tablet: 324 mg [65 mg]

Feratab®: 187 mg [60 mg]

Tablet, exsiccated (Feosol®): 200 mg [65 mg]

Tablet, exsiccated, timed release (Slow FE®): 160 mg [50 mg]

ferrous sulfate and ascorbic acid (FER us SUL fate & a SKOR bik AS id)

Synonyms ascorbic acid and ferrous sulfate

U.S./Canadian Brand Names Fero-Grad 500® [US-OTC]

Therapeutic Category Vitamin

Use Treatment of iron deficiency in nonpregnant adults; treatment and prevention of iron deficiency in pregnant adults

Usual Dosage Adults: Oral: 1 tablet daily

Dosage Forms Elemental iron listed in brackets:

Tablet (Fero-Grad 500®): Ferrous sulfate 525 mg [105 mg] and ascorbic acid 500 mg

ferrous sulfate, ascorbic acid, and vitamin B-complex

(FER us SUL fate, a SKOR bik AS id, & VYE ta min bee-KOM pleks)

U.S./Canadian Brand Names Iberet®-Liquid 500 [US-OTC]; Iberet®-Liquid [US-OTC]

Therapeutic Category Vitamin

Use Treatment of conditions of iron deficiency with an increased need for B complex vitamins and vitamin C

Usual Dosage Oral:

Children 1-3 years: 5 mL twice daily after meals

Children >4 years and Adults: 10 mL 3 times/day after meals

Dosage Forms Liquid (components all per 15 mL):

Iberet®-Liquid:

Ascorbic acid: 112.5 mg

B_1: 4.5 mg

B_2: 4.5 mg

B_3: 22.5 mg

B_5: 7.5 mg

B_6: 3.75 mg

B_{12}: 18.75 mg

Ferrous sulfate: 78.75 mg

(Continued)

ferrous sulfate, ascorbic acid, and vitamin B-complex
(Continued)

Iberet®-Liquid 500:
Ascorbic acid: 375 mg
B_1: 4.5 mg
B_2: 4.5 mg
B_3: 22.5 mg
B_5: 7.5 mg
B_6: 3.75 mg
B_{12}: 18.75 mg
Ferrous sulfate: 78.75 mg

ferrous sulfate, ascorbic acid, vitamin B-complex, and folic acid
(FER us SUL fate, a SKOR bik AS id, VYE ta min bee-KOM pleks, & FOE lik AS id)
U.S./Canadian Brand Names Iberet-Folic-500® [US]
Therapeutic Category Vitamin
Use Treatment of iron deficiency and prevention of concomitant folic acid deficiency where there is an associated deficient intake or increased need for B complex vitamins
Usual Dosage Adults: Oral: 1 tablet daily
Dosage Forms
Tablet, controlled release:
Ascorbic acid: 500 mg
B_1: 6 mg
B_2: 6 mg
B_3: 30 mg
B_5: 10 mg
B_6: 5 mg
B_{12}: 25 mcg
Ferrous sulfate: 105 mg
Folic acid: 800 mcg

Fertinex® [US] *see* urofollitropin *on page 668*

Fertinorm® H.P. [Can] *see* urofollitropin *on page 668*

ferumoxides (fer yoo MOX ides)
U.S./Canadian Brand Names Feridex I.V.® [US]
Therapeutic Category Radiopaque Agents
Use For I.V. administration as an adjunct to MRI (in adult patients) to enhance the T2 weighted images used in the detection and evaluation of lesions of the liver
Usual Dosage Adults: 0.56 mg of iron (0.05 mL Feridex I.V.®)/kg body weight diluted in 100 mL of 5% dextrose and infused over 30 minutes; a 5-micron filter is recommended; do not administer undiluted
Dosage Forms Injection: Iron 11.2 mg and mannitol per mL (5 mL)

FeSO₄ *see* ferrous sulfate *on previous page*

Feverall® [US-OTC] *see* acetaminophen *on page 3*

fexofenadine (feks oh FEN a deen)
U.S./Canadian Brand Names Allegra® [US/Can]
Therapeutic Category Antihistamine
Use Nonsedating antihistamine indicated for the relief of seasonal allergic rhinitis
Usual Dosage Children ≥12 years and Adults: Oral: 1 capsule (60 mg) twice daily
Dosage Forms
Capsule, as hydrochloride: 60 mg
Tablet, as hydrochloride: 30 mg, 60 mg, 180 mg

fexofenadine and pseudoephedrine
(feks oh FEN a deen & soo doe e FED rin)

U.S./Canadian Brand Names Allegra-D® [US/Can]

Therapeutic Category Antihistamine/Decongestant Combination

Use Relief of symptoms associated with seasonal allergic rhinitis in adults and children ≥12 years. Symptoms treated effectively include sneezing, rhinorrhea, itchy nose/ palate/ and/or throat, itchy/watery/red eyes, and nasal congestion.

Usual Dosage Oral: Adults: 1 tablet twice daily for adults and children ≥12 years of age. It is recommended that the administration with food should be avoided. A dose of 1 tablet once daily is recommended as the starting dose in patients with decreased renal function.

Dosage Forms Tablet, extended release: Fexofenadine hydrochloride 60 mg and pseudoephedrine hydrochloride 120 mg

Fiberall® Chewable Tablet [US-OTC] *see* calcium polycarbophil *on page 108*

Fiberall® Powder [US-OTC] *see* psyllium *on page 554*

Fiberall® Wafer [US-OTC] *see* psyllium *on page 554*

FiberCon® Tablet [US-OTC] *see* calcium polycarbophil *on page 108*

Fiber-Lax® Tablet [US-OTC] *see* calcium polycarbophil *on page 108*

fibrinolysin and desoxyribonuclease
(fye brin oh LYE sin & des oks i rye boe NOO klee ase)

U.S./Canadian Brand Names Elase® [US]

Therapeutic Category Enzyme

Use Debriding agent; cervicitis; and irrigating agent in infected wounds

Usual Dosage
Ointment: 2-3 times/day
Wet dressing: 3-4 times/day

Dosage Forms Ointment: Fibrinolysin 1 unit and desoxyribonuclease 666.6 units per g (10 g, 30 g)

fibrin sealant kit (FI brin SEEL ent kit)

Synonyms FS

U.S./Canadian Brand Names Tisseel® VH Fibrin Sealant Kit [US/Can]

Therapeutic Category Hemostatic Agent

Use Adjunct to hemostasis in cardiopulmonary bypass surgery and splenic injury (due to blunt or penetrating trauma to the abdomen) when the control of bleeding by conventional surgical techniques is ineffective or impractical; adjunctive sealant for closure of colostomies; hemostatic agent in heparinized patients undergoing cardiopulmonary bypass

Usual Dosage Adjunct to hemostasis: Adults: Apply topically; actual dose is based on size of surface to be covered:
Maximum area to be sealed: 4 cm^2
 Required size of Tisseel® VH kit: 0.5 mL
Maximum area to be sealed: 8 cm^2
 Required size of Tisseel® VH kit: 1 mL
Maximum area to be sealed: 16 cm^2
 Required size of Tisseel® VH kit: 2 mL
Maximum area to be sealed: 40 cm^2
 Required size of Tisseel® VH kit: 5 mL

Apply in thin layers to avoid excess formation of granulation tissue and slow absorption of the sealant. Following application, hold the sealed parts in the desired position for 3-5 minutes. To prevent sealant from adhering to gloves or surgical instruments, wet them with saline prior to contact.

Dosage Forms Tisseel® VH Kit: Fibrin sealant, two-component fibrin sealant, vapor-heated, kit (0.5 mL, 1 mL, 2 mL, 5 mL)

filgrastim (fil GRA stim)

Synonyms G-CSF; granulocyte colony-stimulating factor

U.S./Canadian Brand Names Neupogen® [US/Can]

Therapeutic Category Colony-Stimulating Factor

Use To reduce the duration of neutropenia and the associated risk of infection in patients with nonmyeloid malignancies receiving myelosuppressive chemotherapeutic regimens associated with a significant incidence of severe neutropenia with fever; it has also been used in AIDS patients on zidovudine and in patients with noncancer chemotherapy-induced neutropenia

Usual Dosage Children and Adults (refer to individual protocols): I.V., S.C.: 5-10 mcg/kg/day (~150-300 mcg/m^2/day) once daily for up to 14 days until ANC = 10,000/mm^3; dose escalations at 5 mcg/kg/day may be required in some individuals when response at 5 mcg/kg/day is not adequate; dosages of 0.6-120 mcg/kg/day have been used in children ranging in age from 3 months to 18 years

Dosage Forms

Injection, solution [preservative free]: 300 mcg/mL (1 mL, 1.6 mL)

Neupogen® Singleject® [prefilled syringe]: 600 mcg/mL (0.5 mL, 0.8 mL)

finasteride (fi NAS teer ide)

U.S./Canadian Brand Names Propecia® [US/Can]; Proscar® [US/Can]

Therapeutic Category Antiandrogen

Use Early data indicate that finasteride is useful in the treatment of benign prostatic hyperplasia

Usual Dosage Benign prostatic hyperplasia: Adults: Oral: 5 mg/day as a single dose; clinical responses occur within 12 weeks to 6 months of initiation of therapy; long-term administration is recommended for maximal response

Dosage Forms

Tablet, film coated:

Propecia®: 1 mg

Proscar®: 5 mg

Finevin™ [US] *see* azelaic acid *on page 65*

Fiorgen PF® *(Discontinued)* *see page 814*

Fioricet® [US] *see* butalbital, acetaminophen, and caffeine *on page 99*

Fiorinal® [US/Can] *see* butalbital, aspirin, and caffeine *on page 100*

Fiorinal®-C 1/2 [Can] *see* butalbital compound and codeine *on page 100*

Fiorinal®-C 1/4 [Can] *see* butalbital compound and codeine *on page 100*

Fiorinal® With Codeine [US] *see* butalbital compound and codeine *on page 100*

Fiorital® *(Discontinued)* *see page 814*

fisalamine *see* mesalamine *on page 411*

FK506 *see* tacrolimus *on page 617*

Flagyl® [US/Can] *see* metronidazole *on page 426*

Flagyl ER® [US] *see* metronidazole *on page 426*

Flamazine® [Can] *see* silver sulfadiazine *on page 590*

Flarex® [US/Can] *see* fluorometholone *on page 278*

Flatulex® [US-OTC] *see* simethicone *on page 591*

Flavorcee® *(Discontinued)* *see page 814*

flavoxate (fla VOKS ate)

U.S./Canadian Brand Names Urispas® [US/Can]

Therapeutic Category Antispasmodic Agent, Urinary

Use Antispasmodic to provide symptomatic relief of dysuria, nocturia, suprapubic pain, urgency, and incontinence

Usual Dosage Children >12 years and Adults: Oral: 100-200 mg 3-4 times/day

Dosage Forms Tablet, film coated, as hydrochloride: 100 mg

Flaxedil® *(Discontinued)* see page 814

flecainide (fle KAY nide)

U.S./Canadian Brand Names Tambocor™ [US/Can]

Therapeutic Category Antiarrhythmic Agent, Class I-C

Use Prevention and suppression of documented life-threatening ventricular arrhythmias (ie, sustained ventricular tachycardia); prevention of symptomatic, disabling supraventricular tachycardias in patients without structural heart disease

Usual Dosage Oral:

Children: Initial: 3 mg/kg/day in 3 divided doses; usual 3-6 mg/kg/day in 3 divided doses; up to 11 mg/kg/day for uncontrolled patients with subtherapeutic levels

Adults: Initial: 100 mg every 12 hours, increase by 100 mg/day (administer in 2 doses/day) every 4 days to maximum of 400 mg/day; for patients receiving 400 mg/day who are not controlled and have trough concentrations <0.6 mcg/mL, dosage may be increased to 600 mg/day

Dosage Forms Tablet, as acetate: 50 mg, 100 mg, 150 mg

Fleet® **Babylax**® **[US-OTC]** see glycerin on page 302

Fleet® **Bisacodyl Enema [US-OTC]** see bisacodyl on page 87

Fleet® **Enema [US/Can]** see sodium phosphates on page 598

Fleet® **Flavored Castor Oil** *(Discontinued)* see page 814

Fleet® **Glycerin Suppositories Maximum Strength [US-OTC]** see glycerin on page 302

Fleet® **Glycerin Suppositories [US-OTC]** see glycerin on page 302

Fleet® **Laxative** *(Discontinued)* see page 814

Fleet® **Liquid Glycerin Suppositories [US-OTC]** see glycerin on page 302

Fleet® **Pain Relief [US-OTC]** see pramoxine on page 534

Fleet® **Phospho**®**-Soda [US/Can]** see sodium phosphates on page 598

Fleet® **Stimulant Laxative [US-OTC]** see bisacodyl on page 87

Flexaphen® *(Discontinued)* see page 814

Flexeril® **[US/Can]** see cyclobenzaprine on page 168

Flexitec [Can] see cyclobenzaprine on page 168

Flo-Coat® **[US]** see radiological/contrast media (ionic) on page 561

floctafenine *(Canada only)* (flok ta FEN een)

U.S./Canadian Brand Names Idarac® [Can]

Therapeutic Category Nonsteroidal Anti-inflammatory Drug (NSAID), Oral

Use Short-term use in acute pain of mild and moderate severity

Usual Dosage Adults: Oral: 200-400 mg every 6-8 hours as required; maximum recommended daily dose: 1200 mg

Dosage Forms Tablet: 200 mg, 400 mg

Flolan® **[US/Can]** see epoprostenol on page 231

Flomax® **[US/Can]** see tamsulosin on page 618

Flonase® **[US]** see fluticasone (nasal) on page 283

Flonase® **9 g** *(Discontinued)* see page 814

Florical® **[US-OTC]** see calcium carbonate on page 104

Florinef® **Acetate [US/Can]** see fludrocortisone on page 275

Florone® *(Discontinued)* see page 814

Florone E® *(Discontinued)* see page 814

Floropryl® Ophthalmic *(Discontinued)* see page 814

Flovent® [US] see fluticasone (oral inhalation) on page 283

Flovent® Rotadisk® [US] see fluticasone (oral inhalation) on page 283

Floxin® [US/Can] see ofloxacin on page 475

floxuridine (floks YOOR i deen)

Synonyms fluorodeoxyuridine

U.S./Canadian Brand Names FUDR® [US/Can]

Therapeutic Category Antineoplastic Agent

Use Palliative management of carcinomas of head, neck, and brain as well as liver, gallbladder, and bile ducts

Usual Dosage Adults:

Intra-arterial infusion: 0.1-0.6 mg/kg/day for 14 days followed by heparinized saline for 14 days

Investigational: I.V.: 0.5-1 mg/kg/day for 6-15 days

Dosage Forms Injection, powder for reconstitution: 500 mg (5 mL, 10 mL)

Fluanxol® Depot [Can] see flupenthixol *(Canada only)* on page 280

Fluanxol® Tablet [Can] see flupenthixol *(Canada only)* on page 280

flubenisolone see betamethasone (topical) on page 83

fluconazole (floo KOE na zole)

U.S./Canadian Brand Names Apo®-Fluconazole [Can]; Diflucan® [US/Can]

Therapeutic Category Antifungal Agent

Use Treatment of susceptible fungal infections including oropharyngeal, esophageal, and vaginal candidiasis; treatment of systemic candidal infections including urinary tract infection, peritonitis, cystitis, and pneumonia; treatment and suppression of cryptococcal meningitis; prophylaxis of candidiasis in patients undergoing bone marrow transplantation; alternative to amphotericin B in patients with pre-existing renal impairment or when requiring concomitant therapy with other potentially nephrotoxic drugs

Usual Dosage Daily dose of fluconazole is the same for oral and I.V. administration

Infants and Children: Oral, I.V.: Safety profile of fluconazole has been studied in 577 children, ages 1 day to 17 years; doses as high as 12 mg/kg/day once daily (equivalent to adult doses of 400 mg/day) have been used to treat candidiasis in immunocompromised children; 10-12 mg/kg/day doses once daily have been used prophylactically against fungal infections in pediatric bone marrow transplantation patients. Do not exceed 600 mg/day.

Adults:

Vaginal candidiasis: Oral: 150 mg single dose

Prophylaxis against fungal infections in bone marrow transplantation patients: Oral, I.V.: 400 mg/day once daily

Dosage Forms

Injection: 2 mg/mL (100 mL, 200 mL)

Powder for oral suspension: 10 mg/mL (35 mL); 40 mg/mL (35 mL)

Tablet: 50 mg, 100 mg, 150 mg, 200 mg

flucytosine (floo SYE toe seen)

Synonyms 5-FC; 5-flurocytosine

U.S./Canadian Brand Names Ancobon® [US/Can]

Therapeutic Category Antifungal Agent

Use In combination with amphotericin B in the treatment of serious *Candida*, *Aspergillus*, *Cryptococcus*, and *Torulopsis* infections

Usual Dosage Children and Adults: Oral: 50-150 mg/kg/day in divided doses every 6 hours

Dosage Forms Capsule: 250 mg, 500 mg

Fludara® **[US/Can]** *see* fludarabine *on this page*

fludarabine (floo DARE a been)

U.S./Canadian Brand Names Fludara® [US/Can]

Therapeutic Category Antineoplastic Agent

Use Treatment of B-cell chronic lymphocytic leukemia unresponsive to previous therapy with an alkylating agent containing regimen. Fludarabine has been tested in patients with refractory acute lymphocytic leukemia and acute nonlymphocytic leukemia, but required a highly toxic dose to achieve response.

Usual Dosage Adults: I.V.:

Chronic lymphocytic leukemia: 25 mg/m^2/day over a 30-minute period for 5 days

Non-Hodgkin's lymphoma: Loading dose: 20 mg/m^2 followed by 30 mg/m^2/day for 48 hours

Dosage Forms Injection, powder for reconstitution, as phosphate: 50 mg (6 mL)

fludrocortisone (floo droe KOR ti sone)

Synonyms fluohydrocortisone; 9α-fluorohydrocortisone

U.S./Canadian Brand Names Florinef® Acetate [US/Can]

Therapeutic Category Adrenal Corticosteroid (Mineralocorticoid)

Use Addison's disease; partial replacement therapy for adrenal insufficiency; treatment of salt-losing forms of congenital adrenogenital syndrome; has been used with increased sodium intake for the treatment of idiopathic orthostatic hypotension

Usual Dosage Oral:

Infants and Children: 0.05-0.1 mg/day

Adults: 0.05-0.2 mg/day

Dosage Forms Tablet, as acetate: 0.1 mg

Flumadine® **[US/Can]** *see* rimantadine *on page 573*

flumazenil (FLO may ze nil)

U.S./Canadian Brand Names Anexate® [Can]; Romazicon® [US/Can]

Therapeutic Category Antidote

Use Benzodiazepine antagonist; reverses sedative effects of benzodiazepines used in general anesthesia or conscious sedation; management of benzodiazepine overdose; not indicated for ethanol, barbiturate, general anesthetic or narcotic overdose

Usual Dosage Reversal of conscious sedation or general anesthesia: 0.2 mg (2 mL) administered I.V. over 15 seconds; if desired effect is not achieved after 60 seconds, repeat in 0.2 mg (2 mL) increments every 60 seconds up to a total of 1 mg (10 mL); in event of resedation, repeat doses may be administered at 20-minute intervals with no more than 1 mg (10 mL) administered at any one time, with a maximum of 3 mg in any 1 hour

Dosage Forms Injection: 0.1 mg/mL (5 mL, 10 mL)

flunarizine *(Canada only)* (floo NAR i zeen)

U.S./Canadian Brand Names Sibelium® [Can]

Therapeutic Category Calcium-Entry Blocker (Selective)

Use Prophylaxis of migraine with and without aura; the safety of flunarizine in long-term use (ie, >4 months) has not been systematically evaluated in controlled clinical trials. Flunarizine is not indicated in the treatment of acute migraine attacks.

Usual Dosage The usual adult dosage is 10 mg/day administered in the evening. Patients who experience side effects may be maintained on 5 mg at bedtime.

Duration of therapy: Clinical experience indicates that the onset of effect of flunarizine is gradual and maximum benefits may not be seen before the patient has completed (Continued)

flunarizine *(Canada only)* *(Continued)*

several weeks of continuous treatment. Therapy, therefore, should not be discontinued for lack of response before an adequate time period has elapsed (ie, 6-8 weeks).

Dosage Forms Capsule, as hydrochloride: 5 mg

flunisolide (floo NIS oh lide)

U.S./Canadian Brand Names AeroBid®-M [US]; AeroBid® [US]; Alti-Flunisolide [Can]; Apo®-Flunisolide [Can]; Nasalide® [US/Can]; Nasarel® [US]; Rhinalar® [Can]

Therapeutic Category Adrenal Corticosteroid

Use Steroid-dependent asthma; nasal solution is used for seasonal or perennial rhinitis

Usual Dosage

Children:

Oral inhalation: >6 years: 2 inhalations twice daily up to 4 inhalations/day

Nasal: 6-14 years: 1 spray each nostril 2-3 times/day, not to exceed 4 sprays/day each nostril

Adults:

Oral inhalation: 2 inhalations twice daily up to 8 inhalations/day

Nasal: 2 sprays each nostril twice daily; maximum dose: 8 sprays/day in each nostril

Dosage Forms

Aerosol for oral inhalation:

AeroBid® Aerosol: 250 mcg/actuation [100 metered doses] (7 g)

AeroBid-M® Aerosol: 250 mcg/actuation [100 metered doses] (7 g) [menthol flavor]

Nasal spray:

Nasalide®: 25 mcg/actuation [200 sprays] (25 mL)

Nasarel®: 0.025% [200 actuations] (25 mL)

fluocinolone (floo oh SIN oh lone)

U.S./Canadian Brand Names Capex™ [US/Can]; Derma-Smoothe/FS® [US/Can]; Fluoderm [Can]; Synalar® [US/Can]

Therapeutic Category Corticosteroid, Topical

Use Relief of susceptible inflammatory dermatosis

Usual Dosage Children and Adults: Topical: Apply 2-4 times/day. Therapy should be discontinued when control is achieved. If no improvement is seen, reassessment of diagnosis may be necessary.

Dosage Forms

Cream, as acetonide: 0.01% (15 g, 60 g); 0.025% (15 g, 60 g)

Synalar®: 0.025% (15 g, 60 g)

Oil, topical, as acetonide (Derma-Smoothe/FS®): 0.01% (120 mL) [contains peanut oil]

Ointment, as acetonide: 0.025% (15 g, 60 g)

Synalar®: 0.025% (15 g, 30 g, 60 g)

Shampoo, as acetonide (Capex™): 0.01% (120 mL)

Solution, topical, as acetonide: 0.01% (20 mL, 60 mL)

Synalar®: 0.01% (20 mL, 60 mL)

fluocinolone, hydroquinone, and tretinoin

(floo oh SIN oh lone, HYE droe kwin one, & TRET i noyn)

U.S./Canadian Brand Names Tri-Luma™ [US]

Therapeutic Category Corticosteroid, Topical; Depigmenting Agent; Retinoic Acid Derivative

Use Short-term treatment of moderate to severe melasma of the face

Usual Dosage Topical: Adults: Melasma: Apply a thin film once daily to hyperpigmented areas of melasma (including 1/2 inch of normal-appearing surrounding skin). Apply 30 minutes prior to bedtime; not indicated for use beyond 8 weeks. Do not use occlusive dressings.

Dosage Forms Cream, topical: Hydroquinone 4%, tretinoin 0.05%, fluocinolone acetonide 0.01% (30 g) [contains sodium bisulfite]

fluocinonide (floo oh SIN oh nide)

U.S./Canadian Brand Names Lidemol® [Can]; Lidex-E® [US]; Lidex® [US/Can]; Lyderm® [Can]; Lydonide [Can]; Tiamol® [Can]; Topsyn® [Can]

Therapeutic Category Corticosteroid, Topical

Use Inflammation of corticosteroid-responsive dermatoses

Usual Dosage Children and Adults: Topical: Apply thin layer to affected area 2-4 times/day depending on the severity of the condition. Therapy should be discontinued when control is achieved. If no improvement is seen, reassessment of diagnosis may be necessary.

Dosage Forms

Cream: 0.05% (15 g, 30 g, 60 g, 120 g)

Cream, anhydrous, emollient (Lidex®): 0.05% (15 g, 30 g, 60 g, 120 g)

Cream, aqueous, emollient (Lidex-E®): 0.05% (15 g, 30 g, 60 g, 120 g)

Gel: 0.05% (15 g, 60 g)

Lidex®: 0.05% (15 g, 30 g, 60 g, 120 g)

Ointment: 0.05% (15 g, 30 g, 60 g)

Lidex®: 0.05% (15 g, 30 g, 60 g, 120 g)

Solution, topical: 0.05% (20 mL, 60 mL)

Lidex®: 0.05% (20 mL, 60 mL)

Fluoderm [Can] see fluocinolone on previous page

fluohydrocortisone see fludrocortisone on page 275

Fluonid® Topical (Discontinued) see page 814

Fluoracaine® [US] see proparacaine and fluorescein on page 547

Fluor-A-Day® [Can] see fluoride on next page

FluorCare® Neutral (Discontinued) see page 814

fluorescein sodium (FLURE e seen SOW dee um)

Synonyms soluble fluorescein

U.S./Canadian Brand Names AK-Fluor [US]; Diofluor™ [Can]; Fluorescite® [US/Can]; Fluorets® Ophthalmic Strips [US/Can]; Fluor-I-Strip-AT® [US]; Fluor-I-Strip® [US]; Fluress® [US]; Ful-Glo® Ophthalmic Strips [US]; Ophthifluor® [US]

Therapeutic Category Diagnostic Agent

Use Demonstrates defects of corneal epithelium; diagnostic aid in ophthalmic angiography

Usual Dosage

Injection: Perform intradermal skin test before use to avoid possible allergic reaction

Children: 3.5 mg/lb (7.5 mg/kg) injected rapidly into antecubital vein

Adults: 500-750 mg injected rapidly into antecubital vein

Strips: Moisten with sterile water or irrigating solution, touch conjunctiva with moistened tip, blink several times after application

Topical solution: Instill 1-2 drops, allow a few seconds for staining, then wash out excess with sterile irrigation solution

Dosage Forms

Injection (AK-Fluor, Fluorescite®, Ophthifluor®): 10% [100 mg/mL] (5 mL); 25% [250 mg/mL] (2 mL, 3 mL)

Solution, ophthalmic: 2% [20 mg/mL] (1 mL, 2 mL, 15 mL)

Fluress®: 0.25% [2.5 mg/mL] (5 mL) [contains benoxinate 0.4%]

Strip, ophthalmic:

Fluorets®, Fluor-I-Strip-AT®: 1 mg

Fluor-I-Strip®: 9 mg

Ful-Glo®: 0.6 mg

Fluorescite® [US/Can] see fluorescein sodium on this page

Fluorets® Ophthalmic Strips [US/Can] see fluorescein sodium on this page

fluoride (FLOR ide)

U.S./Canadian Brand Names Fluor-A-Day® [Can]; Fluorigard® [US-OTC]; Fluorinse® [US]; Fluotic® [Can]; Flura-Drops® [US]; Flura-Loz® [US]; Gel-Kam® [US]; Luride® [US]; Luride® Lozi-Tab® [US]; Pediaflor® [US]; Pharmaflur® [US]; Phos-Flur® [US]; PreviDent® [US]; PreviDent® 5000 Plus™ [US]; Stop® [US-OTC]; Thera-Flur-N® [US]

Therapeutic Category Mineral, Oral

Use Prevention of dental caries

Usual Dosage Oral: Dental rinse or gel:

Children 6-12 years: 5-10 mL rinse or apply to teeth and spit daily after brushing

Adults: 10 mL rinse or apply to teeth and spit daily after brushing

Dosage Forms Fluoride ion content listed in brackets:

Cream, oral topical, as sodium (PreviDent® 5000 Plus™): 1.1% [2.5 mg per dose] (51 g)

Gel, oral topical, acidulated phosphate fluoride (Minute-Gel®): 1.23% (480 mL)

Gel, oral topical, sodium fluoride (Karigel®, Karigel®-N, PreviDent®): 1.1% [0.5%] (24 g, 30 g, 60 g, 120 g, 130 g, 250 g)

Gel, oral topical, stannous fluoride (Gel Kam®, Stop®): 0.4% [0.1%] (60 g, 65 g, 105 g, 120 g)

Lozenge, as sodium (Flura-Loz®): 2.2 mg [1 mg] [raspberry flavor]

Solution, oral, as sodium (Phos-Flur®): 0.44 mg/mL [0.2 mg/mL] (250 mL, 500 mL, 3780 mL)

Solution, oral drops, as sodium:

Flura-Drops®: 0.55 mg/drop [0.25 mg/drop] (22.8 mL, 24 mL)

Karidium®: 0.275 mg/drop [0.125 mg/drop] (30 mL, 60 mL)

Luride®, Pediaflor®: 1.1 mg/mL [0.5 mg/mL] (50 mL)

Solution, oral rinse, as sodium:

Fluorigard®: 0.05% [0.02%] (90 mL, 180 mL, 300 mL, 360 mL, 480 mL)

Fluorinse®, Point-Two®, 0.2% [0.09%] (240 mL, 480 mL, 3780 mL)

PreviDent®: 0.2% [9 mg per dose] (250 mL)

Tablet, as sodium (Flura®, Karidium®): 2.2 mg [1 mg]

Tablet, chewable:

Luride® Lozi-Tabs®, Pharmaflur®: 1.1 mg [0.5 mg]

Karidium®, Luride® Lozi-Tabs®, Luride®-SF Lozi-Tabs®, Pharmaflur®: 2.2 mg [1 mg]

Fluorigard® [US-OTC] *see* fluoride *on this page*

Fluori-Methane® [US] *see* dichlorodifluoromethane and trichloromonofluoromethane *on page 193*

Fluorinse® [US] *see* fluoride *on this page*

Fluor-I-Strip® [US] *see* fluorescein sodium *on previous page*

Fluor-I-Strip-AT® [US] *see* fluorescein sodium *on previous page*

Fluoritab® *(Discontinued)* *see page 814*

fluorodeoxyuridine *see* floxuridine *on page 274*

9α-fluorohydrocortisone *see* fludrocortisone *on page 275*

fluorometholone (flure oh METH oh lone)

U.S./Canadian Brand Names Flarex® [US/Can]; Fluor-Op® [US]; FML® Forte [US/Can]; FML® [US/Can]

Therapeutic Category Adrenal Corticosteroid

Use Inflammatory conditions of the eye, including keratitis, iritis, cyclitis, and conjunctivitis

Usual Dosage Children >2 years and Adults: Ophthalmic: 1-2 drops into conjunctival sac every hour during day, every 2 hours at night until favorable response is obtained, then use 1 drop every 4 hours; in mild or moderate inflammation: 1-2 drops into conjunctival sac 2-4 times/day. Ointment may be applied every 4 hours in severe cases or 1-3 times/day in mild to moderate cases.

Dosage Forms

Ointment, ophthalmic (FML®): 0.1% (3.5 g)

Suspension, ophthalmic:
Flarex®: 0.1% (2.5 mL, 5 mL, 10 mL)
Fluor-Op®: 0.1% (5 mL, 10 mL, 15 mL)
FML®: 0.1% (1 mL, 5 mL, 10 mL, 15 mL)
FML® Forte: 0.25% (2 mL, 5 mL, 10 mL, 15 mL)

fluorometholone and sulfacetamide *see* sulfacetamide sodium and fluorometholone *on page 611*

Fluor-Op® [US] *see* fluorometholone *on previous page*

Fluoroplex® [US] *see* fluorouracil *on this page*

fluorouracil (flure oh YOOR a sil)
Synonyms 5-fluorouracil; 5-FU
U.S./Canadian Brand Names Adrucil® [US/Can]; Carac™ [US]; Efudex® [US/Can]; Fluoroplex® [US]
Therapeutic Category Antineoplastic Agent
Use Treatment of carcinoma of stomach, colon, rectum, breast, and pancreas; also used topically for management of multiple actinic keratoses and superficial basal cell carcinomas
Usual Dosage Children and Adults (refer to individual protocols):
I.V.: Initial: 12 mg/kg/day (maximum: 800 mg/day) for 4-5 days; maintenance: 6 mg/kg every other day for 4 doses
Single weekly bolus dose of 15 mg/kg can be administered depending on the patient's reaction to the previous course of treatment; maintenance dose of 5-15 mg/kg/week as a single dose not to exceed 1 g/week
I.V. infusion: 15 mg/kg/day (maximum daily dose: 1 g) has been administered by I.V. infusion over 4 hours for 5 days
Oral: 20 mg/kg/day for 5 days every 5 weeks for colorectal carcinoma; 15 mg/kg/week for hepatoma
Topical: 5% cream twice daily
Dosage Forms
Cream:
Carac™: 0.5% (30 g)
Efudex®: 5% (25 g)
Fluoroplex®: 1% (30 g)
Injection (Adrucil®): 50 mg/mL (10 mL, 20 mL, 50 mL, 100 mL)
Solution, topical:
Efudex®: 2% (10 mL); 5% (10 mL)
Fluoroplex®: 1% (30 mL)

5-fluorouracil *see* fluorouracil *on this page*

Fluothane® *(Discontinued)* *see page 814*

Fluotic® [Can] *see* fluoride *on previous page*

fluoxetine (floo OKS e teen)
Synonyms fluoxetine hydrochloride
U.S./Canadian Brand Names Alti-Fluoxetine [Can]; Apo®-Fluoxetine [Can]; Gen-Fluoxetine [Can]; Novo-Fluoxetine [Can]; Nu-Fluoxetine [Can]; PMS-Fluoxetine [Can]; Prozac® [US/Can]; Prozac® Weekly™ [US]; Rhoxal-fluoxetine [Can]; Sarafem™ [US]
Therapeutic Category Antidepressant, Selective Serotonin Reuptake Inhibitor
Use Treatment of major depression; geriatric depression; treatment of binge-eating and vomiting in patients with moderate-to-severe bulimia nervosa; obsessive-compulsive disorder (OCD); premenstrual dysphoric disorder (PMDD)
Usual Dosage Oral:
Children:
<5 years: No dosing information available
(Continued)

fluoxetine *(Continued)*

5-18 years: Initial: 5-10 mg/day; titrate upwards as needed (usual maximum dose: 60 mg/day)

Adults: 20 mg/day in the morning; may increase after several weeks by 20 mg/day increments; maximum: 80 mg/day; doses >20 mg should be divided into morning and noon dose. **Note:** Lower doses of 5-10 mg/day have been used for initial treatment.

Usual dosage range:

Bulimia nervosa: 60-80 mg/day

Depression: 20-40 mg/day; patients maintained on Prozac® 20 mg/day may be changed to Prozac® Weekly™ 90 mg/week, starting dose 7 days after the last 20 mg/day dose

Obesity: 20-60 mg/day

OCD: 40-80 mg/day

PMDD (Sarafem™): 20 mg/day

Dosage Forms

Capsule, as hydrochloride:

Prozac®: 10 mg, 20 mg, 40 mg

Sarafem™: 10 mg, 20 mg

Capsule, sustained release, as hydrochloride (Prozac® Weekly™): 90 mg

Solution, oral, as hydrochloride (Prozac®): 20 mg/5 mL (120 mL) [contains alcohol 0.23%] [mint flavor]

Tablet, scored, as hydrochloride (Prozac®): 10 mg

fluoxetine hydrochloride *see* fluoxetine *on previous page*

fluoxymesterone (floo oks i MES te rone)

U.S./Canadian Brand Names Halotestin® [US]

Therapeutic Category Androgen

Use Replacement of endogenous testicular hormone; in female used as palliative treatment of breast cancer, postpartum breast engorgement

Usual Dosage Adults: Oral:

Male:

Hypogonadism: 5-20 mg/day

Delayed puberty: 2.5-20 mg/day for 4-6 months

Female:

Breast carcinoma: 10-40 mg/day in divided doses for 1-3 months

Breast engorgement: 2.5 mg after delivery, 5-10 mg/day in divided doses for 4-5 days

Dosage Forms Tablet: 2 mg, 5 mg, 10 mg

flupenthixol *(Canada only)* (floo pen THIKS ol)

U.S./Canadian Brand Names Fluanxol® Depot [Can]; Fluanxol® Tablet [Can]

Therapeutic Category Antipsychotic Agent; Thioxanthene Derivative

Use Maintenance therapy of chronic schizophrenic patients whose main manifestations do not include excitement, agitation, or hyperactivity

Usual Dosage

Injection: Flupenthixol is administered by deep I.M. injection, preferably in the gluteus maximus, NOT for I.V. use

Patients not previously treated with long-acting depot neuroleptics should be given an initial test dose of 5 mg (0.25 mL) to 20 mg (1 mL). An initial dose of 20 mg (1 mL) is usually well tolerated; however, a 5 mg (0.25 mL) test dose is recommended in elderly, frail and cachectic patients, and in patients whose individual or family history suggests a predisposition to extrapyramidal reactions. In the subsequent 5-10 days, the therapeutic response and the appearance of extrapyramidal symptoms should be carefully monitored. Oral neuroleptic drugs may be continued, but in diminishing dosage, during this period.

Tablets: The dosage should be individualized and adjusted according to the severity of symptoms and tolerance to the drug. Initial recommended dose: 1 mg, 3 times/day. This may be increased, if necessary by 1 mg every 2-3 days until there is effective control of psychotic symptoms. The usual maintenance dosage: 3-6 mg/day in divided doses, although doses of up to 12 mg/day or more have been used in some patients.

Dosage Forms
Injection, solution, as decanoate [depot]: 20 mg/mL (10 mL); 100 mg/mL (2 mL)
Tablet, as dihydrochloride: 0.5 mg, 3 mg

fluphenazine (floo FEN a zeen)

U.S./Canadian Brand Names Apo®-Fluphenazine [Can]; Modecate® [Can]; Moditen® Enanthate [Can]; Moditen® HCl [Can]; PMS-Fluphenazine Decanoate [Can]; Prolixin® [US]; Prolixin Decanoate® [US]; Prolixin Enanthate® [US]; Rho®-Fluphenazin Decanoate [Can]

Therapeutic Category Phenothiazine Derivative

Use Management of manifestations of psychotic disorders

Usual Dosage Adults:
Oral: 0.5-10 mg/day in divided doses every 6-8 hours; usual maximum dose 20 mg/day
I.M.: 2.5-10 mg/day in divided doses every 6-8 hours; usual maximum dose 10 mg/day
I.M., S.C. (Decanoate®): Oral to I.M., S.C. conversion ratio = 12.5 mg, I.M., S.C. every 3 weeks for every 10 mg of oral fluphenazine

Dosage Forms
Elixir, as hydrochloride (Prolixin®): 2.5 mg/5 mL (60 mL, 473 mL) [contains alcohol 14%]
Injection, as decanoate (Prolixin Decanoate®): 25 mg/mL (1 mL, 5 mL)
Injection, as enanthate (Prolixin Enanthate®): 25 mg/mL (5 mL)
Injection, as hydrochloride (Prolixin®): 2.5 mg/mL (10 mL)
Solution, oral concentrate, as hydrochloride (Prolixin®): 5 mg/mL (120 mL) [contains alcohol 14%]
Tablet, as hydrochloride (Prolixin®): 1 mg, 2.5 mg, 5 mg, 10 mg

Flura® *(Discontinued)* see page 814

Flura-Drops® **[US]** *see* fluoride on page 278

Flura-Loz® **[US]** *see* fluoride on page 278

flurandrenolide (flure an DREN oh lide)

Synonyms flurandrenolone

U.S./Canadian Brand Names Cordran® SP [US]; Cordran® [US/Can]

Therapeutic Category Corticosteroid, Topical

Use Inflammation of corticosteroid-responsive dermatoses

Usual Dosage Topical:
Children:
Ointment or cream: Apply 1-2 times/day
Tape: Apply once daily
Adults: Cream, lotion, ointment: Apply 2-3 times/day; therapy should be discontinued when control is achieved. If no improvement is seen, reassessment of diagnosis may be necessary.

Dosage Forms
Cream, emulsified, as base (Cordran® SP): 0.025% (30 g, 60 g); 0.05% (15 g, 30 g, 60 g)
Lotion (Cordran®): 0.05% (15 mL, 60 mL)
Ointment (Cordran®): 0.025% (30 g, 60 g); 0.05% (15 g, 30 g, 60 g)
Tape, topical (Cordran®): 4 mcg/cm^2 (7.5 cm x 60 cm, 7.5 cm x 200 cm rolls)

flurandrenolone *see* flurandrenolide on this page

Flurate® Ophthalmic Solution *(Discontinued)* see page 814

flurazepam (flure AZ e pam)

U.S./Canadian Brand Names Apo®-Flurazepam [Can]; Dalmane® [US/Can]

Therapeutic Category Benzodiazepine

Controlled Substance C-IV

(Continued)

flurazepam *(Continued)*

Use Short-term treatment of insomnia

Usual Dosage Oral:

Children:

<15 years: Dose not established

>15 years: 15 mg at bedtime

Adults: 15-30 mg at bedtime

Dosage Forms Capsule, as hydrochloride: 15 mg, 30 mg

flurbiprofen (flure BI proe fen)

U.S./Canadian Brand Names Alti-Flurbiprofen [Can]; Ansaid® Oral [US/Can]; Apo®-Flurbiprofen [Can]; Froben® [Can]; Froben-SR® [Can]; Novo-Flurprofen [Can]; Nu-Flurprofen [Can]; Ocufen® Ophthalmic [US/Can]

Therapeutic Category Analgesic, Non-narcotic; Nonsteroidal Anti-inflammatory Drug (NSAID)

Use

Ophthalmic: For inhibition of intraoperative trauma-induced miosis; the value of flurbiprofen for the prevention and management of postoperative ocular inflammation and postoperative cystoid macular edema remains to be determined

Systemic: Management of inflammatory disease and rheumatoid disorders; dysmenorrhea; pain

Usual Dosage

Oral: Rheumatoid arthritis and osteoarthritis: 200-300 mg/day in 2, 3, or 4 divided doses

Ophthalmic: Instill 1 drop every 30 minutes, 2 hours prior to surgery (total of 4 drops to each affected eye)

Dosage Forms

Solution, ophthalmic, as sodium [with thimerosal 0.005% as preservative] (Ocufen®): 0.03% (2.5 mL, 5 mL, 10 mL)

Tablet, as sodium (Ansaid®): 50 mg, 100 mg

Fluress® [US] *see* fluorescein sodium *on page 277*

5-flurocytosine *see* flucytosine *on page 274*

Fluro-Ethyl® Aerosol [US] *see* ethyl chloride and dichlorotetrafluoroethane *on page 257*

Flurosyn® Topical *(Discontinued) see page 814*

FluShield® [US] *see* influenza virus vaccine *on page 350*

flutamide (FLOO ta mide)

U.S./Canadian Brand Names Apo-Flutamide [Can]; Euflex® [Can]; Eulexin® [US/Can]; Novo-Flutamide [Can]; PMS-Flutamide [Can]

Therapeutic Category Antiandrogen

Use In combination with LHRH agonistic analogs for the treatment of metastatic prostatic carcinoma

Usual Dosage Oral: 2 capsules every 8 hours

Dosage Forms Capsule: 125 mg

Flutex® Topical *(Discontinued) see page 814*

fluticasone and salmeterol (floo TIK a sone & sal ME te role)

Synonyms salmeterol and fluticasone

U.S./Canadian Brand Names Advair™ Diskus® [US/Can]

Therapeutic Category Beta$_2$-Adrenergic Agonist Agent; Corticosteroid, Inhalant

Use Maintenance treatment of asthma in adults and children ≥12 years; **not** for use for relief of acute bronchospasm

Usual Dosage Do not use to transfer patients from systemic corticosteroid therapy

Children ≥12 and Adults: Oral inhalation: One inhalation twice daily, morning and evening, 12 hours apart

Advair™ Diskus® is available in 3 strengths, initial dose prescribed should be based upon previous asthma therapy. Dose should be increased after 2 weeks if adequate response is not achieved. Patients should be titrated to lowest effective dose once stable. (Because each strength contains salmeterol 50 mcg/inhalation, dose adjustments should be made by changing inhaler strength. No more than 1 inhalation of any strength should be taken more than twice a day). Maximum dose: Fluticasone 500 mcg/salmeterol 50 mcg, one inhalation twice daily.

Patients not currently on inhaled corticosteroids: Fluticasone 100 mcg/salmeterol 50 mcg

Patients currently using inhaled beclomethasone dipropionate:
≤420 mcg/day: Fluticasone 100 mcg/salmeterol 50 mcg
462-840 mcg/day: Fluticasone 250 mcg/salmeterol 50 mcg
Patients currently using inhaled budesonide:
≤400 mcg/day: Fluticasone 100 mcg/salmeterol 50 mcg
800-1200 mcg/day: Fluticasone 250 mcg/salmeterol 50 mcg
1600 mcg/day: Fluticasone 500 mcg/salmeterol 50 mcg
Patients currently using inhaled flunisolide:
≤1000 mcg/day: Fluticasone 100 mcg/salmeterol 50 mcg
1250-2000 mcg/day: Fluticasone 250 mcg/salmeterol 50 mcg
Patients currently using inhaled fluticasone propionate aerosol:
≤176 mcg/day: Fluticasone 100 mcg/salmeterol 50 mcg
440 mcg/day: Fluticasone 250 mcg/salmeterol 50 mcg
660-880 mcg/day: Fluticasone 500 mcg/salmeterol 50 mcg
Patients currently using inhaled fluticasone propionate powder:
≤200 mcg/day: Fluticasone 100 mcg/salmeterol 50 mcg
500 mcg/day: Fluticasone 250 mcg/salmeterol 50 mcg
1000 mcg/day: Fluticasone 500 mcg/salmeterol 50 mcg
Patients currently using inhaled triamcinolone acetonide:
≤1000 mcg/day: Fluticasone 100 mcg/salmeterol 50 mcg
1100-1600 mcg/day: Fluticasone 250 mcg/salmeterol 50 mcg

Dosage Forms
Powder for oral inhalation (Advair™ Diskus®):
Fluticasone 100 mcg and salmeterol 50 mcg
Fluticasone 250 mcg and salmeterol 50 mcg
Fluticasone 500 mcg and salmeterol 50 mcg

fluticasone (nasal) (floo TIK a sone NAY sal)

U.S./Canadian Brand Names Flonase® [US]
Therapeutic Category Adrenal Corticosteroid
Use Management of seasonal and perennial allergic rhinitis in patients ≥12 years of age
Usual Dosage
Adolescents:
Intranasal: Initial: 1 spray (50 mcg/spray) per nostril once daily. Patients not adequately responding or patients with more severe symptoms may use 2 sprays (100 mcg) per nostril. Depending on response, dosage may be reduced to 100 mcg daily. Total daily dosage should not exceed 4 sprays (200 mcg)/day.
Adults:
Intranasal: Initial: 2 sprays (50 mcg/spray) per nostril once daily. After the first few days, dosage may be reduced to 1 spray per nostril once daily for maintenance therapy. Maximum total daily dose should not exceed 4 sprays (200 mcg)/day.
Dosage Forms Nasal spray: 50 mcg/actuation (16 g = 120 actuations)

fluticasone (oral inhalation) (floo TIK a sone OR al in hil LA shun)

U.S./Canadian Brand Names Flovent® Rotadisk® [US]; Flovent® [US]
Therapeutic Category Adrenal Corticosteroid
(Continued)

fluticasone (oral inhalation) *(Continued)*

Use Inhalation: Maintenance treatment of asthma as prophylactic therapy. It is also indicated for patients requiring oral corticosteroid therapy for asthma to assist in total discontinuation or reduction of total oral dose. NOT indicated for the relief of acute bronchospasm.

Usual Dosage Oral inhalation: If adequate response is not seen after 2 weeks of initial dosage, increase dosage; doses should be titrated to the lowest effective dose once asthma is controlled; Manufacturer recommendations:

Inhalation aerosol (Flovent®): Children ≥12 years and Adults:

Patients previously treated with bronchodilators only: Initial: 88 mcg twice daily; maximum dose: 440 mcg twice daily

Patients treated with an inhaled corticosteroid: Initial: 88-220 mcg twice daily; maximum dose: 440 mcg twice daily; may start doses above 88 mcg twice daily in poorly controlled patients or in those who previously required higher doses of inhaled corticosteroids

Patients previously treated with oral corticosteroids: Initial: 880 mcg twice daily; maximum dose: 880 mcg twice daily

Inhalation powder (Flovent® Rotadisk®):

Children 4-11 years: Patients previously treated with bronchodilators alone or inhaled corticosteroids: Initial: 50 mcg twice daily; maximum dose: 100 mcg twice daily; may start higher initial dose in poorly controlled patients or in those who previously required higher doses of inhaled corticosteroids

Adolescents and Adults:

Patients previously treated with bronchodilators alone: Initial: 100 mcg twice daily; maximum dose: 500 mcg twice daily

Patients previously treated with inhaled corticosteroids: Initial: 100-250 mcg twice daily; maximum dose: 500 mcg twice daily; may start doses above 100 mcg twice daily in poorly controlled patients or in those who previously required higher doses of inhaled corticosteroids

Patients previously treated with oral corticosteroids: Initial: 1000 mcg twice daily; maximum dose: 1000 mcg twice daily

Dosage Forms

Powder (in 4 blisters containing 15 Rotodisk® with inhalation device): 50 mcg, 100 mcg, 250 mcg

Spray, aerosol, oral inhalation (Flovent®): 44 mcg/actuation (7.9 g = 60 actuations or 13 g = 120 actuations), 110 mcg/actuation (13 g = 120 actuations); 220 mcg/actuation (13 g = 120 actuations)

fluticasone (topical) (floo TIK a sone TOP i kal)

U.S./Canadian Brand Names Cutivate™ [US]

Therapeutic Category Adrenal Corticosteroid; Corticosteroid, Topical

Use Relief of inflammation and pruritus associated with corticosteroid-responsive dermatoses [medium potency topical corticosteroid]

Usual Dosage Topical:

Children: Cutivate™ approved for use in patients ≥3 months of age

Adolescents and Adults: Apply sparingly in a thin film twice daily

Note: Therapy should be discontinued when control is achieved. If no improvement is seen, reassessment of diagnosis may be necessary.

Dosage Forms

Cream: 0.05% (15 g, 30 g, 60 g)

Ointment: 0.005% (15 g, 60 g)

fluvastatin (FLOO va sta tin)

U.S./Canadian Brand Names Lescol® [US/Can]; Lescol® XL [US]

Therapeutic Category HMG-CoA Reductase Inhibitor

Use To be used as a component of multiple risk factor intervention in patients at risk for atherosclerosis vascular disease due to hypercholesterolemia

Adjunct to dietary therapy to reduce elevated total cholesterol (total-C), LDL-C, triglyceride, and apolipoprotein B (apo-B) levels and to increase HDL-C in primary hypercholesterolemia and mixed dyslipidemia (Fredrickson types IIa and IIb); to slow the progression of coronary atherosclerosis in patients with coronary heart disease

Usual Dosage Adults: Oral:

Patients requiring ≥25% decrease in LDL-C: 40 mg capsule or 80 mg extended release tablet once daily in the evening; may also use 40 mg capsule twice daily

Patients requiring < 25% decrease in LDL-C: 20 mg capsule once daily in the evening

Note: Dosing range: 20-80 mg/day; adjust dose based on response to therapy; maximum response occurs within 4-6 weeks

Dosage Forms

Capsule: 20 mg, 40 mg

Tablet, extended release: 80 mg

Fluviral S/F® [Can] *see* influenza virus vaccine *on page 350*

Fluvirin® [US] *see* influenza virus vaccine *on page 350*

fluvoxamine (floo VOKS ah meen)

U.S./Canadian Brand Names Alti-Fluvoxamine [Can]; Apo®-Fluvoxamine [Can]; Gen-Fluvoxamine [Can]; Luvox® [Can]; Novo-Fluvoxamine [Can]; Nu-Fluvoxamine [Can]; PMS-Fluvoxamine [Can]

Therapeutic Category Antidepressant, Selective Serotonin Reuptake Inhibitor

Use Treatment of major depression and obsessive-compulsive disorder (OCD)

Usual Dosage Adults: Initial: 50 mg at bedtime; adjust in 50 mg increments at 4- to 7-day intervals; usual dose range: 100-300 mg/day; divide total daily dose into 2 doses; administer larger portion at bedtime

Dosage Forms Tablet: 25 mg, 50 mg, 100 mg

Fluzone® [US/Can] *see* influenza virus vaccine *on page 350*

FML® [US/Can] *see* fluorometholone *on page 278*

FML® Forte [US/Can] *see* fluorometholone *on page 278*

FML-S® [US] *see* sulfacetamide sodium and fluorometholone *on page 611*

Focalin™ [US] *see* dexmethylphenidate *on page 186*

Foille® Medicated First Aid [US-OTC] *see* benzocaine *on page 77*

Foille® Plus [US-OTC] *see* benzocaine *on page 77*

Foille® [US-OTC] *see* benzocaine *on page 77*

folacin *see* folic acid *on this page*

folacin, vitamin B$_{12}$, and vitamin B$_6$ *see* folic acid, cyanocobalamin, and pyridoxine *on next page*

folate *see* folic acid *on this page*

Folex® Injection *(Discontinued)* *see page 814*

Folex® PFS™ *(Discontinued)* *see page 814*

folic acid (FOE lik AS id)

Synonyms folacin; folate; pteroylglutamic acid

U.S./Canadian Brand Names Apo®-Folic [Can]; Folvite® [US]

Therapeutic Category Vitamin, Water Soluble

Use Treatment of megaloblastic and macrocytic anemias due to folate deficiency

Usual Dosage Folic acid deficiency:

Infants: 15 mcg/kg/dose daily or 50 mcg/day

Children: Oral, I.M., I.V., S.C.: 1 mg/day initial dosage; maintenance dose: 1-10 years: 0.1-0.3 mg/day

Children >11 years and Adults: Oral, I.M., I.V., S.C.: 1 mg/day initial dosage; maintenance dose: 0.5 mg/day

(Continued)

folic acid *(Continued)*

Dosage Forms
Injection, as sodium folate: 5 mg/mL (10 mL)
Folvite®: 5 mg/mL (10 mL)
Tablet: 0.4 mg, 0.8 mg, 1 mg
Folvite®: 1 mg

folic acid, cyanocobalamin, and pyridoxine
(FOE lik AS id, sye an oh koe BAL a min, & peer i DOKS een)

Synonyms cyanocobalamin, folic acid, and pyridoxine; folacin, vitamin B_{12}, and vitamin B_6; pyridoxine, folic acid, and cyanocobalamin

U.S./Canadian Brand Names Foltx™ [US]

Therapeutic Category Vitamin

Use Nutritional supplement in end-stage renal failure, dialysis, hyperhomocystinemia, homocystinemia, malabsorption syndromes, dietary deficiencies

Usual Dosage Oral: Adults: 1 tablet daily

Dosage Forms Tablet: Folic acid 2.5 mg, cyanocobalamin 1 mg, and pyridoxine 25 mg

folinic acid *see* leucovorin *on page 377*

Follistim® [US] *see* follitropin beta *on this page*

follitropin alfa (foe li TRO pin AL fa)

U.S./Canadian Brand Names Gonal-F® [US]

Therapeutic Category Ovulation Stimulator

Use Induction of ovulation in the anovulatory infertile patient in whom the cause of infertility is functional and not caused by primary ovarian failure

Usual Dosage Adults (women): S.C.: Initial: 75 units/day for the first cycle; an incremental dose adjustment of up to 37.5 units may be considered after 14 days; treatment duration should not exceed 35 days unless an E2 rise indicates follicular development

Dosage Forms Injection: 37.5 FSH units, 75 FSH units, 150 FSH units

follitropin beta (foe li TRO pin BAY ta)

U.S./Canadian Brand Names Follistim® [US]

Therapeutic Category Ovulation Stimulator

Use The development of multiple follicles in infertility patients treated in Assisted Reproductive Technology (ART) program and for the induction of ovulation

Usual Dosage Adults (female): I.M./S.C.:
Ovulation: In general, a sequential treatment scheme is recommended. This usually starts with daily administration of 75 int. units (International Units) FSH activity. The starting dose is maintained for at least seven days. If there is no ovarian response, the daily dose is then gradually increased until follicle growth and/or plasma estradiol levels indicate an adequate pharmacodynamic response. A daily increase in estradiol levels of 40% to 100% is considered to be optimal. The daily dose is then maintained until preovulatory conditions are reached. Preovulatory conditions are reached when there ultrasonographic evidence of a dominant follicle of at least 18 mm in diameter and/or when plasma estradiol levels of 300-900 picograms/mL (1000-3000 pmol/L) are attained; usually, 7-14 days of treatment are sufficient to reach this state. The administration is then discontinued and ovulation can be induced by administering human chorionic gonadotropin (hCG). If the number of responding follicles is too high or estradiol levels increase too rapidly (ie, more than a daily doubling of estradiol for 2-3 consecutive days), the daily dose should be decreased. Since follicles of >14 mm may lead to pregnancies, multiple preovulatory follicles exceeding 14 mm carry the risk of multiple gestations. In that case, hCG should be withheld and pregnancy should be avoided in order to prevent multiple gestations.
ART: Various stimulation protocols are applied; starting dose of 150-225 units is recommended for at least the first four days; thereafter, the dose may be adjusted individually, based upon ovarian response. In clinical studies, it was shown that maintenance

dosages ranging from 75-375 units for 6-12 days are sufficient, although longer treatment may be necessary. May be given either alone, or in combination with a GnRH agonist to prevent premature luteinization; in the latter case, a higher total treatment dose of Follistim® may be required. Ovarian response is monitored by ultrasonography and measurement of plasma estradiol levels; when ultrasonographic evaluation indicates the presence of at least three follicles of 16-20 mm, and there is evidence of a good estradiol (plasma levels of about 300-400 picogram/mL (1000-1300 pmol/L) for each follicle with a diameter >18 mm), the final phase of maturation of the follicles is induced by administration of hCG. Oocyte retrieval is performed 34-35 hours later.

Dosage Forms Injection: 75 FSH units

Follutein® *(Discontinued)* see page 814

Foltx™ [US] see folic acid, cyanocobalamin, and pyridoxine on previous page

Folvite® [US] see folic acid on page 285

fomepizole (foe ME pi zole)

Synonyms 4-methylpyrazole; 4-MP

U.S./Canadian Brand Names Antizol® [US]

Therapeutic Category Antidote

Use Ethylene glycol and methanol toxicity (antifreeze); may be useful in propylene glycol; unclear whether it is useful in disulfiram-ethanol reactions

Usual Dosage Oral: 15 mg/kg followed by 5 mg/kg in 12 hours and then 10 mg/kg every 12 hours until levels of toxin are not present

One other protocol (from France) suggests an infusion of 10-20 mg/kg before dialysis and intravenous infusion of 1-1.5 mg/kg/hour during hemodialysis

META (methylpyrazole for toxic alcohol) study in U.S. (investigational): Loading I.V. dose of 15 mg/kg followed by 10 mg/kg I.V. every 12 hours for 48 hours; continue treatment until methanol or ethylene glycol levels are <20 mg/dL; supplemental doses required during dialysis; contact your local poison center regarding this study

Dosage Forms Injection: 1 g/mL (1.5 mL)

fomivirsen (foe MI vir sen)

U.S./Canadian Brand Names Vitravene™ [US/Can]

Therapeutic Category Antiviral Agent, Ophthalmic

Use Treatment of cytomegalovirus (CMV); CMV can affect one or both eyes in patients with acquired immunodeficiency syndrome (AIDS) who cannot take other treatment(s) for CMV retinitis or who did not respond to other treatments for CMV retinitis; the diagnosis should be made after a comprehensive eye exam, including indirect ophthalmoscopy

Usual Dosage Treatment with Vitravene™ consists of two phases:

Phase I (induction phase): One injection (6.6 mg) every other week for 2 doses

Phase II (maintenance phase): One injection (6.6 mg) once every 4 weeks

Dosage Forms Injection, intravitreal: 6.6 mg/mL (0.25 mL)

fondaparinux (fon da PARE i nuks)

U.S./Canadian Brand Names Arixtra® [US]

Therapeutic Category Factor Xa Inhibitor

Use Prophylaxis of deep vein thrombosis (DVT) in patients undergoing surgery for hip fracture or hip or knee replacement

Usual Dosage S.C.:

Adults: ≥50 kg: Usual dose: 2.5 mg once daily. **Note:** Initiate dose after hemostasis has been established, 6-8 hours postoperatively.

Dosage Forms Injection, solution, as sodium [prefilled syringe]: 2.5 mg/0.5 mL

Foradil® Aerolizer™ [US/Can] see formoterol on next page

Forane® [US/Can] see isoflurane on page 361

formoterol (for MOT ter ol)

U.S./Canadian Brand Names Foradil® Aerolizer™ [US/Can]

Therapeutic Category Beta$_2$-Adrenergic Agonist Agent

Use Maintenance treatment of asthma and prevention of bronchospasm in patients ≥5 years of age with reversible obstructive airway disease, including patients with symptoms of nocturnal asthma, who require regular treatment with inhaled, short-acting beta$_2$ agonists; maintenance treatment of bronchoconstriction in patients with chronic obstructive pulmonary disease (COPD); prevention of exercise-induced bronchospasm in patients ≥12 years of age

Usual Dosage Inhalation:

Children ≥5 years and Adults: Asthma maintenance: 12 mcg capsule every 12 hours

Children ≥12 years and Adults: Exercise-induced bronchospasm: 12 mcg capsule at least 15 minutes before exercise on an "as needed" basis; additional doses should not be used for another 12 hours. **Note:** If already using for asthma maintenance then should not use additional doses for exercise-induced bronchospasm.

Adults: Maintenance treatment for COPD: 12 mcg capsule every 12 hours

Dosage Forms Powder for oral inhalation, as fumarate [capsule]: 12 mcg [contains lactose 25 mg] (18s, 60s)

Formula Q® *(Discontinued)* see page 814

Formulex® **[Can]** see dicyclomine on page 194

5-formyl tetrahydrofolate see leucovorin on page 377

Fortabs® **[US]** see butalbital, aspirin, and caffeine on page 100

Fortaz® **[US/Can]** see ceftazidime on page 125

Fortovase® **[US/Can]** see saquinavir on page 583

Fosamax® **[US/Can]** see alendronate on page 21

foscarnet (fos KAR net)

Synonyms PFA; phosphonoformic acid

U.S./Canadian Brand Names Foscavir® [US/Can]

Therapeutic Category Antiviral Agent

Use Alternative to ganciclovir for treatment of CMV infections and is possibly the preferred initial agent for the treatment of CMV retinitis except for those patients with decreased renal function; treatment of acyclovir-resistant mucocutaneous herpes simplex virus infections in immunocompromised patients; and acyclovir-resistant herpes zoster infections

Usual Dosage

Induction treatment: 60 mg/kg 3 times/day for 14-21 days

Maintenance therapy: 90-120 mg/kg/day

Dosage Forms Injection: 24 mg/mL (250 mL, 500 mL)

Foscavir® **[US/Can]** see foscarnet on this page

fosfomycin (fos foe MYE sin)

U.S./Canadian Brand Names Monurol™ [US/Can]

Therapeutic Category Antibiotic, Miscellaneous

Use Treatment of uncomplicated urinary tract infections

Usual Dosage Adults: Oral: Single dose of 3 g in 4 oz of water

Dosage Forms Powder, as tromethamine: 3 g [mix in 4 oz water]

fosinopril (foe SIN oh pril)

U.S./Canadian Brand Names Monopril® [US/Can]

Therapeutic Category Angiotensin-Converting Enzyme (ACE) Inhibitor

Use Treatment of hypertension, either alone or in combination with other antihypertensive agents

Usual Dosage Adults: Oral: 20-40 mg/day

Dosage Forms Tablet: 10 mg, 20 mg, 40 mg

fosinopril and hydrochlorothiazide
(foe SIN oh pril & hye droe klor oh THYE a zide)

U.S./Canadian Brand Names Monopril-HCT® [US/Can]

Therapeutic Category Angiotensin-Converting Enzyme (ACE) Inhibitor

Use Treatment of hypertension

Usual Dosage Adults: Oral: Dose is individualized; not for initial therapy

Dosage Forms
Tablet:
Fosinopril 10 mg and hydrochlorothiazide 12.5 mg
Fosinopril 20 mg and hydrochlorothiazide 12.5 mg

fosphenytoin (FOS fen i toyn)

U.S./Canadian Brand Names Cerebyx® [US/Can]

Therapeutic Category Hydantoin

Use Indicated for short-term parenteral administration when other means of phenytoin administration are unavailable, inappropriate or deemed less advantageous; the safety and effectiveness of fosphenytoin in this use has not been systematically evaluated for more than 5 days; may be used for the control of generalized convulsive status epilepticus and prevention and treatment of seizures occurring during neurosurgery

Usual Dosage The dose, concentration in solutions, and infusion rates for fosphenytoin are expressed as phenytoin sodium equivalents; fosphenytoin should always be prescribed and dispensed in phenytoin sodium equivalents

Status epilepticus: I.V.: Adults: Loading dose: Phenytoin equivalent 15-20 mg/kg I.V. administered at 100-150 mg/minute

Nonemergent loading and maintenance dosing: I.V. or I.M.: Adults:
Loading dose: Phenytoin equivalent 10-20 mg/kg I.V. or I.M. (max I.V. rate 150 mg/minute)
Initial daily maintenance dose: Phenytoin equivalent 4-6 mg/kg/day I.V. or I.M.

I.M. or I.V. substitution for oral phenytoin therapy: May be substituted for oral phenytoin sodium at the same total daily dose, however, Dilantin® capsules are ~90% bioavailable by the oral route; phenytoin, supplied as fosphenytoin, is 100% bioavailable by both the I.M. and I.V. routes; for this reason, plasma phenytoin concentrations may increase when I.M. or I.V. fosphenytoin is substituted for oral phenytoin sodium therapy; in clinical trials I.M. fosphenytoin was administered as a single daily dose utilizing either 1 or 2 injection sites; some patients may require more frequent dosing

Dosage Forms Injection, as sodium: 75 mg/mL [equivalent to 50 mg/mL phenytoin sodium] (2 mL, 10 mL)

Fostex® 10% BPO [US-OTC] *see* benzoyl peroxide *on page 79*

Fostex® [US-OTC] *see* sulfur and salicylic acid *on page 614*

Fototar® [US-OTC] *see* coal tar *on page 158*

Fragmin® [US/Can] *see* dalteparin *on page 174*

framycetin *(Canada only)* (fra mye CEE tin)

U.S./Canadian Brand Names Sofra-Tulle® [Can]

Therapeutic Category Antibiotic, Topical

Use Treatment of infected or potentially infected burns, wounds, ulcers, and graft sites

Usual Dosage A single layer to be applied directly to the wound and covered with an appropriate dressing. If exudative, dressings should be changed at least daily. In case of leg ulcers, cut dressing accurately to size of ulcer to decrease the risk of sensitization and to avoid contact with surrounding healthy skin.

Dosage Forms Dressing, gauze: 1% (10 cm x 10 cm, 10 cm x 30 cm)

Fraxiparine™ [Can] *see* nadroparin *(Canada only) on page 443*

Freezone® **[US-OTC]** *see* salicylic acid *on page 581*

Frisium® **[Can]** *see* clobazam *(Canada only) on page 152*

Froben® **[Can]** *see* flurbiprofen *on page 282*

Froben-SR® **[Can]** *see* flurbiprofen *on page 282*

Frova™ **[US]** *see* frovatriptan *on this page*

frovatriptan (froe va TRIP tan)
Synonyms frovatriptan succinate
U.S./Canadian Brand Names Frova™ [US]
Therapeutic Category Antimigraine Agent; Serotonin 5-HT$_{1B, 1D}$ Receptor Agonist
Use Acute treatment of migraine with or without aura in adults
Usual Dosage Oral: Adults: Migraine: 2.5 mg; if headache recurs, a second dose may be given if first dose provided some relief and at least 2 hours have elapsed since the first dose (maximum daily dose: 7.5 mg)
Dosage Forms Tablet, as base: 2.5 mg

frovatriptan succinate *see* frovatriptan *on this page*

frusemide *see* furosemide *on next page*

FS *see* fibrin sealant kit *on page 271*

FS Shampoo® **Topical** *(Discontinued) see page 814*

5-FU *see* fluorouracil *on page 279*

Fucidin® **[Can]** *see* fusidic acid *(Canada only) on next page*

FUDR® **[US/Can]** *see* floxuridine *on page 274*

Ful-Glo® **Ophthalmic Strips [US]** *see* fluorescein sodium *on page 277*

fulvestrant (fool VES trant)
Synonyms ICI 182,780
U.S./Canadian Brand Names Faslodex® [US]
Therapeutic Category Antineoplastic Agent, Estrogen Receptor Antagonist
Use Treatment of hormone receptor positive metastatic breast cancer in postmenopausal women with disease progression following anti-estrogen therapy.
Usual Dosage I.M.: Adults (postmenopausal women): 250 mg at 1-month intervals
Dosage Forms Injection, solution [prefilled syringe]: 50 mg/mL (2.5 mL, 5 mL) [contains alcohol, benzyl alcohol, benzyl stearate, castor oil]

Fulvicin® **P/G [US]** *see* griseofulvin *on page 306*

Fulvicin-U/F® **[US/Can]** *see* griseofulvin *on page 306*

Fumasorb® *(Discontinued) see page 814*

Fumerin® *(Discontinued) see page 814*

Funduscein® **Injection** *(Discontinued) see page 814*

Fungi-Nail® **[US-OTC]** *see* undecylenic acid and derivatives *on page 665*

Fungizone® **[US/Can]** *see* amphotericin B (conventional) *on page 39*

Fungoid® **Tincture [US-OTC]** *see* miconazole *on page 427*

Furacin® **Topical** *(Discontinued) see page 814*

Furadantin® **[US]** *see* nitrofurantoin *on page 461*

Furalan® *(Discontinued) see page 814*

Furamide® *(Discontinued) see page 814*

Furan® *(Discontinued) see page 814*

Furanite® *(Discontinued) see page 814*

furazolidone (fyoor a ZOE li done)

U.S./Canadian Brand Names Furoxone® [US/Can]

Therapeutic Category Antiprotozoal

Use Treatment of bacterial or protozoal diarrhea and enteritis caused by susceptible organisms: *Giardia lamblia* and *Vibrio cholerae*

Usual Dosage Oral:

Children >1 month: 5-8.8 mg/kg/day in 3-4 divided doses for 7-10 days, not to exceed 400 mg/day

Adults: 100 mg 4 times/day for 7-10 days

Dosage Forms

Liquid: 50 mg/15 mL (60 mL, 473 mL)

Tablet: 100 mg

furazosin *see* prazosin *on page 536*

Furocot® [US] *see* furosemide *on this page*

furosemide (fyoor OH se mide)

Synonyms frusemide

U.S./Canadian Brand Names Apo®-Furosemide [Can]; Furocot® [US]; Lasix® Special [Can]; Lasix® [US/Can]

Therapeutic Category Diuretic, Loop

Use Management of edema associated with congestive heart failure and hepatic or renal disease; used alone or in combination with antihypertensives in treatment of hypertension

Usual Dosage

Infants and Children:

Oral: 2 mg/kg/dose increased in increments of 1 mg/kg/dose with each succeeding dose until a satisfactory effect is achieved to a maximum of 6 mg/kg/dose no more frequently than 6 hours

I.M., I.V.: 1 mg/kg/dose, increasing by each succeeding dose at 1 mg/kg/dose at intervals of 6-12 hours until a satisfactory response up to 6 mg/kg/dose

Adults:

Oral: Initial: 20-80 mg/dose, increase in increments of 20-40 mg/dose at intervals of 6-8 hours; usual maintenance dose interval is twice daily or every day

I.M., I.V.: 20-40 mg/dose, may be repeated in 1-2 hours as needed and increased by 20 mg/dose with each succeeding dose up to 600 mg/day; usual dosing interval: 6-12 hours

Dosage Forms

Injection: 10 mg/mL (2 mL, 4 mL, 5 mL, 6 mL, 8 mL, 10 mL, 12 mL)

Solution, oral: 10 mg/mL (60 mL, 120 mL); 40 mg/5 mL (5 mL, 10 mL, 500 mL)

Tablet: 20 mg, 40 mg, 80 mg

Furoxone® [US/Can] *see* furazolidone *on this page*

fusidic acid *(Canada only)* (fyoo SI dik AS id)

Synonyms sodium fusidate

U.S./Canadian Brand Names Fucidin® [Can]

Therapeutic Category Antifungal Agent, Systemic

Use The treatment of the following infections when due to susceptible strains of *S. aureus*, both penicillinase producing and nonpenicillinase producing: skin and soft tissue infections, osteomyelitis. For patients with staphylococcal infections where other antibiotics have failed (ie, patients with staphylococcal septicemia, burns, endocarditis, pneumonia, cystic fibrosis). Appropriate culture and susceptibility studies should be performed. Fucidin® may be administered to those patients in whom a staphylococcal infection is suspected. This antibiotic treatment may subsequently require modification once these results become available.

Usual Dosage Adults:

I.V.: 500 mg 3 times/day

(Continued)

291

fusidic acid *(Canada only)* *(Continued)*
Oral: 500 mg 3 times/day
Dosage Forms
Powder for injection: 500 mg
Suspension, oral (banana flavor): 246 mg/5 mL (50 mL)
Tablet, sodium fusidate: 250 mg (equivalent to 240 mg fusidic acid)

G-1® *(Discontinued)* see page 814

gabapentin (GA ba pen tin)
U.S./Canadian Brand Names Neurontin® [US/Can]
Therapeutic Category Anticonvulsant
Use Adjunct for treatment of drug-refractory partial and secondarily generalized seizures
Usual Dosage Adults: Oral: 900-1800 mg/day administered in 3 divided doses; therapy is initiated with a rapid titration, beginning with 300 mg on day 1, 300 mg twice daily on day 2, and 300 mg 3 times/day on day 3

Discontinuing therapy or replacing with an alternative agent should be done gradually over a minimum of 7 days
Dosage Forms
Capsule: 100 mg, 300 mg, 400 mg
Solution, oral: 250 mg/5 mL (480 mL) [cool strawberry anise flavor]
Tablet: 600 mg, 800 mg

Gabitril® **[US/Can]** see tiagabine on page 637

galantamine (ga LAN ta meen)
Synonyms galantamine hydrobromide
U.S./Canadian Brand Names Reminyl® [US]
Therapeutic Category Acetylcholinesterase Inhibitor (Central)
Use Treatment of mild to moderate dementia of Alzheimer's disease
Usual Dosage Note: Take with breakfast and dinner. If therapy is interrupted for ≥3 days, restart at the lowest dose and increase to current dose.
Oral: Adults: Mild to moderate dementia of Alzheimer's: Initial: 4 mg twice a day for 4 weeks
If 8 mg per day tolerated, increase to 8 mg twice daily for ≥4 weeks
If 16 mg per day tolerated, increase to 12 mg twice daily
Range: 16-24 mg/day in 2 divided doses
Dosage Forms
Solution, oral, as hydrobromide: 4 mg/mL (100 mL) [with calibrated pipette]
Tablet, as hydrobromide: 4 mg, 8 mg, 12 mg

galantamine hydrobromide see galantamine on this page

gallium nitrate (GAL ee um NYE trate)
U.S./Canadian Brand Names Ganite™ [US]
Therapeutic Category Antidote
Use Treatment of clearly symptomatic cancer-related hypercalcemia that has not responded to adequate hydration
Usual Dosage Adults: I.V. infusion: 200 mg/m^2 for 5 consecutive days
Dosage Forms Injection: 25 mg/mL (20 mL)

Gamastan® *(Discontinued)* see page 814

Gamimune® **N [US/Can]** see immune globulin (intravenous) on page 347

gamma benzene hexachloride see lindane on page 385

Gammagard® **Injection** *(Discontinued)* see page 814

Gammagard® **S/D [US/Can]** see immune globulin (intravenous) on page 347

gamma globulin *see* immune globulin (intramuscular) *on page 346*

gammaphos *see* amifostine *on page 31*

Gammar® *(Discontinued) see page 814*

Gammar®**-P I.V. [US]** *see* immune globulin (intravenous) *on page 347*

Gamulin® **Rh** *(Discontinued) see page 814*

ganciclovir (gan SYE kloe veer)

Synonyms DHPG sodium; GCV sodium; nordeoxyguanosine

U.S./Canadian Brand Names Cytovene® [US/Can]; Vitrasert® [US/Can]

Therapeutic Category Antiviral Agent

Use

Parenteral: Treatment of CMV retinitis in immunocompromised individuals, including patients with acquired immunodeficiency syndrome; prophylaxis of CMV infection in transplant patients

Oral: Alternative to the I.V. formulation for maintenance treatment of CMV retinitis in immunocompromised patients, including patients with AIDS, in whom retinitis is stable following appropriate induction therapy and for whom the risk of more rapid progression is balanced by the benefit associated with avoiding daily I.V. infusions.

Usual Dosage Slow I.V. infusion:

Retinitis: Children >3 months and Adults: Induction therapy: 5 mg/kg/dose every 12 hours for 14-21 days followed by maintenance therapy; maintenance therapy: 5 mg/kg/day as a single daily dose for 7 days/week or 6 mg/kg/day for 5 days/week

Other CMV infections: 5 mg/kg/dose every 12 hours for 14-21 days or 2.5 mg/kg/dose every 8 hours; maintenance therapy: 5 mg/kg/day as a single daily dose for 7 days/week or 6 mg/kg/day for 5 days/week

Dosage Forms

Capsule (Cytovene®): 250 mg, 500 mg

Implant, intravitreal (Vitrasert®): 4.5 mg [released gradually over 5-8 months]

Injection, powder for reconstitution, as sodium (Cytovene®): 500 mg

Ganite™ **[US]** *see* gallium nitrate *on previous page*

Gani-Tuss® **NR [US]** *see* guaifenesin and codeine *on page 308*

Gantanol® *(Discontinued) see page 814*

Gantrisin® **Ophthalmic** *(Discontinued) see page 814*

Gantrisin® **Pediatric Suspension [US]** *see* sulfisoxazole *on page 614*

Gantrisin® **Tablet** *(Discontinued) see page 814*

Garamycin® **[US/Can]** *see* gentamicin *on page 297*

Garatec [Can] *see* gentamicin *on page 297*

Gas-Ban DS® *(Discontinued) see page 814*

Gastrocrom® **[US]** *see* cromolyn sodium *on page 166*

Gastrografin® **[US]** *see* radiological/contrast media (ionic) *on page 561*

Gastrosed™ *(Discontinued) see page 814*

Gas-X® **[US-OTC]** *see* simethicone *on page 591*

gatifloxacin (ga ti FLOKS a sin)

U.S./Canadian Brand Names Tequin® [US/Can]

Therapeutic Category Antibiotic, Quinolone

Use Treatment of the following infections when caused by susceptible bacteria: Acute bacterial exacerbation of chronic bronchitis due to *S. pneumoniae*, *H. influenzae*, *H. parainfluenzae*, *M. catarrhalis*, or *S. aureus*; acute sinusitis due to *S. pneumoniae*, *H. influenzae*; community acquired pneumonia due to *S. pneumoniae*, *H. influenzae*, *H. parainfluenzae*, *M. catarrhalis*, *S. aureus*, *M. pneumoniae*, *C. pneumoniae*, or *L.* (Continued)

gatifloxacin *(Continued)*

pneumophilia; uncomplicated urinary tract infections (cystitis) due to *E. coli*, *K. pneumoniae*, or *P. mirabilis*; complicated urinary tract infections due to *E. coli*, *K. pneumoniae*, or *P. mirabilis*; pyelonephritis due to *E. coli*; uncomplicated urethral and cervical gonorrhea; acute, uncomplicated rectal infections in women due to *N. gonorrhoeae*

Usual Dosage Adult: Oral, I.V.:

Acute bacterial exacerbation of chronic bronchitis: 400 mg every 24 hours for 5 days

Acute sinusitis: 400 mg every 24 hours for 10 days

Community-acquired pneumonia: 400 mg every 24 hours for 7-14 days

Uncomplicated urinary tract infections (cystitis): 400 mg single dose or 200 mg every 24 hours for 3 days

Complicated urinary tract infections: 400 mg every 24 hours for 7-10 days

Acute pyelonephritis: 400 mg every 24 hours for 7-10 days

Uncomplicated urethral gonorrhea in men, cervical or rectal gonorrhea in women: 400 mg single dose

Dosage Forms

Injection, solution: 10 mg/mL (20 mL, 40 mL)

Injection, infusion [premixed in D_5W]: 200 mg (100 mL); 400 mg (200 mL)

Tablet: 200 mg, 400 mg

Gaviscon® Extra Strength [US-OTC] *see* aluminum hydroxide and magnesium carbonate *on page 28*

Gaviscon® Liquid [US-OTC] *see* aluminum hydroxide and magnesium carbonate *on page 28*

G-CSF *see* filgrastim *on page 272*

GCV sodium *see* ganciclovir *on previous page*

Gee Gee® *(Discontinued)* *see page 814*

gelatin (absorbable) (JEL a tin ab SORB a ble)

Synonyms absorbable gelatin sponge

U.S./Canadian Brand Names Gelfilm® [US]; Gelfoam® [US]

Therapeutic Category Hemostatic Agent

Use Adjunct to provide hemostasis in surgery; also used in oral and dental surgery; in open prostatic surgery

Usual Dosage Topical: Hemostasis: Apply packs or sponges dry or saturated with sodium chloride. When applied dry, hold in place with moderate pressure. When applied wet, squeeze to remove air bubbles. Prostatectomy cones are designed for use with the Foley bag catheter. The powder is applied as a paste prepared by adding approximately 4 mL of sterile saline solution to the powder.

Dosage Forms

Film, ophthalmic (Gelfilm®): 25 mm x 50 mm (6s)

Film, topical (Gelfilm®): 100 mm x 125 mm (1s)

Powder, topical (Gelfoam®): 1 g

Sponge, dental (Gelfoam®): Size 4 (12s)

Sponge, topical (Gelfoam®):

Size 50 (4s)

Size 100 (6s)

Size 200 (6s)

Size 2 cm (1s)

Size 6 cm (6s)

Size 12-7 mm (12s)

gelatin, pectin, and methylcellulose

(JEL a tin, PEK tin, & meth il SEL yoo lose)

U.S./Canadian Brand Names Orabase® Plain [US-OTC]

Therapeutic Category Protectant, Topical

Use Temporary relief from minor oral irritations

Usual Dosage Oral: Press small dabs into place until the involved area is coated with a thin film; do not try to spread onto area; may be used as often as needed
Dosage Forms Paste, oral: 5 g, 15 g

Gelfilm®️ [US] *see* gelatin (absorbable) *on previous page*

Gelfoam®️ [US] *see* gelatin (absorbable) *on previous page*

Gel-Kam®️ [US] *see* fluoride *on page 278*

Gel-Tin®️ *(Discontinued)* *see page 814*

Gelucast®️ [US] *see* zinc gelatin *on page 690*

Gelusil®️ [Can] *see* aluminum hydroxide and magnesium hydroxide *on page 29*

Gelusil®️ Extra Strength [Can] *see* aluminum hydroxide and magnesium hydroxide *on page 29*

Gelusil®️ Liquid *(Discontinued)* *see page 814*

gemcitabine (jem SIT a been)
U.S./Canadian Brand Names Gemzar®️ [US/Can]
Therapeutic Category Antineoplastic Agent
Use Treatment of patients with inoperable pancreatic cancer
Usual Dosage Adults: I.V.: 1000 mg/^{2} over 30 minutes once weekly for up to 7 weeks
Dosage Forms Injection, powder for reconstitution, as hydrochloride: 200 mg, 1 g

gemfibrozil (jem FI broe zil)
Synonyms CI-719
U.S./Canadian Brand Names Apo®️-Gemfibrozil [Can]; Gen-Gemfibrozil [Can]; Lopid®️ [US/Can]; Novo-Gemfibrozil [Can]; Nu-Gemfibrozil [Can]; PMS-Gemfibrozil [Can]
Therapeutic Category Antihyperlipidemic Agent, Miscellaneous
Use Hypertriglyceridemia in types IV and V hyperlipidemia; increases HDL cholesterol
Usual Dosage Oral: 1200 mg/day in 2 divided doses, 30 minutes before breakfast and supper
Dosage Forms Tablet, film coated: 600 mg

gemtuzumab ozogamicin (gem TUZ yu mab oh zog a MY sin)
U.S./Canadian Brand Names Mylotarg™️ [US/Can]
Therapeutic Category Antineoplastic Agent, Natural Source (Plant) Derivative
Use Treatment of acute myeloid leukemia (CD33 positive) in first relapse in patients who are 60 years of age or older and who are not considered candidates for cytotoxic chemotherapy.
Usual Dosage Adults ≥60 years: I.V.: 9 mg/m^2, infused over 2 hours. The patient should receive diphenhydramine 50 mg and acetaminophen 650-1000 mg orally 1 hour prior to administration of each dose. Acetaminophen dosage should be repeated as needed every 4 hours for two additional doses. A full treatment course is a total of two doses administered with 14 days between doses. Full hematologic recovery is not necessary for administration of the second dose. There has been only limited experience with repeat courses of gemtuzumab ozogamicin.
Dosage Forms Injection, powder for reconstitution: 5 mg

Gemzar®️ [US/Can] *see* gemcitabine *on this page*

Genabid®️ *(Discontinued)* *see page 814*

Gen-Acebutolol [Can] *see* acebutolol *on page 3*

Genaced [US-OTC] *see* acetaminophen, aspirin, and caffeine *on page 7*

Genac®️ Tablet [US-OTC] *see* triprolidine and pseudoephedrine *on page 659*

Gen-Acyclovir [Can] *see* acyclovir *on page 13*

Genagesic®️ *(Discontinued)* *see page 814*

Genahist® **[US-OTC]** *see* diphenhydramine *on page 202*

Gen-Alprazolam [Can] *see* alprazolam *on page 24*

Genamin® **Cold Syrup** *(Discontinued) see page 814*

Genamin® **Expectorant** *(Discontinued) see page 814*

Gen-Amiodarone [Can] *see* amiodarone *on page 34*

Gen-Amoxicillin [Can] *see* amoxicillin *on page 37*

Genapap® **Children [US-OTC]** *see* acetaminophen *on page 3*

Genapap® **Extra Strength [US-OTC]** *see* acetaminophen *on page 3*

Genapap® **Infant [US-OTC]** *see* acetaminophen *on page 3*

Genapap® **[US-OTC]** *see* acetaminophen *on page 3*

Genaphed® **[US-OTC]** *see* pseudoephedrine *on page 552*

Genasal [US-OTC] *see* oxymetazoline *on page 486*

Genasoft® **Plus [US-OTC]** *see* docusate and casanthranol *on page 209*

Genaspor® **[US-OTC]** *see* tolnaftate *on page 644*

Genatap® **Elixir** *(Discontinued) see page 814*

Gen-Atenolol [Can] *see* atenolol *on page 60*

Genatuss® *(Discontinued) see page 814*

Genatuss DM® **[US-OTC]** *see* guaifenesin and dextromethorphan *on page 308*

Gen-Azathioprine [Can] *see* azathioprine *on page 65*

Gen-Baclofen [Can] *see* baclofen *on page 70*

Gen-Beclo [Can] *see* beclomethasone *on page 73*

Gen-Bromazepam [Can] *see* bromazepam *(Canada only) on page 92*

Gen-Budesonide AQ [Can] *see* budesonide *on page 95*

Gen-Buspirone [Can] *see* buspirone *on page 98*

Gencalc® **600** *(Discontinued) see page 814*

Gen-Captopril [Can] *see* captopril *on page 112*

Gen-Carbamazepine CR [Can] *see* carbamazepine *on page 113*

Gen-Cimetidine [Can] *see* cimetidine *on page 146*

Gen-Clobetasol [Can] *see* clobetasol *on page 152*

Gen-Clomipramine [Can] *see* clomipramine *on page 154*

Gen-Clonazepam [Can] *see* clonazepam *on page 154*

Gen-Cyclobenzaprine [Can] *see* cyclobenzaprine *on page 168*

Gen-Cyproterone [Can] *see* cyproterone *(Canada only) on page 170*

Gen-Diltiazem [Can] *see* diltiazem *on page 199*

Gen-Divalproex [Can] *see* valproic acid and derivatives *on page 670*

Gen-Doxazosin [Can] *see* doxazosin *on page 213*

Gen-D-phen® *(Discontinued) see page 814*

Genebs® **Extra Strength [US-OTC]** *see* acetaminophen *on page 3*

Genebs® **[US-OTC]** *see* acetaminophen *on page 3*

Generlac® **[US]** *see* lactulose *on page 372*

Genesec® **[US-OTC]** *see* acetaminophen and phenyltoloxamine *on page 6*

Gen-Etodolac [Can] *see* etodolac *on page 258*

Geneye® **[US-OTC]** *see* tetrahydrozoline *on page 629*

Gen-Famotidine [Can] *see* famotidine *on page 262*

Gen-Fenofibrat Micro [Can] *see* fenofibrate *on page 265*
Gen-Fluoxetine [Can] *see* fluoxetine *on page 279*
Gen-Fluvoxamine [Can] *see* fluvoxamine *on page 285*
Gen-Gemfibrozil [Can] *see* gemfibrozil *on page 295*
Gen-Gliclazide [Can] *see* gliclazide *(Canada only) on page 299*
Gen-Glybe [Can] *see* glyburide *on page 301*
Gengraf™ [US] *see* cyclosporine *on page 169*
Gen-Indapamide [Can] *see* indapamide *on page 348*
Gen-Ipratropium [Can] *see* ipratropium *on page 358*
Gen-K® *(Discontinued)* *see page 814*
Gen-Medroxy [Can] *see* medroxyprogesterone acetate *on page 404*
Gen-Metformin [Can] *see* metformin *on page 414*
Gen-Metoprolol [Can] *see* metoprolol *on page 425*
Gen-Minocycline [Can] *see* minocycline *on page 431*
Gen-Naproxen EC [Can] *see* naproxen *on page 447*
Gen-Nortriptyline [Can] *see* nortriptyline *on page 466*
Genoptic® [US] *see* gentamicin *on this page*
Genora® 0.5/35 *(Discontinued)* *see page 814*
Genora® 1/35 *(Discontinued)* *see page 814*
Genora® 1/50 *(Discontinued)* *see page 814*
Genotropin® [US] *see* human growth hormone *on page 324*
Genotropin Miniquick® [US] *see* human growth hormone *on page 324*
Gen-Oxybutynin [Can] *see* oxybutynin *on page 484*
Gen-Pindolol [Can] *see* pindolol *on page 516*
Gen-Piroxicam [Can] *see* piroxicam *on page 517*
Genpril® [US-OTC] *see* ibuprofen *on page 342*
Gen-Ranitidine [Can] *see* ranitidine hydrochloride *on page 564*
Gen-Selegiline [Can] *see* selegiline *on page 586*
Gen-Sotalol [Can] *see* sotalol *on page 602*
Gentacidin® [US] *see* gentamicin *on this page*
Gentak® [US] *see* gentamicin *on this page*

gentamicin (jen ta MYE sin)
  U.S./Canadian Brand Names Alcomicin® [Can]; Diogent® [Can]; Garamycin® [US/
    Can]; Garatec [Can]; Genoptic® [US]; Gentacidin® [US]; Gentak® [US]
  Therapeutic Category Aminoglycoside (Antibiotic); Antibiotic, Ophthalmic; Antibiotic,
    Topical
  Use Treatment of susceptible bacterial infections, normally due to gram-negative orga-
    nisms including *Pseudomonas*, *Proteus*, *Serratia*, and gram-positive *Staphylococcus*;
    treatment of bone infections, CNS infections, respiratory tract infections, skin and soft
    tissue infections, as well as abdominal and urinary tract infections, endocarditis, and
    septicemia; used in combination with ampicillin as empiric therapy for sepsis in
    newborns; used topically to treat superficial infections of the skin or ophthalmic infec-
    tions caused by susceptible bacteria
  Usual Dosage Dosage should be based on an estimate of ideal body weight
    Infants and Children >3 months: Intrathecal: 1-2 mg/day
    Infants and Children <5 years: 2.5 mg/kg/dose every 8 hours
    Children >5 years: 1.5-2.5 mg/kg/dose every 8 hours
    (Continued)

gentamicin *(Continued)*

Ophthalmic: Solution: 1-2 drops every 2-4 hours, up to 2 drops every hour for severe infections; ointment: 2-3 times/day

Topical: Apply 3-4 times/day

Adults:

I.M., I.V.: 3-5 mg/kg/day in divided doses every 8 hours

Topical: Apply 3-4 times/day

Ophthalmic: Solution: 1-2 drops every 2-4 hours; ointment: 2-3 times/day

Dosage Forms

Cream, topical, as sulfate (Garamycin®): 0.1% (15 g)

Infusion, as sulfate [premixed in NS]: 40 mg (50 mL); 60 mg (50 mL, 100 mL); 70 mg (50 mL); 80 mg (50 mL, 100 mL); 90 mg (100 mL); 100 mg (50 mL, 100 mL); 120 mg (100 mL)

Injection, solution, as sulfate [ADD-Vantage® vial]: 10 mg/mL (6 mL, 8 mL, 10 mL)

Injection, solution, as sulfate: 40 mg/mL (2 mL, 20 mL) [may contain sodium metabisulfite]

Garamycin®: 40 mg/mL (2 mL) [contains sodium bisulfite]

Injection, solution, pediatric, as sulfate: 10 mg/mL (2 mL) [may contain sodium metabisulfite]

Injection, solution, pediatric, as sulfate [preservative free]: 10 mg/mL (2 mL)

Ointment, ophthalmic, as sulfate: 0.3% [3 mg/g] (3.5 g)

Ointment, topical, as sulfate (Garamycin®): 0.1% (15 g)

Solution, ophthalmic, as sulfate: 0.3% (5 mL, 15 mL) [contains benzalkonium chloride]

Garamycin®, Gentacidin®: 0.3% (5 mL) [contains benzalkonium chloride]

Genoptic®: 0.3% (1 mL, 5 mL) [contains benzalkonium chloride]

Gentak®: 0.3% (5 mL, 15 mL) [contains benzalkonium chloride]

gentamicin and prednisolone *see* prednisolone and gentamicin *on page 537*

Gen-Tamoxifen [Can] *see* tamoxifen *on page 618*

GenTeal™ [US/Can] *see* hydroxypropyl methylcellulose *on page 337*

Gen-Temazepam [Can] *see* temazepam *on page 621*

Gen-Ticlopidine [Can] *see* ticlopidine *on page 639*

Gen-Timolol [Can] *see* timolol *on page 639*

Gentran® [US/Can] *see* dextran *on page 187*

Gentrasul® *(Discontinued)* *see page 814*

Gen-Trazodone [Can] *see* trazodone *on page 649*

Gen-Triazolam [Can] *see* triazolam *on page 653*

Gen-Verapamil [Can] *see* verapamil *on page 675*

Gen-Verapamil SR [Can] *see* verapamil *on page 675*

Gen-Zopiclone [Can] *see* zopiclone *(Canada only) on page 693*

Geocillin® [US] *see* carbenicillin *on page 114*

Geodon® [US] *see* ziprasidone *on page 692*

Geone® [US] *see* butalbital, acetaminophen, and caffeine *on page 99*

Geref® [US] *see* sermorelin acetate *on page 588*

Geref® Diagnostic [US] *see* sermorelin acetate *on page 588*

Geridium® *(Discontinued)* *see page 814*

Geridryl® [US-OTC] *see* diphenhydramine *on page 202*

German measles vaccine *see* rubella virus vaccine (live) *on page 579*

Germinal® [US] *see* ergoloid mesylates *on page 233*

Gevrabon® [US-OTC] *see* vitamin B complex *on page 681*

GG *see* guaifenesin *on page 307*

GG-Cen® *(Discontinued)* see page 814

glatiramer acetate (gla TIR a mer AS e tate)

Synonyms copolymer-1

U.S./Canadian Brand Names Copaxone® [US/Can]

Therapeutic Category Biological, Miscellaneous

Use Reduce the frequency of relapses in relapsing-remitting multiple sclerosis (MS)

Usual Dosage Adults: S.C.: 20 mg/day

Dosage Forms Injection, powder for reconstitution: 20 mg [contains mannitol 40 mg; packaged with sterile water for injection]

Glaucon® *(Discontinued)* see page 814

Gleevec™ **[US]** see imatinib on page 345

Gliadel® **[US]** see carmustine on page 118

glibenclamide see glyburide on page 301

gliclazide *(Canada only)* (GLYE kla zide)

U.S./Canadian Brand Names Diamicron® [Can]; Gen-Gliclazide [Can]; Novo-Gliclazide [Can]

Therapeutic Category Antidiabetic Agent; Hypoglycemic Agent, Oral; Sulfonylurea Agent

Use Control of hyperglycemia in gliclazide-responsive diabetes mellitus of stable, mild, nonketosis prone, maturity onset or adult type which cannot be controlled by proper dietary management and exercise, or when insulin therapy is not appropriate.

Usual Dosage Adults: Oral: There is no fixed dosage regimen for the management of diabetes mellitus with gliclazide or any other hypoglycemic agent. Determination of the proper dosage for gliclazide for each patient should be made on the basis of frequent determinations of blood glucose during dose titration and throughout maintenance.

Recommended daily dosage: 80-320 mg; dosage of ≥160 mg should be divided into 2 equal parts for twice daily administration. Gliclazide should be taken preferentially with meals.

Recommended starting dose: 160 mg/day taken as 1 tablet twice daily with meals; total daily dose should not exceed 320 mg

Dosage Forms

Tablet (Diamicron®): 80 mg

Tablet, sustained release (Diamicron® MR): 30 mg

glimepiride (GLYE me pye ride)

U.S./Canadian Brand Names Amaryl® [US/Can]

Therapeutic Category Antidiabetic Agent, Oral

Use

Management of noninsulin-dependent diabetes mellitus (type II) as an adjunct to diet and exercise to lower blood glucose

In combination with insulin to lower blood glucose in patients whose hyperglycemia cannot be controlled by diet and exercise in conjunction with an oral hypoglycemic agent

Usual Dosage Oral (allow several days between dose titrations):

Adults: Initial: 1-2 mg once daily, administered with breakfast or the first main meal; usual maintenance dose: 1-4 mg once daily; after a dose of 2 mg once daily, increase in increments of 2 mg at 1- to 2-week intervals based upon the patient's blood glucose response to a maximum of 8 mg once daily

Combination with insulin therapy (fasting glucose level for instituting combination therapy is in the range of >150 mg/dL in plasma or serum depending on the patient): 8 mg once daily with the first main meal

After starting with low-dose insulin, upward adjustments of insulin can be done approximately weekly as guided by frequent measurements of fasting blood glucose. Once (Continued)

glimepiride *(Continued)*

stable, combination-therapy patients should monitor their capillary blood glucose on an ongoing basis, preferably daily.

Dosage Forms Tablet: 1 mg, 2 mg, 4 mg

glipizide (GLIP i zide)

Synonyms glydiazinamide

Tall-Man glipiZIDE

U.S./Canadian Brand Names Glucotrol® [US]; Glucotrol® XL [US]

Therapeutic Category Antidiabetic Agent, Oral

Use Management of noninsulin-dependent diabetes mellitus (type II)

Usual Dosage Adults: Oral: 2.5-40 mg/day; doses larger than 15-20 mg/day should be divided and administered twice daily

Dosage Forms

Tablet (Glucotrol®): 5 mg, 10 mg

Tablet, extended release (Glucotrol® XL): 2.5 mg, 5 mg, 10 mg

glivec *see* imatinib *on page 345*

GlucaGen® [US] *see* glucagon *on this page*

GlucaGen® Diagnostic Kit [US] *see* glucagon *on this page*

glucagon (GLOO ka gon)

U.S./Canadian Brand Names GlucaGen® Diagnostic Kit [US]; GlucaGen® [US]; Glucagon Diagnostic Kit [US]; Glucagon Emergency Kit [US]

Therapeutic Category Antihypoglycemic Agent

Use Hypoglycemia; diagnostic aid in the radiologic examination of GI tract when a hypotonic state is needed; used with some success as a cardiac stimulant in management of severe cases of beta-adrenergic blocking agent overdosage

Usual Dosage

Hypoglycemia or insulin shock therapy: I.M., I.V., S.C.:

Children: 0.025-0.1 mg/kg/dose, not to exceed 1 mg/dose, repeated in 20 minutes as needed

Adults: 0.5-1 mg, may repeat in 20 minutes as needed

Diagnostic aid: Adults: I.M., I.V.: 0.25-2 mg 10 minutes prior to procedure

Dosage Forms

Injection, powder for reconstitution, as hydrochloride:

GlucaGen®, Glucagon: 1 mg [1 unit]

GlucaGen® Diagnostic Kit: 1 mg [1 unit] [packaged with sterile water]

Glucagon Diagnostic Kit, Glucagon Emergency Kit: 1 mg [1 unit] [packaged with diluent syringe containing glycerin 12 mg/mL and water for injection]

Glucagon Diagnostic Kit [US] *see* glucagon *on this page*

Glucagon Emergency Kit [US] *see* glucagon *on this page*

glucocerebrosidase *see* alglucerase *on page 22*

GlucoNorm® [Can] *see* repaglinide *on page 567*

Glucophage® [US/Can] *see* metformin *on page 414*

Glucophage® XR [US] *see* metformin *on page 414*

glucose (instant) (GLOO kose IN stant)

U.S./Canadian Brand Names B-D™ Glucose [US-OTC]; Dex4 Glucose [US-OTC]; Glutol™ [US-OTC]; Glutose™ [US-OTC]; Insta-Glucose® [US-OTC]

Therapeutic Category Antihypoglycemic Agent

Use Management of hypoglycemia

Usual Dosage Oral: 10-20 g

Dosage Forms
Gel, oral:
Glutose™: 40% (15 g, 45 g)
Insta-Glucose®: 40% (30 g)
Solution, oral (Glutol™): 55% [100 g dextrose/180 mL] (180 mL)
Tablet, chewable:
B-D™ Glucose: 5 g
Dex4 Glucose: 4 g

glucose polymers (GLOO kose POL i merz)
U.S./Canadian Brand Names Moducal® [US-OTC]; Polycose® [US-OTC]
Therapeutic Category Nutritional Supplement
Use Supplies calories for those persons not able to meet the caloric requirement with usual food intake
Usual Dosage Adults: Oral: Add to foods or beverages or mix in water
Dosage Forms
Liquid (Polycose®): 43% (126 mL)
Powder:
Moducal®: 368 g
Polycose®: 350 g

Glucotrol® [US] *see* glipizide *on previous page*

Glucotrol® XL [US] *see* glipizide *on previous page*

Glucovance™ [US] *see* glyburide and metformin *on next page*

Glukor® (Discontinued) *see page 814*

Glu-K® [US-OTC] *see* potassium gluconate *on page 531*

glutamic acid (gloo TAM ik AS id)
U.S./Canadian Brand Names Feracid® [US]
Therapeutic Category Gastrointestinal Agent, Miscellaneous
Use Treatment of hypochlorhydria and achlorhydria
Usual Dosage Adults: Oral: 340 mg to 1.02 g 3 times/day before meals or food
Dosage Forms
Capsule, as hydrochloride: 340 mg
Tablet: 500 mg

Glutol™ [US-OTC] *see* glucose (instant) *on previous page*

Glutose™ [US-OTC] *see* glucose (instant) *on previous page*

Glyate® (Discontinued) *see page 814*

glyburide (GLYE byoor ide)
Synonyms glibenclamide
Tall-Man glyBURIDE
U.S./Canadian Brand Names Albert® Glyburide [Can]; Apo®-Glyburide [Can]; DiaBeta® [US/Can]; Euglucon® [Can]; Gen-Glybe [Can]; Glynase™ PresTab™ [US]; Micronase® [US]; Novo-Glyburide [Can]; Nu-Glyburide [Can]; PMS-Glyburide [Can]
Therapeutic Category Antidiabetic Agent, Oral
Use Management of noninsulin-dependent diabetes mellitus (type II)
Usual Dosage Oral:
Diaβeta®, Micronase®:
Adults: Initial: 1.25-5 mg, then increase at weekly intervals to 1.25-20 mg maintenance dose/day divided in 1-2 doses
Glynase™ PresTab™: Adults: Initial: 0.75-3 mg/day, increase by 1.5 mg/day in weekly intervals, maximum: 12 mg/day
Dosage Forms
Tablet (Diaβeta®, Micronase®): 1.25 mg, 2.5 mg, 5 mg
(Continued)

glyburide *(Continued)*

Tablet, micronized (Glynase™ PresTab™): 1.5 mg, 3 mg, 6 mg

glyburide and metformin (GLYE byoor ide & met FOR min)

U.S./Canadian Brand Names Glucovance™ [US]

Therapeutic Category Antidiabetic Agent, Oral; Antidiabetic Agent (Sulfonylurea)

Use Initial therapy for management of type 2 (noninsulin-dependent) diabetes mellitus when hyperglycemia cannot be managed with diet and exercise alone. Second-line therapy for management of type 2 (noninsulin-dependent) diabetes mellitus when hyperglycemia cannot be managed with a sulfonylurea or metformin along with diet and exercise.

Usual Dosage Adults: Oral: Dose should be individualized based on effectiveness and tolerance; titrate to minimum effective dose needed to achieve blood glucose control; **do not exceed maximum recommended doses**

Initial therapy: Glucovance™ 1.25 mg/250 mg once daily with a meal; patients with Hb A_{1c} >9% or fasting plasma glucose (FPG) >200 mg/dL may start with Glucovance™ 1.25 mg/250 mg twice daily with meals

Dosage increases may be made every 2 weeks, in increments of Glucovance™ 1.25 mg/250 mg, until a dose of glyburide 10 mg/metformin 2000 mg per day has been reached

Due to increased risk of hypoglycemia, do not start with Glucovance™ 5 mg/500 mg.

Second-line therapy: Patients previously treated with a sulfonylurea or metformin alone: Starting dose: Glucovance™ 2.5 mg/500 mg or Glucovance™ 5 mg/500 mg twice daily with the morning and evening meals; doses may be increased in increments no larger than glyburide 5 mg/metformin 500 mg, up to a maximum dose of glyburide 20 mg/metformin 2000 mg.

When switching patients previously on a sulfonylurea and metformin together, do not exceed the daily dose of glyburide (or glyburide equivalent) or metformin.

Dosage Forms

Tablet, film coated:

1.25 mg/250 mg: Glyburide 1.25 mg and metformin hydrochloride 250 mg

2.5 mg/500 mg: Glyburide 2.5 mg and metformin hydrochloride 500 mg

5 mg/500 mg: Glyburide 5 mg and metformin hydrochloride 500 mg

glycerin (GLIS er in)

Synonyms glycerol

U.S./Canadian Brand Names Bausch & Lomb® Computer Eye Drops [US-OTC]; Fleet® Babylax® [US-OTC]; Fleet® Glycerin Suppositories Maximum Strength [US-OTC]; Fleet® Glycerin Suppositories [US-OTC]; Fleet® Liquid Glycerin Suppositories [US-OTC]; Osmoglyn® [US]; Sani-Supp® [US-OTC]

Therapeutic Category Laxative; Ophthalmic Agent, Miscellaneous

Use Constipation; reduction of intraocular pressure; reduction of corneal edema; glycerin has been administered orally to reduce intracranial pressure

Usual Dosage

Constipation: Rectal:

Children <6 years: 1 infant suppository 1-2 times/day as needed or 2-5 mL as an enema

Children >6 years and Adults: 1 adult suppository 1-2 times/day as needed or 5-15 mL as an enema

Children and Adults:

Reduction of intraocular pressure: Oral: 1-1.8 g/kg 1-1½ hours preoperatively; additional doses may be administered at 5-hour intervals

Reduction of corneal edema: Instill 1-2 drops in eye(s) every 3-4 hours

Reduction of intracranial pressure: Oral: 1.5 g/kg/day divided every 4 hours; dose of 1 g/kg/dose every 6 hours has also been used

Dosage Forms
Solution, ophthalmic, sterile (Bausch & Lomb® Computer Eye Drops): 1% (15 mL) [contains benzalkonium chloride]
Solution, oral (Osmoglyn®): 50% (220 mL) [lime flavor]
Solution, rectal:
Fleet® Babylax®: 2.3 g/2.3 mL (4 mL) [6 units per box]
Fleet® Liquid Glycerin Suppositories: 5.6 g/5.5 mL (7.5 mL) [4 units per box]
Suppository, rectal: 12s, 24s, 25s, 50s [pediatric and adult sizes]:
Fleet® Glycerin Suppositories: 1 g (12s) [pediatric size]; 2g (12s, 24s, 50s) [adult size]
Fleet® Glycerin Suppositories Maximum Strength: 3g (18s) [adult size]
Sani-Supp®: 82.5% (10s, 25s) [pediatric size]; 82.5% (10s, 25s, 50s) [adult size]

glycerin, lanolin, and peanut oil (GLIS er in, LAN oh lin, & PEE nut oyl)

U.S./Canadian Brand Names Massé® Breast Cream [US-OTC]
Therapeutic Category Topical Skin Product
Use Nipple care of pregnant and nursing women
Usual Dosage Topical: Apply as often as needed
Dosage Forms Cream: 2 oz

glycerol *see* glycerin *on previous page*

glycerol guaiacolate *see* guaifenesin *on page 307*

Glycerol-T® *(Discontinued) see page 814*

glycerol triacetate *see* triacetin *on page 650*

glyceryl trinitrate *see* nitroglycerin *on page 462*

Glycofed® *(Discontinued) see page 814*

Glycon [Can] *see* metformin *on page 414*

glycopyrrolate (glye koe PYE roe late)

U.S./Canadian Brand Names Robinul® Forte [US]; Robinul® [US]
Therapeutic Category Anticholinergic Agent
Use Adjunct in treatment of peptic ulcer disease; inhibit salivation and excessive secretions of the respiratory tract; reversal of cholinergic agents such as neostigmine and pyridostigmine; control of upper airway secretions
Usual Dosage
Children: Control of secretions:
Oral: 40-100 mcg/kg/dose 3-4 times/day
I.M., I.V.: 4-10 mcg/kg/dose every 3-4 hours; maximum: 0.2 mg/dose or 0.8 mg/24 hours
Children:
Intraoperative: I.V.: 4 mcg/kg not to exceed 0.1 mg; repeat at 2- to 3-minute intervals as needed
Preoperative: I.M.:
<2 years: 4.4-8.8 mcg/kg 30-60 minutes before procedure
>2 years: 4.4 mcg/kg 30-60 minutes before procedure
Children and Adults: Reverse neuromuscular blockade: I.V.: 0.2 mg for each 1 mg of neostigmine or 5 mg of pyridostigmine administered
Adults:
Intraoperative: I.V.: 0.1 mg repeated as needed at 2- to 3-minute intervals
Peptic ulcer:
Oral: 1-2 mg 2-3 times/day
I.M., I.V.: 0.1-0.2 mg 3-4 times/day
Preoperative: I.M.: 4.4 mcg/kg 30-60 minutes before procedure
Dosage Forms
Injection, solution (Robinul®): 0.2 mg/mL (1 mL, 2 mL, 5 mL, 20 mL) [contains benzyl alcohol]
(Continued)

glycopyrrolate *(Continued)*
Tablet:
Robinul®: 1 mg
Robinul® Forte: 2 mg

Glycotuss® *(Discontinued)* see page 814

Glycotuss-dM® *(Discontinued)* see page 814

glydiazinamide see glipizide on page 300

Glynase™ PresTab™ [US] see glyburide on page 301

Gly-Oxide® Oral [US-OTC] see carbamide peroxide on page 113

Glyset™ [US/Can] see miglitol on page 430

Glytuss® [US-OTC] see guaifenesin on page 307

GM-CSF see sargramostim on page 583

G-myticin® *(Discontinued)* see page 814

GnRH see gonadorelin on this page

gold sodium thiomalate (gold SOW dee um thye oh MAL ate)
U.S./Canadian Brand Names Aurolate® [US]; Myochrysine® [Can]
Therapeutic Category Gold Compound
Use Treatment of progressive rheumatoid arthritis
Usual Dosage I.M.:
Children: Initial: Test dose of 10 mg I.M. is recommended, followed by 1 mg/kg I.M. weekly for 20 weeks; not to exceed 50 mg in a single injection; maintenance: 1 mg/kg/dose at 2- to 4-week intervals thereafter for as long as therapy is clinically beneficial and toxicity does not develop. Administration for 2-4 months is usually required before clinical improvement is observed.
Adults: 10 mg first week; 25 mg second week; then 25-50 mg/week until 1 g cumulative dose has been administered. If improvement occurs without adverse reactions, administer 25-50 mg every 2-3 weeks, then every 3-4 weeks.
Dosage Forms Injection, solution: 50 mg/mL (1 mL, 10 mL) [contains benzyl alcohol]

GoLYTELY® [US] see polyethylene glycol-electrolyte solution on page 525

gonadorelin (goe nad oh REL in)
Synonyms GnRH; gonadotropin-releasing hormone; LHRH; LRH; luteinizing hormone-releasing hormone
U.S./Canadian Brand Names Factrel® [US]; Lutrepulse™ [Can]
Therapeutic Category Diagnostic Agent; Gonadotropin
Use Evaluation of hypothalamic-pituitary gonadotropic function; used to evaluate abnormal gonadotropin regulation as in precocious puberty and delayed puberty; treatment of primary hypothalamic amenorrhea
Usual Dosage Female:
Diagnostic test: Children >12 years and Adults: I.V., S.C. hydrochloride salt: 100 mcg administered in women during early phase of menstrual cycle (day 1-7)
Primary hypothalamic amenorrhea: Adults: Acetate: I.V.: 5 mcg every 90 minutes via Lutrepulse® pump kit at treatment intervals of 21 days (pump will pulsate every 90 minutes for 7 days)
Dosage Forms Injection, powder for reconstitution, as hydrochloride (Factrel®): 100 mcg [diluent contains benzyl alcohol]

gonadotropin-releasing hormone see gonadorelin on this page

Gonak™ [US-OTC] see hydroxypropyl methylcellulose on page 337

Gonal-F® [US] see follitropin alfa on page 286

Gonic® *(Discontinued)* see page 814

gonioscopic ophthalmic solution *see* hydroxypropyl methylcellulose *on page 337*

Goniosol® [US-OTC] *see* hydroxypropyl methylcellulose *on page 337*

Goody's® Extra Strength Headache Powder [US-OTC] *see* acetaminophen, aspirin, and caffeine *on page 7*

Goody's PM® Powder [US-OTC] *see* acetaminophen and diphenhydramine *on page 5*

Gordofilm® [US-OTC] *see* salicylic acid *on page 581*

Gormel® [US-OTC] *see* urea *on page 666*

goserelin (GOE se rel in)
   U.S./Canadian Brand Names Zoladex® LA [Can]; Zoladex® [US/Can]
   Therapeutic Category Gonadotropin-Releasing Hormone Analog
   Use Palliative treatment of advanced prostate cancer and breast cancer
   Usual Dosage Adults: S.C.:
      Breast/prostatic cancer: 3.6 mg as a depot injection every 28 days into upper abdominal wall using sterile technique under the supervision of a physician. At the physician's option, local anesthesia may be used prior to injection. The injection should be repeated every 28 days as long as the patient can tolerate the side effects and there is satisfactory disease regression. While a delay of a few days is permissible, every effort should be made to adhere to the 28-day schedule.
      Prostatic cancer: 10.8 mg as a depot injection every 12 weeks into upper abdominal wall using sterile technique under the supervision of a physician. At the physician's option, local anesthesia may be used prior to injection. The injection should be repeated every 12 weeks as long as the patient can tolerate the side effects and there is satisfactory disease regression. While a delay of a few days is permissible, every effort should be made to adhere to the 12-week schedule.
   Dosage Forms
      Injection, solution, 1-month implant [disposable syringe; single-dose]: 3.6 mg [with 16-gauge hypodermic needle]
      Injection, solution, 3-month implant [disposable syringe; single-dose]: 10.8 mg [with 14-gauge hypodermic needle]

GP 47680 *see* oxcarbazepine *on page 482*

G-Phed [US] *see* guaifenesin and pseudoephedrine *on page 310*

G-Phed-PD [US] *see* guaifenesin and pseudoephedrine *on page 310*

gramicidin, neomycin, and polymyxin B *see* neomycin, polymyxin B, and gramicidin *on page 453*

granisetron (gra NI se tron)
   U.S./Canadian Brand Names Kytril™ [US/Can]
   Therapeutic Category Selective 5-HT$_3$ Receptor Antagonist
   Use
      Oral: Prophylaxis of chemotherapy-related emesis; prophylaxis of nausea and vomiting associated with radiation therapy, including total body irradiation and fractionated abdominal radiation
      I.V.: Prophylaxis of chemotherapy-related emesis; prophylaxis and treatment of postoperative nausea and vomiting (PONV)
   Usual Dosage
      Oral: Adults:
         Prophylaxis of chemotherapy-related emesis: 2 mg once daily up to 1 hour before chemotherapy or 1 mg twice daily; the first 1 mg dose should be given up to 1 hour before chemotherapy. **Note:** Administer granisetron on day(s) of chemotherapy.
         Prophylaxis of radiation therapy-associated emesis: 2 mg once daily given 1 hour before radiation therapy.
      (Continued)

granisetron *(Continued)*

I.V.:

Children ≥2 years and Adults: Prophylaxis of chemotherapy-related emesis:

Within U.S.: 10 mcg/kg/dose (or 1 mg/dose) administered IVPB over 5 minutes given within 30 minutes of chemotherapy: for some drugs (eg, carboplatin, cyclophosphamide) with a later onset of emetic action, 10 mcg/kg every 12 hours may be necessary.

Outside U.S.: 40 mcg/kg/dose (or 3 mg/dose); maximum: 9 mg/24 hours

Breakthrough: Repeat the dose 2-3 times within the first 24 hours as necessary (suggested by anecdotal information; not based on controlled trials, or generally recommended).

Note: Administer granisetron on the day(s) of chemotherapy

Adults: PONV:

Prevention: 1 mg given undiluted over 30 seconds; administer before induction of anesthesia or before reversal of anesthesia

Treatment: 1 mg given undiluted over 30 seconds

Dosage Forms

Injection, solution, as hydrochloride: 1 mg/mL (4 mL) [contains benzyl alcohol]

Injection, solution, as hydrochloride [preservative free]: 1 mg/mL (1 mL)

Tablet, as hydrochloride: 1 mg

Granulex [US] *see* trypsin, balsam Peru, and castor oil *on page 662*

granulocyte colony-stimulating factor *see* filgrastim *on page 272*

granulocyte colony stimulating factor (PEG Conjugate) *see* pegfilgrastim *on page 496*

granulocyte-macrophage colony-stimulating factor *see* sargramostim *on page 583*

Gravol® [Can] *see* dimenhydrinate *on page 200*

Grifulvin® V [US] *see* griseofulvin *on this page*

Grisactin® *(Discontinued)* *see page 814*

Grisactin® Ultra *(Discontinued)* *see page 814*

griseofulvin (gri see oh FUL vin)

Synonyms griseofulvin microsize; griseofulvin ultramicrosize

U.S./Canadian Brand Names Fulvicin® P/G [US]; Fulvicin-U/F® [US/Can]; Grifulvin® V [US]; Gris-PEG® [US]

Therapeutic Category Antifungal Agent

Use Treatment of tinea infections of the skin, hair, and nails caused by susceptible species of *Microsporum*, *Epidermophyton*, or *Trichophyton*

Usual Dosage Oral:

Children:

Microsize: 10-15 mg/kg/day in single or divided doses;

Ultramicrosize: >2 years: 5.5-7.3 mg/kg/day in single or divided doses

Adults:

Microsize: 500-1000 mg/day in single or divided doses

Ultramicrosize: 330-375 mg/day in single or divided doses; doses up to 750 mg/day have been used for infections more difficult to eradicate such as tinea unguium

Duration of therapy depends on the site of infection:

Tinea corporis: 2-4 weeks

Tinea capitis: 4-6 weeks or longer

Tinea pedis: 4-8 weeks

Tinea unguium: 3-6 months

Dosage Forms

Suspension, oral, microsize (Grifulvin® V): 125 mg/5 mL (120 mL) [contains alcohol 0.2%]

Tablet, microsize (Fulvicin-U/F®): 250 mg, 500 mg

Tablet, ultramicrosize: 125 mg, 250 mg, 330 mg
Fulvicin® P/G: 125 mg, 165 mg, 250 mg, 330 mg
Gris-PEG®: 125 mg, 250 mg

griseofulvin microsize *see* griseofulvin *on previous page*

griseofulvin ultramicrosize *see* griseofulvin *on previous page*

Gris-PEG® [US] *see* griseofulvin *on previous page*

Guaifed-PD® [US] *see* guaifenesin and pseudoephedrine *on page 310*

Guaifed® [US-OTC] *see* guaifenesin and pseudoephedrine *on page 310*

guaifenesin (gwye FEN e sin)

Synonyms GG; glycerol guaiacolate

U.S./Canadian Brand Names Amibid LA [US]; Balminil Expectorant [Can]; Benylin® E Extra Strength [Can]; Diabetic Tussin® EX [US-OTC]; Duratuss-G® [US]; Fenesin™ [US]; Glytuss® [US-OTC]; Guaifenex® G [US]; Guaifenex® LA [US]; Guiatuss® [US-OTC]; Humibid® L.A. [US]; Humibid® Pediatric [US]; Hytuss-2X® [US-OTC]; Hytuss® [US-OTC]; Koffex Expectorant [Can]; Liquibid® 1200 [US]; Liquibid® [US]; Mucinex™ [US-OTC]; Organidin® NR [US]; Phanasin [US-OTC]; Respa-GF® [US]; Robitussin® [US/Can]; Scot-Tussin® Sugar Free Expectorant [US-OTC]; Touro Ex® [US]

Therapeutic Category Expectorant

Use Temporary control of cough due to minor throat and bronchial irritation

Usual Dosage Oral:

Children:

<2 years: 12 mg/kg/day in 6 divided doses

2-5 years: 50-100 mg (2.5-5 mL) every 4 hours, not to exceed 600 mg/day

6-11 years: 100-200 mg (5-10 mL) every 4 hours, not to exceed 1.2 g/day

Children >12 years and Adults: 200-400 mg (10-20 mL) every 4 hours to a maximum of 2.4 g/day (60 mL/day)

Dosage Forms

Caplet, sustained release (Touro Ex®): 575 mg

Capsule (Hytuss-2X®): 200 mg

Capsule, sustained release (Humibid® Pediatric): 300 mg

Liquid: 100 mg/5 mL (120 mL, 240 mL, 480 mL)

Diabetic Tussin EX®: 100 mg/5 mL (120 mL) [alcohol free, sugar free, dye free; contains phenylalanine 8.4 mg/5 mL]

Organidin NR®: 100 mg/5 mL (480 mL) [contains sodium benzoate; raspberry flavor]

Syrup: 100 mg/5 mL (120 mL, 240 mL, 480 mL)

Guiatuss®: 100 mg/5 mL (120 mL, 240 mL, 480 mL, 3840 mL) [alcohol free; fruit-mint flavor]

Phanasin: 100 mg/5 mL (120 mL, 240 mL) [alcohol free, sugar free, sodium free]

Robitussin®: 100 mg/5 mL (5 mL, 10 mL, 15 mL, 30 mL, 120 mL, 240 mL, 480 mL) [alcohol free]

Scot-Tussin® Sugar Free Expectorant: 100 mg/5 mL (120 mL) [alcohol free, dye free; contains benzoic acid; grape flavor]

Tablet: 200 mg

Glytuss®, Organidin® NR: 200 mg

Hytuss®: 100 mg

Tablet, extended release (Mucinex™): 600 mg

Tablet, sustained release 600 mg, 1200 mg

Amibid LA, Fenesin™; Guafenex® LA, Humibid® LA, Liquibid®, Respa-GF®: 600 mg

Duratuss G, Liquibid® 1200: 1200 mg

Guaifenex® G: 1200 mg [dye free, film coated]

guaifenesin and codeine (gwye FEN e sin & KOE deen)

Synonyms codeine and guaifenesin

U.S./Canadian Brand Names Brontex® [US]; Cheracol® [US]; Gani-Tuss® NR [US]; Guaituss AC® [US]; Mytussin® AC [US]; Robafen® AC [US]; Romilar® AC [US]; Tussi-Organidin® NR [US]; Tussi-Organidin® S-NR [US]

Therapeutic Category Antitussive/Expectorant

Controlled Substance C-V

Use Temporary control of cough due to minor throat and bronchial irritation

Usual Dosage Oral:

Children:

2-6 years: 1-1.5 mg/kg codeine/day divided into 4 doses administered every 4-6 hours

6-12 years: 5 mL every 4 hours, not to exceed 30 mL/24 hours

>12 years: 10 mL every 4 hours, up to 60 mL/24 hours

Adults: 10 mL or 1 tablet every 6-8 hours

Dosage Forms

Liquid: Guaifenesin 100 mg and codeine phosphate 10 mg per 5 mL (120 mL, 480 mL)

Brontex®: Guaifenesin 75 mg and codeine phosphate 2.5 mg per 5 mL (480 mL) [alcohol free; mint flavor]

Gani-Tuss® NR: Guaifenesin 100 mg and codeine phosphate 10 mg per 5 mL (480 mL) [sugar free, alcohol free; raspberry flavor]

Tussi-Organidin® NR: Guaifenesin 100 mg and codeine phosphate 10 mg per 5 mL (480 mL) [contains sodium benzoate; raspberry flavor]

Tussi-Organidin® S-NR: Guaifenesin 100 mg and codeine phosphate 10 mg per 5 mL (120 mL) [contains sodium benzoate; raspberry flavor]

Syrup: Guaifenesin 100 mg and codeine phosphate 10 mg per 5 mL (120 mL, 480 mL)

Cheracol®: Guaifenesin 100 mg and codeine phosphate 10 mg per 5 mL (120 mL) [contains alcohol 4.75% and benzoic acid]

Guaituss AC®: Guaifenesin 100 mg and codeine phosphate 10 mg per 5 mL (120 mL, 480 mL, 3840 mL) [contains alcohol; sugar free; fruit-mint flavor]

Mytussin® AC: Guaifenesin 100 mg and codeine phosphate 10 mg per 5 mL (120 mL, 480 mL, 3840 mL) [contains alcohol; sugar free; fruit flavor]

Robafen AC: Guaifenesin 100 mg and codeine phosphate 10 mg per 5 mL (120 mL, 480 mL, 3840 mL)

Robitussin® AC: Guaifenesin 100 mg and codeine phosphate 10 mg per 5 mL (120 mL) [contains alcohol 3.5%; contains sodium benzoate]

Romilar® AC: Guaifenesin 100 mg and codeine phosphate 10 mg per 5 mL (480 mL) [contains phenylalanine; alcohol free, sugar free, dye free]

Tablet (Brontex®): Guaifenesin 300 mg and codeine phosphate 10 mg

guaifenesin and dextromethorphan
(gwye FEN e sin & deks troe meth OR fan)

Synonyms dextromethorphan and guaifenesin

U.S./Canadian Brand Names Aquatab® DM [US]; Balminil DM E [Can]; Benylin® DM-E [Can]; Benylin® Expectorant [US-OTC]; Cheracol® D [US-OTC]; Cheracol® Plus [US-OTC]; Diabetic Tussin® DM Maximum Strength [US-OTC]; Diabetic Tussin® DM [US-OTC]; Duratuss® DM [US]; Fenesin™ DM [US]; Genatuss DM® [US-OTC]; Guaifenex® DM [US]; Guaituss-DM® [US-OTC]; Humibid® DM [US]; Hydro-Tussin™ DM [US]; Koffex DM-Expectorant; Kolephrin® GG/DM [US-OTC]; Mytussin® DM [US-OTC]; Respa® DM [US]; Robitussin® DM [US/Can]; Robitussin® Sugar Free Cough [US-OTC]; Safe Tussin® 30 [US-OTC]; Silexin® [US-OTC]; Tolu-Sed® DM [US-OTC]; Touro® DM [US]; Tussi-Organidin® DM NR [US]; Vicks® 44E [US-OTC]; Vicks® Pediatric Formula 44E [US-OTC]

Therapeutic Category Antitussive/Expectorant

Use Temporary control of cough due to minor throat and bronchial irritation

Usual Dosage Oral:

Children:

2-5 years: 2.5 mL every 6-8 hours; maximum: 10 mL/day

6-12 years: 5 mL every 6-8 hours; maximum: 20 mL/24 hours

>12 years: 10 mL every 6-8 hours; maximum: 40 mL/24 hours
Alternatively: 0.1-0.15 mL/kg/dose every 6-8 hours as needed
Adults: 10 mL every 6-8 hours

Dosage Forms

Liquid: Guaifenesin 100 mg and dextromethorphan hydrobromide 10 mg per 5 mL (120 mL, 240 mL)

Diabetic Tussin® DM: Guaifenesin 100 mg and dextromethorphan hydrobromide 10 mg per 5 mL (120 mL) [alcohol free, sugar free, dye free; contains phenylalanine 8.4 mg/5 mL]

Diabetic Tussin® DM Maximum Strength: Guaifenesin 200 mg and dextromethorphan hydrobromide 10 mg per 5 mL (120 mL) [alcohol free, sugar free, dye free; contains phenylalanine 8.4 mg/5 mL]

Duratuss® DM: Guaifenesin 200 mg and dextromethorphan hydrobromide 20 mg per 5 mL (480 mL, 3840 mL) [contains alcohol 5%, sodium benzoate; fruit flavor]

Hydro-Tussin™ DM: Guaifenesin 200 mg and dextromethorphan hydrobromide 20 mg per 5 mL (480 mL) [alcohol free, sugar free]

Robitussin® Sugar Free Cough: Guaifenesin 100 mg and dextromethorphan hydrobromide 10 mg per 5 mL (120 mL) [alcohol free, sugar free]

Safe Tussin® 30: Guaifenesin 100 mg and dextromethorphan hydrobromide 15 mg per 5 mL (120 mL) [alcohol free, sugar free, dye free; mint flavor]

Tussi-Organidin® DM NR: Guaifenesin 100 mg and dextromethorphan hydrobromide 10 mg per 5 mL (120 mL, 480 mL) [contains sodium benzoate; raspberry flavor]

Vicks® 44E: Guaifenesin 200 mg and dextromethorphan hydrobromide 20 mg per 15 mL (120 mL, 235 mL) [contains sodium 31 mg/15 mL, alcohol, sodium benzoate]

Vicks® Pediatric Formula 44E: Guaifenesin 100 mg and dextromethorphan hydrobromide 10 mg per 15 mL (120 mL) [alcohol free; contains sodium 30 mg/15 mL, sodium benzoate; cherry flavor]

Syrup: Guaifenesin 100 mg and dextromethorphan hydrobromide 10 mg per 5 mL (120 mL, 240 mL, 480 mL)

Benylin® Expectorant: Guaifenesin 100 mg and dextromethorphan hydrobromide 5 mg per 5 mL (120 mL) [alcohol free, sugar free; contains sodium benzoate; raspberry flavor]

Cheracol® D: Guaifenesin 100 mg and dextromethorphan hydrobromide 10 mg per 5 mL (120 mL, 180 mL) [contains alcohol, benzoic acid]

Cheracol® Plus: Guaifenesin 100 mg and dextromethorphan hydrobromide 10 mg per 5 mL (120 mL)

Genatuss DM®: Guaifenesin 100 mg and dextromethorphan hydrobromide 10 mg per 5 mL (120 mL) [cherry flavor]

Guiatuss® DM: Guaifenesin 100 mg and dextromethorphan hydrobromide 10 mg per 5 mL (120 mL, 240 mL, 480 mL, 3840 mL) [alcohol free; fruit-mint flavor]

Kolephrin® GG/DM: Guaifenesin 150 mg and dextromethorphan hydrobromide 10 mg per 5 mL (120 mL) [alcohol free; cherry flavor]

Mytussin® DM: Guaifenesin 100 mg and dextromethorphan hydrobromide 10 mg per 5 mL (120 mL, 480 mL) [alcohol free; cherry flavor]

Robitussin®-DM: Guaifenesin 100 mg and dextromethorphan hydrobromide 10 mg per 5 mL (5 mL, 120 mL, 360 mL, 480 mL) [alcohol free]

Silexin®: Guaifenesin 100 mg and dextromethorphan hydrobromide 10 mg per 5 mL (45 mL, 480 mL)

Tolu-Sed®: Guaifenesin 100 mg and dextromethorphan hydrobromide 10 mg per 5 mL (120 mL)

Tablet (Silexin®): Guaifenesin 100 mg and dextromethorphan hydrobromide 10 mg

Tablet, extended release: Guaifenesin 600 mg and dextromethorphan hydrobromide 30 mg

Aquatab® DM: Guaifenesin 1200 mg and dextromethorphan hydrobromide 60 mg

Fenesin™ DM, Guaifenex® DM, Humibid® DM, Respa DM®: Guaifenesin 600 mg and dextromethorphan hydrobromide 30 mg

Touro® DM: Guaifenesin 575 mg and dextromethorphan hydrobromide 30 mg

guaifenesin and hydrocodone *see* hydrocodone and guaifenesin *on page 331*

guaifenesin and phenylephrine (gwye FEN e sin & fen il EF rin)

Synonyms phenylephrine and guaifenesin

U.S./Canadian Brand Names Endal® [US]; Entex® LA [US]; Liquibid-D [US]; Prolex-D [US]

Therapeutic Category Cold Preparation

Use Symptomatic relief of those respiratory conditions where tenacious mucous plugs and congestion complicate the problem such as sinusitis, pharyngitis, bronchitis, asthma, and as an adjunctive therapy in serous otitis media

Usual Dosage Adults: Oral: 1-2 tablets/capsules every 12 hours

Dosage Forms

Tablet, extended release: Guaifenesin 600 mg and phenylephrine hydrochloride 20 mg

Endal®: Guaifenesin 300 mg and phenylephrine hydrochloride 20 mg

Liquibid-D: Guaifenesin 600 mg and phenylephrine hydrochloride 40 mg

Tablet, sustained release (Entex® LA): Guaifenesin 600 mg and phenylephrine hydrochloride 30 mg

guaifenesin and pseudoephedrine (gwye FEN e sin & soo doe e FED rin)

Synonyms pseudoephedrine and guaifenesin

U.S./Canadian Brand Names Ami-Tex PSE [US]; Anatuss LA [US]; Aquatab® D Dose Pack [US]; Aquatab® [US]; Congestac® [US]; Deconsal® II [US]; Defen-LA® [US]; Duratuss™ GP [US]; Duratuss™ [US]; Entex® PSE [US]; Eudal®-SR [US]; G-Phed-PD [US]; G-Phed [US]; Guaifed-PD® [US]; Guaifed® [US-OTC]; Guaifenex® GP [US]; Guaifenex® PSE [US]; Guaifen PSE [US]; Guai-Vent™/PSE [US]; Maxifed-G® [US]; Maxifed® [US]; Miraphen PSE [US]; Novahistex® Expectorant With Decongestant [Can]; PanMist® Jr. [US]; PanMist® LA [US]; PanMist® S [US]; Profen® II [US-OTC]; Pseudo GG TR [US]; Pseudovent™ [US]; Pseudovent™-Ped [US]; Respa-1st® [US]; Respaire®-60 SR [US]; Respaire®-120 SR [US]; Robitussin-PE® [US-OTC]; Robitussin® Severe Congestion [US-OTC]; Touro LA® [US]; V-Dec-M® [US]; Versacaps® [US]; Zephrex LA® [US]; Zephrex® [US]

Therapeutic Category Expectorant/Decongestant

Use Enhance the output of respiratory tract fluid and reduce mucosal congestion and edema in the nasal passage

Usual Dosage Oral:

Children:

2-6 years: 2.5 mL every 4 hours not to exceed 15 mL/24 hours

6-12 years: 5 mL every 4 hours not to exceed 30 mL/24 hours

Children >12 years and Adults: 10 mL every 4 hours not to exceed 60 mL/24 hours

Dosage Forms

Caplet (Congestac®): Guaifenesin 400 mg and pseudoephedrine hydrochloride 60 mg

Caplet, long acting (Touro LA®): Guaifenesin 500 mg and pseudoephedrine hydrochloride 120 mg

Capsule:

Pseudovent™: Guaifenesin 250 mg and pseudoephedrine hydrochloride 120 mg

Pseudovent™-Ped: Guaifenesin 300 mg and pseudoephedrine hydrochloride 60 mg

Robitussin® Severe Congestion: Guaifenesin 200 mg and pseudoephedrine hydrochloride 30 mg

Capsule, extended release:

G-Phed, Guaifed®, Respaire®-120 SR: Guaifenesin 250 mg and pseudoephedrine hydrochloride 120 mg

G-Phed-PD, Guaifed-PD®, Versacaps®: Guaifenesin 300 mg and pseudoephedrine hydrochloride 60 mg

Respaire®-60 SR: Guaifenesin 200 mg and pseudoephedrine hydrochloride 60 mg

Syrup:

PanMist®-S: Guaifenesin 200 mg and pseudoephedrine hydrochloride 45 mg per 5 mL (480 mL) [grape flavor]

Robitussin-PE®: Guaifenesin 100 mg and pseudoephedrine hydrochloride 30 mg per 5 mL (120 mL, 240 mL) [alcohol free]

Tablet: Zephrex®: Guaifenesin 400 mg and pseudoephedrine hydrochloride 60 mg

Tablet, extended release: Guaifenesin 600 mg and pseudoephedrine hydrochloride 60 mg; guaifenesin 600 mg and pseudoephedrine hydrochloride 120 mg; guaifenesin 1200 mg and pseudoephedrine hydrochloride 60 mg; guaifenesin 1200 mg and pseudoephedrine hydrochloride 120 mg

Amitex PSE, Duratuss®, Entex® PSE, Guaifen PSE, Guaifenex PSE® 120, Guai-Vent™/PSE, Miraphen PSE, Zephrex LA®: Guaifenesin 600 mg and pseudoephedrine hydrochloride 120 mg

Anatuss LA, Eudal®-SR: Guaifenesin 400 mg and pseudoephedrine hydrochloride 120 mg

Aquatab® D: Guaifenesin 1200 mg and pseudoephedrine hydrochloride 60 mg

Aquatab® D Dose Pack, Deconsal® II, Defen-LA®, Guaifenex PSE® 60, Respa-1st®: Guaifenesin 600 mg and pseudoephedrine hydrochloride 60 mg

Duratuss™ GP, Guaifenex® GP: Guaifenesin 1200 mg and pseudoephedrine hydrochloride 120 mg [dye free]

Maxifed®: Guaifenesin 700 mg and pseudoephedrine hydrochloride 80 mg

Maxifed-G®: Guaifenesin 550 mg and pseudoephedrine hydrochloride 60 mg

PanMist®-JR, Pseudo GG TR: Guaifenesin 600 mg and pseudoephedrine hydrochloride 45 mg

Profen® II: Guaifenesin 800 mg and pseudoephedrine hydrochloride 45 mg

PanMist®-LA: Guaifenesin 800 mg and pseudoephedrine hydrochloride 80 mg

V-Dec-M®: Guaifenesin 500 mg and pseudoephedrine hydrochloride 120 mg

guaifenesin and theophylline *see* theophylline and guaifenesin *on page 631*

guaifenesin, hydrocodone, and pseudoephedrine *see* hydrocodone, pseudoephedrine, and guaifenesin *on page 332*

guaifenesin, pseudoephedrine, and codeine
(gwye FEN e sin, soo doe e FED rin, & KOE deen)

Synonyms codeine, guaifenesin, and pseudoephedrine; pseudoephedrine, guaifenesin, and codeine

U.S./Canadian Brand Names Benylin® 3.3 mg-D-E [Can]; Calmylin with Codeine [Can]; Cheratussin DAC [US]; Codafed® Expectorant [US]; Codafed® Pediatric Expectorant [US]; Dihistine® Expectorant [US]; Guiatuss™ DAC® [US]; Halotussin® DAC [US]; Mytussin® DAC [US]; Nucofed® Expectorant [US]; Nucofed® Pediatric Expectorant [US]; Nucotuss® [US]

Therapeutic Category Antitussive/Decongestant/Expectorant

Controlled Substance C-III; C-V

Use Temporarily relieves nasal congestion and controls cough due to minor throat and bronchial irritation; helps loosen phlegm and thin bronchial secretions to make coughs more productive

Usual Dosage Oral:

Children 6-12 years: 5 mL every 4 hours, not to exceed 40 mL/24 hours

Children >12 years and Adults: 10 mL every 4 hours, not to exceed 40 mL/24 hours

Dosage Forms

Liquid:

Cheratussin DAC: Guaifenesin 100 mg, pseudoephedrine hydrochloride 30 mg, and codeine phosphate 10 mg per 5 mL (480 mL) [sugar free]

Dihistine® Expectorant: Guaifenesin 100 mg, pseudoephedrine hydrochloride 30 mg, and codeine phosphate 10 mg per 5 mL (120 mL) [contains alcohol 7.5%; fruit flavor]

Halotussin DAC: Guaifenesin 100 mg, pseudoephedrine hydrochloride 30 mg, and codeine phosphate 10 mg per 5 mL (480 mL) [sugar free; cherry-raspberry flavor]

Syrup:

Codafed® Expectorant: Guaifenesin 200 mg, pseudoephedrine hydrochloride 60 mg, and codeine phosphate 20 mg per 5 mL (480 mL) [wintergreen flavor]

Codafed® Pediatric Expectorant: Guaifenesin 100 mg, pseudoephedrine hydrochloride 30 mg, and codeine phosphate 10 mg per 5 mL (480 mL) [strawberry flavor]

Guiatuss™ DAC: Guaifenesin 100 mg, pseudoephedrine hydrochloride 30 mg, and codeine phosphate 10 mg per 5 mL (480 mL) [may contain codeine]

(Continued)

311

guaifenesin, pseudoephedrine, and codeine *(Continued)*

Mytussin® DAC: Guaifenesin 100 mg, pseudoephedrine hydrochloride 30 mg, and codeine phosphate 10 mg per 5 mL (120 mL, 480 mL) [sugar free; contains alcohol 1.7%; strawberry-raspberry flavor]

Nucofed® Expectorant, Nucotuss® Expectorant: Guaifenesin 200 mg, pseudoephedrine hydrochloride 60 mg, and codeine phosphate 20 mg per 5 mL (480 mL) [contains alcohol 12.5%; cherry flavor]

Nucofed® Pediatric Expectorant: Guaifenesin 100 mg, pseudoephedrine hydrochloride 30 mg, and codeine phosphate 10 mg per 5 mL (480 mL) [contains alcohol 6%; strawberry flavor]

guaifenesin, pseudoephedrine, and dextromethorphan

(gwye FEN e sin, soo doe e FED rin, & deks troe meth OR fan)

Synonyms dextromethorphan, guaifenesin, and pseudoephedrine; pseudoephedrine, dextromethorphan, and guaifenesin

U.S./Canadian Brand Names Aquatab® C [US]; Balminil DM + Decongestant + Expectorant [Can]; Benylin® DM-D-E [Can]; Guiatuss™ CF [US]; Koffex DM + Decongestant + Expectorant [Can]; Maxifed® DM [US]; Novahistex® DM Decongestant Expectorant [Can]; Novahistine® DM Decongestant Expectorant [Can]; PanMist®-DM [US]; Robitussin® Cold and Congestion [US-OTC]; Robitussin® Cough and Cold Infant [US-OTC]; Touro™ CC [US]

Therapeutic Category Cold Preparation

Use Temporarily relieves nasal congestion and controls cough due to minor throat and bronchial irritation; helps loosen phlegm and thin bronchial secretions to make coughs more productive

Usual Dosage Adults: Oral: 2 capsules (caplets) or 10 mL every 4 hours

Dosage Forms

Caplet (Robitussin® Cold and Congestion): Guaifenesin 200 mg, pseudoephedrine hydrochloride 30 mg, and dextromethorphan hydrobromide 10 mg

Caplet, sustained release (Touro™ CC): Guaifenesin 575 mg, pseudoephedrine hydrochloride 60 mg, and dextromethorphan hydrobromide 30 mg [dye free]

Capsule (Robitussin® Cold and Congestion): Guaifenesin 200 mg, pseudoephedrine hydrochloride 30 mg, and dextromethorphan hydrobromide 10 mg [softgel]

Liquid, oral drops (Robitussin® Cough and Cold Infant): Guaifenesin 100 mg, pseudoephedrine hydrochloride 15 mg, and dextromethorphan hydrobromide 5 mg per 2.5 mL (30 mL) [alcohol free]

Syrup: Guaifenesin 100 mg, pseudoephedrine hydrochloride 45 mg, and dextromethorphan hydrobromide 15 mg per 5 mL (480 mL)

Guiatuss™ CF: Guaifenesin 100 mg, pseudoephedrine hydrochloride 30 mg, and dextromethorphan hydrobromide 10 mg per 5 mL (120 mL) [alcohol free; cherry flavor]

PanMist®-DM: Guaifenesin 100 mg, pseudoephedrine hydrochloride 45 mg, and dextromethorphan hydrobromide 15 mg per 5 mL (480 mL) [alcohol free, dye free, sugar free; strawberry flavor]

Tablet, extended release: Guaifenesin 600 mg, pseudoephedrine hydrochloride 45 mg, and dextromethorphan hydrobromide 30 mg; guaifenesin 800 mg, pseudoephedrine hydrochloride 45 mg, and dextromethorphan hydrobromide 30 mg; guaifenesin 1200 mg, pseudoephedrine hydrochloride 120 mg, and dextromethorphan hydrobromide 60 mg

Aquatab® C: Guaifenesin 1200 mg, pseudoephedrine hydrochloride 120 mg, and dextromethorphan hydrobromide 60 mg

PanMist®-DM: Guaifenesin 600 mg, pseudoephedrine hydrochloride 45 mg, and dextromethorphan hydrobromide 30 mg

Tablet, sustained release (Maxifed® DM): Guaifenesin 550 mg, pseudoephedrine hydrochloride 60 mg, and dextromethorphan hydrobromide 30 mg

Guaifenex® *(Discontinued)* see page 814

Guaifenex® DM [US] see guaifenesin and dextromethorphan on page 308

Guaifenex® G [US] see guaifenesin on page 307

Guaifenex® GP [US] *see* guaifenesin and pseudoephedrine *on page 310*

Guaifenex® LA [US] *see* guaifenesin *on page 307*

Guaifenex® PPA 75 *(Discontinued)* *see page 814*

Guaifenex® PSE [US] *see* guaifenesin and pseudoephedrine *on page 310*

Guaifen PSE [US] *see* guaifenesin and pseudoephedrine *on page 310*

Guaipax® *(Discontinued)* *see page 814*

Guaitab® *(Discontinued)* *see page 814*

Guaituss AC® [US] *see* guaifenesin and codeine *on page 308*

Guaivent® *(Discontinued)* *see page 814*

Guai-Vent™/PSE [US] *see* guaifenesin and pseudoephedrine *on page 310*

guanabenz (GWAHN a benz)
Therapeutic Category Alpha-Adrenergic Agonist
Use Management of hypertension
Usual Dosage Adults: Oral: Initial: 4 mg twice daily, increase in increments of 4-8 mg/day every 1-2 weeks to a maximum of 32 mg twice daily
Dosage Forms Tablet, as acetate: 4 mg, 8 mg

guanadrel (GWAHN a drel)
U.S./Canadian Brand Names Hylorel® [US/Can]
Therapeutic Category Alpha-Adrenergic Agonist
Use Step 2 agent in stepped-care treatment of hypertension, usually with a diuretic
Usual Dosage Oral: Initial: 10 mg/day (5 mg twice daily); adjust dosage until blood pressure is controlled, usual dosage: 20-75 mg/day, administered twice daily
Dosage Forms Tablet, as sulfate: 10 mg, 25 mg

guanethidine (gwahn ETH i deen)
U.S./Canadian Brand Names Ismelin® [US]
Therapeutic Category Alpha-Adrenergic Agonist
Use Treatment of moderate to severe hypertension
Usual Dosage Oral:
  Children:
   Initial: 0.2 mg/kg/day administered daily
   Maximum dose: Up to 3 mg/kg/24 hours
  Adults: Initial: 10-12.5 mg/day, then 25-50 mg/day in 3 divided doses
Dosage Forms Tablet, as monosulfate: 10 mg, 25 mg

guanfacine (GWAHN fa seen)
U.S./Canadian Brand Names Tenex® [US/Can]
Therapeutic Category Alpha-Adrenergic Agonist
Use Management of hypertension
Usual Dosage Adults: Oral: 1 mg (usually at bedtime), may increase if needed at 3- to 4-week intervals to a maximum of 3 mg/day; 1 mg/day is most common dose
Dosage Forms Tablet, as hydrochloride: 1 mg, 2 mg

guanidine (GWAHN i deen)
Therapeutic Category Cholinergic Agent
Use Reduction of the symptoms of muscle weakness associated with the myasthenic syndrome of Eaton-Lambert, not for myasthenia gravis
Usual Dosage Adults: Oral: Initial: 10-15 mg/kg/day in 3-4 divided doses, gradually increase to 35 mg/kg/day
Dosage Forms Tablet, as hydrochloride: 125 mg

GuiaCough® *(Discontinued)* *see page 814*

GuiaCough® Expectorant *(Discontinued)* see page 814

Guiatex® *(Discontinued)* see page 814

Guiatuss™ CF [US] see guaifenesin, pseudoephedrine, and dextromethorphan on page 312

Guiatuss™ DAC® [US] see guaifenesin, pseudoephedrine, and codeine on page 311

Guiatuss-DM® [US-OTC] see guaifenesin and dextromethorphan on page 308

Guiatuss® [US-OTC] see guaifenesin on page 307

gum benjamin see benzoin on page 79

GVG see vigabatrin *(Canada only)* on page 678

G-well® *(Discontinued)* see page 814

Gynazole-1™ [US] see butoconazole on page 101

Gynecort® [US-OTC] see hydrocortisone (topical) on page 334

GyneCure™ [Can] see tioconazole on page 640

Gyne-Lotrimin® 3 [US-OTC] see clotrimazole on page 156

Gyne-Lotrimin® [US-OTC] see clotrimazole on page 156

Gyne-Sulf® *(Discontinued)* see page 814

Gynix® [US-OTC] see clotrimazole on page 156

Gynodiol™ [US] see estradiol on page 238

Gynogen® Injection *(Discontinued)* see page 814

Gynogen L.A.® Injection *(Discontinued)* see page 814

Gynol II® [US-OTC] see nonoxynol 9 on page 464

Habitrol® [Can] see nicotine on page 458

Haemophilus B conjugate and hepatitis B vaccine
(hem OF fi lus bee KON joo gate & hep a TYE tis bee vak SEEN)
U.S./Canadian Brand Names Comvax® [US]
Therapeutic Category Vaccine, Inactivated Virus
Use For vaccination against *Haemophilus influenzae* type B and hepatitis B virus in infants 6 weeks to 15 months old of HGsAG-negative mothers
Usual Dosage Children: I.M.: 0.5 mL as a single dose should be administered
Dosage Forms Injection: 7.5 mcg *Haemophilus* b PRP and 5 mcg $HB_sAg/0.5$ mL

Haemophilus B conjugate vaccine
(hem OF fi lus bee KON joo gate vak SEEN)
Synonyms HIB polysaccharide conjugate; PRP-D
U.S./Canadian Brand Names ActHIB® [US/Can]; HibTITER® [US]; PedvaxHIB® [US/Can]
Therapeutic Category Vaccine, Inactivated Bacteria
Use Immunization of children 24 months to 6 years of age against diseases caused by *H. influenzae* type B
Usual Dosage Children: I.M.: 0.5 mL as a single dose should be administered
Dosage Forms
Injection:
ActHIB® [with 0.4% sodium chloride diluent]: Capsular polysaccharide 10 mcg and tetanus toxoid 24 mcg per 0.5 mL
HibTITER®: Capsular oligosaccharide 10 mcg and diphtheria CRM_{197} protein ~25 mcg per 0.5 mL (0.5 mL, 2.5 mL, 5 mL)
PedvaxHIB®: Purified capsular polysaccharide 15 mcg and *Neisseria meningitidis* OMPC 250 mcg per dose (0.5 mL)

halazepam (hal AZ e pam)

U.S./Canadian Brand Names Paxipam® [US/Can]
Therapeutic Category Benzodiazepine
Controlled Substance C-IV
Use Management of anxiety disorders; short-term relief of the symptoms of anxiety
Usual Dosage Adults: Oral: 20-40 mg 3 or 4 times/day
Dosage Forms Tablet: 20 mg, 40 mg

halazone tablet *(Discontinued)* *see page 814*

halcinonide (hal SIN oh nide)

U.S./Canadian Brand Names Halog®-E [US]; Halog® [US/Can]
Therapeutic Category Corticosteroid, Topical
Use Inflammation of corticosteroid-responsive dermatoses
Usual Dosage Children and Adults: Topical: Apply sparingly 1-3 times/day; occlusive dressing may be used for severe or resistant dermatoses. Therapy should be discontinued when control is achieved. If no improvement is seen, reassessment of diagnosis may be necessary.
Dosage Forms
Cream (Halog®): 0.1% (15 g, 30 g, 60 g, 240 g)
Cream, emollient base (Halog®-E): 0.1% (30 g, 60 g)
Ointment (Halog®): 0.1% (15 g, 30 g, 60 g, 240 g)
Solution, topical (Halog®): 0.1% (20 mL, 60 mL)

Halcion® [US/Can] *see* triazolam *on page 653*

Haldol® [US/Can] *see* haloperidol *on next page*

Haldol® Decanoate [US] *see* haloperidol *on next page*

Haldrone® *(Discontinued)* *see page 814*

Halenol® Tablet *(Discontinued)* *see page 814*

Haley's M-O® [US-OTC] *see* magnesium hydroxide and mineral oil emulsion *on page 398*

Halfan® [US] *see* halofantrine *on this page*

Halfprin® [US-OTC] *see* aspirin *on page 58*

halobetasol (hal oh BAY ta sol)

U.S./Canadian Brand Names Ultravate™ [US/Can]
Therapeutic Category Corticosteroid, Topical
Use Relief of inflammatory and pruritic manifestations of corticosteroid-response dermatoses
Usual Dosage Children and Adults: Topical: Apply sparingly to skin twice daily; rub in gently and completely. Therapy should be discontinued when control is achieved. If no improvement is seen, reassessment of diagnosis may be necessary.
Dosage Forms
Cream, as propionate: 0.05% (15 g, 45 g)
Ointment, as propionate: 0.05% (15 g, 45 g)

halofantrine (ha loe FAN trin)

U.S./Canadian Brand Names Halfan® [US]
Therapeutic Category Antimalarial Agent
Use Treatment of mild to moderate acute malaria caused by susceptible strains of *Plasmodium falciparum* and *Plasmodium vivax*
Usual Dosage Oral:
Children <40 kg: 8 mg/kg every 6 hours for 3 doses
Adults: 500 mg every 6 hours for 3 doses
Dosage Forms Tablet, as hydrochloride: 250 mg

Halog® **[US/Can]** *see* halcinonide *on previous page*

Halog®-E [US] *see* halcinonide *on previous page*

haloperidol (ha loe PER i dole)

U.S./Canadian Brand Names Apo®-Haloperidol [Can]; Haldol® Decanoate [US]; Haldol® [US/Can]; Novo-Peridol [Can]; Peridol [Can]; PMS-Haloperidol LA [Can]; Rho®-Haloperidol Decanoate [Can]

Therapeutic Category Antipsychotic Agent, Butyrophenone

Use Treatment of psychoses, Tourette's disorder, and severe behavioral problems in children

Usual Dosage

Children:

<3 years: Not recommended

3-6 years: Dose and indications are not well established

Control of agitation or hyperkinesia in disturbed children: Oral: 0.01-0.03 mg/kg/day once daily

Infantile autism: Oral: Daily doses of 0.5-4 mg have been reported to be helpful in this disorder

6-12 years: Dose not well established

I.M.: 1-3 mg/dose every 4-8 hours, up to a maximum of 0.1 mg/kg/day

Acute psychoses: Oral: Begin with 0.5-1.5 mg/day and increase gradually in increments of 0.5 mg/day, to a maintenance dose of 2-4 mg/day (0.05-0.1 mg/kg/day).

Tourette's syndrome and mental retardation with hyperkinesia: Oral: Begin with 0.5 mg/day and increase by 0.5 mg/day each day until symptoms are controlled or a maximum dose of 15 mg is reached

Children >12 years and Adults:

I.M.:

Acute psychoses: 2-5 mg/dose every 1-8 hours PRN up to a total of 10-30 mg, until control of symptoms is achieved

Mental retardation with hyperkinesia: Begin with 20 mg/day in divided doses, then increase slowly, up to a maximum of 60 mg/day; change to oral administration as soon as symptoms are controlled

Oral:

Acute psychoses: Begin with 1-15 mg/day in divided doses, then gradually increase until symptoms are controlled, up to a maximum of 100 mg/day; after control of symptoms is achieved, reduce dose to the minimal effective dose

Tourette's syndrome: Begin with 6-15 mg/day in divided doses, increase in increments of 2-10 mg/day until symptoms are controlled or adverse reactions become disabling; when symptoms are controlled, reduce to approximately 9 mg/day for maintenance

Dosage Forms

Injection, as decanoate: 50 mg/mL (1 mL, 5 mL); 100 mg/mL (1 mL, 5 mL)

Injection, as lactate: 5 mg/mL (1 mL, 2 mL, 2.5 mL, 10 mL)

Solution, oral concentrate, as lactate: 2 mg/mL (5 mL, 10 mL, 15 mL, 120 mL, 240 mL)

Tablet: 0.5 mg, 1 mg, 2 mg, 5 mg, 10 mg, 20 mg

Halotestin® **[US]** *see* fluoxymesterone *on page 280*

Halotex® *(Discontinued)* *see page 814*

halothane (HA loe thane)

Therapeutic Category General Anesthetic

Use General induction and maintenance of anesthesia (inhalation)

Usual Dosage Maintenance concentration varies from 0.5% to 1.5%

Dosage Forms Liquid: 125 mL, 250 mL

Halotussin® *(Discontinued)* *see page 814*

Halotussin® **DAC [US]** *see* guaifenesin, pseudoephedrine, and codeine *on page 311*

Halotussin® DM *(Discontinued)* *see page 814*

Halotussin® PE *(Discontinued)* *see page 814*

Haltran® [US-OTC] *see* ibuprofen *on page 342*

hamamelis water *see* witch hazel *on page 686*

Haponal® [US] *see* hyoscyamine, atropine, scopolamine, and phenobarbital *on page 340*

Harmonyl® *(Discontinued)* *see page 814*

Havrix® [US/Can] *see* hepatitis A vaccine *on page 319*

Hayfebrol® [US-OTC] *see* chlorpheniramine and pseudoephedrine *on page 138*

H-BIG® *(Discontinued)* *see page 814*

HBIG *see* hepatitis B immune globulin *on page 320*

hBNP *see* nesiritide *on page 455*

HCG *see* chorionic gonadotropin (human) *on page 144*

HCTZ *see* hydrochlorothiazide *on page 328*

HD 85® [US] *see* radiological/contrast media (ionic) *on page 561*

HD 200 Plus® [US] *see* radiological/contrast media (ionic) *on page 561*

HDA® Toothache [US-OTC] *see* benzocaine *on page 77*

HDCV *see* rabies virus vaccine *on page 561*

HDRS *see* rabies virus vaccine *on page 561*

Head & Shoulders® Intensive Treatment [US-OTC] *see* selenium sulfide *on page 587*

Head & Shoulders® [US-OTC] *see* pyrithione zinc *on page 557*

Healon® *(Discontinued)* *see page 814*

Healon® [Can] *see* sodium hyaluronate *on page 597*

Healon® GV *(Discontinued)* *see page 814*

Healon® GV [Can] *see* sodium hyaluronate *on page 597*

Heartburn 200® [US-OTC] *see* cimetidine *on page 146*

Heartburn Relief 200® [US-OTC] *see* cimetidine *on page 146*

Hectorol® [US/Can] *see* doxercalciferol *on page 214*

Helidac™ [US] *see* bismuth subsalicylate, metronidazole, and tetracycline *on page 88*

Helistat® [US] *see* microfibrillar collagen hemostat *on page 428*

Helixate® FS [US] *see* antihemophilic factor (recombinant) *on page 46*

Hemabate™ [US/Can] *see* carboprost tromethamine *on page 116*

HemFe® *(Discontinued)* *see page 814*

hemiacidrin *see* citric acid bladder mixture *on page 149*

hemin (HEE min)
  U.S./Canadian Brand Names Panhematin® [US]
  Therapeutic Category Blood Modifiers
  Use Treatment of recurrent attacks of acute intermittent porphyria (AIP) only after an appropriate period of alternate therapy has been tried
  Usual Dosage I.V.: 1-4 mg/kg/day administered over 10-15 minutes for 3-14 days; may be repeated no earlier than every 12 hours; not to exceed 6 mg/kg in any 24-hour period
  Dosage Forms Powder for injection, preservative free: 313 mg/vial [hematin 7 mg/mL] (43 mL)

Hemocyte® [US-OTC] *see* ferrous fumarate *on page 268*

Hemofil® M [US/Can] *see* antihemophilic factor (human) *on page 45*

Hemonyne® [US] *see* factor IX complex (human) *on page 261*

Hemotene® [US] *see* microfibrillar collagen hemostat *on page 428*

Hepalean® [Can] *see* heparin *on this page*

Hepalean® Leo [Can] *see* heparin *on this page*

Hepalean®-LOK [Can] *see* heparin *on this page*

heparin (HEP a rin)

Synonyms heparin lock flush

U.S./Canadian Brand Names Hepalean® [Can]; Hepalean® Leo [Can]; Hepalean®-LOK [Can]; Hep-Lock® [US]

Therapeutic Category Anticoagulant (Other)

Use Prophylaxis and treatment of thromboembolic disorders

Usual Dosage Note: For full-dose heparin (ie, nonlow-dose), the dose should be titrated according to PTT results. For anticoagulation, an APTT 1.5-2.5 times normal is usually desired. APTT is usually measured prior to heparin therapy, 6-8 hours after initiation of a continuous infusion (following a loading dose), and 6-8 hours after changes in the infusion rate; increase or decrease infusion by 2-4 units/kg/hour dependent on PTT. Continuous I.V. infusion is preferred vs I.V. intermittent injections. For intermittent I.V. injections, PTT is measured 3.5-4 hours after I.V. injection.

Children:
Intermittent I.V.: Initial: 50-100 units/kg, then 50-100 units/kg every 4 hours
I.V. infusion: Initial: 50 units/kg, then 15-25 units/kg/hour; increase dose by 2-4 units/kg/hour every 6-8 hours as required

Adults:
Prophylaxis (low-dose heparin): S.C.: 5000 units every 8-12 hours
Intermittent I.V.: Initial: 10,000 units, then 50-70 units/kg (5000-10,000 units) every 4-6 hours
I.V. infusion: Initial: 75-100 units/kg, then 15 units/kg/hour with dose adjusted according to PTT results; usual range: 10-30 units/kg/hour

Dosage Forms

Infusion, porcine intestinal mucosa, as sodium:
D_5W: 40 units/mL (500 mL); 50 units/mL (250 mL, 500 mL); 100 units/mL (100 mL, 250 mL)
NaCl 0.45%: 2 units/mL (500 mL, 1000 mL); 50 units/mL (250 mL); 100 units/mL (250 mL)
NaCl 0.9%: 2 units/mL (500 mL, 1000 mL); 5 units/mL (1000 mL); 50 units/mL (250 mL, 500 mL, 1000 mL)

Injection, as sodium [lock flush] [**Note:** Heparin lock flush solution is intended only to maintain patency of I.V. devices and is **not** to be used for anticoagulant therapy]:
Beef lung source: 10 units/mL (1 mL, 2 mL, 2.5 mL, 3 mL, 5 mL, 10 mL, 30 mL); 100 units/mL (1 mL, 2 mL, 2.5 mL, 3 mL, 5 mL, 10 mL, 30 mL)
Porcine intestinal mucosa: 10 units/mL (1 mL, 2 mL, 10 mL, 30 mL); 100 units/mL (1 mL, 2 mL, 10 mL, 30 mL)
Porcine intestinal mucosa [preservative free]: 10 units/mL (1 mL); 100 units/mL (1 mL)

Injection, as sodium [multidose vial]:
Beef lung source [with preservative]: 1000 units/mL (5 mL, 10 mL, 30 mL); 5000 units/mL (10 mL); 10,000 units/mL (1 mL, 4 mL, 5 mL, 10 mL); 20,000 units/mL (2 mL, 5 mL); 40,000 units/mL (2 mL, 5 mL)
Porcine intestinal mucosa [with preservative]: 1000 units/mL (10 mL, 30 mL); 5000 units/mL (10 mL); 10,000 units/mL (4 mL); 20,000 units/mL (2 mL, 5 mL)

Injection, as sodium [single-dose vial]:
Beef lung: 1000 units/mL (1 mL); 5000 units/mL (1 mL); 10,000 units/mL (1 mL); 20,000 units/mL (1 mL); 40,000 units/mL (1 mL)
Porcine intestinal mucosa: 1000 units/mL (1 mL); 5000 units/mL (1 mL); 10,000 units/mL (1 mL); 20,000 units/mL (1 mL); 40,000 units/mL (1 mL)

Injection, porcine intestinal mucosa, as calcium [preservative free] [unit dose] (Calciparine®): 5000 units/dose (0.2 mL); 12,500 units/dose (0.5 mL); 20,000 units/dose (0.8 mL)

Injection, porcine intestinal mucosa, as sodium [with preservative] [unit dose]: 1000 units/dose (1 mL, 2 mL); 2500 units/dose (1 mL); 5000 units/dose (0.5 mL, 1 mL); 7500 units/dose (1 mL); 10,000 units/dose (1 mL); 15,000 units/dose (1 mL); 20,000 units/dose (1 mL)

heparin cofactor I *see* antithrombin III *on page 47*

heparin lock flush *see* heparin *on previous page*

hepatitis A inactivated and hepatitis B (recombinant) vaccine
(hep a TYE tis aye in ak ti VAY ted & hep a TYE tis bee (ree KOM be nant) vak SEEN)

Synonyms hepatitis B (recombinant) and hepatitis A inactivated vaccine

U.S./Canadian Brand Names Twinrix® [US/Can]

Therapeutic Category Vaccine

Use Active immunization against disease caused by hepatitis A virus and hepatitis B virus (all known subtypes) in populations desiring protection against or at high risk of exposure to these viruses.

Populations include travelers to areas of intermediate/high endemicity for **both** HAV and HBV; those at increased risk of HBV infection due to behavioral or occupational factors; patients with chronic liver disease; laboratory workers who handle live HAV and HBV; healthcare workers, police, and other personnel who render first-aid or medical assistance; workers who come in contact with sewage; employees of day care centers and correctional facilities; patients/staff of hemodialysis units; male homosexuals; patients frequently receiving blood products; military personnel; users of injectable illicit drugs; close household contacts of patients with hepatitis A and hepatitis B infection.

Usual Dosage I.M.: Adults: Primary immunization: Three doses (1 mL each) given on a 0-, 1-, and 6-month schedule

Dosage Forms

Injection [single-dose vial]: Inactivated hepatitis A virus 720 ELISA units and hepatitis B surface antigen 20 mcg per mL (1 mL)

Injection [prefilled syringe; single-dose vial]: Inactivated hepatitis A virus 720 ELISA units and hepatitis B surface antigen 20 mcg per mL (1 mL)

hepatitis A vaccine (hep a TYE tis aye vak SEEN)

U.S./Canadian Brand Names Avaxim® [Can]; Epaxal Berna® [Can]; Havrix® [US/Can]; VAQTA® [US/Can]

Therapeutic Category Vaccine, Inactivated Virus

Use For populations desiring protection against hepatitis A or for populations at high risk of exposure to hepatitis A virus (travelers to developing countries, household and sexual contacts of persons infected with hepatitis A), child day care employees, illicit drug users, male homosexuals, institutional workers (eg, institutions for the mentally and physically handicapped persons, prisons, etc), and healthcare workers who may be exposed to hepatitis A virus (eg, laboratory employees)

Usual Dosage I.M.:

Children: 0.5 mL (360 units) on days 1 and 30, with a booster dose 6-12 months late; completion of the first 2 doses (ie, the primary series) should be accomplished at least 2 weeks before anticipated exposure to hepatitis A

Adults: 1 mL (1440 units), with a booster dose at 6-12 months

Dosage Forms

Injection, adult [prefilled syringe; single-dose vial]:

Havrix®: 1440 ELISA units/mL

VAQTA®: 50 units/mL HAV protein

Injection, pediatric [prefilled syringe; single-dose vial] (Havrix®): 720 ELISA units/0.5 mL

Injection, pediatric/adolescent [prefilled syringe; single-dose vial] (VAQTA®): 25 units/0.5 mL HAV protein

hepatitis B immune globulin (hep a TYE tis bee i MYUN GLOB yoo lin)

Synonyms HBIG

U.S./Canadian Brand Names BayHep B™ [US/Can]; Nabi-HB® [US]

Therapeutic Category Immune Globulin

Use Provide prophylactic passive immunity to hepatitis B infection to those individuals exposed. Hepatitis B immune globulin is not indicated for treatment of active hepatitis B infections and is ineffective in the treatment of chronic active hepatitis B infection.

Usual Dosage I.M.:

Newborns: Hepatitis B: 0.5 mL as soon after birth as possible (within 12 hours)

Adults: Postexposure prophylaxis: 0.06 mL/kg; usual dose: 3-5 mL; repeat at 28-30 days after exposure

Dosage Forms

Injection, neonatal [single-dose vial] (BayHep B™): 0.5 mL

Injection [single-dose vial] (BayHep B™, Nabi-HB®): 1 mL, 5 mL

hepatitis B inactivated virus vaccine (plasma derived) *see* hepatitis B vaccine *on this page*

hepatitis B inactivated virus vaccine (recombinant DNA) *see* hepatitis B vaccine *on this page*

hepatitis B (recombinant) and hepatitis A inactivated vaccine *see* hepatitis A inactivated and hepatitis B (recombinant) vaccine *on previous page*

hepatitis B vaccine (hep a TYE tis bee vak SEEN)

Synonyms hepatitis B inactivated virus vaccine (plasma derived); hepatitis B inactivated virus vaccine (recombinant DNA)

U.S./Canadian Brand Names Engerix-B® [US/Can]; Recombivax HB® [US/Can]

Therapeutic Category Vaccine, Inactivated Virus

Use Immunization against infection caused by all known subtypes of hepatitis B virus in individuals considered at high risk of potential exposure to hepatitis B virus or HB_sAg-positive materials

Usual Dosage I.M.:

Children:

≤11 years: 2.5 mcg doses

11-19 years: 5 mcg doses

Adults >20 years: 10 mcg doses

Dosage Forms

Injection, suspension [recombinant DNA]:

Engerix-B®:

Adult: Hepatitis B surface antigen 20 mcg/mL (1 mL) [contains trace amounts of thimerosal]

Pediatric/adolescent: Hepatitis B surface antigen 10 mcg/0.5 mL (0.5 mL) [contains trace amounts of thimerosal]

Recombivax HB®:

Adult [with preservative]: Hepatitis B surface antigen 10 mcg/mL (1 mL, 3 mL)

Dialysis [with preservative]: Hepatitis B surface antigen 40 mcg/mL (1 mL)

Pediatric/adolescent [preservative free]: Hepatitis B surface antigen 5 mcg/0.5 mL (0.5 mL)

Pediatric/adolescent [with preservative]: Hepatitis B surface antigen 5 mcg/0.5 mL (0.5 mL)

Hep-B-Gammagee® *(Discontinued) see page 814*

Hep-Lock® [US] *see* heparin *on page 318*

Hepsera™ [US] *see* adefovir *on page 15*

Heptalac® *(Discontinued) see page 814*

Heptovir® [Can] *see* lamivudine *on page 373*

Herceptin® [US/Can] *see* trastuzumab *on page 648*

Herplex® *(Discontinued)* see page 814

HES see hetastarch on this page

Hespan® **[US]** see hetastarch on this page

hetastarch (HET a starch)
Synonyms HES; hydroxyethyl starch
U.S./Canadian Brand Names Hespan® [US]; Hextend® [US]
Therapeutic Category Plasma Volume Expander
Use Blood volume expander used in treatment of shock or impending shock when blood or blood products are not available (does not have oxygen-carrying capacity and is not a substitute for blood or plasma)
Usual Dosage I.V. infusion (requires an infusion pump):
Children: Safety and efficacy have not been established
Shock:
Adults: 500-1000 mL (up to 1500 mL/day) or 20 mL/kg/day (up to 1500 mL/day); larger volumes (15,000 mL/24 hours) have been used safely in small numbers of patients
Leukapheresis: 250-700 mL hetastarch
Dosage Forms
Infusion [in lactated electrolyte injection] (Hextend®): 6% (500 mL, 1000 mL)
Infusion [in sodium chloride 0.9%] (Hespan®): 6% (500 mL)

Hetrazan® *(Discontinued)* see page 814

Hexabrix™ **[US]** see radiological/contrast media (ionic) on page 561

hexachlorocyclohexane see lindane on page 385

hexachlorophene (heks a KLOR oh feen)
U.S./Canadian Brand Names pHisoHex® [US/Can]
Therapeutic Category Antibacterial, Topical
Use Surgical scrub and as a bacteriostatic skin cleanser; to control an outbreak of gram-positive staphylococcal infection when other infection control procedures have been unsuccessful
Usual Dosage Children and Adults: Topical: Apply 5 mL cleanser and water to area to be cleansed; lather and rinse thoroughly under running water
Dosage Forms Liquid, topical (pHisoHex®): 3% (8 mL, 150 mL, 500 mL, 3840 mL)

Hexadrol® **[US/Can]** see dexamethasone (systemic) on page 184

Hexalen® **[US/Can]** see altretamine on page 27

hexamethylenetetramine see methenamine on page 416

hexamethylmelamine see altretamine on page 27

Hexit™ **[Can]** see lindane on page 385

Hextend® **[US]** see hetastarch on this page

hexylresorcinol (heks il re ZOR si nole)
U.S./Canadian Brand Names Sucrets® Sore Throat [US-OTC]
Therapeutic Category Local Anesthetic
Use Minor antiseptic and local anesthetic for sore throat
Usual Dosage May be used as needed, allow to dissolve slowly in mouth
Dosage Forms Lozenge: 2.4 mg

Hibiclens® **[US-OTC]** see chlorhexidine gluconate on page 134

Hibistat® **[US-OTC]** see chlorhexidine gluconate on page 134

HIB polysaccharide conjugate see Haemophilus B conjugate vaccine on page 314

HibTITER® **[US]** see Haemophilus B conjugate vaccine on page 314

Hi-Cor-1.0® **[US]** *see* hydrocortisone (topical) *on page 334*

Hi-Cor-2.5® **[US]** *see* hydrocortisone (topical) *on page 334*

Hip-Rex™ **[Can]** *see* methenamine *on page 416*

Hiprex® **[US/Can]** *see* methenamine *on page 416*

hirulog *see* bivalirudin *on page 89*

Hismanal® *(Discontinued) see page 814*

Histafed® **[US-OTC]** *see* triprolidine and pseudoephedrine *on page 659*

Histaject® *(Discontinued) see page 814*

Histalet Forte® **Tablet** *(Discontinued) see page 814*

Histalet® **[US-OTC]** *see* chlorpheniramine and pseudoephedrine *on page 138*

Histalet® **X** *(Discontinued) see page 814*

histamine (HIS ta meen)

U.S./Canadian Brand Names Histatrol® [US]

Therapeutic Category Diagnostic Agent

Use To test the ability of the gastric mucosa to produce hydrochloric acid

Usual Dosage Adults: S.C.: Gastric acid test:

The patient fasts for 12 hours. A plastic duodenal tube is passed into the stomach, the gastric content withdrawn, and its acidity determined. Care should be taken to prevent the patient from swallowing salivary secretions during administration of the test results. The alkalinity of the saliva may interfere with the test results. Histamine phosphate 500 to 750 mcg is then injected.

Gastric content is again removed after 5 minutes and at 15 minute intervals thereafter on 3 occasions

The volume and acidity of each specimen is determined. If no acidity is detected, a maximum histamine stimulation test can be performed using 40 mcg/kg histamine phosphate. Pulse rate and blood pressure should be determined immediately after histamine injection.

Dosage Forms Injection, as phosphate: 0.275 mg/mL (5 mL)

Histatab® **Plus [US-OTC]** *see* chlorpheniramine and phenylephrine *on page 138*

Hista-Tabs® **[US-OTC]** *see* triprolidine and pseudoephedrine *on page 659*

Histatrol® **[US]** *see* histamine *on this page*

Hista-Vadrin® **Tablet** *(Discontinued) see page 814*

Histerone® **Injection** *(Discontinued) see page 814*

Histinex® **D Liquid** *(Discontinued) see page 814*

Histolyn-CYL® **[US]** *see* histoplasmin *on this page*

histoplasmin (his toe PLAZ min)

Synonyms histoplasmosis skin test antigen

U.S./Canadian Brand Names Histolyn-CYL® [US]

Therapeutic Category Diagnostic Agent

Use Diagnosing histoplasmosis; to assess cell-mediated immunity

Usual Dosage Adults: Intradermally: 0.1 mL of 1:100 dilution 5-10 cm apart into volar surface of forearm; induration of ≥5 mm in diameter indicates a positive reaction

Dosage Forms Injection: 1:100 (0.1 mL, 1.3 mL)

histoplasmosis skin test antigen *see* histoplasmin *on this page*

Histor-D® **Syrup** *(Discontinued) see page 814*

Histor-D® **Timecelles**® *(Discontinued) see page 814*

histrelin (his TREL in)
U.S./Canadian Brand Names Supprelin™ [US]
Therapeutic Category Gonadotropin-Releasing Hormone Analog
Use Central idiopathic precocious puberty; also used to treat estrogen-associated gyne-cological disorders (ie, endometriosis, intermittent porphyria, possibly premenstrual syndrome, leiomyomata uteri [uterine fibroids])
Usual Dosage
Central idiopathic precocious puberty: S.C.: Usual dose is 10 mcg/kg/day administered as a single daily dose at the same time each day
Acute intermittent porphyria in women:
S.C.: 5 mcg/day
Intranasal: 400-800 mcg/day
Endometriosis: S.C.: 100 mcg/day
Leiomyomata uteri: S.C.: 20-50 mcg/day or 4 mcg/kg/day
Dosage Forms Injection [single-use; 7-day kit]: 120 mcg/0.6 mL; 300 mcg/0.6 mL; 600 mcg/0.6 mL

Histrodrix® [US] *see* dexbrompheniramine and pseudoephedrine *on page 185*

Histussin D® Liquid [US] *see* hydrocodone and pseudoephedrine *on page 331*

Hivid® [US/Can] *see* zalcitabine *on page 688*

HMS Liquifilm® [US] *see* medrysone *on page 405*

HN₂ *see* mechlorethamine *on page 403*

Hold® DM [US-OTC] *see* dextromethorphan *on page 189*

homatropine (hoe MA troe peen)
U.S./Canadian Brand Names Isopto® Homatropine [US]
Therapeutic Category Anticholinergic Agent
Use Producing cycloplegia and mydriasis for refraction; treatment of acute inflammatory conditions of the uveal tract
Usual Dosage Ophthalmic:
Children:
Mydriasis and cycloplegia for refraction: 1 drop of 2% solution immediately before the procedure; repeat at 10-minute intervals as needed
Uveitis: 1 drop of 2% solution 2-3 times/day
Adults:
Mydriasis and cycloplegia for refraction: 1-2 drops of 2% solution or 1 drop of 5% solution before the procedure; repeat at 5- to 10-minute intervals as needed
Uveitis: 1-2 drops 2-3 times/day up to every 3-4 hours as needed
Dosage Forms
Solution, ophthalmic, as hydrobromide: 2% (1 mL, 5 mL); 5% (1 mL, 2 mL, 5 mL)
Isopto® Homatropine: 2% (5 mL, 15 mL); 5% (5 mL, 15 mL)

homatropine and hydrocodone *see* hydrocodone and homatropine *on page 331*

Honvol® [Can] *see* diethylstilbestrol *on page 196*

horse antihuman thymocyte gamma globulin *see* lymphocyte immune globulin *on page 395*

H.P. Acthar® Gel [US] *see* corticotropin *on page 164*

Hp-PAC® [Can] *see* lansoprazole, amoxicillin, and clarithromycin *on page 375*

HTF919 *see* tegaserod *on page 620*

Humalog® [US/Can] *see* insulin preparations *on page 352*

Humalog® Mix 75/25™ [US] *see* insulin preparations *on page 352*

human growth hormone (HYU man grothe HOR mone)

Synonyms somatrem; somatropin

U.S./Canadian Brand Names Genotropin® [US]; Genotropin Miniquick® [US]; Humatrope® [US/Can]; Norditropin® [US/Can]; Norditropin® Cartridges [US]; Nutropin® [US]; Nutropin AQ® [US/Can]; Nutropin Depot® [US]; Protropin® [US/Can]; Saizen® [US/Can]; Serostim® [US/Can]

Therapeutic Category Growth Hormone

Use

Children:

Long-term treatment of growth failure due to lack of adequate endogenous growth hormone secretion (Genotropin®, Humatrope®, Norditropin®, Nutropin®, Nutropin AQ®, Nutropin® Depot™, Protropin®, Saizen®)

Long-term treatment of short stature associated with Turner syndrome (Humatrope®, Nutropin®, Nutropin AQ®)

Treatment of Prader-Willi syndrome (Genotropin®)

Treatment of growth failure associated with chronic renal insufficiency (CRI) up until the time of renal transplantation (Nutropin®, Nutropin AQ®)

Long-term treatment of growth failure in children born small for gestational age who fail to manifest catch-up growth by 2 years of age (Genotropin®)

Adults:

AIDS wasting or cachexia with concomitant antiviral therapy (Serostim®)

Replacement of endogenous growth hormone in patients with adult growth hormone deficiency who meet both of the following criteria (Genotropin®, Humatrope®, Nutropin®, Nutropin AQ®):

Biochemical diagnosis of adult growth hormone deficiency by means of a subnormal response to a standard growth hormone stimulation test (peak growth hormone ≤5 μg/L)

and

Adult-onset: Patients who have adult growth hormone deficiency whether alone or with multiple hormone deficiencies (hypopituitarism) as a result of pituitary disease, hypothalamic disease, surgery, radiation therapy, or trauma

or

Childhood-onset: Patients who were growth hormone deficient during childhood, confirmed as an adult before replacement therapy is initiated

Usual Dosage

Children (individualize dose):

Growth hormone deficiency:

Somatrem: Protropin®: I.M., S.C.: Weekly dosage: 0.3 mg/kg divided into daily doses

Somatropin:

Genotropin®: S.C.: Weekly dosage: 0.16-0.24 mg/kg divided into 6-7 doses

Humatrope®: I.M., S.C.: Weekly dosage: 0.18 mg/kg; maximum replacement dose: 0.3 mg/kg/week; dosing should be divided into equal doses given 3 times/week on alternating days, 6 times/week, or daily

Norditropin®: S.C.: Weekly dosage: 0.024-0.034 mg/kg administered in the evening, divided into doses 6-7 times/week; cartridge and vial formulations are bioequivalent; cartridge formulation does not need to be reconstituted prior to use; cartridges must be administered using the corresponding color-coded NordiPen® injection pen

Nutropin® Depot™: S.C.:

Once-monthly injection: 1.5 mg/kg administered on the same day of each month; patients >15 kg will require more than 1 injection per dose

Twice-monthly injection: 0.75 mg/kg administered twice each month on the same days of each month (eg, days 1 and 15 of each month); patients >30 kg will require more than 1 injection per dose

Nutropin®, Nutropin® AQ: S.C.: Weekly dosage: 0.3 mg/kg divided into daily doses; pubertal patients: ≤0.7 mg/kg/week divided daily

Saizen®: I.M., S.C.: Weekly dosage: 0.06 mg/kg administered 3 times/week

Note: Therapy should be discontinued when patient has reached satisfactory adult height, when epiphyses have fused, or when the patient ceases to respond. Growth of 5 cm/year or more is expected, if growth rate does not exceed 2.5 cm in a 6-month period, double the dose for the next 6 months; if there is still no satisfactory response, discontinue therapy

Chronic renal insufficiency (CRI): Nutropin®, Nutropin® AQ: S.C.: Weekly dosage: 0.35 mg/kg divided into daily injections; continue until the time of renal transplantation

Dosage recommendations in patients treated for CRI who require dialysis:

Hemodialysis: Administer dose at night prior to bedtime or at least 3-4 hours after hemodialysis to prevent hematoma formation from heparin

CCPD: Administer dose in the morning following dialysis

CAPD: Administer dose in the evening at the time of overnight exchange

Turner syndrome: Humatrope®, Nutropin®, Nutropin® AQ: S.C.: Weekly dosage: ≤0.375 mg/kg divided into equal doses 3-7 times per week

Prader-Willi syndrome: Genotropin®: S.C.: Weekly dosage: 0.24 mg/kg divided into 6-7 doses

Small for gestational age: Genotropin®: S.C.: Weekly dosage: 0.48 mg/kg divided into 6-7 doses

Adults:

Growth hormone deficiency: To minimize adverse events in older or overweight patients, reduced dosages may be necessary. During therapy, dosage should be decreased if required by the occurrence of side effects or excessive IGF-I levels.

Somatropin:

Nutropin®, Nutropin® AQ: S.C.: ≤0.006 mg/kg/day; dose may be increased according to individual requirements, up to a maximum of 0.025 mg/kg/day in patients <35 years of age, or up to a maximum of 0.0125 mg/kg/day in patients ≥35 years of age

Humatrope®: S.C.: ≤0.006 mg/kg/day; dose may be increased according to individual requirements, up to a maximum of 0.0125 mg/kg/day

Genotropin®: S.C.: Weekly dosage: ≤0.04 mg/kg divided into 6-7 doses; dose may be increased at 4- to 8-week intervals according to individual requirements, to a maximum of 0.08 mg/kg/week

AIDS wasting or cachexia:

Serostim®: S.C.: Dose should be given once daily at bedtime; patients who continue to lose weight after 2 weeks should be re-evaluated for opportunistic infections or other clinical events; rotate injection sites to avoid lipodystrophy

Daily dose based on body weight:

<35 kg: 0.1 mg/kg

35-45 kg: 4 mg

45-55 kg: 5 mg

>55 kg: 6 mg

Dosage Forms

Injection, powder for reconstitution [rDNA origin]:

Somatrem: Protropin® [diluent contains benzyl alcohol]: 5 mg [~15 int. units]; 10 mg [~30 int. units]

Somatropin:

Genotropin® [preservative free]: 1.5 mg [4 int. units/mL] [delivers 1.3 mg/mL]

Genotropin® [with preservative]:

5.8 mg [15 int. units/mL] [delivers 5 mg/mL]

13.8 mg [36 int. units/mL] [delivers 12 mg/mL]

Genotropin Miniquick® [preservative free]: 0.2 mg, 0.4 mg, 0.6 mg, 0.8 mg, 1 mg, 1.2 mg, 1.4 mg, 1.6 mg, 1.8 mg, 2 mg [each strength delivers 0.25 mL]

Humatrope®: 5 mg [~15 int. units], 6 mg [18 int. units], 12 mg [36 int. units], 24 mg [72 int. units]

Norditropin® [diluent contains benzyl alcohol]: 4 mg [~12 int. units]; 8 mg [~24 int. units]

Nutropin® [diluent contains benzyl alcohol]: 5 mg [~15 int. units]; 10 mg [~30 int. units]

Nutropin Depot® [preservative free]: 13.5 mg; 18 mg; 22.5 mg

Saizen® [diluent contains benzyl alcohol]: 5 mg [~15 int. units]

Serostim®: 4 mg [12 int. units]; 5 mg [15 int. units]; 6 mg [18 int. units]

(Continued)

human growth hormone *(Continued)*

Solution, injection [rDNA origin]:
Somatropin:
Norditropin® Cartridges: 5 mg/1.5 mL (1.5 mL); 10 mg/1.5 mL (1.5 mL); 15 mg/1.5 mL (1.5 mL)
Nutropin AQ®: 5 mg/mL [~30 int. units/2 mL] (2 mL)

humanized IgG1 anti-CD52 monoclonal antibody *see* alemtuzumab *on page 21*

human thyroid-stimulating hormone *see* thyrotropin alpha *on page 637*

Humate-P® [US/Can] *see* antihemophilic factor (human) *on page 45*

Humatin® [US/Can] *see* paromomycin *on page 493*

Humatrope® [US/Can] *see* human growth hormone *on page 324*

Humegon™ [US] *see* menotropins *on page 407*

Humibid® DM [US] *see* guaifenesin and dextromethorphan *on page 308*

Humibid® L.A. [US] *see* guaifenesin *on page 307*

Humibid® Pediatric [US] *see* guaifenesin *on page 307*

Humibid® Sprinkle *(Discontinued)* *see page 814*

Humorsol® Ophthalmic *(Discontinued)* *see page 814*

Humulin® 50/50 [US] *see* insulin preparations *on page 352*

Humulin® 70/30 [US/Can] *see* insulin preparations *on page 352*

Humulin® 80/20 [Can] *see* insulin preparations *on page 352*

Humulin® L [US/Can] *see* insulin preparations *on page 352*

Humulin® N [US/Can] *see* insulin preparations *on page 352*

Humulin® R [US/Can] *see* insulin preparations *on page 352*

Humulin® R (Concentrated) U-500 [US] *see* insulin preparations *on page 352*

Humulin® U [US/Can] *see* insulin preparations *on page 352*

Hurricaine® [US] *see* benzocaine *on page 77*

Hyalgan® [US] *see* sodium hyaluronate *on page 597*

hyaluronic acid *see* sodium hyaluronate *on page 597*

hyaluronidase *(hye al yoor ON i dase)*

U.S./Canadian Brand Names Kinerase® [US]
Therapeutic Category Enzyme
Use Improving the appearance and texture of sun-damaged facial skin and providing gentle moisturization for a variety of skin types
Usual Dosage Adults: Topical: Apply twice daily
Dosage Forms Ointment: 0.1% (40 g, 80 g)

Hyate®:C [US] *see* antihemophilic factor (porcine) *on page 45*

hycamptamine *see* topotecan *on page 645*

Hycamtin™ [US/Can] *see* topotecan *on page 645*

HycoClear Tuss® *(Discontinued)* *see page 814*

Hycodan® [US] *see* hydrocodone and homatropine *on page 331*

Hycomine® *(Discontinued)* *see page 814*

Hycomine® Compound [US] *see* hydrocodone, chlorpheniramine, phenylephrine, acetaminophen, and caffeine *on page 332*

Hycomine® Pediatric *(Discontinued)* *see page 814*

Hycort® [US] *see* hydrocortisone (rectal) *on page 333*

Hycotuss® Expectorant Liquid [US] *see* hydrocodone and guaifenesin *on page 331*

Hydeltra-T.B.A.® *(Discontinued) see page 814*

Hydergine® [US/Can] *see* ergoloid mesylates *on page 233*

Hydergine® LC [US] *see* ergoloid mesylates *on page 233*

Hyderm [Can] *see* hydrocortisone (topical) *on page 334*

hydralazine (hye DRAL a zeen)

Tall-Man hydrALAZINE

U.S./Canadian Brand Names Apo®-Hydralazine [Can]; Apresoline® [US/Can]; Novo-Hylazin [Can]; Nu-Hydral [Can]

Therapeutic Category Vasodilator

Use Management of moderate to severe hypertension, congestive heart failure, hypertension secondary to pre-eclampsia/eclampsia, primary pulmonary hypertension

Usual Dosage

Children:

Oral: Initial: 0.75-1 mg/kg/day in 2-4 divided doses; increase over 3-4 weeks to maximum of 7.5 mg/kg/day in 2-4 divided doses; maximum daily dose: 200 mg/day

I.M., I.V.: 0.1-0.2 mg/kg/dose (not to exceed 20 mg) every 4-6 hours as needed, up to 1.7-3.5 mg/kg/day in 4-6 divided doses

Adults:

Oral: Hypertension:

Initial dose: 10 mg 4 times/day for first 2-4 days; increase to 25 mg 4 times/day for the balance of the first week

Increase by 10-25 mg/dose gradually to 50 mg 4 times/day; 300 mg/day may be required for some patients

Oral: Congestive heart failure:

Initial dose: 10-25 mg 3-4 times/day

Adjustment: Dosage must be adjusted based on individual response

Target dose: 75 mg 4 times/day in combination with isosorbide dinitrate (40 mg 4 times a day)

Range: Typically 200-600 mg daily in 2-4 divided doses. Dosages as high as 3 g/day have been used in some patients for symptomatic and hemodynamic improvement. Hydralazine 75 mg 4 times a day combined with isosorbide dinitrate 40 mg 4 times a day were shown in clinical trials to provide a mortality benefit in the treatment of CHF. Higher doses may be used for symptomatic and hemodynamic improvement following optimization of standard therapy.

I.M., I.V.:

Hypertension: Initial: 10-20 mg/dose every 4-6 hours as needed, may increase to 40 mg/dose; change to oral therapy as soon as possible.

Pre-eclampsia/eclampsia: 5 mg/dose then 5-10 mg every 20-30 minutes as needed.

Hemodialysis: Supplemental dose is not necessary.

Peritoneal dialysis: Supplemental dose is not necessary.

Dosage Forms

Injection, as hydrochloride: 20 mg/mL (1 mL)

Tablet, as hydrochloride: 10 mg, 25 mg, 50 mg, 100 mg

hydralazine and hydrochlorothiazide

(hye DRAL a zeen & hye droe klor oh THYE a zide)

Synonyms hydrochlorothiazide and hydralazine

U.S./Canadian Brand Names Hydra-Zide® [US]

Therapeutic Category Antihypertensive Agent, Combination

Use Management of moderate to severe hypertension and treatment of congestive heart failure

Usual Dosage Adults: Oral: 1 capsule twice daily

(Continued)

hydralazine and hydrochlorothiazide *(Continued)*

Dosage Forms
Capsule:
25/25: Hydralazine hydrochloride 25 mg and hydrochlorothiazide 25 mg
50/50: Hydralazine hydrochloride 50 mg and hydrochlorothiazide 50 mg
100/50: Hydralazine hydrochloride 100 mg and hydrochlorothiazide 50 mg

hydralazine, hydrochlorothiazide, and reserpine

(hye DRAL a zeen, hye droe klor oh THYE a zide, & re SER peen)
Synonyms hydrochlorothiazide, hydralazine, and reserpine; reserpine, hydralazine, and hydrochlorothiazide
U.S./Canadian Brand Names Hyserp® [US]
Therapeutic Category Antihypertensive Agent, Combination
Use Hypertensive disorders
Usual Dosage Adults: Oral: 1-2 tablets 3 times/day
Dosage Forms Tablet: Hydralazine 25 mg, hydrochlorothiazide 15 mg, and reserpine 0.1 mg

Hydramine® [US-OTC] *see* diphenhydramine *on page 202*

Hydramyn® Syrup *(Discontinued)* *see page 814*

Hydrate® [US] *see* dimenhydrinate *on page 200*

Hydra-Zide® [US] *see* hydralazine and hydrochlorothiazide *on previous page*

Hydrea® [US/Can] *see* hydroxyurea *on page 338*

Hydrobexan® Injection *(Discontinued)* *see page 814*

Hydrocet® [US] *see* hydrocodone and acetaminophen *on next page*

hydrochlorothiazide (hye droe klor oh THYE a zide)

Synonyms HCTZ
U.S./Canadian Brand Names Apo®-Hydro [Can]; Aquazide H® [US]; Ezide® [US]; Hydrocot® [US]; HydroDIURIL® [US/Can]; Microzide™ [US]; Oretic® [US]; Zide® [US]
Therapeutic Category Diuretic, Thiazide
Use Management of mild to moderate hypertension; treatment of edema in congestive heart failure and nephrotic syndrome
Usual Dosage Oral:
Children (daily dosages should be decreased if used with other antihypertensives):
<6 months: 2-3 mg/kg/day in 2 divided doses
>6 months: 2 mg/kg/day in 2 divided doses
Adults: 25-50 mg/day in 1-2 doses; maximum: 200 mg/day
Dosage Forms
Capsule: 12.5 mg
Solution, oral (mint flavor): 50 mg/5 mL (50 mL)
Tablet: 25 mg, 50 mg, 100 mg

hydrochlorothiazide and amiloride *see* amiloride and hydrochlorothiazide *on page 32*

hydrochlorothiazide and benazepril *see* benazepril and hydrochlorothiazide *on page 75*

hydrochlorothiazide and bisoprolol *see* bisoprolol and hydrochlorothiazide *on page 88*

hydrochlorothiazide and captopril *see* captopril and hydrochlorothiazide *on page 112*

hydrochlorothiazide and enalapril *see* enalapril and hydrochlorothiazide *on page 226*

hydrochlorothiazide and hydralazine *see* hydralazine and hydrochlorothiazide *on previous page*

hydrochlorothiazide and lisinopril *see* lisinopril and hydrochlorothiazide *on page 388*

hydrochlorothiazide and losartan *see* losartan and hydrochlorothiazide *on page 392*

hydrochlorothiazide and methyldopa *see* methyldopa and hydrochlorothiazide *on page 421*

hydrochlorothiazide and propranolol *see* propranolol and hydrochlorothiazide *on page 550*

hydrochlorothiazide and spironolactone
(hye droe klor oh THYE a zide & speer on oh LAK tone)
Synonyms spironolactone and hydrochlorothiazide
U.S./Canadian Brand Names Aldactazide® [US/Can]; Novo-Spirozine [Can]
Therapeutic Category Antihypertensive Agent, Combination
Use Management of mild to moderate hypertension; treatment of edema in congestive heart failure and nephrotic syndrome
Usual Dosage Oral:
Children: 1.66-3.3 mg/kg/day (of spironolactone) in 2-4 divided doses
Adults: 1-8 tablets in 1-2 divided doses
Dosage Forms
Tablet:
25/25: Hydrochlorothiazide 25 mg and spironolactone 25 mg
50/50: Hydrochlorothiazide 50 mg and spironolactone 50 mg

hydrochlorothiazide and triamterene
(hye droe klor oh THYE a zide & trye AM ter een)
Synonyms triamterene and hydrochlorothiazide
U.S./Canadian Brand Names Apo®-Triazide [Can]; Dyazide® [US]; Maxzide® [US]; Novo-Triamzide [Can]; Nu-Triazide [Can]
Therapeutic Category Antihypertensive Agent, Combination
Use Management of mild to moderate hypertension; treatment of edema in congestive heart failure and nephrotic syndrome
Usual Dosage Adults: Oral:
Triamterene/hydrochlorothiazide 37.5 mg/25 mg: 1-2 tablets/capsules once daily
Triamterene/hydrochlorothiazide 75 mg/50 mg: 1 tablet daily
Dosage Forms
Capsule (Dyazide®): Hydrochlorothiazide 25 mg and triamterene 37.5 mg
Tablet:
Maxzide®: Hydrochlorothiazide 25 mg and triamterene 37.5 mg; hydrochlorothiazide 50 mg and triamterene 75 mg

hydrochlorothiazide, hydralazine, and reserpine *see* hydralazine, hydrochlorothiazide, and reserpine *on previous page*

Hydrocil® [US-OTC] *see* psyllium *on page 554*

Hydro Cobex® *(Discontinued)* *see page 814*

hydrocodone and acetaminophen
(hye droe KOE done & a seet a MIN oh fen)
Synonyms acetaminophen and hydrocodone
U.S./Canadian Brand Names Anexsia® [US]; Bancap HC® [US]; Co-Gesic® [US]; DHC® [US]; Dolacet® [US]; Hydrocet® [US]; Hydrogesic® [US]; Lorcet® 10/650 [US]; Lorcet®-HD [US]; Lorcet® Plus [US]; Lortab® [US]; Margesic® H [US]; Norco® [US]; Stagesic® [US]; T-Gesic® [US]; Vicodin® [US]; Vicodin® ES [US]; Vicodin® HP [US]; Zydone® [US]
Therapeutic Category Analgesic, Narcotic
Controlled Substance C-III
Use Relief of moderate to severe pain; antitussive (hydrocodone)
(Continued)

329

hydrocodone and acetaminophen *(Continued)*

Usual Dosage Doses should be titrated to appropriate analgesic effect
Adults: Oral: 1-2 tablets or capsules every 4-6 hours

Dosage Forms
Capsule: Bancap HC®, Dolacet®, Hydrocet®, Hydrogesic®, Lorcet®-HD, Margesic® H, Norcet®, Stagesic®, T-Gesic®, Zydone®: Hydrocodone bitartrate 5 mg and acetaminophen 500 mg

Elixir (Lortab®): Hydrocodone bitartrate 2.5 mg and acetaminophen 167 mg per 5 mL (480 mL) [contains alcohol 7%; tropical fruit punch flavor]

Solution, oral (Lortab®): Hydrocodone bitartrate 2.5 mg and acetaminophen 167 mg per 5 mL (480 mL) [contains alcohol 7%; tropical fruit punch flavor]

Tablet:
Hydrocodone bitartrate 5 mg and acetaminophen 400 mg
Hydrocodone bitartrate 5 mg and acetaminophen 500 mg
Hydrocodone bitartrate 7.5 mg and acetaminophen 400 mg
Hydrocodone bitartrate 7.5 mg and acetaminophen 500 mg
Hydrocodone bitartrate 7.5 mg and acetaminophen 650 mg
Hydrocodone bitartrate 7.5 mg and acetaminophen 750 mg
Hydrocodone bitartrate 10 mg and acetaminophen 400 mg
Hydrocodone bitartrate 10 mg and acetaminophen 650 mg
Anexsia® 5/500, Co-Gesic®, DHC®; Lorcet®-HD, Lortab® 5/500, Vicodin®: Hydrocodone bitartrate 5 mg and acetaminophen 500 mg
Anexsia® 7.5/650, Lorcet® Plus: Hydrocodone bitartrate 7.5 mg and acetaminophen 650 mg
Lorcet® 10/650: Hydrocodone bitartrate 10 mg and acetaminophen 650 mg
Lortab® 2.5/500: Hydrocodone bitartrate 2.5 mg and acetaminophen 500 mg
Lortab® 7.5/500: Hydrocodone bitartrate 7.5 mg and acetaminophen 500 mg
Lortab® 10/500: Hydrocodone bitartrate 10 mg and acetaminophen 500 mg
Norco®: Hydrocodone bitartrate 10 mg and acetaminophen 325 mg
Vicodin® ES: Hydrocodone bitartrate 7.5 mg and acetaminophen 750 mg
Vicodin® HP: Hydrocodone bitartrate 10 mg and acetaminophen 660 mg
Zydone®:
Hydrocodone bitartrate 5 mg and acetaminophen 400 mg
Hydrocodone bitartrate 7.5 mg and acetaminophen 400 mg
Hydrocodone bitartrate 10 mg and acetaminophen 400 mg

hydrocodone and aspirin *(hye droe KOE done & AS pir in)*

Synonyms aspirin and hydrocodone
U.S./Canadian Brand Names Lortab® ASA [US]
Therapeutic Category Analgesic, Narcotic
Controlled Substance C-III
Use Relief of moderate to moderately severe pain
Usual Dosage Adults: Oral: 1-2 tablets every 4-6 hours as needed for pain
Dosage Forms Tablet: Hydrocodone bitartrate 5 mg and aspirin 500 mg

hydrocodone and chlorpheniramine
(hye droe KOE done & klor fen IR a meen)

Synonyms chlorpheniramine and hydrocodone
U.S./Canadian Brand Names Tussionex® [US]
Therapeutic Category Antihistamine/Antitussive
Controlled Substance C-III
Use Symptomatic relief of cough
Usual Dosage Oral:
Children 6-12 years: 2.5 mL every 12 hours; do not exceed 5 mL/24 hours
Adults: 5 mL every 12 hours; do not exceed 10 mL/24 hours
Dosage Forms Syrup: Hydrocodone polistirex 10 mg and chlorpheniramine polistirex 8 mg per 5 mL (480 mL, 900 mL) [alcohol free]

hydrocodone and guaifenesin (hye droe KOE done & gwye FEN e sin)

Synonyms guaifenesin and hydrocodone

U.S./Canadian Brand Names Codiclear® DH [US]; Hycotuss® Expectorant Liquid [US]; Kwelcof® [US]; Vicodin Tuss™ [US]

Therapeutic Category Antitussive/Expectorant

Controlled Substance C-III

Use Symptomatic relief of nonproductive coughs associated with upper and lower respiratory tract congestion

Usual Dosage Oral:

Children:

<2 years: 0.3 mg/kg/day (hydrocodone) in 4 divided doses

2-12 years: 2.5 mL every 4 hours, after meals and at bedtime

>12 years: 5 mL every 4 hours, after meals and at bedtime

Adults: 5 mL every 4 hours, after meals and at bedtime, up to 30 mL/24 hours

Dosage Forms Liquid: Hydrocodone bitartrate 5 mg and guaifenesin 100 mg per 5 mL (120 mL, 480 mL)

hydrocodone and homatropine (hye droe KOE done & hoe MA troe peen)

Synonyms homatropine and hydrocodone

U.S./Canadian Brand Names Hycodan® [US]; Hydromet® [US]; Hydropane® [US]; Hydrotropine® [US]; Tussigon® [US]

Therapeutic Category Antitussive

Controlled Substance C-III

Use Symptomatic relief of cough

Usual Dosage Oral (based on hydrocodone component):

Children: 0.6 mg/kg/day in 3-4 divided doses; do not administer more frequently than every 4 hours

A single dose should not exceed 10 mg in children >12 years, 5 mg in children 2-12 years, and 1.25 mg in children <2 years of age

Adults: 5-10 mg every 4-6 hours, a single dose should not exceed 15 mg; do not administer more frequently than every 4 hours

Dosage Forms

Syrup (Hycodan®, Hydromet®, Hydropane®, Hydrotropine®): Hydrocodone bitartrate 5 mg and homatropine methylbromide 1.5 mg per 5 mL (120 mL, 480 mL, 4000 mL)

Tablet (Hycodan®, Tussigon®): Hydrocodone bitartrate 5 mg and homatropine methylbromide 1.5 mg

hydrocodone and ibuprofen (hye droe KOE done & eye byoo PROE fen)

Synonyms ibuprofen and hydrocodone

U.S./Canadian Brand Names Vicoprofen® [US/Can]

Therapeutic Category Analgesic, Narcotic

Controlled Substance C-III

Use Relief of moderate to moderately severe pain (short-term, less than 10 days)

Usual Dosage Adults: Oral: 1-2 tablets every 4-6 hours as needed for pain

Dosage Forms Tablet: Hydrocodone bitartrate 7.5 mg and ibuprofen 200 mg

hydrocodone and pseudoephedrine

(hye droe KOE done & soo doe e FED rin)

U.S./Canadian Brand Names Detussin® Liquid [US]; Histussin D® Liquid [US]

Therapeutic Category Cough and Cold Combination

Use Symptomatic relief of cough due to colds, etc

Usual Dosage Oral: Adults: 5 mL or one tablet 4 times/day

Dosage Forms Liquid (Detussin®, Histussin D®): Hydrocodone bitartrate 5 mg and pseudoephedrine hydrochloride 60 mg per 5 mL

hydrocodone, chlorpheniramine, phenylephrine, acetaminophen, and caffeine

(hye droe KOE done, klor fen IR a meen, fen il EF rin, a seet a MIN oh fen, & KAF een)

Synonyms acetaminophen, caffeine, hydrocodone, chlorpheniramine, and phenylephrine; caffeine, hydrocodone, chlorpheniramine, phenylephrine, and acetaminophen; chlorpheniramine, hydrocodone, phenylephrine, acetaminophen, and caffeine; phenylephrine, hydrocodone, chlorpheniramine, acetaminophen, and caffeine

U.S./Canadian Brand Names Hycomine® Compound [US]

Therapeutic Category Antitussive

Use Symptomatic relief of cough and symptoms of upper respiratory infections

Usual Dosage Adults: Oral: 1 tablet every 4 hours, up to 4 times/day

Dosage Forms Tablet: Hydrocodone bitartrate 5 mg, chlorpheniramine maleate 2 mg, phenylephrine hydrochloride 10 mg, acetaminophen 250 mg, and caffeine 30 mg

Hydrocodone PA® Syrup *(Discontinued)* see page 814

hydrocodone, pseudoephedrine, and guaifenesin

(hye droe KOE done, soo doe e FED rin, & gwye FEN e sin)

Synonyms guaifenesin, hydrocodone, and pseudoephedrine; pseudoephedrine, hydrocodone, and guaifenesin

U.S./Canadian Brand Names Duratuss® HD [US]; Hydro-Tussin™ HD [US]; Hydro-Tussin™ XP [US]; Pancof®-XP [US]; Su-Tuss®-HD [US]; Tussend® Expectorant [US]

Therapeutic Category Antitussive/Decongestant/Expectorant

Controlled Substance C-III

Use Symptomatic relief of irritating, nonproductive cough associated with respiratory conditions such as bronchitis, bronchial asthma, tracheobronchitis, and the common cold

Usual Dosage Adults: Oral: 5 mL every 4-6 hours

Dosage Forms

Elixir: Hydrocodone bitartrate 2.5 mg, pseudoephedrine hydrochloride 30 mg, and guaifenesin 100 mg per 5 mL (480 mL)

Duratuss® HD: Hydrocodone bitartrate 2.5 mg, pseudoephedrine hydrochloride 30 mg, and guaifenesin 100 mg per 5 mL (480 mL, 3785 mL) [contains alcohol; fruit punch flavor]

Su-Tuss® HD: Hydrocodone bitartrate 2.5 mg, pseudoephedrine hydrochloride 30 mg, and guaifenesin 100 mg per 5 mL (480 mL) [contains alcohol; fruit punch flavor]

Liquid: Hydrocodone bitartrate 2.5 mg, pseudoephedrine hydrochloride 30 mg, and guaifenesin 100 mg per 5 mL (480 mL)

Hydro-Tussin™ HD: Hydrocodone bitartrate 2.5 mg, pseudoephedrine hydrochloride 30 mg, and guaifenesin 100 mg per 5 mL [alcohol free; contains sodium benzoate]

Hydro-Tussin™ XP: Hydrocodone bitartrate 3 mg, pseudoephedrine hydrochloride 15 mg, and guaifenesin 100 mg per 5 mL (480 mL) [alcohol free, dye free]

Pancof®-XP: Hydrocodone bitartrate 3 mg, pseudoephedrine hydrochloride 15 mg, and guaifenesin 100 mg per 5 mL (25 mL, 480 mL) [alcohol free, dye free]

Tussend® Expectorant: Hydrocodone bitartrate 2.5 mg, pseudoephedrine hydrochloride 30 mg, and guaifenesin 100 mg per 5 mL (480 mL) [contains alcohol; fruit punch flavor]

Hydrocort® [US] see hydrocortisone (topical) on page 334

hydrocortisone and benzoyl peroxide see benzoyl peroxide and hydrocortisone on page 80

hydrocortisone and clioquinol see clioquinol and hydrocortisone on page 152

hydrocortisone and dibucaine see dibucaine and hydrocortisone on page 193

hydrocortisone and iodoquinol see iodoquinol and hydrocortisone on page 358

hydrocortisone and lidocaine *see* lidocaine and hydrocortisone *on page 384*

hydrocortisone and neomycin *see* neomycin and hydrocortisone *on page 452*

hydrocortisone and pramoxine *see* pramoxine and hydrocortisone *on page 535*

hydrocortisone and urea *see* urea and hydrocortisone *on page 667*

hydrocortisone, bacitracin, neomycin, and polymyxin B *see* bacitracin, neomycin, polymyxin B, and hydrocortisone *on page 69*

hydrocortisone, neomycin, and polymyxin B *see* neomycin, polymyxin B, and hydrocortisone *on page 453*

hydrocortisone (rectal) (hye droe KOR ti sone REK tal)

U.S./Canadian Brand Names Anusol-HC® Suppository [US]; Colocort™ [US]; Cortenema® [US/Can]; Cortifoam® [US/Can]; Emo-Cort® [Can]; Hycort® [US]; Proctocort™ Rectal [US]; ProctoCream ® HC Cream [US]

Therapeutic Category Adrenal Corticosteroid

Use Management of adrenocortical insufficiency; adjunctive treatment of ulcerative colitis

Usual Dosage Ulcerative colitis: Adults: Rectal: 10-100 mg 1-2 times/day for 2-3 weeks

Dosage Forms
Acetate:
Aerosol, rectal: 10% [90 mg/applicatorful] 20 g
Suppository, rectal: 25 mg
Base:
Cream: 2.5% (30 g)
Rectal: 1% (30 g)
Suspension, rectal: 100 mg/60 mL (7s)

hydrocortisone (systemic) (hye droe KOR ti sone sis TEM ik)

Synonyms compound F

U.S./Canadian Brand Names A-HydroCort® [US/Can]; Cortef® [US/Can]; Hydrocortone® Acetate [US]; Solu-Cortef® [US/Can]

Therapeutic Category Adrenal Corticosteroid

Use Management of adrenocortical insufficiency; relief of inflammation of corticosteroid-responsive dermatoses

Usual Dosage Dose should be based on severity of disease and patient response
Acute adrenal insufficiency: I.M., I.V.:
Infants and young Children: Succinate: 1-2 mg/kg/dose bolus, then 25-150 mg/day in divided doses every 6-8 hours
Older Children: Succinate: 1-2 mg/kg bolus then 150-250 mg/day in divided doses every 6-8 hours
Adults: Succinate: 100 mg I.V. bolus, then 300 mg/day in divided doses every 8 hours or as a continuous infusion for 48 hours; once patient is stable change to oral, 50 mg every 8 hours for 6 doses, then taper to 30-50 mg/day in divided doses
Chronic adrenal corticoid insufficiency: Adults: Oral: 20-30 mg/day

Anti-inflammatory or immunosuppressive:
Infants and Children:
Oral: 2.5-10 mg/kg/day **or** 75-300 mg/m^2/day every 6-8 hours
I.M., I.V.: Succinate: 1-5 mg/kg/day **or** 30-150 mg/m^2/day divided every 12-24 hours
Adolescents and Adults: Oral, I.M., I.V.: Succinate: 15-240 mg every 12 hours
Congenital adrenal hyperplasia: Oral: Initial: 10-20 mg/m^2/day in 3 divided doses; a variety of dosing schedules have been used. **Note:** Inconsistencies have occurred with liquid formulations; tablets may provide more reliable levels. Doses must be individualized by monitoring growth, bone age, and hormonal levels. Mineralcorticoid and sodium supplementation may be required based upon electrolyte regulation and plasma renin activity.
Physiologic replacement: Children:
Oral: 0.5-0.75 mg/kg/day **or** 20-25 mg/m^2/day every 8 hours
(Continued)

hydrocortisone (systemic) *(Continued)*

I.M.: Succinate: 0.25-0.35 mg/kg/day **or** 12-15 mg/m^2/day once daily

Shock: I.M., I.V.: Succinate:

Children: Initial: 50 mg/kg, then repeated in 4 hours and/or every 24 hours as needed

Adolescents and Adults: 500 mg to 2 g every 2-6 hours

Status asthmaticus: Children and Adults: I.V.: Succinate: 1-2 mg/kg/dose every 6 hours for 24 hours, then maintenance of 0.5-1 mg/kg every 6 hours

Rheumatic diseases:

Adults: Intralesional, intra-articular, soft tissue injection: Acetate:

Large joints: 25 mg (up to 37.5 mg)

Small joints: 10-25 mg

Tendon sheaths: 5-12.5 mg

Soft tissue infiltration: 25-50 mg (up to 75 mg)

Bursae: 25-37.5 mg

Ganglia: 12.5-25 mg

Dermatosis: Children >2 years and Adults: Topical: Apply to affected area 3-4 times/day (Buteprate: Apply once or twice daily)

Ulcerative colitis: Adults: Rectal: 10-100 mg 1-2 times/day for 2-3 weeks

Dosage Forms

Injection, suspension: 25 mg/mL (5 mL, 10 mL); 50 mg/mL (5 mL, 10 mL)

Suspension, oral: 10 mg/5 mL (120 mL)

Tablet: 5 mg, 10 mg, 20 mg

hydrocortisone (topical) (hye droe KOR ti sone TOP i kal)

U.S./Canadian Brand Names Acticort® [US]; Aeroseb-HC® [US]; Ala-Cort® [US]; Ala-Scalp® [US]; Anusol® HC-1 [US-OTC]; Anusol® HC-2.5% [US-OTC]; Aquacort® [Can]; Bactine® Hydrocortisone [US-OTC]; CaldeCORT® Anti-Itch Spray [US]; CaldeCORT® [US-OTC]; Cetacort®; Clocort® Maximum Strength [US-OTC]; CortaGel® [US-OTC]; Cortaid® Maximum Strength [US-OTC]; Cortaid® with Aloe [US-OTC]; Cort-Dome® [US]; Cortizone®-5 [US-OTC]; Cortizone®-10 [US-OTC]; Cortoderm [Can]; Delcort® [US]; Dermacort® [US]; Dermarest Dricort® [US]; Dermolate® [US-OTC]; Dermtex® HC with Aloe [US-OTC]; Eldecort® [US]; Gynecort® [US-OTC]; Hi-Cor-1.0® [US]; Hi-Cor-2.5® [US]; Hyderm [Can]; Hydrocort® [US]; Hydro-Tex® [US-OTC]; Hytone® [US]; LactiCare-HC® [US]; Lanacort® [US-OTC]; Locoid® [US/Can]; Nutracort® [US]; Orabase® HCA [US]; Penecort® [US]; Prevex® HC [Can]; Sarna® HC [Can]; Scalpicin® [US]; S-T Cort® [US]; Synacort® [US]; Tegrin®-HC [US-OTC]; Texacort® [US]; U-Cort™ [US]; Westcort® [US/Can]

Therapeutic Category Corticosteroid, Topical

Use Management of adrenocortical insufficiency; relief of inflammation of corticosteroid-responsive dermatoses; adjunctive treatment of ulcerative colitis

Usual Dosage Children >2 years and Adults: Topical: Apply to affected area 3-4 times/day (Buteprate: Apply once or twice daily). Therapy should be discontinued when control is achieved. If no improvement is seen, reassessment of diagnosis may be necessary.

Dosage Forms

Aerosol, topical:

Cream: 0.5%, 1%, 2.5%

Gel: 0.5%

Lotion: 0.5%, 1%, 2.5%

Ointment, topical: 0.5%, 1%, 2.5%

Paste: 0.5% (5 g)

Solution, topical; 1%

Butyrate:

Cream: 0.1%

Ointment, topical: 0.1%

Solution, topical: 0.1%

Valerate:

Cream: 0.2%

Ointment, topical: 0.2%

Hydrocortone® **Acetate [US]** *see* hydrocortisone (systemic) *on page 333*
Hydrocot® **[US]** *see* hydrochlorothiazide *on page 328*
Hydro-Crysti-12® *(Discontinued) see page 814*
HydroDIURIL® **[US/Can]** *see* hydrochlorothiazide *on page 328*
hydrogenated ergot alkaloids *see* ergoloid mesylates *on page 233*
Hydrogesic® **[US]** *see* hydrocodone and acetaminophen *on page 329*
hydromagnesium aluminate *see* magaldrate *on page 396*
Hydromet® **[US]** *see* hydrocodone and homatropine *on page 331*
Hydromorph Contin® **[Can]** *see* hydromorphone *on this page*

hydromorphone (hye droe MOR fone)

Synonyms dihydromorphinone
U.S./Canadian Brand Names Dilaudid-5® [US]; Dilaudid-HP-Plus® [Can]; Dilaudid-HP® [US/Can]; Dilaudid® [US/Can]; Dilaudid-XP® [Can]; Hydromorph Contin® [Can]; PMS-Hydromorphone [Can]
Therapeutic Category Analgesic, Narcotic
Controlled Substance C-II
Use Management of moderate to severe pain; antitussive at lower doses
Usual Dosage
Acute pain (moderate to severe): **Note:** These are guidelines and do not represent the maximum doses that may be required in all patients. Doses should be titrated to pain relief/prevention.
Young Children ≥6 months and <50 kg:
Oral: 0.03-0.08 mg/kg/dose every 3-4 hours as needed
I.V.: 0.015 mg/kg/dose ever 3-6 hours as needed
Older Children >50 kg and Adults:
Oral: Initial: Opiate-naive: 2-4 mg every 3-4 hours as needed; patients with prior opiate exposure may require higher initial doses; usual dosage range: 2-8 mg every 3-4 hours as needed
I.V.: Initial: Opiate-naive: 0.2-0.6 mg every 2-3 hours as needed; patients with prior opiate exposure may tolerate higher initial doses **Note:** More frequent dosing may be needed. Mechanically-ventilated patients (based on 70 kg patient): 0.7-2 mg every 1-2 hours as needed; infusion (based on 70 kg patient): 0.5-1 mg/hour
Patient-controlled analgesia (PCA): Initial: Opiate-naive: Consider lower end of dosing range; after loading: 0.05-0.4 mg/dose; usual lockout range: 5-10 minutes
Epidural: Initial: 0.8-1.5 mg/dose; infusion: 0.15-0.3 mg/hour
I.M., S.C.: **Note:** I.M. use may result in variable absorption and a lag time to peak effect. Initial: Opiate-naive: 0.8-1 mg every 4-6 hours; patients with prior opiate exposure may require higher initial doses; usual dosage range: 1-2 mg every 3-6 hours as needed
Rectal: 3 mg every 4-8 hours as needed

Chronic pain: Patients taking opioids chronically may become tolerant and require doses higher than the usual dosage range to maintain the desired effect. Tolerance can be managed by appropriate dose titration. There is no optimal or maximal dose for hydromorphone in chronic pain. The appropriate dose is one that relieves pain throughout its dosing interval without causing unmanageable side effects.

Antitussive: Oral:
Children 6-12 years: 0.5 mg every 3-4 hours as needed
Children >12 years and Adults: 1 mg every 3-4 hours as needed
Dosage Forms
Injection, as hydrochloride:
Dilaudid®: 1 mg/mL (1 mL); 2 mg/mL (1 mL, 20 mL); 4 mg/mL (1 mL)
Dilaudid-HP®: 10 mg/mL (1 mL, 2 mL, 5 mL)
(Continued)

hydromorphone *(Continued)*

Injection, powder for reconstitution, as hydrochloride (Dilaudid-HP®): 250 mg
Liquid, as hydrochloride (Dilaudid-5®): 1 mg/mL (1 mL, 4 mL, 8 mL, 120 mL, 250 mL, 480 mL, 500 mL)
Solution, oral, as hydrochloride: 5 mg/mL (120 mL, 250 mL, 500 mL) [raspberry flavor]
Suppository, rectal, as hydrochloride: 3 mg (6s)
Tablet, as hydrochloride: 2 mg, 4 mg, 8 mg

Hydromox® *(Discontinued)* see page 814

Hydropane® [US] see hydrocodone and homatropine on page 331

Hydro-Par® *(Discontinued)* see page 814

Hydrophed® *(Discontinued)* see page 814

Hydropres® *(Discontinued)* see page 814

hydroquinol see hydroquinone on this page

hydroquinone (HYE droe kwin one)

Synonyms hydroquinol; quinol
U.S./Canadian Brand Names Eldopaque Forte® [US]; Eldopaque® [US-OTC]; Eldoquin® Forte® [US]; Eldoquin® [US/Can]; Esoterica® Facial [US-OTC]; Esoterica® Regular [US-OTC]; Esoterica® Sensitive Skin Formula [US-OTC]; Esoterica® Sunscreen [US-OTC]; Melanex® [US]; Melpaque HP® [US]; Melquin-3® [US-OTC]; Melquin HP® [US]; Neostrata® HQ [Can]; Nuquin® Gel [US]; Nuquin HP® Cream [US]; Solaquin Forte® [US/Can]; Solaquin® [US/Can]; Ultraquin™ [Can]
Therapeutic Category Topical Skin Product
Use Gradual bleaching of hyperpigmented skin conditions
Usual Dosage Topical: Apply thin layer and rub in twice daily
Dosage Forms
Cream:
Eldopaque®, Eldoquin®, Esoterica® Facial, Esoterica® Regular: 2% (14.2 g, 28.4 g, 60 g, 85 g, 120 g)
Eldopaque Forte®, Eldoquin® Forte®, Melquin HP®: 4% (14.2 g, 28.4 g)
Esoterica® Sensitive Skin Formula: 1.5% (85 g)
Cream [with sunscreen]:
Esoterica® Sunscreen, Solaquin®: 2% (28.4 g, 120 g)
Melpaque HP®, Nuquin HP®, Solaquin Forte®: 4% (14.2 g, 28.4 g)
Gel [with sunscreen] (Nuquin® Gel, Solaquin Forte® Gel): 4% (14.2 g, 28.4 g)
Solution, topical (Melanex®, Melquin-3®): 3% (30 mL)

Hydro-Tex® [US-OTC] see hydrocortisone (topical) on page 334

Hydrotropine® [US] see hydrocodone and homatropine on page 331

Hydro-Tussin™-CBX [US] see carbinoxamine and pseudoephedrine on page 115

Hydro-Tussin™ DM [US] see guaifenesin and dextromethorphan on page 308

Hydro-Tussin™ HD [US] see hydrocodone, pseudoephedrine, and guaifenesin on page 332

Hydro-Tussin™ XP [US] see hydrocodone, pseudoephedrine, and guaifenesin on page 332

Hydroxacen® *(Discontinued)* see page 814

hydroxycarbamide see hydroxyurea on page 338

hydroxychloroquine (hye droks ee KLOR oh kwin)

U.S./Canadian Brand Names Plaquenil® [US/Can]
Therapeutic Category Aminoquinoline (Antimalarial)
Use Suppression or chemoprophylaxis of malaria caused by susceptible *P. vivax*, *P. ovale*, *P. malariae*, and some strains of *P. falciparum* (not active against pre-erythrocytic

or exoerythrocytic tissue stages of *Plasmodium*); treatment of systemic lupus erythematosus (SLE) and rheumatoid arthritis

Usual Dosage Oral:

Children:

Chemoprophylaxis of malaria: 5 mg/kg (base) once weekly; should not exceed the recommended adult dose; begin 2 weeks before exposure; continue for 8 weeks after leaving endemic area

Acute attack: 10 mg/kg (base) initial dose; followed by 5 mg/kg in 6 hours on day 1; 5 mg/kg in 1 dose on day 2 and on day 3

Juvenile rheumatoid arthritis or SLE: 3-5 mg/kg/day divided 1-2 times/day to a maximum of 400 mg/day; not to exceed 7 mg/kg/day

Adults:

Chemoprophylaxis of malaria: 2 tablets weekly on same day each week; begin 2 weeks before exposure; continue for 6-8 weeks after leaving epidemic area

Acute attack: 4 tablets first dose day 1; 2 tablets in 6 hours day 1; 2 tablets in 1 dose day 2; and 2 tablets in 1 dose on day 3

Rheumatoid arthritis: 2-3 tablets/day to start with food or milk; increase dose until optimum response level is reached; usually after 4-12 weeks dose should be reduced by ½ and a maintenance dose of 1-2 tablets/day

Lupus erythematosus: 2 tablets every day or twice daily for several weeks depending on response; 1-2 tablets/day for prolonged maintenance therapy

Dosage Forms Tablet, as sulfate: 200 mg [base 155 mg]

25-hydroxycholecalciferol *see* calcifediol *on page 103*

hydroxydaunomycin *see* doxorubicin *on page 214*

hydroxyethyl starch *see* hetastarch *on page 321*

hydroxyprogesterone caproate (hye droks ee proe JES te rone KAP roe ate)

U.S./Canadian Brand Names Hylutin® [US]; Prodrox® [US]

Therapeutic Category Progestin

Use Treatment of amenorrhea, abnormal uterine bleeding, submucous fibroids, endometriosis, uterine carcinoma, and testing of estrogen production

Usual Dosage Adults: I.M.:

Amenorrhea: 375 mg; if no bleeding, begin cyclic treatment with estradiol valerate

Endometriosis: Start cyclic therapy with estradiol valerate

Uterine carcinoma: 1 g one or more times/day (1-7 g/week) for up to 12 weeks

Test for endogenous estrogen production: 250 mg anytime; bleeding 7-14 days after injection indicate positive test

Dosage Forms Injection, as caproate (Hylutin®, Prodrox®): 250 mg/mL (5 mL)

hydroxypropyl cellulose (hye droks ee PROE pil SEL yoo lose)

U.S./Canadian Brand Names Lacrisert® [US/Can]

Therapeutic Category Ophthalmic Agent, Miscellaneous

Use Dry eyes

Usual Dosage Adults: Ophthalmic: Apply once daily into the inferior cul-de-sac beneath the base of tarsus, not in apposition to the cornea nor beneath the eyelid at the level of the tarsal plate

Dosage Forms Insert, ophthalmic: 5 mg

hydroxypropyl methylcellulose (hye droks ee PROE pil meth il SEL yoo lose)

Synonyms gonioscopic ophthalmic solution

U.S./Canadian Brand Names GenTeal™ [US/Can]; Gonak™ [US-OTC]; Goniosol® [US-OTC]

Therapeutic Category Ophthalmic Agent, Miscellaneous

(Continued)

hydroxypropyl methylcellulose *(Continued)*

Use Ophthalmic surgical aid in cataract extraction and intraocular implantation; gonioscopic examinations

Usual Dosage Introduced into anterior chamber of eye with 20-gauge or larger cannula

Dosage Forms
Gel, ophthalmic: 0.3% (10 mL)
Solution, ophthalmic: 0.3% (15 mL, 25 mL); 2.5% (15 mL)

hydroxyurea (hye droks ee yoor EE a)

Synonyms hydroxycarbamide

U.S./Canadian Brand Names Droxia™ [US]; Hydrea® [US/Can]; Mylocel™ [US]

Therapeutic Category Antineoplastic Agent

Use CML in chronic phase; radiosensitizing agent in the treatment of primary brain tumors, head and neck tumors, uterine cervix and nonsmall cell lung cancer, and psoriasis; treatment of hematologic conditions such as essential thrombocythemia, polycythemia vera, hypereosinophilia, and hyperleukocytosis due to acute leukemia. Has shown activity against renal cell cancer, melanoma, ovarian cancer, head and neck cancer, and prostate cancer.

Sickle cell anemia: Specifically for patients >18 years of age who have had at least three "painful crises" in the previous year - to reduce frequency of these crises and the need for blood transfusions

Unlabeled use: Thrombocythemia

Usual Dosage Oral (refer to individual protocols): All dosage should be based on ideal or actual body weight, whichever is less:

Children:
No FDA-approved dosage regimens have been established; dosages of 1500-3000 mg/m^2 as a single dose in combination with other agents every 4-6 weeks have been used in the treatment of pediatric astrocytoma, medulloblastoma, and primitive neuroectodermal tumors
CML: Initial: 10-20 mg/kg/day once daily; adjust dose according to hematologic response

Adults: Dose should always be titrated to patient response and WBC counts; usual oral doses range from 10-30 mg/kg/day or 500-3000 mg/day; if WBC count falls to <2500 cells/mm^3, or the platelet count to <100,000/mm^3, therapy should be stopped for at least 3 days and resumed when values rise toward normal

Solid tumors:
Intermittent therapy: 80 mg/kg as a single dose every third day
Continuous therapy: 20-30 mg/kg/day given as a single dose/day

Concomitant therapy with irradiation: 80 mg/kg as a single dose every third day starting at least 7 days before initiation of irradiation

Resistant chronic myelocytic leukemia: 20-30 mg/kg/day divided daily

HIV: 1000-1500 mg daily in a single dose or divided doses

Sickle cell anemia (moderate/severe disease): Initial: 15 mg/kg/day, increased by 5 mg/kg every 12 weeks if blood counts are in an acceptable range until the maximum tolerated dose of 35 mg/kg/day is achieved or the dose that does not produce toxic effects

Acceptable range:
Neutrophils ≥2500 cells/mm^3
Platelets ≥95,000/mm^3
Hemoglobin >5.3 g/dL, and
Reticulocytes ≥95,000/mm^3 if the hemoglobin concentration is <9 g/dL

Toxic range:
Neutrophils <2000 cells/mm^3
Platelets <80,000/mm^3
Hemoglobin <4.5 g/dL
Reticulocytes <80,000/mm^3 if the hemoglobin concentration is <9 g/dL

Monitor for toxicity every 2 weeks; if toxicity occurs, stop treatment until the bone marrow recovers; restart at 2.5 mg/kg/day less than the dose at which toxicity occurs; if no toxicity occurs over the next 12 weeks, then the subsequent dose should be increased by 2.5 mg/kg/day; reduced dosage of hydroxyurea alternating with erythropoietin may decrease myelotoxicity and increase levels of fetal hemoglobin in patients who have not been helped by hydroxyurea alone

Dosage Forms
Capsule: 500 mg
Droxia™: 200 mg, 300 mg, 400 mg
Hydrea®: 500 mg
Tablet (Mylocel™): 1000 mg

25-hydroxyvitamin D₃ *see* calcifediol *on page 103*

hydroxyzine (hye DROKS i zeen)

Tall-Man hydrOXYzine

U.S./Canadian Brand Names ANX® [US]; Apo®-Hydroxyzine [Can]; Atarax® [US/Can]; Hyzine-50® [US]; Novo-Hydroxyzin [Can]; PMS-Hydroxyzine [Can]; Restall® [US]; Vistacot® [US]; Vistaril® [US/Can]

Therapeutic Category Antiemetic; Antihistamine

Use Treatment of anxiety; preoperative sedative; antipruritic; antiemetic

Usual Dosage
Children:
Oral: 2 mg/kg/day divided every 6-8 hours
I.M.: 0.5-1 mg/kg/dose every 4-6 hours as needed
Adults:
Antiemetic: I.M.: 25-100 mg/dose every 4-6 hours as needed
Anxiety: Oral: 25-100 mg 4 times/day; maximum dose: 600 mg/day
Preoperative sedation:
Oral: 50-100 mg
I.M.: 25-100 mg
Management of pruritus: Oral: 25 mg 3-4 times/day

Dosage Forms
Capsule, as pamoate: 25 mg, 50 mg, 100 mg
Injection, as hydrochloride: 25 mg/mL (1 mL, 2 mL, 10 mL); 50 mg/mL (1 mL, 2 mL, 10 mL)
Suspension, oral, as pamoate: 25 mg/5 mL (120 mL, 480 mL)
Syrup, as hydrochloride: 10 mg/5 mL (120 mL, 480 mL, 4000 mL)
Tablet, as hydrochloride: 10 mg, 25 mg, 50 mg, 100 mg

Hygroton® *(Discontinued) see page 814*

Hylorel® [US/Can] *see guanadrel on page 313*

Hylutin® [US] *see hydroxyprogesterone caproate on page 337*

Hyonatol® [US] *see hyoscyamine, atropine, scopolamine, and phenobarbital on next page*

hyoscine *see scopolamine on page 585*

hyoscyamine (hye oh SYE a meen)

Synonyms *l*-hyoscyamine sulfate

U.S./Canadian Brand Names Anaspaz® [US]; A-Spas® S/L [US]; Cystospaz-M® [US]; Cystospaz® [US/Can]; Hyosine [US]; Levbid® [US]; Levsinex® [US]; Levsin/SL® [US]; Levsin® [US/Can]; NuLev™ [US]; Spacol T/S [US]; Spacol [US]; Symax SL [US]; Symax SR [US]

Therapeutic Category Anticholinergic Agent

Use GI tract disorders caused by spasm, adjunctive therapy for peptic ulcers
(Continued)

hyoscyamine *(Continued)*

Usual Dosage
Children:
<2 years: $1/4$ adult dosage
2-10 years: $1/2$ adult dosage
Adults:
Oral, S.L.: 0.125-0.25 mg 3-4 times/day before meals or food and at bedtime; 0.375-0.75 mg (timed release) every 12 hours
I.M., I.V., S.C.: 0.25-0.5 mg every 6 hours

Dosage Forms
Capsule, timed release, as sulfate (Cystospaz-M®, Levsinex®): 0.375 mg
Elixir, as sulfate (Hyosine, Levsin®): 0.125 mg/5 mL [contains alcohol 20%; orange flavor] (480 mL)
Injection, as sulfate (Levsin®): 0.5 mg/mL (1 mL)
Liquid, as sulfate (Spacol): 0.125 mg/5 mL (120 mL) [alcohol free; bubblegum flavor; simethicone based; sugar free]
Solution, oral drops, as sulfate (Hyosine, Levsin®): 0.125 mg/mL (15 mL) [contains alcohol 5%; orange flavor]
Tablet (Cystospaz®): 0.15 mg
Tablet, as sulfate (Anaspaz®, ED-SPAZ®, Levsin®, Spacol): 0.125 mg
Tablet, extended release, as sulfate (Levbid®, Symax SR, Spacol T/S): 0.375 mg
Tablet, orally-disintegrating, as sulfate (NuLev™): 0.125 mg [contains phenylalanine 1.7 mg/tablet; mint flavor]
Tablet, sublingual, as sulfate:
A-Spas® S/L, Symax SL: 0.125 mg
Levsin/SL®: 0.125 mg [peppermint flavor]

hyoscyamine, atropine, scopolamine, and phenobarbital
(hye oh SYE a meen, A troe peen, skoe POL a meen, & fee noe BAR bi tal)
Synonyms antispasmodic compound; atropine, hyoscyamine, scopolamine, and phenobarbital; phenobarbital, hyoscyamine, atropine, and scopolamine; scopolamine, hyoscyamine, atropine, and phenobarbital
U.S./Canadian Brand Names Antispas® Tablet [US]; Donnapine® [US]; Donnatal® [US]; Haponal® [US]; Hyonatol® [US]; Hypersed® [US]
Therapeutic Category Anticholinergic Agent
Use Adjunct in treatment of peptic ulcer disease, irritable bowel, spastic colitis, spastic bladder, and renal colic
Usual Dosage Oral:
Children 2-12 years:
Kinesed® dose: $1/2$ to 1 tablet 3-4 times/day
Donnatal®: 0.1 mL/kg/dose every 4 hours; maximum dose: 5 mL
Adults: 0.125-0.25 mg (1-2 capsules or tablets) 3-4 times/day; or 0.375-0.75 mg (1 Donnatal® Extentab®) in sustained release form every 12 hours; or 5-10 mL elixir 3-4 times/day or every 8 hours
Dosage Forms
Capsule: Hyoscyamine sulfate 0.1037 mg, atropine sulfate 0.0194 mg, scopolamine hydrobromide 0.0065 mg, and phenobarbital 16.2 mg
Elixir: Hyoscyamine sulfate 0.1037 mg, atropine sulfate 0.0194 mg, scopolamine hydrobromide 0.0065 mg, and phenobarbital 16.2 mg per 5 mL (120 mL, 480 mL, 4000 mL)
Tablet:
Tablet, long-acting: Hyoscyamine sulfate 0.3111 mg, atropine sulfate 0.0582 mg, scopolamine hydrobromide 0.0195 mg, and phenobarbital 48.6 mg

hyoscyamine, atropine, scopolamine, kaolin, and pectin
(hye oh SYE a meen, A troe peen, skoe POL a meen, KAY oh lin, & PEK tin)
Therapeutic Category Anticholinergic Agent
Use Antidiarrheal; also used in gastritis, enteritis, colitis, and acute gastrointestinal upsets, and nausea which may accompany any of these conditions

Usual Dosage Oral:
Children:
10-20 lb: 2.5 mL
20-30 lb: 5 mL
>30 lb: 5-10 mL
Adults:
Diarrhea: 30 mL at once and 15-30 mL with each loose stool
Other conditions: 15 mL every 3 hours as needed
Dosage Forms Suspension, oral: Hyoscyamine sulfate 0.1037 mg, atropine sulfate 0.0194 mg, scopolamine hydrobromide 0.0065 mg, kaolin 6 g, and pectin 142.8 mg per 30 mL

hyoscyamine, atropine, scopolamine, kaolin, pectin, and opium
(hye oh SYE a meen, A troe peen, skoe POL a meen, KAY oh lin, PEK tin, & OH pee um)
U.S./Canadian Brand Names Donnapectolin-PG® [US]; Kapectolin PG® [US]
Therapeutic Category Anticholinergic Agent
Controlled Substance C-V
Use Treatment of diarrhea
Usual Dosage Oral:
Children 6-12 years: Initial: 10 mL, then 5-10 mL every 3 hours thereafter
Dosage recommendations (body weight/dosage): 10 lb/2.5 mL; 20 lb/5 mL; 30 lb and over/5-10 mL; do not administer more than 4 doses in any 24-hour period
Children >12 years and Adults: Initial: 30 mL (1 fluid oz) followed by 15 mL every 3 hours
Dosage Forms Suspension, oral: Hyoscyamine sulfate 0.1037 mg, atropine sulfate 0.0194 mg, scopolamine hydrobromide 0.0065 mg, kaolin 6 g, pectin 142.8 mg, and powdered opium 24 mg per 30 mL with alcohol 5%

Hyosine [US] *see* hyoscyamine *on page 339*

Hy-Pam® Oral *(Discontinued)* *see page 814*

Hypaque-Cysto® [US] *see* radiological/contrast media (ionic) *on page 561*

Hypaque® Meglumine [US] *see* radiological/contrast media (ionic) *on page 561*

Hypaque® Sodium [US] *see* radiological/contrast media (ionic) *on page 561*

Hyperab® *(Discontinued)* *see page 814*

Hypersed® [US] *see* hyoscyamine, atropine, scopolamine, and phenobarbital *on previous page*

Hyperstat® I.V. [US/Can] *see* diazoxide *on page 192*

Hyper-Tet® *(Discontinued)* *see page 814*

Hy-Phen® *(Discontinued)* *see page 814*

HypoTears PF [US-OTC] *see* artificial tears *on page 56*

HypoTears [US-OTC] *see* artificial tears *on page 56*

HypRho®-D *(Discontinued)* *see page 814*

HypRho®-D Mini-Dose *(Discontinued)* *see page 814*

Hyprogest® 250 *(Discontinued)* *see page 814*

Hyrexin® [US-OTC] *see* diphenhydramine *on page 202*

Hyserp® [US] *see* hydralazine, hydrochlorothiazide, and reserpine *on page 328*

Hytakerol® [US/Can] *see* dihydrotachysterol *on page 198*

Hytinic® [US-OTC] *see* polysaccharide-iron complex *on page 527*

Hytone® [US] *see* hydrocortisone (topical) *on page 334*

Hytrin® [US/Can] *see* terazosin *on page 622*

Hytuss-2X® [US-OTC] *see* guaifenesin *on page 307*

Hytuss® **[US-OTC]** *see* guaifenesin *on page 307*

Hyzaar® **[US/Can]** *see* losartan and hydrochlorothiazide *on page 392*

Hyzine-50® **[US]** *see* hydroxyzine *on page 339*

ibenzmethyzin *see* procarbazine *on page 542*

Iberet-Folic-500® **[US]** *see* ferrous sulfate, ascorbic acid, vitamin B-complex, and folic acid *on page 270*

Iberet®-Liquid 500 **[US-OTC]** *see* ferrous sulfate, ascorbic acid, and vitamin B-complex *on page 269*

Iberet®-Liquid **[US-OTC]** *see* ferrous sulfate, ascorbic acid, and vitamin B-complex *on page 269*

ibidomide *see* labetalol *on page 370*

ibritumomab (ib ri TYOO mo mab)

Synonyms ibritumomab tiuxetan; In-111 zevalin; Y-90 zevalin

U.S./Canadian Brand Names Zevalin™ [US]

Therapeutic Category Antineoplastic Agent, Monoclonal Antibody; Radiopharmaceutical

Use Treatment of relapsed or refractory low-grade, follicular, or transformed B-cell non-Hodgkin's lymphoma (including rituximab-refractory follicular non-Hodgkin's lymphoma) as part of a therapeutic regimen with rituximab (Zevalin™ therapeutic regimen); **not to be used as single-agent therapy**; must be radiolabeled prior to use

Usual Dosage I.V.: Adults: Ibritumomab is administered **only** as part of the Zevalin™ therapeutic regimen (a combined treatment regimen with rituximab). The regimen consists of two steps:

Step 1:
Rituximab infusion: 250 mg/m² at an initial rate of 50 mg/hour. If hypersensitivity or infusion-related events do not occur, increase infusion in increments of 50 mg/hour every 30 minutes, to a maximum of 400 mg/hour. Infusions should be temporarily slowed or interrupted if hypersensitivity or infusion-related events occur. The infusion may be resumed at one-half the previous rate upon improvement of symptoms.

In-111 ibritumomab infusion: Within 4 hours of the completion of rituximab infusion, inject 5 mCi (1.6 mg total antibody dose) over 10 minutes.

Biodistribution of In-111 ibritumomab should be assessed by imaging at 2-24 hours and at 48-72 hours post-injection. An optional third imaging may be performed 90-120 hours following injection. If biodistribution is not acceptable, the patient should not proceed to Step 2.

Step 2 (initiated 7-9 days following Step 1):
Rituximab infusion: 250 mg/m² at an initial rate of 100 mg/hour (50 mg/hour if infusion-related events occurred with the first infusion). If hypersensitivity or infusion-related events do not occur, increase infusion in increments of 100 mg/hour every 30 minutes, to a maximum of 400 mg/hour, as tolerated.

Y-90 ibritumomab infusion: Within 4 hours of the completion of rituximab infusion:

Dosage Forms Each kit contains 4 vials for preparation of either In-111 or Y-90 conjugate (as indicated on container label)

Injection, solution: 1.6 mg/mL (2 mL) [supplied with sodium acetate solution, formulation buffer vial (includes albumin 750 mg), and an empty reaction vial]

ibritumomab tiuxetan *see* ibritumomab *on this page*

Ibuprin® *(Discontinued)* *see page 814*

ibuprofen (eye byoo PROE fen)

Synonyms p-isobutylhydratropic acid

U.S./Canadian Brand Names Advil® [US/Can]; Advil® Children's [US-OTC]; Advil® Infants' Concentrated Drops [US-OTC]; Advil® Junior [US-OTC]; Advil® Migraine [US-OTC]; Apo®-Ibuprofen [Can]; Genpril® [US-OTC]; Haltran® [US-OTC]; Ibu-Tab® [US]; I-

Prin [US-OTC]; Menadol® [US-OTC]; Midol® Maximum Strength Cramp Formula [US-OTC]; Motrin® [US/Can]; Motrin® Children's [US/Can]; Motrin® IB [US/Can]; Motrin® Infants' [US-OTC]; Motrin® Junior Strength [US-OTC]; Motrin® Migraine Pain [US-OTC]; Novo-Profen® [Can]; Nu-Ibuprofen [Can]

Therapeutic Category Analgesic, Non-narcotic; Antipyretic; Nonsteroidal Anti-inflammatory Drug (NSAID)

Use Inflammatory diseases and rheumatoid disorders including juvenile rheumatoid arthritis (JRA); mild to moderate pain; fever; dysmenorrhea; gout

Usual Dosage Oral:

Children:

Antipyretic: 6 months to 12 years: Temperature <102.5°F (39°C): 5 mg/kg/dose; temperature >102.5°F: 10 mg/kg/dose administered every 6-8 hours; maximum daily dose: 40 mg/kg/day

Juvenile rheumatoid arthritis: 30-50 mg/kg/day in 4 divided doses; start at lower end of dosing range and titrate upward; maximum: 2.4 g/day

Analgesic: 4-10 mg/kg/dose every 6-8 hours

Adults:

Inflammatory disease: 400-800 mg/dose 3-4 times/day; maximum dose: 3.2 g/day

Pain/fever/dysmenorrhea: 200-400 mg/dose every 4-6 hours; maximum daily dose: 1.2 g

Dosage Forms

Caplet: 200 mg [OTC]

Advil®: 200 mg [contains sodium benzoate]

Menadol®, Motrin® IB, Motrin® Migraine Pain: 200 mg

Motrin® Junior Strength: 100 mg [contains tartrazine]

Capsule, liqui-gel:

Advil®: 200 mg

Advil® Migraine: 200 mg [solubilized ibuprofen]

Gelcap:

Advil®: 200 mg

Motrin® IB: 200 mg [contains benzyl alcohol]

Suspension, oral: 100 mg/5 mL (5 mL, 120 mL, 480 mL)

Advil® Children's: 100 mg/5 mL (60 mL, 120 mL) [contains sodium benzoate; blue raspberry, fruit, and grape flavors]

Motrin® Children's: 100 mg/5 mL (60 mL, 120 mL) [contains sodium benzoate; berry, dye-free berry, bubble gum, and grape flavors]

Suspension, oral drops:

Advil® Infants' Concentrated Drops: 40 mg/mL (15 mL) [contains sodium benzoate; fruit and grape flavors]

Motrin® Infants': 40 mg/mL (15 mL) [contains sodium benzoate; berry and dye-free berry flavors]

Tablet: 200 mg [OTC], 400 mg, 600 mg, 800 mg

Advil®: 200 mg [contains sodium benzoate]

Advil® Junior: 100 mg [contains sodium benzoate; coated tablets]

Genpril®, Haltran®, I-Prin, Midol® Maximum Strength Cramp Formula, Motrin® IB: 200 mg

Ibu-Tab®, Motrin®: 400 mg, 600 mg, 800 mg

Tablet, chewable:

Advil® Children's: 50 mg [contains phenylalanine 2.1 mg; fruit and grape flavors]

Advil® Junior: 100 mg [contains phenylalanine 2.1 mg; fruit and grape flavors]

Motrin® Children's: 50 mg [contains phenylalanine 1.4 mg; orange flavor]

Motrin® Junior Strength: 100 mg [contains phenylalanine 2.1 mg; grape and orange flavors]

ibuprofen and hydrocodone see hydrocodone and ibuprofen on page 331

Ibu-Tab® [US] see ibuprofen on previous page

ibutilide (i BYOO ti lide)

U.S./Canadian Brand Names Corvert® [US]

Therapeutic Category Antiarrhythmic Agent, Class III

Use Acute termination of atrial fibrillation or flutter of recent onset; the effectiveness of ibutilide has not been determined in patients with arrhythmias of >90 days in duration

Usual Dosage I.V.: Initial:

<60 kg: 0.01 mg/kg over 10 minutes

≥60 kg: 1 mg over 10 minutes

If the arrhythmia does not terminate within 10 minutes after the end of the initial infusion, a second infusion of equal strength may be infused over a 10-minute period

Dosage Forms Injection, solution, as fumarate: 0.1 mg/mL (10 mL)

IC-Green® [US] see indocyanine green on page 349

ICI 182,780 see fulvestrant on page 290

ICI 204, 219 see zafirlukast on page 688

ICRF-187 see dexrazoxane on page 187

Icy Hot Arthritis Therapy® [US] see capsaicin on page 111

Idamycin® [Can] see idarubicin on this page

Idamycin® (Discontinued) see page 814

Idamycin PFS® [US] see idarubicin on this page

Idarac® [Can] see floctafenine (Canada only) on page 273

idarubicin (eye da ROO bi sin)

Synonyms 4-demethoxydaunorubicin; 4-dmdr

U.S./Canadian Brand Names Idamycin® [Can]; Idamycin PFS® [US]

Therapeutic Category Antineoplastic Agent

Use In combination with other antineoplastic agents for treatment of acute myelogenous leukemia (AML) in adults and acute lymphocytic leukemia (ALL) in children

Usual Dosage I.V.:

Children:

Leukemia: 10-12 mg/m^2 once daily for 3 days and repeat every 3 weeks

Solid tumors: 5 mg/m^2 once daily for 3 days and repeat every 3 weeks

Adults: 12 mg/m^2/day for 3 days by slow I.V. injection (10-15 minutes) in combination with Ara-C. The Ara-C may be given as 100 mg/m^2/day by continuous infusion for 7 days or 25 mg/m^2 bolus followed by Ara-C 200 mg/m^2/day for 5 days continuous infusion.

Dosage Forms

Injection, solution, as hydrochloride [preservative free] (Idamycin PFS®): 1 mg/mL (5 mL, 10 mL, 20 mL)

Ifex® [US/Can] see ifosfamide on this page

IFLrA see interferon alfa-2a on page 353

ifosfamide (eye FOSS fa mide)

U.S./Canadian Brand Names Ifex® [US/Can]

Therapeutic Category Antineoplastic Agent

Use In combination with other antineoplastics in treatment of lung cancer, Hodgkin's and non-Hodgkin's lymphoma, breast cancer, acute and chronic lymphocytic leukemia, ovarian cancer, testicular cancer, and sarcomas

Usual Dosage I.V. (refer to individual protocols):

Children: 1800 mg/m^2/day for 3-5 days every 21-28 days or 5000 mg/m^2 as a single 24-hour infusion or 3 g/m^2/day for 2 days

Adults: 700-2000 mg/m^2/day for 5 days or 2400 mg/m^2/day for 3 days every 21-28 days; 5000 mg/m^2 as a single dose over 24 hours

Dosage Forms Injection, powder for reconstitution: 1 g, 3 g [packaged with Mesnex® (mesna) 1 g]

IG *see* immune globulin (intramuscular) *on next page*

IGIM *see* immune globulin (intramuscular) *on next page*

IGIV *see* immune globulin (intravenous) *on page 347*

IL-1Ra *see* anakinra *on page 42*

IL-11 *see* oprelvekin *on page 478*

Ilopan-Choline® Oral *(Discontinued)* *see page 814*

Ilopan® Injection *(Discontinued)* *see page 814*

Ilosone® Pulvules® *(Discontinued)* *see page 814*

Ilozyme® *(Discontinued)* *see page 814*

imatinib (eye MAT eh nib)
Synonyms CGP 57148B; glivec; imatinib mesylate; ST1571
U.S./Canadian Brand Names Gleevec™ [US]
Therapeutic Category Antineoplastic, Tyrosine Kinase Inhibitor
Use Treatment of patients with chronic myeloid leukemia (CML) in blast crisis, accelerated phase, or in chronic phase after failure of interferon-alpha therapy
Usual Dosage Oral: Adults: Dose should be taken with food and large glass of water:
Chronic myeloid leukemia (CML):
Chronic phase: 400 mg once daily; may be increased to 600 mg daily in the event of disease progression, loss of previously achieved response, or failure to achieve response after at least 3 months of therapy and in the absence of severe adverse reaction
Accelerated phase or blast crisis: 600 mg once daily; may be increased to 800 mg daily (400 mg twice daily) in the event of disease progression, loss of previously achieved response, or failure to achieve response after at least 3 months of therapy and in the absence of severe adverse reaction
Dosage Forms Capsule, as mesylate: 100 mg

imatinib mesylate *see* imatinib *on this page*

Imdur® [US/Can] *see* isosorbide mononitrate *on page 362*

imidazole carboxamide *see* dacarbazine *on page 172*

imiglucerase (i mi GLOO ser ace)
U.S./Canadian Brand Names Cerezyme® [US]
Therapeutic Category Enzyme
Use Long-term enzyme replacement therapy for patients with Type 1 Gaucher's disease
Usual Dosage I.V.: 2.5 units/kg 3 times/week up to as much as 60 units/kg administered as frequently as once weekly or as infrequently as every 4 weeks; 60 units/kg administered every 2 weeks is the most common dose
Dosage Forms Injection, powder for reconstitution [preservative free]: 200 units, 400 units

imipemide *see* imipenem and cilastatin *on this page*

imipenem and cilastatin (i mi PEN em & sye la STAT in)
Synonyms cilastatin and imipenem; imipemide
U.S./Canadian Brand Names Primaxin® [US/Can]
Therapeutic Category Carbapenem (Antibiotic)
Use Treatment of documented multidrug resistant gram-negative infection due to organisms proven or suspected to be susceptible to imipenem/cilastatin; treatment of multiple organism infection in which other agents have an insufficient spectrum of
(Continued)

imipenem and cilastatin *(Continued)*

activity or are contraindicated due to toxic potential; therapeutic alternative for treatment of gram negative sepsis in immunocompromised patients

Usual Dosage I.V. infusion (dosage recommendation based on imipenem component):
Children: 60-100 mg/kg/day in 4 divided doses
Adults:
Serious infection: 2-4 g/day in 3-4 divided doses
Mild to moderate infection: 1-2 g/day in 3-4 divided doses

Dosage Forms
Injection, powder for reconstitution [I.M.]: Imipenem 500 mg and cilastatin 500 mg
Injection, powder for reconstitution [I.V.]: Imipenem 250 mg and cilastatin 250 mg; Imipenem 500 mg and cilastatin 500 mg

imipramine (im IP ra meen)

U.S./Canadian Brand Names Apo®-Imipramine [Can]; Tofranil-PM® [US]; Tofranil® [US/Can]

Therapeutic Category Antidepressant, Tricyclic (Tertiary Amine)

Use Treatment of various forms of depression, often in conjunction with psychotherapy; enuresis in children; analgesic for certain chronic and neuropathic pain

Usual Dosage
Children: Oral (safety and efficacy of imipramine therapy for treatment of depression in children <12 years have not been established):
Enuresis: ≥6 years: Initial: 10-25 mg at bedtime, if inadequate response still seen after 1 week of therapy, increase by 25 mg/day; dose should not exceed 2.5 mg/kg/day or 50 mg at bedtime if 6-12 years of age or 75 mg at bedtime if ≥12 years of age
Adjunct in the treatment of cancer pain: Initial: 0.2-0.4 mg/kg at bedtime; dose may be increased by 50% every 2-3 days up to 1-3 mg/kg/dose at bedtime
Adolescents: Oral: Initial: 25-50 mg/day; increase gradually; maximum: 100 mg/day in single or divided doses
Adults:
Oral: Initial: 25 mg 3-4 times/day, increase dose gradually, total dose may be administered at bedtime; maximum: 300 mg/day
I.M.: Initial: Up to 100 mg/day in divided doses; change to oral as soon as possible

Dosage Forms
Capsule, as pamoate (Tofranil-PM®): 75 mg, 100 mg, 125 mg, 150 mg
Tablet, as hydrochloride (Tofranil®): 10 mg, 25 mg, 50 mg [generic tablets may contain sodium benzoate]

imiquimod (i mi KWI mod)

U.S./Canadian Brand Names Aldara™ [US/Can]

Therapeutic Category Immune Response Modifier

Use Treatment of external genital and perianal warts/condyloma acuminata in children ≥12 years of age and adults

Usual Dosage Adults: Topical: Apply 3 times/week, prior to bedtime, leave on for 6-10 hours; remove cream by washing area with mild soap and water

Dosage Forms Cream: 5% (12s) [contains benzyl alcohol; single-dose packets]

Imitrex® [US/Can] *see* sumatriptan succinate *on page 615*

ImmuCyst® [Can] *see* BCG vaccine *on page 72*

immune globulin (intramuscular)

(i MYUN GLOB yoo lin IN tra MUS kyoo ler)

Synonyms gamma globulin; IG; IGIM; immune serum globulin; ISG

U.S./Canadian Brand Names BayGam® [US/Can]

Therapeutic Category Immune Globulin

Use Prophylaxis against hepatitis A, measles, varicella, and possibly rubella and immunoglobulin deficiency, idiopathic thrombocytopenia purpura, Kawasaki syndrome, lymphocytic leukemia

Usual Dosage I.M.:
Hepatitis A: 0.02 mL/kg
IgG: 1.3 mL/kg then 0.66 mL/kg in 3-4 weeks
Measles: 0.25 mL/kg
Rubella: 0.55 mL/kg
Varicella: 0.6-1.2 mL/kg

Dosage Forms Injection, solution [preservative free]: 15% to 18% (2 mL, 10 mL)

immune globulin (intravenous) (i MYUN GLOB yoo lin IN tra VEE nus)

Synonyms IGIV; IVIG

U.S./Canadian Brand Names Carimune™ [US]; Gamimune® N [US/Can]; Gammagard® S/D [US/Can]; Gammar®-P I.V. [US]; Iveegam EN [US]; Iveegam Immuno® [Can]; Panglobulin® [US]; Polygam® S/D [US]; Venoglobulin®-S [US]

Therapeutic Category Immune Globulin

Use Immunodeficiency syndrome, idiopathic thrombocytopenic purpura (ITP) and B-cell chronic lymphocytic leukemia (CLL); used in conjunction with appropriate anti-infective therapy to prevent or modify acute bacterial or viral infections in patients with iatrogenically-induced or disease-associated immunodepression; autoimmune neutropenia, bone marrow transplantation patients, Kawasaki disease, Guillain-Barré syndrome, demyelinating polyneuropathies

Usual Dosage Children and Adults: I.V. infusion:
Immunodeficiency syndrome: 100-200 mg/kg/dose every month; may increase to 400 mg/kg/dose as needed
Idiopathic thrombocytopenic purpura: 400-1000 mg/kg/dose for 2-5 consecutive days; maintenance dose: 400-1000 mg/kg/dose every 3-6 weeks based on clinical response and platelet count
Kawasaki disease: 400 mg/kg/day for 4 days or 2 g/kg as a single dose
Congenital and acquired antibody deficiency syndrome: 100-400 mg/kg/dose every 3-4 weeks
Bone marrow transplant: 500 mg/kg/week
Severe systemic viral and bacterial infections: Children: 500-1000 mg/kg/week

Dosage Forms
Injection, solution [preservative free; solvent detergent-treated]:
Gamimune® N: 10% [100 mg/mL] (10 mL, 50 mL, 100 mL, 200 mL)
Venoglobulin® S: 5% [50 mg/mL] (50 mL, 100 mL, 200 mL); 10% [100 mg/mL] (50 mL, 100 mL, 200 mL) [stabilized with human albumin]
Injection, powder for reconstitution [preservative free]:
Carimune™, Panglobulin®: 1 g, 3 g, 6 g, 12 g
Gammar®-P I.V.: 1 g, 2.5 g, 5 g, 10 g [stabilized with human albumin and sucrose]
Iveegam EN: 0.5 g, 1 g, 2.5 g, 5 g [stabilized with glucose]
Injection, powder for reconstitution [preservative free, solvent detergent treated] (Gammagard® S/D): 2.5 g, 5 g, 10 g [stabilized with human albumin, glycine, glucose, and polyethylene glycol]

immune serum globulin *see* immune globulin (intramuscular) *on previous page*

Immunine® VH [Can] *see* factor IX (purified/human) *on page 261*

Imodium® [US/Can] *see* loperamide *on page 390*

Imodium® A-D [US-OTC] *see* loperamide *on page 390*

Imogam® [US] *see* rabies immune globulin (human) *on page 561*

Imogam® Rabies Pasteurized [Can] *see* rabies immune globulin (human) *on page 561*

Imogen® [US] *see* loperamide *on page 390*

Imotil® [US] *see* loperamide *on page 390*

Imovane® [Can] *see* zopiclone *(Canada only) on page 693*

Imovax® Rabies [US/Can] *see* rabies virus vaccine *on page 561*

Imperim® [US-OTC] *see* loperamide *on page 390*

Imuran® [US/Can] *see* azathioprine *on page 65*

In-111 zevalin *see* ibritumomab *on page 342*

inamrinone (eye NAM ri none)
Synonyms amrinone; inamrinone lactate
Therapeutic Category Adrenergic Agonist Agent
Use Treatment of low cardiac output states (sepsis, congestive heart failure); adjunctive therapy of pulmonary hypertension

To avoid confusion with amiodarone, the generic name "amrinone" changed to "inamrinone" on July, 2000

Usual Dosage Dosage is based on clinical response. **Note:** Dose should not exceed 10 mg/kg/24 hours.

Children: 0.75 mg/kg I.V. bolus over 2-3 minutes followed by maintenance infusion 5-10 mcg/kg/minute; I.V. bolus may need to be repeated in 30 minutes
Adults: 0.75 mg/kg I.V. bolus over 2-3 minutes followed by maintenance infusion of 5-10 mcg/kg/minute

Dosage Forms Injection, as lactate: 5 mg/mL (20 mL)

inamrinone lactate *see* inamrinone *on this page*

I-Naphline® Ophthalmic *(Discontinued) see page 814*

Inapsine® [US] *see* droperidol *on page 217*

indapamide (in DAP a mide)
U.S./Canadian Brand Names Apo®-Indapamide [Can]; Gen-Indapamide [Can]; Lozide® [Can]; Lozol® [US/Can]; Novo-Indapamide [Can]; Nu-Indapamide [Can]; PMS-Indapamide [Can]
Therapeutic Category Diuretic, Miscellaneous
Use Management of mild to moderate hypertension; treatment of edema in congestive heart failure and nephrotic syndrome
Usual Dosage Adults: Oral: 2.5-5 mg/day
Dosage Forms Tablet: 1.25 mg, 2.5 mg

Inderal® [US/Can] *see* propranolol *on page 549*

Inderal® LA [US/Can] *see* propranolol *on page 549*

Inderide® [US] *see* propranolol and hydrochlorothiazide *on page 550*

Inderide® LA [US] *see* propranolol and hydrochlorothiazide *on page 550*

indinavir (in DIN a veer)
U.S./Canadian Brand Names Crixivan® [US/Can]
Therapeutic Category Antiviral Agent
Use Treatment of HIV infection, especially advanced disease; usually administered as part of a three-drug regimen (two nucleosides plus a protease inhibitor) or double therapy (one nucleoside plus a protease inhibitor)
Usual Dosage Adults: Oral: 800 mg every 8 hours
Dosage Forms Capsule, as sulfate: 100 mg, 200 mg, 333 mg, 400 mg

Indocid® [Can] *see* indomethacin *on next page*

Indocid® P.D.A. [Can] *see* indomethacin *on next page*

Indocin® [US] *see* indomethacin *on next page*

Indocin® I.V. [US] *see* indomethacin *on next page*

Indocin® SR [US] *see* indomethacin *on this page*

indocyanine green (in doe SYE a neen green)
U.S./Canadian Brand Names IC-Green® [US]
Therapeutic Category Diagnostic Agent
Use Determining hepatic function, cardiac output and liver blood flow and for ophthalmic angiography
Usual Dosage Dilute dose in sterile water for injection or 0.9% NaCl to final volume of 1 mL if necessary doses may be repeated periodically; total dose should not exceed 2 mg/kg

Infants: 1.25 mg
Children: 2.5 mg
Adults: 5 mg

Dosage Forms Injection, powder for reconstitution: 25 mg [supplied with diluent]

Indo-Lemmon [Can] *see* indomethacin *on this page*

indometacin *see* indomethacin *on this page*

indomethacin (in doe METH a sin)
Synonyms indometacin
U.S./Canadian Brand Names Apo®-Indomethacin [Can]; Indocid® [Can]; Indocid® P.D.A. [Can]; Indocin® I.V. [US]; Indocin® SR [US]; Indocin® [US]; Indo-Lemmon [Can]; Indotec [Can]; Novo-Methacin [Can]; Nu-Indo [Can]; Rhodacine® [Can]
Therapeutic Category Analgesic, Non-narcotic; Nonsteroidal Anti-inflammatory Drug (NSAID)
Use Management of inflammatory diseases and rheumatoid disorders; moderate pain; acute gouty arthritis, acute bursitis/tendonitis, moderate to severe osteoarthritis, rheumatoid arthritis, ankylosing spondylitis; I.V. form used as alternative to surgery for closure of patent ductus arteriosus in neonates
Usual Dosage
Patent ductus arteriosus:
Neonates: I.V.: Initial: 0.2 mg/kg, followed by 2 doses depending on postnatal age (PNA):
PNA **at time of first dose** <48 hours: 0.1 mg/kg at 12- to 24-hour intervals
PNA **at time of first dose** 2-7 days: 0.2 mg/kg at 12- to 24-hour intervals
PNA **at time of first dose** >7 days: 0.25 mg/kg at 12- to 24-hour intervals
In general, may use 12-hour dosing interval if urine output >1 mL/kg/hour after prior dose; use 24-hour dosing interval if urine output is <1 mL/kg/hour but >0.6 mL/kg/hour; doses should be withheld if patient has oliguria (urine output <0.6 mL/kg/hour) or anuria
Inflammatory/rheumatoid disorders: Oral:
Children: 1-2 mg/kg/day in 2-4 divided doses; maximum dose: 4 mg/kg/day; not to exceed 150-200 mg/day
Adults: 25-50 mg/dose 2-3 times/day; maximum dose: 200 mg/day; extended release capsule should be given on a 1-2 times/day schedule
Dosage Forms
Capsule (Indocin®): 25 mg, 50 mg
Capsule, sustained release (Indocin® SR): 75 mg
Injection, powder for reconstitution, as sodium trihydrate (Indocin® I.V.): 1 mg
Suspension, oral (Indocin®): 25 mg/5 mL (237 mL) [contains alcohol 1%; pineapple-coconut-mint flavor]

Indotec [Can] *see* indomethacin *on this page*

INF-alpha 2 *see* interferon alfa-2b *on page 354*

Infanrix® [US] *see* diphtheria, tetanus toxoids, and acellular pertussis vaccine *on page 204*

Infantaire [US-OTC] *see* acetaminophen *on page 3*

infliximab (in FLIKS e mab)

U.S./Canadian Brand Names Remicade® [US]

Therapeutic Category Monoclonal Antibody

Use

Crohn's disease: Reduce the signs and symptoms of moderate to severe disease in patients who have an inadequate response to conventional therapy; reduce the number of draining enterocutaneous fistulas in fistulizing disease

Rheumatoid arthritis: Used with methotrexate in patients who have had an inadequate response to methotrexate alone; used with methotrexate to inhibit the progression of structural damage and improve physical function in patients with moderate to severe disease

Usual Dosage

Moderately to severely active Crohn's disease: Adults: I.V.: 5 mg/kg as a single infusion over a minimum of 2 hours

Fistulizing Crohn's disease: 5 mg/kg as an infusion over a minimum of 2 hours, dose repeated at 2 and 6 weeks after the initial infusion

Dosage Forms Injection, powder for reconstitution: 100 mg

influenza virus vaccine (in floo EN za VYE rus vak SEEN)

Synonyms influenza virus vaccine (inactivated whole-virus); influenza virus vaccine (purified surface antigen); influenza virus vaccine (split-virus)

U.S./Canadian Brand Names FluShield® [US]; Fluviral S/F® [Can]; Fluvirin® [US]; Fluzone® [US/Can]; Vaxigrip® [Can]

Therapeutic Category Vaccine, Inactivated Virus

Use Provide active immunity to influenza virus strains contained in the vaccine; for high-risk persons, previous year vaccines should not be used to prevent present year influenza

Groups at Increased Risk for Influenza-Related Complications:

- Persons ≥65 years of age
- Residents of nursing homes and other chronic-care facilities that house persons of any age with chronic medical conditions
- Adults and children with chronic disorders of the pulmonary or cardiovascular systems, including children with asthma
- Adults and children who have required regular medical follow-up or hospitalization during the preceding year because of chronic metabolic diseases (including diabetes mellitus), renal dysfunction, hemoglobinopathies, or immunosuppression (including immunosuppression caused by medications)
- Children and adolescents (6 months to 18 years of age) who are receiving long-term aspirin therapy and therefore, may be at risk for developing Reye's syndrome after influenza
- Women who will be in the 2nd or 3rd trimester of pregnancy during the influenza season

Otherwise healthy children aged 6-23 months, healthy persons who may transmit influenza to those at risk, and others who are interested in immunization to influenza virus should receive the vaccine as long as supply is available.

Usual Dosage Annual vaccination with current vaccine; either whole- or split-virus vaccine may be used

Dosage Forms

Injection, solution, purified split-virus (FluShield®): (5 mL) [contains thimerosal; packaging contains dry natural rubber; manufactured with gentamicin]

Injection, solution, purified split-virus surface antigen [preservative free, prefilled syringe] (Fluvirin®): (0.5 mL) [contains thimerosal (trace amounts); manufactured using neomycin and polymyxin]

Injection, suspension, purified split-virus:

Fluzone®: (0.5 mL) [prefilled syringe; contains thimerosal]; (5 mL) [vial; contains thimerosal]

Fluzone® [preservative free, prefilled syringe]: (0.25 mL, 0.5 mL) [contains thimerosal (trace amount)]

influenza virus vaccine (inactivated whole-virus) *see* influenza virus vaccine *on previous page*

influenza virus vaccine (purified surface antigen) *see* influenza virus vaccine *on previous page*

influenza virus vaccine (split-virus) *see* influenza virus vaccine *on previous page*

Infufer® **[Can]** *see* iron dextran complex *on page 360*

Infumorph® **[US]** *see* morphine sulfate *on page 437*

INH *see* isoniazid *on page 361*

inhalation devices (in hal LAY shun deh VYE sez)

U.S./Canadian Brand Names AeroChamber™ [US]; InspirEase™ [US]

Therapeutic Category Inhalation, Miscellaneous

Use Improves the distribution and deposition in the lungs of aerosolized medication from metered dose inhalers (MDIs)

Dosage Forms

AeroChamber™, AeroChamber™ with mask (small, medium)

Inhalation kit (InspirEase™)

Replacement bags (InspirEase™)

Inhibace® **[Can]** *see* cilazapril *(Canada only) on page 146*

Innohep® **[US/Can]** *see* tinzaparin *on page 640*

Innovar® **[US]** *see* droperidol and fentanyl *on page 217*

Inocor® ***(Discontinued)*** *see page 814*

INOmax® **[US/Can]** *see* nitric oxide *on page 461*

insect sting kit (IN sekt sting kit)

U.S./Canadian Brand Names Ana-Kit® [US]

Therapeutic Category Antidote

Use Anaphylaxis emergency treatment of insect bites or stings by the sensitive patient that may occur within minutes of insect sting or exposure to an allergic substance

Usual Dosage Children and Adults:

Epinephrine:

<2 years: 0.05-0.1 mL

2-6 years: 0.15 mL

6-12 years: 0.2 mL

>12 years : 0.3 mL

Chlorpheniramine:

<6 years: 1 tablet

6-12 years: 2 tablets

>12 years: 4 tablets

Dosage Forms Kit: Epinephrine hydrochloride 1:1000 (1 mL syringe), chlorpheniramine maleate chewable tablet 2 mg (4), sterile alcohol pads (2), tourniquet

InspirEase™ [US] *see* inhalation devices *on previous page*
Insta-Glucose® [US-OTC] *see* glucose (instant) *on page 300*

insulin preparations (IN su lin prep a RAY shuns)

U.S./Canadian Brand Names Humalog® Mix 75/25™ [US]; Humalog® [US/Can]; Humulin® 50/50 [US]; Humulin® 70/30 [US/Can]; Humulin® 80/20 [Can]; Humulin® L [US/Can]; Humulin® N [US/Can]; Humulin® R (Concentrated) U-500 [US]; Humulin® R [US/Can]; Humulin® U [US/Can]; Lantus® [US]; Lente® Iletin® II [US]; Novolin® 70/30 [US]; Novolin®ge [Can]; Novolin® L [US]; Novolin® N [US]; Novolin® R [US]; NovoLog® [US]; NPH Iletin® II [US]; Regular Iletin® II [US]; Velosulin® BR (Buffered) [US]

Therapeutic Category Antidiabetic Agent, Parenteral

Use Treatment of insulin-dependent diabetes mellitus, also noninsulin-dependent diabetes mellitus unresponsive to treatment with diet and/or oral hypoglycemics; to assure proper utilization of glucose and reduce glucosuria in nondiabetic patients receiving parenteral nutrition whose glucosuria cannot be adequately controlled with infusion rate adjustments or those who require assistance in achieving optimal caloric intakes; hyperkalemia (regular insulin only; use with glucose to shift potassium into cells to lower serum potassium levels)

Usual Dosage Dose requires continuous medical supervision; may administer I.V. (regular), I.M., S.C.

Diabetes mellitus: The number and size of daily doses, time of administration, and diet and exercise require continuous medical supervision. In addition, specific formulations may require distinct administration procedures.

Lispro should be given within 15 minutes before or immediately after a meal

Human regular insulin should be given within 30-60 minutes before a meal.

Intermediate-acting insulins may be administered 1-2 times/day.

Long-acting insulins may be administered once daily.

Insulin glargine (Lantus®) should be administered subcutaneously once daily at bedtime. Maintenance doses should be administered subcutaneously and sites should be rotated to prevent lipodystrophy.

Children and Adults: 0.5-1 unit/kg/day in divided doses

Adolescents (growth spurts): 0.8-1.2 units/kg/day in divided doses

Adjust dose to maintain premeal and bedtime blood glucose of 80-140 mg/dL (children <5 years: 100-200 mg/dL)

Insulin glargine (Lantus®):

Type 2 diabetes (patient not already on insulin): 10 units once daily, adjusted according to patient response (range in clinical study 2-100 units/day)

Patients already receiving insulin: In clinical studies, when changing to insulin glargine from once-daily NPH or Ultralente® insulin, the initial dose was not changed; when changing from twice-daily NPH to once daily insulin glargine, the total daily dose was reduced by 20% and adjusted according to patient response

Hyperkalemia: Administer calcium gluconate and $NaHCO_3$ first then 50% dextrose at 0.5-1 mL/kg and insulin 1 unit for every 4-5 g dextrose given

Diabetic ketoacidosis: Children and Adults: Regular insulin: I.V. loading dose: 0.1 unit/kg, then maintenance continuous infusion: 0.1 unit/kg/hour (range: 0.05-0.2 units/kg/hour depending upon the rate of decrease of serum glucose - too rapid decrease of serum glucose may lead to cerebral edema)

Optimum rate of decrease (serum glucose): 80-100 mg/dL/hour

Note: Newly diagnosed patients with IDDM presenting in DKA and patients with blood sugars <800 mg/dL may be relatively "sensitive" to insulin and should receive loading and initial maintenance doses approximately ½ of those indicated above.

Dosage Forms

RAPID-ACTING:

Injection, solution, aspart, human:

NovoLog®: 100 units/mL (10 mL vial)

NovoLog® [PenFill®]: 100 units/mL (3 mL cartridge)

Injection, solution, lispro, human (Humalog®): 100 units/mL (1.5 mL cartridge, 3 mL disposable pen, 10 mL vial)

SHORT-ACTING:
Injection, solution, regular, human:
Humulin® R: 100 units/mL (10 mL vial)
Novolin® R: 100 units/mL (1.5 mL prefilled syringe, 10 mL vial)
Novolin® R [PenFill®]: 100 units/mL (1.5 mL cartridge, 3 mL cartridge)
Injection, solution, regular, human, buffered (Velosulin® BR): 100 units/mL (10 mL vial)
Injection, solution, regular, human, concentrate (Humulin® R U-500): 500 units/mL (20 mL vial)
Injection, solution, regular, purified pork (Regular Iletin II): 100 units/mL (10 mL vial)

INTERMEDIATE-ACTING:
Injection, suspension, lente, human [zinc] (Humulin® L, Novolin® L): 100 units/mL (10 mL vial)
Injection, suspension, lente, purified pork [zinc] (Lente® Iletin II): 100 units/mL (10 mL vial)
Injection, suspension, NPH, human [isophane]:
Humulin® N: 100 units/mL (3 mL disposable pen, 10 mL vial)
Novolin® N: 100 units/mL (1.5 mL prefilled syringe, 10 mL vial)
Novolin® N [PenFill®]: 100 units/mL (1.5 mL cartridge, 3 mL cartridge)
Injection, suspension, NPH, purified pork [isophane] (NPH Iletin® II): 100 units/mL (10 mL vial)

LONG-ACTING:
Injection, suspension, Ultralente®, human [zinc] (Humulin U Ultralente®): 100 units/mL (10 mL vial)
Injection, solution, glargine, human (Lantus®): 100 unit/mL (10 mL vial)

COMBINATION, INTERMEDIATE-ACTING:
Injection, lispro human suspension 75% and rapid-acting lispro human solution 25% (Humalog® Mix 75/25™): 100 units/mL (3 mL disposable pen, 10 mL vial)
Injection, NPH human insulin suspension 50% and short-acting regular human insulin solution 50% (Humulin® 50/50): 100 units/mL (10 mL vial)
Injection, NPH human insulin suspension 70% and short-acting regular human insulin solution 30%:
Humulin® 70/30: 100 units/mL (3 mL disposable pen, 10 mL vial)
Humulin® 80/20: 100 units/mL (3 mL disposable pen, 10 mL vial)
Novolin® 70/30: 100 units/mL (1.5 mL prefilled syringe, 10 mL vial)
Novolin® 70/30 [PenFill®]: 100 units/mL (1.5 mL cartridge, 3 mL cartridge)

Intal® [US/Can] *see* cromolyn sodium *on page 166*

Intal® Inhalation Capsule *(Discontinued)* *see page 814*

Integrilin® [US/Can] *see* eptifibatide *on page 232*

Intercept™ *(Discontinued)* *see page 814*

α-2-interferon *see* interferon alfa-2b *on next page*

interferon alfa-2a (in ter FEER on AL fa-too aye)

Synonyms IFLrA; rIFN-A
U.S./Canadian Brand Names Roferon-A® [US/Can]
Therapeutic Category Biological Response Modulator
Use Hairy cell leukemia, AIDS-related Kaposi's sarcoma in patients >18 years of age, multiple unlabeled uses
Usual Dosage
Children: S.C.: Pulmonary hemangiomatosis: 1-3 million units/m²/day once daily
Adults >18 years:
Hairy cell leukemia: I.M., S.C.: Induction dose is 3 million units/day for 16-24 weeks; maintenance: 3 million units 3 times/week
AIDS-related Kaposi's sarcoma: I.M., S.C.: Induction dose is 36 million units for 10-12 weeks; maintenance: 36 million units 3 times/week (may begin with dose escalation
(Continued)

interferon alfa-2a *(Continued)*

from 3-9-18 million units each day over 3 consecutive days followed by 36 million units daily for the remainder of the 10-12 weeks of induction)

Dosage Forms

Injection, solution [multidose vial]: 6 million units/mL (3 mL) [contains benzyl alcohol]

Injection, solution, [single-dose prefilled syringe; S.C. use only]: 3 million units/0.5 mL (0.5 mL); 6 million units/0.5 mL (0.5 mL); 9 million units/0.5 mL (0.5 mL) [contains benzyl alcohol]

Injection, solution [single-dose vial]: 36 million units/mL (1 mL) [contains benzyl alcohol]

interferon alfa-2b (in ter FEER on AL fa-too bee)

Synonyms INF-alpha 2; α-2-interferon; rLFN-α2

U.S./Canadian Brand Names Intron® A [US/Can]

Therapeutic Category Biological Response Modulator

Use AIDS-related thrombocytopenia, cutaneous ulcerations of Behçet's disease, carcinoid syndrome, cervical cancer, lymphomatoid granulomatosis, genital herpes, hepatitis D, chronic myelogenous leukemia (CML), non-Hodgkin's lymphomas (other than follicular lymphoma, see approved use), polycythemia vera, medullary thyroid carcinoma, multiple myeloma, renal cell carcinoma, basal and squamous cell skin cancers, essential thrombocytopenia, thrombocytopenic purpura

Investigational: West Nile virus

Usual Dosage Refer to individual protocols

Children 1-17 years: Chronic hepatitis B: S.C.: 3 million units/m² 3 times/week for 1 week; then 6 million units/m² 3 times/week; maximum: 10 million units 3 times/week; total duration of therapy 16-24 weeks

Adults:

Hairy cell leukemia: I.M., S.C.: 2 million units/m² 3 times/week for 2-6 months

Lymphoma (follicular): S.C.: 5 million units 3 times/week for up to 18 months

Malignant melanoma: 20 million units/m² I.V. for 5 consecutive days per week for 4 weeks, then 10 million units/m² S.C. 3 times/week for 48 weeks

AIDS-related Kaposi's sarcoma: I.M., S.C.: 30 million units/m² 3 times/week

Chronic hepatitis B: I.M., S.C.: 5 million units/day or 10 million units 3 times/week for 16 weeks

Chronic hepatitis C: I.M., S.C.: 3 million units 3 times/week for 16 weeks. In patients with normalization of ALT at 16 weeks, continue treatment for 18-24 months; consider discontinuation if normalization does not occur at 16 weeks. **Note:** May be used in combination therapy with ribavirin in previously untreated patients or in patients who relapse following alpha interferon therapy; refer to Interferon Alfa-2b and Ribavirin Combination Pack monograph.

Condyloma acuminata: Intralesionally: 1 million units/lesion (maximum: 5 lesions/treatment) 3 times/week (on alternate days) for 3 weeks. Use 1 million unit per 0.1 mL concentration.

Dosage Forms

Injection, powder for reconstitution: 3 million units; 5 million units; 10 million units; 18 million units; 25 million units; 50 million units [contains human albumin; diluent contains benzyl alcohol]

Injection, solution [multidose prefilled pen]:

Delivers 3 million units/0.2 mL (1.5 mL) [delivers 6 doses; 18 million units]

Delivers 5 million units/0.2 mL (1.5 mL) [delivers 6 doses; 30 million units]

Delivers 10 million units/0.2 mL (1.5 mL) [delivers 6 doses; 60 million units]

Injection, solution [multidose vial]: 6 million units/mL (3 mL); 10 million units/mL (2.5 mL)

Injection, solution [single-dose vial]: 3 million units/ 0.5 mL (0.5 mL); 5 million units/0.5 mL (0.5 mL); 10 million units/ mL (1 mL)

See also interferon alfa-2b and ribavirin combination pack monograph.

interferon alfa-2b and ribavirin combination pack

(in ter FEER on AL fa-too bee & rye ba VYE rin com bi NAY shun pak)

U.S./Canadian Brand Names Rebetron™ [US/Can]

Therapeutic Category Antiviral Agent; Biological Response Modulator

Use The combination therapy is indicated for the treatment of chronic hepatitis C in patients with compensated liver disease who have relapsed following alpha interferon therapy

Usual Dosage The recommended dosage of combination therapy is 3 million int. units of Intron® A injected subcutaneously three times per week and 1000-1200 mg of Rebetrol® capsules administered orally in a divided daily (morning and evening) dose for 24 weeks; patients weighing 75 kg (165 pounds) or less should receive 1000 mg of Rebetrol® daily, while patients weighing more than 75 kg should receive 1200 mg of Rebetrol® daily

Dosage Forms

Combination package for patients ≥75 kg:

Injection, solution: Interferon alfa-2b (Intron® A): 3 million int. units/0.5 mL (0.5 mL) [6 vials (3 million int. units/vial), 6 syringes and alcohol swabs]
Capsules: Ribavirin (Rebetol®): 200 mg (70s)

Injection, solution: Interferon alfa-2b (Intron® A): 3 million int. units/0.5 mL (3.8 mL) [1 multidose vial (18 million int. units/vial), 6 syringes and alcohol swabs]
Capsules: Ribavirin (Rebetol®): 200 mg (70s)

Injection, solution: Interferon alfa-2b (Intron® A): 3 million int. units/0.2 mL (1.5 mL) [1 multidose pen (18 million int. units/pen), 6 needles and alcohol swabs]
Capsules: Ribavirin (Rebetol®): 200 mg (70s)

Combination package for patients >75 kg:

Injection, solution: Interferon alfa-2b (Intron® A): 3 million int. units/0.5 mL (0.5 mL) [6 vials (3 million int. units/vial), 6 syringes and alcohol swabs]
Capsules: Ribavirin (Rebetol®): 200 mg (84s)

Injection, solution: Interferon alfa-2b (Intron® A): 3 million int. units/0.5 mL (3.8 mL) [1 multidose vial (18 million int. units/vial), 6 syringes and alcohol swabs]
Capsules: Ribavirin (Rebetol®): 200 mg (84s)

Injection, solution: Interferon alfa-2b (Intron® A): 3 million int. units/0.2 mL (1.5 mL) [1 multidose pen (18 million int. units/pen), 6 needles and alcohol swabs]
Capsules: Ribavirin (Rebetol®): 200 mg (84s)

Combination package for Rebetol® dose reduction:

Injection, solution: Interferon alfa-2b (Intron® A): 3 million int. units/0.5 mL (0.5 mL) [6 vials (3 million int. units/vial), 6 syringes and alcohol swabs]
Capsules: Ribavirin (Rebetol®): 200 mg (42s)

Injection, solution: Interferon alfa-2b (Intron® A): 3 million int. units/0.5 mL (3.8 mL) [1 multidose vial (18 million int. units/vial), 6 syringes and alcohol swabs]
Capsules: Ribavirin (Rebetol®): 200 mg (42s)

Injection, solution: Interferon alfa-2b (Intron® A): 3 million int. units/0.2 mL (1.5 mL) [1 multidose pen (18 million int. units/pen), 6 needles and alcohol swabs]
Capsules: Ribavirin (Rebetol®): 200 mg (42s)

interferon alfacon-1 (in ter FEER on AL fa con-one)

U.S./Canadian Brand Names Infergen® [US/Can]

Therapeutic Category Interferon

Use Treatment of chronic hepatitis C virus (HCV) infection in patients ≥18 years of age with compensated liver disease and anti-HCV serum antibodies or HCV RNA.

Usual Dosage Adults ≥18 years: S.C.:

Chronic HCV infection: 9 mcg 3 times/week for 24 weeks; allow 48 hours between doses

(Continued)

interferon alfacon-1 *(Continued)*

Patients who have previously tolerated interferon therapy but did not respond or relapsed: 15 mcg 3 times/week for 6 months

Dose reduction for toxicity: Dose should be held in patients who experience a severe adverse reaction, and treatment should be stopped or decreased if the reaction does not become tolerable

Doses were reduced from 9 mcg to 7.5 mcg in the pivotal study

For patients receiving 15 mcg/dose, doses were reduced in 3 mcg increments. Efficacy is decreased with doses <7.5 mcg

Dosage Forms Injection, solution [preservative free; prefilled syringe or single-dose vial]; 30 mcg/mL (0.3 mL, 0.5 mL)

interferon alfa-n3 (in ter FEER on AL fa-en three)

U.S./Canadian Brand Names Alferon® N [US/Can]

Therapeutic Category Biological Response Modulator

Use Intralesional treatment of refractory or recurring genital or venereal warts; useful in patients who do not respond or are not candidates for usual treatments; indications and dosage regimens are specific for a particular brand of interferon

Usual Dosage Adults: Inject 250,000 units (0.05 mL) in each wart twice weekly for a maximum of 8 weeks; therapy should not be repeated for at least 3 months after the initial 8-week course of therapy

Dosage Forms Injection, solution: 5 million int. units (1 mL) [contains albumin]

interferon beta-1a (in ter FEER on BAY-ta won aye)

U.S./Canadian Brand Names Avonex® [US/Can]; Rebif® [US/Can]

Therapeutic Category Biological Response Modulator

Use Treatment of relapsing forms of multiple sclerosis (MS); to slow the accumulation of physical disability and decrease the frequency of clinical exacerbations

Usual Dosage Adults >18 years: I.M.: 30 mcg once weekly

Dosage Forms

Injection, powder for reconstitution (Avonex®): 33 mcg [6.6 million units] [contains albumin; packaged with diluent, alcohol wipes, and access pin and needle]

Injection, solution [preservative free; prefilled syringe] (Rebif®): 22 mcg/mL (0.5 mL); 44 mcg/mL (0.5 mL) [contains albumin]

interferon beta-1b (in ter FEER on BAY ta-won bee)

U.S./Canadian Brand Names Betaseron® [US/Can]

Therapeutic Category Biological Response Modulator

Use Reduce the frequency of clinical exacerbations in ambulatory patients with relapsing-remitting multiple sclerosis

Usual Dosage Adults: S.C.: 0.25 mg every other day

Dosage Forms Injection, powder for reconstitution: 0.3 mg [9.6 million units] [contains albumin; packaged with diluent]

interferon gamma-1b (in ter FEER on GAM ah-won bee)

U.S./Canadian Brand Names Actimmune® [US/Can]

Therapeutic Category Biological Response Modulator

Use Reduce the frequency and severity of serious infections associated with chronic granulomatous disease

Usual Dosage If severe reactions occur, modify dose (50% reduction) or therapy should be discontinued until adverse reactions abate.

Chronic granulomatous disease: Children >1 year and Adults: S.C.:

BSA ≤0.5 m^2: 1.5 mcg/kg/dose 3 times/week

BSA >0.5 m^2: 50 mcg/m^2 (1 million int. units/m^2) 3 times/week

Severe, malignant osteopetrosis: Children >1 year: S.C.:

BSA ≤0.5 m^2: 1.5 mcg/kg/dose 3 times/week

BSA >0.5 m^2: 50 mcg/m^2 (1 million int. units/m^2) 3 times/week

Note: Previously expressed as 1.5 million units/m^2, 50 mcg is equivalent to 1 million int. units/m^2.

Dosage Forms Injection, solution [preservative free]: 100 mcg [2 million int. units] (0.5 mL)

Previously, 100 mcg was expressed as 3 million units. This is equivalent to 2 million int. units.

interleukin-1 receptor antagonist *see* anakinra *on page 42*

interleukin-2 *see* aldesleukin *on page 20*

interleukin-11 *see* oprelvekin *on page 478*

Intralipid® **[US/Can]** *see* fat emulsion *on page 263*

intravenous fat emulsion *see* fat emulsion *on page 263*

Intron® **A [US/Can]** *see* interferon alfa-2b *on page 354*

Intropin® **[Can]** *see* dopamine *on page 211*

Intropin® *(Discontinued) see page 814*

Invanz™ **[US]** *see* ertapenem *on page 234*

Inversine® **[US/Can]** *see* mecamylamine *on page 403*

Invirase® **[US/Can]** *see* saquinavir *on page 583*

Iodex-p® *(Discontinued) see page 814*

Iodex [US-OTC] *see* iodine *on this page*

iodine (EYE oh dyne)
U.S./Canadian Brand Names Iodex [US-OTC]; Iodoflex™ [US]; Iodosorb® [US]
Therapeutic Category Topical Skin Product
Use Topically as an antiseptic in the management of minor, superficial skin wounds and has been used to disinfect the skin preoperatively
Usual Dosage Topical: Apply as necessary to affected areas of skin
Dosage Forms
Dressing, topical [gel pad] (Iodoflex™): 0.9% (5 g, 10 g)
Gel, topical (Iodosorb®): 0.9% (40 g)
Solution, topical: 2% (500 mL, 4000 mL); 5% (100 mL, 500 mL, 4000 mL)
Ointment (Iodex): 4.7% (30 g, 720 g)
Tincture, topical: 2% (30 mL, 480 mL, 500 mL, 4000 mL); 7% (30 mL, 100 mL, 480 mL, 500 mL, 4000 mL)

iodochlorhydroxyquin and hydrocortisone *see* clioquinol and hydrocortisone *on page 152*

Iodoflex™ **[US]** *see* iodine *on this page*

Iodo-Niacin® **Tablet** *(Discontinued) see page 814*

Iodopen® **[US]** *see* trace metals *on page 646*

iodoquinol (eye oh doe KWIN ole)
Synonyms diiodohydroxyquin
U.S./Canadian Brand Names Diodoquin® [Can]; Diquinol® [US]; Yodoxin® [US]
Therapeutic Category Amebicide
Use Treatment of acute and chronic intestinal amebiasis due to *Entamoeba histolytica*; asymptomatic cyst passers; *Blastocystis hominis* infections; iodoquinol alone is ineffective for amebic hepatitis or hepatic abscess
Usual Dosage Oral:
Children: 30-40 mg/kg/day in 3 divided doses for 20 days; not to exceed 1.95 g/day
Adults: 650 mg 3 times/day after meals for 20 days; not to exceed 2 g/day
(Continued)

iodoquinol *(Continued)*

Dosage Forms
Powder: 25 g, 100 g
Tablet: 210 mg, 650 mg

iodoquinol and hydrocortisone

(eye oh doe KWIN ole & hye droe KOR ti sone)
Synonyms hydrocortisone and iodoquinol
U.S./Canadian Brand Names Dermazene® [US]; Vytone® [US]
Therapeutic Category Antifungal/Corticosteroid
Use Treatment of eczema; infectious dermatitis; chronic eczematoid otitis externa; mycotic dermatoses
Usual Dosage Topical: Apply 3-4 times/day
Dosage Forms Cream: Iodoquinol 1% and hydrocortisone acetate 1% (30 g)
Dermazene®: Iodoquinol 1% and hydrocortisone acetate 1% (30 g, 45 g)
Vytone®: Iodoquinol 1% and hydrocortisone acetate 1% (30 g)

Iodosorb® [US] *see* iodine *on previous page*

Ionamin® [US/Can] *see* phentermine *on page 509*

Iophen® *(Discontinued)* *see page 814*

Iophen-C® *(Discontinued)* *see page 814*

Iophen-DM® *(Discontinued)* *see page 814*

Iophylline® *(Discontinued)* *see page 814*

Iopidine® [US/Can] *see* apraclonidine *on page 53*

Iosopan® Plus [US] *see* magaldrate and simethicone *on page 396*

Iotuss® *(Discontinued)* *see page 814*

Iotuss-DM® *(Discontinued)* *see page 814*

ipecac syrup (IP e kak SIR up)

Therapeutic Category Antidote
Use Treatment of acute oral drug overdosage and certain poisonings
Usual Dosage Oral:
Children:
6-12 months: 5-10 mL followed by 10-20 mL/kg of water; repeat dose one time if vomiting does not occur within 20 minutes
1-12 years: 15 mL followed by 10-20 mL/kg of water; repeat dose one time if vomiting does not occur within 20 minutes
Adults: 30 mL followed by 200-300 mL of water; repeat dose one time if vomiting does not occur within 20 minutes
Dosage Forms Syrup: 70 mg/mL (30 mL) [contains alcohol]

I-Pentolate® *(Discontinued)* *see page 814*

I-Phrine® Ophthalmic Solution *(Discontinued)* *see page 814*

I-Picamide® *(Discontinued)* *see page 814*

IPOL™ [US/Can] *see* poliovirus vaccine (inactivated) *on page 524*

ipratropium (i pra TROE pee um)

U.S./Canadian Brand Names Alti-Ipratropium [Can]; Apo®-Ipravent [Can]; Atrovent® [US/Can]; Gen-Ipratropium [Can]; Novo-Ipramide [Can]; Nu-Ipratropium [Can]; PMS-Ipratropium [Can]
Therapeutic Category Anticholinergic Agent
Use Bronchodilator used in bronchospasm associated with asthma, COPD, bronchitis, and emphysema; nasal spray used for symptomatic relief of rhinorrhea

Usual Dosage Children >12 years and Adults: 2 inhalations 4 times/day up to 12 inhalations/24 hours

Dosage Forms
Solution for nebulization, as bromide: 0.02% (2.5 mL)
Solution for oral inhalation, as bromide: 18 mcg/actuation (14 g)
Nasal spray, as bromide: 0.03% (30 mL); 0.06% (15 mL)

ipratropium and albuterol (i pra TROE pee um & al BYOO ter ole)
U.S./Canadian Brand Names Combivent® [US/Can]; DuoNeb™ [US]
Therapeutic Category Bronchodilator
Use Treatment of chronic obstructive pulmonary disease (COPD) in those patients that are currently on a regular bronchodilator who continue to have bronchospasms and require a second bronchodilator
Usual Dosage Adults:
Inhalation: 2 inhalations 4 times/day (maximum: 12 inhalations/24 hours)
Inhalation via nebulization: Initial: 3 mL every 6 hours (maximum: 3 mL every 4 hours)
Dosage Forms
Aerosol for oral inhalation (Combivent®): Ipratropium bromide 18 mcg and albuterol sulfate 103 mcg per actuation [200 doses] (14.7 g)
Solution for oral inhalation (DuoNeb™): Ipratropium bromide 0.5 mg [0.017%] and albuterol base 2.5 mg [0.083%] per 3 mL vial (30s, 60s)

I-Prin [US-OTC] *see* ibuprofen *on page 342*

iproveratril *see* verapamil *on page 675*

IPV *see* poliovirus vaccine (inactivated) *on page 524*

irbesartan (ir be SAR tan)
U.S./Canadian Brand Names Avapro® [US/Can]
Therapeutic Category Angiotensin II Receptor Antagonist
Use Treatment of hypertension alone or in combination with other antihypertensives
Usual Dosage Adults: Oral: 150 mg once daily with or without food; patients may be titrated to 300 mg once daily
Dosage Forms Tablet: 75 mg, 150 mg, 300 mg

irbesartan and hydrochlorothiazide
(ir be SAR tan & hye droe klor oh THYE a zide)
U.S./Canadian Brand Names Avalide® [US/Can]
Therapeutic Category Antihypertensive Agent, Combination
Use Combination therapy for the management of hypertension
Dosage Forms
Tablet:
Irbesartan 150 mg and hydrochlorothiazide 12.5 mg
Irbesartan 300 mg and hydrochlorothiazide 12.5 mg

Ircon® [US-OTC] *see* ferrous fumarate *on page 268*

irinotecan (eye rye no TEE kan)
U.S./Canadian Brand Names Camptosar® [US/Can]
Therapeutic Category Antineoplastic Agent
Use Treatment of patients with metastatic carcinoma of the colon or rectum whose disease has progressed following 5-FU based therapy
Usual Dosage Adults: I.V.: The recommended starting dose is 125 mg/m^2 (I.V. infusion over 90 minutes) once a week for 4 weeks, followed by a 2-week rest period; additional 6-week cycles of treatment may be repeated indefinitely in patients who remain stable or do not develop intolerable toxicities
Dosage Forms Injection, solution, as hydrochloride: 20 mg/mL (2 mL, 5 mL)

iron dextran complex (EYE ern DEKS tran KOM pleks)

U.S./Canadian Brand Names Dexferrum® [US]; Dexiron™ [Can]; INFeD® [US]; Infufer® [Can]

Therapeutic Category Electrolyte Supplement, Oral

Use Treatment of microcytic, hypochromic anemia resulting from iron deficiency when oral iron administration is infeasible or ineffective

Usual Dosage I.M., I.V.:

A 0.5 mL test dose (0.25 mL in infants) should be administered prior to starting iron dextran therapy

Iron deficiency anemia: Dose (mL) = 0.0476 x LBW (kg) x (normal hemoglobin - observed hemoglobin) + (1 mL/5 kg of LBW to maximum of 14 mL for iron stores)

Hb_n = desired hemoglobin (g/dL)

Hb_o = measured hemoglobin (g/dL)

Maximum daily dose:

Infants <5 kg: 25 mg iron

Children:

5-10 kg: 50 mg iron

10-50 kg: 100 mg iron

Adults >50 kg: 100 mg iron

Dosage Forms Injection, solution:

Dexferrum®: 50 mg/mL (1 mL, 2 mL)

INFeD®: 50 mg/mL (2 mL)

iron sucrose (EYE ern SOO krose)

U.S./Canadian Brand Names Venofer® [US]

Therapeutic Category Iron Salt

Use Treatment of iron-deficiency anemia in patients undergoing chronic hemodialysis who are receiving supplemental erythropoietin therapy

Usual Dosage Doses expressed in mg of **elemental** iron

Iron-deficiency anemia: I.V.: 100 mg (5 mL of iron sucrose injection) administered 1-3 times/week during dialysis, to a total dose of 1000 mg (10 doses); administer no more than 3 times/week; may continue to administer at lowest dose necessary to maintain target hemoglobin, hematocrit, and iron storage parameters

Test dose: Product labeling does not indicate need for a test dose in product-naive patients; test doses were administered in some clinical trials as 50 mg (2.5 mL) in 50 mL 0.9% NaCl administered over 3-10 minutes

Dosage Forms Injection, solution: 20 mg of elemental iron/mL (5 mL)

ISD see isosorbide dinitrate on page 362

ISDN see isosorbide dinitrate on page 362

ISG see immune globulin (intramuscular) on page 346

Ismelin® [US] see guanethidine on page 313

ISMN see isosorbide mononitrate on page 362

Ismo® [US] see isosorbide mononitrate on page 362

Ismotic® *(Discontinued)* see page 814

isoamyl nitrite see amyl nitrite on page 41

isobamate see carisoprodol on page 117

Iso-Bid® *(Discontinued)* see page 814

Isocaine® HCl [US] see mepivacaine on page 409

Isocal® [US-OTC] see nutritional formula, enteral/oral on page 472

isocarboxazid (eye soe kar BOKS a zid)

U.S./Canadian Brand Names Marplan® [US]

Therapeutic Category Antidepressant, Monoamine Oxidase Inhibitor

Use Symptomatic treatment of atypical, nonendogenous or neurotic depression
Usual Dosage Adults: Oral: 10 mg 3 times/day; reduce to 10-20 mg/day in divided doses when condition improves
Dosage Forms Tablet: 10 mg

isoetharine (eye soe ETH a reen)

Therapeutic Category Adrenergic Agonist Agent
Use Bronchodilator used in asthma and for the reversible bronchospasm occurring with bronchitis and emphysema
Usual Dosage Treatments are usually not repeated more often than every 4 hours, except in severe cases, and may be repeated up to 5 times/day if necessary

Nebulizer: Children: 0.1-0.2 mg/kg/dose every 2-6 hours as needed; adult: 0.5 mL diluted in 2-3 mL normal saline or 4 inhalations of undiluted 1% solution
Dosage Forms Solution for oral inhalation, as hydrochloride: 1% (10 mL) [contains sodium sulfite and sodium bisulfite]

isoflurane (eye soe FLURE ane)

U.S./Canadian Brand Names Forane® [US/Can]
Therapeutic Category General Anesthetic
Use General induction and maintenance of anesthesia (inhalation)
Usual Dosage 1.5% to 3%
Dosage Forms Solution: 100 mL, 250 mL

Isollyl® Improved *(Discontinued)* see page 814

isoniazid (eye soe NYE a zid)

Synonyms INH; isonicotinic acid hydrazide
U.S./Canadian Brand Names Isotamine® [Can]; Nydrazid® [US]; PMS-Isoniazid [Can]
Therapeutic Category Antitubercular Agent
Use Treatment of susceptible mycobacterial infection due to *M. tuberculosis* and prophylactically to those individuals exposed to tuberculosis
Usual Dosage Oral, I.M.:
Children: 10-20 mg/kg/day in 1-2 divided doses (maximum: 300 mg total dose)
Prophylaxis: 10 mg/kg/day administered daily (up to 300 mg total dose) for 12 months
Adults: 5 mg/kg/day administered daily (usual dose: 300 mg)
Disseminated disease: 10 mg/kg/day in 1-2 divided doses
Treatment should be continued for 9 months with rifampin or for 6 months with rifampin and pyrazinamide
Prophylaxis: 300 mg/day administered daily for 12 months

American Thoracic Society and CDC currently recommend twice weekly therapy as part of a short-course regimen which follows 1-2 months of daily treatment for uncomplicated pulmonary tuberculosis in compliant patients
Children: 20-40 mg/kg/dose (up to 900 mg) twice weekly
Adults: 15 mg/kg/dose (up to 900 mg) twice weekly
Dosage Forms
Injection, solution (Nydrazid®): 100 mg/mL (10 mL)
Syrup: 50 mg/5 mL (473 mL) [orange flavor]
Tablet: 100 mg, 300 mg

isoniazid and rifampin *see* rifampin and isoniazid *on page 572*

isoniazid, rifampin, and pyrazinamide *see* rifampin, isoniazid, and pyrazinamide *on page 573*

isonicotinic acid hydrazide *see* isoniazid *on this page*

isonipecaine *see* meperidine *on page 408*

isoproterenol (eye soe proe TER e nole)

U.S./Canadian Brand Names Isuprel® [US]

Therapeutic Category Adrenergic Agonist Agent

Use Asthma or COPD (reversible airway obstruction); ventricular arrhythmias due to A-V nodal block; hemodynamically compromised bradyarrhythmias or atropine-resistant bradyarrhythmias, temporary use in third degree A-V block until pacemaker insertion; low cardiac output or vasoconstrictive shock states

Usual Dosage

Children: I.V. infusion: 0.05-2 mcg/kg/minute; rate (mL/hour) = dose (mcg/kg/minute) x weight (kg) x 60 minutes/hour divided by concentration (mcg/mL)

Adults: A-V nodal block: I.V. infusion: 2-20 mcg/minute

Dosage Forms Injection, solution, as hydrochloride: 0.02 mg/mL (10 mL); 0.2 mg/mL (1:5000) (1 mL, 5 mL) [contains sodium metabisulfite]

Isoptin® [US/Can] *see* verapamil *on page 675*

Isoptin® SR [US/Can] *see* verapamil *on page 675*

Isopto® Atropine [US/Can] *see* atropine *on page 62*

Isopto® Carbachol [US/Can] *see* carbachol *on page 112*

Isopto® Carpine [US/Can] *see* pilocarpine *on page 514*

Isopto® Cetapred® *(Discontinued)* *see page 814*

Isopto® Eserine *(Discontinued)* *see page 814*

Isopto® Frin Ophthalmic Solution *(Discontinued)* *see page 814*

Isopto® Homatropine [US] *see* homatropine *on page 323*

Isopto® Hyoscine [US] *see* scopolamine *on page 585*

Isopto® P-ES *(Discontinued)* *see page 814*

Isopto® Plain Solution *(Discontinued)* *see page 814*

Isopto® Tears [US/Can] *see* artificial tears *on page 56*

Isordil® [US] *see* isosorbide dinitrate *on this page*

isosorbide dinitrate (eye soe SOR bide dye NYE trate)

Synonyms ISD; ISDN

U.S./Canadian Brand Names Apo®-ISDN [Can]; Cedocard®-SR [Can]; Dilatrate®-SR [US]; Isordil® [US]

Therapeutic Category Vasodilator

Use Prevention and treatment of angina pectoris; for congestive heart failure; to relieve pain, dysphagia, and spasm in esophageal spasm with GE reflux

Usual Dosage Adults:

Oral: 5-30 mg 4 times/day or 40 mg every 6-12 hours in sustained-released dosage form

Chewable: 5-10 mg every 2-3 hours

Sublingual: 2.5-10 mg every 4-6 hours

Dosage Forms

Capsule, sustained release (Dilatrate®-SR): 40 mg

Tablet: 5 mg, 10 mg, 20 mg, 30 mg,

Isordil®: 5 mg, 10 mg, 20 mg, 30mg, 40 mg

Tablet, chewable: 5 mg, 10 mg

Tablet, sublingual (Isordil®): 2.5 mg, 5 mg, 10 mg

isosorbide mononitrate (eye soe SOR bide mon oh NYE trate)

Synonyms ISMN

U.S./Canadian Brand Names Imdur® [US/Can]; Ismo® [US]; Monoket® [US]

Therapeutic Category Vasodilator

Use Long-acting metabolite of the vasodilator isosorbide dinitrate used for the prophylactic treatment of angina pectoris

Usual Dosage Adults: Oral:

Regular tablet: 20 mg twice daily separated by 7 hours

Extended-release tablet: 30 mg (½ of 60 mg tablet) or 60 mg (administered as a single tablet) once daily; after several days the dosage may be increased to 120 mg (administered as two 60 mg tablets) once daily; the daily dose should be administered in the morning upon arising

Dosage Forms

Tablet: 10 mg, 20 mg

Ismo®: 20 mg

Monoket®: 10 mg, 20 mg

Tablet, extended release (Imdur®): 30 mg, 60 mg, 120 mg

Isotamine® [Can] *see* isoniazid *on page 361*

isotretinoin (eye soe TRET i noyn)

Synonyms 13-*cis*-retinoic acid

U.S./Canadian Brand Names Accutane® [US/Can]; Isotrex® [Can]

Therapeutic Category Retinoic Acid Derivative

Use Treatment of severe recalcitrant nodular acne unresponsive to conventional therapy

Usual Dosage Oral:

Children: Maintenance therapy for neuroblastoma: 100-250 mg/m^2/day in 2 divided doses has been used investigationally

Children and Adults: 0.5-2 mg/kg/day in 2 divided doses for 15-20 weeks

Dosage Forms Capsule: 10 mg, 20 mg, 40 mg

Isotrex® [Can] *see* isotretinoin *on this page*

Isovex® (Discontinued) *see page 814*

Isovue® [US] *see* radiological/contrast media (non-ionic) *on page 563*

isoxsuprine (eye SOKS syoo preen)

U.S./Canadian Brand Names Vasodilan® [US]

Therapeutic Category Vasodilator

Use Treatment of peripheral vascular diseases, such as arteriosclerosis obliterans and Raynaud's disease

Usual Dosage Adults: Oral: 10-20 mg 3-4 times/day

Dosage Forms Tablet, as hydrochloride: 10 mg, 20 mg

isradipine (iz RA di peen)

U.S./Canadian Brand Names DynaCirc® CR [US]; DynaCirc® [US/Can]

Therapeutic Category Calcium Channel Blocker

Use Management of hypertension, alone or concurrently with thiazide-type diuretics

Usual Dosage Adults: 2.5 mg twice daily; antihypertensive response occurs in 2-3 hours; maximal response in 2-4 weeks; increase dose at 2- to 4-week intervals at 2.5-5 mg increments; usual dose range: 5-20 mg/day. **Note:** Most patients show no improvement with doses >10 mg/day except adverse reaction rate increases

Dosage Forms

Capsule (DynaCirc®): 2.5 mg, 5 mg

Tablet, controlled release (DynaCirc® CR): 5 mg, 10 mg

Isuprel® [US] *see* isoproterenol *on previous page*

Isuprel® Glossets® (Discontinued) *see page 814*

Itch-X® [US-OTC] *see* pramoxine *on page 534*

itraconazole (i tra KOE na zole)

U.S./Canadian Brand Names Sporanox® [US/Can]

Therapeutic Category Antifungal Agent

Use Treatment of systemic fungal infections in immunocompromised and nonimmunocompromised patients including the treatment of susceptible blastomycosis, histoplasmosis, and aspergillosis in patients who do not respond to or cannot tolerate amphotericin B; it also has activity against *Cryptococcus*, *Coccidioides*, and sporotrichosis species; has also been used for prophylaxis against aspergillosis infection

Usual Dosage Oral: Capsule: Absorption is best if taken with food, therefore, it is best to administer itraconazole after meals; Solution: Should be taken on an empty stomach. Absorption of both products is significantly increased when taken with a cola beverage.

Children: Efficacy and safety have not been established; a small number of patients 3-16 years of age have been treated with 100 mg/day for systemic fungal infections with no serious adverse effects reported

Adults:

Oral:

Blastomycosis/histoplasmosis: 200 mg once daily, if no obvious improvement or there is evidence of progressive fungal disease, increase the dose in 100 mg increments to a maximum of 400 mg/day; doses >200 mg/day are given in 2 divided doses; length of therapy varies from 1 day to >6 months depending on the condition and mycological response

Aspergillosis: 200-400 mg/day

Onychomycosis: 200 mg once daily for 12 consecutive weeks

Life-threatening infections: Loading dose: 200 mg 3 times/day (600 mg/day) should be given for the first 3 days of therapy

Oropharyngeal and esophageal candidiasis: Oral solution: 100-200 mg once daily

I.V.: 200 mg twice daily for 4 doses, followed by 200 mg daily

Dosage Forms

Capsule: 100 mg

Injection, solution: 10 mg/mL (25 mL) [packaged in a kit containing sodium chloride 0.9% (50 mL); filtered infusion set (1)]

Solution, oral: 100 mg/10 mL (150 mL) [cherry flavor]

I-Tropine® *(Discontinued)* see page 814

Iveegam EN [US] see immune globulin (intravenous) on page 347

Iveegam Immuno® [Can] see immune globulin (intravenous) on page 347

ivermectin (eye ver MEK tin)

U.S./Canadian Brand Names Stromectol® [US]

Therapeutic Category Antibiotic, Miscellaneous

Use Treatment of the following infections: Strongyloidiasis of the intestinal tract due the nematode parasite *Strongyloides stercoralis*. Onchocerciasis due to the nematode parasite *Onchocerca volvulus*. Note: Ivermectin is ineffective against adult *Onchocerca volvulus* parasites because they reside in subcutaneous nodules which are infrequently palpable. Surgical excision of these nodules may be considered in the management of patients with onchocerciasis.

Usual Dosage Oral:

Children >5 years: 150 mcg/kg as a single dose once every 12 months

Adults: 150 mcg/kg as a single dose; may be repeated every 6-12 months

Dosage Forms Tablet: 3 mg

IVIG see immune globulin (intravenous) on page 347

IvyBlock® [US-OTC] see bentoquatam on page 76

Janimine® *(Discontinued)* see page 814

Japanese encephalitis virus vaccine (inactivated)
(jap a NEESE en sef a LYE tis VYE rus vak SEEN in ak ti VAY ted)

U.S./Canadian Brand Names JE-VAX® [US/Can]

Therapeutic Category Vaccine, Inactivated Virus

Use Active immunization against Japanese encephalitis for persons spending a month or longer in endemic areas, especially if travel will include rural areas

Usual Dosage S.C. (administered on days 0, 7, and 30):

Children 1-3 years: 3 doses of 0.5 mL; booster doses of 0.5 mL may administer 2 years after primary immunization series

Children >3 years and Adults: 3 doses of 1 mL; booster doses of 1 mL may be administered 2 years after primary immunization series

Dosage Forms Injection, powder for reconstitution: 1 mL, 10 mL

Jenamicin® *(Discontinued)* see page 814

Jenest™-28 [US] see ethinyl estradiol and norethindrone on page 251

JE-VAX® [US/Can] see Japanese encephalitis virus vaccine (inactivated) on this page

Just Tears® Solution *(Discontinued)* see page 814

K+ 10® [US] see potassium chloride on page 530

Kabikinase® *(Discontinued)* see page 814

Kadian® [US/Can] see morphine sulfate on page 437

Kala® [US-OTC] see Lactobacillus on page 372

Kalcinate® *(Discontinued)* see page 814

Kaletra™ [US] see lopinavir and ritonavir on page 390

kanamycin (kan a MYE sin)

U.S./Canadian Brand Names Kantrex® [US/Can]

Therapeutic Category Aminoglycoside (Antibiotic)

Use

Oral: Preoperative bowel preparation in the prophylaxis of infections and adjunctive treatment of hepatic coma (oral kanamycin is not indicated in the treatment of systemic infections)

Parenteral: Initial therapy of severe infections where the strain is thought to be susceptible in patients allergic to other antibiotics, or in mixed staphylococcal or gram-negative infections

Usual Dosage

Children: Infections: I.M., I.V.: 15 mg/kg/day in divided doses every 8-12 hours

Adults:

Infections: I.M., I.V.: 15 mg/kg/day in divided doses every 8-12 hours

Preoperative intestinal antisepsis: Oral: 1 g every 4-6 hours for 36-72 hours

Dosage Forms

Injection, solution, as sulfate: 1 g/3 mL (3 mL) [contains sodium bisulfate]

Kantrex® [US/Can] see kanamycin on this page

Kaochlor® [US] see potassium chloride on page 530

Kaochlor-Eff® *(Discontinued)* see page 814

Kaochlor® SF *(Discontinued)* see page 814

Kaodene® *(Discontinued)* see page 814

Kaodene® A-D [US-OTC] see loperamide on page 390

Kaodene® NN [US-OTC] see kaolin and pectin on next page

kaolin and pectin (KAY oh lin & PEK tin)
Synonyms pectin and kaolin
U.S./Canadian Brand Names Kaodene® NN [US-OTC]; Kaolinpec® [US-OTC]; Kao-Spen® [US-OTC]; Kapectolin® [US-OTC]
Therapeutic Category Antidiarrheal
Use Treatment of uncomplicated diarrhea
Usual Dosage Oral:
  Children:
    <6 years: Do not use
    6-12 years: 30-60 mL after each loose stool
  Adults: 60-120 mL after each loose stool
Dosage Forms
  Suspension, oral: Kaolin 967 mg and pectin 22 mg per 5 mL (30 mL, 180 mL)
    Kaodene® NN: Kaolin 650 mg and pectin 32.4 mg per 5 mL (120 mL) [contains bismuth subsalicylate 2.8 mg/5 mL]
    Kao-Spen®: Kaolin 860 mg and pectin 43 mg per 5 mL (3840 mL)
    Kapectolin®: Kaolin 15 g and pectin 33 mg per 5 mL (120 mL, 240 mL, 480 mL)

Kaolinpec® [US-OTC] *see* kaolin and pectin *on this page*

Kaon® [US/Can] *see* potassium gluconate *on page 531*

Kaon-Cl® [US] *see* potassium chloride *on page 530*

Kaon-Cl-10® [US] *see* potassium chloride *on page 530*

Kao-Paverin® [US-OTC] *see* loperamide *on page 390*

Kaopectate® [US/Can] *see* attapulgite *on page 63*

Kaopectate® Advanced Formula [US-OTC] *see* attapulgite *on page 63*

Kaopectate® Children's Tablet *(Discontinued)* *see page 814*

Kaopectate® II *(Discontinued)* *see page 814*

Kaopectate® Maximum Strength Caplets [US-OTC] *see* attapulgite *on page 63*

Kao-Spen® [US-OTC] *see* kaolin and pectin *on this page*

Kapectolin PG® [US] *see* hyoscyamine, atropine, scopolamine, kaolin, pectin, and opium *on page 341*

Kapectolin® [US-OTC] *see* kaolin and pectin *on this page*

Karidium® *(Discontinued)* *see page 814*

Karigel® *(Discontinued)* *see page 814*

Karigel®-N *(Discontinued)* *see page 814*

Kariva™ [US] *see* ethinyl estradiol and desogestrel *on page 244*

Kasof® *(Discontinued)* *see page 814*

Kato® Powder *(Discontinued)* *see page 814*

Kaybovite-1000® *(Discontinued)* *see page 814*

Kay Ciel® [US] *see* potassium chloride *on page 530*

Kayexalate® [US/Can] *see* sodium polystyrene sulfonate *on page 600*

K+ Care® [US] *see* potassium chloride *on page 530*

K+ Care® ET [US] *see* potassium bicarbonate *on page 529*

KCl *see* potassium chloride *on page 530*

K-Dur® 10 [US/Can] *see* potassium chloride *on page 530*

K-Dur® 20 [US/Can] *see* potassium chloride *on page 530*

Keflex® [US] *see* cephalexin *on page 128*

Keflin® *(Discontinued)* *see page 814*

Keftab® **[US/Can]** *see* cephalexin *on page 128*

Kefurox® **[US/Can]** *see* cefuroxime *on page 126*

Kefzol® **[US/Can]** *see* cefazolin *on page 121*

K-Electrolyte® **Effervescent** *(Discontinued)* *see page 814*

Kemadrin® **[US/Can]** *see* procyclidine *on page 543*

Kemsol® **[Can]** *see* dimethyl sulfoxide *on page 201*

Kenacort® **Oral** *(Discontinued)* *see page 814*

Kenaject® **Injection** *(Discontinued)* *see page 814*

Kenalog® **Injection [US/Can]** *see* triamcinolone (systemic) *on page 651*

Kenalog® **in Orabase**® **[US/Can]** *see* triamcinolone (topical) *on page 652*

Kenalog® **Topical [US/Can]** *see* triamcinolone (topical) *on page 652*

Kenonel® **Topical** *(Discontinued)* *see page 814*

Keppra® **[US/Can]** *see* levetiracetam *on page 378*

Keralyt® **Gel [US-OTC]** *see* salicylic acid and propylene glycol *on page 581*

Kerlone® **[US]** *see* betaxolol *on page 84*

Kestrin® **Injection** *(Discontinued)* *see page 814*

Kestrone® **[US/Can]** *see* estrone *on page 242*

Ketalar® **[US/Can]** *see* ketamine *on this page*

ketamine (KEET a meen)

U.S./Canadian Brand Names Ketalar® [US/Can]
Therapeutic Category General Anesthetic
Controlled Substance C-III
Use Anesthesia, short surgical procedures, dressing changes
Usual Dosage
  Children:
    I.M.: 3-7 mg/kg
    I.V.: Range: 0.5-2 mg/kg, use smaller doses (0.5-1 mg/kg) for sedation for minor procedures; usual induction dosage: 1-2 mg/kg
  Adults:
    I.M.: 3-8 mg/kg
    I.V.: Range: 1-4.5 mg/kg; usual induction dosage: 1-2 mg/kg
  Children and Adults: Maintenance: Supplemental doses of $1/3$ to $1/2$ of initial dose
Dosage Forms Injection, solution, as hydrochloride: 10 mg/mL (20 mL, 25 mL, 50 mL); 50 mg/mL (10 mL); 100 mg/mL (5 mL)

ketoconazole (kee toe KOE na zole)

U.S./Canadian Brand Names Apo®-Ketoconazole [Can]; Nizoral® A-D [US-OTC]; Nizoral® [US/Can]; Novo-Ketoconazole [Can]
Therapeutic Category Antifungal Agent
Use Treatment of susceptible fungal infections, including candidiasis, oral thrush, blastomycosis, histoplasmosis, coccidioidomycosis, paracoccidioidomycosis, chronic mucocutaneous candidiasis, as well as certain recalcitrant cutaneous dermatophytoses; used topically for treatment of tinea corporis, tinea cruris, tinea versicolor, and cutaneous candidiasis; shampoo is used for dandruff
Usual Dosage
  Children: Oral: 5-10 mg/kg/day divided every 12-24 hours until lesions clear
  Adults:
    Oral: 200-400 mg/day as a single daily dose
    Topical: Rub gently into the affected area once daily to twice daily for two weeks
Dosage Forms
  Cream, topical (Nizoral®): 2% (15 g, 30 g, 60 g)
  (Continued)

ketoconazole *(Continued)*

Shampoo, topical (Nizoral® A-D): 1% (6 mL, 120 mL, 207 mL)
Tablet (Nizoral®): 200 mg

ketoprofen (kee toe PROE fen)

U.S./Canadian Brand Names Apo®-Keto [Can]; Apo®-Keto-E [Can]; Apo®-Keto SR [Can]; Novo-Keto [Can]; Novo-Keto-EC [Can]; Nu-Ketoprofen [Can]; Nu-Ketoprofen-E [Can]; Orafen [Can]; Orudis® KT [US-OTC]; Orudis® SR [Can]; Oruvail® [US/Can]; Rhodis™ [Can]; Rhodis-EC™ [Can]; Rhodis SR™ [Can]

Therapeutic Category Analgesic, Non-narcotic; Nonsteroidal Anti-inflammatory Drug (NSAID)

Use Acute or long-term treatment of rheumatoid arthritis and osteoarthritis; primary dysmenorrhea; mild to moderate pain

Usual Dosage Oral:

Children 3 months to 14 years: Fever: 0.5-1 mg/kg

Children >12 years and Adults:

Rheumatoid arthritis or osteoarthritis: 50-75 mg 3-4 times/day up to a maximum of 300 mg/day

Mild to moderate pain: 25-50 mg every 6-8 hours up to a maximum of 300 mg/day

Dosage Forms

Capsule, extended release (Oruvail®): 100 mg, 150 mg, 200 mg

Tablet (Orudis® KT): 12.5 mg

ketorolac (KEE toe role ak)

Synonyms ketorolac tromethamine

U.S./Canadian Brand Names Acular® PF [US]; Acular® [US/Can]; Apo®-Ketorolac [Can]; Novo-Ketorolac [Can]; Toradol® [US/Can]

Therapeutic Category Analgesic, Non-narcotic; Nonsteroidal Anti-inflammatory Drug (NSAID)

Use

Oral, I.M., I.V.,: Short-term (≤5 days) management of moderate to severe pain, including postoperative pain, visceral pain associated with cancer, pain associated with trauma, acute renal colic

Ophthalmic: Ocular itch associated with seasonal allergic conjunctivitis

Usual Dosage Adults (pain relief usually begins within 10 minutes with parenteral forms):

Oral: 10 mg every 4-6 hours as needed for a maximum of 40 mg/day; on day of transition from I.M. to oral: maximum oral dose: 40 mg (or 120 mg combined oral and I.M.); maximum 5 days administration

I.M.: Initial: 30-60 mg, then 15-30 mg every 6 hours as needed for up to 5 days maximum; maximum dose in the first 24 hours: 150 mg with 120 mg/24 hours for up to 5 days total

I.V.: Initial: 30 mg, then 15-30 mg every 6 hours as needed for up to 5 days **maximum**; maximum daily dose: 120 mg for up to 5 days total

Ophthalmic: Instill 1 drop in eye(s) 4 times/day

Dosage Forms

Injection, as tromethamine: 15 mg/mL (1 mL); 30 mg/mL (1 mL, 2 mL)

Solution, ophthalmic, as tromethamine:

Acular®: 0.5% (3 mL, 5 mL, 10 mL) [contains benzalkonium chloride]

Acular® PF [preservative free]: 0.5% (0.4 mL)

Tablet, as tromethamine (Toradol®): 10 mg

ketorolac tromethamine *see* ketorolac *on this page*

ketotifen (kee toe TYE fen)

U.S./Canadian Brand Names Apo®-Ketotifen [Can]; Novo-Ketotifen [Can]; Zaditen® [Can]; Zaditor™ [US/Can]

Therapeutic Category Antihistamine, H₁ Blocker, Ophthalmic
Use Temporary prevention of eye itching due to allergic conjunctivitis
Usual Dosage Adults: Ophthalmic: Instill 1 drop in the affected eye(s) every 8-12 hours
Dosage Forms Solution, ophthalmic, as fumarate: 0.025% (5 mL) [contains benzalkonium chloride]

Keygesic-10® [US] *see* magnesium salicylate *on page 398*

Key-Pred® [US] *see* prednisolone (systemic) *on page 537*

Key-Pred-SP® [US] *see* prednisolone (systemic) *on page 537*

K-G® *(Discontinued)* *see page 814*

K-Gen® Effervescent *(Discontinued)* *see page 814*

KI *see* potassium iodide *on page 531*

K-Ide® *(Discontinued)* *see page 814*

Kidrolase® [Can] *see* asparaginase *on page 58*

Kinerase® [US] *see* hyaluronidase *on page 326*

Kineret™ [US] *see* anakinra *on page 42*

Kinevac® [US] *see* sincalide *on page 591*

Kionex™ [US] *see* sodium polystyrene sulfonate *on page 600*

Klaron® [US] *see* sulfacetamide *on page 610*

Klean-Prep® [Can] *see* polyethylene glycol-electrolyte solution *on page 525*

K-Lease® *(Discontinued)* *see page 814*

Klerist-D® Tablet *(Discontinued)* *see page 814*

Klonopin™ [US/Can] *see* clonazepam *on page 154*

K-Lor™ [US/Can] *see* potassium chloride *on page 530*

Klor-Con® [US] *see* potassium chloride *on page 530*

Klor-Con® 8 [US] *see* potassium chloride *on page 530*

Klor-Con® 10 [US] *see* potassium chloride *on page 530*

Klor-Con®/25 [US] *see* potassium chloride *on page 530*

Klor-Con®/EF [US] *see* potassium bicarbonate and potassium citrate, effervescent *on page 529*

Klorominr® Oral *(Discontinued)* *see page 814*

Klorvess® [US] *see* potassium chloride *on page 530*

Klorvess® Effervescent *(Discontinued)* *see page 814*

Klotrix® [US] *see* potassium chloride *on page 530*

K-Lyte® [US/Can] *see* potassium bicarbonate and potassium citrate, effervescent *on page 529*

K-Lyte/Cl® [US/Can] *see* potassium bicarbonate and potassium chloride, effervescent *on page 529*

K-Lyte® Effervescent *(Discontinued)* *see page 814*

K-Norm® *(Discontinued)* *see page 814*

Koāte®-DVI [US] *see* antihemophilic factor (human) *on page 45*

Koāte®-HS Injection *(Discontinued)* *see page 814*

Koāte®-HT Injection *(Discontinued)* *see page 814*

Koffex DM-D [Can] *see* pseudoephedrine and dextromethorphan *on page 553*

Koffex DM + Decongestant + Expectorant [Can] *see* guaifenesin, pseudoephedrine, and dextromethorphan *on page 312*

Koffex DM-Expectorant *see* guaifenesin and dextromethorphan *on page 308*

Koffex Expectorant [Can] *see* guaifenesin *on page 307*

Kogenate® FS [US/Can] *see* antihemophilic factor (recombinant) *on page 46*

Kolephrin® GG/DM [US-OTC] *see* guaifenesin and dextromethorphan *on page 308*

Kolyum® Powder *(Discontinued) see page 814*

Konakion® Injection *(Discontinued) see page 814*

Kondon's Nasal® *(Discontinued) see page 814*

Konsyl-D® [US-OTC] *see* psyllium *on page 554*

Konsyl® [US-OTC] *see* psyllium *on page 554*

Konȳne® 80 [US] *see* factor IX complex (human) *on page 261*

Konȳne-HT® Injection *(Discontinued) see page 814*

K-Pec® II [US-OTC] *see* loperamide *on page 390*

K-Pek® [US-OTC] *see* attapulgite *on page 63*

K-Phos® MF [US] *see* potassium phosphate and sodium phosphate *on page 533*

K-Phos® Neutral [US] *see* potassium phosphate and sodium phosphate *on page 533*

K-Phos® No. 2 [US] *see* potassium phosphate and sodium phosphate *on page 533*

K-Phos® Original [US] *see* potassium acid phosphate *on page 528*

Kristalose™ [US] *see* lactulose *on page 372*

K-Tab® [US] *see* potassium chloride *on page 530*

Kutrase® [US] *see* pancrelipase *on page 489*

Ku-Zyme® [US] *see* pancrelipase *on page 489*

Ku-Zyme® HP [US] *see* pancrelipase *on page 489*

Kwelcof® [US] *see* hydrocodone and guaifenesin *on page 331*

Kwell® *(Discontinued) see page 814*

Kwellada-P™ [Can] *see* permethrin *on page 505*

Kytril™ [US/Can] *see* granisetron *on page 305*

***L*-3-hydroxytyrosine** *see* levodopa *on page 380*

L-749,345 *see* ertapenem *on page 234*

LA-12® [US] *see* cyanocobalamin *on page 167*

labetalol (la BET a lole)

Synonyms ibidomide

U.S./Canadian Brand Names Normodyne® [US/Can]; Trandate® [US/Can]

Therapeutic Category Alpha-/Beta- Adrenergic Blocker

Use Treatment of mild to severe hypertension; I.V. for hypertensive emergencies

Usual Dosage

Children: Limited information regarding labetalol use in pediatric patients is currently available in literature. Some centers recommend initial oral doses of 4 mg/kg/day in 2 divided doses. Reported oral doses have started at 3 mg/kg/day and 20 mg/kg/day and have increased up to 40 mg/kg/day.

I.V., intermittent bolus doses of 0.3-1 mg/kg/dose have been reported

For treatment of pediatric hypertensive emergencies, initial continuous infusions of 0.4-1 mg/kg/hour with a maximum of 3 mg/kg/hour have been used.

Due to limited documentation of its use, labetalol should be initiated cautiously in pediatric patients with careful dosage adjustment and blood pressure monitoring

Adults:
Oral: Initial: 100 mg twice daily, may increase as needed every 2-3 days by 100 mg until desired response is obtained; usual dose: 200-400 mg twice daily; not to exceed 2.4 g/day
I.V.: 20 mg or 1-2 mg/kg whichever is lower, IVP over 2 minutes, may administer 40-80 mg at 10-minute intervals, up to 300 mg total dose
I.V. infusion: Initial: 2 mg/minute; titrate to response
Dosage Forms
Injection, as hydrochloride: 5 mg/mL (20 mL, 40 mL, 60 mL)
Injection, as hydrochloride [prefilled syringe]: 5 mg/mL (4 mL, 8 mL)
Tablet, as hydrochloride: 100 mg, 200 mg, 300 mg

Lac-Hydrin® [US] *see* lactic acid with ammonium hydroxide *on this page*

Lacril® Ophthalmic Solution *(Discontinued)* *see page 814*

Lacrinorm [Can] *see* carbopol 940 *(Canada only) on page 116*

Lacrisert® [US/Can] *see* hydroxypropyl cellulose *on page 337*

Lactaid® [US-OTC] *see* lactase *on this page*

lactase (LAK tase)
U.S./Canadian Brand Names Dairyaid® [Can]; Dairy Ease® [US-OTC]; Lactaid® [US-OTC]; Lactrase® [US-OTC]
Therapeutic Category Nutritional Supplement
Use Help digest lactose in milk for patients with lactose intolerance
Usual Dosage Oral:
Capsule: 1-2 capsules administered with milk or meal; pretreat milk with 1-2 capsules per quart of milk
Liquid: 5-15 drops per quart of milk
Tablet: 1-3 tablets with meals
Dosage Forms
Caplet: ≥3000 FCC lactase units
Capsule: 250 mg standardized enzyme lactase
Liquid: 1250 neutral lactase units/5 drops
Tablet, chewable: 3000 FCC lactase units, 3300 FCC lactase units

lactic acid and salicylic acid *see* salicylic acid and lactic acid *on page 581*

lactic acid and sodium-PCA (LAK tik AS id & SOW dee um-pee see aye)
Synonyms sodium-pca and lactic acid
U.S./Canadian Brand Names LactiCare® [US-OTC]
Therapeutic Category Topical Skin Product
Use Lubricate and moisturize the skin counteracting dryness and itching
Usual Dosage Topical: Apply as needed
Dosage Forms Lotion: Lactic acid 5% and sodium (PCA) 2.5% (240 mL)

lactic acid with ammonium hydroxide
(LAK tik AS id with a MOE nee um hye DROKS ide)
Synonyms ammonium lactate
U.S./Canadian Brand Names Lac-Hydrin® [US]
Therapeutic Category Topical Skin Product
Use Treatment of moderate to severe xerosis and ichthyosis vulgaris
Usual Dosage Topical: Shake well; apply to affected areas, use twice daily, rub in well
Dosage Forms
Cream, topical: Lactic acid 12% with ammonium hydroxide (280 g, 385 g)
Lotion, topical: Lactic acid 12% with ammonium hydroxide (225 g, 400 g)

LactiCare-HC® [US] *see* hydrocortisone (topical) *on page 334*

LactiCare® [US-OTC] *see* lactic acid and sodium-PCA *on this page*

Lactinex® [US-OTC] *see* Lactobacillus *on this page*

Lactobacillus (lak toe ba SIL us)

Synonyms *Lactobacillus acidophilus*; *Lactobacillus acidophilus* and *Lactobacillus bulgaricus*

U.S./Canadian Brand Names Bacid® [US/Can]; Fermalac [Can]; Kala® [US-OTC]; Lactinex® [US-OTC]; MoreDophilus® [US-OTC]; Pro-Bionate® [US-OTC]; Probiotica® [US-OTC]; Superdophilus® [US-OTC]

Therapeutic Category Gastrointestinal Agent, Miscellaneous

Use Uncomplicated diarrhea particularly that caused by antibiotic therapy; re-establish normal physiologic and bacterial flora of the intestinal tract

Usual Dosage Children >3 years and Adults: Oral:

Capsules: 2 capsules 2-4 times/day

Granules: 1 packet added to or taken with cereal, food, milk, fruit juice, or water, 3-4 times/day

Powder: $1/4$-1 teaspoonful 1-3 times/daily with liquid

Tablet, chewable: 4 tablets 3-4 times/day; may follow each dose with a small amount of milk, fruit juice, or water

Dosage Forms

Capsule:

Bacid®: ≥500 million units [cultured strain *L. acidophilus*] (50s, 100s)

Pro-Bionate®: 2 billion units per g [strain NAS *L. acidophilus*] (30s, 60s)

Granules (Lactinex®): 1 g/packet [mixed culture *L. acidophilus, L. bulgaricus*] (12 packets/box)

Powder:

MoreDophilus®: 4 billion units per g [*L. acidophilus*-carrot derivative] (120 g)

Superdophilus®: 2 billion units per g [strain DDS-1 *L. acidophilus*] (37.5 g, 75 g, 135 g)

Tablet (Kala®): 200 million units [soy-based *L. acidophilus*] (100s, 250s, 500s)

Tablet, chewable

Lactinex®: Mixed culture *L. acidophilus, L. bulgaricus* (50s)

Probiotica®: 100 million units *L. reuteri* (30s, 60s)

Lactobacillus acidophilus *see* Lactobacillus *on this page*

Lactobacillus acidophilus and *Lactobacillus bulgaricus* *see* Lactobacillus *on this page*

lactoflavin *see* riboflavin *on page 571*

Lactrase® [US-OTC] *see* lactase *on previous page*

lactulose (LAK tyoo lose)

U.S./Canadian Brand Names Acilac [Can]; Cholac® [US]; Constilac® [US]; Constulose® [US]; Enulose® [US]; Generlac® [US]; Kristalose™ [US]; Laxilose [Can]; PMS-Lactulose [Can]

Therapeutic Category Ammonium Detoxicant; Laxative

Use Adjunct in the prevention and treatment of portal-systemic encephalopathy (PSE); treatment of chronic constipation

Usual Dosage Oral:

Infants: 2.5-10 mL/day divided 3-4 times/day

Children: 40-90 mL/day divided 3-4 times/day

Adults:

Acute episodes of portal systemic encephalopathy: 30-45 mL at 1- to 2-hour intervals until laxative effect observed

Chronic therapy: 30-45 mL/dose 3-4 times/day; titrate dose to produce 2-3 soft stools per day

Rectal: 300 mL diluted with 700 mL of water or normal saline, and administered via a rectal balloon catheter and retained for 30-60 minutes; may administer every 4-6 hours

Dosage Forms
Crystals for reconstitution (Kristalose™): 10 g, 20 g
Syrup: 10 g/15 mL (15 mL, 30 mL, 237 mL, 473 mL, 946 mL, 1890 mL, 3785 mL)

Lactulose PSE® *(Discontinued) see page 814*

L-AmB *see* amphotericin B liposomal *on page 40*

Lamictal® [US/Can] *see* lamotrigine *on this page*

Lamisil® Cream [US] *see* terbinafine (topical) *on page 623*

Lamisil® Oral [US/Can] *see* terbinafine (oral) *on page 623*

lamivudine (la MI vyoo deen)

U.S./Canadian Brand Names Epivir®-HBV™ [US]; Epivir® [US]; Heptovir® [Can]; 3TC® [Can]
Therapeutic Category Antiviral Agent
Use
Epivir®: In combination with zidovudine for treatment of HIV infection when therapy is warranted based on clinical and/or immunological evidence of disease progression
Epivir®-HBV™: Treatment of chronic hepatitis B associated with evidence of hepatitis B viral replication and active liver inflammation
Usual Dosage Oral:
Hepatitis B virus (HBV): 100 mg once daily
HIV:
Adolescents 12-16 years and Adults: 150 mg twice daily with zidovudine
Adults <50 kg: 2 mg/kg twice daily with zidovudine
Dosage Forms
Solution, oral:
Epivir®: 10 mg/mL (240 mL) [strawberry-banana flavor]
Epivir-HBV®: 5 mg/mL (240 mL) [strawberry-banana flavor]
Tablet:
Epivir®: 150 mg, 300 mg
Epivir-HBV®: 100 mg

lamotrigine (la MOE tri jeen)

Synonyms LTG
U.S./Canadian Brand Names Lamictal® [US/Can]
Therapeutic Category Anticonvulsant
Use Adjunctive treatment of partial seizures, with or without secondary generalized seizures; investigations for absence, generalized tonic-clonic, atypical absence, myoclonic seizures, and Lennox-Gastaut syndrome are in progress
Usual Dosage Oral:
Children: 2-12 years: **Note:** Only whole tablets should be used for dosing, rounded down to the nearest whole tablet
With concomitant antiepileptic drug (AED) regimen with valproic acid (VPA) therapy: 0.15 mg/kg/day in 1-2 divided doses for 2 weeks, then 0.3 mg/kg/day in 1-2 divided doses for 2 weeks; thereafter, titrate by additional 0.3 mg/kg/day every 1-2 weeks; usual maintenance dose: 1-5 mg/kg/day (maximum: 200 mg/day)
With concomitant enzyme-inducing AED regimen without VPA: 0.6 mg/kg/day for 2 weeks, then 1.2 mg/kg/day for 2 weeks; thereafter, titrate by additional 1.2 mg/kg/day every 1-2 weeks; usual maintenance dose: 5-15 mg/kg/day (maximum: 400 mg/day)
Adults: Initial dose: 50 mg/day for 2 weeks, then 100 mg in 2 doses for 2 weeks; thereafter, daily dose can be increased by 100 mg every 1-2 weeks to 300-500 mg/day given in 2 divided doses
With concomitant VPA therapy and other AEDs: 25 mg every other day for 2 weeks; 25 mg/day for 2 weeks; thereafter, dose may be increased by 25-50 mg/day every 1-2 weeks to 150 mg/day given in 2 divided doses
Dosage Forms
Tablet: 25 mg, 100 mg, 150 mg, 200 mg
(Continued)

lamotrigine *(Continued)*

Tablet, dispersible/chewable: 2 mg, 5 mg, 25 mg [black currant flavor]

Lamprene® [US/Can] *see* clofazimine *on page 153*

Lamprene® 100 mg *(Discontinued)* *see page 814*

Lanacane® *(Discontinued)* *see page 814*

Lanacort® [US-OTC] *see* hydrocortisone (topical) *on page 334*

Lanaphilic® [US-OTC] *see* urea *on page 666*

Laniazid® Tablet *(Discontinued)* *see page 814*

Laniroif® [US] *see* butalbital, aspirin, and caffeine *on page 100*

lanolin, cetyl alcohol, glycerin, and petrolatum

(LAN oh lin, SEE til AL koe hol, GLIS er in, & pe troe LAY tum)

U.S./Canadian Brand Names Lubriderm® Fragrance Free [US-OTC]; Lubriderm® [US-OTC]

Therapeutic Category Topical Skin Product

Use Treatment of dry skin

Usual Dosage Topical: Apply to skin as necessary

Dosage Forms

Lotion, bottle, topical: 120 mL, 240 mL, 360 mL, 480 mL

Lotion, tube, topical: 100 mL

Lanorinal® *(Discontinued)* *see page 814*

Lanoxicaps® [US/Can] *see* digoxin *on page 197*

Lanoxin® [US/Can] *see* digoxin *on page 197*

Lanoxin® Pediatric [US] *see* digoxin *on page 197*

lansoprazole (lan SOE pra zole)

U.S./Canadian Brand Names Prevacid® [US/Can]

Therapeutic Category Gastric Acid Secretion Inhibitor

Use Short-term treatment of active duodenal ulcers; maintenance treatment of healed duodenal ulcers; as part of a multidrug regimen for *H. pylori* eradication to reduce the risk of duodenal ulcer recurrence; short-term treatment of active benign gastric ulcer; treatment of NSAID-associated gastric ulcer; to reduce the risk of NSAID-associated gastric ulcer in patients with a history of gastric ulcer who require an NSAID; short-term treatment of symptomatic GERD; short-term treatment for all grades of erosive esophagitis; to maintain healing of erosive esophagitis; long-term treatment of pathological hypersecretory conditions, including Zollinger-Ellison syndrome

Usual Dosage Oral:

Adults:

Duodenal ulcer: Short-term treatment: 15 mg once daily for 4 weeks; maintenance therapy: 15 mg once daily

Gastric ulcer: Short-term treatment: 30 mg once daily for up to 8 weeks

NSAID-associated gastric ulcer (healing): 30 mg once daily for 8 weeks; controlled studies did not extend past 8 weeks of therapy

NSAID-associated gastric ulcer (to reduce risk): Oral: 15 mg once daily for up to 12 weeks; controlled studies did not extend past 12 weeks of therapy

Symptomatic GERD: Short-term treatment: 15 mg once daily for up to 8 weeks

Erosive esophagitis: Short-term treatment: 30 mg once daily for up to 8 weeks; continued treatment for an additional 8 weeks may be considered for recurrence or for patients that do not heal after the first 8 weeks of therapy; maintenance therapy: 15 mg once daily

Hypersecretory conditions: Initial: 60 mg once daily; adjust dose based upon patient response and to reduce acid secretion to <10 mEq/hour (5 mEq/hour in patients with prior gastric surgery); doses of 90 mg twice daily have been used; administer doses >120 mg/day in divided doses

Helicobacter pylori eradication: Currently accepted recommendations (may differ from product labeling): Dose varies with regimen: 30 mg once daily or 60 mg/day in 2 divided doses; requires combination therapy with antibiotics

Dosage Forms

Capsule, delayed release: 15 mg, 30 mg

Granules, oral suspension, delayed release: 15 mg/packet (30s), 30 mg/packet (30s)

lansoprazole, amoxicillin, and clarithromycin

(lan SOE pra zole, a moks i SIL in, & kla RITH roe mye sin)

U.S./Canadian Brand Names Hp-PAC® [Can]; Prevpac™ [US/Can]

Therapeutic Category Antibiotic, Macrolide Combination; Antibiotic, Penicillin; Gastrointestinal Agent, Miscellaneous

Use Eradication of *H. pylori* to reduce the risk of recurrent duodenal ulcer

Dosage Forms The package contains:

Capsule:

Amoxicillin: 500 mg

Lansoprazole: 30 mg

Tablet: Clarithromycin: 500 mg

Lantus® **[US]** *see* insulin preparations *on page 352*

Lanvis® **[Can]** *see* thioguanine *on page 633*

Largactil® **[Can]** *see* chlorpromazine *on page 141*

Largon® *(Discontinued) see page 814*

Lariam® **[US/Can]** *see* mefloquine *on page 405*

Larodopa® *(Discontinued) see page 814*

Lasan™ **HP-1 Topical** *(Discontinued) see page 814*

Lasan™ **Topical** *(Discontinued) see page 814*

Lasix® **[US/Can]** *see* furosemide *on page 291*

Lasix® **Special [Can]** *see* furosemide *on page 291*

Lassar's zinc paste *see* zinc oxide *on page 691*

latanoprost (la TAN oh prost)

U.S./Canadian Brand Names Xalatan® [US/Can]

Therapeutic Category Prostaglandin

Use Reduction of elevated intraocular pressure in patients with open-angle glaucoma and ocular hypertension who are intolerant of the other IOP lowering medications or insufficiently responsive (failed to achieve target IOP determined after multiple measurements over time) to another IOP lowering medication

Usual Dosage Ophthalmic:

Children: Not recommended

Adults: 1 drop in affected eye(s) once daily in the evening

Dosage Forms Solution, ophthalmic: 0.005% (2.5 mL)

***Latrodectus mactans* antivenin** *see* antivenin *(Latrodectus mactans) on page 48*

Lavacol® **[US-OTC]** *see* alcohol (ethyl) *on page 20*

Laxilose [Can] *see* lactulose *on page 372*

l-bunolol *see* levobunolol *on page 379*

l-carnitine *see* levocarnitine *on page 379*

LCD *see* coal tar *on page 158*

LCR *see* vincristine *on page 678*

l-deprenyl *see* selegiline *on page 586*

l-dopa *see* levodopa *on page 380*

Lectopam® **[Can]** *see* bromazepam *(Canada only) on page 92*

Ledercillin VK® *(Discontinued) see page 814*

leflunomide (le FLU no mide)

U.S./Canadian Brand Names Arava™ [US/Can]

Therapeutic Category Anti-inflammatory Agent

Use Treatment of active rheumatoid arthritis to reduce signs and symptoms and to retard structural damage as evidenced by X-ray erosions and joint space narrowing

Usual Dosage Oral:

Adults: Initial: 100 mg/day for 3 days, followed by 20 mg/day; dosage may be decreased to 10 mg/day in patients who have difficulty tolerating the 20 mg dose. Due to the long half-life of the active metabolite, plasma levels may require a prolonged period to decline after dosage reduction.

Guidelines for dosage adjustment or discontinuation based on the severity and persistence of ALT elevation have been developed. For ALT elevations >2 times the upper limit of normal, dosage reduction to 10 mg/day may allow continued administration. Cholestyramine 8 g 3 times/day for 1-3 days may be administered to decrease plasma levels. If elevations >2 times but less than or equal to 3 times the upper limit of normal persist, liver biopsy is recommended. If elevations >3 times the upper limit of normal persist despite cholestyramine administration and dosage reduction, leflunomide should be discontinued and drug elimination should be enhanced with additional cholestyramine as indicated.

Dosage Forms Tablet: 10 mg, 20 mg, 100 mg

Legatrin PM® **[US-OTC]** *see* acetaminophen and diphenhydramine *on page 5*

Lenoltec [Can] *see* acetaminophen and codeine *on page 5*

Lente® **Iletin**® **II [US]** *see* insulin preparations *on page 352*

Lente® **Insulin** *(Discontinued) see page 814*

Lente® **L** *(Discontinued) see page 814*

lepirudin (leh puh ROO din)

U.S./Canadian Brand Names Refludan® [US/Can]

Therapeutic Category Anticoagulant (Other)

Use Indicated for anticoagulation in patient with heparin-induced thrombocytopenia (HIT) and associated thromboembolic disease in order to prevent further thromboembolic complications

Usual Dosage Maximum dose: Do not exceed 0.21 mg/kg/hour unless an evaluation of coagulation abnormalities limiting response has been completed; dosing is weight-based, however patients weighing >110 kg should not receive doses greater than the recommended dose for a patient weighing 110 kg (44 mg bolus and initial maximal infusion rate of 16.5 mg/hour)

Use in patients with heparin-induced thrombocytopenia: Bolus dose: 0.4 mg/kg IVP (over 15-20 seconds), followed by continuous infusion at 0.15 mg/kg/hour; bolus and infusion must be reduced in renal insufficiency

Concomitant use with thrombolytic therapy: Bolus dose: 0.2 mg/kg IVP (over 15-20 seconds), followed by continuous infusion at 0.1 mg/kg/hour

Dosing adjustments during infusions: Monitor first APTT 4 hours after the start of the infusion; subsequent determinations of APTT should be obtained at least once daily during treatment; more frequent monitoring is recommended in renally impaired patients; any APTT out of range should be confirmed prior to adjusting dose, unless a clinical need for immediate reaction exists; if the APTT is below target range, increase infusion by 20%; if the APTT is in excess of the target range, decrease infusion rate by 50%; a repeat APTT should be obtained 4 hours after any dosing change

Dosage Forms Injection: 50 mg

Lescol® **[US/Can]** *see* fluvastatin *on page 284*

Lescol® **XL [US]** *see* fluvastatin *on page 284*

Lessina™ [US] *see* ethinyl estradiol and levonorgestrel *on page 248*

letrozole (LET roe zole)

U.S./Canadian Brand Names Femara® [US/Can]

Therapeutic Category Antineoplastic Agent, Hormone (Antiestrogen)

Use Treatment of advanced breast cancer in postmenopausal women with disease progression following tamoxifen therapy. Patients with ER-negative disease and patients who did not respond to tamoxifen therapy rarely responded to anastrozole.

Usual Dosage Adults: Oral: 2.5 mg once/day, without regard to meals

Dosage Forms Tablet: 2.5 mg

leucovorin (loo koe VOR in)

Synonyms citrovorum factor; folinic acid; 5-formyl tetrahydrofolate

U.S./Canadian Brand Names Wellcovorin® [US]

Therapeutic Category Folic Acid Derivative

Use Antidote for folic acid antagonists; treatment of folate deficient megaloblastic anemias of infancy, sprue, pregnancy; nutritional deficiency when oral folate therapy is not possible

Usual Dosage Children and Adults:

Adjunctive therapy with antimicrobial agents (pyrimethamine): Oral: 2-15 mg/day for 3 days or until blood counts are normal or 5 mg every 3 days; doses of 6 mg/day are needed for patients with platelet counts <100,000/mm^3

Folate-deficient megaloblastic anemia: I.M.: 1 mg/day

Megaloblastic anemia secondary to congenital deficiency of dihydrofolate reductase: I.M.: 3-6 mg/day

Rescue dose: I.V.: 10 mg/m^2 to start, then 10 mg/m^2 every 6 hours orally for 72 hours; if serum creatinine 24 hours after methotrexate is elevated 50% or more **or** the serum MTX concentration is >5 x 10^{-6}M, increase dose to 100 mg/m^2/dose every 3 hours until serum methotrexate level is less than 1 x 10^{-8}M

Dosage Forms

Injection, as calcium: 3 mg/mL (1 mL)

Injection, powder for reconstitution, as calcium: 50 mg, 100 mg, 350 mg

Tablet, as calcium: 5 mg, 10 mg, 15 mg, 25 mg

Leukeran® **[US/Can]** *see* chlorambucil *on page 133*

Leukine™ [US/Can] *see* sargramostim *on page 583*

leuprolide acetate (loo PROE lide AS e tate)

U.S./Canadian Brand Names Eligard™ [US]; Lupron Depot-Ped® [US]; Lupron Depot® [US/Can]; Lupron® [US/Can]; Viadur® [US/Can]

Therapeutic Category Antineoplastic Agent; Luteinizing Hormone-Releasing Hormone Analog

Use Treatment of precocious puberty; palliative treatment of advanced prostate carcinoma

Usual Dosage

Children: S.C.: Precocious puberty: 20-45 mcg/kg/day

Adults:

Advanced prostatic carcinoma:

S.C.: 1 mg/day **or**

I.M. (suspension): 7.5 mg/dose administered monthly

Endometriosis: ≥18 years: I.M.: 3.75 mg/month for 6 months

Dosage Forms

Implant, as acetate (Viadur®): 65 mg [released over 12 months]

(Continued)

leuprolide acetate *(Continued)*

Injection, solution, as acetate (Lupron®): 5 mg/mL (2.8 mL) [contains benzyl alcohol]
Injection, powder for reconstitution, as acetate [depot formulation]:
Eligard™:
  7.5 mg [released over 1 month]
  22.5 mg [released over 3 months]
Lupron Depot®: 3.75 mg, 7.5 mg
Lupron Depot®-3 Month: 11.25 mg, 22.5 mg
Lupron Depot®-4 Month: 30 mg
Lupron Depot-Ped®: 7.5 mg, 11.25 mg, 15 mg

leurocristine *see* vincristine *on page 678*

Leustatin™ **[US/Can]** *see* cladribine *on page 149*

levalbuterol (leve al BYOO ter ole)

Synonyms R-albuterol
U.S./Canadian Brand Names Xopenex™ [US/Can]
Therapeutic Category Adrenergic Agonist Agent; Beta$_2$-Adrenergic Agonist Agent; Bronchodilator
Use Treatment or prevention of bronchospasm in adults and adolescents ≥12 years of age with reversible obstructive airway disease
Usual Dosage
Children: Safety and efficacy in patients <12 years of age not established
Children >12 years and Adults: Inhalation: 0.63 mg 3 times/day at intervals of 6-8 hours, via nebulization. Dosage may be increased to 1.25 mg 3 times/day with close monitoring for adverse effects. Most patients gain optimal benefit from regular use
Dosage Forms Solution for nebulization: 0.31 mg/3 mL (24s); 0.63 mg/3 mL (24s); 1.25 mg/3 mL (24s)

levamisole (lee VAM i sole)

U.S./Canadian Brand Names Ergamisol® [US/Can]
Therapeutic Category Immune Modulator
Use Adjuvant treatment with fluorouracil in Dukes stage C colon cancer
Usual Dosage Oral: Initial: 50 mg every 8 hours for 3 days, then 50 mg every 8 hours for 3 days every 2 weeks (fluorouracil is always administered concomitantly)
Dosage Forms Tablet, as base: 50 mg

Levaquin® **[US/Can]** *see* levofloxacin *on page 380*

Levatol® **[US/Can]** *see* penbutolol *on page 497*

Levbid® **[US]** *see* hyoscyamine *on page 339*

levetiracetam (lev e tir AS e tam)

U.S./Canadian Brand Names Keppra® [US/Can]
Therapeutic Category Anticonvulsant, Miscellaneous
Use Indicated as adjunctive therapy in the treatment of partial onset seizures in adults with epilepsy
Usual Dosage Adults: Initial: 500 mg twice daily; additional dosing increments may be given (1000 mg/day additional every 2 weeks) to a maximum recommended daily dose of 3000 mg
Dosage Forms Tablet: 250 mg, 500 mg, 750 mg

Levlen® **[US]** *see* ethinyl estradiol and levonorgestrel *on page 248*

Levlite™ **[US]** *see* ethinyl estradiol and levonorgestrel *on page 248*

levobetaxolol (lee voe be TAX oh lol)

U.S./Canadian Brand Names Betaxon® [US/Can]

Therapeutic Category Beta-Adrenergic Blocker, Ophthalmic

Use Lowers intraocular pressure in patients with chronic open-angle glaucoma or ocular hypertension

Usual Dosage Adults: Ophthalmic: Instill 1 drop in affected eye(s) twice daily

Dosage Forms Solution, ophthalmic: 0.5% (5 mL, 10 mL, 15 mL)

levobunolol (lee voe BYOO noe lole)

Synonyms l-bunolol

U.S./Canadian Brand Names Betagan® [US/Can]; Novo-Levobunolol [Can]; Optho-Bunolol® [Can]; PMS-Levobunolol [Can]

Therapeutic Category Beta-Adrenergic Blocker

Use To lower intraocular pressure in chronic open-angle glaucoma or ocular hypertension

Usual Dosage Adults: Ophthalmic: 1-2 drops of 0.5% solution in eye(s) once daily or 1-2 drops of 0.25% solution twice daily

Dosage Forms Solution, ophthalmic, as hydrochloride: 0.25% (5 mL, 10 mL, 15 mL); 0.5% (2 mL, 5 mL, 10 mL, 15 mL)

levobupivacaine (LEE voe byoo PIV a kane)

U.S./Canadian Brand Names Chirocaine® [US/Can]

Therapeutic Category Local Anesthetic, Amide Derivative; Local Anesthetic, Injectable

Use Production of local or regional anesthesia for surgery and obstetrics, and for postoperative pain management

Usual Dosage Adults: **Note:** Rapid injection of a large volume of local anesthetic solution should be avoided. Fractional (incremental) doses are recommended.

Maximum dosage: Epidural doses up to 375 mg have been administered incrementally to patients during a surgical procedure

Intraoperative block and postoperative pain: 695 mg in 24 hours

Postoperative epidural infusion over 24 hours: 570 mg

Single-fractionated injection for brachial plexus block: 300 mg

Dosage Forms Injection: 2.5 mg/mL (10 mL, 30 mL); 5 mg/mL (10 mL, 30 mL); 7.5 mg/mL (10 mL, 30 mL)

levocabastine (LEE voe kab as teen)

U.S./Canadian Brand Names Livostin® [US/Can]

Therapeutic Category Antihistamine

Use Temporary relief of the signs and symptoms of seasonal allergic conjunctivitis

Usual Dosage Adults: Ophthalmic: Instill 1 drop in affected eye 4 times/day for up to 2 weeks

Dosage Forms Suspension, ophthalmic, as hydrochloride: 0.05% (2.5 mL, 5 mL, 10 mL)

levocarnitine (lee voe KAR ni teen)

Synonyms l-carnitine

U.S./Canadian Brand Names Carnitor® [US/Can]; Mito-Carn® [US]

Therapeutic Category Dietary Supplement

Use Treatment of primary or secondary carnitine deficiency

Usual Dosage Oral:

Children: 50-100 mg/kg/day divided 2-3 times/day, maximum: 3 g/day; dosage must be individualized based upon patient response; higher dosages have been used

Adults: 1-3 g/day for 50 kg subject; start at 1 g/day, increase slowly assessing tolerance and response

Dosage Forms

Capsule: 250 mg

Injection: 200 mg/mL ampul (5 mL)

(Continued)

levocarnitine (Continued)
Solution, oral: 100 mg/mL (118 mL)
Tablet: 330 mg

levodopa (lee voe DOE pa)
Synonyms L-3-hydroxytyrosine; l-dopa
Therapeutic Category Diagnostic Agent; Dopaminergic Agent (Anti-Parkinson's)
Use Diagnostic agent for growth hormone deficiency
Usual Dosage Children: Oral (administered as a single dose to evaluate growth hormone deficiency): 0.5 g/m^2
> **or**
> <30 lbs: 125 mg
> 30-70 lbs: 250 mg
> >70 lbs: 500 mg

Dosage Forms
Capsule: 100 mg, 250 mg, 500 mg
Tablet: 100 mg, 250 mg, 500 mg

levodopa and carbidopa (lee voe DOE pa & kar bi DOE pa)
Synonyms carbidopa and levodopa
U.S./Canadian Brand Names Apo®-Levocarb [Can]; Endo®-Levodopa/Carbidopa [Can]; Nu-Levocarb [Can]; Sinemet® CR [US/Can]; Sinemet® [US/Can]
Therapeutic Category Anti-Parkinson's Agent; Dopaminergic Agent (Anti-Parkinson's)
Use Idiopathic Parkinson's disease; postencephalitic parkinsonism; symptomatic parkinsonism
Usual Dosage Adults: Oral (carbidopa/levodopa): 75/300 to 150/1500 mg/day in 3-4 divided doses; can increase up to 200/2000 mg/day
Dosage Forms
Tablet:
  10/100: Carbidopa 10 mg and levodopa 100 mg
  25/100: Carbidopa 25 mg and levodopa 100 mg
  25/250: Carbidopa 25 mg and levodopa 250 mg
Tablet, sustained release:
  Carbidopa 25 mg and levodopa 100 mg
  Carbidopa 50 mg and levodopa 200 mg

Levo-Dromoran® [US] *see* levorphanol *on page 382* *on page 382*

levofloxacin (lee voe FLOKS a sin)
U.S./Canadian Brand Names Levaquin® [US/Can]; Quixin™ Ophthalmic [US]
Therapeutic Category Antibiotic, Ophthalmic; Antibiotic, Quinolone
Use
Systemic:
Acute bacterial exacerbation of chronic bronchitis and community-acquired pneumonia due to *S. aureus*, *S. pneumoniae* (including penicillin-resistant strains), *H. influenzae*, *H. parainfluenzae*, or *M. catarrhalis*, *C. pneumoniae*, *L. pneumophila*, or *M. pneumoniae*
Acute maxillary sinusitis due to *S. pneumoniae*, *H. influenzae*, or *M. catarrhalis*
Acute pyelonephritis caused by *E. coli*
Skin or skin structure infections:
  Complicated, due to methcillin-susceptible *S. aureus*, *Enterococcus fecalis*, *S. pyogenes*, or *Proteus mirabilis*
  Uncomplicated, due to *S. aureus* or *S. pyogenes*
Urinary tract infections:
  Complicated, due to gram-negative bacteria (*E. coli*, *Enterobacter cloacae*, *Klebsiella pneumoniae*, *Proteus mirabilis*, *Enterococcus fecalis*, or *Pseudomonas aeruginosa*)
  Uncomplicated, due to *E. coli*, *K. pneumoniae*, or *S. saprophyticus*

Ophthalmic: Bacterial conjunctivitis due to *S. aureus* (methicillin-susceptible strains), *S. epidermidis* (methicillin-susceptible strains), *S. pneumoniae*, *Streptococcus* (groups C/F), *Streptococcus* (group G), Viridans group streptococci, *Corynebacterium* spp, *H. influenzae*, *Acinetobacter lwoffii*, or *Serratia marcescens*

Usual Dosage
Adults: Oral, I.V. (infuse I.V. solution over 60 minutes):
Acute bacterial exacerbation of chronic bronchitis: 500 mg every 24 hours for at least 7 days
Community-acquired pneumonia: 500 mg every 24 hours for 7-14 days
Acute maxillary sinusitis: 500 mg every 24 hours for 10-14 days
Uncomplicated skin infections: 500 mg every 24 hours for 7-10 days
Complicated skin infections: 750 mg every 24 hours for 7-14 days
Uncomplicated urinary tract infections: 250 mg once daily for 3 days
Complicated urinary tract infections, including acute pyelonephritis: 250 mg every 24 hours for 10 days

Children ≥1 year and Adults: Ophthalmic:
Treatment day 1 and day 2: Instill 1-2 drops into affected eye(s) every 2 hours while awake, up to 8 times/day
Treatment day 3 through day 7: Instill 1-2 drops into affected eye(s) every 4 hours while awake, up to 4 times/day

Dosage Forms
Infusion [in D$_5$W]: 5 mg/mL (50 mL, 100 mL)
Injection: 25 mg/mL (20 mL)
Solution, ophthalmic: 0.5% (2.5 mL, 5 mL)
Tablet: 250 mg, 500 mg, 750 mg

levomepromazine *see* methotrimeprazine *(Canada only) on page 418*

levomethadyl acetate hydrochloride
(lee voe METH a dil AS e tate hye droe KLOR ide)
U.S./Canadian Brand Names ORLAAM® [US]
Therapeutic Category Analgesic, Narcotic
Controlled Substance C-II
Use Management of opiate dependence
Usual Dosage Adults: Oral: 20-40 mg 3 times/week; range: 10 mg to as high as 140 mg 3 times/week
Dosage Forms Solution, oral: 10 mg/mL (474 mL)

levonorgestrel (LEE voe nor jes trel)
U.S./Canadian Brand Names Mirena® [US]; Norplant® Implant [Can]; Plan B™ [US/Can]
Therapeutic Category Contraceptive, Implant (Progestin); Contraceptive, Progestin Only
Use Prevention of pregnancy
Usual Dosage Adults:
Long-term prevention of pregnancy:
Subdermal capsules: Total administration doses (implanted): 216 mg in 6 capsules which should be implanted during the first 7 days of onset of menses subdermally in the upper arm; each Norplant® silastic capsule releases 80 mcg of levonorgestrel/day for 6-18 months, following which a rate of release of 25-30 mcg/day is maintained for ≤5 years; capsules should be removed by end of 5th year
Intrauterine system: To be inserted into uterine cavity; should be inserted within 7 days of onset of menstruation or immediately after first trimester abortion; releases 20 mcg levonorgestrel/day over 5 years. May be removed and replaced with a new unit at anytime during menstrual cycle; do not leave any one system in place for >5 years
Emergency contraception: Oral tablet: One 0.75 mg tablet as soon as possible within 72 hours of unprotected sexual intercourse; a second 0.75 mg tablet should be taken 12 hours after the first dose; may be used at any time during menstrual cycle
(Continued)

levonorgestrel (Continued)

Dosage Forms
Capsule, subdermal implantation (Norplant® Implant): 36 mg (6s)
Intrauterine device (Mirena®): 52 mg
Tablet (Plan B™): 0.75 mg

levonorgestrel and ethinyl estradiol *see* ethinyl estradiol and levonorgestrel *on page 248*

Levophed® [US/Can] *see* norepinephrine *on page 465*

Levora® [US] *see* ethinyl estradiol and levonorgestrel *on page 248*

levorphanol (lee VOR fa nole)

U.S./Canadian Brand Names Levo-Dromoran® [US]
Therapeutic Category Analgesic, Narcotic
Controlled Substance C-II
Use Relief of moderate to severe pain; also used parenterally for preoperative sedation and an adjunct to nitrous oxide/oxygen anesthesia
Usual Dosage Adults: Oral, S.C.: 2 mg, up to 3 mg if necessary
Dosage Forms
Injection, as tartrate: 2 mg/mL (1 mL, 10 mL)
Tablet, as tartrate: 2 mg

Levo-T™ [US] *see* levothyroxine *on this page*

Levothroid® [US] *see* levothyroxine *on this page*

levothyroxine (lee voe thye ROKS een)

Synonyms *l*-thyroxine; t_4 thyroxine
U.S./Canadian Brand Names Eltroxin® [Can]; Levothroid® [US]; Levo-T™ [US]; Levoxyl® [US]; Novothyrox [US]; Synthroid® [US/Can]; Unithroid™ [US]
Therapeutic Category Thyroid Product
Use Replacement or supplemental therapy in hypothyroidism; management of nontoxic goiter, chronic lymphocytic thyroiditis, as an adjunct to thyrotoxicosis
Usual Dosage
Children:
Oral:
0-6 months: 8-10 mcg/kg/day
6-12 months: 6-8 mcg/kg/day
1-5 years: 5-6 mcg/kg/day
6-12 years: 4-5 mcg/kg/day
>12 years: 2-3 mcg/kg/day
I.M., I.V.: 75% of the oral dose
Adults:
Oral: 12.5-50 mcg/day to start, then increase by 25-50 mcg/day at intervals of 2-4 weeks; average adult dose: 100-200 mcg/day
I.M., I.V.: 50% of the oral dose
Myxedema coma or stupor: I.V.: 200-500 mcg one time, then 100-300 mcg the next day if necessary
Dosage Forms
Injection, powder for reconstitution, as sodium (Synthroid®): 0.2 mg, 0.5 mg
Tablet, as sodium: 25 mcg, 50 mcg, 75 mcg, 88 mcg, 100 mcg, 112 mcg, 125 mcg, 150 mcg, 175 mcg, 200 mcg, 300 mcg
Levothroid®, Levoxyl®, Synthroid®: 25 mcg, 50 mcg, 75 mcg, 88 mcg, 100 mcg, 112 mcg, 125 mcg, 137 mcg, 150 mcg, 175 mcg, 200 mcg, 300 mcg
Levo-T™, Unithroid™: 25 mcg, 50 mcg, 75 mcg, 88 mcg, 100 mcg, 112 mcg, 125 mcg, 150 mcg, 175 mcg, 200 mcg, 300 mcg
Novothyrox: 25 mcg, 50 mcg, 75 mcg, 88 mcg, 100 mcg, 112 mcg, 125 mcg, 137 mcg, 150 mcg, 175 mcg, 200 mcg, 300 mcg [dye free]

Levoxyl® **[US]** *see* levothyroxine *on previous page*

Levsin® **[US/Can]** *see* hyoscyamine *on page 339*

Levsinex® **[US]** *see* hyoscyamine *on page 339*

Levsin/SL® **[US]** *see* hyoscyamine *on page 339*

Levulan® **Kerastick™** **[US/Can]** *see* aminolevulinic acid *on page 33*

levulose, dextrose and phosphoric acid *see* phosphorated carbohydrate solution *on page 512*

Lexapro™ **[US]** *see* escitalopram *on page 236*

Lexxel™ **[US/Can]** *see* enalapril and felodipine *on page 226*

LHRH *see* gonadorelin *on page 304*

l-hyoscyamine sulfate *see* hyoscyamine *on page 339*

Librax® **[US/Can]** *see* clidinium and chlordiazepoxide *on page 151*

Libritabs® **(all products)** *(Discontinued)* *see page 814*

Librium® **[US]** *see* chlordiazepoxide *on page 134*

Lice-Enz® Shampoo *(Discontinued)* *see page 814*

Lida-Mantle HC® **[US]** *see* lidocaine and hydrocortisone *on next page*

Lidemol® **[Can]** *see* fluocinonide *on page 277*

Lidex® **[US/Can]** *see* fluocinonide *on page 277*

Lidex-E® **[US]** *see* fluocinonide *on page 277*

lidocaine (LYE doe kane)

Synonyms lignocaine

U.S./Canadian Brand Names Anestacon® [US]; Dermaflex® Gel [US]; ELA-Max® [US-OTC]; Lidodan™ [Can]; Lidoderm® [US/Can]; LidoPen® Auto-Injector [US]; Solarcaine® Aloe Extra Burn Relief [US-OTC]; Xylocaine® [US/Can]; Xylocard® [Can]; Zilactin® [Can]; Zilactin-L® [US-OTC]

Therapeutic Category Analgesic, Topical; Antiarrhythmic Agent, Class I-B; Local Anesthetic

Use Drug of choice for ventricular ectopy, ventricular tachycardia (VT), ventricular fibrillation (VF); for pulseless VT or VF preferably administer **after** defibrillation and epinephrine; control of premature ventricular contractions, wide-complex PSVT; local anesthetic

Usual Dosage

Topical: Apply to affected area as needed; maximum: 3 mg/kg/dose; do not repeat within 2 hours

Injectable local anesthetic: Varies with procedure, degree of anesthesia needed, vascularity of tissue, duration of anesthesia required, and physical condition of patient; maximum: 4.5 mg/kg/dose; do not repeat within 2 hours

Children: Endotracheal, I.O., I.V.: Loading dose: 1 mg/kg; may repeat in 10-15 minutes to a maximum total dose of 5 mg/kg; after loading dose, start I.V. continuous infusion 20-50 mcg/kg/minute. Use 20 mcg/kg/minute in patients with shock, hepatic disease, mild congestive heart failure (CHF); moderate to severe CHF may require 1/2 loading dose and lower infusion rates to avoid toxicity. Endotracheal doses should be diluted to 1-2 mL with normal saline prior to endotracheal administration and may need 2-3 times the I.V. dose.

Adults: Antiarrhythmic:

Endotracheal: Total dose: 5 mg/kg; follow with 0.5 mg/kg in 10 minutes if effective

I.M.: 300 mg may be repeated in 1-1 1/2 hours

I.V.: Loading dose: 1 mg/kg/dose, then 50-100 mg bolus over 2-3 minutes; may repeat in 5-10 minutes up to 200-300 mg in a 1-hour period; continuous infusion of 20-50 mcg/kg/minute or 1-4 mg/minute; decrease the dose in patients with CHF, shock, or hepatic disease

(Continued)

lidocaine *(Continued)*

Dosage Forms
Cream, as hydrochloride: 2% (56 g); 4% (5 g, 30 g)
Gel, as hydrochloride: 0.5% (15 mL); 2.5% (15 mL)
Injection, I.M.: 10% [100 mg/mL] (3 mL)
Injection, as hydrochloride:
  0.5% [5 mg/mL] (50 mL)
  1% [10 mg/mL] (2 mL, 5 mL, 10 mL, 20 mL, 30 mL, 50 mL)
  1.5% [15 mg/mL] (20 mL)
  2% [20 mg/mL] (2 mL, 5 mL, 10 mL, 20 mL, 30 mL, 50 mL)
  4% [40 mg/mL] (5 mL); 10% [100 mg/mL] (10 mL)
  20% [200 mg/mL] (10 mL, 20 mL)
Injection, I.V. direct:
  1% [10 mg/mL] (5 mL, 20 mL, 30 mL, 50 mL)
  2% [20 mg/mL] (5 mL, 10 mL, 20 mL, 30 mL, 50 mL)
Injection, I.V. admixture [preservative free]:
  4% [40 mg/mL] (5 mL, 25 mL, 50 mL)
  10% [100 mg/mL] (10 mL)
  20% [200 mg/mL] (5 mL, 10 mL)
Injection, I.V. infusion [in D_5W]:
  0.2% [2 mg/mL] (500 mL)
  0.4% [4 mg/mL] (250 mL, 500 mL, 1000 mL)
  0.8% [8 mg/mL] (250 mL, 500 mL)
Jelly, as hydrochloride: 2%
Liquid, topical, as hydrochloride: 2.5% (7.5 mL)
Liquid, viscous, as hydrochloride: 2% (20 mL, 100 mL)
Ointment, as hydrochloride: 2.5% [OTC], 5% (35 g)
Patch, transdermal: 5%
Solution, topical, as hydrochloride: 2% (15 mL, 240 mL); 4% (50 mL)

lidocaine and epinephrine (LYE doe kane & ep i NEF rin)

Synonyms epinephrine and lidocaine
U.S./Canadian Brand Names Xylocaine® With Epinephrine [US/Can]
Therapeutic Category Local Anesthetic
Use Local infiltration anesthesia
Usual Dosage Children (dosage varies with the anesthetic procedure): Use lidocaine concentrations of 0.5% or 1% (or even more dilute) to decrease possibility of toxicity; lidocaine dose should not exceed 4.5 mg/kg/dose; do not repeat within 2 hours
Dosage Forms
Injection with epinephrine:
  Epinephrine 1:200,000: Lidocaine hydrochloride 0.5% [5 mg/mL] (50 mL); 1% [10 mg/mL] (30 mL); 1.5% [15 mg/mL] (5 mL, 10 mL, 30 mL); 2% [20 mg/mL] (20 mL)
  Epinephrine 1:100,000: Lidocaine hydrochloride 1% [10 mg/mL] (20 mL, 50 mL); 2% [20 mg/mL] (1.8 mL, 20 mL, 30 mL, 50 mL)
  Epinephrine 1:50,000: Lidocaine hydrochloride 2% [20 mg/mL] (1.8 mL)

lidocaine and hydrocortisone (LYE doe kane & hye droe KOR ti sone)

Synonyms hydrocortisone and lidocaine
U.S./Canadian Brand Names Lida-Mantle HC® [US]
Therapeutic Category Anesthetic/Corticosteroid
Use Topical anti-inflammatory and anesthetic for skin disorders
Usual Dosage Topical: Apply 2-4 times/day
Dosage Forms Cream: Lidocaine 3% and hydrocortisone 0.5% (15 g, 30 g)

lidocaine and prilocaine (LYE doe kane & PRIL oh kane)

Synonyms prilocaine and lidocaine
U.S./Canadian Brand Names EMLA® [US/Can]

Therapeutic Category Analgesic, Topical

Use Topical anesthetic for use on normal intact skin to provide local analgesia for minor procedures such as I.V. cannulation or venipuncture; has also been used for painful procedures such as lumbar puncture and skin graft harvesting

Usual Dosage Children and Adults: Topical: Apply a thick layer of cream to intact skin and cover with an occlusive dressing; for minor procedures, apply 2.5 g/site for at least 60 minutes; for painful procedures, apply 2 g/10 cm^2 of skin and leave on for at least 2 hours

Dosage Forms

Cream: Lidocaine 2.5% and prilocaine 2.5% [2 Tegaderm® dressings] (5 g, 30 g)

Disc, anesthetic: 1 g (25 mg lidocaine and 25 mg prilocaine in each 10 square centimeter disc)

Lidodan™ [Can] *see* lidocaine *on page 383*

Lidoderm® [US/Can] *see* lidocaine *on page 383*

LidoPen® Auto-Injector [US] *see* lidocaine *on page 383*

LidoPen® I.M. Injection Auto-Injector *(Discontinued)* *see page 814*

LID-Pack® [Can] *see* bacitracin and polymyxin B *on page 68*

lignocaine *see* lidocaine *on page 383*

Limbitrol® [US/Can] *see* amitriptyline and chlordiazepoxide *on page 35*

Limbitrol® DS [US] *see* amitriptyline and chlordiazepoxide *on page 35*

Lin-Amox [Can] *see* amoxicillin *on page 37*

Lin-Buspirone [Can] *see* buspirone *on page 98*

Lincocin® [US/Can] *see* lincomycin *on this page*

lincomycin (lin koe MYE sin)

U.S./Canadian Brand Names Lincocin® [US/Can]; Lincorex® [US]

Therapeutic Category Macrolide (Antibiotic)

Use Treatment of susceptible bacterial infections, mainly those caused by streptococci and staphylococci

Usual Dosage

Children >1 month:

I.M.: 10 mg/kg every 12-24 hours

I.V.: 10-20 mg/kg/day in divided doses 2-3 times/day

Adults:

I.M.: 600 mg every 12-24 hours

I.V.: 600-1 g every 8-12 hours up to 8 g/day

Dosage Forms

Capsule, as hydrochloride: 250 mg, 500 mg

Injection, as hydrochloride: 300 mg/mL (2 mL, 10 mL)

Lincorex® [US] *see* lincomycin *on this page*

lindane (LIN dane)

Synonyms benzene hexachloride; gamma benzene hexachloride; hexachlorocyclohexane

U.S./Canadian Brand Names Hexit™ [Can]; PMS-Lindane [Can]

Therapeutic Category Scabicides/Pediculicides

Use Treatment of scabies (*Sarcoptes scabiei*), *Pediculus capitis* (head lice), and *Pediculus pubis* (crab lice)

Usual Dosage Children and Adults: Topical:

Scabies: Apply a thin layer of lotion and massage it on skin from the neck to the toes. For adults, bathe and remove the drug after 8-12 hours; for children, wash off 6 hours after application.

(Continued)

lindane *(Continued)*

Pediculosis: 15-30 mL of shampoo is applied and lathered for 4-5 minutes; rinse hair thoroughly and comb with a fine tooth comb to remove nits; repeat treatment in 7 days if lice or nits are still present

Dosage Forms

Lotion: 1% (60 mL, 473 mL, 4000 mL)

Shampoo: 1% (60 mL, 473 mL, 4000 mL)

linezolid (li NE zoh lid)

U.S./Canadian Brand Names Zyvox™ [US]

Therapeutic Category Antibiotic, Oxazolidinone

Use Treatment of vancomycin-resistant *Enterococcus faecium* (VRE) infections, nosocomial pneumonia caused by *Staphylococcus aureus* including MRSA or *Streptococcus pneumoniae* (penicillin-susceptible strains only), complicated and uncomplicated skin and skin structure infections, and community-acquired pneumonia caused by susceptible gram-positive organisms.

Usual Dosage Adult:

Oral, I.V.:

VRE infections: 600 mg every 12 hours for 14-28 days

Nosocomial pneumonia, complicated skin and skin structure infections, community-acquired pneumonia including concurrent bacteremia: 600 mg every 12 hours for 10-14 days

Oral: Uncomplicated skin and skin structure infections: 400 mg every 12 hours for 10-14 days

Dosage Forms

Injection [premixed]: 200 mg (100 mL); 400 mg (200 mL); 600 mg (300 mL)

Suspension, oral: 20 mg/mL (150 mL) [orange flavor]

Tablet: 400 mg, 600 mg

Lin-Megestrol [Can] *see* megestrol acetate *on page 405*

Lin-Pravastatin [Can] *see* pravastatin *on page 535*

Lioresal® [US/Can] *see* baclofen *on page 70*

Liotec [Can] *see* baclofen *on page 70*

liothyronine (lye oh THYE roe neen)

Synonyms *l*-triiodothyronine; t_3 thyronine

U.S./Canadian Brand Names Cytomel® [US/Can]; Triostat™ [US]

Therapeutic Category Thyroid Product

Use Replacement or supplemental therapy in hypothyroidism, management of nontoxic goiter, chronic lymphocytic thyroiditis, as an adjunct in thyrotoxicosis and as a diagnostic aid; levothyroxine is recommended for chronic therapy; (if rapid correction of thyroid is needed, T_3 is preferred, but use cautiously and with lower recommended doses)

Usual Dosage

Mild hypothyroidism: 25 mcg/day; daily dosage may then be increased by 12.5 or 25 mcg/day every 1 or 2 weeks; maintenance: 25-75 mcg/day

Myxedema: 5mcg/day; may be increased by 5-10 mcg/day every 1-2 weeks; when 25 mcg is reached, dosage may often be increased by 12.5 or 25 mcg every 1 or 2 weeks; maintenance: 50-100 mcg/day

Cretinism: 5 mcg/day with a 5 mcg increment every 3-4 days until the desired response is achieved

Simple (nontoxic) goiter: 5 mcg/day; may be increased every week or two by 5 or 10 mcg; when 25 mcg/day is reached, dosage may be increased every week or two by 12.5 or 25 mcg; maintenance: 75 mcg/day

T_3 suppression test: I^{131} thyroid uptake is in the borderline-high range, administer 75-100 mcg/day for 7 days then repeat I^{131} thyroid uptake test

Children and Elderly: Start therapy with 5 mcg/day; increase only by 5 mcg increments at the recommended intervals

Dosage Forms

Injection, solution, as sodium (Triostar®): 10 mcg/mL (1 mL) [contains alcohol 6.8%]

Tablet, as sodium (Cytomel®): 5 mcg, 25 mcg, 50 mcg

liotrix (LYE oh triks)

Synonyms t_3/t_4 liotrix

U.S./Canadian Brand Names Thyrolar® [US/Can]

Therapeutic Category Thyroid Product

Use Replacement or supplemental therapy in hypothyroidism

Usual Dosage Congenital hypothyroidism: Oral:

Children (dose/day):

0-6 months: 8-10 mcg/kg

6-12 months: 6-8 mcg/kg

1-5 years: 5-6 mcg/kg

6-12 years: 4-5 mcg/kg

>12 years: 2-3 mcg/kg

Adults: 30 mg/day, increasing by 15 mg/day at 2- to 3-week intervals to a maximum of 180 mg/day

Dosage Forms

Tablet (in mg of thyroid equivalent):

15 mg [levothyroxine sodium 12.5 mcg and liothyronine sodium 3.1 mcg]

30 mg [levothyroxine sodium 25 mcg and liothyronine sodium 6.25 mcg]

60 mg [levothyroxine sodium 50 mcg and liothyronine sodium 12.5 mcg]

120 mg [levothyroxine sodium 100 mcg and liothyronine sodium 25 mcg]

180 mg [levothyroxine sodium 150 mcg and liothyronine sodium 37.5 mcg]

lipancreatin see pancrelipase on page 489

lipase, protease, and amylase see pancrelipase on page 489

Lipidil Micro® [Can] see fenofibrate on page 265

Lipidil Supra® [Can] see fenofibrate on page 265

Lipitor® [US/Can] see atorvastatin on page 61

Liposyn® [US] see fat emulsion on page 263

Lipram® [US] see pancrelipase on page 489

Liquaemin® (Discontinued) see page 814

Liquibid® [US] see guaifenesin on page 307

Liquibid® 1200 [US] see guaifenesin on page 307

Liquibid-D [US] see guaifenesin and phenylephrine on page 310

Liqui-Char® [US/Can] see charcoal on page 131

liquid antidote see charcoal on page 131

Liquid Barosperse® [US] see radiological/contrast media (ionic) on page 561

Liquid Pred® (Discontinued) see page 814

Liqui-E® [US] see tocophersolan on page 642

Liquifilm® Forte Solution (Discontinued) see page 814

Liquifilm® Tears Solution (Discontinued) see page 814

Liquifilm® Tears [US-OTC] see artificial tears on page 56

Liquipake® [US] see radiological/contrast media (ionic) on page 561

Liquiprin® for Children [US-OTC] see acetaminophen on page 3

lisinopril (lyse IN oh pril)

U.S./Canadian Brand Names Apo®-Lisinopril [Can]; Prinivil® [US/Can]; Zestril® [US/Can]

Therapeutic Category Angiotensin-Converting Enzyme (ACE) Inhibitor

Use Treatment of hypertension, either alone or in combination with other antihypertensive agents

Usual Dosage Adults: Oral: 10-40 mg/day in a single dose

Dosage Forms Tablet: 2.5 mg, 5 mg, 10 mg, 20 mg, 30 mg, 40 mg

lisinopril and hydrochlorothiazide

(lyse IN oh pril & hye droe klor oh THYE a zide)

Synonyms hydrochlorothiazide and lisinopril

U.S./Canadian Brand Names Prinzide® [US/Can]; Zestoretic® [US/Can]

Therapeutic Category Antihypertensive Agent, Combination

Use Treatment of hypertension

Usual Dosage Adults: Oral: Dosage is individualized; see each component for appropriate dosing suggestions

Dosage Forms
Tablet:
Lisinopril 10 mg and hydrochlorothiazide 12.5 mg
Lisinopril 20 mg and hydrochlorothiazide 12.5 mg
Lisinopril 20 mg and hydrochlorothiazide 25 mg

Listerex® Scrub *(Discontinued)* *see page 814*

Listermint® With Fluoride *(Discontinued)* *see page 814*

Lithane™ [Can] *see* lithium *on this page*

Lithane® (Discontinued) *see page 814*

lithium (LITH ee um)

U.S./Canadian Brand Names Carbolith™ [Can]; Duralith® [Can]; Eskalith CR® [US]; Eskalith® [US]; Lithane™ [Can]; Lithobid® [US]; PMS-Lithium Carbonate [Can]; PMS-Lithium Citrate [Can]

Therapeutic Category Antimanic Agent

Use Management of acute manic episodes, bipolar disorders, and depression

Usual Dosage Oral: Monitor serum concentrations and clinical response (efficacy and toxicity) to determine proper dose

Children: 15-60 mg/kg/day in 3-4 divided doses; dose not to exceed usual adult dosage
Adults: 300 mg 3-4 times/day; usual maximum maintenance dose: 2.4 g/day

Dosage Forms
Capsule, as carbonate: 150 mg, 300 mg, 600 mg
Syrup, as citrate: 300 mg/5 mL (5 mL, 10 mL, 480 mL)
Tablet, as carbonate: 300 mg
Tablet, controlled release, as carbonate: 450 mg
Tablet, extended release, as carbonate: 300 mg

Lithobid® [US] *see* lithium *on this page*

Lithonate® (Discontinued) *see page 814*

Lithostat® [US] *see* acetohydroxamic acid *on page 11*

Lithotabs® (Discontinued) *see page 814*

Livostin® [US/Can] *see* levocabastine *on page 379*

LKV-Drops® [US-OTC] *see* vitamin (multiple/pediatric) *on page 683*

l-lysine (el-LYE seen)

U.S./Canadian Brand Names Lysinyl® [US-OTC]

Therapeutic Category Dietary Supplement

Use Improves utilization of vegetable proteins
Usual Dosage Adults: Oral: 334-1500 mg/day
Dosage Forms
  Capsule, as hydrochloride: 500 mg
  Tablet, as hydrochloride: 312 mg, 334 mg, 500 mg, 1000 mg

LMD®️ [US] *see* dextran *on page 187*

LoCHOLEST®️ [US] *see* cholestyramine resin *on page 143*

LoCHOLEST®️ Light [US] *see* cholestyramine resin *on page 143*

Locoid®️ [US/Can] *see* hydrocortisone (topical) *on page 334*

Lodine®️ [US/Can] *see* etodolac *on page 258*

Lodine®️ XL [US] *see* etodolac *on page 258*

Lodosyn®️ [US] *see* carbidopa *on page 114*

Iodoxamide tromethamine (loe DOKS a mide troe METH a meen)
  U.S./Canadian Brand Names Alomide®️ [US/Can]
  Therapeutic Category Mast Cell Stabilizer
  Use Symptomatic treatment of vernal keratoconjunctivitis, vernal conjunctivitis, and vernal keratitis
  Usual Dosage Children >2 years and Adults: Ophthalmic: Instill 1-2 drops in eye(s) 4 times/day for up to 3 months
  Dosage Forms Solution, ophthalmic: 0.1% (10 mL)

Lodrane®️ 12 Hour [US-OTC] *see* brompheniramine *on page 93*

Loestrin®️ [US/Can] *see* ethinyl estradiol and norethindrone *on page 251*

Loestrin®️ Fe [US] *see* ethinyl estradiol and norethindrone *on page 251*

Logen®️ *(Discontinued)* *see page 814*

Lomanate®️ *(Discontinued)* *see page 814*

lomefloxacin (loe me FLOKS a sin)
  U.S./Canadian Brand Names Maxaquin®️ [US]
  Therapeutic Category Quinolone
  Use Quinolone antibiotic for skin and skin structure, lower respiratory and urinary tract infections, and sexually transmitted diseases
  Usual Dosage Adults: Oral: 400 mg once daily for 10-14 days
  Dosage Forms Tablet, as hydrochloride: 400 mg

Lomine [Can] *see* dicyclomine *on page 194*

Lomocot®️ [US] *see* diphenoxylate and atropine *on page 203*

Lomotil®️ [US/Can] *see* diphenoxylate and atropine *on page 203*

lomustine (loe MUS teen)
  Synonyms CCNU
  U.S./Canadian Brand Names CeeNU®️ [US/Can]
  Therapeutic Category Antineoplastic Agent
  Use Treatment of brain tumors, Hodgkin's and non-Hodgkin's lymphomas, melanoma, renal carcinoma, lung cancer, colon cancer
  Usual Dosage Oral (refer to individual protocols):
    Children: 75-150 mg/m^2 as a single dose every 6 weeks. Subsequent doses are readjusted after initial treatment according to platelet and leukocyte counts
    Adults: 100-130 mg/m^2 as a single dose every 6 weeks; readjust after initial treatment according to platelet and leukocyte counts
  Dosage Forms
    Capsule: 10 mg, 40 mg, 100 mg
    (Continued)

lomustine *(Continued)*
Dose pack: 10 mg (2s); 40 mg (2s); 100 mg (2s)

Loniten® **[US]** *see* minoxidil *on page 432*

Lonox® **[US]** *see* diphenoxylate and atropine *on page 203*

Lo/Ovral® **[US]** *see* ethinyl estradiol and norgestrel *on page 255*

loperamide (loe PER a mide)
U.S./Canadian Brand Names Apo®-Loperamide [Can]; Diamode® [US-OTC]; Diarr-Eze [Can]; Imodium® [US/Can]; Imodium® A-D [US-OTC]; Imogen® [US]; Imotil® [US]; Imperim® [US-OTC]; Kaodene® A-D [US-OTC]; Kao-Paverin® [US-OTC]; K-Pec® II [US-OTC]; Lopercap [Can]; Novo-Loperamide [Can]; PMS-Loperamine [Can]; Rhoxal-loperamine [Can]; Riva-Loperamine [Can]
Therapeutic Category Antidiarrheal
Use Treatment of acute diarrhea and chronic diarrhea associated with inflammatory bowel disease; chronic functional diarrhea (idiopathic), chronic diarrhea caused by bowel resection or organic lesions; to decrease the volume of ileostomy discharge
Usual Dosage Oral:
Children:
Acute diarrhea: 0.4-0.8 mg/kg/day divided every 6-12 hours, maximum: 2 mg/dose
Chronic diarrhea: 0.08-0.24 mg/kg/day divided 2-3 times/day, maximum: 2 mg/dose
Adults: Initial: 4 mg (2 capsules), followed by 2 mg after each loose stool, up to 16 mg/day (8 capsules)
Dosage Forms
Caplet, as hydrochloride: 2 mg
Capsule, as hydrochloride: 2 mg
Liquid, oral, as hydrochloride: 1 mg/5 mL (60 mL, 90 mL, 120 mL)
Tablet, as hydrochloride: 2 mg

Lopercap [Can] *see* loperamide *on this page*

Lopid® **[US/Can]** *see* gemfibrozil *on page 295*

lopinavir *see* lopinavir and ritonavir *on this page*

lopinavir and ritonavir (loe PIN a veer & rye TON a veer)
Synonyms lopinavir
U.S./Canadian Brand Names Kaletra™ [US]
Therapeutic Category Antiretroviral Agent, Non-nucleoside Reverse Transcriptase Inhibitor (NNRTI)
Use For use in combination with other antiretroviral agents in the treatment of HIV infection
Usual Dosage Oral (take with food):
Children 6 months to 12 years: Dosage based on weight, presented based on mg of lopinavir (maximum dose: 400 mg lopinavir/100 mg ritonavir)
7-<15 kg: 12 mg/kg twice daily
15-40 kg: 10 mg/kg twice daily
>40 kg: Refer to adult dosing
Children >12 years and Adults: 400 mg lopinavir/100 mg ritonavir twice daily

Dosage adjustment when taken with efavirenz or nevirapine:
Children 6 months to 12 years:
7-<15 kg: 13 mg/kg twice daily
15-50 kg: 11 mg/kg twice daily
>50 kg: Refer to adult dosing
Children >12 years and Adults: 533 mg lopinavir/133 mg ritonavir twice daily
Dosage Forms
Capsule: Lopinavir 133.3 mg and ritonavir 33.3 mg
Solution, oral: Lopinavir 80 mg and ritonavir 20 mg per mL [contains alcohol 42.4%]

lopremone *see* protirelin *on page 551*
Lopressor® **[US/Can]** *see* metoprolol *on page 425*
Loprox® **[US/Can]** *see* ciclopirox *on page 145*
Lorabid™ **[US/Can]** *see* loracarbef *on this page*

loracarbef (lor a KAR bef)
U.S./Canadian Brand Names Lorabid™ [US/Can]
Therapeutic Category Antibiotic, Carbacephem
Use Treatment of mild to moderate community-acquired infections of the respiratory tract, skin and skin structure, and urinary tract that are caused by susceptible *S. pneumoniae, H. influenzae, B. catarrhalis, S. aureus,* and *E. coli*
Usual Dosage Oral:
Acute otitis media: Children: 15 mg/kg twice a day for 10 days
Urinary tract infections: Women: 200 mg once a day for 7 days
Dosage Forms
Capsule: 200 mg, 400 mg
Suspension, oral: 100 mg/5 mL (50 mL, 100 mL); 200 mg/5 mL (50 mL, 100 mL)

loratadine (lor AT a deen)
U.S./Canadian Brand Names Claritin® RediTabs® [US]; Claritin® [US/Can]
Therapeutic Category Antihistamine
Use Relief of nasal and non-nasal symptoms of seasonal allergic rhinitis; treatment of chronic idiopathic urticaria
Usual Dosage
Children 2-5 years: Seasonal allergic rhinitis, chronic idiopathic urticaria: Oral: 5 mg once daily
Children ≥6 years and Adults: Seasonal allergic rhinitis, chronic idiopathic urticaria: Oral: 10 mg once daily
Dosage Forms
Syrup: 1 mg/mL (480 mL)
Tablet: 10 mg
Tablet, rapidly-disintegrating (RediTabs®): 10 mg

loratadine and pseudoephedrine (lor AT a deen & soo doe e FED rin)
Synonyms pseudoephedrine and loratadine
U.S./Canadian Brand Names Chlor-Tripolon ND® [Can]; Claritin-D® 12-Hour [US]; Claritin-D® 24-Hour [US]; Claritin® Extra [Can]
Therapeutic Category Antihistamine/Decongestant Combination
Use Temporary relief of symptoms of seasonal and perennial allergic rhinitis, and vasomotor rhinitis, including nasal obstruction
Usual Dosage Adults: Oral: 1 tablet every 12 hours
Dosage Forms
Tablet:
Extended release, 12-hour: Loratadine 5 mg and pseudoephedrine sulfate 120 mg
Extended release, 24-hour: Loratadine 10 mg and pseudoephedrine sulfate 240 mg

lorazepam (lor A ze pam)
U.S./Canadian Brand Names Apo®-Lorazepam [Can]; Ativan® [US/Can]; Novo-Lorazem® [Can]; Nu-Loraz [Can]; Riva-Lorazepam [Can]
Therapeutic Category Benzodiazepine
Controlled Substance C-IV
Use Management of anxiety; status epilepticus; preoperative sedation and amnesia
Usual Dosage
Anxiety and sedation:
Infants and Children: Oral, I.V.: Usual: 0.05 mg/kg/dose (range: 0.02-0.09 mg/kg) every 4-8 hours
(Continued)

lorazepam *(Continued)*

Adults: Oral: 1-10 mg/day in 2-3 divided doses; usual dose: 2-6 mg/day in divided doses

Insomnia: Adults: Oral: 2-4 mg at bedtime

Preoperative: Adults:
I.M.: 0.05 mg/kg administered 2 hours before surgery; maximum: 4 mg/dose
I.V.: 0.044 mg/kg 15-20 minutes before surgery; usual maximum: 2 mg/dose
Operative amnesia: Adults: I.V.: up to 0.05 mg/kg; maximum: 4 mg/dose
Status epilepticus: I.V.:
Infants and Children: 0.1 mg/kg slow I.V. over 2-5 minutes, do not exceed 4 mg/single dose; may repeat second dose of 0.05 mg/kg slow I.V. in 10-15 minutes if needed
Adolescents: 0.07 mg/kg slow I.V. over 2-5 minutes; maximum: 4 mg/dose; may repeat in 10-15 minutes
Adults: 4 mg/dose administered slowly over 2-5 minutes; may repeat in 10-15 minutes; usual maximum dose: 8 mg

Dosage Forms
Injection: 2 mg/mL (1 mL, 10 mL); 4 mg/mL (1 mL, 10 mL)
Solution, oral concentrate: 2 mg/mL (30 mL) [alcohol free, dye free]
Tablet: 0.5 mg, 1 mg, 2 mg

Lorcet® *(Discontinued)* see page 814

Lorcet® 10/650 [US] see hydrocodone and acetaminophen on page 329

Lorcet®-HD [US] see hydrocodone and acetaminophen on page 329

Lorcet® Plus [US] see hydrocodone and acetaminophen on page 329

Lorelco® *(Discontinued)* see page 814

Loroxide® [US-OTC] see benzoyl peroxide on page 79

Lorsin® *(Discontinued)* see page 814

Lortab® [US] see hydrocodone and acetaminophen on page 329

Lortab® ASA [US] see hydrocodone and aspirin on page 330

losartan (loe SAR tan)

Synonyms DuP 753; MK594
U.S./Canadian Brand Names Cozaar® [US/Can]
Therapeutic Category Angiotensin II Receptor Antagonist
Use Treatment of hypertension alone or in combination with other antihypertensives; in considering the use of monotherapy with Cozaar®, it should be noted that in controlled trials Cozaar® had an effect on blood pressure that was notably less in black patients than in nonblacks, a finding similar to the small effect of ACE inhibitors in blacks
Usual Dosage Adults: Oral: Initial: 50 mg once daily, with 25 mg used in patients with possible depletion of intravascular volume (eg, patients treated with diuretics) and patients with a history of hepatic impairment; can be administered once or twice daily with total daily doses ranging from 25-100 mg; if the antihypertensive effect measured at trough using once daily dosing is inadequate, a twice daily regimen at the same total daily dose or an increase in dose may give a more satisfactory response; if blood pressure is not controlled by Cozaar® alone, a low dose of a diuretic may be added; hydrochlorothiazide has been shown to have an additive effect
Dosage Forms Tablet, film coated, as potassium: 25 mg, 50 mg, 100 mg

losartan and hydrochlorothiazide

(loe SAR tan & hye droe klor oh THYE a zide)
Synonyms hydrochlorothiazide and losartan
U.S./Canadian Brand Names Hyzaar® [US/Can]
Therapeutic Category Antihypertensive Agent, Combination
Use Treatment of hypertension
Usual Dosage Adults: Oral: 1 tablet daily

Dosage Forms
Tablet:
Losartan potassium 50 mg and hydrochlorothiazide 12.5 mg
Losartan potassium 100 mg and hydrochlorothiazide 25 mg

Losopan® *(Discontinued)* *see page 814*

Lotemax™ [US/Can] *see* loteprednol *on this page*

Lotensin® [US/Can] *see* benazepril *on page 75*

Lotensin® HCT [US] *see* benazepril and hydrochlorothiazide *on page 75*

loteprednol (loe te PRED nol)

U.S./Canadian Brand Names Alrex™ [US/Can]; Lotemax™ [US/Can]
Therapeutic Category Corticosteroid, Ophthalmic
Use Temporary relief of signs and symptoms of seasonal allergic conjunctivitis
Usual Dosage Adults: Ophthalmic: Instill 1 drop in eye(s) 4 times/day
Dosage Forms
Suspension, ophthalmic, as etabonate:
(Alrex™): 0.2% (5 mL, 10 mL)
(Lotemax™): 0.5% (2.5 mL, 5 mL, 10 mL, 15 mL)

Lotrel® [US/Can] *see* amlodipine and benazepril *on page 36*

Lotrimin® [US] *see* clotrimazole *on page 156*

Lotrimin® AF Cream *(Discontinued)* *see page 814*

Lotrimin® AF Lotion *(Discontinued)* *see page 814*

Lotrimin® AF Powder/Spray [US-OTC] *see* miconazole *on page 427*

Lotrimin® AF Solution *(Discontinued)* *see page 814*

Lotrimin® Ultra™ [US-OTC] *see* butenafine *on page 100*

Lotrisone® [US/Can] *see* betamethasone and clotrimazole *on page 83*

lovastatin (LOE va sta tin)

Synonyms mevinolin; monacolin k
U.S./Canadian Brand Names Altocor™ [US]; Apo®-Lovastatin [Can]; Mevacor® [US/Can]
Therapeutic Category HMG-CoA Reductase Inhibitor
Use
Adjunct to dietary therapy to decrease elevated serum total and LDL-cholesterol concentrations in primary hypercholesterolemia
Primary prevention of coronary artery disease (patients without symptomatic disease with average to moderately elevated total and LDL-cholesterol and below average HDL-cholesterol); slow progression of coronary atherosclerosis in patients with coronary heart disease
Adjunct to dietary therapy in adolescent patients (10-17 years of age, females >1 year post-menarche) with heterozygous familial hypercholesterolemia having LDL >189 mg/dL, **or** LDL >160 mg/dL with positive family history of premature cardiovascular disease (CVD), **or** LDL >160 mg/dL with the presence of at least two other CVD risk factors
Usual Dosage Oral:
Adolescents 10-17 years: Immediate release tablet:
LDL reduction <20%: Initial: 10 mg/day with evening meal
LDL reduction ≥20%: Initial: 20 mg/day with evening meal
Usual range: 10-40 mg with evening meal, then adjust dose at 4-week intervals
Adults: Initial: 20 mg with evening meal, then adjust at 4-week intervals; maximum dose: 80 mg/day immediate release tablet **or** 60 mg/day extended release tablet; before initiation of therapy, patients should be placed on a standard cholesterol-lowering diet for 3-6 months and the diet should be continued during drug therapy
(Continued)

lovastatin *(Continued)*

Dosage Forms
Tablet (Mevacor®): 10 mg, 20 mg, 40 mg
Tablet, extended release (Altocor™): 10 mg, 20 mg, 40 mg, 60 mg

lovastatin and niacin *see* niacin and lovastatin *on page 457*

Lovenox® **[US/Can]** *see* enoxaparin *on page 227*

Low-Ogestrel® **[US]** *see* ethinyl estradiol and norgestrel *on page 255*

Lowsium® **Plus [US]** *see* magaldrate and simethicone *on page 396*

loxapine (LOKS a peen)

Synonyms oxilapine
U.S./Canadian Brand Names Apo®-Loxapine [Can]; Loxitane® C [US]; Loxitane® I.M. [US]; Loxitane® [US]; Nu-Loxapine [Can]; PMS-Loxapine [Can]
Therapeutic Category Antipsychotic Agent, Dibenzoxazepine
Use Management of psychotic disorders
Usual Dosage Adults:
Oral: 10 mg twice daily, increase dose until psychotic symptoms are controlled; usual dose range: 60-100 mg/day in divided doses 2-4 times/day; dosages >250 mg/day are not recommended
I.M.: 12.5-50 mg every 4-6 hours or longer as needed and change to oral therapy as soon as possible
Dosage Forms
Capsule, as succinate (Loxitane®): 5 mg, 10 mg, 25 mg, 50 mg
Injection, as hydrochloride (Loxitane® IM): 50 mg/mL (1 mL)
Solution, oral concentrate, as hydrochloride (Loxitane® C): 25 mg/mL [120 mL dropper bottle]

Loxitane® **[US]** *see* loxapine *on this page*

Loxitane® **C [US]** *see* loxapine *on this page*

Loxitane® **I.M. [US]** *see* loxapine *on this page*

Lozide® **[Can]** *see* indapamide *on page 348*

Lozi-Tab® *(Discontinued) see page 814*

Lozol® **[US/Can]** *see* indapamide *on page 348*

l-PAM *see* melphalan *on page 406*

LRH *see* gonadorelin *on page 304*

l-sarcolysin *see* melphalan *on page 406*

LTG *see* lamotrigine *on page 373*

l-thyroxine *see* levothyroxine *on page 382*

l-triiodothyronine *see* liothyronine *on page 386*

Lu-26-054 *see* escitalopram *on page 236*

Lubriderm® **Fragrance Free [US-OTC]** *see* lanolin, cetyl alcohol, glycerin, and petrolatum *on page 374*

Lubriderm® **[US-OTC]** *see* lanolin, cetyl alcohol, glycerin, and petrolatum *on page 374*

LubriTears® **Solution** *(Discontinued) see page 814*

Ludiomil® **[US/Can]** *see* maprotiline *on page 401*

Lufyllin® **[US/Can]** *see* dyphylline *on page 221*

Lugol's solution *see* potassium iodide *on page 531*

Lumigan™ **[US]** *see* bimatoprost *on page 86*

Luminal® **Sodium [US]** *see* phenobarbital *on page 507*

Lumitene™ **[US]** *see* beta-carotene *on page 82*

Lunelle™ **[US]** *see* estradiol cypionate and medroxyprogesterone acetate *on page 240*

Lupron® **[US/Can]** *see* leuprolide acetate *on page 377*

Lupron Depot® **[US/Can]** *see* leuprolide acetate *on page 377*

Lupron Depot-Ped® **[US]** *see* leuprolide acetate *on page 377*

Luride® **[US]** *see* fluoride *on page 278*

Luride® **Lozi-Tab**® **[US]** *see* fluoride *on page 278*

Luride®-**SF** *(Discontinued)* *see page 814*

luteinizing hormone-releasing hormone *see* gonadorelin *on page 304*

Lutrepulse™ **[Can]** *see* gonadorelin *on page 304*

Luvox® **[Can]** *see* fluvoxamine *on page 285*

Luvox® *(Discontinued)* *see page 814*

Luxiq™ **[US]** *see* betamethasone (topical) *on page 83*

LY170053 *see* olanzapine *on page 475*

Lycolan® **Elixir** *(Discontinued)* *see page 814*

Lyderm® **[Can]** *see* fluocinonide *on page 277*

Lydonide [Can] *see* fluocinonide *on page 277*

LYMErix™ *(Discontinued)* *see page 814*

Lymphazurin® **[US]** *see* radiological/contrast media (ionic) *on page 561*

lymphocyte immune globulin (LIM foe site i MYUN GLOB yoo lin)

Synonyms antithymocyte globulin (equine); ATG; horse antihuman thymocyte gamma globulin

U.S./Canadian Brand Names Atgam® [US/Can]

Therapeutic Category Immunosuppressant Agent

Use Prevention and treatment of acute allograft rejection; treatment of moderate to severe aplastic anemia in patients not considered suitable candidates for bone marrow transplantation; prevention of graft-vs-host disease following bone marrow transplantation

Usual Dosage An intradermal skin test is recommended prior to administration of the initial dose of ATG. Use 0.1 mL of a 1:1000 dilution of ATG in normal saline

Aplastic anemia protocol: I.V.: 10-20 mg/kg/day for 8-14 days, then administer every other day for 7 more doses

Rejection prevention: Children and Adults: I.V.: 15 mg/kg/day for 14 days, then administer every other day for 7 more doses; initial dose should be administered within 24 hours before or after transplantation

Rejection treatment: Children and Adults: I.V. 10-15 mg/kg/day for 14 days, then administer every other day for 7 more doses

Dosage Forms Injection: 50 mg of equine IgG/mL (5 mL)

Lyphocin® **Injection** *(Discontinued)* *see page 814*

Lysinyl® **[US-OTC]** *see* l-lysine *on page 388*

Lysodren® **[US/Can]** *see* mitotane *on page 433*

Lyteprep™ **[Can]** *see* polyethylene glycol-electrolyte solution *on page 525*

Maalox® **Anti-Gas [US-OTC]** *see* simethicone *on page 591*

Maalox® **Fast Release Liquid [US-OTC]** *see* aluminum hydroxide, magnesium hydroxide, and simethicone *on page 29*

Maalox® **Max [US-OTC]** *see* aluminum hydroxide, magnesium hydroxide, and simethicone *on page 29*

Maalox® Plus *(Discontinued)* see page 814

Maalox® TC (Therapeutic Concentrate) [US-OTC] *see* aluminum hydroxide and magnesium hydroxide *on page 29*

Maalox® [US-OTC] *see* aluminum hydroxide and magnesium hydroxide *on page 29*

Macrobid® [US/Can] *see* nitrofurantoin *on page 461*

Macrodantin® [US/Can] *see* nitrofurantoin *on page 461*

Macrodex® [US] *see* dextran *on page 187*

mafenide (MA fe nide)
Synonyms succinate mafenide acetate
U.S./Canadian Brand Names Sulfamylon® [US]
Therapeutic Category Antibacterial, Topical
Use Adjunct in the treatment of second and third degree burns to prevent septicemia caused by susceptible organisms such as *Pseudomonas aeruginosa*
Usual Dosage Children and Adults: Topical: Apply once or twice daily with a sterile gloved hand; apply to a thickness of approximately 16 mm; the burned area should be covered with cream at all times
Dosage Forms
Cream, as acetate: 85 mg/g (56.7 g, 113.4 g, 411 g)
Powder: 5% (50 g)

magaldrate (MAG al drate)
Synonyms hydromagnesium aluminate
U.S./Canadian Brand Names Riopan® [US-OTC]
Therapeutic Category Antacid
Use Symptomatic relief of hyperacidity associated with peptic ulcer, gastritis, peptic esophagitis and hiatal hernia
Usual Dosage Adults: Oral: 540-1080 mg between meals and at bedtime
Dosage Forms Suspension, oral: 540 mg/5 mL (360 mL)

magaldrate and simethicone (MAG al drate & sye METH i kone)
Synonyms simethicone and magaldrate
U.S./Canadian Brand Names Iosopan® Plus [US]; Lowsium® Plus [US]; Riopan Plus® Double Strength [US-OTC]; Riopan Plus® [US-OTC]
Therapeutic Category Antacid; Antiflatulent
Use Relief of hyperacidity associated with peptic ulcer, gastritis, peptic esophagitis and hiatal hernia which are accompanied by symptoms of gas
Usual Dosage Adults: Oral: 5-10 mL between meals and at bedtime
Dosage Forms
Suspension, oral:
Magaldrate 540 mg and simethicone 20 mg per 5 mL (360 mL, 420 mL)
Magaldrate 540 mg and simethicone 40 mg per 5 mL (360 mL)
Magaldrate 1080 mg and simethicone 40 mg per 5 mL (360 mL)
Tablet, chewable:
Magaldrate 540 mg and simethicone 20 mg
Magaldrate 1080 mg and simethicone 20 mg

Magalox Plus® *(Discontinued)* see page 814

Magan® *(Discontinued)* see page 814

Mag Delay® [US] *see* magnesium chloride *on next page*

Mag-Gel® 600 [US] *see* magnesium oxide *on page 398*

Magnacal® [US-OTC] *see* nutritional formula, enteral/oral *on page 472*

magnesia magma *see* magnesium hydroxide *on next page*

magnesium chloride (mag NEE zhum KLOR ide)

U.S./Canadian Brand Names Chloromag® [US]; Mag Delay® [US]; Mag-SR® [US]; Slow-Mag® [US/Can]

Therapeutic Category Electrolyte Supplement, Oral

Use Correct or prevent hypomagnesemia

Usual Dosage I.V. in TPN:

Children: 2-10 mEq/day; the usual recommended pediatric maintenance intake of magnesium ranges from 0.2-0.6 mEq/kg/day. The dose of magnesium may also be based on the caloric intake; on that basis, 3-10 mEq/day of magnesium are needed; maximum maintenance dose: 8-16 mEq/day

Adults: 8-24 mEq/day

Dosage Forms

Injection: 200 mg/mL [1.97 mEq/mL] (50 mL)

Tablet, extended release: 535 mg [elemental magnesium 64 mg]

magnesium citrate (mag NEE zhum SIT rate)

Synonyms citrate of magnesia

U.S./Canadian Brand Names Citro-Mag® [Can]

Therapeutic Category Laxative

Use Evacuation of bowel prior to certain surgical and diagnostic procedures

Usual Dosage Cathartic: Oral:

Children:

<6 years: 2-4 mL/kg administered as a single daily dose or in divided doses

6-12 years: $^1/_3$ to $^1/_2$ bottle

Children ≥12 years and Adults: $^1/_2$ to 1 full bottle

Dosage Forms Solution, oral: 300 mL (1.75 g/30 mL)

magnesium gluconate (mag NEE zhum GLOO koe nate)

U.S./Canadian Brand Names Magonate® [US-OTC]

Therapeutic Category Electrolyte Supplement, Oral

Use Dietary supplement for treatment of magnesium deficiencies

Usual Dosage The recommended dietary allowance (RDA) of magnesium is 4.5 mg/kg which is a total daily allowance of 350-400 mg for adult men and 280-300 mg for adult women. During pregnancy the RDA is 300 mg and during lactation the RDA is 355 mg. Average daily intakes of dietary magnesium have declined in recent years due to processing of food. The latest estimate of the average American dietary intake was 349 mg/day.

Dietary supplement: Oral:

Children: 3-6 mg/kg/day in divided doses 3-4 times/day; maximum: 400 mg/day

Adults: 27-54 mg 2-3 times/day or 100 mg 4 times/day

Dosage Forms

Liquid:

326 mg [elemental magnesium 17.6 mg] per 5 mL

1000 mg [elemental magnesium 54 mg] per 5 mL

Tablet: 500 mg [elemental magnesium 27 mg]

magnesium hydroxide (mag NEE zhum hye DROKS ide)

Synonyms magnesia magma; milk of magnesia; MOM

U.S./Canadian Brand Names Phillips'® Milk of Magnesia [US-OTC]

Therapeutic Category Antacid; Electrolyte Supplement, Oral; Laxative

Use Short-term treatment of occasional constipation and symptoms of hyperacidity

Usual Dosage Oral:

Laxative:

<2 years: 0.5 mL/kg/dose

2-5 years: 5-15 mL/day or in divided doses

6-12 years: 15-30 mL/day or in divided doses

≥12 years: 30-60 mL/day or in divided doses

(Continued)

magnesium hydroxide *(Continued)*

Antacid:
Children: 2.5-5 mL as needed
Adults: 5-15 mL as needed

Dosage Forms
Liquid, oral: 400 mg/5 mL (15 mL, 30 mL, 100 mL, 120 mL, 180 mL, 360 mL, 720 mL)
Liquid, oral concentrate: 800 mg/5 mL (240 mL) [10 mL equivalent to 30 mL milk of magnesia USP]
Tablet: 300 mg, 600 mg

magnesium hydroxide and aluminum hydroxide *see* aluminum hydroxide and magnesium hydroxide *on page 29*

magnesium hydroxide and mineral oil emulsion

(mag NEE zhum hye DROKS ide & MIN er al oyl e MUL shun)
Synonyms mom/mineral oil emulsion
U.S./Canadian Brand Names Haley's M-O® [US-OTC]
Therapeutic Category Laxative
Use Short-term treatment of occasional constipation
Usual Dosage Adults: Oral: 5-45 mL at bedtime
Dosage Forms Suspension, oral: Magnesium hydroxide 300 mg and mineral oil 1.25 mL per 5 mL (12 oz, 29 oz) [equivalent to magnesium hydroxide 24 mL/mineral oil emulsion 6 mL]

magnesium oxide (mag NEE zhum OKS ide)

U.S./Canadian Brand Names Mag-Gel® 600 [US]; Mag-Ox® 400 [US-OTC]; Uro-Mag® [US-OTC]
Therapeutic Category Antacid; Electrolyte Supplement, Oral; Laxative
Use Treatment of magnesium deficiencies, short-term treatment of occasional constipation, and symptoms of hyperacidity
Usual Dosage Oral:
Antacid: 250 mg to 1.5 g with water or milk 4 times/day after meals and at bedtime
Laxative: 2-4 g at bedtime with full glass of water
Dosage Forms
Capsule: 140 mg [elemental magnesium 84.5 mg]
Tablet: 400 mg [elemental magnesium 241.3 mg]

magnesium salicylate (mag NEE zhum sa LIS i late)

U.S./Canadian Brand Names Backache Pain Relief Extra Strength [US]; Doan's®, Original [US-OTC]; Extra Strength Doan's® [US-OTC]; Keygesic-10® [US]; Mobidin® [US]; Momentum® [US-OTC]
Therapeutic Category Nonsteroidal Anti-inflammatory Drug (NSAID)
Use Mild to moderate pain, fever, various inflammatory conditions
Usual Dosage Adults: Oral: 650 mg 4 times/day or 1090 mg 3 times/day; may increase to 3.6-4.8 mg/day in 3-4 divided doses
Dosage Forms
Tablet, as anhydrous magnesium salicylate:
Backache Pain Relief Extra Strength, Momentum®: 467 mg
Doan's®, Original: 325 mg
Extra Strength Doan's®: 500 mg
Keygesic-10®: 650 mg
Mobidin®: 600 mg

magnesium sulfate (mag NEE zhum SUL fate)

Synonyms epsom salts
Therapeutic Category Anticonvulsant; Electrolyte Supplement, Oral; Laxative

Use Treatment and prevention of hypomagnesemia; hypertension; encephalopathy and seizures associated with acute nephritis in children; also used as a cathartic

Usual Dosage Dose represented as $MgSO_4$ unless stated otherwise

Hypomagnesemia:

Children:

I.M., I.V.: 25-50 mg/kg/dose (0.2-0.4 mEq/kg/dose) every 4-6 hours for 3-4 doses, maximum single dose: 2000 mg (16 mEq), may repeat if hypomagnesemia persists (higher dosage up to 100 mg/kg/dose $MgSO_4$ I.V. has been used)

Oral: 100-200 mg/kg/dose 4 times/day

Maintenance: I.V.: 30-60 mg/kg/day (0.25-0.5 mEq/kg/day)

Adults: I.M., I.V.: 1 g every 6 hours for 4 doses or 250 mg/kg over a 4-hour period; for severe hypomagnesemia: 8-12 g $MgSO_4$/day in divided doses has been used; Oral: 3 g every 6 hours for 4 doses as needed

Management of seizures and hypertension: Children: I.M., I.V.: 20-100 mg/kg/dose every 4-6 hours as needed; in severe cases doses as high as 200 mg/kg/dose have been used

Cathartic: Oral:

Children: 0.25 g/kg/dose

Adults: 10-30 g

Dosage Forms

Granules: ~40 mEq magnesium/5 g (120 g, 240 g)

Injection: 100 mg/mL (20 mL); 125 mg/mL (8 mL); 200 mg/mL (50 mL); 500 mg/mL (2 mL, 5 mL, 10 mL, 50 mL)

Magnevist® [US] see radiological/contrast media (ionic) on page 561

Magonate® [US-OTC] see magnesium gluconate on page 397

Mag-Ox® 400 [US-OTC] see magnesium oxide on previous page

Magsal® (Discontinued) see page 814

Mag-SR® [US] see magnesium chloride on page 397

Majeptil® [Can] see thioproperazine (Canada only) on page 634

Malarone™ [US/Can] see atovaquone and proguanil on page 61

Malatal® (Discontinued) see page 814

malathion (mal a THYE on)

U.S./Canadian Brand Names Ovide™ [US]

Therapeutic Category Scabicides/Pediculicides

Use Treatment of head lice and their ova

Usual Dosage Topical: Sprinkle Ovide™ lotion on dry hair and rub gently until the scalp is thoroughly moistened; pay special attention to the back of the head and neck. Allow to dry naturally, use no heat and leave uncovered. After 8-12 hours, the hair should be washed with a nonmedicated shampoo; rinse and use a fine-toothed comb to remove dead lice and eggs. If required, repeat with second application in 7-9 days. Further treatment is generally not necessary. Other family members should be evaluated to determine if infested and if so, receive treatment.

Dosage Forms Lotion: 0.5% (59 mL)

Mallamint® [US-OTC] see calcium carbonate on page 104

Mallazine® Eye Drops [US-OTC] see tetrahydrozoline on page 629

Mallisol® (Discontinued) see page 814

Malotuss® Syrup (Discontinued) see page 814

malt soup extract (malt soop EKS trakt)

U.S./Canadian Brand Names Maltsupex® [US-OTC]

Therapeutic Category Laxative

Use Short-term treatment of constipation

(Continued)

malt soup extract *(Continued)*

Usual Dosage Oral:

Infants >1 month:

Breast fed: 1-2 teaspoonfuls in 2-4 oz of water or fruit juice 1-2 times/day

Bottle fed: $1/2$ to 2 tablespoonfuls/day in formula for 3-4 days, then 1-2 teaspoonfuls/day

Children 2-11 years: 1-2 tablespoonfuls 1-2 times/day

Adults ≥12 years: 2 tablespoonfuls twice daily for 3-4 days, then 1-2 tablespoonfuls every evening

Dosage Forms

Liquid: Nondiastatic barley malt extract 16 g/15 mL

Powder: Nondiastatic barley malt extract 8 g/heaping tablespoonful

Tablet: Nondiastatic barley malt extract 750 mg

Maltsupex® [US-OTC] *see* malt soup extract *on previous page*

Mandelamine® [Can] *see* methenamine *on page 416*

Mandol® [US] *see* cefamandole *on page 121*

mandrake *see* podophyllum resin *on page 523*

Manerix® [Can] *see* moclobemide *(Canada only) on page 434*

manganese injection *see* trace metals *on page 646*

mannitol (MAN i tole)

Synonyms *d*-mannitol

U.S./Canadian Brand Names Osmitrol® [US/Can]; Resectisol® Irrigation Solution [US]

Therapeutic Category Diuretic, Osmotic

Use Reduction of increased intracranial pressure (ICP) associated with cerebral edema; promotion of diuresis in the prevention and/or treatment of oliguria or anuria due to acute renal failure; reduction of increased intraocular pressure; promotion of urinary excretion of toxic substances

Usual Dosage

Children:

Test dose (to assess adequate renal function): 200 mg/kg over 3-5 minutes to produce a urine flow of at least 1 mL/kg/hour for 1-3 hours

Initial: 0.5-1 g/kg

Maintenance: 0.25-0.5 g/kg/hour administered every 4-6 hours

Adults:

Test dose: 12.5 g (200 mg/kg) over 3-5 minutes to produce a urine flow of at least 30-50 mL of urine per hour over the next 2-3 hours

Initial: 0.5-1 g/kg

Maintenance: 0.25-0.5 g/kg every 4-6 hours

Dosage Forms

Injection: 5% [50 mg/mL] (1000 mL); 10% [100 mg/mL] (500 mL, 1000 mL); 15% [150 mg/mL] (500 mL); 20% [200 mg/mL] (250 mL, 500 mL); 25% [250 mg/mL] (50 mL)

Solution, urogenital: 0.5% [5 mg/mL] (2000 mL); 0.54% [5.4 mg/mL] (1500 mL, 3000 mL) [with sorbitol 2.7 g/mL]

Mantadil® Cream *(Discontinued) see page 814*

Mantoux *see* tuberculin tests *on page 662*

Maolate® *(Discontinued) see page 814*

Maox® *(Discontinued) see page 814*

Mapap® Children's [US-OTC] *see* acetaminophen *on page 3*

Mapap® Extra Strength [US-OTC] *see* acetaminophen *on page 3*

Mapap® Infants [US-OTC] *see* acetaminophen *on page 3*

Mapap® [US-OTC] *see* acetaminophen *on page 3*

maprotiline (ma PROE ti leen)
U.S./Canadian Brand Names Ludiomil® [US/Can]
Therapeutic Category Antidepressant, Tetracyclic
Use Treatment of depression and anxiety associated with depression
Usual Dosage Oral:
Children 6-14 years: 10 mg/day, increase to a maximum daily dose of 75 mg
Adults: 75 mg/day to start, increase by 25 mg every 2 weeks up to 150-225 mg/day; administered in 3 divided doses or in a single daily dose
Dosage Forms Tablet, as hydrochloride: 25 mg, 50 mg, 75 mg

Marax® *(Discontinued)* *see page 814*

Marcaine® **[US/Can]** *see* bupivacaine *on page 97*

Marcaine® **Spinal [US]** *see* bupivacaine *on page 97*

Marcillin® **[US]** *see* ampicillin *on page 40*

Marezine® **Injection** *(Discontinued)* *see page 814*

Margesic® **[US]** *see* butalbital, acetaminophen, and caffeine *on page 99*

Margesic® **H [US]** *see* hydrocodone and acetaminophen *on page 329*

Marinol® **[US/Can]** *see* dronabinol *on page 217*

Marmine® **Injection** *(Discontinued)* *see page 814*

Marmine® **Oral** *(Discontinued)* *see page 814*

Marplan® **[US]** *see* isocarboxazid *on page 360*

Marten-Tab® **[US]** *see* butalbital, acetaminophen, and caffeine *on page 99*

Marthritic® *(Discontinued)* *see page 814*

Marvelon® **[Can]** *see* ethinyl estradiol and desogestrel *on page 244*

Massé® **Breast Cream [US-OTC]** *see* glycerin, lanolin, and peanut oil *on page 303*

Matulane® **[US/Can]** *see* procarbazine *on page 542*

Mavik® **[US/Can]** *see* trandolapril *on page 647*

Maxair™ **[US]** *see* pirbuterol *on page 517*

Maxair™ **Autohaler™ [US]** *see* pirbuterol *on page 517*

Maxalt® **[US/Can]** *see* rizatriptan *on page 575*

Maxalt-MLT™ **[US]** *see* rizatriptan *on page 575*

Maxalt RPD™ **[Can]** *see* rizatriptan *on page 575*

Maxaquin® **[US]** *see* lomefloxacin *on page 389*

Max-Caro® *(Discontinued)* *see page 814*

Maxidex® **[US/Can]** *see* dexamethasone (ophthalmic) *on page 184*

Maxifed® **[US]** *see* guaifenesin and pseudoephedrine *on page 310*

Maxifed® **DM [US]** *see* guaifenesin, pseudoephedrine, and dextromethorphan *on page 312*

Maxifed-G® **[US]** *see* guaifenesin and pseudoephedrine *on page 310*

Maxiflor® **[US]** *see* diflorasone *on page 196*

Maximum Strength Desenex® **Antifungal Cream** *(Discontinued)* *see page 814*

Maximum Strength Dex-A-Diet® *(Discontinued)* *see page 814*

Maximum Strength Dexatrim® *(Discontinued)* *see page 814*

Maxipime® **[US/Can]** *see* cefepime *on page 122*

Maxitrol® **[US/Can]** *see* neomycin, polymyxin B, and dexamethasone *on page 452*

Maxivate® **[US]** *see* betamethasone (topical) *on page 83*

Maxolon® *(Discontinued) see page 814*

Maxzide® **[US]** *see* hydrochlorothiazide and triamterene *on page 329*

Maxzide®-25 *(Discontinued) see page 814*

may apple *see* podophyllum resin *on page 523*

Mazanor® *(Discontinued) see page 814*

3M™ Cavilon™ Skin Cleanser [US-OTC] *see* benzalkonium chloride *on page 76*

MCH *see* microfibrillar collagen hemostat *on page 428*

m-cresyl acetate (em-KREE sil AS e tate)
U.S./Canadian Brand Names Cresylate® [US]
Therapeutic Category Otic Agent, Anti-infective
Use Provides an acid medium; for external otitis infections caused by susceptible bacteria or fungus
Usual Dosage Otic: Instill 2-4 drops as required
Dosage Forms Solution: 25% with isopropanol 25%, chlorobutanol 1%, benzyl alcohol 1%, and castor oil 5% in propylene glycol (15 mL dropper bottle)

MCT Oil® **[US/Can]** *see* medium chain triglycerides *on page 404*

MD-Gastroview® **[US]** *see* radiological/contrast media (ionic) *on page 561*

MDL-71754 *see* vigabatrin *(Canada only) on page 678*

ME-500® **[US]** *see* methionine *on page 416*

measles and rubella vaccines, combined
(MEE zels & roo BEL a vak SEENS, kom BINED)
Synonyms rubella and measles vaccines, combined
U.S./Canadian Brand Names M-R-VAX® II [US]
Therapeutic Category Vaccine, Live Virus
Use Simultaneous immunization against measles and rubella
Usual Dosage S.C.: Inject into outer aspect of upper arm
Dosage Forms Injection: 1000 $TCID_{50}$ each of live attenuated measles virus vaccine and live rubella virus vaccine

measles, mumps, and rubella vaccines, combined
(MEE zels, mumpz, & roo BEL a vak SEENS, kom BINED)
Synonyms MMR
U.S./Canadian Brand Names M-M-R® II [US/Can]; Priorix™ [Can]
Therapeutic Category Vaccine, Live Virus
Use Measles, mumps, and rubella prophylaxis
Usual Dosage S.C.: Inject in outer aspect of the upper arm to children ≥15 months of age; each dose contains 1000 $TCID_{50}$ (tissue culture infectious doses) of live attenuated measle virus vaccine, 5000 $TCID_{50}$ of live mumps virus vaccine and 1000 $TCID_{50}$ of live rubella virus vaccine
Dosage Forms Injection, powder for reconstitution [preservative free]: 1000 $TCID_{50}$ each of measles virus and rubella virus, and 20,000 $TCID_{50}$ mumps virus [contains neomycin 25 mcg, gelatin, human albumin; produced in chick embryo cell culture]

measles virus vaccine (live) (MEE zels VYE rus vak SEEN live)
Synonyms more attenuated enders strain; rubeola vaccine
U.S./Canadian Brand Names Attenuvax® [US]
Therapeutic Category Vaccine, Live Virus
Use Immunization against measles (rubeola) in persons ≥15 months of age

Usual Dosage Children >15 months and Adults: S.C.: 0.5 mL in outer aspect of the upper arm

Dosage Forms Injection: 1000 $TCID_{50}$ per dose

Measurin® *(Discontinued)* *see page 814*

Mebaral® [US/Can] *see* mephobarbital *on page 409*

mebendazole (me BEN da zole)

U.S./Canadian Brand Names Vermox® [US/Can]

Therapeutic Category Anthelmintic

Use Treatment of enterobiasis (pinworm infection), trichuriasis (whipworm infections), ascariasis (roundworm infection), and hookworm infections caused by *Necator americanus* or *Ancylostoma duodenale*; drug of choice in the treatment of capillariasis

Usual Dosage Children and Adults: Oral:

Pinworms: Single chewable tablet; may need to repeat after 2 weeks

Whipworms, roundworms, hookworms: 1 tablet twice daily, morning and evening on 3 consecutive days; if patient is not cured within 3-4 weeks, a second course of treatment may be administered

Dosage Forms Tablet, chewable: 100 mg

mecamylamine (mek a MIL a meen)

U.S./Canadian Brand Names Inversine® [US/Can]

Therapeutic Category Ganglionic Blocking Agent

Use Treatment of moderately severe to severe hypertension and in uncomplicated malignant hypertension

Usual Dosage Adults: Oral: 2.5 mg twice daily after meals for 2 days; increased by increments of 2.5 mg at intervals of ≥2 days until desired blood pressure response is achieved

Dosage Forms Tablet, as hydrochloride: 2.5 mg

mechlorethamine (me klor ETH a meen)

Synonyms HN_2; mustine; nitrogen mustard

U.S./Canadian Brand Names Mustargen® [US/Can]

Therapeutic Category Antineoplastic Agent

Use Combination therapy of Hodgkin's disease, brain tumors, non-Hodgkin's lymphoma, and malignant lymphomas; palliative treatment of bronchogenic, breast, and ovarian carcinoma; sclerosing agent in intracavitary therapy of pleural, pericardial, and other malignant effusions

Usual Dosage Refer to individual protocols.

Children: MOPP: I.V.: 6 mg/m² on days 1 and 8 of a 28-day cycle

Adults:

I.V.: 0.4 mg/kg or 12-16 mg/m² for one dose or divided into 0.1 mg/kg/day for 4 days

Intracavitary: 10-20 mg or 0.2-0.4 mg/kg

Dosage Forms Injection, powder for reconstitution, as hydrochloride: 10 mg

Meclan® Topical *(Discontinued)* *see page 814*

meclizine (MEK li zeen)

Synonyms meclozine

U.S./Canadian Brand Names Antivert® [US/Can]; Bonamine™ [Can]; Bonine® [US/Can]; Dramamine® II [US-OTC]; Meni-D® [US]

Therapeutic Category Antihistamine

Use Prevention and treatment of motion sickness; management of vertigo

Usual Dosage Children >12 years and Adults: Oral:

Motion sickness: 25-50 mg 1 hour before travel, repeat dose every 24 hours if needed

Vertigo: 25-100 mg/day in divided doses

(Continued)

meclizine *(Continued)*

Dosage Forms
Capsule, as hydrochloride: 25 mg, 30 mg
Tablet, as hydrochloride: 12.5 mg, 25 mg, 50 mg
Tablet, chewable, as hydrochloride: 25 mg

meclofenamate (me kloe fen AM ate)

Therapeutic Category Analgesic, Non-narcotic; Nonsteroidal Anti-inflammatory Drug (NSAID)
Use Treatment of inflammatory disorders
Usual Dosage Adults: Oral: 200-300 mg 3-4 times/day
Dosage Forms Capsule, as sodium: 50 mg, 100 mg

Meclomen® *(Discontinued)* see page 814

meclozine see meclizine on previous page

medicinal carbon see charcoal on page 131

Medidin® **Liquid** *(Discontinued)* see page 814

Medigesic® **[US]** see butalbital, acetaminophen, and caffeine on page 99

Medihaler-Epi® *(Discontinued)* see page 814

Medihaler Ergotamine® *(Discontinued)* see page 814

Medihaler-Iso® *(Discontinued)* see page 814

Medipain 5® *(Discontinued)* see page 814

Mediphedryl® **[US-OTC]** see diphenhydramine on page 202

Mediplast® **Plaster [US-OTC]** see salicylic acid on page 581

Medipren® *(Discontinued)* see page 814

Medi-Quick® **Topical Ointment** *(Discontinued)* see page 814

Medi-Sleep® **[US-OTC]** see doxylamine on page 216

Medi-Synal [US-OTC] see acetaminophen and pseudoephedrine on page 6

Medi-Tuss® *(Discontinued)* see page 814

medium chain triglycerides (mee DEE um chane trye GLIS er ides)

Synonyms triglycerides, medium chain
U.S./Canadian Brand Names MCT Oil® [US/Can]
Therapeutic Category Nutritional Supplement
Use Dietary supplement for those who cannot digest long chain fats; malabsorption associated with disorders such as pancreatic insufficiency, bile salt deficiency, and bacterial overgrowth of the small bowel; induce ketosis as a prevention for seizures (akinetic, clonic, and petit mal)
Usual Dosage Oral: 15 mL 3-4 times/day
Dosage Forms Oil: 14 g/15 mL (960 mL)

Medralone® **Injection** *(Discontinued)* see page 814

Medrapred® *(Discontinued)* see page 814

Medrol® **Acetate Topical** *(Discontinued)* see page 814

Medrol® **Tablet [US/Can]** see methylprednisolone on page 423

medroxyprogesterone acetate (me DROKS ee proe JES te rone AS e tate)

Synonyms acetoxymethylprogesterone; methylacetoxyprogesterone
Tall-Man medroxyPROGESTERone acetate
U.S./Canadian Brand Names Alti-MPA [Can]; Depo-Provera® [US/Can]; Gen-Medroxy [Can]; Novo-Medrone [Can]; Provera® [US/Can]
Therapeutic Category Contraceptive, Progestin Only; Progestin

Use Secondary amenorrhea or abnormal uterine bleeding due to hormonal imbalance

Usual Dosage

Adolescents and Adults: Oral:

Amenorrhea: 5-10 mg/day for 5-10 days or 2.5 mg/day

Abnormal uterine bleeding: 5-10 mg for 5-10 days starting on day 16 or 21 of cycle

Accompanying cyclic estrogen therapy, postmenopausal: 2.5-10 mg the last 10-13 days of estrogen dosing each month

Adults:

Contraception: Deep I.M.: 150 mg every 3 months or 450 mg every 6 months

Endometrial or renal carcinoma: I.M.: 400-1000 mg/week

Dosage Forms

Injection, suspension, as acetate (Depot-Provera®): 150 mg/mL (1 mL); 400 mg/mL (1 mL, 2.5 mL, 10 mL)

Tablet, as acetate (Provera®): 2.5 mg, 5 mg, 10 mg

medroxyprogesterone and estrogens *see* estrogens and medroxyprogesterone *on page 241*

medroxyprogesterone and estrogens

medrysone (ME dri sone)

U.S./Canadian Brand Names HMS Liquifilm® [US]

Therapeutic Category Adrenal Corticosteroid

Use Treatment of allergic conjunctivitis, vernal conjunctivitis, episcleritis, ophthalmic epinephrine sensitivity reaction

Usual Dosage Children and Adults: Ophthalmic: 1 drop in conjunctival sac 2-4 times/day up to every 4 hours; may use every 1-2 hours during first 1-2 days

Dosage Forms Solution, ophthalmic: 1% (5 mL, 10 mL) [contains benzalkonium chloride]

mefenamic acid (me fe NAM ik AS id)

U.S./Canadian Brand Names Apo®-Mefenamic [Can]; Nu-Mefenamic [Can]; PMS-Mefenamic Acid [Can]; Ponstan® [Can]; Ponstel® [US/Can]

Therapeutic Category Analgesic, Non-narcotic; Nonsteroidal Anti-inflammatory Drug (NSAID)

Use Short-term relief of mild to moderate pain including primary dysmenorrhea

Usual Dosage Children >14 years and Adults: Oral: 500 mg to start then 250 mg every 4 hours as needed; maximum therapy: 1 week

Dosage Forms Capsule: 250 mg

mefloquine (ME floe kwin)

U.S./Canadian Brand Names Lariam® [US/Can]

Therapeutic Category Antimalarial Agent

Use Treatment of acute malarial infections and prevention of malaria

Usual Dosage Adults: Oral:

Mild to moderate malaria infection: 5 tablets (1250 mg) as a single dose with at least 8 oz of water

Malaria prophylaxis: 1 tablet (250 mg) weekly starting 1 week before travel, continuing weekly during travel and for 4 weeks after leaving endemic area

Dosage Forms Tablet, as hydrochloride: 250 mg

Mefoxin® [US/Can] *see* cefoxitin *on page 124*

Mega B® [US-OTC] *see* vitamin B complex *on page 681*

Megace® [US/Can] *see* megestrol acetate *on this page*

Megace® OS *see* megestrol acetate *on this page*

megestrol acetate (me JES trole AS e tate)

U.S./Canadian Brand Names Apo®-Megestrol [Can]; Lin-Megestrol [Can]; Megace® OS; Megace® [US/Can]; Nu-Megestrol [Can]

Therapeutic Category Antineoplastic Agent; Progestin

(Continued)

megestrol acetate *(Continued)*

Use Palliative treatment of breast and endometrial carcinomas, appetite stimulation and promotion of weight gain in cachexia

Usual Dosage Adults: Oral:

Breast carcinoma: 40 mg 4 times/day

Endometrial: 40-320 mg/day in divided doses

Dosage Forms

Suspension, oral, as acetate: 40 mg/mL (240 mL) [contains alcohol 0.06%]

Tablet, as acetate: 20 mg, 40 mg

Melanex® **[US]** *see* hydroquinone *on page 336*

Melfiat® **[US]** *see* phendimetrazine *on page 507*

Mellaril® **[US/Can]** *see* thioridazine *on page 635*

Mellaril-S® *(Discontinued) see page 814*

meloxicam (mel OX ee cam)

U.S./Canadian Brand Names Mobicox® [Can]; MOBIC® [US/Can]

Therapeutic Category Nonsteroidal Anti-inflammatory Drug (NSAID)

Use Relief of signs and symptoms of osteoarthritis

Usual Dosage Adult: Oral: Initial: 7.5 mg once daily; some patients may receive additional benefit from an increased dose of 15 mg once daily

Dosage Forms Tablet: 7.5 mg, 15 mg

Melpaque HP® **[US]** *see* hydroquinone *on page 336*

melphalan (MEL fa lan)

Synonyms l-PAM; l-sarcolysin; phenylalanine mustard

U.S./Canadian Brand Names Alkeran® [US/Can]

Therapeutic Category Antineoplastic Agent

Use Palliative treatment of multiple myeloma and nonresectable epithelial ovarian carcinoma; neuroblastoma, rhabdomyosarcoma, breast cancer, sarcoma; I.V. formulation: Use in patients in whom oral therapy is not appropriate

Usual Dosage Refer to individual protocols.

Children: I.V. (investigational, distributed under the auspices of the NCI for authorized studies):

Pediatric rhabdomyosarcoma: 10-35 mg/m^2 bolus every 21-28 days

Chemoradiotherapy supported by marrow infusions for neuroblastoma: 70-140 mg/m^2 on day 7 and 6 before BMT

Adults: Oral:

Multiple myeloma: 6 mg/day or 10 mg/day for 7-10 days, or 0.15 mg/kg/day for 7 days

Ovarian carcinoma: 0.2 mg/kg/day for 5 days, repeat in 4-5 weeks

Dosage Forms

Injection, powder for reconstitution: 50 mg

Tablet: 2 mg

Melquin-3® **[US-OTC]** *see* hydroquinone *on page 336*

Melquin HP® **[US]** *see* hydroquinone *on page 336*

Menadol® **[US-OTC]** *see* ibuprofen *on page 342*

Menest® **[US]** *see* estrogens (esterified) *on page 242*

Meni-D® **[US]** *see* meclizine *on page 403*

meningococcal polysaccharide vaccine (groups A, C, Y and W-135)

(me NIN joe kok al pol i SAK a ride vak SEEN groops aye, see, why, & dubl yoo-won thur tee fyve)

U.S./Canadian Brand Names Menomune®-A/C/Y/W-135 [US]

Therapeutic Category Vaccine, Live Bacteria

Use Immunization against infection caused by *Neisseria meningitidis* groups A,C,Y, and W-135 in persons ≥2 years

Usual Dosage S.C.: 0.5 mL; do not inject intradermally or I.V.

Dosage Forms Injection, powder for reconstitution: Polysaccharide antigen groups A, C, Y, and W-135 (50 mcg of each antigen/0.5 mL following reconstitution) (1 mL, 6 mL) [contains lactose; 6 mL vial contains thimerosal; vial stoppers contain dry, natural latex rubber]

Menomune®-A/C/Y/W-135 [US] *see* meningococcal polysaccharide vaccine (groups A, C, Y and W-135) *on this page*

menotropins (men oh TROE pins)

U.S./Canadian Brand Names Humegon™ [US]; Pergonal® [US/Can]; Repronex® [US]

Therapeutic Category Gonadotropin

Use Sequentially with hCG to induce ovulation and pregnancy in the infertile woman with functional anovulation or in patients who have previously received pituitary suppression; used with hCG in men to stimulate spermatogenesis in those with primary hypogonadotropic hypogonadism

Usual Dosage Adults: I.M.:

Male: Following pretreatment with hCG, 1 ampul 3 times/week and hCG 2000 units twice weekly until sperm is detected in the ejaculate (4-6 months) then may be increased to 2 ampuls of menotropins (150 units FSH/150 units LH) 3 times/week

Female: 1 ampul/day (75 units of FSH and LH) for 9-12 days followed by 10,000 units hCG 1 day after the last dose; repeated at least twice at same level before increasing dosage to 2 ampuls (150 units FSH/150 units LH)

Repronex®: I.M., S.C.:

Infertile patients with oligo-anovulation: Initial: 150 int. units daily for the first 5 days of treatment. Adjustments should not be made more frequently than once every 2 days and should not exceed 75-150 int. units per adjustment. Maximum daily dose should not exceed 450 int. units and dosing beyond 12 days is not recommended. If patient's response to Repronex® is appropriate, hCG 5000-10,000 units should be given one day following the last dose of Repronex®.

Assisted reproductive technologies: Initial (in patients who have received GnRH agonist or antagonist pituitary suppression): 225 int. units; adjustments in dose should not be made more frequently than once every 2 days and should not exceed more than 75-50 int. units per adjustment. The maximum daily doses of Repronex® given should not exceed 450 int. units and dosing beyond 12 days is not recommended. Once adequate follicular development is evident, hCG (5000-10,000 units) should be administered to induce final follicular maturation in preparation for oocyte retrieval.

Dosage Forms

Injection:

Follicle stimulating hormone activity 75 units and luteinizing hormone activity 75 units per 2 mL ampul

Follicle stimulating hormone activity 150 units and luteinizing hormone activity 150 units per 2 mL ampul

Mentax® [US] *see* butenafine *on page 100*

292 MEP® [Can] *see* aspirin and meprobamate *on page 59*

mepenzolate (me PEN zoe late)
U.S./Canadian Brand Names Cantil® [US/Can]
Therapeutic Category Anticholinergic Agent
Use Management of peptic ulcer disease; inhibit salivation and excessive secretions in respiratory tract preoperatively
Usual Dosage Adults: Oral: 25-50 mg 4 times/day with meals and at bedtime
Dosage Forms Tablet, as bromide: 25 mg

Mepergan® [US] *see* meperidine and promethazine *on this page*

meperidine (me PER i deen)
Synonyms isonipecaine; pethidine
U.S./Canadian Brand Names Demerol® [US/Can]; Meperitab® [US]
Therapeutic Category Analgesic, Narcotic
Controlled Substance C-II
Use Management of moderate to severe pain; adjunct to anesthesia and preoperative sedation
Usual Dosage Doses should be titrated to appropriate analgesic effect; when changing route of administration, note that oral doses are about half as effective as parenteral dose

Oral, I.M., I.V., S.C.:
Children: 1-1.5 mg/kg/dose every 3-4 hours as needed; 1-2 mg/kg as a single dose preoperative medication may be used; maximum 100 mg/dose
Adults: 50-150 mg/dose every 3-4 hours as needed
Dosage Forms
Infusion, as hydrochloride: 10 mg/mL (30 mL) [via compatible infusion device only]
Injection, as hydrochloride [multidose vial]: 50 mg/mL (30 mL); 100 mg/mL (20 mL)
Injection, as hydrochloride [single-dose]: 25 mg/dose (1 mL); 50 mg/dose (1 mL); 75 mg/dose (1 mL); 100 mg/dose (1 mL)
Syrup, as hydrochloride: 50 mg/5 mL (500 mL)
Tablet, as hydrochloride: 50 mg, 100 mg

meperidine and promethazine (me PER i deen & proe METH a zeen)
Synonyms promethazine and meperidine
U.S./Canadian Brand Names Mepergan® [US]
Therapeutic Category Analgesic, Narcotic
Controlled Substance C-II
Use Management of moderate to severe pain
Usual Dosage Adults:
Oral: 1 capsule every 4-6 hours
I.M.: 1-2 mL every 3-4 hours
Dosage Forms Capsule: Meperidine hydrochloride 50 mg and promethazine hydrochloride 25 mg

Meperitab® [US] *see* meperidine *on this page*

mephentermine (me FEN ter meen)
U.S./Canadian Brand Names Wyamine® Sulfate [US]
Therapeutic Category Adrenergic Agonist Agent
Use Treatment of hypotension secondary to ganglionic blockade or spinal anesthesia; may be used as an emergency measure to maintain blood pressure until whole blood replacement becomes available
Usual Dosage
Hypotension: I.M., I.V.:
Children: 0.4 mg/kg
Adults: 0.5 mg/kg
Hypotensive emergency: I.V. infusion: 20-60 mg

Dosage Forms Injection, as sulfate: 15 mg/mL (2 mL, 10 mL)

mephobarbital (me foe BAR bi tal)
Synonyms methylphenobarbital
U.S./Canadian Brand Names Mebaral® [US/Can]
Therapeutic Category Barbiturate
Controlled Substance C-IV
Use Treatment of generalized tonic-clonic and simple partial seizures
Usual Dosage Epilepsy: Oral:
  Children: 4-10 mg/kg/day in 2-4 divided doses
  Adults: 200-600 mg/day in 2-4 divided doses
Dosage Forms Tablet: 32 mg, 50 mg, 100 mg

Mephyton® [US/Can] *see* phytonadione *on page 513*

mepivacaine (me PIV a kane)
U.S./Canadian Brand Names Carbocaine® [US/Can]; Isocaine® HCl [US]; Polocaine® [US/Can]
Therapeutic Category Local Anesthetic
Use Local anesthesia by nerve block; infiltration in dental procedures
Usual Dosage
  Injectable local anesthetic: Varies with procedure, degree of anesthesia needed, vascularity of tissue, duration of anesthesia required, and physical condition of patient
  Topical: Apply to affected area as needed
Dosage Forms Injection, as hydrochloride: 1% [10 mg/mL] (30 mL, 50 mL); 1.5% [15 mg/mL] (30 mL); 2% [20 mg/mL] (20 mL, 50 mL); 3% [30 mg/mL] (1.8 mL)

meprobamate (me proe BA mate)
U.S./Canadian Brand Names Apo®-Meprobamate [Can]; Miltown® [US]
Therapeutic Category Antianxiety Agent, Miscellaneous
Controlled Substance C-IV
Use Management of anxiety disorders
Usual Dosage Oral:
  Children 6-12 years: 100-200 mg 2-3 times/day
    Sustained release: 200 mg twice daily
  Adults: 400 mg 3-4 times/day, up to 2400 mg/day
    Sustained release: 400-800 mg twice daily
Dosage Forms Tablet: 200 mg, 400 mg

meprobamate and aspirin *see* aspirin and meprobamate *on page 59*
Mepron™ [US/Can] *see* atovaquone *on page 61*
Meprospan® (Discontinued) *see page 814*

mequinol and tretinoin (ME kwi nol & TRET i noyn)
U.S./Canadian Brand Names Solagé™ [US/Can]
Therapeutic Category Retinoic Acid Derivative; Vitamin A Derivative; Vitamin, Topical
Use Treatment of solar lentigines; the efficacy of using Solagé™ daily for >24 weeks has not been established. The local cutaneous safety of Solagé™ in non-Caucasians has not been adequately established.
Usual Dosage Adults: Topical: Apply twice daily to solar lentigines using the applicator tip while avoiding application to the surrounding skin. Separate application by at least 8 hours or as directed by physician.
Dosage Forms Liquid, topical: Mequinol 2% and tretinoin 0.01% (30 mL)

merbromin (mer BROE min)
U.S./Canadian Brand Names Mercurochrome® [US]
Therapeutic Category Topical Skin Product
  (Continued)

merbromin (Continued)
Use Topical antiseptic
Usual Dosage Topical: Apply freely, until injury has healed
Dosage Forms Solution, topical: 2%

mercaptopurine (mer kap toe PYOOR een)
Synonyms 6-mercaptopurine; 6-MP
U.S./Canadian Brand Names Purinethol® [US/Can]
Therapeutic Category Antineoplastic Agent
Use Treatment of acute leukemias (ALL, CML)
Usual Dosage Oral (refer to individual protocols):
Induction: 2.5 mg/kg/day for several weeks or more; if, after 4 weeks there is no improvement and no myelosuppression, increase dosage up to 5 mg/kg/day
Maintenance: 1.5-2.5 mg/kg/day
Dosage Forms Tablet, scored: 50 mg

6-mercaptopurine see mercaptopurine on this page

mercapturic acid see acetylcysteine on page 11

mercuric oxide (mer KYOOR ik OKS ide)
Synonyms yellow mercuric oxide
U.S./Canadian Brand Names Ocu-Merox® [US]
Therapeutic Category Antibiotic, Ophthalmic
Use Treatment of irritation and minor infections of the eyelids
Usual Dosage Ophthalmic: Apply small amount to inner surface of lower eyelid once or twice daily
Dosage Forms Ointment, ophthalmic: 1%, 2% [OTC]

Mercurochrome® [US] see merbromin on previous page

Meridia™ [US/Can] see sibutramine on page 589

meropenem (mer oh PEN em)
U.S./Canadian Brand Names Merrem® I.V. [US/Can]
Therapeutic Category Carbapenem (Antibiotic)
Use Meropenem is indicated as single agent therapy for the treatment of intra-abdominal infections including complicated appendicitis and peritonitis in adults and bacterial meningitis in pediatric patients >3 months of age caused by *S. pneumoniae, H. influenzae,* and *N. meningitidis* (penicillin-resistant pneumococci have not been studied in clinical trials); it is better tolerated than imipenem and highly effective against a broad range of bacteria
Usual Dosage
Children:
Intra-abdominal infections: 20 mg/kg every 8 hours (maximum dose: 1 g every 8 hours)
Meningitis: 40 mg/kg every 8 hours (maximum dose: 2 g every 8 hours)
Adults: 1 g every 8 hours
Dosage Forms
Injection, powder for reconstitution: 500 mg, 1 g
ADD-Vantage®: 500 mg, 1 g

Merrem® I.V. [US/Can] see meropenem on this page

Mersol® [US-OTC] see thimerosal on page 633

Merthiolate® [US-OTC] see thimerosal on page 633

Meruvax® II [US] see rubella virus vaccine (live) on page 579

mesalamine (me SAL a meen)

Synonyms 5-aminosalicylic acid; 5-ASA; fisalamine; mesalazine

U.S./Canadian Brand Names Asacol® [US/Can]; Canasa™ [US]; Mesasal® [Can]; Novo-ASA [Can]; Pentasa® [US/Can]; Quintasa® [Can]; Rowasa® [US/Can]; Salofalk® [Can]

Therapeutic Category 5-Aminosalicylic Acid Derivative

Use Treatment of ulcerative colitis, proctosigmoiditis, and proctitis

Usual Dosage Adults (usual course of therapy is 3-6 weeks): Oral: 800 mg 3 times/day
Retention enema: 60 mL (4 g) at bedtime, retained overnight, approximately 8 hours
Rectal suppository: Insert 1 suppository in rectum twice daily

Dosage Forms
Capsule, controlled release (Pentasa®): 250 mg
Suppository, rectal (Canasa™, Rowasa®): 500 mg
Suspension, rectal (Rowasa®): 4 g/60 mL [contains potassium metabisulphite] (7s)
Tablet, delayed release, enteric coated (Asacol®): 400 mg

mesalazine see mesalamine on this page

Mesantoin® *(Discontinued)* see page 814

Mesasal® [Can] see mesalamine on this page

M-Eslon® [Can] see morphine sulfate on page 437

mesna (MES na)

Synonyms sodium 2-mercaptoethane sulfonate

U.S./Canadian Brand Names Mesnex™ [US/Can]; Uromitexan™ [Can]

Therapeutic Category Antidote

Use Detoxifying agent used as a protectant against hemorrhagic cystitis induced by ifosfamide and cyclophosphamide

Usual Dosage Refer to individual protocols.
Children and Adults:
I.V. regimen: Recommended dose is 60% of the ifosfamide dose given in 3 divided doses, with ifosfamide, and 4 hours and 8 hours after the ifosfamide dose.
Note: Other I.V. doses/regimens include 4 divided doses of mesna (0, 3, 6, and 9 hours after the start of ifosfamide) and continuous infusions. Continuous infusions commonly employ doses equal to the dose of ifosfamide or cyclophosphamide. It has been suggested that continuous infusions provide more consistent urinary free thiol levels. Infusions are continued for 8-24 hours after completion of ifosfamide or cyclophosphamide.
I.V./Oral regimen: Commonly, the first dose is I.V. and the 2-hour and 6-hour doses are oral. I.V. dose is 20% of the ifosfamide dose at the time of ifosfamide dosing. Oral doses are 40% of the ifosfamide dose and are given 2 hours and 6 hours after the ifosfamide dose. **Note:** Total dose equal 100% of the ifosfamide dose.

Dosage Forms
Injection: 100 mg/mL (2 mL, 4 mL, 10 mL)
Tablet: 400 mg

Mesnex™ [US/Can] see mesna on this page

mesoridazine (mez oh RID a zeen)

U.S./Canadian Brand Names Serentil® [US/Can]

Therapeutic Category Phenothiazine Derivative

Use Symptomatic management of psychotic disorders, including schizophrenia, behavioral problems, alcoholism as well as reducing anxiety and tension occurring in neurosis

Usual Dosage Initial: 25 mg for most patients; may repeat dose in 30-60 minutes, if necessary; usual optimum dosage range: 25-200 mg/day. Concentrate may be diluted just prior to administration with distilled water, acidified tap water, orange or grape juice; do not prepare and store bulk dilutions.
(Continued)

mesoridazine *(Continued)*

Dosage Forms
Injection, as besylate: 25 mg/mL (1 mL)
Liquid, oral, as besylate: 25 mg/mL (118 mL)
Tablet, as besylate: 10 mg, 25 mg, 50 mg, 100 mg

Mestinon® [US/Can] *see* pyridostigmine *on page 556*
Mestinon®-SR [Can] *see* pyridostigmine *on page 556*
Mestinon® Timespan® [US] *see* pyridostigmine *on page 556*

mestranol and norethindrone (MES tra nole & nor eth IN drone)

Synonyms norethindrone and mestranol
U.S./Canadian Brand Names Necon® 1/50 [US]; Norinyl® 1+50 [US]; Ortho-Novum® 1/50 [US/Can]
Therapeutic Category Contraceptive, Oral
Use Prevention of pregnancy; treatment of hypermenorrhea, endometriosis, female hypogonadism
Usual Dosage Oral: Adults: Female: Contraception:
Schedule 1 (Sunday starter): Dose begins on first Sunday after onset of menstruation; if the menstrual period starts on Sunday, take first tablet that very same day. **With a Sunday start, an additional method of contraception should be used until after the first 7 days of consecutive administration.**
For 21-tablet package: Dosage is 1 tablet daily for 21 consecutive days, followed by 7 days off of the medication; a new course begins on the 8th day after the last tablet is taken.
For 28-tablet package: Dosage is 1 tablet daily without interruption.
Schedule 2 (Day 1 starter): Dose starts on first day of menstrual cycle taking 1 tablet daily.
For 21-tablet package: Dosage is 1 tablet daily for 21 consecutive days, followed by 7 days off of the medication; a new course begins on the 8th day after the last tablet is taken.
For 28-tablet package: Dosage is 1 tablet daily without interruption.
If all doses have been taken on schedule and one menstrual period is missed, continue dosing cycle. If two consecutive menstrual periods are missed, pregnancy test is required before new dosing cycle is started.
Missed doses monophasic formulations (refer to package insert for complete information):
One dose missed: Take as soon as remembered or take 2 tablets next day
Two consecutive doses missed in the first 2 weeks: Take 2 tablets as soon as remembered or 2 tablets next 2 days. **An additional method of contraception should be used for 7 days after missed dose.**
Two consecutive doses missed in week 3 or three consecutive doses missed at any time: **An additional method of contraception must be used for 7 days after a missed dose:**
Schedule 1 (Sunday starter): Continue dose of 1 tablet daily until Sunday, then discard the rest of the pack, and a new pack should be started that same day.
Schedule 2 (Day 1 starter): Current pack should be discarded, and a new pack should be started that same day.
Dosage Forms Tablet, monophasic formulations:
Necon® 1/50-21: Norethindrone 1 mg and mestranol 0.05 mg [light blue tablets] (21s)
Necon® 1/50-28: Norethindrone 1 mg and mestranol 0.05 mg [21 light blue tablets and 7 white inactive tablets] (28s)
Norinyl® 1+50: Norethindrone 1 mg and mestranol 0.05 mg [21 white tablets and 7 orange inactive tablets] (28s)
Ortho-Novum® 1/50: Norethindrone 1 mg and mestranol 0.05 mg [21 yellow tablets and 7 green inactive tablets] (28s)

metacortandralone *see* prednisolone (systemic) *on page 537*

Metadate® CD [US] *see* methylphenidate *on page 422*

Metadate™ ER [US] *see* methylphenidate *on page 422*

Metadol™ [Can] *see* methadone *on page 415*

Metahydrin® *(Discontinued) see page 814*

Metamucil® [US/Can] *see* psyllium *on page 554*

Metamucil® Smooth Texture [US-OTC] *see* psyllium *on page 554*

Metaprel® Aerosol *(Discontinued) see page 814*

Metaprel® Inhalation Solution *(Discontinued) see page 814*

Metaprel® Syrup *(Discontinued) see page 814*

Metaprel® Tablet *(Discontinued) see page 814*

metaproterenol (met a proe TER e nol)
Synonyms orciprenaline
U.S./Canadian Brand Names Alupent® [US]
Therapeutic Category Adrenergic Agonist Agent
Use Bronchodilator in reversible airway obstruction due to asthma or COPD
Usual Dosage
Oral:
Children:
<2 years: 0.4 mg/kg/dose administered 3-4 times/day; in infants, the dose can be administered every 8-12 hours
2-6 years: 1-2.6 mg/kg/day divided every 6-8 hours
6-9 years: 10 mg/dose administered 3-4 times/day
Children >9 years and Adults: 20 mg/dose administered 3-4 times/day
Inhalation: Children >12 years and Adults: 2-3 inhalations every 3-4 hours, up to 12 inhalations in 24 hours
Nebulizer:
Infants: 6 mg/dose administered over 5 minutes
Children <12 years: 0.01-0.02 mL/kg of 5% solution; diluted in 2-3 mL normal saline every 4-6 hours (may be administered more frequently according to need), maximum dose: 15 mg/dose every 4-6 hours
Adolescents and Adults: 5-20 breaths of full strength 5% metaproterenol **or** 0.2-0.3 mL of 5% metaproterenol in 2.5-3 mL normal saline nebulized every 4-6 hours (can be administered more frequently according to need)
Dosage Forms
Aerosol for oral inhalation, as sulfate: 0.65 mg/dose (14 g) [200 actuations]
Solution for oral inhalation, as sulfate [preservative free]: 0.4% [4 mg/mL] (2.5 mL); 0.6% [6 mg/mL] (2.5 mL); 5% [50 mg/mL] (10 mL, 30 mL)
Syrup, as sulfate: 10 mg/5 mL (120 mL, 480 mL)
Tablet, as sulfate: 10 mg, 20 mg

metaraminol (met a RAM i nole)
U.S./Canadian Brand Names Aramine® [US/Can]
Therapeutic Category Adrenergic Agonist Agent
Use Acute hypotensive crisis in the treatment of shock
Usual Dosage Adults:
Prevention of hypotension: I.M., S.C.: 2-10 mg
Adjunctive treatment of hypotension: I.V.: 15-100 mg in 250-500 mL NS or 5% dextrose in water
Severe shock: I.V.: 0.5-5 mg direct I.V. injection then use I.M. dose
Dosage Forms Injection, as bitartrate: 10 mg/mL (10 mL)

Metasep® [US-OTC] *see* parachlorometaxylenol *on page 492*

Metastron® [US/Can] *see* strontium-89 *on page 608*

Metatensin® [Can] *see* trichlormethiazide *on page 653*

metaxalone (me TAKS a lone)
U.S./Canadian Brand Names Skelaxin® [US/Can]
Therapeutic Category Skeletal Muscle Relaxant
Use Relief of discomfort associated with acute, painful musculoskeletal conditions
Usual Dosage Children >12 years and Adults: Oral: 800 mg 3-4 times/day
Dosage Forms Tablet: 400 mg

metformin (met FOR min)
U.S./Canadian Brand Names Apo®-Metformin [Can]; Gen-Metformin [Can]; Glucophage® [US/Can]; Glucophage® XR [US]; Glycon [Can]; Novo-Metformin [Can]; Nu-Metformin [Can]; Rho®-Metformin [Can]
Therapeutic Category Antidiabetic Agent, Oral
Use Management of noninsulin-dependent diabetes mellitus (type II) as monotherapy when hyperglycemia cannot be managed on diet alone. May be used concomitantly with a sulfonylurea when diet and metformin or sulfonylurea alone do not result in adequate glycemic control.
Usual Dosage Oral (allow 1-2 weeks between dose titrations):
Adults:
500 mg tablets: Initial: 500 mg twice daily (administered with the morning and evening meals). Dosage increases should be made in increments of one tablet every week, administered in divided doses, up to a maximum of 2,500 mg/day. Doses of up to 2000 mg/day may be administered twice daily. If a dose of 2,500 mg/day is required, it may be better tolerated 3 times/day (with meals).
850 mg tablets: Initial: 850 mg once daily (administered with the morning meal). Dosage increases should be made in increments of one tablet every OTHER week, administered in divided doses, up to a maximum of 2550 mg/day. The usual maintenance dose is 850 mg twice daily (with the morning and evening meals). Some patients may be administered 850 mg 3 times/day (with meals).

Transfer from other antidiabetic agents: No transition period is generally necessary except when transferring from chlorpropamide. When transferring from chlorproPA-MIDE, care should be exercised during the first 2 weeks because of the prolonged retention of chlorpropamide in the body, leading to overlapping drug effects and possible hypoglycemia.

Concomitant metformin and oral sulfonylurea therapy: If patients have not responded to 4 weeks of the maximum dose of metformin monotherapy, consideration to a gradually addition of an oral sulfonylurea while continuing metformin at the maximum dose, even if prior primary or secondary failure to a sulfonylurea has occurred.
Dosage Forms
Tablet, as hydrochloride: 500 mg, 850 mg, 1000 mg
Tablet, extended release, as hydrochloride: 500 mg

methacholine (meth a KOLE leen)
U.S./Canadian Brand Names Provocholine® [US/Can]
Therapeutic Category Diagnostic Agent
Use Diagnosis of bronchial airway hyperactivity in subjects who do not have clinically apparent asthma

Vial	Serial Concentration (mg/mL)	No. of Breaths	Cumulative Units per Concentration	Total Cumulative Units
E	0.025	5	0.125	0.125
D	0.25	5	1.25	1.375
C	2.5	5	12.5	13.88
B	10	5	50	63.88
A	25	5	125	188.88

Usual Dosage The table is a suggested schedule for administration of methacholine challenge. Calculate cumulative units by multiplying number of breaths by concentration given. Total cumulative units is the sum of cumulative units for each concentration given.

Dosage Forms Powder for oral inhalation, as chloride: 100 mg/5 mL [when reconstituted]

methadone (METH a done)
U.S./Canadian Brand Names Dolophine® [US/Can]; Metadol™ [Can]; Methadose® [US/Can]
Therapeutic Category Analgesic, Narcotic
Controlled Substance C-II
Use Management of severe pain, used in narcotic detoxification maintenance programs and for the treatment of iatrogenic narcotic dependency
Usual Dosage Doses should be titrated to appropriate effects:
Children: Analgesia:
Oral, I.M., S.C.: 0.7 mg/kg/24 hours divided every 4-6 hours as needed or 0.1-0.2 mg/kg every 4-12 hours as needed; maximum: 10 mg/dose
I.V.: Initial: 0.1 mg/kg every 4 hours for 2-3 doses, then every 6-12 hours as needed; maximum: 10 mg/dose
Adults:
Analgesia: Oral, I.M., S.C.: 2.5-10 mg every 3-8 hours as needed, up to 5-20 mg every 6-8 hours
Detoxification: Oral: 15-40 mg/day
Maintenance of opiate dependence: Oral: 20-120 mg/day
Dosage Forms
Injection, as hydrochloride: 10 mg/mL (20 mL)
Solution, oral, as hydrochloride: 5 mg/5 mL (5 mL, 500 mL); 10 mg/5 mL (500 mL)
Solution, oral concentrate, as hydrochloride: 10 mg/mL (30 mL)
Tablet, as hydrochloride: 5 mg, 10 mg
Tablet, dispersible, as hydrochloride: 40 mg

Methadose® [US/Can] see methadone on this page

methaminodiazepoxide see chlordiazepoxide on page 134

methamphetamine (meth am FET a meen)
Synonyms desoxyephedrine
U.S./Canadian Brand Names Desoxyn® Gradumet® [US]; Desoxyn® [US/Can]
Therapeutic Category Amphetamine
Controlled Substance C-II
Use Narcolepsy; exogenous obesity; abnormal behavioral syndrome in children (minimal brain dysfunction)
Usual Dosage Oral:
Attention deficit disorder: Children >6 years: 2.5-5 mg 1-2 times/day, may increase by 5 mg increments weekly until optimum response is achieved, usually 20-25 mg/day
Exogenous obesity: Children >12 years and Adults: 5 mg, 30 minutes before each meal, 10-15 mg in morning; treatment duration should not exceed a few weeks
Dosage Forms
Tablet, as hydrochloride: 5 mg
Tablet, extended release, as hydrochloride (Desoxyn® Gradumet®): 5 mg, 10 mg, 15 mg

methazolamide (meth a ZOE la mide)
U.S./Canadian Brand Names Neptazane® [US/Can]
Therapeutic Category Carbonic Anhydrase Inhibitor
Use Adjunctive treatment of open-angle or secondary glaucoma; short-term therapy of narrow-angle glaucoma when delay of surgery is desired
Usual Dosage Adults: Oral: 50-100 mg 2-3 times/day
(Continued)

methazolamide *(Continued)*

Dosage Forms Tablet: 25 mg, 50 mg

methenamine (meth EN a meen)

Synonyms hexamethylenetetramine

U.S./Canadian Brand Names Dehydral® [Can]; Hip-Rex™ [Can]; Hiprex® [US/Can]; Mandelamine® [Can]; Urasal® [Can]; Urex® [US/Can]

Therapeutic Category Antibiotic, Miscellaneous

Use Prophylaxis or suppression of recurrent urinary tract infections

Usual Dosage Oral:

Children:

Hippurate: 6-12 years: 25-50 mg/kg/day divided every 12 hours

Mandelate: 50-75 mg/kg/day divided every 6 hours

Adults:

Hippurate: 1 g twice daily

Mandelate: 1 g 4 times/day after meals and at bedtime

Dosage Forms

Suspension, oral, as mandelate: 0.5 g/5 mL (480 mL)

Tablet, as hippurate (Hiprex®, Urex®): 1 g [Hiprex® contains tartrazine dye]

Tablet, enteric coated, as mandelate: 500 mg, 1 g

methenamine, phenyl salicylate, atropine, hyoscyamine, benzoic acid, and methylene blue

(meth EN a meen, fen nil sa LIS i late, A troe peen, hye oh SYE a meen, ben ZOE ik AS id, & METH i leen bloo)

U.S./Canadian Brand Names Atrosept® [US]; Dolsed® [US]; UAA® [US]; Uridon Modified® [US]; Urised® [US]; Uritin® [US]

Therapeutic Category Antibiotic, Urinary Anti-infective; Urinary Tract Product

Usual Dosage Adults: Oral: Two tablets four/daily

Dosage Forms Tablet: Methenamine 40.8 mg, phenyl salicylate 18.1 mg, atropine sulfate 0.03 mg, hyoscyamine sulfate 0.03 mg, benzoic acid 4.5 mg, and methylene blue 5.4 mg

Methergine® [US/Can] *see* methylergonovine *on page 421*

methimazole (meth IM a zole)

Synonyms thiamazole

U.S./Canadian Brand Names Tapazole® [US/Can]

Therapeutic Category Antithyroid Agent

Use Palliative treatment of hyperthyroidism, to return the hyperthyroid patient to a normal metabolic state prior to thyroidectomy, and to control thyrotoxic crisis that may accompany thyroidectomy

Usual Dosage Oral:

Children: Initial: 0.4 mg/kg/day in 3 divided doses; maintenance: 0.2 mg/kg/day in 3 divided doses

Adults: Initial: 10 mg every 8 hours; maintenance dose ranges from 5-30 mg/day

Dosage Forms Tablet: 5 mg, 10 mg

methionine (me THYE oh neen)

U.S./Canadian Brand Names ME-500® [US]; Pedameth® [US]

Therapeutic Category Dietary Supplement

Use Treatment of diaper rash and control of odor, dermatitis and ulceration caused by ammoniacal urine

Usual Dosage Oral:

Children: Control of diaper rash: 75 mg in formula or other liquid 3-4 times/day for 3-5 days

Adults:
Control of odor in incontinent adults: 200-400 mg 3-4 times/day
Dietary supplement: 500 mg/day
Dosage Forms
Capsule (ME-500®): 500 mg
Liquid (Pedameth®): 75 mg/5 mL (480 mL)
Tablet: 500 mg

Methitest® [US] *see* methyltestosterone *on page 423*

methocarbamol (meth oh KAR ba mole)
U.S./Canadian Brand Names Robaxin® [US/Can]
Therapeutic Category Skeletal Muscle Relaxant
Use Treatment of muscle spasm associated with acute painful musculoskeletal conditions; supportive therapy in tetanus
Usual Dosage
Children: Recommended **only** for use in tetanus I.V.: 15 mg/kg/dose or 500 mg/m^2/dose, may repeat every 6 hours if needed; maximum dose: 1.8 g/m^2/day for 3 days only
Adults: Muscle spasm:
Oral: 1.5 g 4 times/day for 2-3 days, then decrease to 4-4.5 g/day in 3-6 divided doses
I.M., I.V.: 1 g every 8 hours if oral not possible
Dosage Forms
Injection: 100 mg/mL [in polyethylene glycol 50%] (10 mL)
Tablet: 500 mg, 750 mg

methocarbamol and aspirin (meth oh KAR ba mole & AS pir in)
Synonyms aspirin and methocarbamol
U.S./Canadian Brand Names Aspirin® Backache [Can]; Methoxisal [Can]; Methoxisal-C [Can]; Robaxisal® Extra Strength [Can]; Robaxisal® [US/Can]
Therapeutic Category Skeletal Muscle Relaxant
Use Adjunct to rest, physical therapy, and other measures for the relief of discomfort associated with acute, painful musculoskeletal disorders
Usual Dosage Children >12 years and Adults: Oral: 2 tablets 4 times/day
Dosage Forms Tablet: Methocarbamol 400 mg and aspirin 325 mg

methohexital (meth oh HEKS i tal)
U.S./Canadian Brand Names Brevital® Sodium [US/Can]
Therapeutic Category Barbiturate
Controlled Substance C-IV
Use Induction and maintenance of general anesthesia for short procedures
Usual Dosage Doses must be titrated to effect
Children:
I.M.: Preop: 5-10 mg/kg/dose
I.V.: Induction: 1-2 mg/kg/dose
Rectal: Preop/induction: 20-35 mg/kg/dose; usual: 25 mg/kg/dose; administer as 10% aqueous solution
Adults: I.V.: Induction: 50-120 mg to start; 20-40 mg every 4-7 minutes
Dosage Forms Injection, as sodium: 500 mg, 2.5 g, 5 g

methotrexate (meth oh TREKS ate)
Synonyms amethopterin; MTX
U.S./Canadian Brand Names Rheumatrex® [US]; Trexall™ [US]
Therapeutic Category Antineoplastic Agent
Use Treatment of trophoblastic neoplasms, leukemias, osteosarcoma, non-Hodgkin's lymphoma; psoriasis, rheumatoid arthritis
Usual Dosage Refer to individual protocols.
(Continued)

methotrexate *(Continued)*

Children:

High-dose MTX for acute lymphocytic leukemia: I.V.: Loading dose of 200 mg/m² and a 24-hour infusion of 1200 mg/m²/day

Induction of remission in acute lymphoblastic leukemias: Oral, I.M., I.V.: 3.3 mg/m²/day for 4-6 weeks

Leukemia: Remission maintenance: Oral, I.M.: 20-30 mg/m² 2 times/week

Juvenile rheumatoid arthritis: Oral: 5-15 mg/m²/week as a single dose or as 3 divided doses administered 12 hours apart

Osteosarcoma:

I.T.: 10-15 mg/m² (maximum dose: 15 mg) by protocol

I.V.: <12 years: 12 g/m² (12-18 g); >12 years: 8 g/m² (maximum dose: 18 g)

Non-Hodgkin's lymphoma: I.V.: 200-300 mg/m²

Adults:

Trophoblastic neoplasms: Oral, I.M.: 15-30 mg/day for 5 days, repeat in 7 days for 3-5 courses

Rheumatoid arthritis: Oral: 7.5 mg once weekly or 2.5 mg every 12 hours for 3 doses/ week; not to exceed 20 mg/week

Dosage Forms

Injection, as sodium: 25 mg/mL (2 mL, 10 mL) [with benzyl alcohol 0.9%]

Injection, as sodium [preservative free]: 25 mg/mL (2 mL, 4 mL, 8 mL, 10 mL)

Injection, powder for reconstitution: 20 mg, 1 g

Tablet, as sodium: 2.5 mg

Rheumatrex®: 25 mg

Trexall™: 5 mg, 7.5 mg, 10 mg, 15 mg

Tablet, as sodium [dose pack] (Rheumatrex® Dose Pack): 2.5 mg (4 cards with 2, 3, 4, 5, or 6 tablets each)

methotrimeprazine *(Canada only)* (meth oh trye MEP ra zeen)

Synonyms levomepromazine

U.S./Canadian Brand Names Apo®-Methoprazine [Can]; Novo-Meprazine [Can]; Nozinan® [Can]

Therapeutic Category Neuroleptic Agent

Use Acute and chronic schizophrenia, senile psychoses, manic-depressive syndromes. Conditions associated with anxiety and tension: autonomic disturbances, personality disturbances, emotional troubles secondary to such physical conditions as resistant pruritus. Methotrimeprazine is also employed: As an analgesic: In pain due to cancer, zona, trigeminal neuralgia and neurocostal neuralgia and in phantom limb pains and muscular discomforts.

Usual Dosage Adults: I.M.:

Sedation analgesia: 10-20 mg every 4-6 hours as needed

Preoperative medication: 2-20 mg, 45 minutes to 3 hours before surgery

Postoperative analgesia: 2.5-7.5 mg every 4-6 hours is suggested as necessary since residual effects of anesthetic may be present

Pre- and postoperative hypotension: I.M.: 5-10 mg

Dosage Forms Injection, as hydrochloride: 20 mg/mL (10 mL)

Methoxisal [Can] *see* methocarbamol and aspirin *on previous page*

Methoxisal-C [Can] *see* methocarbamol and aspirin *on previous page*

methoxsalen (meth OKS a len)

Synonyms methoxypsoralen

U.S./Canadian Brand Names 8-MOP® [US/Can]; Oxsoralen® Lotion [US/Can]; Oxsor-alen-Ultra® [US/Can]; Ultramop™ [Can]; Uvadex® [US/Can]

Therapeutic Category Psoralen

Use Symptomatic control of severe, recalcitrant, disabling psoriasis in conjunction with long wave ultraviolet radiation; induce repigmentation in vitiligo topical repigmenting agent in conjunction with controlled doses of ultraviolet A (UVA) or sunlight

Usual Dosage

Psoriasis: Adults: Oral: 10-70 mg 1½-2 hours before exposure to UVA light, 2-3 times at least 48 hours apart; dosage is based upon patient's body weight and skin type

<30 kg: 10 mg

30-50 kg: 20 mg

51-65 kg: 30 mg

66-80 kg: 40 mg

81-90 kg: 50 mg

91-115 kg: 60 mg

>115 kg: 70 mg

Vitiligo: Children >12 years and Adults:

Oral: 20 mg 2-4 hours before exposure to UVA light or sunlight; limit exposure to 15-40 minutes based on skin basic color and exposure

Topical: Apply lotion 1-2 hours before exposure to UVA light, no more than once weekly

Dosage Forms

Capsule (8-MOP®): 10 mg

Gelcap (Oxsoralen-Ultra®): 10 mg

Lotion (Oxsoralen®): 1% (30 mL)

Solution, sterile (Uvadex®): 20 mcg/mL (10 mL) [**not for injection**]

methoxycinnamate and oxybenzone

(meth OKS ee SIN a mate & oks i BEN zone)

Synonyms sunscreen (paba-free)

U.S./Canadian Brand Names PreSun® 29 [US-OTC]; Ti-Screen® [US-OTC]

Therapeutic Category Sunscreen

Use Reduce the chance of premature aging of the skin and skin cancer from overexposure to the sun

Usual Dosage Adults: Topical: Apply liberally to all exposed areas at least 30 minutes prior to sun exposure

Dosage Forms Lotion:

SPF 15: 120 mL

SPF 29: 120 mL

methoxyflurane (meth oks ee FLOO rane)

U.S./Canadian Brand Names Penthrane® [US/Can]

Therapeutic Category General Anesthetic

Use Adjunct to provide anesthesia procedures <4 hours in duration

Usual Dosage 0.3% to 0.8% for analgesia and anesthesia, with 0.1% to 2% for maintenance when used with nitrous oxide

Dosage Forms Liquid: 15 mL, 125 mL

methoxypsoralen *see* methoxsalen *on previous page*

methscopolamine (meth skoe POL a meen)

Synonyms methscopolamine bromide

U.S./Canadian Brand Names Pamine® [US/Can]

Therapeutic Category Anticholinergic Agent

Use Adjunctive therapy in the treatment of peptic ulcer

Usual Dosage Adults: Oral: 2.5 mg 30 minutes before meals or food and 2.5-5 mg at bedtime

Dosage Forms Tablet, as bromide: 2.5 mg

methscopolamine bromide *see* methscopolamine *on this page*

methsuximide (meth SUKS i mide)
U.S./Canadian Brand Names Celontin® [US/Can]
Therapeutic Category Anticonvulsant
Use Control of absence (petit mal) seizures; useful adjunct in refractory, partial complex (psychomotor) seizures
Usual Dosage Oral:
Children: Initial: 10-15 mg/kg/day in 3-4 divided doses; increase weekly up to maximum of 30 mg/kg/day
Adults: 300 mg/day for the first week; may increase by 300 mg/day at weekly intervals up to 1.2 g in 2-4 divided doses/day
Dosage Forms Capsule: 150 mg, 300 mg

methyclothiazide (meth i kloe THYE a zide)
U.S./Canadian Brand Names Aquatensen® [US/Can]; Enduron® [US/Can]
Therapeutic Category Diuretic, Thiazide
Use Management of mild to moderate hypertension; treatment of edema in congestive heart failure and nephrotic syndrome
Usual Dosage Adults: Oral:
Edema: 2.5-10 mg/day
Hypertension: 2.5-5 mg/day
Dosage Forms Tablet: 2.5 mg, 5 mg

methyclothiazide and deserpidine
(meth i kloe THYE a zide & de SER pi deen)
Synonyms deserpidine and methyclothiazide
U.S./Canadian Brand Names Enduronyl® Forte [US/Can]; Enduronyl® [US/Can]
Therapeutic Category Antihypertensive Agent, Combination
Use Management of mild to moderately severe hypertension
Usual Dosage Oral: Individualized, normally 1-4 tablets/day
Dosage Forms Tablet: Methyclothiazide 5 mg and deserpidine 0.25 mg; methyclothiazide 5 mg and deserpidine 0.5 mg

methylacetoxyprogesterone *see* medroxyprogesterone acetate *on page 404*

methylbenzethonium chloride (meth il ben ze THOE nee um KLOR ide)
U.S./Canadian Brand Names Puri-Clens™ [US-OTC]; Sween Cream® [US-OTC]
Therapeutic Category Topical Skin Product
Use Treatment of diaper rash and ammonia dermatitis
Usual Dosage Topical: Apply to area as needed
Dosage Forms
Cream, topical: 0.1% (30 g, 60 g, 120 g)
Ointment, topical: 0.1% (30 g, 60 g, 120 g)
Powder, topical: 0.055% (120 g, 270 g, 420 g)

methylcellulose (meth il SEL yoo lose)
U.S./Canadian Brand Names Citrucel® [US-OTC]
Therapeutic Category Laxative
Use Adjunct in treatment of constipation
Usual Dosage Oral:
Children: 5-10 mL 1-2 times/day
Adults: 5-20 mL 3 times/day
Dosage Forms Powder: 105 mg/g

methyldopa (meth il DOE pa)
U.S./Canadian Brand Names Aldomet® [US/Can]; Apo®-Methyldopa [Can]; Nu-Medopa [Can]
Therapeutic Category Alpha-Adrenergic Blocking Agent

Use Management of moderate to severe hypertension
Usual Dosage
Children:
Oral: Initial: 10 mg/kg/day in 2-4 divided doses; increase every 2 days as needed to maximum dose of 65 mg/kg/day; do not exceed 3 g/day
I.V.: 5-10 mg/kg/dose every 6-8 hours
Adults:
Oral: Initial: 250 mg 2-3 times/day; increase every 2 days as needed; usual dose 1-1.5 g/day in 2-4 divided doses; maximum dose: 3 g/day
I.V.: 250-1000 mg every 6-8 hours
Dosage Forms
Injection, as methyldopate hydrochloride: 50 mg/mL (5 mL, 10 mL)
Suspension, oral: 250 mg/5 mL (5 mL, 473 mL)
Tablet: 125 mg, 250 mg, 500 mg

methyldopa and hydrochlorothiazide
(meth il DOE pa & hye droe klor oh THYE a zide)
Synonyms hydrochlorothiazide and methyldopa
U.S./Canadian Brand Names Aldoril® [US]; Apo®-Methazide [Can]
Therapeutic Category Antihypertensive Agent, Combination
Use Management of moderate to severe hypertension
Usual Dosage Oral: 1 tablet 2-3 times/day for first 48 hours, then decrease or increase at intervals of not less than 2 days until an adequate response is achieved
Dosage Forms
Tablet:
Aldoril® 15: Methyldopa 250 mg and hydrochlorothiazide 15 mg
Aldoril® 25: Methyldopa 250 mg and hydrochlorothiazide 25 mg
Aldoril® D30: Methyldopa 500 mg and hydrochlorothiazide 30 mg
Aldoril® D50: Methyldopa 500 mg and hydrochlorothiazide 50 mg

methylene blue (METH i leen bloo)
U.S./Canadian Brand Names Urolene Blue® [US]
Therapeutic Category Antidote
Use Antidote for cyanide poisoning and drug-induced methemoglobinemia, indicator dye, bacteriostatic genitourinary antiseptic
Usual Dosage
Children:
NADH-methemoglobin reductase deficiency: Oral: 1.5-5 mg/kg/day (maximum: 300 mg/day) administered with 5-8 mg/kg/day of ascorbic acid
Methemoglobinemia: I.V.: 1-2 mg/kg over several minutes
Adults:
Genitourinary antiseptic: Oral: 55-130 mg 3 times/day (maximum: 390 mg/day)
Methemoglobinemia: I.V.: 1-2 mg/kg over several minutes; may be repeated in 1 hour if necessary
Dosage Forms
Injection: 10 mg/mL (1 mL, 10 mL)
Tablet: 65 mg

methylergonovine (meth il er goe NOE veen)
U.S./Canadian Brand Names Methergine® [US/Can]
Therapeutic Category Ergot Alkaloid and Derivative
Use Prevention and treatment of postpartum and postabortion hemorrhage caused by uterine atony or subinvolution
Usual Dosage Adults:
Oral: 0.2-0.4 mg every 6-12 hours for 2-7 days
I.M., I.V.: 0.2 mg every 2-4 hours for 5 doses then change to oral dosage
Dosage Forms
Injection, as maleate: 0.2 mg/mL (1 mL)
(Continued)

methylergonovine *(Continued)*

Tablet, as maleate: 0.2 mg

Methylin™ [US] *see* methylphenidate *on this page*

Methylin™ ER [US] *see* methylphenidate *on this page*

methylmorphine *see* codeine *on page 159*

methylphenidate (meth il FEN i date)

U.S./Canadian Brand Names Concerta™ [US]; Metadate® CD [US]; Metadate™ ER [US]; Methylin™ [US]; Methylin™ ER [US]; PMS-Methylphenidate [Can]; Riphenidate [Can]; Ritalin® [US/Can]; Ritalin® LA [US]; Ritalin-SR® [US/Can]

Therapeutic Category Central Nervous System Stimulant, Nonamphetamine

Controlled Substance C-II

Use Treatment of attention-deficit/hyperactivity disorder (ADHD); symptomatic management of narcolepsy

Unlabeled use: Depression (especially elderly or medically ill)

Usual Dosage Oral (discontinue periodically to re-evaluate or if no improvement occurs within 1 month):

Children ≥6 years: ADHD: Initial: 0.3 mg/kg/dose or 2.5-5 mg/dose given before breakfast and lunch; increase by 0.1 mg/kg/dose or by 5-10 mg/day at weekly intervals; usual dose: 0.5-1 mg/kg/day; maximum dose: 2 mg/kg/day or 90 mg/day

Extended release products:

Metadate™ ER, Methylin™ ER, Ritalin® SR: Duration of action is 8 hours. May be given in place of regular tablets, once the daily dose is titrated using the regular tablets and the titrated 8-hour dosage corresponds to sustained release tablet size.

Metadate® CD, Ritalin® LA: Initial: 20 mg once daily; may be adjusted in 10-20 mg increments at weekly intervals; maximum: 60 mg/day

Concerta™: Duration of action is 12 hours:

Children not currently taking methylphenidate:

Initial: 18 mg once daily in the morning

Adjustment: May increase to maximum of 54 mg/day in increments of 18 mg/day; dose may be adjusted at weekly intervals

Children currently taking methylphenidate: **Note:** Dosing based on current regimen and clinical judgment; suggested dosing listed below:

Patients taking methylphenidate 5 mg 2-3 times/day or 20 mg/day sustained release formulation: Initial dose: 18 mg once every morning (maximum: 54 mg/day)

Patients taking methylphenidate 10 mg 2-3 times/day or 40 mg/day sustained release formulation: Initial dose: 36 mg once every morning (maximum: 54 mg/day)

Patients taking methylphenidate 15 mg 2-3 times/day or 60 mg/day sustained release formulation: Initial dose: 54 mg once every morning (maximum: 54 mg/day)

Note: A 27 mg dosage strength is available for situations in which a dosage between 18 mg and 36 mg is desired.

Adults:

Narcolepsy: 10 mg 2-3 times/day, up to 60 mg/day

Depression (unlabeled use): Initial: 2.5 mg every morning before 9 AM; dosage may be increased by 2.5-5 mg every 2-3 days as tolerated to a maximum of 20 mg/day; may be divided (ie, 7 AM and 12 noon), but should not be given after noon; do not use sustained release product

Dosage Forms

Capsule, extended release, as hydrochloride

Metadate® CD: 20 mg

Ritalin® LA: 20 mg, 30 mg, 40 mg

Tablet, as hydrochloride: 5 mg, 10 mg, 20 mg

Methylin™, Ritalin®: 5 mg, 10 mg, 20 mg

Tablet, extended release, as hydrochloride (Metadate™ ER): 10 mg, 20 mg

Tablet, osmotic controlled release, as hydrochloride (Concerta™): 18 mg, 27 mg, 36 mg, 54 mg

Tablet, sustained release, as hydrochloride: 20 mg
Methylin™ ER: 10 mg, 20 mg
Ritalin-SR®: 20 mg

methylphenobarbital *see* mephobarbital *on page 409*

methylphenyl isoxazolyl penicillin *see* oxacillin *on page 481*

methylphytyl napthoquinone *see* phytonadione *on page 513*

methylprednisolone (meth il pred NIS oh lone)
Tall-Man methyl**PREDNIS**olone
U.S./Canadian Brand Names A-methaPred® [US]; Depo-Medrol® [US/Can]; Depopred® [US]; Medrol® Tablet [US/Can]; Solu-Medrol® [US/Can]
Therapeutic Category Adrenal Corticosteroid
Use Anti-inflammatory or immunosuppressant agent in the treatment of a variety of diseases including those of hematologic, allergic, inflammatory, neoplastic, and autoimmune origin
Usual Dosage Methylprednisolone sodium succinate is highly soluble and has a rapid effect by I.M. and I.V. routes. Methyl**PREDNIS**olone acetate has a low solubility and has a sustained I.M. effect.

Children:
Anti-inflammatory or immunosuppressive: Oral, I.M., I.V. (sodium succinate): 0.16-0.8 mg/kg/day or 5-25 mg/m^2/day in divided doses every 6-12 hours
Status asthmaticus: I.V. (sodium succinate): Loading dose: 2 mg/kg/dose, then 0.5-1 mg/kg/dose every 6 hours for up to 5 days
Lupus nephritis: I.V. (sodium succinate): 30 mg/kg every other day for 6 doses
Adults:
Anti-inflammatory or immunosuppressive: Oral: 4-48 mg/day to start, followed by gradual reduction in dosage to the lowest possible level consistent with maintaining an adequate clinical response
I.M. (sodium succinate): 10-80 mg/day once daily
I.M. (acetate): 40-120 mg every 1-2 weeks
I.V. (sodium succinate): 10-40 mg over a period of several minutes and repeated I.V. or I.M. at intervals depending on clinical response; when high dosages are needed, administer 30 mg/kg over a period of 10-20 minutes and may be repeated every 4-6 hours for 48 hours
Status asthmaticus: I.V. (sodium succinate): Loading dose: 2 mg/kg/dose, then 0.5-1 mg/kg/dose every hours for up to 5 days
Lupus nephritis:
I.V. (sodium succinate): 1 g/day for 3 days
Intra-articular (acetate):
Large joints: 20-80 mg
Small joints: 4-10 mg
Intralesional (acetate): 20-60 mg
Dosage Forms
Injection, as acetate: 20 mg/mL (5 mL, 10 mL); 40 mg/mL (1 mL, 5 mL, 10 mL); 80 mg/mL (1 mL, 5 mL)
Injection, as sodium succinate: 40 mg (1 mL, 3 mL); 125 mg (2 mL, 5 mL); 500 mg (1 mL, 4 mL, 8 mL, 20 mL); 1000 mg (1 mL, 8 mL, 50 mL); 2000 mg (30.6 mL)
Tablet: 2 mg, 4 mg, 8 mg, 16 mg, 24 mg, 32 mg
Tablet [dose pack]: 4 mg (21s)

4-methylpyrazole *see* fomepizole *on page 287*

methyltestosterone (meth il tes TOS te rone)
Tall-Man methyl**TESTOSTER**one
U.S./Canadian Brand Names Android® [US]; Methitest® [US]; Testred® [US]; Virilon® [US]
Therapeutic Category Androgen
(Continued)

methyltestosterone *(Continued)*

Use
Male: Hypogonadism; delayed puberty; impotence and climacteric symptoms
Female: Palliative treatment of metastatic breast cancer; postpartum breast pain and/or engorgement

Usual Dosage Adults:
Male:
Oral: 10-40 mg/day
Buccal: 5-20 mg/day
Female:
Breast pain/engorgement:
Oral: 80 mg/day for 3-5 days
Buccal: 40 mg/day for 3-5 days
Breast cancer:
Oral: 200 mg/day
Buccal: 100 mg/day

Dosage Forms
Capsule: 10 mg
Tablet: 10 mg, 25 mg

methysergide (meth i SER jide)
U.S./Canadian Brand Names Sansert® [US/Can]
Therapeutic Category Ergot Alkaloid and Derivative
Use Prophylaxis of vascular headache
Usual Dosage Oral: 4-8 mg/day with meals; if no improvement is noted after 3 weeks, drug is unlikely to be beneficial; must not be administered continuously for longer than 6 months, and a drug-free interval of 3-4 weeks must follow each 6-month course; dosage should be tapered over the 2- to 3-week period before drug discontinuation to avoid rebound headaches
Dosage Forms Tablet, as maleate: 2 mg

Meticorten® [US] *see* prednisone *on page 538*
Metimyd® [US] *see* sulfacetamide and prednisolone *on page 611*

metipranolol (met i PRAN oh lol)
U.S./Canadian Brand Names OptiPranolol® [US/Can]
Therapeutic Category Beta-Adrenergic Blocker
Use Agent for lowering intraocular pressure
Usual Dosage Adults: Ophthalmic: 1 drop in the affected eye(s) twice daily
Dosage Forms Solution, ophthalmic, as hydrochloride: 0.3% (5 mL, 10 mL)

Metizol® Tablet *(Discontinued)* *see page 814*

metoclopramide (met oh kloe PRA mide)
U.S./Canadian Brand Names Apo®-Metoclop [Can]; Nu-Metoclopramide [Can]; Reglan® [US]
Therapeutic Category Gastrointestinal Agent, Prokinetic
Use Gastroesophageal reflux; prevention of nausea associated with chemotherapy; facilitates intubation of the small intestine and symptomatic treatment of diabetic gastric stasis
Usual Dosage
Children:
Gastroesophageal reflux: Oral: 0.1 mg/kg/dose up to 4 times/day; efficacy of continuing metoclopramide beyond 12 weeks in reflux has not been determined; total daily dose should not exceed 0.5 mg/kg/day
Gastrointestinal hypomotility: Oral, I.M., I.V.: 0.1 mg/kg/dose up to 4 times/day, not to exceed 0.5 mg/kg/day

Antiemetic: I.V.: 1-2 mg/kg 30 minutes before chemotherapy and every 2-4 hours
Facilitate intubation: I.V.: <6 years: 0.1 mg/kg; 6-14 years: 2.5-5 mg
Adults:
Stasis/reflux: Oral: 10-15 mg/dose up to 4 times/day 30 minutes before meals or food and at bedtime; efficacy of continuing metoclopramide beyond 12 weeks in reflux has not been determined
Gastrointestinal hypomotility: Oral, I.M., I.V.: 10 mg 30 minutes before each meal and at bedtime
Antiemetic: I.V.: 1-2 mg/kg 30 minutes before chemotherapy and every 2-4 hours
Facilitate intubation: I.V.: 10 mg

Dosage Forms
Injection, as hydrochloride: 5 mg/mL (2 mL, 10 mL, 30 mL, 50 mL, 100 mL)
Solution, as hydrochloride, oral, concentrated: 10 mg/mL (10 mL, 30 mL)
Syrup, as hydrochloride, sugar free: 5 mg/5 mL (10 mL, 480 mL)
Tablet, as hydrochloride: 5 mg, 10 mg

metolazone (me TOLE a zone)
U.S./Canadian Brand Names Mykrox® [US/Can]; Zaroxolyn® [US/Can]
Therapeutic Category Diuretic, Miscellaneous
Use Management of mild to moderate hypertension; treatment of edema in congestive heart failure, nephrotic syndrome, and impaired renal function
Usual Dosage Oral:
Children: 0.2-0.4 mg/kg/day divided every 12-24 hours
Adults:
Edema: 5-20 mg/dose every 24 hours
Hypertension: 2.5-5 mg/dose every 24 hours
Dosage Forms
Tablet, rapid acting (Mykrox®): 0.5 mg
Tablet, slow acting (Zaroxolyn®): 2.5 mg, 5 mg, 10 mg

Metopirone® [US] see metyrapone on next page

metoprolol (me toe PROE lole)
U.S./Canadian Brand Names Apo®-Metoprolol [Can]; Betaloc® [Can]; Betaloc® Durules®; Gen-Metoprolol [Can]; Lopressor® [US/Can]; Novo-Metoprolol [Can]; Nu-Metop [Can]; PMS-Metoprolol [Can]; Toprol-XL® [US/Can]
Therapeutic Category Beta-Adrenergic Blocker
Use Treatment of hypertension and angina pectoris; prevention of myocardial infarction; selective inhibitor of beta$_1$-adrenergic receptors
Usual Dosage Safety and efficacy in children have not been established.
Children: Oral: 1-5 mg/kg/24 hours divided twice daily; allow 3 days between dose adjustments
Adults:
Oral: 100-450 mg/day in 2-3 divided doses, begin with 50 mg twice daily and increase doses at weekly intervals to desired effect
I.V.: 5 mg every 2 minutes for 3 doses in early treatment of myocardial infarction; thereafter administer 50 mg orally every 6 hours 15 minutes after last I.V. dose and continue for 48 hours; then administer a maintenance dose of 100 mg twice daily
Dosage Forms
Injection, as tartrate: 1 mg/mL (5 mL)
Tablet, as tartrate: 25 mg, 50 mg, 100 mg
Tablet, sustained release, as succinate [equivalent to tartrate]: 25 mg, 50 mg, 100 mg, 200 mg

Metra® (Discontinued) see page 814
Metreton® [US] see prednisolone (ophthalmic) on page 537
MetroCream® [US/Can] see metronidazole on next page
Metrodin® [US] see urofollitropin on page 668

MetroGel® Topical [US/Can] *see* metronidazole *on this page*

MetroGel®-Vaginal [US] *see* metronidazole *on this page*

Metro I.V.® Injection *(Discontinued)* *see page 814*

MetroLotion® [US] *see* metronidazole *on this page*

metronidazole (me troe NI da zole)

U.S./Canadian Brand Names Apo®-Metronidazole [Can]; Flagyl® [US/Can]; Flagyl ER® [US]; MetroCream® [US/Can]; MetroGel® Topical [US/Can]; MetroGel®-Vaginal [US]; MetroLotion® [US]; Nidagel™ [Can]; Noritate™ [US/Can]; Novo-Nidazol [Can]

Therapeutic Category Amebicide; Antibiotic, Topical; Antibiotic, Miscellaneous; Antiprotozoal

Use Treatment of susceptible anaerobic bacterial and protozoal infections in the following conditions: amebiasis (liver abscess, dysentery), giardiasis, symptomatic and asymptomatic trichomoniasis; skin and skin structure infections, CNS infections, intra-abdominal infections, and systemic anaerobic bacterial infections; topically for the treatment of acne rosacea; treatment of antibiotic-associated pseudomembranous colitis (AAPC) caused by *C. difficile*; bacterial vaginosis

Usual Dosage

Infants and Children:

Amebiasis: Oral: 35-50 mg/kg/day in divided doses every 8 hours

Other parasitic infections: Oral: 15-30 mg/kg/day in divided doses every 8 hours

Anaerobic infections: Oral, I.V.: 30 mg/kg/day in divided doses every 6 hours

Clostridium difficile (antibiotic-associated colitis): Oral: 20 mg/kg/day divided every 6 hours

Maximum dose: 2 g/day

Adults:

Amebiasis: Oral: 500-750 mg every 8 hours

Other parasitic infections: Oral: 250 mg every 8 hours or 2 g as a single dose

Anaerobic infections: Oral, I.V.: 30 mg/kg/day in divided doses every 6 hours; not to exceed 4 g/day

AAPC: Oral: 250-500 mg 3-4 times/day for 10-14 days

Topical: Apply a thin film twice daily to affected areas

Vaginal: One applicatorful in vagina each morning and evening or given once daily at bedtime

Dosage Forms

Capsule: 375 mg

Cream: 0.75% (45 g), 1% (30 g)

Gel: 0.75% [7.5 mg/mL] (30 g)

Gel, vaginal: 0.75% [5 g applicator delivering 37.5 mg] (70 g tube)

Injection, powder for reconstitution, as hydrochloride: 500 mg

Injection [ready-to-use]: 5 mg/mL (100 mL)

Lotion: 0.75%

Tablet: 250 mg, 500 mg

Tablet, extended release: 750 mg

Metubine® Iodide *(Discontinued)* *see page 814*

metyrapone (me TEER a pone)

U.S./Canadian Brand Names Metopirone® [US]

Therapeutic Category Diagnostic Agent

Use Diagnostic test for hypothalamic-pituitary ACTH function

Usual Dosage Oral:

Children: 15 mg/kg every 4 hours for 6 doses; minimum dose: 250 mg

Adults: 750 mg every 4 hours for 6 doses

Dosage Forms Capsule: 250 mg

metyrosine (me TYE roe seen)

Synonyms AMPT; OGMT

U.S./Canadian Brand Names Demser® [US/Can]

Therapeutic Category Tyrosine Hydroxylase Inhibitor

Use Short-term management of pheochromocytoma before surgery, long-term management when surgery is contraindicated or when malignant

Usual Dosage Children >12 years and Adults: Oral: Initial: 250 mg 4 times/day, increased by 250-500 mg/day up to 4 g/day; maintenance: 2-3 g/day in 4 divided doses; for preoperative preparation, administer optimum effective dosage for 5-7 days

Dosage Forms Capsule: 250 mg

Mevacor® [US/Can] *see* lovastatin *on page 393*

mevinolin *see* lovastatin *on page 393*

mexiletine (MEKS i le teen)

U.S./Canadian Brand Names Mexitil® [US/Can]; Novo-Mexiletine [Can]

Therapeutic Category Antiarrhythmic Agent, Class I-B

Use Management of serious ventricular arrhythmias; suppression of PVCs

Unlabeled use: Diabetic neuropathy

Usual Dosage Oral:

Children: Range: 1.4-5 mg/kg/dose (mean: 3.3 mg/kg/dose) administered every 8 hours; start with lower initial dose and increase according to effects and serum concentrations

Adults: Initial: 200 mg every 8 hours (may load with 400 mg if necessary); adjust dose every 2-3 days; usual dose: 200-300 mg every 8 hours; maximum dose: 1.2 g/day (some patients respond to every 12-hour dosing)

Dosage Forms Capsule: 150 mg, 200 mg, 250 mg

Mexitil® [US/Can] *see* mexiletine *on this page*

Miacalcin® [US/Can] *see* calcitonin *on page 103*

Micanol® [US/Can] *see* anthralin *on page 44*

Micardis® [US/Can] *see* telmisartan *on page 620*

Micardis® HCT [US] *see* telmisartan and hydrochlorothiazide *on page 620*

Micatin® [US/Can] *see* miconazole *on this page*

miconazole (mi KON a zole)

U.S./Canadian Brand Names Aloe Vesta® 2-n-1 Antifungal [US-OTC]; Baza® Antifungal [US-OTC]; Carrington Antifungal [US-OTC]; Fungoid® Tincture [US-OTC]; Lotrimin® AF Powder/Spray [US-OTC]; Micatin® [US/Can]; Micozole [Can]; Micro-Guard® [US-OTC]; Mitrazol® [US-OTC]; Monistat® 1 Combination Pack [US-OTC]; Monistat® 3 [US-OTC]; Monistat® 7 [US-OTC]; Monistat® [Can]; Monistat-Derm® [US]; Zeasorb®-AF [US-OTC]

Therapeutic Category Antifungal Agent

Use Treatment of vulvovaginal candidiasis and a variety of skin and mucous membrane fungal infections

Usual Dosage

Topical: Children and Adults: **Note:** Not for OTC use in children <2 years:

Tinea pedis and tinea corporis: Apply twice daily for 4 weeks

Tinea cruris: Apply twice daily for 2 weeks

Vaginal: Adults: Vulvovaginal candidiasis:

Cream, 2%: Insert 1 applicatorful at bedtime for 7 days

Cream, 4%: Insert 1 applicatorful at bedtime for 3 days

Suppository, 100 mg: Insert 1 suppository at bedtime for 7 days

Suppository, 200 mg: Insert 1 suppository at bedtime for 3 days

Suppository, 1200 mg: Insert 1 suppository at bedtime (a one-time dose)

(Continued)

miconazole *(Continued)*

Note: Many products are available as a combination pack, with a suppository for vaginal instillation and cream to relieve external symptoms.

Dosage Forms

Aerosol, powder, as nitrate (Lotrimin® AF): 2% (100 g)

Combination products:

Monistat® 1 Combination Pack: Miconazole nitrate vaginal insert 1200 mg (1) and miconazole external cream 2% (5 g) [Note: Do not confuse with 1-Day™ (formerly Monistat® 1) which contains tioconazole]

Monistat® 3 Combination Pack: Miconazole nitrate vaginal suppository 200 mg (3s) and miconazole nitrate external cream 2%

Monistat® 3 Cream Combination Pack: Miconazole nitrate vaginal cream 4% and miconazole nitrate external cream 2%

Monistat® 7 Combination Pack: Miconazole nitrate vaginal suppository 100 mg (7s) and miconazole nitrate external cream 2%

Cream, as nitrate:

Baza® Antifungal: 2% (4 g, 57 g, 142 g) [zinc oxide based formula]

Carrington Antifungal: 2% (150 g)

Micatin® [OTC], Monistat-Derm® [Rx]: 2% (15 g, 30 g)

Micro-Guard®: 2% (60 g)

Triple Care Antifungal: 2% (60 g, 98 g)

Cream, vaginal, as nitrate [available in prefilled applicators or single refillable applicator]:

Monistat® 3: 4% (15 g, 25 g)

Monistat® 7: 2% (45 g)

Liquid, spray, as nitrate (Micatin®): 2% (90 mL, 105 mL)

Lotion powder, as nitrate (Zeasorb®-AF): 2% (56 g) [contains alcohol 36%]

Ointment, as nitrate: (Aloe Vesta® 2-n-1 Antifungal): 2% (60 g, 150 g)

Powder, as nitrate:

Lotrimin® AF, Micatin®, Micro-Guard®: 2% (90 g)

Zeasorb®-AF: 2% (70 g)

Suppository, vaginal, as nitrate:

Monistat® 3: 200 mg (3s)

Monistat® 7: 100 mg (7s)

Tincture, topical, as nitrate (Fungoid®): 2% (30 mL, 473 mL)

Micozole [Can] *see* miconazole *on previous page*

microfibrillar collagen hemostat

(mye kro FI bri lar KOL la jen HEE moe stat)

Synonyms MCH

U.S./Canadian Brand Names Avitene® [US]; Helistat® [US]; Hemotene® [US]

Therapeutic Category Hemostatic Agent

Use Adjunct to hemostasis when control of bleeding by ligature is ineffective or impractical

Usual Dosage Apply dry directly to source of bleeding

Dosage Forms

Fibrous: 1 g

Web, nonwoven: 2.5 cm x 5 cm; 5 cm x 8 cm; 8 cm x 10 cm; 35 mm x 35 mm x 1 mm; 70 mm x 70 mm x 1 mm; 70 mm x 35 mm x 1 mm

Microgestin™ Fe [US] *see* ethinyl estradiol and norethindrone *on page 251*

Micro-Guard® [US-OTC] *see* miconazole *on previous page*

Micro-K® 10 Extencaps® [US] *see* potassium chloride *on page 530*

Micro-K® Extencaps [US/Can] *see* potassium chloride *on page 530*

Micro-K® LS *(Discontinued)* *see page 814*

Microlipid™ [US-OTC] *see* nutritional formula, enteral/oral *on page 472*

Micronase® **[US]** *see* glyburide *on page 301*

microNefrin® *(Discontinued) see page 814*

Micronor® **[US/Can]** *see* norethindrone *on page 465*

Microzide™ **[US]** *see* hydrochlorothiazide *on page 328*

Midamor® **[US/Can]** *see* amiloride *on page 31*

midazolam (MID aye zoe lam)

Synonyms midazolam hydrochloride

U.S./Canadian Brand Names Versed® [Can]

Therapeutic Category Benzodiazepine

Controlled Substance C-IV

Use Preoperative sedation; conscious sedation prior to diagnostic or radiographic procedures

Usual Dosage

Preoperative sedation: Children:

Oral:

<5 years: 0.5 mg/kg;

>5 years: 0.4-0.5 mg/kg; doses as high as 0.5-0.75 mg/kg have provided effective preanesthetic sedation

I.M.: 0.07-0.08 mg/kg 30 minutes to 1 hour before surgery; range: 0.05-0.1 mg/kg

I.V.: 0.035 mg/kg/dose, repeat over several minutes as required to achieve the desired sedative effect up to a total dose of 0.1-0.2 mg/kg or 5 mg total

Conscious sedation during mechanical ventilation:

Neonates: I.V. continuous infusion: 0.15-1 mcg/kg/minute

Children:

I.V.: 0.1-0.2 mg/kg; follow loading dose with a 1-2 mcg/kg/minute continuous infusion; titrate to the desired effect; range: 0.4-6 mcg/kg/minute

I.V. intermittent infusion: 0.05-0.2 mg/kg every 1-2 hours as needed

Conscious sedation for procedures:

Children:

Oral: 0.2-0.4 mg/kg; dose as high as 1 mg/kg have been used in younger (6 months to <6 years of age) and less cooperative patients; (maximum: 20 mg) 30-45 minutes before the procedure

Intranasal: 0.2-0.4 mg/kg (use undiluted 5 mg/mL injectable drug for intranasal administration)

I.V.: 0.05-0.1 mg/kg 3 minutes before procedure

Adolescents >12 years:

Sedation for procedure: I.V.: 0.5 mg every 3-4 minutes until effect achieved

Preoperative sedation: I.M.: 0.07-0.08 mg/kg 30-60 minutes before surgery; usual dose: 5 mg

Conscious sedation: I.V.: Initial: 0.5-2 mg; slowly titrate to effect by repeating doses every 2-3 minutes; usual total dose: 2.5-5 mg

Adults, healthy <60 years: Some patients respond to doses as low as 1 mg; no more than 2.5 mg should be administered over a period of 2 minutes. Additional doses of midazolam may be administered after a 2-minute waiting period and evaluation of sedation after each dose increment. A total dose >5 mg is generally not needed. If narcotics or other CNS depressants are administered concomitantly, the midazolam dose should be reduced by 30%.

Dosage Forms

Injection, as hydrochloride: 1 mg/mL (2 mL, 5 mL, 10 mL); 5 mg/mL (1 mL, 2 mL, 5 mL, 10 mL)

Syrup, as hydrochloride: 2 mg/mL (118 mL)

midazolam hydrochloride *see* midazolam *on this page*

midodrine (MI doe dreen)

U.S./Canadian Brand Names Amatine® [Can]; ProAmatine [US]

Therapeutic Category Alpha-Adrenergic Agonist

Use Treatment of symptomatic orthostatic hypotension in patients whose lives are considerably impaired despite standard clinical care.

Usual Dosage Adults: Oral: 10 mg 3 times/day (every 3-4 hours); dosing should take place during daytime hours when the patient needs to be upright, pursuing activities of daily living; a suggested dosing schedule is as follows:

Dose 1: Shortly before or upon rising in the morning

Dose 2: At midday

Dose 3: In the late afternoon (not later than 6 PM)

Dosage Forms Tablet, as hydrochloride: 2.5 mg, 5 mg

Midol® Maximum Strength Cramp Formula [US-OTC] *see* ibuprofen *on page 342*

Midrin® [US] *see* acetaminophen, isometheptene, and dichloralphenazone *on page 9*

Mifeprex® [US] *see* mifepristone *on this page*

mifepristone (mi fe PRIS tone)

Synonyms RU-486; RU-38486

U.S./Canadian Brand Names Mifeprex® [US]

Therapeutic Category Abortifacient; Antineoplastic Agent, Hormone Antagonist; Anti-progestin

Use Medical termination of intrauterine pregnancy, through day 49 of pregnancy. Patients may need treatment with misoprostol and possibly surgery to complete therapy

Unlabeled uses: Treatment of unresectable meningioma; has been studied in the treatment of breast cancer, ovarian cancer, and adrenal cortical carcinoma

Usual Dosage Oral:

Adults: Termination of pregnancy: Treatment consists of three office visits by the patient; the patient must read medication guide and sign patient agreement prior to treatment:

Day 1: 600 mg (three 200 mg tablets) taken as a single dose under physician supervision

Day 3: Patient must return to the healthcare provider 2 days following administration of mifepristone; if termination of pregnancy cannot be confirmed using ultrasound or clinical examination: 400 mcg (two 200 mcg tablets) of misoprostol; patient may need treatment for cramps or gastrointestinal symptoms at this time

Day 14: Patient must return to the healthcare provider ~14 days after administration of mifepristone; confirm complete termination of pregnancy by ultrasound or clinical exam. Surgical termination is recommended to manage treatment failures.

Dosage Forms Tablet: 200 mg

Miflex® Tablet *(Discontinued)* *see page 814*

miglitol (MIG li tol)

U.S./Canadian Brand Names Glyset™ [US/Can]

Therapeutic Category Antidiabetic Agent, Oral

Use As an adjunct to diet to lower blood glucose in patients with noninsulin-dependent diabetes mellitus (NIDDM)

Usual Dosage Adults: Oral: 25 mg 3 times/day with the first bite of food at each meal; dose may be increased to 50 mg 3 times/day after 4-8 weeks; maximum recommended dose: 100 mg 3 times/day

Dosage Forms Tablet: 25 mg, 50 mg, 100 mg

Migranal® [US/Can] *see* dihydroergotamine *on page 198*

Migrapap® *(Discontinued)* *see page 814*

Migratine® **[US]** *see* acetaminophen, isometheptene, and dichloralphenazone *on page 9*

MIH *see* procarbazine *on page 542*

Miles® Nervine [US-OTC] *see* diphenhydramine *on page 202*

Milkinol® *(Discontinued)* *see page 814*

milk of magnesia *see* magnesium hydroxide *on page 397*

Milontin® *(Discontinued)* *see page 814*

Milophene® *(Discontinued)* *see page 814*

Milprem® *(Discontinued)* *see page 814*

milrinone (MIL ri none)
    U.S./Canadian Brand Names Primacor® [US/Can]
    Therapeutic Category Cardiovascular Agent, Other
    Use Short-term I.V. therapy of congestive heart failure
    Usual Dosage Adults: I.V.: Loading dose: 50 mcg/kg administered over 10 minutes, then 0.375-0.75 mcg/kg/min as a continuous infusion for a total daily dose of 0.59-1.13 mg/kg
    Dosage Forms
        Infusion, as lactate [in D_5W]: 200 mcg/mL (100 mL, 200 mL)
        Injection, as lactate: 1 mg/mL (5 mL, 10 mL, 20 mL, 50 mL)

Miltown® **[US]** *see* meprobamate *on page 409*

Minestrin™ 1/20 [Can] *see* ethinyl estradiol and norethindrone *on page 251*

Minidyne® **[US-OTC]** *see* povidone-iodine *on page 533*

Mini-Gamulin® Rh *(Discontinued)* *see page 814*

Minipress® **[US/Can]** *see* prazosin *on page 536*

Minitran™ [US/Can] *see* nitroglycerin *on page 462*

Minizide® **[US]** *see* prazosin and polythiazide *on page 536*

Minocin® **[US/Can]** *see* minocycline *on this page*

Minocin® Tablet *(Discontinued)* *see page 814*

minocycline (mi noe SYE kleen)
    U.S./Canadian Brand Names Alti-Minocycline [Can]; Apo®-Minocycline [Can]; Dynacin® [US]; Gen-Minocycline [Can]; Minocin® [US/Can]; Novo-Minocycline [Can]; Rhoxal-Minocycline [Can]
    Therapeutic Category Tetracycline Derivative
    Use Treatment of susceptible bacterial infections of both gram-negative and gram-positive organisms; acne
    Usual Dosage
        Children 8-12 years: 4 mg/kg stat, then 4 mg/kg/day (maximum: 200 mg/day) in divided doses every 12 hours
        Adults:
        Infection: Oral, I.V.: 200 mg stat, 100 mg every 12 hours
        Acne: Oral: 50 mg 1-3 times/day
    Dosage Forms
        Capsule, as hydrochloride: 50 mg, 75 mg, 100 mg
        Dynacin®: 50 mg, 75 mg, 100 mg
        Capsule, pellet-filled, as hydrochloride (Minocin®): 50 mg, 100 mg
        Injection, powder for reconstitution, as hydrochloride (Minocin®): 100 mg

Min-Ovral® **[Can]** *see* ethinyl estradiol and levonorgestrel *on page 248*

Minox [Can] *see* minoxidil *on next page*

minoxidil (mi NOKS i dil)
U.S./Canadian Brand Names Apo®-Gain [Can]; Loniten® [US]; Minox [Can]; Rogaine® [Can]; Rogaine® Extra Strength for Men [US-OTC]; Rogaine® for Men [US-OTC]; Rogaine® for Women [US-OTC]

Therapeutic Category Topical Skin Product; Vasodilator

Use Management of severe hypertension; topically for management of alopecia or male pattern alopecia

Usual Dosage
Children <12 years: Hypertension: Oral: Initial: 0.1-0.2 mg/kg once daily; maximum: 5 mg/day; increase gradually every 3 days; usual dosage: 0.25-1 mg/kg/day in 1-2 divided doses; maximum: 50 mg/day

Adults:
Hypertension: Oral: Initial: 5 mg once daily, increase gradually every 3 days; usual dose: 10-40 mg/day in 1-2 divided doses; maximum: 100 mg/day
Alopecia: Topical: Apply twice daily

Dosage Forms
Solution, topical: 2% = 20 mg/metered dose (60 mL); 5% = 50 mg/metered dose (60 mL)
Tablet: 2.5 mg, 10 mg

Mintezol® [US] *see* thiabendazole *on page 632*

Minute-Gel® (Discontinued) *see page 814*

Miocarpine® [Can] *see* pilocarpine *on page 514*

Miochol® (Discontinued) *see page 814*

Miochol-E® [US/Can] *see* acetylcholine *on page 11*

Miostat® Intraocular [US/Can] *see* carbachol *on page 112*

Miradon® [US] *see* anisindione *on page 44*

MiraLax™ [US] *see* polyethylene glycol-electrolyte solution *on page 525*

Mirapex® [US/Can] *see* pramipexole *on page 534*

Miraphen PSE [US] *see* guaifenesin and pseudoephedrine *on page 310*

Mircette® [US] *see* ethinyl estradiol and desogestrel *on page 244*

Mirena® [US] *see* levonorgestrel *on page 381*

mirtazapine (mir TAZ a peen)
U.S./Canadian Brand Names Remeron® SolTab™ [US]; Remeron® [US]

Therapeutic Category Antidepressant, Alpha-2 Antagonist

Use Treatment of depression, works through noradrenergic and serotonergic pharmacologic action

Usual Dosage Adults: Oral: Initial: 15 mg/day, then 15-45 mg/day

Dosage Forms
Tablet: 15 mg, 30 mg, 45 mg
Tablet, orally-disintegrating:
15 mg [phenylalanine 2.6 mg/tablet] [orange flavor]
30 mg [phenylalanine 5.2 mg/tablet] [orange flavor]
45 mg [phenylalanine 7.8 mg/tablet] [orange flavor]

misoprostol (mye soe PROST ole)
U.S./Canadian Brand Names Cytotec® [US/Can]

Therapeutic Category Prostaglandin

Use Prevention of NSAID-induced gastric ulcers

Usual Dosage Oral: 200 mcg 4 times/day with food

Dosage Forms Tablet: 100 mcg, 200 mcg

misoprostol and diclofenac *see* diclofenac and misoprostol *on page 194*

Mithracin® **[US/Can]** *see* plicamycin *on page 519*

mithramycin *see* plicamycin *on page 519*

Mito-Carn® **[US]** *see* levocarnitine *on page 379*

mitomycin (mye toe MYE sin)

Synonyms mitomycin-c; MTC

U.S./Canadian Brand Names Mutamycin® [US/Can]

Therapeutic Category Antineoplastic Agent

Use Therapy of disseminated adenocarcinoma of stomach, colon, or pancreas in combination with other approved chemotherapeutic agents; bladder cancer, breast cancer

Usual Dosage Children and Adults (refer to individual protocols): I.V.: 10-20 mg/m²/dose every 6-8 weeks, or 2 mg/m²/day for 5 days, stop for 2 days then repeat; subsequent doses should be adjusted to platelet and leukocyte response

Dosage Forms Powder for injection: 5 mg, 20 mg, 40 mg

mitomycin-c *see* mitomycin *on this page*

mitotane (MYE toe tane)

Synonyms o,p'-DDD

U.S./Canadian Brand Names Lysodren® [US/Can]

Therapeutic Category Antineoplastic Agent

Use Treatment of inoperable adrenal cortical carcinoma

Usual Dosage Adults: Oral: 8-10 g/day in 3-4 divided doses; dose is changed based on side effects with aim of administering as high a dose as tolerated

Dosage Forms Tablet, scored: 500 mg

mitoxantrone (mye toe ZAN trone)

Synonyms DHAD

U.S./Canadian Brand Names Novantrone® [US/Can]

Therapeutic Category Antineoplastic Agent

Use FDA approved for remission-induction therapy of acute nonlymphocytic leukemia (ANLL); mitoxantrone is also active against other various leukemias, lymphoma, and breast cancer, and moderately active against pediatric sarcoma

Usual Dosage I.V. (refer to individual protocols):

Leukemias:

Children ≤2 years: 0.4 mg/kg/day once daily for 3-5 days

Children >2 years and Adults: 8-12 mg/m²/day once daily for 5 days or 12 mg/m²/day once daily for 3 days

Solid tumors:

Children: 18-20 mg/m² every 3-4 weeks

Adults: 12-14 mg/m² every 3-4 weeks

Dosage Forms Injection, as base: 2 mg/mL (10 mL, 12.5 mL, 15 mL)

Mitran® **Oral *(Discontinued)*** *see page 814*

Mitrazol® **[US-OTC]** *see* miconazole *on page 427*

Mitrolan® **Chewable Tablet [US-OTC]** *see* calcium polycarbophil *on page 108*

Mivacron® **[US/Can]** *see* mivacurium *on this page*

mivacurium (mye va KYOO ree um)

U.S./Canadian Brand Names Mivacron® [US/Can]

Therapeutic Category Skeletal Muscle Relaxant

Use Short-acting nondepolarizing neuromuscular blocking agent; an adjunct to general anesthesia; facilitates endotracheal intubation; provides skeletal muscle relaxation during surgery or mechanical ventilation

Usual Dosage I.V.:

Children 2-12 years: 0.2 mg/kg over 5-15 seconds; continuous infusion: 14 mcg/kg

(Continued)

mivacurium *(Continued)*

Adults: Initial: 0.15 mg/kg administered over 5-15 seconds
Dosage Forms
Infusion, as chloride [in D₅W]: 0.5 mg/mL (50 mL)
Injection, as chloride: 2 mg/mL (5 mL, 10 mL)

MK594 *see* losartan *on page 392*

MK-0826 *see* ertapenem *on page 234*

MMR *see* measles, mumps, and rubella vaccines, combined *on page 402*

M-M-R® II [US/Can] *see* measles, mumps, and rubella vaccines, combined *on page 402*

Moban® [US/Can] *see* molindone *on next page*

MOBIC® [US/Can] *see* meloxicam *on page 406*

Mobicox® [Can] *see* meloxicam *on page 406*

Mobidin® [US] *see* magnesium salicylate *on page 398*

moclobemide *(Canada only)* (moe KLOE be mide)

Synonyms Ro 11-1163
U.S./Canadian Brand Names Alti-Moclobemide [Can]; Apo®-Moclobemide [Can]; Manerix® [Can]; Novo-Moclobemide [Can]; Nu-Moclobemide [Can]
Therapeutic Category Antidepressant, Monoamine Oxidase Inhibitor
Use Depression; smoking cessation
Usual Dosage Oral:
Depression: Initial: 100 mg 3 times/day immediately following a meal; maximum dose/day: 600 mg; reduce dosage by 30% to 50% in patients with hepatic disease
Smoking cessation: 400 mg/day for 2 months, then, 200 mg/day for 1 month
Dosage Forms Tablet: 150 mg, 300 mg

Moctanin® [US/Can] *see* monoctanoin *on page 436*

modafinil (moe DAF i nil)

U.S./Canadian Brand Names Alertec® [Can]; Provigil® [US/Can]
Therapeutic Category Central Nervous System Stimulant, Nonamphetamine
Controlled Substance C-IV
Use Indicated to improve wakefulness in patients with excessive daytime sleepiness associated with narcolepsy
Usual Dosage Adults: Oral: Initial: 200 mg as a single daily dose
Dosage Forms Tablet: 100 mg, 200 mg

Modane® Bulk [US-OTC] *see* psyllium *on page 554*

Modane® Soft *(Discontinued)* *see page 814*

Modane Tablets® [US-OTC] *see* bisacodyl *on page 87*

Modecate® [Can] *see* fluphenazine *on page 281*

Modicon® [US] *see* ethinyl estradiol and norethindrone *on page 251*

modified Dakin's solution *see* sodium hypochlorite solution *on page 597*

Moditen® Enanthate [Can] *see* fluphenazine *on page 281*

Moditen® HCl [Can] *see* fluphenazine *on page 281*

Moducal® [US-OTC] *see* glucose polymers *on page 301*

Modulon® [Can] *see* trimebutine *(Canada only)* *on page 656*

Moduret® [Can] *see* amiloride and hydrochlorothiazide *on page 32*

Moduretic® [US/Can] *see* amiloride and hydrochlorothiazide *on page 32*

moexipril (mo EKS i pril)

U.S./Canadian Brand Names Univasc® [US]

Therapeutic Category Angiotensin-Converting Enzyme (ACE) Inhibitor

Use Treatment of hypertension, alone or in combination with thiazide diuretics

Usual Dosage Oral:

Patients not receiving diuretics: Initial: 7.5 mg 1 hour prior to meals once daily; if antihypertensive effect diminishes toward end of dosing interval, increase or divide dose; maintenance dose of 7.5-30 mg/day in 1 or 2 divided doses

Patients receiving diuretics: Discontinue diuretic 2-3 days before starting moexipril to avoid symptomatic hypotension; if blood pressure is not controlled, resume diuretic therapy; if diuretic cannot be held, initiate moexipril at 3.75 mg/day

Dosage Forms Tablet, as hydrochloride: 7.5 mg, 15 mg

moexipril and hydrochlorothiazide

(mo EKS i pril & hye droe klor oh THYE a zide)

U.S./Canadian Brand Names Uniretic™ [US/Can]

Therapeutic Category Angiotensin-Converting Enzyme (ACE) Inhibitor; Diuretic, Thiazide

Use Treatment of hypertension

Usual Dosage Adults: Oral: 7.5-30 mg of moexipril, taken either in a single or divided dose one hour before meals

Dosage Forms Tablet:

Moexipril hydrochloride 7.5 mg and hydrochlorothiazide 12.5 mg

Moexipril hydrochloride 15 mg and hydrochlorothiazide 12.5 mg

Moexipril hydrochloride 15 mg and hydrochlorothiazide 25 mg

Moi-Stir® [US-OTC] *see* saliva substitute *on page 582*

Moisture® Eyes PM [US-OTC] *see* artificial tears *on page 56*

Moisture® Eyes [US-OTC] *see* artificial tears *on page 56*

Moisturel® Lotion *(Discontinued)* *see page 814*

molindone (moe LIN done)

U.S./Canadian Brand Names Moban® [US/Can]

Therapeutic Category Antipsychotic Agent, Dihydroindoline

Use Management of psychotic disorder

Usual Dosage Oral: 50-75 mg/day; up to 225 mg/day

Dosage Forms

Solution, oral concentrate, as hydrochloride: 20 mg/mL (120 mL)

Tablet, as hydrochloride: 5 mg, 10 mg, 25 mg, 50 mg, 100 mg

Mollifene® Ear Wax Removing Formula [US-OTC] *see* carbamide peroxide *on page 113*

molybdenum injection *see* trace metals *on page 646*

Molypen® [US] *see* trace metals *on page 646*

MOM *see* magnesium hydroxide *on page 397*

Momentum® [US-OTC] *see* magnesium salicylate *on page 398*

mometasone furoate (moe MET a sone FYOOR oh ate)

U.S./Canadian Brand Names Elocon® [US/Can]; Nasonex® [US/Can]

Therapeutic Category Corticosteroid, Intranasal; Corticosteroid, Topical

Use Topical forms for the relief of the inflammatory and pruritic manifestations of corticosteroid-responsive dermatoses (medium potency topical corticosteroid); nasal spray used for the prophylaxis and treatment of nasal symptoms of seasonal allergic rhinitis and the treatment of nasal symptoms of perennial allergic rhinitis in adults and children 12 years of age and older

(Continued)

mometasone furoate *(Continued)*

Usual Dosage Adults:
Nasally: 200 mcg (two sprays per nostril) once daily
Topical: Apply sparingly to area once daily, do not use occlusive dressings
Dosage Forms
Cream, topical (Elocon®): 0.1% (15 g, 45 g)
Lotion, topical (Elocon®): 0.1% (30 mL, 60 mL)
Ointment, topical (Elocon®): 0.1% (15 g, 45 g)
Suspension, intranasal spray (Nasonex®): 50 mcg/spray (17 g) [delivers 120 sprays; contains benzalkonium chloride]

mom/mineral oil emulsion *see* magnesium hydroxide and mineral oil emulsion *on page 398*

monacolin k *see* lovastatin *on page 393*

Monafed® *(Discontinued) see page 814*

Monafed® DM *(Discontinued) see page 814*

Monarc® M [US] *see* antihemophilic factor (human) *on page 45*

***Monilia* skin test** *see* Candida albicans (Monilia) *on page 110*

Monistat® [Can] *see* miconazole *on page 427*

Monistat® 1 Combination Pack [US-OTC] *see* miconazole *on page 427*

Monistat® 3 [US-OTC] *see* miconazole *on page 427*

Monistat® 7 [US-OTC] *see* miconazole *on page 427*

Monistat-Derm® [US] *see* miconazole *on page 427*

Monistat i.v.™ Injection *(Discontinued) see page 814*

Monitan® [Can] *see* acebutolol *on page 3*

monobenzone *(mon oh BEN zone)*

U.S./Canadian Brand Names Benoquin® [US]
Therapeutic Category Topical Skin Product
Use Final depigmentation in extensive vitiligo
Usual Dosage Adults: Topical: Apply 2-3 times/day
Dosage Forms Cream, topical: 20% (35.4 g)

Monocete® Topical Liquid *(Discontinued) see page 814*

Monocid® *(Discontinued) see page 814*

Monoclate-P® [US] *see* antihemophilic factor (human) *on page 45*

monoclonal antibody *see* muromonab-CD3 *on page 440*

monoclonal antibody purified *see* factor IX (purified/human) *on page 261*

Monocor® [Can] *see* bisoprolol *on page 88*

monoctanoin *(mon OK ta noyn)*

Synonyms monooctanoin
U.S./Canadian Brand Names Moctanin® [US/Can]
Therapeutic Category Gallstone Dissolution Agent
Use Solubilize cholesterol gallstones that are retained in the biliary tract after cholecystectomy
Usual Dosage Administer via T-tube into common bile duct at rate of 3-5 mL/hour at pressure of 10 mL water for 7-21 days
Dosage Forms Solution: 120 mL

Monodox® [US] *see* doxycycline *on page 215*

Mono-Gesic® [US] *see* salsalate *on page 583*

Monoket® **[US]** *see* isosorbide mononitrate *on page 362*

Mononine® **[US]** *see* factor IX (purified/human) *on page 261*

monooctanoin *see* monoctanoin *on previous page*

Monopril® **[US/Can]** *see* fosinopril *on page 288*

Monopril-HCT® **[US/Can]** *see* fosinopril and hydrochlorothiazide *on page 289*

montelukast (mon te LOO kast)
U.S./Canadian Brand Names Singulair® [US/Can]
Therapeutic Category Leukotriene Receptor Antagonist
Use Prophylaxis and chronic treatment of asthma in adults and children ≥6 years
Usual Dosage Oral:
   Children 6-14 years: 5 mg once daily
   Children >14 years and Adults: 10 mg once daily
Dosage Forms
   Granules, as sodium: 4 mg/packet
   Tablet, as sodium: 10 mg
   Tablet, chewable, as sodium: 4 mg [cherry flavor; contains phenylalanine 0.674 mg]; 5 mg [cherry flavor; contains phenylalanine 0.842 mg]

Monurol™ **[US/Can]** *see* fosfomycin *on page 288*

8-MOP® **[US/Can]** *see* methoxsalen *on page 418*

more attenuated enders strain *see* measles virus vaccine (live) *on page 402*

MoreDophilus® **[US-OTC]** *see* Lactobacillus *on page 372*

moricizine (mor EYE siz een)
U.S./Canadian Brand Names Ethmozine® [US/Can]
Therapeutic Category Antiarrhythmic Agent, Class I
Use Treatment of ventricular tachycardia and life-threatening ventricular arrhythmias; a Class I antiarrhythmic agent
Usual Dosage Adults: Oral: 200-300 mg every 8 hours, adjust dosage at 150 mg/day at 3-day intervals
Dosage Forms Tablet, as hydrochloride: 200 mg, 250 mg, 300 mg

Morphine HP® **[Can]** *see* morphine sulfate *on this page*

morphine sulfate (MOR feen SUL fate)
Synonyms MS
U.S./Canadian Brand Names Astramorph™ PF [US]; Avinza™ [US]; Duramorph® [US]; Infumorph® [US]; Kadian® [US/Can]; M-Eslon® [Can]; Morphine HP® [Can]; M.O.S.-Sulfate® [Can]; MS Contin® [US/Can]; MSIR® [US/Can]; Oramorph SR® [US/Can]; RMS® [US]; Roxanol® [US]; Roxanol 100® [US]; Roxanol®-T [US]; Statex® [Can]
Therapeutic Category Analgesic, Narcotic
Controlled Substance C-II
Use Relief of moderate to severe acute and chronic pain; pain of myocardial infarction; relieves dyspnea of acute left ventricular failure and pulmonary edema; preanesthetic medication
Usual Dosage Doses should be titrated to appropriate effect; when changing routes of administration in chronically treated patients, please note that oral doses are approximately $\frac{1}{6}$ as effective as parenteral dose

Infants and Children:
   Oral: Tablet and solution (prompt-release): 0.2-0.5 mg/kg/dose every 4-6 hours as needed; tablet (controlled-release): 0.3-0.6 mg/kg/dose every 12 hours
   I.M., I.V., S.C.: 0.1-0.2 mg/kg/dose every 2-4 hours as needed; usual maximum: 15 mg/dose; may initiate at 0.05 mg/kg/dose
(Continued)

morphine sulfate *(Continued)*

I.V., S.C. continuous infusion: Sickle cell or cancer pain: 0.025-2 mg/kg/hour; postoperative pain: 0.01-0.04 mg/kg/hour

Sedation/analgesia for procedures: I.V.: 0.05-0.1 mg/kg 5 minutes before the procedure

Adolescents >12 years: Sedation/analgesia for procedures: I.V.: 3-4 mg and repeat in 5 minutes if necessary

Adults:

Oral: Prompt-release: 10-30 mg every 4 hours as needed; controlled release: 15-30 mg every 8-12 hours

I.M., I.V., S.C.: 2.5-20 mg/dose every 2-6 hours as needed; usual: 10 mg/dose every 4 hours as needed

I.V., S.C. continuous infusion: 0.8-10 mg/hour; may increase depending on pain relief/adverse effects; usual range up to 80 mg/hour

Epidural: Initial: 5 mg in lumbar region; if inadequate pain relief within 1 hour, administer 1-2 mg, maximum dose: 10 mg/24 hours

Intrathecal ($^1/_{10}$ of epidural dose): 0.2-1 mg/dose; repeat doses **not** recommended

Dosage Forms

Capsule (MSIR®): 15 mg, 30 mg

Capsule, extended release (Avinza™): 30 mg, 60 mg, 90 mg, 120 mg

Capsule, sustained release (Kadian®): 20 mg, 30 mg, 50 mg, 60 mg, 100 mg

Infusion [premixed in dextrose]: 0.2 mg/mL (250 mL, 500 mL); 1 mg/mL (100 mL, 250 mL, 500 mL)

Injection, solution: 0.5 mg/mL (10 mL); 1 mg/mL (10 mL, 30 mL, 50 mL); 2 mg/mL (1 mL); 4 mg/mL (1 mL); 5 mg/mL (1 mL, 30 mL, 50 mL); 8 mg/mL (1 mL); 10 mg/mL (1 mL, 2 mL, 10 mL); 15 mg/mL (1 mL, 20 mL); 25 mg/mL (4 mL, 10 mL, 20 mL, 40 mL, 50 mL); 50 mg/mL (10 mL, 20 mL, 40 mL, 50 mL)

Astramorph™ PF [preservative free]: 0.5 mg/mL (2 mL, 10 mL); 1 mg/mL (2 mL, 10 mL)

Infumorph® [preservative free]: 10 mg/mL (20 mL); 25 mg/mL (20 mL)

Duramorph® [preservative free]: 0.5 mg/mL (10 mL); 1 mg/mL (10 mL)

Solution, oral: 10 mg/5 mL (5 mL, 100 mL, 500 mL); 20 mg/5 mL (30 mL, 100 mL, 120 mL, 240 mL); 20 mg/5 mL (5 mL, 100 mL, 120 mL, 500 mL)

MSIR®: 10 mg/5 mL (120 mL); 20 mg/mL (30 mL, 120 mL) [contains sodium benzoate]

Roxanol®: 20 mg/mL (30 mL, 120 mL)

Roxanol® T: 20 mg/mL (30 mL, 120 mL) [flavored; tinted]

Roxanol 100®: 100 mg/5 mL (240 mL) [with calibrated spoon]

Suppository, rectal (RMS®): 5 mg, 10 mg, 20 mg, 30 mg

Tablet: 15 mg, 30 mg

MSIR®: 15 mg, 30 mg

Tablet, controlled release: MS Contin®: 15 mg, 30 mg, 60 mg, 100 mg, 200 mg

Tablet, extended release: 15 mg, 30 mg, 60 mg, 100 mg, 200 mg

Tablet, sustained release (Oramorph SR®): 15 mg, 30 mg, 60 mg, 100 mg

morrhuate sodium *(MOR yoo ate SOW dee um)*

U.S./Canadian Brand Names Scleromate™ [US]

Therapeutic Category Sclerosing Agent

Use Treatment of small, uncomplicated varicose veins of the lower extremities

Usual Dosage I.V.:

Children 1-18 years: Esophageal hemorrhage: 2, 3, or 4 mL of 5% solution repeated every 3-4 days until bleeding is controlled, then every 6 weeks until varices obliterated

Adults: 50-250 mg, repeat at 5- to 7-day intervals (50-100 mg for small veins, 150-250 mg for large veins)

Dosage Forms Injection: 50 mg/mL (30 mL)

Mosco® [US-OTC] *see* salicylic acid *on page 581*

M.O.S.-Sulfate® [Can] *see* morphine sulfate *on previous page*

Motilium® [Can] *see* domperidone *(Canada only) on page 211*

Motofen® **[US]** *see* difenoxin and atropine *on page 196*

Motrin® **[US/Can]** *see* ibuprofen *on page 342*

Motrin® Children's [US/Can] *see* ibuprofen *on page 342*

Motrin® IB [US/Can] *see* ibuprofen *on page 342*

Motrin® IB Sinus *(Discontinued) see page 814*

Motrin® Infants' [US-OTC] *see* ibuprofen *on page 342*

Motrin® Junior Strength [US-OTC] *see* ibuprofen *on page 342*

Motrin® Migraine Pain [US-OTC] *see* ibuprofen *on page 342*

MouthKote® [US-OTC] *see* saliva substitute *on page 582*

Moxam® Injection *(Discontinued) see page 814*

moxifloxacin (mox i FLOX a sin)
  U.S./Canadian Brand Names ABC Pack™ (Avelox®) [US]; Avelox® [US/Can]
  Therapeutic Category Antibiotic, Quinolone
  Use Treatment of mild to moderate community-acquired pneumonia, acute bacterial exacerbation of chronic bronchitis, acute bacterial sinusitis, uncomplicated skin infections
  Usual Dosage Adults: Oral:
    Community-acquired pneumonia or acute bacterial sinusitis: 400 mg every 24 hours for 10 days
    Chronic bronchitis, acute bacterial exacerbation: 400 mg every 24 hours for 5 days
    Uncomplicated skin infections: 400 mg every 24 hours for 7 days
  Dosage Forms
    Solution for infusion, as hydrochloride [premixed in sodium chloride 0.8%]: 400 mg/250 mL
    Tablet, as hydrochloride: 400 mg
    Tablet, as hydrochloride [dose pack] (Avelox® ABC Pack™): 400 mg (5/card)

Moxilin® [US] *see* amoxicillin *on page 37*

4-MP *see* fomepizole *on page 287*

6-MP *see* mercaptopurine *on page 410*

M-Prednisol® Injection *(Discontinued) see page 814*

M-R-VAX® II [US] *see* measles and rubella vaccines, combined *on page 402*

MS *see* morphine sulfate *on page 437*

MS Contin® [US/Can] *see* morphine sulfate *on page 437*

MSIR® [US/Can] *see* morphine sulfate *on page 437*

MSTA® Mumps [US/Can] *see* mumps skin test antigen *on next page*

MTC *see* mitomycin *on page 433*

M.T.E.-4® [US] *see* trace metals *on page 646*

M.T.E.-5® [US] *see* trace metals *on page 646*

M.T.E.-6® [US] *see* trace metals *on page 646*

MTX *see* methotrexate *on page 417*

Mucinex™ [US-OTC] *see* guaifenesin *on page 307*

Mucomyst® [US/Can] *see* acetylcysteine *on page 11*

MulTE-PAK-4® [US] *see* trace metals *on page 646*

MulTE-PAK-5® [US] *see* trace metals *on page 646*

Multitest CMI® [US] *see* skin test antigens, multiple *on page 592*

multivitamins/fluoride *see* vitamin (multiple/pediatric) *on page 683*

Multi Vit® Drops [US-OTC] *see* vitamin (multiple/pediatric) *on page 683*

mumps skin test antigen (mumpz skin test AN ti jen)
U.S./Canadian Brand Names MSTA® Mumps [US/Can]
Therapeutic Category Diagnostic Agent
Use Assess the status of cell-mediated immunity
Usual Dosage Children and Adults: 0.1 mL intradermally into flexor surface of the forearm; examine reaction site in 24-48 hours; a positive reaction is ≥1.5 mm diameter induration
Dosage Forms Injection: 1 mL (10 tests)

Mumpsvax® [US/Can] *see* mumps virus vaccine, live, attenuated *on this page*

mumps virus vaccine, live, attenuated
(mumpz VYE rus vak SEEN, live, a ten YOO ate ed)
U.S./Canadian Brand Names Mumpsvax® [US/Can]
Therapeutic Category Vaccine, Live Virus
Use Immunization against mumps in children ≥12 months and adults
Usual Dosage S.C.: 1 vial (5000 units) in outer aspect of the upper arm
Dosage Forms Injection, powder for reconstitution [single dose; with diluent]: 20,000 $TCID_{50}$

mupirocin (myoo PEER oh sin)
Synonyms pseudomonic acid A
U.S./Canadian Brand Names Bactroban® Nasal [US]; Bactroban® [US/Can]
Therapeutic Category Antibiotic, Topical
Use Topical treatment of impetigo caused by *Staphylococcus aureus* and *Streptococcus pyogenes*; also effective for the topical treatment of folliculitis, furunculosis, minor wounds, burns, and ulcers caused by susceptible organisms; used as a prophylactic agent applied to intravenous catheter exit sites; used for eradication of *S. aureus* from nasal and perineal carriage sites
Usual Dosage
  Children and Adults: Topical: Apply small amount to affected area 2-5 times/day for 5-14 days
  Children ≥12 years and Adults: Intranasal: ~1/2 of a single-use tube (0.5 g) to each nostril twice daily for 5 days
Dosage Forms
  Cream, as calcium: 2% (15 g, 30 g)
  Ointment: 2% (22 g)
  Ointment, as calcium: 2% (15 g, 30 g)
  Ointment, intranasal, as calcium [single-use tube]: 2% (1 g)

Murine® Ear Drops [US-OTC] *see* carbamide peroxide *on page 113*

Murine® Plus Ophthalmic [US-OTC] *see* tetrahydrozoline *on page 629*

Murine® Tears [US-OTC] *see* artificial tears *on page 56*

Muro 128® [US-OTC] *see* sodium chloride *on page 595*

Murocel® [US-OTC] *see* artificial tears *on page 56*

Murocoll-2® [US] *see* phenylephrine and scopolamine *on page 511*

muromonab-CD3 (myoo roe MOE nab-see dee three)
Synonyms monoclonal antibody; OKT3
U.S./Canadian Brand Names Orthoclone OKT® 3 [US/Can]
Therapeutic Category Immunosuppressant Agent
Use Treatment of acute allograft rejection in renal transplant patients; effective in reversing acute hepatic, cardiac, and bone marrow transplant rejection episodes resistant to conventional treatment
Usual Dosage I.V. (refer to individual protocols):
  Children <30 kg: 2.5 mg/day once daily for 10-14 days

Adults: 5 mg/day once daily for 10-14 days

Children and Adults: Methylprednisolone sodium succinate 1 mg/kg I.V. administered prior to first muromonab-CD3 administration and I.V. hydrocortisone sodium succinate 50-100 mg administered 30 minutes after administration are strongly recommended to decrease the incidence of reactions to the first dose; patient temperature should not exceed 37.8°C (100°F) at time of administration

Dosage Forms Injection: 1 mg/mL (5 mL)

Muroptic-5® *(Discontinued)* see page 814

Muse® Pellet [US] see alprostadil on page 25

Mus-Lax® *(Discontinued)* see page 814

Mustargen® [US/Can] see mechlorethamine on page 403

mustine see mechlorethamine on page 403

Mutacol Berna® [Can] see cholera vaccine on page 143

Mutamycin® [US/Can] see mitomycin on page 433

M.V.C.® 9 + 3 [US] see vitamin (multiple/injectable) on page 682

M.V.I.®-12 [US] see vitamin (multiple/injectable) on page 682

M.V.I.® Concentrate [US] see vitamin (multiple/injectable) on page 682

M.V.I.® Pediatric [US] see vitamin (multiple/injectable) on page 682

Myambutol® [US] see ethambutol on page 243

Mycelex® [US] see clotrimazole on page 156

Mycelex®-3 [US-OTC] see butoconazole on page 101

Mycelex®-7 [US-OTC] see clotrimazole on page 156

Mycelex®-G *(Discontinued)* see page 814

Mycelex® Twin Pack [US-OTC] see clotrimazole on page 156

Mycifradin® Sulfate *(Discontinued)* see page 814

Myciguent [US-OTC] see neomycin on page 451

Mycinettes® [US-OTC] see benzocaine on page 77

Mycitracin® [US-OTC] see bacitracin, neomycin, and polymyxin B on page 69

Mycobutin® [US/Can] see rifabutin on page 571

Mycolog®-II [US] see nystatin and triamcinolone on page 473

Myconel® Topical *(Discontinued)* see page 814

mycophenolate (mye koe FEN oh late)

U.S./Canadian Brand Names CellCept® [US/Can]

Therapeutic Category Immunosuppressant Agent

Use Prophylaxis of organ rejection concomitantly with cyclosporine and corticosteroids in patients receiving allogenic renal, cardiac, or hepatic transplants. Intravenous formulation is an alternative dosage form to oral capsules, suspension, and tablets.

Unlabeled uses: Treatment of rejection in liver transplant patients unable to tolerate tacrolimus or cycloSPORINE due to neurotoxicity; mild rejection in heart transplant patients; treatment of moderate-severe psoriasis

Usual Dosage Adults: I.V./Oral: 1 g twice daily (2 g daily dose), administered within 72 hours of transplantation, when administered in combination with corticosteroids and cyclosporine

Dosage Forms

Capsule, as mofetil: 250 mg

Injection: 500 mg

Suspension, oral, as mofetil: 200 mg/mL (225 mL)

Tablet, film coated, as mofetil: 500 mg

Mycostatin® **[US/Can]** *see* nystatin *on page 473*

Mydfrin® **Ophthalmic** **[US/Can]** *see* phenylephrine *on page 510*

Mydriacyl® **[US/Can]** *see* tropicamide *on page 661*

Mykrox® **[US/Can]** *see* metolazone *on page 425*

Mylanta® **[Can]** *see* aluminum hydroxide, magnesium hydroxide, and simethicone *on page 29*

Mylanta AR® *(Discontinued)* *see page 814*

Mylanta™ **Double Strength** *see* aluminum hydroxide, magnesium hydroxide, and simethicone *on page 29*

Mylanta™ **Extra Strength** **[Can]** *see* aluminum hydroxide, magnesium hydroxide, and simethicone *on page 29*

Mylanta® **Extra Strength Liquid** **[US-OTC]** *see* aluminum hydroxide, magnesium hydroxide, and simethicone *on page 29*

Mylanta® **Gas** **[US-OTC]** *see* simethicone *on page 591*

Mylanta® **Gelcaps®** **[US-OTC]** *see* calcium carbonate and magnesium hydroxide *on page 105*

Mylanta®-II *(Discontinued)* *see page 814*

Mylanta® **Liquid** **[US-OTC]** *see* aluminum hydroxide, magnesium hydroxide, and simethicone *on page 29*

Mylanta™ **Regular Strength** **[Can]** *see* aluminum hydroxide, magnesium hydroxide, and simethicone *on page 29*

Mylanta® **Tablets** **[US-OTC]** *see* calcium carbonate and magnesium hydroxide *on page 105*

Mylanta® **Ultra Tablet** **[US-OTC]** *see* calcium carbonate and magnesium hydroxide *on page 105*

Mylaxen® **Injection** *(Discontinued)* *see page 814*

Myleran® **[US/Can]** *see* busulfan *on page 99*

Mylicon® **[US-OTC]** *see* simethicone *on page 591*

Mylocel™ **[US]** *see* hydroxyurea *on page 338*

Mylotarg™ **[US/Can]** *see* gemtuzumab ozogamicin *on page 295*

Myminic® **Expectorant** *(Discontinued)* *see page 814*

Myobloc® **[US]** *see* botulinum toxin type B *on page 91*

Myochrysine® **[Can]** *see* gold sodium thiomalate *on page 304*

Myochrysine® *(Discontinued)* *see page 814*

Myoflex® **[US/Can]** *see* triethanolamine salicylate *on page 654*

Myotonachol™ **[Can]** *see* bethanechol *on page 84*

Myotonachol™ *(Discontinued)* *see page 814*

Myphetane DC® *(Discontinued)* *see page 814*

Mysoline® **[US/Can]** *see* primidone *on page 540*

Mytelase® **[US/Can]** *see* ambenonium *on page 30*

Mytrex® **[US]** *see* nystatin and triamcinolone *on page 473*

Mytussin® **AC** **[US]** *see* guaifenesin and codeine *on page 308*

Mytussin® **DAC** **[US]** *see* guaifenesin, pseudoephedrine, and codeine *on page 311*

Mytussin® **DM** **[US-OTC]** *see* guaifenesin and dextromethorphan *on page 308*

Nabi-HB® **[US]** *see* hepatitis B immune globulin *on page 320*

nabumetone (na BYOO me tone)
U.S./Canadian Brand Names Apo®-Nabumetone [Can]; Relafen® [US/Can]

Therapeutic Category Analgesic, Non-narcotic; Nonsteroidal Anti-inflammatory Drug (NSAID)

Use Management of osteoarthritis and rheumatoid arthritis

Usual Dosage Adults: Oral: 1000 mg/day; an additional 500-1000 mg may be needed in some patients to obtain more symptomatic relief; may be administered once or twice daily

Dosage Forms Tablet: 500 mg, 750 mg

NAC *see* acetylcysteine *on page 11*

N-acetylcysteine *see* acetylcysteine *on page 11*

N-acetyl-L-cysteine *see* acetylcysteine *on page 11*

n-acetyl-p-aminophenol *see* acetaminophen *on page 3*

NaCl *see* sodium chloride *on page 595*

nadolol (nay DOE lole)
U.S./Canadian Brand Names Alti-Nadolol [Can]; Apo®-Nadol [Can]; Corgard® [US/Can]; Novo-Nadolol [Can]

Therapeutic Category Beta-Adrenergic Blocker

Use Treatment of hypertension and angina pectoris; prevention of myocardial infarction; prophylaxis of migraine headaches

Usual Dosage Adults: Oral: Initial: 40 mg once daily; increase gradually; usual dosage: 40-80 mg/day; may need up to 240-320 mg/day; doses as high as 640 mg/day have been used

Dosage Forms Tablet: 20 mg, 40 mg, 80 mg, 120 mg, 160 mg

Nadopen-V® [Can] *see* penicillin V potassium *on page 499*

nadroparin *(Canada only)* (nad roe PA rin)
U.S./Canadian Brand Names Fraxiparine™ [Can]

Therapeutic Category Low Molecular Weight Heparin

Use Prevention of clotting during hemodialysis; Prophylaxis of thromboembolic disorders (particularly deep vein thrombosis and pulmonary embolism) in general surgery and in orthopedic surgery; treatment of deep vein thrombosis

Usual Dosage Adult: S.C.:
Thromboembolism prophylaxis: 0.3 mL daily S.C for 7 days.

Orthopedic surgery: 0.2-0.4 mL daily for 3 days then 0.3-0.6 mL daily; doses should be adjusted for body weight.

Thromboembolism treatment: 0.4-0.9 mL twice daily for 10 days. Doses should be adjusted for body weight.

Hemodialysis: 0.3-0.6 mL into the arterial line at start of 4 hour session. Dose should be adjusted for body weight.

Child: Hemodialysis: 60-120 int. units/kg at the start of 4 hour session. Duration of therapy should be determined by the clinical need. Dosage should be individualized.

Dosage Forms Injection, solution, as calcium:
Fraxiparine™:
9500 anti-Xa int. units/mL (0.2 mL, 0.3 mL, 0.4 mL) [ungraduated prefilled syringe]
9500 anti-Xa int. units/mL (0.6 mL, 0.8 mL, 1 mL) [graduated prefilled syringe]
Fraxiparine™ Forte: 19,000 anti-Xa int. units/mL (0.6 mL, 0.8 mL, 1 mL) [graduated prefilled syringe]

nafarelin (NAF a re lin)
U.S./Canadian Brand Names Synarel® [US/Can]

Therapeutic Category Hormone, Posterior Pituitary
(Continued)

nafarelin (Continued)

Use Treatment of endometriosis, including pain and reduction of lesions; treatment of central precocious puberty (gonadotropin-dependent precocious puberty) in children of both sexes

Usual Dosage Adults: 1 spray in one nostril each morning and evening for 6 months

Dosage Forms Nasal spray, as acetate: 2 mg/mL (8 mL) [200 mcg/spray: 60 metered doses]

Nafazair® Ophthalmic (Discontinued) see page 814

Nafcil™ (Discontinued) see page 814

nafcillin (naf SIL in)

Synonyms ethoxynaphthamido penicillin sodium

Therapeutic Category Penicillin

Use Treatment of bacterial infections such as osteomyelitis, septicemia, endocarditis, and CNS infections due to susceptible penicillinase-producing strains of *Staphylococcus*

Usual Dosage

Children:
I.M.: 25 mg/kg twice daily
I.V.:
 Mild to moderate infections: 50-100 mg/kg/day in divided doses every 6 hours
 Severe infections: 100-200 mg/kg/day in divided doses every 4-6 hours
 Maximum dose: 12 g/day
Adults:
I.M.: 500 mg every 4-6 hours
I.V.: 500-2000 mg every 4-6 hours

Dosage Forms
Infusion [premixed iso-osmotic dextrose solution]: 1 g (50 mL); 2 g (100 mL)
Injection, powder for reconstitution, as sodium: 1 g, 2 g, 10 g

naftifine (NAF ti feen)

U.S./Canadian Brand Names Naftin® [US]

Therapeutic Category Antifungal Agent

Use Topical treatment of tinea cruris and tinea corporis

Usual Dosage Adults: Topical: Apply twice daily

Dosage Forms
Cream, as hydrochloride: 1% (15 g, 30 g, 60 g) [contains alcohol]
Gel, as hydrochloride: 1% (20 g, 40 g, 60 g) [contains alcohol]

Naftin® [US] see naftifine on this page

NaHCO₃ see sodium bicarbonate on page 594

nalbuphine (NAL byoo feen)

U.S./Canadian Brand Names Nubain® [US/Can]

Therapeutic Category Analgesic, Narcotic

Use Relief of moderate to severe pain

Usual Dosage I.M., I.V., S.C.: 10 mg/70 kg every 3-6 hours

Dosage Forms Injection, solution, as hydrochloride: 10 mg/mL (1 mL, 10 mL); 20 mg/mL (1 mL, 10 mL)

Nalcrom® [Can] see cromolyn sodium on page 166

Naldecon® (Discontinued) see page 814

Naldecon® DX Adult Liquid (Discontinued) see page 814

Naldecon-EX® Children's Syrup (Discontinued) see page 814

Naldelate® (Discontinued) see page 814

Nalfon® **[US/Can]** *see* fenoprofen *on page 265*

Nalgest® *(Discontinued) see page 814*

nalidixic acid (nal i DIKS ik AS id)

Synonyms nalidixinic acid

U.S./Canadian Brand Names NegGram® [US/Can]

Therapeutic Category Quinolone

Use Lower urinary tract infections due to susceptible gram-negative organisms including *E. coli, Enterobacter, Klebsiella*, and *Proteus* (inactive against *Pseudomonas*)

Usual Dosage Oral:

Children: 55 mg/kg/day divided every 6 hours; suppressive therapy is 33 mg/kg/day divided every 6 hours

Adults: 1 g 4 times/day for 2 weeks; then suppressive therapy of 500 mg 4 times/day

Dosage Forms

Suspension, oral: 250 mg/5 mL (473 mL) [raspberry flavor]

Tablet: 250 mg, 500 mg, 1 g

nalidixinic acid *see* nalidixic acid *on this page*

Nallpen® *(Discontinued) see page 814*

***n*-allylnoroxymorphone** *see* naloxone *on this page*

nalmefene (NAL me feen)

U.S./Canadian Brand Names Revex® [US]

Therapeutic Category Antidote

Use Complete or partial of opioid drug effects; management of known or suspected opioid overdose

Usual Dosage Titrate to reverse the undesired effects of opioids; once adequate reversal has been established, additional administration is not required and may actually be harmful due to unwanted reversal of analgesia or precipitated withdrawal; the recommended initial dose for nonopioid dependent patient is 0.5 mg/70 kg, a second dose of 1 mg/70 kg 2-5 minutes later may be administered, after a total dose of 1.5 mg/70 kg has been administered with no clinical response, additional nalmefene is not likely to have an effect

Dosage Forms Injection, solution, as hydrochloride: 100 mcg/mL [blue label] (1 mL); 1000 mcg/mL [green label] (2 mL)

naloxone (nal OKS one)

Synonyms *n*-allylnoroxymorphone

U.S./Canadian Brand Names Narcan® [US/Can]

Therapeutic Category Antidote

Use Reverses CNS and respiratory depression in suspected narcotic overdose; neonatal opiate depression; coma of unknown etiology

Investigational use: Shock, phencyclidine, and alcohol ingestion

Usual Dosage I.M., I.V. (preferred), intratracheal, S.C. (administer undiluted injection):

Infants and Children:

Postanesthesia narcotic reversal: 0.01 mg/kg; may repeat every 2-3 minutes as needed based on response

Opiate intoxication:

Birth (including premature infants) to 5 years or <20 kg: 0.1 mg/kg; repeat every 2-3 minutes if needed; may need to repeat doses every 20-60 minutes

>5 years or ≥20 kg: 2 mg/dose; if no response, repeat every 2-3 minutes; may need to repeat doses every 20-60 minutes

Children and Adults: Continuous infusion: I.V.: If continuous infusion is required, calculate dosage/hour based on effective intermittent dose used and duration of adequate response seen, titrate dose 0.04-0.16 mg/kg/hour for 2-5 days in children, adult dose typically 0.25-6.25 mg/hour (short-term infusions as high as 2.4 mg/kg/hour have been

(Continued)

naloxone *(Continued)*

tolerated in adults during treatment for septic shock); alternatively, continuous infusion utilizes $^2/_3$ of the initial naloxone bolus on an hourly basis; add 10 times this dose to each liter of D_5W and infuse at a rate of 100 mL/hour; $^1/_2$ of the initial bolus dose should be readministered 15 minutes after initiation of the continuous infusion to prevent a drop in naloxone levels; increase infusion rate as needed to assure adequate ventilation

Adults: 0.4-2 mg every 2-3 minutes as needed; may need to repeat doses every 20-60 minutes; if no response is observed for a total of 10 mg, re-evaluate patient for possibility of a drug or disease process unresponsive to naloxone. **Note:** Use 0.1-0.2 mg increments in patients who are opioid dependent and in postoperative patients to avoid large cardiovascular changes

Dosage Forms

Injection, neonatal solution, as hydrochloride: 0.02 mg/mL (2 mL)

Injection, solution, as hydrochloride: 0.4 mg/mL (1 mL, 10 mL); 1 mg/mL (2 mL, 10 mL)

Nalspan® *(Discontinued)* see page 814

naltrexone (nal TREKS one)

U.S./Canadian Brand Names ReVia® [US/Can]

Therapeutic Category Antidote

Use Adjunct to the maintenance of an opioid-free state in detoxified individual

Usual Dosage Do not administer until patient is opioid-free for 7-10 days as required by urine analysis

Adults: Oral: 25 mg; if no withdrawal signs within 1 hour administer another 25 mg; maintenance regimen is flexible, variable and individualized (50 mg/day to 100-150 mg 3 times/week)

Dosage Forms Tablet, as hydrochloride: 50 mg

Nandrobolic® Injection *(Discontinued)* see page 814

nandrolone (NAN droe lone)

U.S./Canadian Brand Names Deca-Durabolin® [US/Can]; Durabolin® [Can]

Therapeutic Category Androgen

Controlled Substance C-III

Use Control of metastatic breast cancer; management of anemia of renal insufficiency

Usual Dosage

Children 2-13 years: 25-50 mg every 3-4 weeks

Adults:

Male: 100-200 mg/week

Female: 50-100 mg/week

Dosage Forms Injection, solution, as decanoate [in sesame oil]: 100 mg/mL (2 mL); 200 mg/mL (1 mL) [contains benzyl alcohol]

naphazoline (naf AZ oh leen)

U.S./Canadian Brand Names AK-Con™ [US]; Albalon® [US]; Allersol® [US]; Clear Eyes® ACR [US-OTC]; Clear Eyes® [US-OTC]; Naphcon Forte® [Can]; Naphcon® [US-OTC]; Privine® [US-OTC]; VasoClear® [US-OTC]; Vasocon® [Can]

Therapeutic Category Adrenergic Agonist Agent

Use Topical ocular vasoconstrictor (to soothe, refresh, moisturize, and relieve redness due to minor eye irritation); temporarily relieves nasal congestion associated with rhinitis, sinusitis, hay fever, or the common cold

Usual Dosage

Nasal:

Children:

<6 years: Not recommended (especially infants) due to CNS depression

6-12 years: 1 spray of 0.05% into each nostril, repeat in 3 hours if necessary

Children >12 years and Adults: 0.05%, instill 2 drops or sprays every 3-6 hours if needed; therapy should not exceed 3-5 days or more frequently than every 3 hours
Ophthalmic:
Children <6 years: Not recommended for use due to CNS depression (especially in infants)
Children >6 years and Adults: Instill 1-2 drops into conjunctival sac of affected eye(s) every 3-4 hours; therapy generally should not exceed 3-4 days

Dosage Forms
Solution, intranasal drops, as hydrochloride (Privine®): 0.05% (25 mL)
Nasal spray, as hydrochloride (Privine®): 0.05% (20 mL, 480 mL)
Solution, ophthalmic, as hydrochloride: 0.1% (15 mL)
AK-Con™, Albalon®, Allersol®: 0.1% (15 mL) [contains benzalkonium chloride]
Clear Eyes®: 0.012% (6 mL, 15 mL, 30 mL) [contains glycerin 0.2% and benzalkonium chloride]
Clear Eyes® ACR: 0.012% (15 mL, 30 mL) [contains glycerin 0.2%, zinc sulfate 0.25%, and benzalkonium chloride]
Naphcon®: 0.012% (15 mL) [contains benzalkonium chloride]
VasoClear®: 0.02% (15 mL) [contains benzalkonium chloride]

naphazoline and antazoline (naf AZ oh leen & an TAZ oh leen)
U.S./Canadian Brand Names Albalon®-A Liquifilm [Can]; Vasocon-A® [US/Can]
Therapeutic Category Antihistamine/Decongestant Combination
Use Topical ocular congestion, irritation, and itching
Usual Dosage Ophthalmic: 1-2 drops every 3-4 hours
Dosage Forms Solution, ophthalmic: Naphazoline hydrochloride 0.05% and antazoline phosphate 0.5% (15 mL) [contains benzalkonium chloride]

naphazoline and pheniramine (naf AZ oh leen & fen NIR a meen)
Synonyms pheniramine and naphazoline
U.S./Canadian Brand Names Naphcon-A® [US/Can]; Opcon-A® [US-OTC]; Visine-A™ [US-OTC]
Therapeutic Category Antihistamine/Decongestant Combination
Use Topical ocular vasoconstrictor
Usual Dosage Ophthalmic: 1-2 drops every 3-4 hours
Dosage Forms Solution, ophthalmic: Naphazoline hydrochloride 0.025% and pheniramine 0.3% (15 mL) [contains benzalkonium chloride]

Naphcon-A® [US/Can] *see* naphazoline and pheniramine *on this page*
Naphcon Forte® [Can] *see* naphazoline *on previous page*
Naphcon Forte® Ophthalmic (Discontinued) *see page 814*
Naphcon® [US-OTC] *see* naphazoline *on previous page*
Naprelan® [US] *see* naproxen *on this page*
Naprosyn® [US/Can] *see* naproxen *on this page*

naproxen (na PROKS en)
U.S./Canadian Brand Names Aleve® [US-OTC]; Anaprox® DS [US/Can]; Anaprox® [US/Can]; Apo®-Napro-Na [Can]; Apo®-Napro-Na DS [Can]; Apo®-Naproxen [Can]; Apo®-Naproxen SR [Can]; EC-Naprosyn® [US]; Gen-Naproxen EC [Can]; Naprelan® [US]; Naprosyn® [US/Can]; Naxen® [Can]; Novo-Naprox [Can]; Novo-Naprox Sodium [Can]; Novo-Naprox Sodium DS [Can]; Novo-Naprox SR [Can]; Nu-Naprox [Can]; Riva-Naproxen [Can]; Synflex® [Can]; Synflex® DS [Can]
Therapeutic Category Analgesic, Non-narcotic; Antipyretic; Nonsteroidal Anti-inflammatory Drug (NSAID)
Use Management of inflammatory disease and rheumatoid disorders (including juvenile rheumatoid arthritis); acute gout; mild to moderate pain; dysmenorrhea; fever
(Continued)

447

naproxen *(Continued)*

Usual Dosage Oral (as naproxen):

Children >2 years:

Antipyretic or analgesic: 5-7 mg/kg/dose every 8-12 hours

Juvenile rheumatoid arthritis: 10 mg/kg/day, up to a maximum of 1000 mg/day divided twice daily

Adults:

Rheumatoid arthritis, osteoarthritis, and ankylosing spondylitis: 500-1000 mg/day in 2 divided doses

Mild to moderate pain or dysmenorrhea: Initial: 500 mg, then 250 mg every 6-8 hours; maximum: 1250 mg/day

Dosage Forms

Caplet, as sodium (Aleve®): 220 mg [equivalent to naproxen 200 mg and sodium 20 mg]

Gelcap, as sodium (Aleve®): 220 mg [equivalent to naproxen 200 mg and sodium 20 mg]

Suspension, oral (Naprosyn®): 125 mg/5 mL (480 mL) [contains sodium 0.3 mEq/mL; orange-pineapple flavor]

Tablet (Naprosyn®): 250 mg, 375 mg, 500 mg

Tablet, as sodium: 220 mg [equivalent to naproxen 200 mg and sodium 20 mg]; 275 mg [equivalent to naproxen 250 mg and sodium 25 mg]; 550 mg [equivalent to naproxen 500 mg and sodium 50 mg]

Aleve®: 220 mg [equivalent to naproxen 200 mg and sodium 20 mg]

Anaprox®: 275 mg [equivalent to naproxen 250 mg and sodium 25 mg]

Anaprox® DS: 550 mg [equivalent to naproxen 500 mg and sodium 50 mg]

Tablet, controlled release, as sodium (Naprelan®): 421.5 mg [equivalent to naproxen 375 mg and sodium 37.5 mg]; 550 mg [equivalent to naproxen 500 mg and sodium 50 mg]

Tablet, delayed release (EC-Naprosyn®): 375 mg, 500 mg

Naqua® **[US/Can]** *see* trichlormethiazide *on page 653*

naratriptan *(NAR a trip tan)*

U.S./Canadian Brand Names Amerge® [US/Can]

Therapeutic Category Antimigraine Agent; Serotonin Agonist

Use Acute treatment of migraine with or without aura

Usual Dosage Oral: Adults: 1 mg or 2.5 mg (maximum dose: 5 mg); if no response, dose may be repeated in 4 hours

Dosage Forms Tablet: 1 mg, 2.5 mg

Narcan® **[US/Can]** *see* naloxone *on page 445*

Nardil® **[US/Can]** *see* phenelzine *on page 507*

Naropin™ **[US/Can]** *see* ropivacaine *on page 578*

Nasacort® **[US/Can]** *see* triamcinolone (inhalation, nasal) *on page 651*

Nasacort® AQ **[US/Can]** *see* triamcinolone (inhalation, nasal) *on page 651*

Nasahist B® *(Discontinued) see page 814*

Nasalcrom® **[US-OTC]** *see* cromolyn sodium *on page 166*

Nasalide® **[US/Can]** *see* flunisolide *on page 276*

Nasal Moist® **[US-OTC]** *see* sodium chloride *on page 595*

NāSal™ **[US-OTC]** *see* sodium chloride *on page 595*

Nasarel® **[US]** *see* flunisolide *on page 276*

Nascobal® **[US]** *see* cyanocobalamin *on page 167*

Nasonex® **[US/Can]** *see* mometasone furoate *on page 435*

Natabec® *(Discontinued) see page 814*

Natabec® FA *(Discontinued) see page 814*

Natabec® **Rx** *(Discontinued)* *see page 814*

Natacyn® **[US/Can]** *see* natamycin *on this page*

Natalins® **Rx** *(Discontinued)* *see page 814*

Natalins® **[US-OTC]** *see* vitamin (multiple/prenatal) *on page 683*

natamycin (na ta MYE sin)

Synonyms pimaricin

U.S./Canadian Brand Names Natacyn® [US/Can]

Therapeutic Category Antifungal Agent

Use Treatment of blepharitis, conjunctivitis, and keratitis caused by susceptible fungi (*Aspergillus, Candida, Cephalosporium, Curvularia, Fusarium, Penicillium, Microsporum, Epidermophyton, Blastomyces dermatitidis, Coccidioides immitis, Cryptococcus neoformans, Histoplasma capsulatum, Sporothrix schenckii, Trichomonas vaginalis*)

Usual Dosage Adults: Ophthalmic: 1 drop in conjunctival sac every 1-2 hours, after 3-4 days dose may be reduced to one drop 6-8 times/day; usual course of therapy: 2-3 weeks

Dosage Forms Suspension, ophthalmic: 5% (15 mL) [contains benzalkonium chloride]

nateglinide (na TEG li nide)

U.S./Canadian Brand Names Starlix® [US]

Therapeutic Category Antidiabetic Agent

Use Management of type 2 diabetes mellitus (noninsulin dependent, NIDDM) as monotherapy when hyperglycemia cannot be managed by diet and exercise alone; in combination with metformin to lower blood glucose in patients whose hyperglycemia cannot be controlled by exercise, diet, and metformin alone.

Usual Dosage

Children: Safety and efficacy have not been established

Adults: Management of type 2 diabetes mellitus: Oral: Initial and maintenance dose: 120 mg 3 times/day, 1-30 minutes before meals; may be given alone or in combination with metformin; patients close to Hb A_{1c} goal may be started at 60 mg 3 times/day

Dosage Forms Tablet: 60 mg, 120 mg

Natrecor® **[US]** *see* nesiritide *on page 455*

natriuretic peptide *see* nesiritide *on page 455*

Natulan® **[Can]** *see* procarbazine *on page 542*

natural lung surfactant *see* beractant *on page 81*

Nature's Tears® **[US-OTC]** *see* artificial tears *on page 56*

Nature-Throid® **NT [US]** *see* thyroid *on page 636*

Naturetin® **[US]** *see* bendroflumethiazide *on page 75*

Naus-A-Way® *(Discontinued)* *see page 814*

Nausetrol® **[US-OTC]** *see* phosphorated carbohydrate solution *on page 512*

Navane® **[US/Can]** *see* thiothixene *on page 635*

Navelbine® **[US/Can]** *see* vinorelbine *on page 679*

Naxen® **[Can]** *see* naproxen *on page 447*

Na-Zone® **[US-OTC]** *see* sodium chloride *on page 595*

N-B-P® **Ointment** *(Discontinued)* *see page 814*

ND-Stat® **Solution [US-OTC]** *see* brompheniramine *on page 93*

Nebcin® **[US/Can]** *see* tobramycin *on page 641*

NebuPent™ **[US]** *see* pentamidine *on page 500*

Necon® **0.5/35 [US]** *see* ethinyl estradiol and norethindrone *on page 251*

Necon® **1/35 [US]** *see* ethinyl estradiol and norethindrone *on page 251*

Necon® 1/50 [US] *see* mestranol and norethindrone *on page 412*

Necon® 10/11 [US] *see* ethinyl estradiol and norethindrone *on page 251*

nedocromil (inhalation) (ne doe KROE mil in hil LA shun)

U.S./Canadian Brand Names Tilade® [US/Can]
Therapeutic Category Mast Cell Stabilizer
Use Maintenance therapy in patients with mild to moderate bronchial asthma
Usual Dosage Adults: Inhalation: 2 inhalations 4 times/day
Dosage Forms Aerosol, as sodium: 1.75 mg/activation (16.2 g)

nedocromil (ophthalmic) (ne doe KROE mil op THAL mik)

U.S./Canadian Brand Names Alocril™ [US/Can]
Therapeutic Category Mast Cell Stabilizer
Use Treatment of itching associated with allergic conjunctivitis
Usual Dosage Adults: Ophthalmic: 1-2 drops in eye(s) twice daily
Dosage Forms Solution, ophthalmic, as sodium: 2% (5 mL)

nefazodone (nef AY zoe done)

U.S./Canadian Brand Names Serzone® [US/Can]
Therapeutic Category Antidepressant, Miscellaneous
Use Treatment of depression
Usual Dosage Adults: Oral: Initial: 200 mg/day administered in two divided doses with a range of 300-600 mg/day in two divided doses thereafter
Dosage Forms Tablet, as hydrochloride: 50 mg, 100 mg, 150 mg, 200 mg, 250 mg

NegGram® [US/Can] *see* nalidixic acid *on page 445*

nelfinavir (nel FIN a veer)

U.S./Canadian Brand Names Viracept® [US/Can]
Therapeutic Category Antiviral Agent
Use As monotherapy or preferably in combination with nucleoside analogs in the treatment of HIV infection, in adults and children, when antiretroviral therapy is warranted
Usual Dosage Oral:
Children 2-13 years: 20-30 mg/kg 3 times/day with a meal or light snack; if tablets are unable to be taken, use oral powder in small amount of water, milk, formula, or dietary supplements; do not use acidic food/juice or store for >6 hours
Adults: 750 mg 3 times/day with meals
Dosage Forms
Powder, oral: 50 mg/g (144 g) [contains phenylalanine 11.2 mg]
Tablet, film coated: 250 mg

Nelova™ 0.5/35E *(Discontinued) see page 814*

Nelova™ 1/35E *(Discontinued) see page 814*

Nelova™ 1/50M *(Discontinued) see page 814*

Nelova™ 10/11 *(Discontinued) see page 814*

Nemasol® Sodium [Can] *see* aminosalicylate sodium *on page 34*

Nembutal® [US/Can] *see* pentobarbital *on page 501*

Neoasma® [US] *see* theophylline and guaifenesin *on page 631*

Neo-Calglucon® *(Discontinued) see page 814*

Neo-Castaderm® *(Discontinued) see page 814*

Neo-Cortef® [Can] *see* neomycin and hydrocortisone *on page 452*

Neo-Cortef® *(Discontinued) see page 814*

NeoDecadron® Ocumeter® [US] *see* neomycin and dexamethasone *on next page*

NeoDecadron® Topical *(Discontinued)* *see page 814*

Neo-Dexameth® Ophthalmic *(Discontinued)* *see page 814*

Neo-Durabolic® *(Discontinued)* *see page 814*

Neofed® *(Discontinued)* *see page 814*

Neo-Fradin™ [US] *see* neomycin *on this page*

Neoloid® [US-OTC] *see* castor oil *on page 119*

Neo-Medrol® Acetate Topical *(Discontinued)* *see page 814*

Neomixin® Topical *(Discontinued)* *see page 814*

neomycin (nee oh MYE sin)

U.S./Canadian Brand Names Myciguent [US-OTC]; Neo-Fradin™ [US]; Neo-Rx [US]

Therapeutic Category Aminoglycoside (Antibiotic); Antibiotic, Topical

Use Administered orally to prepare GI tract for surgery; treat minor skin infections; treat diarrhea caused by *E. coli*; adjunct in the treatment of hepatic encephalopathy

Usual Dosage

Children: Oral:

Preoperative intestinal antisepsis: 90 mg/kg/day divided every 4 hours for 2 days; or 25 mg/kg at 1 PM, 2 PM, and 11 PM on the day preceding surgery as an adjunct to mechanical cleansing of the intestine and in combination with erythromycin base

Hepatic coma: 50-100 mg/kg/day in divided doses every 6-8 hours or 2.5-7 g/m^2/day divided every 4-6 hours for 5-6 days not to exceed 12 g/day

Children and Adults: Topical: Apply ointment 1-4 times/day; topical solutions containing 0.1% to 1% neomycin have been used for irrigation

Adults: Oral:

Preoperative intestinal antisepsis: 1 g each hour for 4 doses then 1 g every 4 hours for 5 doses; or 1 g at 1 PM, 2 PM, and 11 PM on day preceding surgery as an adjunct to mechanical cleansing of the bowel and oral erythromycin; or 6 g/day divided every 4 hours for 2-3 days

Hepatic coma: 500-2000 mg every 6-8 hours or 4-12 g/day divided every 4-6 hours for 5-6 days

Chronic hepatic insufficiency: Oral: 4 g/day for an indefinite period

Dosage Forms

Ointment, topical, as sulfate (Myciguent): 3.5 mg/g (15 g, 30 g)

Powder, micronized, as sulfate [for prescription compounding] (Neo-Rx): (10 g, 100 g)

Solution, oral, as sulfate (Neo-Fradin™): 125 mg/5 mL (480 mL) [contains benzoic acid; cherry flavor]

Tablet, as sulfate: 500 mg

neomycin and dexamethasone (nee oh MYE sin & deks a METH a sone)

Synonyms dexamethasone and neomycin

U.S./Canadian Brand Names NeoDecadron® Ocumeter® [US]

Therapeutic Category Antibiotic/Corticosteroid, Ophthalmic; Antibiotic/Corticosteroid, Topical

Use Treatment of steroid responsive inflammatory conditions of the palpebral and bulbar conjunctiva, lid, cornea, and anterior segment of the globe

Usual Dosage

Ophthalmic: Instill 1-2 drops in eye(s) every 3-4 hours

Topical: Apply thin coat 3-4 times/day until favorable response is observed, then reduce dose to one application/day. Therapy should be discontinued when control is achieved. If no improvement is seen, reassessment of diagnosis may be necessary.

Dosage Forms Solution, ophthalmic: Neomycin sulfate 0.35% [3.5 mg/mL] and dexamethasone sodium phosphate 0.1% [1 mg/mL] (5 mL) [contains benzalkonium chloride and sodium bisulfite]

neomycin and hydrocortisone (nee oh MYE sin & hye droe KOR ti sone)

Synonyms hydrocortisone and neomycin

U.S./Canadian Brand Names Neo-Cortef® [Can]

Therapeutic Category Antibiotic/Corticosteroid, Ophthalmic; Antibiotic/Corticosteroid, Topical

Use Treatment of susceptible topical bacterial infections with associated inflammation

Usual Dosage Topical: Apply to area in a thin film 2-4 times/day. Therapy should be discontinued when control is achieved. If no improvement is seen, reassessment of diagnosis may be necessary.

Dosage Forms Ointment, topical: Neomycin sulfate 0.5% and hydrocortisone 1% (20 g)

neomycin and polymyxin B (nee oh MYE sin & pol i MIKS in bee)

Synonyms polymyxin B and neomycin

U.S./Canadian Brand Names Neosporin® Cream [Can]; Neosporin® G.U. Irrigant [US/Can]

Therapeutic Category Antibiotic, Topical; Genitourinary Irrigant

Use Short-term use as a continuous irrigant or rinse in the urinary bladder to prevent bacteriuria and gram-negative rod septicemia associated with the use of indwelling catheters; to help prevent infection in minor cuts, scrapes, and burns

Usual Dosage Children and Adults:

Topical: Apply cream 2-4 times/day

Bladder irrigation: Continuous irrigant or rinse in the urinary bladder for up to 10 days where 1 mL is added to 1 L of normal saline with administration rate adjusted to patient's urine output; usually no more than 1 L of irrigant is used per day

Dosage Forms

Cream: Neomycin sulfate 3.5 mg and polymyxin B sulfate 10,000 units per g (0.94 g, 15 g)

Solution, irrigant: Neomycin sulfate 40 mg and polymyxin B sulfate 200,000 units per mL (1 mL, 20 mL)

neomycin, bacitracin, and polymyxin B *see* bacitracin, neomycin, and polymyxin B *on page 69*

neomycin, bacitracin, polymyxin B, and hydrocortisone *see* bacitracin, neomycin, polymyxin B, and hydrocortisone *on page 69*

neomycin, colistin, hydrocortisone, and thonzonium

(nee oh MYE sin, koe LIS tin, hye droe KOR ti sone, & thon ZOE nee um)

U.S./Canadian Brand Names Coly-Mycin® S Otic [US]; Cortisporin®-TC Otic [US]

Therapeutic Category Antibiotic/Corticosteroid, Otic

Use Treatment of superficial and susceptible bacterial infections of the external auditory canal; for treatment of susceptible bacterial infections of mastoidectomy and fenestration cavities

Usual Dosage

Children: 4 drops in affected ear 3-4 times/day

Adults: 5 drops in affected ear 3-4 times/day

Dosage Forms Suspension, otic:

Coly-Mycin® S: Neomycin sulfate 3.3 mg, colistin sulfate 3 mg, hydrocortisone acetate 10 mg, and thonzonium bromide 0.5 mg per mL (5 mL)

Cortisporin®-TC: Neomycin sulfate 3.3 mg, colistin sulfate 3 mg, hydrocortisone acetate 10 mg, and thonzonium bromide 0.5 mg per mL (10 mL)

neomycin, polymyxin B, and dexamethasone

(nee oh MYE sin, pol i MIKS in bee, & deks a METH a sone)

Synonyms dexamethasone, neomycin, and polymyxin B; polymyxin B, neomycin, and dexamethasone

U.S./Canadian Brand Names AK-Trol® [US]; Dexacidin® [US]; Dexacine™ [US]; Dioptrol® [Can]; Maxitrol® [US/Can]

Therapeutic Category Antibiotic/Corticosteroid, Ophthalmic

Use Steroid-responsive inflammatory ocular conditions in which a corticosteroid is indicated and where bacterial infection or a risk of bacterial infection exists

Usual Dosage Children and Adults: Ophthalmic:

Ointment: Place a small amount (~½") in the affected eye 3-4 times/day or apply at bedtime as an adjunct with drops

Solution: Instill 1-2 drops into affected eye(s) every 4-6 hours; in severe disease, drops may be used hourly and tapered to discontinuation

Dosage Forms

Ointment, ophthalmic (Dexacine™, Maxitrol®): Neomycin sulfate 3.5 mg, polymyxin B sulfate 10,000 units, and dexamethasone 0.1% per g (3.5 g)

Suspension, ophthalmic (AK-Trol®, Dexacidin®, Maxitrol®): Neomycin sulfate 3.5 mg, polymyxin B sulfate 10,000 units, and dexamethasone 0.1% per mL (5 mL) [contains benzalkonium chloride]

neomycin, polymyxin B, and gramicidin

(nee oh MYE sin, pol i MIKS in bee, & gram i SYE din)

Synonyms gramicidin, neomycin, and polymyxin B; polymyxin B, neomycin, and gramicidin

U.S./Canadian Brand Names AK-Spore® Ophthalmic Solution [US]; Neosporin® Ophthalmic Solution [US/Can]; Optimyxin Plus® [Can]

Therapeutic Category Antibiotic, Ophthalmic

Use Treatment of superficial ocular infection, infection prophylaxis in minor skin abrasions

Usual Dosage Ophthalmic: Drops: 1-2 drops 4-6 times/day or more frequently as required for severe infections

Dosage Forms Solution, ophthalmic: Neomycin sulfate 1.75 mg, polymyxin B sulfate 10,000 units, and gramicidin 0.025 mg per mL (2 mL, 10 mL)

neomycin, polymyxin B, and hydrocortisone

(nee oh MYE sin, pol i MIKS in bee, & hye droe KOR ti sone)

Synonyms hydrocortisone, neomycin, and polymyxin B; polymyxin B, neomycin, and hydrocortisone

U.S./Canadian Brand Names AntibiOtic® Ear [US]; Cortimyxin® [Can]; Cortisporin® Cream [US]; Cortisporin® Ophthalmic [US/Can]; Cortisporin® Otic [US/Can]; PediOtic® [US]

Therapeutic Category Antibiotic/Corticosteroid, Ophthalmic; Antibiotic/Corticosteroid, Otic; Antibiotic/Corticosteroid, Topical

Use Steroid-responsive inflammatory condition for which a corticosteroid is indicated and where bacterial infection or a risk of bacterial infection exists

Usual Dosage Duration of use should be limited to 10 days unless otherwise directed by the physician

Ophthalmic: Adults and Children:

Ointment: Apply to the affected eye every 3-4 hours

Suspension: 1 drop every 3-4 hours

Otic: Solution/suspension:

Children: 3 drops into affected ear 3-4 times/day

Adults: 4 drops into affected ear 3-4 times/day

Dosage Forms

Cream, topical (Cortisporin®): Neomycin sulfate 5 mg [equivalent to 3.5 mg base], polymyxin B sulfate 10,000 units, and hydrocortisone 5 mg per g (7.5 g)

Solution, otic (AntibiOtic® Ear; Cortisporin®): Neomycin sulfate 5 mg [equivalent to 3.5 mg base], polymyxin B sulfate 10,000 units, and hydrocortisone 10 mg per mL (10 mL) [contains potassium metabisulfite]

Suspension, ophthalmic (Cortisporin®): Neomycin sulfate 5 mg [equivalent to 3.5 mg base], polymyxin B sulfate 10,000 units, and hydrocortisone 10 mg per mL (7.5 mL) [contains thimerosal]

(Continued)

453

neomycin, polymyxin B, and hydrocortisone *(Continued)*

Suspension, otic: Neomycin sulfate 5 mg [equivalent to 3.5 mg base], polymyxin B sulfate 10,000 units, and hydrocortisone 10 mg per mL (10 mL)

AntibiOtic® Ear, Cortisporin®: Neomycin sulfate 5 mg [equivalent to 3.5 mg base], polymyxin B sulfate 10,000 units, and hydrocortisone 10 mg per mL (10 mL)

PediOtic®: Neomycin sulfate 5 mg [equivalent to 3.5 mg base], polymyxin B sulfate 10,000 units, and hydrocortisone 10 mg per mL (7.5 mL)

neomycin, polymyxin B, and prednisolone

(nee oh MYE sin, pol i MIKS in bee, & pred NIS oh lone)

Synonyms polymyxin B, neomycin, and prednisolone; prednisolone, neomycin, and polymyxin B

U.S./Canadian Brand Names Poly-Pred® [US]

Therapeutic Category Antibiotic/Corticosteroid, Ophthalmic

Use Steroid-responsive inflammatory ocular condition in which bacterial infection or a risk of bacterial ocular infection exists

Usual Dosage Children and Adults: Ophthalmic: Instill 1-2 drops every 3-4 hours; acute infections may require every 30-minute instillation initially with frequency of administration reduced as the infection is brought under control. To treat the lids: Instill 1-2 drops every 3-4 hours, close the eye and rub the excess on the lids and lid margins.

Dosage Forms Suspension, ophthalmic: Neomycin sulfate 0.35%, polymyxin B sulfate 10,000 units, and prednisolone acetate 0.5% per mL (5 mL, 10 mL)

neonatal trace metals *see* trace metals *on page 646*

Neoquess® Injection *(Discontinued)* *see page 814*

Neoquess® Tablet *(Discontinued)* *see page 814*

Neoral® [US/Can] *see* cyclosporine *on page 169*

Neo-Rx [US] *see* neomycin *on page 451*

Neosar® [US] *see* cyclophosphamide *on page 169*

Neosporin® Cream [Can] *see* neomycin and polymyxin B *on page 452*

Neosporin® G.U. Irrigant [US/Can] *see* neomycin and polymyxin B *on page 452*

Neosporin® Ophthalmic Ointment [US/Can] *see* bacitracin, neomycin, and polymyxin B *on page 69*

Neosporin® Ophthalmic Solution [US/Can] *see* neomycin, polymyxin B, and gramicidin *on previous page*

Neosporin® Topical [US/Can] *see* bacitracin, neomycin, and polymyxin B *on page 69*

neostigmine (nee oh STIG meen)

U.S./Canadian Brand Names Prostigmin® [US/Can]

Therapeutic Category Cholinergic Agent

Use Treatment of myasthenia gravis; prevention and treatment of postoperative bladder distention and urinary retention; reversal of the effects of nondepolarizing neuromuscular blocking agents after surgery

Usual Dosage

Myasthenia gravis: Diagnosis: I.M.:

Children: 0.04 mg/kg as a single dose

Adults: 0.02 mg/kg as a single dose

Myasthenia gravis: Treatment:

Children:

Oral: 2 mg/kg/day divided every 3-4 hours

I.M., I.V., S.C.: 0.01-0.04 mg/kg every 2-4 hours

Adults:

Oral: 15 mg/dose every 3-4 hours

I.M., I.V., S.C.: 0.5-2.5 mg every 1-3 hours
Reversal of nondepolarizing neuromuscular blockade after surgery in conjunction with atropine or glycopyrrolate: I.V.:
Infants: 0.025-0.1 mg/kg/dose
Children: 0.025-0.08 mg/kg/dose
Adults: 0.5-2.5 mg; total dose not to exceed 5 mg
Bladder atony: Adults: I.M., S.C.:
Prevention: 0.25 mg every 4-6 hours for 2-3 days
Treatment: 0.5-1 mg every 3 hours for 5 doses after bladder has emptied

Dosage Forms
Injection, solution, as methylsulfate: 0.5 mg/mL (1 mL, 10 mL); 1 mg/mL (10 mL)
Tablet, as bromide: 15 mg

Neostrata®️ HQ [Can] see hydroquinone on page 336

Neo-Synalar®️ Topical (Discontinued) see page 814

Neo-Synephrine®️ 12 Hour Extra Moisturizing [US-OTC] see oxymetazoline on page 486

Neo-Synephrine®️ 12 Hour [US-OTC] see oxymetazoline on page 486

Neo-Synephrine®️ Injection [US/Can] see phenylephrine on page 510

Neo-Synephrine®️ Nasal [US-OTC] see phenylephrine on page 510

Neo-Synephrine®️ Ophthalmic [US] see phenylephrine on page 510

Neo-Tabs®️ (Discontinued) see page 814

Neotopic®️ [Can] see bacitracin, neomycin, and polymyxin B on page 69

Neotrace-4®️ [US] see trace metals on page 646

NeoVadrin®️ (Discontinued) see page 814

Nephro-Calci®️ [US-OTC] see calcium carbonate on page 104

Nephrocaps®️ [US] see vitamin B complex with vitamin C and folic acid on page 681

Nephro-Fer™️ [US-OTC] see ferrous fumarate on page 268

Nephrox Suspension (Discontinued) see page 814

Neptazane®️ [US/Can] see methazolamide on page 415

Nervocaine®️ Injection (Discontinued) see page 814

Nesacaine®️ [US] see chloroprocaine on page 136

Nesacaine®️-CE [Can] see chloroprocaine on page 136

Nesacaine®️-MPF [US] see chloroprocaine on page 136

nesiritide (ni SIR i tide)
Synonyms B-type natriuretic peptide (human); hBNP; natriuretic peptide
U.S./Canadian Brand Names Natrecor®️ [US]
Therapeutic Category Natriuretic Peptide, B-type, Human; Vasodilator
Use Treatment of acutely decompensated congestive heart failure (CHF) in patients with dyspnea at rest or with minimal activity
Usual Dosage Adults: I.V.: Initial: 2 mcg/kg (bolus); followed by continuous infusion at 0.01 mcg/kg/minute; **Note:** Should not be initiated at a dosage higher than initial recommended dose. At intervals of ≥3 hours, the dosage may be increased by 0.005 mcg/kg/minute (preceded by a bolus of 1 mcg/kg), up to a maximum of 0.03 mcg/kg/minute. Increases beyond the initial infusion rate should be limited to selected patients and accompanied by hemodynamic monitoring.
Patients experiencing hypotension during the infusion: Infusion should be interrupted. May attempt to restart at a lower dose (reduce initial infusion dose by 30% and omit bolus).
Dosage Forms Injection, powder for reconstitution: 1.5 mg

Nestrex® *(Discontinued)* see page 814

Netromycin® *(Discontinued)* see page 814

Neucalm-50® **Injection** *(Discontinued)* see page 814

Neulasta™ **[US]** see pegfilgrastim on page 496

Neuleptil® **[Can]** see pericyazine *(Canada only)* on page 504

Neumega® **[US]** see oprelvekin on page 478

Neupogen® **[US/Can]** see filgrastim on page 272

Neuramate® *(Discontinued)* see page 814

Neuroforte-R® **[US]** see cyanocobalamin on page 167

Neurontin® **[US/Can]** see gabapentin on page 292

Neut® **[US]** see sodium bicarbonate on page 594

Neutra-Phos® **Capsule** *(Discontinued)* see page 814

Neutra-Phos®**-K [US]** see potassium phosphate on page 532

Neutra-Phos® **Powder [US]** see potassium phosphate and sodium phosphate on page 533

Neutrexin® **[US]** see trimetrexate glucuronate on page 657

Neutrogena® **Acne Mask [US-OTC]** see benzoyl peroxide on page 79

Neutrogena® **On The Spot**® **Acne Treatment [US-OTC]** see benzoyl peroxide on page 79

Neutrogena® **T/Derm [US]** see coal tar on page 158

Neutrogena® **T/Sal [US-OTC]** see coal tar and salicylic acid on page 158

nevirapine (ne VYE ra peen)
  U.S./Canadian Brand Names Viramune® [US/Can]
  Therapeutic Category Antiviral Agent
  Use In combination therapy with nucleoside antiretroviral agents in HIV-1 infected adults previously treated for whom current therapy is deemed inadequate
  Usual Dosage Adults: Oral: 200 mg once daily for 2 weeks followed by 200 mg twice daily
  Dosage Forms
    Suspension, oral: 50 mg/5 mL (240 mL)
    Tablet: 200 mg

New Decongestant® *(Discontinued)* see page 814

Nexium™ **[US]** see esomeprazole on page 237

N.G.A.® **Topical** *(Discontinued)* see page 814

Niac® *(Discontinued)* see page 814

Niacels™ *(Discontinued)* see page 814

niacin (NYE a sin)
  Synonyms nicotinic acid; vitamin B_3
  U.S./Canadian Brand Names Niacor® [US]; Niaspan® [US/Can]; Nicotinex [US-OTC]; Slo-Niacin® [US-OTC]
  Therapeutic Category Vitamin, Water Soluble
  Use Adjunctive treatment of hyperlipidemias; peripheral vascular disease and circulatory disorders; treatment of pellagra; dietary supplement
  Usual Dosage
    Children: Pellagra: Oral, I.M., I.V.: 50-100 mg/dose 3 times/day
    Oral: Recommended daily allowances:
      0-1 year: 6-8 mg/day
      2-6 years: 9-11 mg/day

7-10 years: 16 mg/day
>10 years: 15-18 mg/day
Adults: Oral:
  Hyperlipidemia: 1.5-6 g/day in 3 divided doses with or after meals
  Pellagra: 50 mg 3-10 times/day, maximum: 500 mg/day
  Niacin deficiency: 10-20 mg/day, maximum: 100 mg/day

Dosage Forms
  Capsule, extended release: 125 mg, 250 mg, 400 mg, 500 mg
  Capsule, timed release: 250 mg
  Elixir (Nicotinex): 50 mg/5 mL (473 mL) [contains alcohol 10% (sherry wine)]
  Tablet: 50 mg, 100 mg, 250 mg, 500 mg
    Niacor®: 500 mg
  Tablet, controlled release (Slo-Niacin®): 250 mg, 500 mg, 750 mg
  Tablet, extended release (Niaspan®): 500 mg, 750 mg, 1000 mg
  Tablet, timed release: 250 mg, 500 mg, 750 mg, 1000 mg

niacinamide (nye a SIN a mide)
Synonyms nicotinamide
Therapeutic Category Vitamin, Water Soluble
Use Prophylaxis and treatment of pellagra
Usual Dosage Oral:
  Children: Pellagra: 100-300 mg/day
  Adults: 50 mg 3-10 times/day
    Pellagra: 300-500 mg/day
    Hyperlipidemias: 1-2 g 3 times/day
Dosage Forms Tablet: 100 mg, 250 mg, 500 mg

niacin and lovastatin (NYE a sin & LOE va sta tin)
Synonyms lovastatin and niacin
U.S./Canadian Brand Names Advicor™ [US]
Therapeutic Category HMG-CoA Reductase Inhibitor; Vitamin, Water Soluble
Use Treatment of primary hypercholesterolemia (heterozygous familial and nonfamilial) and mixed dyslipidemia (Fredrickson types IIa and IIb) in patients previously treated with either agent alone (patients who require further lowering of triglycerides or increase in HDL-cholesterol from addition of niacin or further lowering of LDL-cholesterol from addition of lovastatin). Combination product; not intended for initial treatment.
Usual Dosage Dosage forms are a fixed combination of niacin and lovastatin.
  Oral: Adults: Lowest dose: Niacin 500 mg/lovastatin 20 mg; may increase by not more than 500 mg (niacin) at 4-week intervals (maximum dose: Niacin 2000 mg/lovastatin 40 mg daily); should be taken at bedtime with a low-fat snack
  Not for use as initial therapy of dyslipidemias. May be substituted for equivalent dose of Niaspan®, however manufacturer does not recommend direct substitution with other niacin products.
Dosage Forms Tablet, extended release (niacin) and immediate release (lovastatin): Niacin 500 mg and lovastatin 20 mg; niacin 750 mg and lovastatin 20 mg; niacin 1000 mg and lovastatin 20 mg

Niacor® [US] see niacin on previous page
Niaspan® [US/Can] see niacin on previous page
NiaStase® [Can] see eptacog alfa (activated) (Canada only) on page 231

nicardipine (nye KAR de peen)
Tall-Man niCARdipine
U.S./Canadian Brand Names Cardene® I.V. [US]; Cardene® SR [US]; Cardene® [US]
Therapeutic Category Calcium Channel Blocker
Use Chronic stable angina; management of essential hypertension
  (Continued)

nicardipine *(Continued)*

Usual Dosage Adults:

Oral: 40 mg 3 times/day (allow 3 days between dose increases)

Oral, sustained release: Initial: 30 mg twice daily, titrate up to 60 mg twice daily

I.V.: (Dilute to 0.1 mg/mL) Initial: 5 mg/hour increased by 2.5 mg/hour every 15 minutes to a maximum of 15 mg/hour

Oral to I.V. dose:

20 mg every 8 hours = I.V. 0.5 mg/hour

30 mg every 8 hours = I.V. 1.2 mg/hour

40 mg every 8 hours = I.V. 2.2 mg/hour

Dosage Forms

Capsule (Cardene®): 20 mg, 30 mg

Capsule, sustained release (Cardene® SR): 30 mg, 45 mg, 60 mg

Injection, solution (Cardene® IV): 2.5 mg/mL (10 mL)

N'ice® *(Discontinued)* see page 814

Niclocide® *(Discontinued)* see page 814

Nicobid® *(Discontinued)* see page 814

Nicoderm® [Can] see nicotine on this page

NicoDerm® CQ® [US-OTC] see nicotine on this page

Nicolar® *(Discontinued)* see page 814

Nicorette® [US/Can] see nicotine on this page

nicotinamide see niacinamide on previous page

nicotine (nik oh TEEN)

U.S./Canadian Brand Names Habitrol® [Can]; Nicoderm® [Can]; NicoDerm® CQ® [US-OTC]; Nicorette® [US/Can]; Nicotrol® Inhaler [US]; Nicotrol® NS [US]; Nicotrol® Patch [US/Can]

Therapeutic Category Smoking Deterrent

Use Treatment aid to giving up smoking while participating in a behavioral modification program, under medical supervision

Usual Dosage

Gum: Chew 1 piece of gum when urge to smoke, up to 30 pieces/day; most patients require 10-12 pieces of gum/day

Inhaler: Usually 6 to 16 cartridges per day; best effect was achieved by frequent continuous puffing (20 minutes); recommended duration of treatment is 3 months, after which patients may be weaned from the inhaler by gradual reduction of the daily dose over 6-12 weeks

Transdermal patch (patients should be advised to completely stop smoking upon initiation of therapy): Apply new patch every 24 hours to nonhairy, clean, dry skin on the upper body or upper outer arm; each patch should be applied to a different site

Initial starting dose: 21 mg/day for 4-8 weeks for most patients

First weaning dose: 14 mg/day for 2-4 weeks

Second weaning dose: 7 mg/day for 2-4 weeks

Initial starting dose for patients <100 pounds, smoke <10 cigarettes/day, have a history of cardiovascular disease: 14 mg/day for 4-8 weeks followed by 7 mg/day for 2-4 weeks

In patients who are receiving >600 mg/day of cimetidine: Decrease to the next lower patch size

Benefits of use of nicotine transdermal patches beyond 3 months have not been demonstrated

Spray: 1-2 sprays/hour; do not exceed more than 5 doses (10 sprays) per hour; each dose (2 sprays) contains 1 mg of nicotine. **Warning:** A dose of 40 mg can cause fatalities

Dosage Forms
Gum, chewing, as polacrilex (Nicorette®): 2 mg/square (48s, 108s, 168s); 4 mg/square (48s, 108s, 168s) [mint, orange, and original flavors]
Oral inhalation system (Nicotrol® Inhaler): 10 mg cartridge [delivering 4 mg nicotine] (42s) [each unit consists of 1 mouthpiece, 7 storage trays each containing 6 cartridges, and 1 storage case]
Patch, transdermal: 7 mg/24 (7s, 30s); 14 mg/24 hours (7s, 14s, 30s); 21 mg/24 hours (7s, 14s, 30s)
Kit: Step 1: 21 mg/24 hours (28s); Step 2: 14 mg/24 hours (14s); Step 3: 7 mg/24 hours (14s) [kit also contains support material]
NicoDerm® CQ® [clear patch]: 7 mg/24 hours (14s); 14 mg/24 hours (14s); 21 mg/24 hours (14s)
NicoDerm® CQ® [tan patch]: 7 mg/24 hours (14s); 14 mg/24 hours (14s); 21 mg/24 hours (7s, 14s)
Nicotrol®: 15 mg/16 hours (7s)
Nasal spray (Nicotrol® NS): 10 mg/mL (10 mL) [delivers 0.5 mg/spray; 200 sprays]

Nicotinex [US-OTC] *see* niacin *on page 456*

nicotinic acid *see* niacin *on page 456*

Nicotrol® Inhaler [US] *see* nicotine *on previous page*

Nicotrol® NS [US] *see* nicotine *on previous page*

Nicotrol® Patch [US/Can] *see* nicotine *on previous page*

Nico-Vert® *(Discontinued)* *see page 814*

Nidagel™ [Can] *see* metronidazole *on page 426*

Nidryl® *(Discontinued)* *see page 814*

Nifedical™ XL [US] *see* nifedipine *on this page*

nifedipine (nye FED i peen)
Tall-Man NIFEdipine
U.S./Canadian Brand Names Adalat® CC [US]; Adalat® XL® [Can]; Apo®-Nifed [Can]; Apo®-Nifed PA [Can]; Nifedical™ XL [US]; Novo-Nifedin [Can]; Nu-Nifed [Can]; Procardia® [US/Can]; Procardia XL® [US]
Therapeutic Category Calcium Channel Blocker
Use Angina, hypertrophic cardiomyopathy, hypertension
Usual Dosage Oral:
Children:
Hypertensive emergencies: 0.25-0.5 mg/kg/dose
Hypertrophic cardiomyopathy: 0.6-0.9 mg/kg/24 hours in 3-4 divided doses
Adults: Initial: 10 mg 3 times/day as capsules or 30-60 mg once daily as sustained release tablet; maintenance: 10-30 mg 3-4 times/day (capsules); maximum: 180 mg/24 hours (capsules) or 120 mg/day (sustained release)
Dosage Forms
Capsule, liquid-filled (Procardia®): 10 mg, 20 mg
Tablet, extended release: 30 mg, 60 mg, 90 mg
Adalat® CC, Procardia XL®: 30 mg, 60 mg, 90 mg
Nifedical™ XL: 30 mg, 60 mg

Niferex Forte® *(Discontinued)* *see page 814*

Niferex®-PN [US] *see* vitamin (multiple/oral) *on page 683*

Niferex® [US-OTC] *see* polysaccharide-iron complex *on page 527*

Night-Time Sleep Aid [US-OTC] *see* doxylamine *on page 216*

Nilandron™ [US] *see* nilutamide *on next page*

Niloric® *(Discontinued)* *see page 814*

Nilstat [Can] *see* nystatin *on page 473*

Nilstat® *(Discontinued)* *see page 814*

nilutamide (ni LU ta mide)
    U.S./Canadian Brand Names Anandron® [Can]; Nilandron™ [US]
    Therapeutic Category Antineoplastic Agent
    Use With orchiectomy (surgical castration) for the treatment of metastatic prostate cancer
    Usual Dosage Adults: Oral: 300 mg (6-50 mg tablets) once daily for 30 days, then 150 mg (3-50 mg tablets) once daily; starting on the same day or day after surgical castration
    Dosage Forms Tablet: 150 mg

Nimbex® **[US/Can]** *see cisatracurium on page 148*

nimodipine (nye MOE di peen)
    U.S./Canadian Brand Names Nimotop® [US/Can]
    Therapeutic Category Calcium Channel Blocker
    Use Improvement of neurological deficits due to spasm following subarachnoid hemorrhage from ruptured congenital intracranial aneurysms who are in good neurological condition postictus
    Usual Dosage Adults: Oral: 60 mg every 4 hours for 21 days, start therapy within 96 hours after subarachnoid hemorrhage
    Dosage Forms Capsule, liquid filled: 30 mg

Nimotop® **[US/Can]** *see nimodipine on this page*
Nipent™ **[US/Can]** *see pentostatin on page 502*
Nipride® **Injection** *(Discontinued)* *see page 814*
Nisaval® *(Discontinued)* *see page 814*

nisoldipine (NYE sole di peen)
    U.S./Canadian Brand Names Sular® [US]
    Therapeutic Category Calcium Channel Blocker
    Use Management of hypertension, may be used alone or in combination with other antihypertensive agents
    Usual Dosage Adults: Oral: Initial: 20 mg once daily, then increase by 10 mg per week (or longer intervals) to attain adequate control of blood pressure; doses >60 mg once daily are not recommended
    Dosage Forms Tablet, extended release: 10 mg, 20 mg, 30 mg, 40 mg

nitalapram *see citalopram on page 148*

nitisinone (ni TIS i known)
    U.S./Canadian Brand Names Orfadin® [US]
    Therapeutic Category 4-Hydroxyphenylpyruvate Dioxygenase Inhibitor
    Use Treatment of hereditary tyrosinemia type 1 (HT-1); to be used with dietary restriction of tyrosine and phenylalanine
    Usual Dosage Oral: **Note:** Must be used in conjunction with a low protein diet restricted in tyrosine and phenylalanine.
    Infants: See dosing for Children and Adults; infants may require maximal dose once liver function has improved
    Children and Adults: Initial: 1 mg/kg/day in divided doses, given in the morning and evening, 1 hour before meals; doses do not need to be divided evenly
    Dosage Forms Capsule: 2 mg, 5 mg, 10 mg

Nitoman® **[Can]** *see tetrabenazine (Canada only) on page 627*
Nitrek® **[US]** *see nitroglycerin on page 462*

nitric oxide (NYE trik OKS ide)

U.S./Canadian Brand Names INOmax® [US/Can]

Therapeutic Category Vasodilator, Pulmonary

Use Treatment of term and near-term (>34 weeks) neonates with hypoxic respiratory failure associated with pulmonary hypertension; used concurrently with ventilatory support and other agents

Usual Dosage Neonates (up to 14 days old): 20 ppm. Treatment should be maintained up to 14 days or until the underlying oxygen desaturation has resolved and the neonate is ready to be weaned from therapy. In the CINRGI trial, patients whose oxygenation improved had their dose reduced to 5 ppm at the end of 4 hours of treatment. Doses above 20 ppm should not be used because of the risk of methemoglobinemia and elevated NO_2.

Dosage Forms Gas, for inhalation:
100 ppm [nitric oxide 0.01% and nitrogen 99.9%] (353 L) [delivers 344 L], (1963 L) [delivers 1918 L]
800 ppm [nitric oxide 0.08% and nitrogen 99.92%] (353 L) [delivers 344 L], (1963 L) [delivers 1918 L]

Nitro-Bid® I.V. Injection *(Discontinued)* see page 814

Nitro-Bid® Ointment [US] see nitroglycerin on next page

Nitro-Bid® Oral *(Discontinued)* see page 814

Nitrocine® Oral *(Discontinued)* see page 814

Nitrodisc® Patch *(Discontinued)* see page 814

Nitro-Dur® [US/Can] see nitroglycerin on next page

nitrofural see nitrofurazone on this page

nitrofurantoin (nye troe fyoor AN toyn)

U.S./Canadian Brand Names Apo®-Nitrofurantoin [Can]; Furadantin® [US]; Macrobid® [US/Can]; Macrodantin® [US/Can]; Novo-Furantoin [Can]

Therapeutic Category Antibiotic, Miscellaneous

Use Prevention and treatment of urinary tract infections caused by susceptible gram-negative and some gram-positive organisms including *E. coli*, *Klebsiella*, *Enterobacter*, *Enterococa*, and *S. aureus*; *Pseudomonas*, *Serratia*, and most species of *Proteus* are generally resistant to nitrofurantoin

Usual Dosage Oral:
Children >1 month: 5-7 mg/kg/day divided every 6 hours; maximum: 400 mg/day
Chronic therapy: 1-2 mg/kg/day in divided doses every 12-24 hours; maximum dose: 400 mg/day
Adults: 50-100 mg/dose every 6 hours (not to exceed 400 mg/24 hours)
Prophylaxis: 50-100 mg/dose at bedtime

Dosage Forms
Capsule, macrocrystal: 50 mg, 100 mg
Macrodantin®: 25 mg, 50 mg, 100 mg
Capsule, macrocrystal/monohydrate (Macrobid®): 100 mg
Suspension, oral (Furadantin®): 25 mg/5 mL (470 mL)

nitrofurazone (nye troe FYOOR a zone)

Synonyms nitrofural

Therapeutic Category Antibacterial, Topical

Use Antibacterial agent used in second- and third-degree burns and skin grafting

Usual Dosage Children and Adults: Topical: Apply once daily or every few days to lesion or place on gauze

Dosage Forms
Cream: 0.2% (28 g)
Ointment, soluble dressing: 0.2% (28 g, 56 g, 454 g, 480 g)
Solution, topical: 0.2% (480 mL)

Nitrogard® [US] *see* nitroglycerin *on this page*

nitrogen mustard *see* mechlorethamine *on page 403*

nitroglycerin (nye troe GLI ser in)

Synonyms glyceryl trinitrate; nitroglycerol; NTG

U.S./Canadian Brand Names Minitran™ [US/Can]; Nitrek® [US]; Nitro-Bid® Ointment [US]; Nitro-Dur® [US/Can]; Nitrogard® [US]; Nitrol® [US/Can]; Nitrolingual® [US]; Nitrong® SR [Can]; NitroQuick® [US]; Nitrostat® [US/Can]; Nitro-Tab® [US]; NitroTime® [US]; Transderm-Nitro® [Can]

Therapeutic Category Vasodilator

Use Angina pectoris; I.V. for congestive heart failure (especially when associated with acute myocardial infarction); pulmonary hypertension; hypertensive emergencies occurring perioperatively (especially during cardiovascular surgery)

Usual Dosage Note: Hemodynamic and antianginal tolerance often develops within 24-48 hours of continuous nitrate administration

Children: Pulmonary hypertension: Continuous infusion: Start 0.25-0.5 mcg/kg/minute and titrate by 1 mcg/kg/minute at 20- to 60-minute intervals to desired effect; usual dose: 1-3 mcg/kg/minute; maximum: 5 mcg/kg/minute

Adults:

Oral: 2.5-9 mg 2-4 times/day (up to 26 mg 4 times/day)

I.V.: 5 mcg/minute, increase by 5 mcg/minute every 3-5 minutes to 20 mcg/minute; if no response at 20 mcg/minute increase by 10 mcg/minute every 3-5 minutes, up to 200 mcg/minute

Sublingual: 0.2-0.6 mg every 5 minutes for maximum of 3 doses in 15 minutes; may also use prophylactically 5-10 minutes prior to activities which may provoke an attack

Ointment: 1" to 2" every 8 hours up to 4" to 5" every 4 hours

Patch, transdermal: 0.2-0.4 mg/hour initially and titrate to doses of 0.4-0.8 mg/hour; tolerance is minimized by using a patch on period of 12-14 hours and patch off period of 10-12 hours

Translingual: 1-2 sprays into mouth under tongue every 3-5 minutes for maximum of 3 doses in 15 minutes, may also be used 5-10 minutes prior to activities which may provoke an attack prophylactically

Buccal: Initial: 1 mg every 3-5 hours while awake (3 times/day); titrate dosage upward if angina occurs with tablet in place

May need to use nitrate-free interval (10-12 hours/day) to avoid tolerance development; tolerance may possibly be reversed with acetylcysteine; gradually decrease dose in patients receiving NTG for prolonged period to avoid withdrawal reaction

Dosage Forms

Aerosol, translingual spray (Nitrolingual®): 0.4 mg/metered spray (12 g) [contains alcohol 20%; 200 metered sprays]

Capsule, extended release (Nitro-Time®): 2.5 mg, 6.5 mg, 9 mg

Infusion [premixed in D_5W]: 0.1 mg/mL (250 mL, 500 mL); 0.2 mg/mL (250 mL); 0.4 mg/mL (250 mL, 500 mL)

Injection, solution: 5 mg/mL (5 mL, 10 mL) [contains alcohol and propylene glycol]

Ointment, topical:

Nitro-Bid®: 2% [20 mg/g] (30 g, 60 g)

Nitrol®: 2% [20 mg/g] (3 g, 60 g)

Tablet, buccal, extended release (Nitrogard®): 2 mg, 3 mg

Tablet, sublingual (NitroQuick®, Nitrostat®, Nitro-Tab®): 0.3 mg, 0.4 mg, 0.6 mg

Transdermal system [once daily patch]: 0.1 mg/hour (30s); 0.2 mg/hour (30s); 0.4 mg/hour (30s); 0.6 mg/hour (30s)

Minitran™: 0.1 mg/hour (30s); 0.2 mg/hour (30s); 0.4 mg/hour (30s); 0.6 mg/hour (30s)

Nitrek®: 0.2 mg/hour (30s); 0.4 mg/hour (30s); 0.6 mg/hour (30s)

Nitro-Dur®: 0.1 mg/hour (30s); 0.2 mg/hour (30s); 0.3 mg/hour (30s); 0.4 mg/hour (30s); 0.6 mg/hour (30s); 0.8 mg/hour (30s)

nitroglycerol *see* nitroglycerin *on this page*

Nitrol® **[US/Can]** *see* nitroglycerin *on previous page*
Nitrolingual® **[US]** *see* nitroglycerin *on previous page*
Nitrong® **Oral Tablet** *(Discontinued)* *see page 814*
Nitrong® **SR [Can]** *see* nitroglycerin *on previous page*
Nitropress® **[US]** *see* nitroprusside *on this page*

nitroprusside (nye troe PRUS ide)
  Synonyms sodium nitroferricyanide
  U.S./Canadian Brand Names Nitropress® [US]
  Therapeutic Category Vasodilator
  Use Management of hypertensive crises; congestive heart failure; used for controlled hypotension during anesthesia
  Usual Dosage I.V.:
    Children: Continuous infusion:
      Initial: 1 mcg/kg/minute by continuous I.V. infusion; increase in increments of 1 mcg/kg/minute at intervals of 20-60 minutes; titrating to the desired response
      Usual dose: 3 mcg/kg/minute; rarely need >4 mcg/kg/minute
      Maximum: 10 mcg/kg/minute. Dilute 15 mg x weight (kg) to 250 mL D_5W, then dose in mcg/kg/minute = infusion rate in mL/hour
    Adults: Begin at 5 mcg/kg/minute; increase in increments of 5 mcg/kg/minute (up to 20 mcg/kg/minute), then in increments of 10-20 mcg/kg/minute; titrating to the desired hemodynamic effect or the appearance of headache or nausea. When >500 mcg/kg is administered by prolonged infusion of faster than 2 mcg/kg/minute, cyanide is generated faster than an unaided patient can handle.
  Dosage Forms
    Injection, powder for reconstitution, as sodium: 50 mg
    Injection, solution, as sodium: 25 mg/mL (2 mL)

NitroQuick® **[US]** *see* nitroglycerin *on previous page*
Nitrostat® **[US/Can]** *see* nitroglycerin *on previous page*
Nitrostat® **0.15 mg Tablet** *(Discontinued)* *see page 814*
Nitro-Tab® **[US]** *see* nitroglycerin *on previous page*
NitroTime® **[US]** *see* nitroglycerin *on previous page*

nitrous oxide (NYE trus OKS ide)
  Therapeutic Category Anesthetic, Gas
  Use Produces sedation and analgesia; principal adjunct to inhalation and intravenous general anesthesia
  Usual Dosage Children and Adults: For sedation and analgesia: Concentrations of 25% to 50% nitrous oxide with oxygen. For general anesthesia, concentrations of 40% to 70% via mask or endotracheal tube. Minimal alveolar concentration or (MAC) ED_{50} is 105%, therefore delivery in a hyperbaric chamber is necessary to use as a complete anesthetic; when administered at 70%, reduces the MAC of other anesthetics by half.

Nix® **[US/Can]** *see* permethrin *on page 505*
Nix® **Dermal Cream [Can]** *see* permethrin *on page 505*

nizatidine (ni ZA ti deen)
  U.S./Canadian Brand Names Apo®-Nizatidine [Can]; Axid® AR [US-OTC]; Axid® [US/Can]; Novo-Nizatidine [Can]
  Therapeutic Category Histamine H_2 Antagonist
  Use Treatment and maintenance of duodenal ulcer; treatment of gastroesophageal reflux disease (GERD)
  Usual Dosage Adults: Active duodenal ulcer: Oral:
    Treatment: 300 mg at bedtime or 150 mg twice daily
    (Continued)

nizatidine *(Continued)*
Maintenance: 150 mg/day
Dosage Forms
Capsule (Axid®): 150 mg, 300 mg
Tablet (Axid® AR): 75 mg

Nizoral® **[US/Can]** *see* ketoconazole *on page 367*

Nizoral® A-D **[US-OTC]** *see* ketoconazole *on page 367*

n-methylhydrazine *see* procarbazine *on page 542*

Noctec® *(Discontinued)* *see page 814*

Nolahist® **[US/Can]** *see* phenindamine *on page 507*

Nolamine® *(Discontinued)* *see page 814*

Nolex® LA *(Discontinued)* *see page 814*

Noludar® *(Discontinued)* *see page 814*

Nolvadex® **[US/Can]** *see* tamoxifen *on page 618*

Nolvadex®-D **[Can]** *see* tamoxifen *on page 618*

Nonbac® **[US]** *see* butalbital, acetaminophen, and caffeine *on page 99*

nonoxynol 9 (non OKS i nole nine)
U.S./Canadian Brand Names Advantage 24™ [Can]; Advantage-S™ [US-OTC]; Aqua Lube Plus [US-OTC]; Conceptrol® [US-OTC]; Delfen® [US-OTC]; Emko® [US-OTC]; Encare® [US-OTC]; Gynol II® [US-OTC]; Semicid® [US-OTC]; Shur-Seal® [US-OTC]; VCF™ [US-OTC]
Therapeutic Category Spermicide
Use Spermatocide in contraception
Usual Dosage Insert into vagina at least 15 minutes before intercourse
Dosage Forms
Film, vaginal (VCF™): 28% (3s, 6s,12s)
Foam, vaginal:
  Delfen: 12.5% (17 g)
  Emko®: 8% (40 g, 90 g)
  VCF™: 12.5% (40 g)
Gel, vaginal:
  Advantage-S™: 3.5% (1.5 g) [packaged in 3s or 6s with reusable applicator]; (30g) [packaged with reusable applicator]
  Aqua Lube Plus: 1% (60 g, 120 g)
  Conceptrol®: 4% (2.7 g) [packaged in 10s with applicator]
  Gynol II: 2% (85 g, 114 g)
  Shur-Seal®: 2% (6 g) [packaged in 24s]
Suppository, vaginal:
  Encare®: 100 mg (12s, 18s)
  Semicid®: 100 mg (9s, 18s)

No Pain-HP® *(Discontinued)* *see page 814*

noradrenaline acid tartrate *see* norepinephrine *on next page*

Norcet® *(Discontinued)* *see page 814*

Norco® **[US]** *see* hydrocodone and acetaminophen *on page 329*

Norcuron® **[US/Can]** *see* vecuronium *on page 674*

nordeoxyguanosine *see* ganciclovir *on page 293*

Nordette® **[US]** *see* ethinyl estradiol and levonorgestrel *on page 248*

Norditropin® **[US/Can]** *see* human growth hormone *on page 324*

Norditropin® Cartridges **[US]** *see* human growth hormone *on page 324*

Nordryl® **Injection** *(Discontinued)* *see page 814*

Nordryl® **Oral** *(Discontinued)* *see page 814*

norelgestromin and ethinyl estradiol *see* ethinyl estradiol and norelgestromin *on page 250*

norepinephrine (nor ep i NEF rin)

Synonyms noradrenaline acid tartrate

U.S./Canadian Brand Names Levophed® [US/Can]

Therapeutic Category Adrenergic Agonist Agent

Use Treatment of shock which persists after adequate fluid volume replacement; severe hypotension; cardiogenic shock

Usual Dosage Note: Dose stated in terms of norepinephrine base. I.V.:
Children: Initial: 0.05-0.1 mcg/kg/minute, titrate to desired effect; rate (mL/hour) = dose (mcg/kg/minute) x weight (kg) x 60 minutes/hour divided by concentration (mcg/mL)
Adults: 8-12 mcg/minute as an infusion; initiate at 4 mcg/minute and titrate to desired response

Dosage Forms Injection, solution, as bitartrate: 1 mg/mL (4 mL) [contains sodium metabisulfite]

Norethin™ 1/35E *(Discontinued)* *see page 814*

norethindrone (nor eth IN drone)

Synonyms norethisterone

U.S./Canadian Brand Names Aygestin® [US]; Micronor® [US/Can]; Norlutate® [Can]; Nor-QD® [US]

Therapeutic Category Contraceptive, Progestin Only; Progestin

Use Treatment of amenorrhea; abnormal uterine bleeding; endometriosis

Usual Dosage Adolescents and Adults: Oral:
Amenorrhea and abnormal uterine bleeding: 2.5-10 mg on days 5-25 of menstrual cycle
Endometriosis: 5 mg/day for 14 days; increase at increments of 2.5 mg/day every 2 weeks up to 15 mg/day

Dosage Forms
Tablet (Micronor®, Nor-QD®): 0.35 mg
Tablet, as acetate (Aygestin®): 5 mg

norethindrone acetate and ethinyl estradiol *see* ethinyl estradiol and norethindrone *on page 251*

norethindrone and mestranol *see* mestranol and norethindrone *on page 412*

norethisterone *see* norethindrone *on this page*

Norflex™ [US/Can] *see* orphenadrine *on page 480*

norfloxacin (nor FLOKS a sin)

U.S./Canadian Brand Names Apo®-Norflox [Can]; Noroxin® [US/Can]; Novo-Norfloxacin [Can]; Riva-Norfloxacin [Can]

Therapeutic Category Quinolone

Use Complicated and uncomplicated urinary tract infections caused by susceptible gram-negative and gram-positive bacteria

Usual Dosage Adults: Oral: 400 mg twice daily for 7-21 days depending on infection

Dosage Forms Tablet: 400 mg

Norgesic™ [US/Can] *see* orphenadrine, aspirin, and caffeine *on page 480*

Norgesic™ Forte [US/Can] *see* orphenadrine, aspirin, and caffeine *on page 480*

norgestimate and estradiol *see* estradiol and norgestimate *on page 239*

norgestimate and ethinyl estradiol *see* ethinyl estradiol and norgestimate *on page 254*

norgestrel (nor JES trel)
U.S./Canadian Brand Names Ovrette® [US/Can]
Therapeutic Category Contraceptive, Progestin Only
Use Prevention of pregnancy; treatment of hypermenorrhea, endometriosis, female hypogonadism
Usual Dosage Oral: Administer daily, starting the first day of menstruation, administer one tablet at the same time each day, every day of the year. If one dose is missed, administer as soon as remembered, then next tablet at regular time; if two doses are missed, administer one tablet and discard the other, then administer daily at usual time; if three doses are missed, use an additional form of birth control until menses or pregnancy is ruled out
Dosage Forms Tablet: 0.075 mg [contains tartrazine]

norgestrel and ethinyl estradiol *see* ethinyl estradiol and norgestrel *on page 255*

Norinyl® 1+35 [US] *see* ethinyl estradiol and norethindrone *on page 251*

Norinyl® 1+50 [US] *see* mestranol and norethindrone *on page 412*

Noritate™ [US/Can] *see* metronidazole *on page 426*

Norlutate® [Can] *see* norethindrone *on previous page*

Norlutate® *(Discontinued) see page 814*

Norlutin® *(Discontinued) see page 814*

normal saline *see* sodium chloride *on page 595*

Normiflo® *(Discontinued) see page 814*

Normodyne® [US/Can] *see* labetalol *on page 370*

Noroxin® [US/Can] *see* norfloxacin *on previous page*

Norpace® [US/Can] *see* disopyramide *on page 207*

Norpace® CR [US] *see* disopyramide *on page 207*

Norplant® Implant [Can] *see* levonorgestrel *on page 381*

Norplant® Implant *(Discontinued) see page 814*

Norpramin® [US/Can] *see* desipramine *on page 181*

Nor-QD® [US] *see* norethindrone *on previous page*

North American coral snake antivenin *see* antivenin *(Micrurus fulvius) on page 48*

North and South American antisnake-bite serum *see* antivenin *(Crotalidae)* polyvalent *on page 48*

Nortrel™ [US] *see* ethinyl estradiol and norethindrone *on page 251*

nortriptyline (nor TRIP ti leen)
U.S./Canadian Brand Names Alti-Nortriptyline [Can]; Apo®-Nortriptyline [Can]; Aventyl® HCl [US/Can]; Gen-Nortriptyline [Can]; Norventyl [Can]; Novo-Nortriptyline [Can]; Nu-Nortriptyline [Can]; Pamelor® [US/Can]; PMS-Nortriptyline [Can]
Therapeutic Category Antidepressant, Tricyclic (Secondary Amine)
Use Treatment of various forms of depression, often in conjunction with psychotherapy; nocturnal enuresis
Usual Dosage Oral:
Adults: 25 mg 3-4 times/day up to 150 mg/day
Adolescents and Elderly: 30-50 mg/day in divided doses
Dosage Forms
Capsule, as hydrochloride: 10 mg, 25 mg, 50 mg, 75 mg
Aventyl® HCl: 10 mg, 25 mg
Pamelor®: 10 mg, 25 mg, 50 mg, 75 mg [may contain benzyl alcohol; 50 mg may also contain sodium bisulfite]

Solution, as hydrochloride (Aventyl® HCl, Pamelor®): 10 mg/5 mL (473 mL) [contains alcohol 4% and benzoic acid]

Norvasc® **[US/Can]** *see* amlodipine *on page 35*

Norventyl [Can] *see* nortriptyline *on previous page*

Norvir® **[US/Can]** *see* ritonavir *on page 575*

Norvir® **SEC [Can]** *see* ritonavir *on page 575*

Norzine® *(Discontinued) see page 814*

Nōstrilla® **[US-OTC]** *see* oxymetazoline *on page 486*

Nostril® **Nasal [US-OTC]** *see* phenylephrine *on page 510*

Novacet® **[US]** *see* sulfur and sulfacetamide *on page 615*

Novafed® *(Discontinued) see page 814*

Novahistex® **DM Decongestant [Can]** *see* pseudoephedrine and dextromethorphan *on page 553*

Novahistex® **DM Decongestant Expectorant [Can]** *see* guaifenesin, pseudoephedrine, and dextromethorphan *on page 312*

Novahistex® **Expectorant With Decongestant [Can]** *see* guaifenesin and pseudoephedrine *on page 310*

Novahistine® **DM Decongestant [Can]** *see* pseudoephedrine and dextromethorphan *on page 553*

Novahistine® **DM Decongestant Expectorant [Can]** *see* guaifenesin, pseudoephedrine, and dextromethorphan *on page 312*

Novahistine DMX® **Liquid** *(Discontinued) see page 814*

Novahistine® **Elixir** *(Discontinued) see page 814*

Novahistine® **Expectorant** *(Discontinued) see page 814*

Novamilor [Can] *see* amiloride and hydrochlorothiazide *on page 32*

Novamoxin® **[Can]** *see* amoxicillin *on page 37*

Novantrone® **[US/Can]** *see* mitoxantrone *on page 433*

Novarel™ **[US]** *see* chorionic gonadotropin (human) *on page 144*

Novasen [Can] *see* aspirin *on page 58*

Novo-Acebutolol [Can] *see* acebutolol *on page 3*

Novo-Alprazol [Can] *see* alprazolam *on page 24*

Novo-Amiodarone [Can] *see* amiodarone *on page 34*

Novo-Ampicillin [Can] *see* ampicillin *on page 40*

Novo-ASA [Can] *see* mesalamine *on page 411*

Novo-Atenol [Can] *see* atenolol *on page 60*

Novo-AZT [Can] *see* zidovudine *on page 689*

Novo-Benzydamine [Can] *see* benzydamine *(Canada only) on page 81*

Novo-Bromazepam [Can] *see* bromazepam *(Canada only) on page 92*

Novo-Buspirone [Can] *see* buspirone *on page 98*

Novocain® **[US/Can]** *see* procaine *on page 541*

Novo-Captopril [Can] *see* captopril *on page 112*

Novo-Carbamaz [Can] *see* carbamazepine *on page 113*

Novo-Cefaclor [Can] *see* cefaclor *on page 120*

Novo-Cefadroxil [Can] *see* cefadroxil *on page 121*

Novo-Cholamine [Can] *see* cholestyramine resin *on page 143*

Novo-Cholamine Light [Can] *see* cholestyramine resin *on page 143*

Novo-Cimetidine [Can] *see* cimetidine *on page 146*

Novo-Clobazam [Can] *see* clobazam *(Canada only) on page 152*

Novo-Clobetasol [Can] *see* clobetasol *on page 152*

Novo-Clonazepam [Can] *see* clonazepam *on page 154*

Novo-Clonidine [Can] *see* clonidine *on page 155*

Novo-Clopate [Can] *see* clorazepate *on page 156*

Novo-Clopramine [Can] *see* clomipramine *on page 154*

Novo-Cloxin [Can] *see* cloxacillin *on page 157*

Novo-Cycloprine [Can] *see* cyclobenzaprine *on page 168*

Novo-Cyproterone [Can] *see* cyproterone *(Canada only) on page 170*

Novo-Desipramine [Can] *see* desipramine *on page 181*

Novo-Difenac® [Can] *see* diclofenac *on page 193*

Novo-Difenac-K [Can] *see* diclofenac *on page 193*

Novo-Difenac® SR [Can] *see* diclofenac *on page 193*

Novo-Diflunisal [Can] *see* diflunisal *on page 196*

Novo-Diltazem [Can] *see* diltiazem *on page 199*

Novo-Diltazem SR [Can] *see* diltiazem *on page 199*

Novo-Dipiradol [Can] *see* dipyridamole *on page 206*

Novo-Divalproex [Can] *see* valproic acid and derivatives *on page 670*

Novo-Domperidone [Can] *see* domperidone *(Canada only) on page 211*

Novo-Doxazosin [Can] *see* doxazosin *on page 213*

Novo-Doxepin [Can] *see* doxepin *on page 213*

Novo-Doxylin [Can] *see* doxycycline *on page 215*

Novo-Famotidine [Can] *see* famotidine *on page 262*

Novo-Fluoxetine [Can] *see* fluoxetine *on page 279*

Novo-Flurprofen [Can] *see* flurbiprofen *on page 282*

Novo-Flutamide [Can] *see* flutamide *on page 282*

Novo-Fluvoxamine [Can] *see* fluvoxamine *on page 285*

Novo-Furantoin [Can] *see* nitrofurantoin *on page 461*

Novo-Gemfibrozil [Can] *see* gemfibrozil *on page 295*

Novo-Gliclazide [Can] *see* gliclazide *(Canada only) on page 299*

Novo-Glyburide [Can] *see* glyburide *on page 301*

Novo-Hydroxyzin [Can] *see* hydroxyzine *on page 339*

Novo-Hylazin [Can] *see* hydralazine *on page 327*

Novo-Indapamide [Can] *see* indapamide *on page 348*

Novo-Ipramide [Can] *see* ipratropium *on page 358*

Novo-Keto [Can] *see* ketoprofen *on page 368*

Novo-Ketoconazole [Can] *see* ketoconazole *on page 367*

Novo-Keto-EC [Can] *see* ketoprofen *on page 368*

Novo-Ketorolac [Can] *see* ketorolac *on page 368*

Novo-Ketotifen [Can] *see* ketotifen *on page 368*

Novo-Levobunolol [Can] *see* levobunolol *on page 379*

Novo-Lexin® [Can] *see* cephalexin *on page 128*

Novolin® 70/30 [US] *see* insulin preparations *on page 352*
Novolin®ge [Can] *see* insulin preparations *on page 352*
Novolin® L [US] *see* insulin preparations *on page 352*
Novolin® N [US] *see* insulin preparations *on page 352*
Novolin® R [US] *see* insulin preparations *on page 352*
NovoLog® [US] *see* insulin preparations *on page 352*
Novo-Loperamide [Can] *see* loperamide *on page 390*
Novo-Lorazem® [Can] *see* lorazepam *on page 391*
Novo-Medrone [Can] *see* medroxyprogesterone acetate *on page 404*
Novo-Meprazine [Can] *see* methotrimeprazine *(Canada only) on page 418*
Novo-Metformin [Can] *see* metformin *on page 414*
Novo-Methacin [Can] *see* indomethacin *on page 349*
Novo-Metoprolol [Can] *see* metoprolol *on page 425*
Novo-Mexiletine [Can] *see* mexiletine *on page 427*
Novo-Minocycline [Can] *see* minocycline *on page 431*
Novo-Moclobemide [Can] *see* moclobemide *(Canada only) on page 434*
Novo-Mucilax [Can] *see* psyllium *on page 554*
Novo-Nadolol [Can] *see* nadolol *on page 443*
Novo-Naprox [Can] *see* naproxen *on page 447*
Novo-Naprox Sodium [Can] *see* naproxen *on page 447*
Novo-Naprox Sodium DS [Can] *see* naproxen *on page 447*
Novo-Naprox SR [Can] *see* naproxen *on page 447*
Novo-Nidazol [Can] *see* metronidazole *on page 426*
Novo-Nifedin [Can] *see* nifedipine *on page 459*
Novo-Nizatidine [Can] *see* nizatidine *on page 463*
Novo-Norfloxacin [Can] *see* norfloxacin *on page 465*
Novo-Nortriptyline [Can] *see* nortriptyline *on page 466*
Novo-Oxybutynin [Can] *see* oxybutynin *on page 484*
Novo-Pen-VK® [Can] *see* penicillin V potassium *on page 499*
Novo-Peridol [Can] *see* haloperidol *on page 316*
Novo-Pindol [Can] *see* pindolol *on page 516*
Novo-Pirocam® [Can] *see* piroxicam *on page 517*
Novo-Prazin [Can] *see* prazosin *on page 536*
Novo-Profen® [Can] *see* ibuprofen *on page 342*
Novo-Ranidine [Can] *see* ranitidine hydrochloride *on page 564*
Novo-Salmol [Can] *see* albuterol *on page 18*
Novo-Selegiline [Can] *see* selegiline *on page 586*
Novo-Sertraline [Can] *see* sertraline *on page 589*
Novo-Seven® [US] *see* factor VIIa (recombinant) *on page 262*
Novo-Sotalol [Can] *see* sotalol *on page 602*
Novo-Spiroton [Can] *see* spironolactone *on page 604*
Novo-Spirozine [Can] *see* hydrochlorothiazide and spironolactone *on page 329*
Novo-Sucralate [Can] *see* sucralfate *on page 609*
Novo-Sundac [Can] *see* sulindac *on page 615*

Novo-Tamoxifen [Can] *see* tamoxifen *on page 618*

Novo-Temazepam [Can] *see* temazepam *on page 621*

Novo-Terazosin [Can] *see* terazosin *on page 622*

Novo-Tetra [Can] *see* tetracycline *on page 628*

Novo-Theophyl SR [Can] *see* theophylline *on page 630*

Novothyrox [US] *see* levothyroxine *on page 382*

Novo-Tiaprofenic [Can] *see* tiaprofenic acid *(Canada only) on page 638*

Novo-Trazodone [Can] *see* trazodone *on page 649*

Novo-Triamzide [Can] *see* hydrochlorothiazide and triamterene *on page 329*

Novo-Trimel [Can] *see* sulfamethoxazole and trimethoprim *on page 612*

Novo-Trimel D.S. [Can] *see* sulfamethoxazole and trimethoprim *on page 612*

Novo-Tripramine [Can] *see* trimipramine *on page 658*

Novo-Veramil [Can] *see* verapamil *on page 675*

Novo-Veramil SR [Can] *see* verapamil *on page 675*

Nozinan® [Can] *see* methotrimeprazine *(Canada only) on page 418*

NP-27® *(Discontinued)* *see page 814*

NPH Iletin® II [US] *see* insulin preparations *on page 352*

NTG *see* nitroglycerin *on page 462*

NTZ® Long Acting Nasal Solution *(Discontinued)* *see page 814*

Nu-Acebutolol [Can] *see* acebutolol *on page 3*

Nu-Acyclovir [Can] *see* acyclovir *on page 13*

Nu-Alprax [Can] *see* alprazolam *on page 24*

Nu-Amilzide [Can] *see* amiloride and hydrochlorothiazide *on page 32*

Nu-Amoxi [Can] *see* amoxicillin *on page 37*

Nu-Ampi [Can] *see* ampicillin *on page 40*

Nu-Atenol *see* atenolol *on page 60*

Nu-Baclo [Can] *see* baclofen *on page 70*

Nubain® [US/Can] *see* nalbuphine *on page 444*

Nu-Beclomethasone [Can] *see* beclomethasone *on page 73*

Nu-Bromazepam [Can] *see* bromazepam *(Canada only) on page 92*

Nu-Buspirone [Can] *see* buspirone *on page 98*

Nu-Capto® [Can] *see* captopril *on page 112*

Nu-Carbamazepine® [Can] *see* carbamazepine *on page 113*

Nu-Cefaclor [Can] *see* cefaclor *on page 120*

Nu-Cephalex® [Can] *see* cephalexin *on page 128*

Nu-Cimet® [Can] *see* cimetidine *on page 146*

Nu-Clonazepam [Can] *see* clonazepam *on page 154*

Nu-Clonidine® [Can] *see* clonidine *on page 155*

Nu-Cloxi® [Can] *see* cloxacillin *on page 157*

Nucofed® Expectorant [US] *see* guaifenesin, pseudoephedrine, and codeine *on page 311*

Nucofed® Pediatric Expectorant [US] *see* guaifenesin, pseudoephedrine, and codeine *on page 311*

Nu-Cotrimox® [Can] *see* sulfamethoxazole and trimethoprim *on page 612*

Nucotuss® [US] *see* guaifenesin, pseudoephedrine, and codeine *on page 311*

Nu-Cromolyn [Can] *see* cromolyn sodium *on page 166*

Nu-Cyclobenzaprine [Can] *see* cyclobenzaprine *on page 168*

Nu-Desipramine [Can] *see* desipramine *on page 181*

Nu-Diclo [Can] *see* diclofenac *on page 193*

Nu-Diclo-SR [Can] *see* diclofenac *on page 193*

Nu-Diflunisal [Can] *see* diflunisal *on page 196*

Nu-Diltiaz [Can] *see* diltiazem *on page 199*

Nu-Diltiaz-CD [Can] *see* diltiazem *on page 199*

Nu-Divalproex [Can] *see* valproic acid and derivatives *on page 670*

Nu-Domperidone [Can] *see* domperidone *(Canada only) on page 211*

Nu-Doxycycline [Can] *see* doxycycline *on page 215*

Nu-Erythromycin-S [Can] *see* erythromycin (systemic) *on page 235*

Nu-Famotidine [Can] *see* famotidine *on page 262*

Nu-Fenofibrate [Can] *see* fenofibrate *on page 265*

Nu-Fluoxetine [Can] *see* fluoxetine *on page 279*

Nu-Flurprofen [Can] *see* flurbiprofen *on page 282*

Nu-Fluvoxamine [Can] *see* fluvoxamine *on page 285*

Nu-Gemfibrozil [Can] *see* gemfibrozil *on page 295*

Nu-Glyburide [Can] *see* glyburide *on page 301*

Nu-Hydral [Can] *see* hydralazine *on page 327*

Nu-Ibuprofen [Can] *see* ibuprofen *on page 342*

Nu-Indapamide [Can] *see* indapamide *on page 348*

Nu-Indo [Can] *see* indomethacin *on page 349*

Nu-Ipratropium [Can] *see* ipratropium *on page 358*

Nu-Iron® [US-OTC] *see* polysaccharide-iron complex *on page 527*

Nu-Ketoprofen [Can] *see* ketoprofen *on page 368*

Nu-Ketoprofen-E [Can] *see* ketoprofen *on page 368*

NuLev™ [US] *see* hyoscyamine *on page 339*

Nu-Levocarb [Can] *see* levodopa and carbidopa *on page 380*

Nullo® [US-OTC] *see* chlorophyll *on page 135*

Nu-Loraz [Can] *see* lorazepam *on page 391*

Nu-Loxapine [Can] *see* loxapine *on page 394*

NuLytely® [US] *see* polyethylene glycol-electrolyte solution *on page 525*

Nu-Medopa [Can] *see* methyldopa *on page 420*

Nu-Mefenamic [Can] *see* mefenamic acid *on page 405*

Nu-Megestrol [Can] *see* megestrol acetate *on page 405*

Nu-Metformin [Can] *see* metformin *on page 414*

Nu-Metoclopramide [Can] *see* metoclopramide *on page 424*

Nu-Metop [Can] *see* metoprolol *on page 425*

Nu-Moclobemide [Can] *see* moclobemide *(Canada only) on page 434*

Numorphan® [US/Can] *see* oxymorphone *on page 487*

Numzident® *(Discontinued)* *see page 814*

Nu-Naprox [Can] *see* naproxen *on page 447*

Nu-Nifed [Can] *see* nifedipine *on page 459*

Nu-Nortriptyline [Can] *see* nortriptyline *on page 466*

Nu-Oxybutyn [Can] *see* oxybutynin *on page 484*

Nu-Pentoxifylline SR [Can] *see* pentoxifylline *on page 502*

Nu-Pen-VK® [Can] *see* penicillin V potassium *on page 499*

Nupercainal® [US-OTC] *see* dibucaine *on page 192*

Nu-Pindol [Can] *see* pindolol *on page 516*

Nu-Pirox [Can] *see* piroxicam *on page 517*

Nu-Prazo [Can] *see* prazosin *on page 536*

Nu-Prochlor [Can] *see* prochlorperazine *on page 542*

Nu-Propranolol [Can] *see* propranolol *on page 549*

Nuquin® Gel [US] *see* hydroquinone *on page 336*

Nuquin HP® Cream [US] *see* hydroquinone *on page 336*

Nu-Ranit [Can] *see* ranitidine hydrochloride *on page 564*

Nuromax® [US/Can] *see* doxacurium *on page 212*

Nursoy® *(Discontinued)* *see page 814*

Nu-Selegiline [Can] *see* selegiline *on page 586*

Nu-Sotalol [Can] *see* sotalol *on page 602*

Nu-Sucralate [Can] *see* sucralfate *on page 609*

Nu-Sulfinpyrazone [Can] *see* sulfinpyrazone *on page 614*

Nu-Sundac [Can] *see* sulindac *on page 615*

Nu-Tears® II [US-OTC] *see* artificial tears *on page 56*

Nu-Tears® [US-OTC] *see* artificial tears *on page 56*

Nu-Temazepam [Can] *see* temazepam *on page 621*

Nu-Terazosin [Can] *see* terazosin *on page 622*

Nu-Tetra [Can] *see* tetracycline *on page 628*

Nu-Tiaprofenic [Can] *see* tiaprofenic acid *(Canada only) on page 638*

Nu-Ticlopidine [Can] *see* ticlopidine *on page 639*

Nu-Timolol [Can] *see* timolol *on page 639*

Nutracort® [US] *see* hydrocortisone (topical) *on page 334*

Nutraplus® [US-OTC] *see* urea *on page 666*

Nu-Trazodone [Can] *see* trazodone *on page 649*

Nu-Triazide [Can] *see* hydrochlorothiazide and triamterene *on page 329*

Nutrilipid® [US] *see* fat emulsion *on page 263*

Nu-Trimipramine [Can] *see* trimipramine *on page 658*

nutritional formula, enteral/oral

(noo TRISH un al FOR myoo la, EN ter al/OR al)

Synonyms dietary supplements

U.S./Canadian Brand Names Carnation Instant Breakfast® [US-OTC]; Citrotein® [US-OTC]; Criticare HN® [US-OTC]; Ensure Plus® [US-OTC]; Ensure® [US-OTC]; Isocal® [US-OTC]; Magnacal® [US-OTC]; Microlipid™ [US-OTC]; Osmolite® HN [US-OTC]; Pedialyte® [US-OTC]; Portagen® [US-OTC]; Pregestimil® [US-OTC]; Propac™ [US-OTC]; Soyalac® [US-OTC]; Vital HN® [US-OTC]; Vitaneed™ [US-OTC]; Vivonex® T.E.N. [US-OTC]; Vivonex® [US-OTC]

Therapeutic Category Nutritional Supplement

Dosage Forms

Liquid: Calcium and sodium caseinate, maltodextrin, sucrose, partially hydrogenated soy oil, soy lecithin

Powder: Amino acids, predigested carbohydrates, safflower oil

Nutropin® **[US]** *see* human growth hormone *on page 324*

Nutropin AQ® **[US/Can]** *see* human growth hormone *on page 324*

Nutropin Depot® **[US]** *see* human growth hormone *on page 324*

NuvaRing® **[US]** *see* ethinyl estradiol and etonogestrel *on page 247*

Nu-Verap [Can] *see* verapamil *on page 675*

Nu-Zopiclone [Can] *see* zopiclone *(Canada only) on page 693*

Nyaderm [Can] *see* nystatin *on this page*

Nydrazid® **[US]** *see* isoniazid *on page 361*

nystatin (nye STAT in)
    U.S./Canadian Brand Names Bio-Statin® [US]; Candistatin® [Can]; Mycostatin® [US/ Can]; Nilstat [Can]; Nyaderm [Can]; Nystat-Rx® [US]; Nystop® [US]; Pedi-Dri® [US]; PMS-Nystatin [Can]
    Therapeutic Category Antifungal Agent
    Use Treatment of susceptible cutaneous, mucocutaneous, oral cavity and vaginal fungal infections normally caused by the *Candida* species
    Usual Dosage
      Oral candidiasis:
        Infants: 200,000 units 4 times/day or 100,000 units to each side of mouth 4 times/day
        Children and Adults: 400,000-600,000 units 4 times/day; troche: 200,000-400,000 units 4-5 times/day
      Cutaneous candidal infections: Children and Adults: Topical: Apply 3-4 times/day
      Intestinal infections: Adults: Oral: 500,000-1,000,000 units every 8 hours
      Vaginal infections: Adults: Vaginal tablets: Insert 1-2 tablets/day at bedtime for 2 weeks
    Dosage Forms
      Capsule (Bio-Statin®): 500,000 units, 1 million units
      Cream: 100,000 units/g (15 g, 30 g)
      Mycostatin®: 100,000 units/g (30 g)
      Lozenge (Mycostatin®): 200,000 units
      Ointment, topical: 100,000 units/g (15 g, 30 g)
      Powder, for prescription compounding: 50 million units (10 g); 150 million units (30 g); 500 million units (100 g); 2 billion units (400 g)
      Nystat-Rx: 50 million units (10 g); 150 million units (30 g); 500 million units (100 g); 1 billion units (190 g); 2 billion units (350 g)
      Powder, topical:
      Mycostatin®, Nystop®: 100,000 units/g (15 g)
      Pedi-Dri®: 100,000 units/g (56.7 g)
      Suspension, oral: 100,000 units/mL (5 mL, 60 mL, 480 mL)
      Mycostatin®: 100,000 units/mL (60 mL, 480 mL) [contains alcohol ≤1%; cherry-mint flavor]
      Tablet (Mycostatin®): 500,000 units
      Tablet, vaginal: 100,000 units (15s) [packaged with applicator]

nystatin and triamcinolone (nye STAT in & trye am SIN oh lone)
    Synonyms triamcinolone and nystatin
    U.S./Canadian Brand Names Mycolog®-II [US]; Mytrex® [US]
    Therapeutic Category Antifungal/Corticosteroid
    Use Treatment of cutaneous candidiasis
    Usual Dosage Topical: Apply twice daily
    Dosage Forms
      Cream (Mycolog®-II, Mytrex®): Nystatin 100,000 units and triamcinolone acetonide 0.1% (15 g, 30 g, 60 g)
      Ointment: Nystatin 100,000 units and triamcinolone acetonide 0.1% (15 g, 30 g, 60 g)
    (Continued)

nystatin and triamcinolone *(Continued)*

Mycolog®-II: Nystatin 100,000 units and triamcinolone acetonide 0.1% (15 g, 30 g, 60 g)

Mytrex®: Nystatin 100,000 units and triamcinolone acetonide 0.1% (15 g, 30 g)

Nystat-Rx® **[US]** *see* nystatin *on previous page*

Nystex® *(Discontinued) see page 814*

Nystop® **[US]** *see* nystatin *on previous page*

Nytol™ **[Can]** *see* diphenhydramine *on page 202*

Nytol™ **Extra Strength [Can]** *see* diphenhydramine *on page 202*

Nytol® **Quickcaps**® **[US-OTC]** *see* diphenhydramine *on page 202*

Obezine® **[US]** *see* phendimetrazine *on page 507*

Occlusal™ **[Can]** *see* salicylic acid *on page 581*

Occlusal®**-HP [US/Can]** *see* salicylic acid *on page 581*

Ocean® **[US-OTC]** *see* sodium chloride *on page 595*

OCL® **[US]** *see* polyethylene glycol-electrolyte solution *on page 525*

Octamide® *(Discontinued) see page 814*

Octicair® **Otic** *(Discontinued) see page 814*

Octocaine® *(Discontinued) see page 814*

Octostim® **[Can]** *see* desmopressin acetate *on page 182*

octreotide (ok TREE oh tide)

U.S./Canadian Brand Names Sandostatin LAR® [US/Can]; Sandostatin® [US/Can]

Therapeutic Category Somatostatin Analog

Use Control of symptoms in patients with metastatic carcinoid and vasoactive intestinal peptide-secreting tumors (VIPomas); acromegaly, insulinomas, Zollinger-Ellison syndrome, pancreatic tumors, gastrinoma, postgastrectomy dumping syndrome, bleeding esophageal varices, small bowel fistulas, AIDS-associated secretory diarrhea, chemotherapy-induced diarrhea, GVHD-induced diarrhea, control of bleeding of esophageal varices; depot suspension is indicated for long term maintenance therapy in acromegalic patients for whom medical treatment is appropriate and who have been shown to respond to and can tolerate the injection

Usual Dosage Adults: S.C.: Initial: 50 mcg 1-2 times/day and titrate dose based on patient tolerance and response

Carcinoid: 100-600 mcg/day in 2-4 divided doses

VIPomas: 200-300 mcg/day in 2-4 divided doses

Diarrhea: Initial: I.V.: 50-100 mcg every 8 hours; increase by 100 mcg/dose at 48-hour intervals; maximum dose: 500 mcg every 8 hours

Dosage Forms

Injection, microspheres for suspension, as acetate [depot formulation] (Sandostatin LAR®): 10 mg, 20 mg, 30 mg [with diluent and syringe]

Injection, solution, as acetate (Sandostatin®): 0.05 mg/mL (1 mL); 0.1 mg/mL (1 mL); 0.2 mg/mL (5 mL); 0.5 mg/mL (1 mL); 1 mg/mL (5 mL)

Ocu-Chlor® **Ophthalmic [US]** *see* chloramphenicol *on page 133*

OcuClear® **[US-OTC]** *see* oxymetazoline *on page 486*

OcuCoat® **[US/Can]** *see* artificial tears *on page 56*

OcuCoat® **PF [US-OTC]** *see* artificial tears *on page 56*

Ocufen® **Ophthalmic [US/Can]** *see* flurbiprofen *on page 282*

Ocuflox® **[US/Can]** *see* ofloxacin *on next page*

Ocu-Merox® **[US]** *see* mercuric oxide *on page 410*

Ocupress® **Ophthalmic [US/Can]** *see* carteolol *on page 118*

Ocusert Pilo-20® *(Discontinued) see page 814*

Ocusert Pilo-40® *(Discontinued) see page 814*

Ocu-Sul® **[US]** *see* sulfacetamide *on page 610*

Ocutricin® **Topical Ointment** *(Discontinued) see page 814*

Oesclim® **[Can]** *see* estradiol *on page 238*

Oestrilin [Can] *see* estrone *on page 242*

Off-Ezy® **Wart Remover [US-OTC]** *see* salicylic acid *on page 581*

ofloxacin (oh FLOKS a sin)

U.S./Canadian Brand Names Apo®-Oflox [Can]; Floxin® [US/Can]; Ocuflox® [US/Can]

Therapeutic Category Antibiotic, Ophthalmic; Antibiotic, Otic; Quinolone

Use Quinolone antibiotic for skin and skin structure, lower respiratory and urinary tract infections, and sexually transmitted diseases; bacterial conjunctivitis caused by susceptible organisms; otitis externa in adults and pediatric ≥1 year of age caused by susceptible organisms; otitis media in patients ≥12 years of age with perforated tympanic membranes caused by susceptible organisms; acute otitis media in pediatric patients ≥1 year of age with tympanostomy tubes caused by susceptible organisms

Usual Dosage

Children >1 year and Adults: Ophthalmic: Instill 1-2 drops in affected eye(s) every 2-4 hours for the first 2 days, then use 4 times/day for an additional 5 days

Children >1 year to 12 years: Otic: Instill 5 drops in affected ear(s) twice daily for 10 days

Children ≥12 years: Otic: Instill 10 drops in affected ear(s) twice daily for 10 days

Adults: Oral, I.V.: 200-400 mg every 12 hours for 7-10 days for most infections or for 6 weeks for prostatitis

Dosage Forms

Infusion [premixed in D_5W] (Floxin®): 200 mg (50 mL); 400 mg (100 mL)

Injection, solution [single-dose vial] (Floxin®): 40 mg/mL (10 mL)

Solution, ophthalmic (Ocuflox®): 0.3% (5 mL, 10 mL) [contains benzalkonium chloride]

Solution, otic (Floxin®[): 0.3% (5 mL, 10 mL)

Tablet (Floxin®): 200 mg, 300 mg, 400 mg

Ogen® **[US/Can]** *see* estropipate *on page 242*

Ogestrel® *see* ethinyl estradiol and norgestrel *on page 255*

OGMT *see* metyrosine *on page 427*

OKT3 *see* muromonab-CD3 *on page 440*

olanzapine (oh LAN za peen)

Synonyms LY170053

U.S./Canadian Brand Names Zyprexa® [US/Can]; Zyprexa® Zydis® [US]

Therapeutic Category Antipsychotic Agent

Use Treatment of the manifestations of psychotic disorders; short-term treatment of acute mania episodes associated with bipolar I disorder

Usual Dosage

Schizophrenia: Usual starting dose: 5-10 mg once daily; increase to 10 mg once daily within 5-7 days, thereafter adjust by 5 mg/day at 1-week intervals, up to a maximum of 20 mg/day; doses of 30-50 mg/day have been used

Bipolar mania: Usual starting dose: 10-15 mg once daily; increase by 5 mg/day at intervals of not less than 24 hours; maximum dose: 20 mg/day

Dosage Forms

Tablet (Zyprexa®): 2.5 mg, 5 mg, 7.5 mg, 10 mg, 15 mg, 20 mg

Tablet, orally-disintegrating (Zyprexa® Zydis®): 5 mg [contains phenylalanine 0.34 mg/tablet], 10 mg [contains phenylalanine 0.45 mg/tablet], 15 mg [contains phenylalanine 0.67 mg/tablet], 20 mg [contains phenylalanine 0.9 mg/tablet]

old tuberculin *see* tuberculin tests *on page 662*

oleovitamin A *see* vitamin A *on page 680*

oleum ricini *see* castor oil *on page 119*

olmesartan (ole me SAR tan)
U.S./Canadian Brand Names Benicar™ [US]
Therapeutic Category Angiotensin II Receptor Antagonist
Use Treatment of hypertension with or without concurrent use of other antihypertensive agents
Usual Dosage Oral:
Adults: Initial: Usual starting dose is 20 mg once daily; if initial response is inadequate, may be increased to 40 mg once daily after 2 weeks. May administer with other antihypertensive agents if blood pressure inadequately controlled with olmesartan. Consider lower starting dose in patients with possible depletion of intravascular volume (eg, patients receiving diuretics).
Dosage Forms Tablet, film coated, as medoxomil: 5 mg, 20 mg, 40 mg

olopatadine (oh LOP ah tah deen)
U.S./Canadian Brand Names Patanol® [US/Can]
Therapeutic Category Antihistamine
Use Allergic conjunctivitis
Usual Dosage Adults: Ophthalmic: 1 drop in affected eye(s) every 6-8 hours (twice daily)
Dosage Forms Solution, ophthalmic: 0.1% (5 mL) [contains benzalkonium chloride]

olsalazine (ole SAL a zeen)
U.S./Canadian Brand Names Dipentum® [US/Can]
Therapeutic Category 5-Aminosalicylic Acid Derivative
Use Maintenance of remission of ulcerative colitis in patients intolerant to sulfasalazine
Usual Dosage Adults: Oral: 1 g daily in 2 divided doses
Dosage Forms Capsule, as sodium: 250 mg

Olux™ [US] *see* clobetasol *on page 152*

omeprazole (oh ME pray zol)
U.S./Canadian Brand Names Prilosec® [US/Can]
Therapeutic Category Gastric Acid Secretion Inhibitor
Use Short-term (4-8 weeks) treatment of active duodenal ulcer disease or active benign gastric ulcer; treatment of heartburn and other symptoms associated with gastroesophageal reflux disease (GERD); short-term (4-8 weeks) treatment of endoscopically-diagnosed erosive esophagitis; maintenance healing of erosive esophagitis; long-term treatment of pathological hypersecretory conditions; as part of a multidrug regimen for *H. pylori* eradication to reduce the risk of duodenal ulcer recurrence
Usual Dosage Adults: Oral:
Duodenal ulcer: 20 mg/day for 4-8 weeks
GERD or erosive esophagitis: 20 mg/day for 4-8 weeks
Maintenance of healing erosive esophagitis: 20 mg/day
Pathological hypersecretory conditions: 60 mg once daily initially; doses up to 120 mg 3 times/day have been administered; administer daily doses >80 mg in divided doses; patients with Zollinger-Ellison syndrome have been treated continuously for over 5 years
Dosage Forms Capsule, delayed release: 10 mg, 20 mg, 40 mg

Omnicef® [US/Can] *see* cefdinir *on page 121*

OmniHIB™ *(Discontinued)* *see page 814*

Omnipaque® [US] *see* radiological/contrast media (non-ionic) *on page 563*

Omnipen® *(Discontinued)* *see page 814*

Omnipen®-N *(Discontinued)* *see page 814*

Oncaspar® [US/Can] *see* pegaspargase *on page 495*

Oncet® *(Discontinued)* *see page 814*

Oncotice™ [Can] *see* BCG vaccine *on page 72*

Oncovin® [US/Can] *see* vincristine *on page 678*

ondansetron (on DAN se tron)

U.S./Canadian Brand Names Zofran® ODT [US/Can]; Zofran® [US/Can]

Therapeutic Category Selective 5-HT₃ Receptor Antagonist

Use Prevention of nausea and vomiting associated with initial and repeat courses of emetogenic cancer chemotherapy and prevention of postoperative nausea and vomiting; prevent postoperative nausea/vomiting (I.M.)

Usual Dosage

Oral:

Children 4-11 years: 4 mg 30 minutes before chemotherapy; repeat 4 and 8 hours after initial dose

Children >11 years and Adults: 8 mg 30 minutes before chemotherapy; repeat 4 and 8 hours after initial dose or every 8 hours for a maximum of 48 hours

I.V.: Administer either three 0.15 mg/kg doses or a single 32 mg dose; with the 3-dose regimen, the initial dose is given 30 minutes prior to chemotherapy with subsequent doses administered 4 and 8 hours after the first dose. With the single-dose regimen 32 mg is infused over 15 minutes beginning 30 minutes before the start of emetogenic chemotherapy. Dosage should be calculated based on weight:

Children: Pediatric dosing should follow the manufacturer's guidelines for 0.15 mg/kg/dose administered 30 minutes prior to chemotherapy, 4 and 8 hours after the first dose. While not as yet FDA-approved, literature supports the day's total dose administered as a single dose 30 minutes prior to chemotherapy.

Adults:

>80 kg: 12 mg IVPB

45-80 kg: 8 mg IVPB

<45 kg: 0.15 mg/kg/dose IVPB

Dosage Forms

Injection, solution, as hydrochloride (Zofran®): 2 mg/mL (2 mL, 20 mL)

Infusion, as hydrochloride [premixed in D₅W] (Zofran®): 32 mg (50 mL)

Solution, as hydrochloride (Zofran®): 4 mg/5 mL (50 mL) [contains sodium benzoate; strawberry flavor]

Tablet, as hydrochloride (Zofran®): 4 mg, 8 mg, 24 mg

Tablet, orally-disintegrating (Zofran® ODT): 4 mg, 8 mg [each strength contains phenylalanine <0.03 mg/tablet; strawberry flavor]

ONTAK® [US] *see* denileukin diftitox *on page 179*

Onxol™ [US] *see* paclitaxel *on page 488*

Ony-Clear® Nail [US-OTC] *see* triacetin *on page 650*

Ony-Clear [US-OTC] *see* benzalkonium chloride *on page 76*

OP-CCK *see* sincalide *on page 591*

Opcon-A® [US-OTC] *see* naphazoline and pheniramine *on page 447*

Opcon® Ophthalmic *(Discontinued)* *see page 814*

o,p'-DDD *see* mitotane *on page 433*

Operand® [US-OTC] *see* povidone-iodine *on page 533*

Ophthaine® *(Discontinued)* *see page 814*

Ophthalgan® Ophthalmic *(Discontinued)* *see page 814*

Ophthetic® [US] *see* proparacaine *on page 547*

Ophthifluor® [US] *see* fluorescein sodium *on page 277*

Ophthochlor® **Ophthalmic** *(Discontinued)* see page 814

Ophthocort® *(Discontinued)* see page 814

Ophtho-Dipivefrin™ **[Can]** see dipivefrin on page 205

Ophtho-Tate® **[Can]** see prednisolone (ophthalmic) on page 537

opium and belladonna see belladonna and opium on page 74

opium tincture (OH pee um TINGK chur)
Synonyms deodorized opium tincture; DTO
Therapeutic Category Analgesic, Narcotic
Controlled Substance C-II
Use Treatment of diarrhea or relief of pain; **a 25-fold dilution with water** (final concentration 0.4 mg/mL morphine) can be used to treat neonatal abstinence syndrome (opiate withdrawal)
Usual Dosage Oral:
Children:
Diarrhea: 0.005-0.01 mL/kg/dose every 3-4 hours
Analgesia: 0.01-0.02 mL/kg/dose every 3-4 hours
Adults: 0.6 mL 4 times/day
Dosage Forms Liquid: 10% (120 mL, 480 mL) [0.6 mL equivalent to morphine 6 mg; contains alcohol 19%]

oprelvekin (oh PREL ve kin)
Synonyms IL-11; interleukin-11; recombinant human interleukin-11; recombinant interleukin-11; rhIL-11; rIL-11
U.S./Canadian Brand Names Neumega® [US]
Therapeutic Category Platelet Growth Factor
Use Prevention and treatment of severe thrombocytopenia following myelosuppressive chemotherapy
Usual Dosage Refer to individual protocols.
Children: 75-100 mcg/kg/day for 10-21 days (until platelet count >50,000/mm^3)
Adults: 50 mcg/kg/day for 10-21 days (until platelet count >50,000/mm^3)
Dosage Forms Injection, powder for reconstitution: 5 mg

Optho-Bunolol® **[Can]** see levobunolol on page 379

Opticrom® **[US/Can]** see cromolyn sodium on page 166

Optigene® **[US-OTC]** see tetrahydrozoline on page 629

Optimine® **[US/Can]** see azatadine on page 65

Optimoist® **Solution** *(Discontinued)* see page 814

Optimyxin® **Ophthalmic [Can]** see bacitracin and polymyxin B on page 68

Optimyxin Plus® **[Can]** see neomycin, polymyxin B, and gramicidin on page 453

OptiPranolol® **[US/Can]** see metipranolol on page 424

Optiray® **[US]** see radiological/contrast media (non-ionic) on page 563

Optivar™ **[US]** see azelastine on page 66

OPV see poliovirus vaccine, live, trivalent, oral on page 524

Orabase®**-B [US-OTC]** see benzocaine on page 77

Orabase® **HCA [US]** see hydrocortisone (topical) on page 334

Orabase®**-O** *(Discontinued)* see page 814

Orabase® **Plain [US-OTC]** see gelatin, pectin, and methylcellulose on page 294

Orabase® **With Benzocaine [US-OTC]** see benzocaine, gelatin, pectin, and sodium carboxymethylcellulose on page 78

Oradex-C® *(Discontinued)* see page 814

Orafen [Can] *see* ketoprofen *on page 368*

Oragrafin® Calcium [US] *see* radiological/contrast media (ionic) *on page 561*

Oragrafin® Sodium [US] *see* radiological/contrast media (ionic) *on page 561*

Orajel® Baby Nighttime [US-OTC] *see* benzocaine *on page 77*

Orajel® Baby [US-OTC] *see* benzocaine *on page 77*

Orajel® Brace-Aid Oral Anesthetic *(Discontinued)* *see page 814*

Orajel® Maximum Strength [US-OTC] *see* benzocaine *on page 77*

Orajel® Perioseptic® [US-OTC] *see* carbamide peroxide *on page 113*

Orajel® [US-OTC] *see* benzocaine *on page 77*

Oramorph SR® [US/Can] *see* morphine sulfate *on page 437*

Orap™ [US/Can] *see* pimozide *on page 515*

Orapred™ [US] *see* prednisolone (systemic) *on page 537*

Orasol® [US-OTC] *see* benzocaine *on page 77*

Orasone® *(Discontinued)* *see page 814*

Oratect® *(Discontinued)* *see page 814*

Orazinc® [US-OTC] *see* zinc sulfate *on page 691*

orciprenaline *see* metaproterenol *on page 413*

Ordrine AT® Extended Release Capsule *(Discontinued)* *see page 814*

Oretic® [US] *see* hydrochlorothiazide *on page 328*

Oreticyl® *(Discontinued)* *see page 814*

Oreton® Methyl *(Discontinued)* *see page 814*

Orexin® [US-OTC] *see* vitamin B complex *on page 681*

Orfadin® [US] *see* nitisinone *on page 460*

Organidin® *(Discontinued)* *see page 814*

Organidin® NR [US] *see* guaifenesin *on page 307*

Orgaran® [US/Can] *see* danaparoid *on page 174*

ORG NC 45 *see* vecuronium *on page 674*

Orimune® [US] *see* poliovirus vaccine, live, trivalent, oral *on page 524*

Orinase® Diagnostic [US] *see* tolbutamide *on page 643*

Orinase® Oral *(Discontinued)* *see page 814*

ORLAAM® [US] *see* levomethadyl acetate hydrochloride *on page 381*

orlistat (OR li stat)
U.S./Canadian Brand Names Xenical® [US/Can]
Therapeutic Category Lipase Inhibitor
Use Management of obesity, including weight loss and weight management when used in conjunction with a reduced-calorie diet; reduce the risk of weight regain after prior weight loss; indicated for obese patients with an initial body mass index (BMI) ≥30 kg/m² or ≥27 kg/m² in the presence of other risk factors
Usual Dosage Adults: Oral: 120 mg 3 times/day with each main meal containing fat (during or up to 1 hour after the meal); omit dose if meal is occasionally missed or contains no fat
Dosage Forms Capsule: 120 mg

Ormazine® *(Discontinued)* *see page 814*

Ornade® Spansule® Capsules *(Discontinued)* *see page 814*

Ornex® Maximum Strength [US-OTC] *see* acetaminophen and pseudoephedrine *on page 6*

Ornex® [US-OTC] *see* acetaminophen and pseudoephedrine *on page 6*

Ornidyl® Injection *(Discontinued)* *see page 814*

orphenadrine (or FEN a dreen)
U.S./Canadian Brand Names Norflex™ [US/Can]; Rhoxal-orphendrine [Can]
Therapeutic Category Skeletal Muscle Relaxant
Use Treatment of muscle spasm associated with acute painful musculoskeletal conditions; supportive therapy in tetanus
Usual Dosage Adults:
Oral: 100 mg twice daily
I.M., I.V.: 60 mg every 12 hours
Dosage Forms
Injection, solution, as citrate: 30 mg/mL (2 mL) [contains sodium bisulfite]
Tablet, extended release, as citrate: 100 mg

orphenadrine, aspirin, and caffeine
(or FEN a dreen, AS pir in, & KAF een)
Synonyms aspirin, orphenadrine, and caffeine; caffeine, orphenadrine, and aspirin
U.S./Canadian Brand Names Norgesic™ Forte [US/Can]; Norgesic™ [US/Can]; Orphengesic Forte [US]; Orphengesic [US]
Therapeutic Category Analgesic, Non-narcotic; Skeletal Muscle Relaxant
Use Relief of discomfort associated with skeletal muscular conditions
Usual Dosage Oral: 1-2 tablets 3-4 times/day
Dosage Forms
Tablet: Orphenadrine citrate 25 mg, aspirin 385 mg, and caffeine 30 mg; orphenadrine citrate 50 mg, aspirin 770 mg, and caffeine 60 mg
Norgesic™, Orphengesic: Orphenadrine citrate 25 mg, aspirin 385 mg, and caffeine 30 mg
Norgesic™ Forte, Orphengesic Forte: Orphenadrine citrate 50 mg, aspirin 770 mg, and caffeine 60 mg

Orphengesic [US] *see* orphenadrine, aspirin, and caffeine *on this page*

Orphengesic Forte [US] *see* orphenadrine, aspirin, and caffeine *on this page*

Ortho-Cept® [US/Can] *see* ethinyl estradiol and desogestrel *on page 244*

Orthoclone OKT® 3 [US/Can] *see* muromonab-CD3 *on page 440*

Ortho-Cyclen® [US/Can] *see* ethinyl estradiol and norgestimate *on page 254*

Ortho-Est® [US] *see* estropipate *on page 242*

Ortho Evra™ [US] *see* ethinyl estradiol and norelgestromin *on page 250*

Ortho-Novum® [US] *see* ethinyl estradiol and norethindrone *on page 251*

Ortho-Novum® 1/50 [US/Can] *see* mestranol and norethindrone *on page 412*

Ortho-Prefest® [US] *see* estradiol and norgestimate *on page 239*

Ortho Tri-Cyclen® [US/Can] *see* ethinyl estradiol and norgestimate *on page 254*

Ortho-Tri-Cyclen® Lo [US] *see* ethinyl estradiol and norgestimate *on page 254*

Or-Tyl® Injection *(Discontinued)* *see page 814*

Orudis® *(Discontinued)* *see page 814*

Orudis® KT [US-OTC] *see* ketoprofen *on page 368*

Orudis® SR [Can] *see* ketoprofen *on page 368*

Oruvail® [US/Can] *see* ketoprofen *on page 368*

Os-Cal® 500 [US/Can] *see* calcium carbonate *on page 104*

oseltamivir (o sel TAM e veer)

U.S./Canadian Brand Names Tamiflu™ [US/Can]

Therapeutic Category Antiviral Agent, Oral

Controlled Substance [FS100]influenza

Use Treatment of uncomplicated acute illness due to influenza (A or B) infection in adults and children >1 year of age who have been symptomatic for no more than 2 days; prophylaxis against influenza (A or B) infection in adults and adolescents ≥13 years of age

Usual Dosage Oral:

Treatment: Initiate treatment within 2 days of onset of symptoms; duration of treatment: 5 days:

Children: 1-12 years:

≤15 kg: 30 mg twice daily

>15 kg - ≤23 kg: 45 mg twice daily

>23 kg - ≤40 kg: 60 mg twice daily

>40 kg: 75 mg twice daily

Adolescents and Adults: 75 mg twice daily

Prophylaxis: Adolescents and Adults: 75 mg once daily for at least 7 days; treatment should begin within 2 days of contact with an infected individual. During community outbreaks, dosing is 75 mg once daily. May be used for up to 6 weeks; duration of protection lasts for length of dosing period

Dosage Forms

Capsule, as phosphate: 75 mg

Powder for oral suspension: 12 mg/mL (25 mL) [contains sodium benzoate; tutti-frutti flavor]

Osmitrol® **[US/Can]** *see* mannitol *on page 400*

Osmoglyn® **[US]** *see* glycerin *on page 302*

Osmolite® **HN [US-OTC]** *see* nutritional formula, enteral/oral *on page 472*

Ostac® **[US/Can]** *see* clodronate disodium *(Canada only) on page 153*

Osteocalcin® *(Discontinued) see page 814*

Ostoforte® **[Can]** *see* ergocalciferol *on page 232*

Otic-Care® **Otic** *(Discontinued) see page 814*

Otic Domeboro® **[US]** *see* aluminum acetate and acetic acid *on page 27*

Otic Tridesilon® *(Discontinued) see page 814*

Otocort® **Otic** *(Discontinued) see page 814*

Otosporin® **Otic** *(Discontinued) see page 814*

Otrivin® *(Discontinued) see page 814*

Otrivin® **Pediatric** *(Discontinued) see page 814*

Ovcon® **[US]** *see* ethinyl estradiol and norethindrone *on page 251*

Ovide™ **[US]** *see* malathion *on page 399*

Ovidrel® **[US]** *see* chorionic gonadotropin (recombinant) *on page 145*

Ovol® **[Can]** *see* simethicone *on page 591*

Ovral® **[US/Can]** *see* ethinyl estradiol and norgestrel *on page 255*

Ovrette® **[US/Can]** *see* norgestrel *on page 466*

O-V Staticin® *(Discontinued) see page 814*

oxacillin (oks a SIL in)

Synonyms methylphenyl isoxazolyl penicillin

Therapeutic Category Penicillin

(Continued)

oxacillin *(Continued)*

Use Treatment of bacterial infections such as osteomyelitis, septicemia, endocarditis, and CNS infections due to susceptible penicillinase-producing strains of *Staphylococcus*

Usual Dosage
Infants and Children:
I.M., I.V.: 150-200 mg/kg/day in divided doses every 6 hours; maximum dose: 12 g/day
Oral: 50-100 mg/kg/day divided every 6 hours
Adults:
Oral: 500-1000 mg every 4-6 hours for at least 5 days
I.M., I.V.: 250 mg to 2 g/dose every 4-6 hours

Dosage Forms
Infusion [premixed iso-osmotic dextrose solution]: 1 g (50 mL); 2 g (50 mL)
Injection, powder for reconstitution, as sodium: 1 g, 2 g, 10 g

Oxandrin® [US] *see* oxandrolone *on this page*

oxandrolone (oks AN droe lone)

U.S./Canadian Brand Names Oxandrin® [US]
Therapeutic Category Androgen
Controlled Substance C-III
Use Treatment of catabolic or tissue-depleting processes
Usual Dosage Adults: Oral: 2.5 mg 2-4 times/day
Dosage Forms Tablet: 2.5 mg

oxaprozin (oks a PROE zin)

U.S./Canadian Brand Names Daypro™ [US/Can]
Therapeutic Category Analgesic, Non-narcotic; Nonsteroidal Anti-inflammatory Drug (NSAID)
Use Acute and long-term use in the management of signs and symptoms of osteoarthritis and rheumatoid arthritis
Usual Dosage Adults: Oral (individualize the dosage to the lowest effective dose to minimize adverse effects):
Osteoarthritis: 600-1200 mg once daily
Rheumatoid arthritis: 1200 mg once daily
Maximum dose: 1800 mg/day or 26 mg/kg (whichever is lower) in divided doses
Dosage Forms Tablet: 600 mg

oxazepam (oks A ze pam)

U.S./Canadian Brand Names Apo®-Oxazepam [Can]; Serax® [US]
Therapeutic Category Anticonvulsant; Benzodiazepine
Controlled Substance C-IV
Use Treatment of anxiety and management of alcohol withdrawal; may also be used as an anticonvulsant in management of simple partial seizures
Usual Dosage Oral:
Children: 1 mg/kg/day has been administered
Adults:
Anxiety: 10-30 mg 3-4 times/day
Alcohol withdrawal: 15-30 mg 3-4 times/day
Hypnotic: 15-30 mg
Dosage Forms
Capsule: 10 mg, 15 mg, 30 mg
Tablet: 15 mg

oxcarbazepine (ox car BAZ e peen)

Synonyms GP 47680
U.S./Canadian Brand Names Trileptal® [US/Can]

Therapeutic Category Anticonvulsant, Miscellaneous

Use Monotherapy or adjunctive therapy in the treatment of partial seizures in adults with epilepsy and as adjunctive therapy in the treatment of partial seizures in children ages 4-16 with epilepsy

Unlabeled use: Antimanic

Usual Dosage

Children:

Adjunctive therapy: 8-10 mg/kg/day, not to exceed 600 mg/day, given in two divided daily doses. Maintenance dose should be achieved over 2 weeks, and is dependent upon patient weight, according to the following:

20-29 kg: 900 mg/day in 2 divided doses

29.1-39 kg: 1200 mg/day in 2 divided doses

>39 kg: 1800 mg/day in 2 divided doses

Adults:

Adjunctive therapy: Initial: 300 mg twice daily; dose may be increased by as much as 600 mg/day at weekly intervals; recommended daily dose: 1200 mg/day in 2 divided doses

Conversion to monotherapy: Oxcarbazepine 600 mg/day in twice daily divided doses while simultaneously initiating the reduction of the dose of the concomitant antiepileptic drug. The concomitant dosage should be withdrawn over 3-6 weeks, while the maximum dose of oxcarbazepine should be reached in about 2-4 weeks. Recommended daily dose: 2400 mg/day.

Initiation of monotherapy: Oxcarbazepine should be initiated at a dose of 600 mg/day in twice daily divided doses; doses may be titrated upward by 300 mg/day every third day to a final dose of 1200 mg/day given in 2 daily divided doses

Dosage Forms

Suspension, oral: 300 mg/5 mL (250 mL) [contains ethanol]

Tablet: 150 mg, 300 mg, 600 mg

oxiconazole (oks i KON a zole)

U.S./Canadian Brand Names Oxistat® [US/Can]; Oxizole® [Can]

Therapeutic Category Antifungal Agent

Use Treatment of tinea pedis, tinea cruris, and tinea corporis

Usual Dosage Topical: Apply once daily to affected areas for 2 weeks to 1 month

Dosage Forms

Cream, as nitrate: 1% (15 g, 30 g, 60 g)

Lotion, as nitrate: 1% (30 mL)

oxilapine *see* loxapine *on page 394*

Oxipor® VHC [US-OTC] *see* coal tar *on page 158*

Oxistat® [US/Can] *see* oxiconazole *on this page*

Oxizole® [Can] *see* oxiconazole *on this page*

oxpentifylline *see* pentoxifylline *on page 502*

oxprenolol *(Canada only)* (ox PREN oh lole)

U.S./Canadian Brand Names Slow-Trasicor® [Can]; Trasicor® [Can]

Therapeutic Category Beta-Adrenergic Blocker

Use Treatment of mild to moderate hypertension

Usual Dosage Adults: Oral: Start with 20 mg three times/day, titrated upward to a maximum dose of 480 mg/day

Dosage Forms

Tablet (Trasicor®): 40 mg, 80 mg

Tablet, slow release (Slow-Trasicor®): 80 mg, 160 mg

Oxsoralen® Lotion [US/Can] *see* methoxsalen *on page 418*

Oxsoralen® Oral *(Discontinued)* *see page 814*

Oxsoralen-Ultra® **[US/Can]** *see* methoxsalen *on page 418*

oxtriphylline (oks TRYE fi lin)
Synonyms choline theophyllinate
U.S./Canadian Brand Names Choledyl SA® [US]
Therapeutic Category Theophylline Derivative
Use Bronchodilator in symptomatic treatment of asthma and reversible bronchospasm
Usual Dosage Oral:
  Children:
    1-9 years: 6.2 mg/kg/dose every 6 hours
    9-16 years: 4.7 mg/kg/dose every 6 hours
  Adults: 4.7 mg/kg every 8 hours; sustained release: administer every 12 hours
Dosage Forms
  Elixir: 100 mg/5 mL (5 mL, 10 mL, 473 mL)
  Syrup: 50 mg/5 mL (473 mL)
  Tablet: 100 mg, 200 mg
    Sustained release: 400 mg, 600 mg

Oxy-5® *(Discontinued)* *see page 814*

Oxy 10® **Balanced Medicated Face Wash [US-OTC]** *see* benzoyl peroxide *on page 79*

oxybutynin (oks i BYOO ti nin)
U.S./Canadian Brand Names Ditropan® [US/Can]; Ditropan® XL [US]; Gen-Oxybutynin [Can]; Novo-Oxybutynin [Can]; Nu-Oxybutyn [Can]; PMS-Oxybutynin [Can]
Therapeutic Category Antispasmodic Agent, Urinary
Use Relief of bladder spasms associated with voiding in patients with uninhibited and reflex neurogenic bladder
Usual Dosage Oral:
  Children:
    1-5 years: 0.2 mg/kg/dose 2-4 times/day
    >5 years: 5 mg twice daily, up to 5 mg 3 times/day
  Adults: 5 mg 2-3 times/day up to 5 mg 4 times/day maximum
Dosage Forms
  Syrup, as chloride (Ditropan®): 5 mg/5 mL (473 mL)
  Tablet, as chloride (Ditropan®): 5 mg
  Tablet, extended release, as chloride (Ditropan® XL): 5 mg, 10 mg, 15 mg

Oxycel® **[US]** *see* cellulose, oxidized *on page 127*

oxychlorosene (oks i KLOR oh seen)
U.S./Canadian Brand Names Clorpactin® WCS-90 [US-OTC]
Therapeutic Category Antibiotic, Topical
Use Treating localized infections
Usual Dosage Topical (0.1% to 0.5% solutions): Apply by irrigation, instillation, spray, soaks, or wet compresses
Dosage Forms Powder for solution, as sodium: 2 g

Oxycodan® **[Can]** *see* oxycodone and aspirin *on next page*

oxycodone (oks i KOE done)
Synonyms dihydrohydroxycodeinone
U.S./Canadian Brand Names OxyContin® [US/Can]; Oxydose™ [US]; OxyFast® [US]; OxyIR® [US/Can]; Roxicodone™ Intensol™ [US]; Roxicodone™ [US]; Supeudol® [Can]
Therapeutic Category Analgesic, Narcotic
Controlled Substance C-II
Use Management of moderate to severe pain, normally used in combination with non-narcotic analgesics

Usual Dosage Oral:
Children:
6-12 years: 1.25 mg every 6 hours as needed
>12 years: 2.5 mg every 6 hours as needed
Adults: 5 mg every 6 hours as needed

Dosage Forms
Capsule, immediate release, as hydrochloride (OxyIR®): 5 mg
Solution, oral, as hydrochloride (Roxicodone™): 5 mg/5 mL (5 mL, 500 mL) [contains alcohol]
Solution, oral concentrate, as hydrochloride:
Oxydose™: 20 mg/mL (30 mL) [contains sodium benzoate; berry flavor]
OxyFast®: 20 mg/mL (30 mL) [contains sodium benzoate]
Roxicodone™ Intensol™: 20 mg/mL (30 mL) [contains sodium benzoate]
Tablet, as hydrochloride: 5 mg
Roxicodone™: 5 mg, 15 mg, 30 mg
Tablet, controlled release, as hydrochloride (OxyContin®): 10 mg, 20 mg, 40 mg, 80 mg, 160 mg

oxycodone and acetaminophen (oks i KOE done & a seet a MIN oh fen)

Synonyms acetaminophen and oxycodone
U.S./Canadian Brand Names Endocet® [US/Can]; Percocet® 2.5/325 [US]; Percocet® 5/325 [US]; Percocet® 7.5/325 [US]; Percocet® 7.5/500 [US]; Percocet® 10/325 [US]; Percocet® 10/650 [US]; Roxicet® 5/500 [US]; Roxicet® [US]; Tylox® [US]
Therapeutic Category Analgesic, Narcotic
Controlled Substance C-II
Use Management of moderate to severe pain
Usual Dosage Oral (doses should be titrated to appropriate analgesic effects):
Children: Oxycodone: 0.05-0.15 mg/kg/dose to 5 mg/dose (maximum) every 4-6 hours as needed
Adults: 1-2 tablets every 4-6 hours as needed for pain
Maximum daily dose of acetaminophen: 4 g/day

Dosage Forms
Caplet (Roxicet® 5/500): Oxycodone hydrochloride 5 mg and acetaminophen 500 mg
Capsule: Oxycodone hydrochloride 5 mg and acetaminophen 500 mg
Tylox®: Oxycodone hydrochloride 5 mg and acetaminophen 500 mg [contains sodium benzoate and sodium metabisulfite]
Solution, oral (Roxicet®): Oxycodone hydrochloride 5 mg and acetaminophen 325 mg per 5 mL (5 mL, 500 mL) [contains alcohol <0.5%]
Tablet: Oxycodone hydrochloride 5 mg and acetaminophen 325 mg; oxycodone hydrochloride 7.5 mg and acetaminophen 500 mg; oxycodone hydrochloride 10 mg and acetaminophen 650 mg
Endocet®: Oxycodone hydrochloride 5 mg and acetaminophen 325 mg
Percocet® 2.5/325: Oxycodone hydrochloride 2.5 mg and acetaminophen 325 mg
Percocet® 5/325: Oxycodone hydrochloride 5 mg and acetaminophen 325 mg
Percocet® 7.5/325: Oxycodone hydrochloride 7.5 mg and acetaminophen 325 mg
Percocet® 7.5/500: Oxycodone hydrochloride 7.5 mg and acetaminophen 500 mg
Percocet® 10/325: Oxycodone hydrochloride 10 mg and acetaminophen 325 mg
Percocet® 10/650: Oxycodone hydrochloride 10 mg and acetaminophen 650 mg
Roxicet®: Oxycodone hydrochloride 5 mg and acetaminophen 325 mg

oxycodone and aspirin (oks i KOE done & AS pir in)

Synonyms aspirin and oxycodone
U.S./Canadian Brand Names Endodan® [US/Can]; Oxycodan® [Can]; Percodan® [US/Can]; Percodan®-Demi® [Can]
Therapeutic Category Analgesic, Narcotic
Controlled Substance C-II
Use Relief of moderate to moderately severe pain
(Continued)

oxycodone and aspirin *(Continued)*

Usual Dosage Oral (based on oxycodone combined salts):
Children: 0.05-0.15 mg/kg/dose every 4-6 hours as needed; maximum: 5 mg/dose (1 tablet Percodan® or 2 tablets Percodan®-Demi/dose) **or**
Alternatively:
6-12 years: Percodan®-Demi: ¹/₄ tablet every 6 hours as needed for pain
>12 years: ¹/₂ tablet every 6 hours as needed for pain
Adults: Percodan®: 1 tablet every 6 hours as needed for pain or Percodan®-Demi: 1-2 tablets every 6 hours as needed for pain

Dosage Forms Tablet:
Percodan®, Endodan®: Oxycodone hydrochloride 4.5 mg, oxycodone terephthalate 0.38 mg, and aspirin 325 mg
Percodan®-Demi: Oxycodone hydrochloride 2.25 mg, oxycodone terephthalate 0.19 mg, and aspirin 325 mg

OxyContin® [US/Can] *see* oxycodone *on page 484*

Oxyderm™ [Can] *see* benzoyl peroxide *on page 79*

Oxydose™ [US] *see* oxycodone *on page 484*

OxyFast® [US] *see* oxycodone *on page 484*

OxyIR® [US/Can] *see* oxycodone *on page 484*

oxymetazoline *(oks i met AZ oh leen)*

U.S./Canadian Brand Names Afrin® Extra Moisturizing [US-OTC]; Afrin® Original [US-OTC]; Afrin® Severe Congestion [US-OTC]; Afrin® Sinus [US-OTC]; Afrin® [US-OTC]; Dristan® Long Lasting Nasal [Can]; Drixoral® Nasal [Can]; Duramist® Plus [US-OTC]; Duration® [US-OTC]; Genasal [US-OTC]; Neo-Synephrine® 12 Hour Extra Moisturizing [US-OTC]; Neo-Synephrine® 12 Hour [US-OTC]; Nōstrilla® [US-OTC]; OcuClear® [US-OTC]; Twice-A-Day® [US-OTC]; Vicks Sinex® 12 Hour Ultrafine Mist [US-OTC]; Visine® L.R. [US-OTC]; 4-Way® Long Acting [US-OTC]

Therapeutic Category Adrenergic Agonist Agent

Use Symptomatic relief of nasal mucosal congestion associated with acute or chronic rhinitis, the common cold, sinusitis, hay fever, or other allergies

Usual Dosage
Intranasal:
Children 2-5 years: 0.025% solution: Instill 2-3 drops in each nostril twice daily
Children ≥6 years and Adults: 0.05% solution: Instill 2-3 drops or 2-3 sprays into each nostril twice daily
Ophthalmic: Adults: Instill 1-2 drops into affected eye(s) every 6 hours

Dosage Forms
Nasal spray, as hydrochloride: 0.05% (15 mL, 30 mL)
Afrin®, Afrin® Extra Moisturizing, Afrin® Sinus: 0.05% (15 mL) [contains benzyl alcohol; no drip formula]
Afrin® Original: 0.05% (15 mL, 30 mL, 45 mL)
Afrin® Severe Congestion: 0.05% (15 mL) [contains benzyl alcohol and menthol; no drip formula]
Duramist® Plus, Neo-Synephrine® 12 Hour, Nōstrilla®, Vicks Sinex® 12 Hour Ultrafine Mist, 4-Way® Long Acting Nasal: 0.05% (15 mL)
Duration®: 0.05% (30 mL)
Genasal: 0.05% (15 mL, 30 mL)
Neo-Synephrine® 12 Hour Extra Moisturizing: 0.05% (15 mL) [contains glycerin]
Solution, ophthalmic, as hydrochloride (OcuClear®, Visine® L.R.): 0.025% (15 mL, 30 mL) [contains benzalkonium chloride]

oxymetholone *(oks i METH oh lone)*

U.S./Canadian Brand Names Anadrol® [US]
Therapeutic Category Anabolic Steroid
Controlled Substance C-III

Use Anemias caused by the administration of myelotoxic drugs
Usual Dosage Erythropoietic effects: 1-5 mg/kg/day as a single dose; maximum: 100 mg/day
Dosage Forms Tablet: 50 mg

oxymorphone (oks i MOR fone)
U.S./Canadian Brand Names Numorphan® [US/Can]
Therapeutic Category Analgesic, Narcotic
Controlled Substance C-II
Use Management of moderate to severe pain and preoperatively as a sedative and a supplement to anesthesia
Usual Dosage Adults:
I.M., S.C.: Initial: 0.5 mg, then 1-1.5 mg every 4-6 hours as needed
I.V.: Initial: 0.5 mg
Rectal: 5 mg every 4-6 hours
Dosage Forms
Injection, solution, as hydrochloride: 1 mg (1 mL); 1.5 mg/mL (10 mL)
Suppository, rectal, as hydrochloride: 5 mg

oxyphenbutazone *(Discontinued)* see page 814

oxytetracycline (oks i tet ra SYE kleen)
U.S./Canadian Brand Names Terramycin® I.M. [US/Can]
Therapeutic Category Tetracycline Derivative
Use Treatment of susceptible bacterial infections; both gram-positive and gram-negative, as well as *Rickettsia* and *Mycoplasma* organisms
Usual Dosage I.M.:
Children >8 years: 15-25 mg/kg/day (maximum: 250 mg/dose) in divided doses every 8-12 hours
Adults: 250-500 mg every 24 hours or 300 mg/day divided every 8-12 hours
Dosage Forms Injection, solution: 5% [50 mg/mL] (10 mL) [contains lidocaine hydrochloride 2%]

oxytetracycline and polymyxin B
(oks i tet ra SYE kleen & pol i MIKS in bee)
Synonyms polymyxin B and oxytetracycline
U.S./Canadian Brand Names Terramycin® w/Polymyxin B Ophthalmic [US]
Therapeutic Category Antibiotic, Ophthalmic
Use Treatment of superficial ocular infections involving the conjunctiva and/or cornea
Usual Dosage Ophthalmic: Apply ½" of ointment onto the lower lid of affected eye 2-4 times/day
Dosage Forms Ointment, ophthalmic: Oxytetracycline hydrochloride 5 mg and polymyxin B 10,000 units per g (3.5 g)

oxytocin (oks i TOE sin)
Synonyms PIT
U.S./Canadian Brand Names Pitocin® [US/Can]
Therapeutic Category Oxytocic Agent
Use Induce labor at term; control postpartum bleeding
Usual Dosage Adults:
Induction of labor: I.V.: 0.001-0.002 unit/minute; increase by 0.001-0.002 units every 15-30 minutes until contraction pattern has been established
Postpartum bleeding: I.V.: 0.001-0.002 unit/minute as needed
Dosage Forms
Injection, solution: 10 units/mL (1 mL, 10 mL)
Pitocin®: 10 units/mL (1 mL)

Oyst-Cal 500 [US-OTC] *see* calcium carbonate *on page 104*

Oystercal® 500 [US] *see* calcium carbonate *on page 104*

P₆E₁® [US] *see* pilocarpine and epinephrine *on page 515*

P-071 *see* cetirizine *on page 129*

Pacaps® [US] *see* butalbital, acetaminophen, and caffeine *on page 99*

Pacerone® [US] *see* amiodarone *on page 34*

Pacis™ [Can] *see* BCG vaccine *on page 72*

paclitaxel (PAK li taks el)
   U.S./Canadian Brand Names Onxol™ [US]; Taxol® [US/Can]
   Therapeutic Category Antineoplastic Agent
   Use Treatment of metastatic carcinoma of the ovary after failure of first-line or subsequent chemotherapy; treatment for AIDS-related Kaposi's sarcoma
   Usual Dosage Adults: I.V.: 135 mg/m² over 24 hours every 3 weeks
   Dosage Forms
     Injection, solution: 6 mg/mL (5 mL, 16.7 mL, 50 mL)
      Onxol™: 6 mg/mL (5 mL, 25 mL, 50 mL) [contains alcohol]
      Taxol®: 6 mg/mL (5 mL, 16.7 mL, 50 mL) [contains alcohol]

Pain Enz® [US] *see* capsaicin *on page 111*

Palafer® [Can] *see* ferrous fumarate *on page 268*

Palgic®-D [US] *see* carbinoxamine and pseudoephedrine *on page 115*

Palgic®-DS [US] *see* carbinoxamine and pseudoephedrine *on page 115*

palivizumab (pah li VIZ u mab)
   U.S./Canadian Brand Names Synagis® [US]
   Therapeutic Category Monoclonal Antibody
   Use Prevention of serious lower respiratory tract disease caused by respiratory syncytial virus (RSV) in pediatric patients at high risk of RSV disease; safety and efficacy were established in infants with bronchopulmonary dysplasia (BPD) and infants with a history of prematurity ≤35 weeks gestational age
   Usual Dosage Children: I.M.: 15 mg/kg of body weight, monthly throughout RSV season (First dose administered prior to commencement of RSV season)
   Dosage Forms Injection: 50 mg, 100 mg

Palmer's® Skin Success Acne [US-OTC] *see* benzoyl peroxide *on page 79*

Palmitate-A® [US-OTC] *see* vitamin A *on page 680*

PALS® [US-OTC] *see* chlorophyll *on page 135*

2-PAM *see* pralidoxime *on page 534*

Pamelor® [US/Can] *see* nortriptyline *on page 466*

pamidronate (pa mi DROE nate)
   U.S./Canadian Brand Names Aredia® [US/Can]
   Therapeutic Category Bisphosphonate Derivative
   Use Symptomatic treatment of Paget's disease; hypercalcemia associated with malignancy
   Usual Dosage Drug must be diluted properly before administration and infused slowly (at least over 2 hours)
     Adults: I.V.:
      Moderate cancer-related hypercalcemia (12-13 mg/dL): 60-90 mg administered as a slow infusion over 2-24 hours
      Severe cancer-related hypercalcemia (>13.5 mg/dL): 90 mg as a slow infusion over 2-24 hours

A period of 7 days should elapse before the use of second course; repeat infusions every 2-3 weeks have been suggested, however, could be administered every 2-3 months according to the degree and of severity of hypercalcemia and/or the type of malignancy

Paget's disease: 60 mg as a single 2- to 24-hour infusion

Dosage Forms Injection, powder for reconstitution: 30 mg, 90 mg

Pamine® [US/Can] *see* methscopolamine *on page 419*

Pamix® [US-OTC] *see* pyrantel pamoate *on page 555*

Pamprin IB® *(Discontinued) see page 814*

Panasal® 5/500 *(Discontinued) see page 814*

Pan-B antibodies *see* rituximab *on page 575*

Pancof®-XP [US] *see* hydrocodone, pseudoephedrine, and guaifenesin *on page 332*

Pancrease® [US] *see* pancrelipase *on this page*

Pancrease® MT 4 [US/Can] *see* pancrelipase *on this page*

Pancrease® MT 10 [US/Can] *see* pancrelipase *on this page*

Pancrease® MT 16 [US/Can] *see* pancrelipase *on this page*

Pancrease® MT 20 [US/Can] *see* pancrelipase *on this page*

Pancrecarb MS-4® [US] *see* pancrelipase *on this page*

Pancrecarb MS-8® [US] *see* pancrelipase *on this page*

pancrelipase (pan kre LI pase)

Synonyms amylase, lipase, and protease; lipancreatin; lipase, protease, and amylase

U.S./Canadian Brand Names Cotazym® [US/Can]; Cotazym-S® [US]; Creon® 5 [US/Can]; Creon® 10 [US/Can]; Creon® 20 [US/Can]; Creon® 25 [Can]; Kutrase® [US]; Ku-Zyme® [US]; Ku-Zyme® HP [US]; Lipram® [US]; Pancrease® [US]; Pancrease® MT 4 [US/Can]; Pancrease® MT 10 [US/Can]; Pancrease® MT 16 [US/Can]; Pancrease® MT 20 [US/Can]; Pancrecarb MS-4® [US]; Pancrecarb MS-8® [US]; Ultrase® [US/Can]; Ultrase® MT12 [US/Can]; Ultrase® MT18 [US/Can]; Ultrase® MT20 [US/Can]; Viokase® [US/Can]

Therapeutic Category Enzyme

Use Replacement therapy in symptomatic treatment of malabsorption syndrome caused by pancreatic insufficiency

Usual Dosage Oral:

Powder: Actual dose depends on the digestive requirements of the patient

Children <1 year: Start with $^1/_8$ teaspoonful with feedings

Enteric coated microspheres and microtablets: The following dosage recommendations are only an approximation for initial dosages. The actual dosage will depend on the digestive requirements of the individual patient.

Children:

<1 year: 2000 units of lipase with meals/feedings

1-6 years: 4000-8000 units of lipase with meals and 4000 units with snacks

7-12 years: 4000-12,000 units of lipase with meals and snacks

Adults: 4000-16,000 units of lipase with meals and with snacks

Dosage Forms

Capsule:

Cotazym®: Lipase 8000 units, protease 30,000 units, amylase 30,000 units

Kutrase®: Lipase 2400 units, protease 30,000 units, amylase 30,000 units

Ku-Zyme®: Lipase 1200 units, protease 15,000 units, amylase 15,000 units

Ku-Zyme® HP: Lipase 8000 units, protease 30,000 units, amylase 30,000 units

Lipram-PN16®: Lipase 16,000 units, protease 48,000 units, amylase 48, 000 units

Lipram-CR20®: Lipase 20,000 units, protease 75,000 units, amylase 66,400 units

Lipram-UL12®: Lipase 12,000 units, protease 39,000 units, amylase 39,000 units

Lipram-PN10®: Lipase 10,000 units, protease 30,000 units, amylase 30,000 units

(Continued)

pancrelipase *(Continued)*

Lipram-UL18®: Lipase 18,000 units, protease 58,500 units, amylase 58,500 units
Lipram-UL20®: Lipase 20,000 units, protease 65,000 units, amylase 65,000 units
Ultrase®: Lipase 4500 units, protease 25,000 units, amylase 20,000 units
Ultrase® MT12: Lipase 12,000 units, protease 39,000 units, amylase 39,000 units
Ultrase® MT18: Lipase 18,000 units, protease 58,500 units, amylase 58,500 units
Ultrase® MT20: Lipase 20,000 units, protease 65,000 units, amylase 65,000 units
Enteric coated microspheres (Pancrease®): Lipase 4000 units, protease 25,000 units, amylase 20,000 units
Enteric coated microtablets:
  Pancrease® MT 4: Lipase 4500 units, protease 12,000 units, amylase 12,000 units
  Pancrease® MT 10: Lipase 10,000 units, protease 30,000 units, amylase 30,000 units
  Pancrease® MT 16: Lipase 16,000 units, protease 48,000 units, amylase 48,000 units
  Pancrease® MT 20: Lipase 20,000 units, protease 44,000 units, amylase 56,000 units
  Pancrecarb MS-4®: Lipase 4000 units, protease 25,000 units, amylase 25,000 units
  Pancrecarb MS-8®: Lipase 8000 units, protease 45,000 units, amylase 40,000 units
Enteric coated spheres:
  Cotazym-S®: Lipase 5000 units, protease 20,000 units, amylase 20,000 units
  Pancrelipase: Lipase 4000 units, protease 25,000 units, amylase 20,000 units
  Zymase®: Lipase 12,000 units, protease 24,000 units, amylase 24,000 units
Delayed release:
  Creon® 5: Lipase 5000 units, protease 18,750 units, amylase 16,600 units
  Creon® 10: Lipase 10,000 units, protease 37,500 units, amylase 33,200 units
  Creon® 20: Lipase 20,000 units, protease 75,000 units, amylase 66,400 units
Powder (Viokase®): Lipase 16,800 units, protease 70,000 units, amylase 70,000 units per 0.7 g
Tablet:
  Viokase®: Lipase 8000 units, protease 30,000 units, amylase 30,000 units

pancuronium *(pan kyoo ROE nee um)*

Therapeutic Category Skeletal Muscle Relaxant

Use Produces skeletal muscle relaxation during surgery after induction of general anesthesia, increases pulmonary compliance during assisted mechanical respiration, facilitates endotracheal intubation

Usual Dosage Administer I.V.; dose to effect; doses will vary due to interpatient variability; use ideal body weight for obese patients
Surgery:
  Neonates <1 month:
    Test dose: 0.02 mg/kg to measure responsiveness
    Initial: 0.03 mg/kg/dose repeated twice at 5- to 10-minute intervals as needed; maintenance: 0.03-0.09 mg/kg/dose every 30 minutes to 4 hours as needed
  Infants >1 month, Children, and Adults: Initial: 0.06-0.1 mg/kg or 0.05 mg/kg after initial dose of succinylcholine for intubation; maintenance dose: 0.01 mg/kg 60-100 minutes after initial dose and then 0.01 mg/kg every 25-60 minutes
  Pretreatment/priming: 10% of intubating dose given 3-5 minutes before initial dose
  ICU: 0.05-0.1 mg/kg bolus followed by 0.8-1.7 mcg/kg/minute once initial recovery from bolus observed or 0.1-0.2 mg/kg every 1-3 hours

Dosage Forms Injection, as bromide: 1 mg/mL (10 mL); 2 mg/mL (2 mL, 5 mL)

Panectyl® [Can] *see* trimeprazine *(Canada only) on page 656*

Panglobulin® [US] *see* immune globulin (intravenous) *on page 347*

Panhematin® [US] *see* hemin *on page 317*

PanMist®-DM [US] *see* guaifenesin, pseudoephedrine, and dextromethorphan *on page 312*

PanMist® Jr. [US] *see* guaifenesin and pseudoephedrine *on page 310*

PanMist® LA [US] *see* guaifenesin and pseudoephedrine *on page 310*

PanMist® S [US] *see* guaifenesin and pseudoephedrine *on page 310*

PanOxyl® [US/Can] *see* benzoyl peroxide *on page 79*

PanOxyl®-AQ [US] *see* benzoyl peroxide *on page 79*

PanOxyl® Bar [US-OTC] *see* benzoyl peroxide *on page 79*

Panretin™ [US] *see* alitretinoin *on page 22*

Panscol® Lotion *(Discontinued)* *see page 814*

Panscol® Ointment *(Discontinued)* *see page 814*

Panthoderm® Cream [US-OTC] *see* dexpanthenol *on page 186*

Panto™ IV [Can] *see* pantoprazole *on this page*

Pantoloc™ [Can] *see* pantoprazole *on this page*

Pantopon® *(Discontinued)* *see page 814*

pantoprazole (pan TOE pra zole)

U.S./Canadian Brand Names Panto™ IV [Can]; Pantoloc™ [Can]; Protonix® [US/Can]
Therapeutic Category Proton Pump Inhibitor
Use
Oral: Treatment and maintenance of healing of erosive esophagitis associated with GERD; reduction in relapse rates of daytime and nighttime heartburn symptoms in GERD
I.V.: As an alternative to oral therapy in patients unable to continue oral pantoprazole; hypersecretory disorders associated with Zollinger-Ellison syndrome or other neoplastic disorders
Unlabeled uses: Hypersecretory disorders (oral), peptic ulcer disease, active ulcer bleeding with parenterally-administered pantoprazole; adjunct treatment with antibiotics for *Helicobacter pylori*
Usual Dosage Adults:
Oral:
Erosive esophagitis associated with GERD:
Treatment: 40 mg once daily for up to 8 weeks; an additional 8 weeks may be used in patients who have not healed after an 8-week course
Maintenance of healing: 40 mg once daily
Note: Lower doses (20 mg once daily) have been used successfully in mild GERD treatment and maintenance of healing
Hypersecretory disorders (unlabeled use): Doses of 40-160 mg/day have been used; adjust dose based on acid output measurements
I.V.:
Erosive esophagitis associated with GERD: 40 mg once daily (infused over 15 minutes) for 7-10 days
Helicobacter pylori eradication (unlabeled use): Doses up to 40 mg twice daily have been used as part of combination therapy
Hypersecretory disorders: 80 mg twice daily; adjust dose based on acid output measurements; 160-240 mg/day in divided doses has been used for a limited period (up to 7 days)
Dosage Forms
Injection, powder for reconstitution: 40 mg
Tablet, enteric coated: 20 mg, 40 mg

pantothenic acid (pan toe THEN ik AS id)

Synonyms calcium pantothenate; vitamin B_5
Therapeutic Category Vitamin, Water Soluble
Use Pantothenic acid deficiency
Usual Dosage Adults: Oral: Recommended daily dose: 4-7 mg/day
Dosage Forms Tablet: 100 mg, 200 mg, 250 mg, 500 mg

pantothenyl alcohol *see* dexpanthenol *on page 186*

Panwarfarin® *(Discontinued)* *see page 814*

Papacon® **[US]** *see* papaverine *on this page*

papain and urea (pa PAY in & yoor EE a)
U.S./Canadian Brand Names Accuzyme™ [US]
Therapeutic Category Enzyme, Topical Debridement; Topical Skin Product
Use Enzymatic debriding ointment for treatment of chronic and acute wounds
Usual Dosage Cleanse wound with cleanser or saline (not hydrogen peroxide); apply directly to the wound, cover with appropriate dressing, secure into place and reapply 1-2 times/day. Irrigate wound at each dressing.
Dosage Forms Ointment, topical: Papain 1.1×10^4 int. units and urea 10% in hydrophilic ointment (30 g)

papaverine (pa PAV er een)
U.S./Canadian Brand Names Papacon® [US]; Para-Time S.R.® [US]; Pavacot® [US]
Therapeutic Category Vasodilator
Use Relief of peripheral and cerebral ischemia associated with arterial spasm

Investigational use: Prophylaxis of migraine headache
Usual Dosage Adults: Oral, sustained release: 150-300 mg every 12 hours; in difficult cases: 150 mg every 8 hours
Dosage Forms
Capsule, sustained release, as hydrochloride: 150 mg
Injection, as hydrochloride: 30 mg/mL (2 mL, 10 mL)

Paplex® *(Discontinued)* *see page 814*

parabromdylamine *see* brompheniramine *on page 93*

paracetaldehyde *see* paraldehyde *on this page*

paracetamol *see* acetaminophen *on page 3*

parachlorometaxylenol (PAIR a klor oh met a ZYE le nol)
Synonyms PCMX
U.S./Canadian Brand Names Metasep® [US-OTC]
Therapeutic Category Antiseborrheic Agent, Topical
Use Aid in relief of dandruff and associated conditions
Usual Dosage Massage to a foamy lather, allow to remain on hair for 5 minutes, rinse thoroughly and repeat
Dosage Forms Shampoo: 2% with isopropyl alcohol 9%

Paradione® *(Discontinued)* *see page 814*

Paraflex® *(Discontinued)* *see page 814*

Parafon Forte® **[Can]** *see* chlorzoxazone *on page 142*

Parafon Forte™ **DSC [US]** *see* chlorzoxazone *on page 142*

Para-Hist AT® *(Discontinued)* *see page 814*

Paral® **[US]** *see* paraldehyde *on this page*

paraldehyde (par AL de hyde)
Synonyms paracetaldehyde
U.S./Canadian Brand Names Paral® [US]
Therapeutic Category Anticonvulsant
Controlled Substance C-IV
Use Treatment of status epilepticus and tetanus-induced seizures; has been used as a sedative/hypnotic and in the treatment of alcohol withdrawal symptoms
Usual Dosage Dilute in milk or iced fruit juice to mask taste and odor

Oral, rectal:
Children: 0.15-0.3 mL/kg
Adults:
Hypnotic: 10-30 mL
Sedative: 5-10 mL
Rectal: Mix paraldehyde 2:1 with oil (cottonseed or olive)
Dosage Forms Liquid, oral or rectal: 1 g/mL (30 mL)

Paraplatin® [US] *see* carboplatin *on page 116*

Paraplatin-AQ [Can] *see* carboplatin *on page 116*

Parathar™ [US] *see* teriparatide *on page 624*

Para-Time S.R.® [US] *see* papaverine *on previous page*

Parcaine® [US] *see* proparacaine *on page 547*

Par Decon® *(Discontinued) see page 814*

Paredrine® *(Discontinued) see page 814*

paregoric (par e GOR ik)
Synonyms camphorated tincture of opium
Therapeutic Category Analgesic, Narcotic
Controlled Substance C-III
Use Treatment of diarrhea or relief of pain; neonatal abstinence syndrome (neonatal opiate withdrawal)
Usual Dosage Oral:
Neonatal opiate withdrawal: 3-6 drops every 3-6 hours as needed, or initially 0.2 mL every 3 hours; increase dosage by approximately 0.05 mL every 3 hours until withdrawal symptoms are controlled; it is rare to exceed 0.7 mL/dose. Stabilize withdrawal symptoms for 3-5 days, then gradually decrease dosage over a 2- to 4-week period.
Children: 0.25-0.5 mL/kg 1-4 times/day
Adults: 5-10 mL 1-4 times/day
Dosage Forms Liquid: 2 mg morphine equivalent/5 mL [equivalent to 20 mg opium powder] (473 mL)

Paremyd® Ophthalmic *(Discontinued) see page 814*

Parepectolin® *(Discontinued) see page 814*

Pargen Fortified® *(Discontinued) see page 814*

Par Glycerol® *(Discontinued) see page 814*

paricalcitol (par eh CAL ci tol)
U.S./Canadian Brand Names Zemplar™ [US/Can]
Therapeutic Category Vitamin D Analog
Use Prevention and treatment of secondary hyperparathyroidism associated with chronic renal failure
Usual Dosage Adults: I.V.: 0.04-0.1 mcg/kg (2.8-7 mcg) given as a bolus dose no more frequently than every other day at any time during dialysis; doses as high as 0.24 mcg/kg (16.8 mcg) have been administered safely
Dosage Forms Injection: 5 mcg/mL (1 mL, 2 mL, 5 mL)

pariprazole *see* rabeprazole *on page 560*

Parlodel® [US/Can] *see* bromocriptine *on page 93*

Parnate® [US/Can] *see* tranylcypromine *on page 648*

paromomycin (par oh moe MYE sin)
U.S./Canadian Brand Names Humatin® [US/Can]
Therapeutic Category Amebicide
(Continued)

paromomycin *(Continued)*

Use Treatment of acute and chronic intestinal amebiasis due to susceptible *Entamoeba histolytica* (not effective in the treatment of extraintestinal amebiasis); tapeworm infestations; adjunctive management of hepatic coma; treatment of cryptosporidial diarrhea

Usual Dosage Oral:

Intestinal amebiasis: Children and Adults: 25-35 mg/kg/day in 3 divided doses for 5-10 days

Tapeworm (fish, dog, bovine, porcine):

Children: 11 mg/kg every 15 minutes for 4 doses

Adults: 1 g every 15 minutes for 4 doses

Hepatic coma: Adults: 4 g/day in 2-4 divided doses for 5-6 days

Dwarf tapeworm: Children and Adults: 45 mg/kg/dose every day for 5-7 days

Dosage Forms Capsule, as sulfate: 250 mg

paroxetine (pa ROKS e teen)

U.S./Canadian Brand Names Paxil® CR™ [US/Can]; Paxil® [US/Can]

Therapeutic Category Antidepressant, Selective Serotonin Reuptake Inhibitor

Use Treatment of depression in adults; treatment of panic disorder with or without agoraphobia; obsessive-compulsive disorder (OCD) in adults; social anxiety disorder (social phobia); generalized anxiety disorder (GAD); post-traumatic stress disorder (PTSD)

Usual Dosage Adults: Oral: 20 mg once daily, preferably in the morning

Dosage Forms

Suspension, oral (Paxil®): 10 mg/5 mL (250 mL) [orange flavor]

Tablet (Paxil®): 10 mg, 20 mg, 30 mg, 40 mg

Tablet, controlled release (Paxil® CR™): 12.5 mg, 25 mg, 37.5 mg

Parsidol® *(Discontinued)* see page 814

Parsitan® [Can] see ethopropazine *(Canada only)* on page 256

Partuss® **LA** *(Discontinued)* see page 814

Parvolex® [Can] see acetylcysteine on page 11

PAS see aminosalicylate sodium on page 34

Patanol® [US/Can] see olopatadine on page 476

Pathilon® *(Discontinued)* see page 814

Pathocil® *(Discontinued)* see page 814

Pavabid® **(all products)** *(Discontinued)* see page 814

Pavacot® [US] see papaverine on page 492

Pavasule® *(Discontinued)* see page 814

Pavatine® *(Discontinued)* see page 814

Pavatym® *(Discontinued)* see page 814

Pavesed® *(Discontinued)* see page 814

Pavulon® *(Discontinued)* see page 814

Paxene® *(Discontinued)* see page 814

Paxil® [US/Can] see paroxetine on this page

Paxil® **CR™** [US/Can] see paroxetine on this page

Paxipam® [US/Can] see halazepam on page 315

PBZ® **(all products)** *(Discontinued)* see page 814

PC-Cap® [US] see propoxyphene and aspirin on page 549

PCE® [US/Can] see erythromycin (systemic) on page 235

PCMX see parachlorometaxylenol on page 492

PCV7 *see* pneumococcal conjugate vaccine (7-valent) *on page 521*

pectin and kaolin *see* kaolin and pectin *on page 366*

Pedameth® **[US]** *see* methionine *on page 416*

PediaCare® Decongestant Infants [US-OTC] *see* pseudoephedrine *on page 552*

Pediacof® **[US]** *see* chlorpheniramine, phenylephrine, and codeine *on page 139*

Pediaflor® **[US]** *see* fluoride *on page 278*

Pedialyte® [US-OTC] *see* nutritional formula, enteral/oral *on page 472*

Pediamist® [US-OTC] *see* sodium chloride *on page 595*

PediaPatch Transdermal Patch *(Discontinued)* *see page 814*

Pediapred® [US/Can] *see* prednisolone (systemic) *on page 537*

Pedia-Profen™ *(Discontinued)* *see page 814*

Pediatric Triban® *(Discontinued)* *see page 814*

Pediatrix [Can] *see* acetaminophen *on page 3*

Pediazole® [US/Can] *see* erythromycin and sulfisoxazole *on page 235*

Pedi-Boro® [US-OTC] *see* aluminum sulfate and calcium acetate *on page 29*

Pedi-Dri® **[US]** *see* nystatin *on page 473*

PediOtic® **[US]** *see* neomycin, polymyxin B, and hydrocortisone *on page 453*

Pedituss® **[US]** *see* chlorpheniramine, phenylephrine, and codeine *on page 139*

PedTE-PAK-4® **[US]** *see* trace metals *on page 646*

Pedtrace-4® **[US]** *see* trace metals *on page 646*

PedvaxHIB® [US/Can] *see* Haemophilus B conjugate vaccine *on page 314*

pegademase (bovine) (peg A de mase BOE vine)
U.S./Canadian Brand Names Adagen™ [US/Can]
Therapeutic Category Enzyme
Use Enzyme replacement therapy for adenosine deaminase (ADA) deficiency in patients with severe combined immunodeficiency disease (SCID) who can not benefit from bone marrow transplant
Usual Dosage Children: I.M.: Dose administered every 7 days, 10 units/kg the first dose, 15 units/kg the second dose, and 20 units/kg the third; maintenance dose: 20 units/kg/week is recommended depending on patient's ADA level
Dosage Forms Injection: 250 units/mL (1.5 mL)

Peganone® [US/Can] *see* ethotoin *on page 257*

pegaspargase (peg AS par jase)
Synonyms PEG-L-asparaginase
U.S./Canadian Brand Names Oncaspar® [US/Can]
Therapeutic Category Antineoplastic Agent
Use Induction treatment of acute lymphoblastic leukemia in combination with other chemotherapeutic agents in patients who have developed hypersensitivity to native forms of asparaginase derived from *E. coli* and/or *Erwinia chrysanthem*, treatment of lymphoma
Usual Dosage Refer to individual protocols; I.M. administration may decrease the risk of anaphylaxis; dose must be individualized based upon clinical response and tolerance of the patient
I.M., I.V.: 2000 units/m^2 every 14 days
Dosage Forms Injection [preservative free]: 750 units/mL

PEG-ES *see* polyethylene glycol-electrolyte solution *on page 525*

pegfilgrastim (peg fil GRA stim)
Synonyms granulocyte colony stimulating factor (PEG Conjugate)
U.S./Canadian Brand Names Neulasta™ [US]
Therapeutic Category Colony-Stimulating Factor
Use Decrease the incidence of infection, by stimulation of granulocyte production, in patients with nonmyeloid malignancies receiving myelosuppressive therapy associated with a significant risk of febrile neutropenia
Usual Dosage S.C.: Adolescents >45 kg and Adults: 6 mg once per chemotherapy cycle; do not administer in the period between 14 days before and 24 hours after administration of cytotoxic chemotherapy; do not use in patients infants, children and smaller adolescents weighing <45 kg
Dosage Forms Injection, solution [prefilled syringe; preservative free]: 10 mg/mL (0.6 mL)

peginterferon alfa-2b (peg in ter FEER on AL fa-too bee)
U.S./Canadian Brand Names PEG-Intron™ [US]
Therapeutic Category Interferon
Use Treatment of chronic hepatitis C in adult patients who have never received interferon alpha and have compensated liver disease
Usual Dosage
Children: Safety and efficacy has not been established
Adults: Chronic hepatitis C: S.C.: Initial:
37-45 kg: 40 mcg
46-56 kg: 50 mcg
57-72 kg: 64 mcg
73-88 kg: 80 mcg
89-106 kg: 96 mcg
107-136 kg: 120 mcg
137-160 kg: 150 mcg
Note: Administer dose once weekly for 1 year; after 24 weeks of treatment, if serum HCV RNA is not below the limit of detection of the assay, consider discontinuation
Dosage Forms Injection, powder for reconstitution: 50 mcg/0.5 mL, 80 mcg/0.5 mL, 120 mcg/0.5 mL, 150 mcg/0.5 mL

PEG-Intron™ [US] *see* peginterferon alfa-2b *on this page*

PEG-L-asparaginase *see* pegaspargase *on previous page*

PegLyte® [Can] *see* polyethylene glycol-electrolyte solution *on page 525*

PemADD® [US] *see* pemoline *on this page*

PemADD CT® [US] *see* pemoline *on this page*

pemirolast (pe MIR oh last)
U.S./Canadian Brand Names Alamast™ [US/Can]
Therapeutic Category Mast Cell Stabilizer; Ophthalmic Agent, Miscellaneous
Use Prevention of itchy eyes due to allergic conjunctivitis.
Dosage Forms Solution, ophthalmic: 0.1% (10 mL)

pemoline (PEM oh leen)
Synonyms phenylisohydantoin; PIO
U.S./Canadian Brand Names Cylert® [US]; PemADD CT® [US]; PemADD® [US]
Therapeutic Category Central Nervous System Stimulant, Nonamphetamine
Controlled Substance C-IV
Use Treatment of attention-deficit/hyperactivity disorder (ADHD); narcolepsy
Usual Dosage Oral:
Children <6 years: Not recommended

Children ≥6 years and Adults: Initial: 37.5 mg administered once daily in the morning, increase by 18.75 mg/day at weekly intervals; effective dose range: 56.25-75 mg/day; maximum: 112.5 mg/day; dosage range: 0.5-3 mg/kg/24 hours

Dosage Forms
Tablet: 18.75 mg, 37.5 mg, 75 mg
Tablet, chewable: 37.5 mg

penbutolol (pen BYOO toe lole)

U.S./Canadian Brand Names Levatol® [US/Can]
Therapeutic Category Beta-Adrenergic Blocker
Use Treatment of mild to moderate arterial hypertension
Usual Dosage Adults: Oral: Initial: 20 mg once daily, full effect of a 20 or 40 mg dose is seen by the end of a 2-week period, doses of 40-80 mg have been tolerated but have shown little additional antihypertensive effects
Dosage Forms Tablet, as sulfate: 20 mg

penciclovir (pen SYE kloe veer)

U.S./Canadian Brand Names Denavir™ [US]
Therapeutic Category Antiviral Agent
Use Antiviral cream for the treatment of recurrent herpes labialis (cold sores) in adults
Usual Dosage Apply cream at the first sign or symptom of cold sore (eg, tingling, swelling); apply every 2 hours during waking hours for 4 days
Dosage Forms Cream: 1% [10 mg/g] (1.5 g)

Penecort® [US] *see* hydrocortisone (topical) *on page 334*

penicillamine (pen i SIL a meen)

Synonyms d-3-mercaptovaline; β,β-dimethylcysteine; d-penicillamine
U.S./Canadian Brand Names Cuprimine® [US/Can]; Depen® [US/Can]
Therapeutic Category Chelating Agent
Use Treatment of Wilson's disease, cystinuria, adjunct in the treatment of severe rheumatoid arthritis; lead poisoning, primary biliary cirrhosis
Usual Dosage Oral:
Rheumatoid arthritis:
Children: Initial: 3 mg/kg/day (≤250 mg/day) for 3 months, then 6 mg/kg/day (≤500 mg/day) in divided doses twice daily for 3 months to a maximum of 10 mg/kg/day in 3-4 divided doses
Adults: 125-250 mg/day, may increase dose at 1- to 3-month intervals up to 1-1.5 g/day
Wilson's disease (doses titrated to maintain urinary copper excretion >1 mg/day):
Infants <6 months: 250 mg/dose once daily
Children <12 years: 250 mg/dose 2-3 times/day
Adults: 250 mg 4 times/day
Cystinuria:
Children: 30 mg/kg/day in 4 divided doses
Adults: 1-4 g/day in divided doses every 6 hours
Lead poisoning (continue until blood lead level is <60 mcg/dL):
Children: 25-40 mg/kg/day in 3 divided doses
Adults: 250 mg/dose every 8-12 hours
Primary biliary cirrhosis: 250 mg/day to start, increase by 250 mg every 2 weeks up to a maintenance dose of 1 g/day, usually administered 250 mg 4 times/day
Arsenic poisoning: Children: 100 mg/kg/day in divided doses every 6 hours for 5 days; maximum: 1 g/day

Dosage Forms
Capsule: 125 mg, 250 mg
Tablet: 250 mg

penicillin G benzathine (pen i SIL in jee BENZ a theen)

Synonyms benzathine benzylpenicillin; benzathine penicillin G; benzylpenicillin benzathine

U.S./Canadian Brand Names Bicillin® L-A [US]; Permapen® [US]

Therapeutic Category Penicillin

Use Active against most gram-positive organisms and some spirochetes; used only for the treatment of mild to moderately severe infections (ie, *Streptococcus* pharyngitis) caused by organisms susceptible to low concentrations of penicillin G, or for prophylaxis of infections caused by these organisms such as rheumatic fever prophylaxis

Usual Dosage I.M.: Administer undiluted injection, very slowly released from site of injection, providing uniform levels over 2-4 weeks; higher doses result in more sustained rather than higher levels. Use a penicillin G benzathine-penicillin G procaine combination to achieve early peak levels in acute infections

Infants and Children:

Group A streptococcal upper respiratory infection: 25,000 units/kg as a single dose; maximum: 1.2 million units

Prophylaxis of recurrent rheumatic fever: 25,000 units/kg every 3-4 weeks; maximum: 1.2 million units/dose

Early syphilis: 50,000 units/kg as a single injection; maximum: 2.4 million units

Syphilis of more than 1-year duration: 50,000 units/kg every week for 3 doses; maximum: 2.4 million units/dose

Adults:

Group A streptococcal upper respiratory infection: 1.2 million units as a single dose

Prophylaxis of recurrent rheumatic fever: 1.2 million units every 3-4 weeks or 600,000 units twice monthly; a single dose of 600,000 to 1,2000,000 units is effective in the prevention of rheumatic fever secondary to streptococcal pharyngitis

Early syphilis: 2.4 million units as a single dose

Syphilis of more than 1-year duration: 2.4 million units once weekly for 3 doses

Dosage Forms Injection, suspension [prefilled syringe]:

Bicillin® L-A: 600,000 units/mL (1 mL, 2 mL, 4 mL)

Permapen® Isoject®: 600,000 units/mL (2 mL)

penicillin G benzathine and procaine combined

(pen i SIL in jee BENZ a theen & PROE kane KOM bined)

Synonyms penicillin G procaine and benzathine combined

U.S./Canadian Brand Names Bicillin® C-R 900/300 [US]; Bicillin® C-R [US]

Therapeutic Category Penicillin

Use Active against most gram-positive organisms, mostly streptococcal and pneumococcal

Usual Dosage I.M.:

Children:

<30 lb: 600,000 units in a single dose

30-60 lb: 900,000 units to 1.2 million units in a single dose

Children >60 lb and Adults: 2.4 million units in a single dose

Dosage Forms Injection, suspension [prefilled syringe]:

Bicillin® C-R:

600,000 units: Penicillin G benzathine 300,000 units and penicillin G 300,000 units (1 mL)

1,200,000 units: Penicillin G benzathine 600,000 units and penicillin G procaine 600,000 units (2 mL)

2,400,000 units: Penicillin G benzathine 1,200,000 units and penicillin G procaine 1,200,000 units (4 mL)

Bicillin® C-R 900/300: 1,200,000 units: Penicillin G benzathine 900,000 units and penicillin G procaine 300,000 units (2 mL)

penicillin G (parenteral/aqueous)
(pen i SIL in jee pa REN ter al/AYE kwee us)

Synonyms benzylpenicillin; crystalline penicillin

U.S./Canadian Brand Names Pfizerpen® [US/Can]

Therapeutic Category Penicillin

Use Active against most gram-positive organisms except *Staphylococcus aureus*; some gram-negative such as *Neisseria gonorrhoeae* and some anaerobes and spirochetes; although ceftriaxone is now the drug of choice for Lyme disease and gonorrhea

Usual Dosage I.M., I.V.:

Infants and Children (sodium salt is preferred in children): 100,000-250,000 units/kg/day in divided doses every 4 hours; maximum: 4.8 million units/24 hours

Severe infections: Up to 400,000 units/kg/day in divided doses every 4 hours; maximum dose: 24 million units/day

Adults: 2-24 million units/day in divided doses every 4 hours

Dosage Forms

Injection, penicillin G potassium [premixed, frozen]: 1 million units, 2 million units, 3 million units

Injection, penicillin G sodium: 5 million units

Injection, powder for reconstitution, penicillin G potassium: 1 million units, 5 million units, 10 million units, 20 million units

penicillin G procaine (pen i SIL in jee PROE kane)

Synonyms APPG; aqueous procaine penicillin G; procaine benzylpenicillin; procaine penicillin G

U.S./Canadian Brand Names Wycillin® [US/Can]

Therapeutic Category Penicillin

Use Moderately severe infections due to *Neisseria gonorrhoeae*, *Treponema pallidum*, and other penicillin G-sensitive microorganisms that are susceptible to low but prolonged serum penicillin concentrations

Usual Dosage I.M.:

Newborns: 50,000 units/kg/day administered every day (avoid using in this age group since sterile abscesses and procaine toxicity occur more frequently with neonates than older patients)

Children: 25,000-50,000 units/kg/day in divided doses 1-2 times/day; not to exceed 4.8 million units/24 hours

Gonorrhea: 100,000 units/kg one time (in 2 injection sites) along with probenecid 25 mg/kg (maximum: 1 g) orally 30 minutes prior to procaine penicillin

Adults: 0.6-4.8 million units/day in divided doses 1-2 times/day

Uncomplicated gonorrhea: 1 g probenecid orally, then 4.8 million units procaine penicillin divided into 2 injection sites 30 minutes later. When used in conjunction with an aminoglycoside for the treatment of endocarditis caused by susceptible *S. viridans*: 1.2 million units every 6 hours for 2-4 weeks

Dosage Forms Injection, suspension: 300,000 units/mL (10 mL); 600,000 units/mL (1 mL, 2 mL, 4 mL)

penicillin G procaine and benzathine combined *see* penicillin G benzathine and procaine combined *on previous page*

penicillin V potassium (pen i SIL in vee poe TASS ee um)

Synonyms pen VK; phenoxymethyl penicillin

U.S./Canadian Brand Names Apo®-Pen VK [Can]; Nadopen-V® [Can]; Novo-Pen-VK® [Can]; Nu-Pen-VK® [Can]; PVF® K [Can]; Suspen® [US]; Truxcillin® [US]; Veetids® [US]

Therapeutic Category Penicillin

Use Treatment of mild to moderately severe susceptible bacterial infections involving the upper respiratory tract, skin, and urinary tract; prophylaxis of pneumococcal infections and rheumatic fever

(Continued)

penicillin V potassium *(Continued)*

Usual Dosage Oral:

Systemic infections:

Children <12 years: 25-50 mg/kg/day in divided doses every 6-8 hours; maximum dose: 3 g/day

Children >12 years and Adults: 125-500 mg every 6-8 hours

Prophylaxis of pneumococcal infections:

Children <5 years: 125 mg twice daily

Children ≥5 years: 250 mg twice daily

Prophylaxis of recurrent rheumatic fever:

Children <5 years: 125 mg

Children ≥5 years and Adults: 250 mg twice daily

Dosage Forms 250 mg = 400,000 units

Powder for oral solution: 125 mg/5 mL (80 mL, 100 mL, 150 mL, 200 mL); 250 mg/5 mL (80 mL, 100 mL, 150 mL, 200 mL)

Tablet: 250 mg, 500 mg

penicilloyl-polylysine *see* benzylpenicilloyl-polylysine *on page 81*

Penlac™ [US/Can] *see* ciclopirox *on page 145*

Penta/3B® [Can] *see* vitamin B complex *on page 681*

Penta/3B®+C [Can] *see* vitamin B complex with vitamin C *on page 681*

Pentacarinat® [Can] *see* pentamidine *on this page*

Pentacarinat® Injection *(Discontinued)* *see page 814*

Pentacel™ [Can] *see* diphtheria, tetanus toxoids, and whole-cell pertussis vaccine *on page 205*

Pentam-300® [US] *see* pentamidine *on this page*

pentamidine (pen TAM i deen)

U.S./Canadian Brand Names NebuPent™ [US]; Pentacarinat® [Can]; Pentam-300® [US]

Therapeutic Category Antiprotozoal

Use Treatment and prevention of pneumonia caused by *Pneumocystis carinii* in patients who cannot tolerate co-trimoxazole or who fail to respond to this drug; treatment of African trypanosomiasis; treatment of visceral leishmaniasis caused by *L. donovani*

Usual Dosage

Children:

Treatment: I.M., I.V. (I.V. preferred): 4 mg/kg/day once daily for 14-21 days

Prevention:

I.M., I.V.: 4 mg/kg monthly or biweekly

Inhalation (aerosolized pentamidine in children ≥5 years): 300 mg/dose administered every 3 weeks or monthly via Respirgard® II inhaler (8 mg/kg dose has also been used in children <5 years)

Treatment of trypanosomiasis: I.V.: 4 mg/kg/day once daily for 10 days

Adults:

Treatment: I.M., I.V. (I.V. preferred): 4 mg/kg/day once daily for 14 days

Prevention: Inhalation: 300 mg every 4 weeks via Respirgard® II nebulizer

Dosage Forms

Injection, powder for reconstitution, as isethionate: 300 mg

Powder for nebulization, as isethionate: 300 mg

Pentamycetin® [Can] *see* chloramphenicol *on page 133*

Pentasa® [US/Can] *see* mesalamine *on page 411*

Pentaspan® [US/Can] *see* pentastarch *on next page*

pentastarch (PEN ta starch)
U.S./Canadian Brand Names Pentaspan® [US/Can]
Therapeutic Category Blood Modifiers
Use Adjunct in leukapheresis to improve the harvesting and increase the yield of leukocytes by centrifugal means
Usual Dosage 250-700 mL to which citrate anticoagulant has been added is administered by adding to the input line of the centrifugation apparatus at a ratio of 1:8-1:13 to venous whole blood
Dosage Forms Injection, in NS: 10%

pentazocine (pen TAZ oh seen)
U.S./Canadian Brand Names Talwin® NX [US]; Talwin® [US/Can]
Therapeutic Category Analgesic, Narcotic
Controlled Substance C-IV
Use Relief of moderate to severe pain; a sedative prior to surgery; supplement to surgical anesthesia
Usual Dosage
Children: I.M., S.C.:
5-8 years: 15 mg
8-14 years: 30 mg
Children >12 years and Adults: Oral: 50 mg every 3-4 hours; may increase to 100 mg/dose if needed, but should not exceed 600 mg/day
Adults:
I.M., S.C.: 30-60 mg every 3-4 hours, not to exceed total daily dose of 360 mg
I.V.: 30 mg every 3-4 hours
Dosage Forms
Injection, as lactate: 30 mg/mL (1 mL, 1.5 mL, 2 mL, 10 mL)
Tablet: Pentazocine hydrochloride 50 mg and naloxone hydrochloride 0.5 mg

pentazocine compound (pen TAZ oh seen KOM pownd)
U.S./Canadian Brand Names Talacen® [US]; Talwin® Compound [US]
Therapeutic Category Analgesic, Narcotic
Use Relief of moderate to severe pain; has also been used as a sedative prior to surgery and as a supplement to surgical anesthesia
Usual Dosage Adults: Oral: 2 tablets 3-4 times/day
Dosage Forms
Tablet:
Talacen®: Pentazocine hydrochloride 25 mg and acetaminophen 650 mg
Talwin® Compound: Pentazocine hydrochloride 12.5 mg and aspirin 325 mg

Penthrane® [US/Can] *see* methoxyflurane *on page 419*
Pentids® (all products) *(Discontinued)* *see page 814*

pentobarbital (pen toe BAR bi tal)
U.S./Canadian Brand Names Nembutal® [US/Can]
Therapeutic Category Barbiturate
Controlled Substance C-II
Use Short-term treatment of insomnia; preoperative sedation; high-dose barbiturate coma for treatment of increased intracranial pressure or status epilepticus unresponsive to other therapy
Usual Dosage
Children:
Sedative: Oral: 2-6 mg/kg/day divided in 3 doses; maximum: 100 mg/day
Hypnotic: I.M.: 2-6 mg/kg; maximum: 100 mg/dose
Rectal:
2 months to 1 year (10-20 lb): 30 mg
1-4 years (20-40 lb): 30-60 mg
(Continued)

pentobarbital *(Continued)*

5-12 years (40-80 lb): 60 mg
12-14 years (80-110 lb): 60-120 mg **or**
<4 years: 3-6 mg/kg/dose
>4 years: 1.5-3 mg/kg/dose
Preoperative/preprocedure sedation: ≥6 months:
Oral, I.M., rectal: 2-6 mg/kg; maximum: 100 mg/dose
I.V.: 1-3 mg/kg to a maximum of 100 mg until asleep
Children 5-12 years: Conscious sedation prior to a procedure: I.V.: 2 mg/kg 5-10 minutes before procedures, may repeat one time
Adolescents: Conscious sedation: Oral, I.V.: 100 mg prior to a procedure

Children and Adults: Barbiturate coma in head injury patients: I.V.:
Loading dose: 5-10 mg/kg administered slowly over 1-2 hours; monitor blood pressure and respiratory rate
Maintenance infusion: Initial: 1 mg/kg/hour; may increase to 2-3 mg/kg/hour; maintain burst suppression on EEG
Adults:
Hypnotic:
Oral: 100-200 mg at bedtime or 20 mg 3-4 times/day for daytime sedation
I.M.: 150-200 mg
I.V.: Initial: 100 mg, may repeat every 1-3 minutes up to 200-500 mg total dose
Rectal: 120-200 mg at bedtime
Preoperative sedation: I.M.: 150-200 mg
Dosage Forms
Capsule, as sodium (C-II): 50 mg, 100 mg
Injection, as sodium (C-II): 50 mg/mL (20 mL, 50 mL)
Suppository, rectal (C-III): 60 mg, 200 mg

pentosan polysulfate sodium (PEN toe san pol i SUL fate SOW dee um)
Synonyms PPS
U.S./Canadian Brand Names Elmiron® [US/Can]
Therapeutic Category Analgesic, Urinary
Use Bladder pain relief or discomfort associated with interstitial cystitis
Usual Dosage Adults: Oral: 100 mg capsule 3 times/day; administer with water at least 1 hour before meals or 2 hours after meals
Dosage Forms Capsule: 100 mg

pentostatin (PEN toe stat in)
Synonyms DCF; 2'-deoxycoformycin
U.S./Canadian Brand Names Nipent™ [US/Can]
Therapeutic Category Antineoplastic Agent
Use Treatment of adult patients with alpha-interferon-refractory hairy cell leukemia; significant antitumor activity in various lymphoid neoplasms has been demonstrated; pentostatin also is known as 2'-deoxycoformycin; it is a purine analogue capable of inhibiting adenosine deaminase
Usual Dosage Refractory hairy cell leukemia: Adults: I.V.: 4 mg/m² every other week
Dosage Forms Injection, powder for reconstitution: 10 mg/vial

Pentothal® Sodium [US/Can] *see* thiopental *on page 634*

pentoxifylline (pen toks I fi leen)
Synonyms oxpentifylline
U.S./Canadian Brand Names Albert® Pentoxifylline [Can]; Apo®-Pentoxifylline SR [Can]; Nu-Pentoxifylline SR [Can]; Trental® [US/Can]
Therapeutic Category Blood Viscosity Reducer Agent
Use Symptomatic management of peripheral vascular disease, mainly intermittent claudication

Investigational use: AIDS patients with increased tumor necrosis factor, cerebrovascular accidents, cerebrovascular diseases, new onset type I diabetes mellitus, diabetic atherosclerosis, diabetic neuropathy, gangrene, cutaneous polyarteritis nodosa, hemodialysis shunt thrombosis, cerebral malaria, septic shock, sepsis in premature neonates, sickle cell syndromes, vasculitis, Kawasaki disease, Raynaud's syndrome, cystic fibrosis, and persistent pulmonary hypertension of the newborn (case report)

Usual Dosage Adults: Oral: 400 mg 3 times/day with meals; may reduce to 400 mg twice daily if GI or CNS side effects occur

Dosage Forms Tablet, controlled release: 400 mg

Pentrax® **[US-OTC]** *see* coal tar *on page 158*

Pen.Vee® **K** *(Discontinued)* *see page 814*

pen VK *see* penicillin V potassium *on page 499*

Pepcid® **[US/Can]** *see* famotidine *on page 262*

Pepcid® **AC [US/Can]** *see* famotidine *on page 262*

Pepcid® **Complete [US-OTC]** *see* famotidine, calcium carbonate, and magnesium hydroxide *on page 263*

Pepcid RPD® *(Discontinued)* *see page 814*

Peptavlon® *(Discontinued)* *see page 814*

Pepto-Bismol® **[US-OTC]** *see* bismuth subsalicylate *on page 87*

Pepto® **Diarrhea Control** *(Discontinued)* *see page 814*

Perchloracap® **[US]** *see* radiological/contrast media (ionic) *on page 561*

Percocet® **2.5/325 [US]** *see* oxycodone and acetaminophen *on page 485*

Percocet® **5/325 [US]** *see* oxycodone and acetaminophen *on page 485*

Percocet® **7.5/325 [US]** *see* oxycodone and acetaminophen *on page 485*

Percocet® **7.5/500 [US]** *see* oxycodone and acetaminophen *on page 485*

Percocet® **10/325 [US]** *see* oxycodone and acetaminophen *on page 485*

Percocet® **10/650 [US]** *see* oxycodone and acetaminophen *on page 485*

Percodan® **[US/Can]** *see* oxycodone and aspirin *on page 485*

Percodan®-**Demi** *(Discontinued)* *see page 814*

Percodan®-**Demi**® **[Can]** *see* oxycodone and aspirin *on page 485*

Percogesic® **[US-OTC]** *see* acetaminophen and phenyltoloxamine *on page 6*

Percolone® *(Discontinued)* *see page 814*

Perdiem® **Plain [US-OTC]** *see* psyllium *on page 554*

Perfectoderm® **Gel** *(Discontinued)* *see page 814*

perflutren lipid microspheres (per FLOO tren LIP id MIKE roe sfeers)
U.S./Canadian Brand Names Definity® [US]
Therapeutic Category Diagnostic Agent
Use Opacification of left ventricular chamber and improvement of delineation of the left ventricular endocardial border in patients with suboptimal echocardiograms
Usual Dosage Adults: Dose should be given following baseline noncontrast echocardiography. Imaging should begin immediately following dose and compared to noncontrast image. Mechanical index for the ultrasound device should be set at ≤0.8.
I.V. bolus: 10 microliters/kg of activated product, followed by 10 mL saline flush. May repeat in 30 minutes if needed (maximum dose: 2 bolus infusions).
I.V. infusion: Initial: 4 mL/minute of prepared infusion; titrate to achieve optimal image; maximum rate: 10 mL/minute (maximum dose: 1 intravenous infusion).
Dosage Forms Injection, solution [preservative free]: OFP 6.52 mg/mL and lipid blend 0.75 mg/mL (2 mL) [following activation, forms a suspension containing perflutren lipid microspheres 1.2 x 10^{10}/mL and OFP 1.1 mg/mL]

pergolide (PER go lide)

U.S./Canadian Brand Names Permax® [US/Can]

Therapeutic Category Anti-Parkinson's Agent; Dopaminergic Agent (Anti-Parkinson's); Ergot Alkaloid and Derivative

Use Adjunctive treatment to levodopa/carbidopa in the management of Parkinson's Disease

Usual Dosage Adults: Oral: Initial: 0.05 mg/day for 2 days, then increase dosage by 0.1 or 0.15 mg/day every 3 days over next 12 days, increase dose by 0.25 mg/day every 3 days until optimal therapeutic dose is achieved

Dosage Forms Tablet, as mesylate: 0.05 mg, 0.25 mg, 1 mg

Pergonal® [US/Can] *see* menotropins *on page 407*

Periactin® [US/Can] *see* cyproheptadine *on page 170*

Peri-Colace® [US/Can] *see* docusate and casanthranol *on page 209*

pericyazine *(Canada only)* (per ee CYE ah zeen)

U.S./Canadian Brand Names Neuleptil® [Can]

Therapeutic Category Phenothiazine Derivative

Use As adjunctive medication in some psychotic patients, for the control of residual prevailing hostility, impulsiveness and aggressiveness

Usual Dosage Oral:

Children and adolescents (5 years of age and over): 2.5-10 mg in the morning and 5-30 mg in the evening. These dosages approximate a daily dosage range of 1-3 mg/year of age.

Adults: 5-20 mg in the morning and 10-40 mg in the evening. For maintenance therapy, the dosage should be reduced to the minimum effective dose. Lower doses of 2.5-15 mg in the morning, and 5-30 mg in the evening have been suggested. For elderly patients the initial total daily dosage should be in the order of 5 mg and increased gradually as tolerated, until an adequate response is obtained. A daily dosage of more than 30 mg will rarely be needed. Children and adolescents (5 years of age and over): 2.5-10 mg in the morning and 5-30 mg in the evening. These dosages approximate a daily dosage range of 1-3 mg/year of age.

Dosage Forms

Capsule: 5 mg, 10 mg, 20 mg

Drops, oral: 10 mg/mL (100 mL)

Peridex® [US] *see* chlorhexidine gluconate *on page 134*

Peridol [Can] *see* haloperidol *on page 316*

perindopril erbumine (per IN doe pril er BYOO meen)

U.S./Canadian Brand Names Aceon® [US]; Coversyl® [Can]

Therapeutic Category Miscellaneous Product

Use Treatment of hypertension

Usual Dosage Adults: Oral: 4 mg once daily; usual range: 4-8 mg/day; maximum: 16 mg/day

Dosage Forms Tablet: 2 mg, 4 mg, 8 mg

Periochip® [US] *see* chlorhexidine gluconate *on page 134*

PerioGard® [US] *see* chlorhexidine gluconate *on page 134*

Periostat® [US] *see* doxycycline *on page 215*

Peritrate® *(Discontinued)* *see page 814*

Peritrate® SA *(Discontinued)* *see page 814*

Permapen® [US] *see* penicillin G benzathine *on page 498*

Permax® [US/Can] *see* pergolide *on this page*

permethrin (per METH rin)

U.S./Canadian Brand Names A-200™ Lice [US-OTC]; Acticin® [US]; Elimite® [US]; Kwellada-P™ [Can]; Nix® [US/Can]; Nix® Dermal Cream [Can]; R & C® Lice [US]; RID® Spray [US-OTC]

Therapeutic Category Scabicides/Pediculicides

Use Single application treatment of infestation with *Pediculus humanus capitis* (head louse) and its nits, or *Sarcoptes scabiei* (scabies)

Usual Dosage

Head lice: Children >2 months and Adults: Topical: After hair has been washed with shampoo, rinsed with water and towel-dried, apply a sufficient volume to saturate the hair and scalp. Leave on hair for 10 minutes before rinsing off with water; remove remaining nits.

Scabies: Apply cream from head to toe; leave on for 8-14 hours before washing off with water

Dosage Forms

Cream, topical (Acticin®, Elimite®): 5% (60 g) [contains coconut oil]

Liquid, topical (Nix®): 1% (60 mL) [contains isopropyl alcohol 20%; creme rinse formulation]

Lotion, topical: 1% (59 mL)

Shampoo (A-200™ Lice): 0.33% (60 mL, 120 mL) [contains benzyl alcohol]

Solution, spray [for bedding and furniture]

A-200™ Lice: 0.5% (180 mL)

Nix®: 0.25% (148 mL)

RID®: 0.5% (150 mL)

Permitil® Oral *(Discontinued)* see page 814

Pernox® [US-OTC] *see* sulfur and salicylic acid on page 614

Peroxin A5® *(Discontinued)* see page 814

Peroxin A10® *(Discontinued)* see page 814

perphenazine (per FEN a zeen)

U.S./Canadian Brand Names Apo®-Perphenazine [Can]; Trilafon® [US/Can]

Therapeutic Category Phenothiazine Derivative

Use Symptomatic management of psychotic disorders, as well as severe nausea and vomiting

Usual Dosage

Children:

Psychoses: Oral:

1-6 years: 4-6 mg/day in divided doses

6-12 years: 6 mg/day in divided doses

>12 years: 4-16 mg 2-4 times/day

I.M.: 5 mg every 6 hours

Nausea/vomiting: I.M.: 5 mg every 6 hours

Adults:

Psychoses:

Oral: 4-16 mg 2-4 times/day not to exceed 64 mg/day

I.M.: 5 mg every 6 hours up to 15 mg/day in ambulatory patients and 30 mg/day in hospitalized patients

Nausea/vomiting:

Oral: 8-16 mg/day in divided doses up to 24 mg/day

I.M.: 5-10 mg every 6 hours as necessary up to 15 mg/day in ambulatory patients and 30 mg/day in hospitalized patients

I.V. (severe): 1 mg at 1- to 2-minute intervals up to a total of 5 mg

Dosage Forms

Injection: 5 mg/mL (1 mL)

Solution, oral concentrate: 16 mg/5 mL (118 mL) [berry flavor]

Tablet: 2 mg, 4 mg, 8 mg, 16 mg

perphenazine and amitriptyline *see* amitriptyline and perphenazine *on page 35*

Persa-Gel® *(Discontinued)* *see page 814*

Persantine® [US/Can] *see* dipyridamole *on page 206*

Pertussin® CS [US-OTC] *see* dextromethorphan *on page 189*

Pertussin® ES [US-OTC] *see* dextromethorphan *on page 189*

pethidine *see* meperidine *on page 408*

Pexicam® [Can] *see* piroxicam *on page 517*

PFA *see* foscarnet *on page 288*

Pfizerpen® [US/Can] *see* penicillin G (parenteral/aqueous) *on page 499*

Pfizerpen-AS® *(Discontinued)* *see page 814*

PGE₁ *see* alprostadil *on page 25*

PGE₂ *see* dinoprostone *on page 201*

Phanasin [US-OTC] *see* guaifenesin *on page 307*

Pharmacist's Capsaicin® [US] *see* capsaicin *on page 111*

Pharmaflur® [US] *see* fluoride *on page 278*

Pharmorubicin® [Can] *see* epirubicin *on page 230*

Phazyme® *(Discontinued)* *see page 814*

Phazyme® [Can] *see* simethicone *on page 591*

Phenadex® Senior *(Discontinued)* *see page 814*

Phenahist-TR® *(Discontinued)* *see page 814*

Phenameth® DM *(Discontinued)* *see page 814*

Phenaphen® *(Discontinued)* *see page 814*

Phenaphen®/Codeine #4 *(Discontinued)* *see page 814*

Phenaphen® With Codeine [US] *see* acetaminophen and codeine *on page 5*

Phenaseptic® *(Discontinued)* *see page 814*

Phenazine® Injection *(Discontinued)* *see page 814*

Phenazo™ [Can] *see* phenazopyridine *on this page*

phenazopyridine (fen az oh PEER i deen)
  Synonyms phenylazo diamino pyridine hydrochloride
  U.S./Canadian Brand Names Azo-Dine® [US-OTC]; Azo-Gesic® [US-OTC]; Azo-Standard® [US]; Baridium® [US]; Phenazo™ [Can]; Prodium™ [US-OTC]; Pyridiate® [US]; Pyridium® [US/Can]; Uristat® [US-OTC]; Urodol® [US-OTC]; Urofemme® [US-OTC]; Urogesic® [US]
  Therapeutic Category Analgesic, Urinary
  Use Symptomatic relief of urinary burning, itching, frequency and urgency in association with urinary tract infection, or following urologic procedures
  Usual Dosage Oral:
    Children 6-12 years: 12 mg/kg/day in 3 divided doses administered after meals for 2 days
    Adults: 100-200 mg 3-4 times/day for 2 days
  Dosage Forms Tablet, as hydrochloride: 95 mg, 97.2 mg, 100 mg, 200 mg

phenazopyridine and sulfisoxazole *see* sulfisoxazole and phenazopyridine *on page 614*

Phencen-50® *(Discontinued)* *see page 814*

Phenclor® S.H.A. *(Discontinued)* *see page 814*

Phendiet® [US] *see* phendimetrazine *on next page*

Phendiet®-105 [US] *see phendimetrazine on this page*

phendimetrazine (fen dye ME tra zeen)
Synonyms phendimetrazine tartrate
U.S./Canadian Brand Names Bontril PDM® [US]; Bontril® Slow-Release [US]; Melfiat® [US]; Obezine® [US]; Phendiet®-105 [US]; Phendiet® [US]; Prelu-2® [US]
Therapeutic Category Anorexiant
Controlled Substance C-III
Use Appetite suppressant during the first few weeks of dieting to help establish new eating habits; its effectiveness lasts only for short periods 3-12 weeks
Usual Dosage Adults: Oral:
  Regular capsule or tablet: 35 mg 2-3 times/day one hour before meals
  Sustained release: 105 mg once daily in the morning before breakfast
Dosage Forms
  Capsule, as tartrate: 35 mg
  Capsule, sustained release, as tartrate: 105 mg
  Tablet, as tartrate: 35 mg

phendimetrazine tartrate *see phendimetrazine on this page*

Phendry® Oral *(Discontinued) see page 814*

phenelzine (FEN el zeen)
U.S./Canadian Brand Names Nardil® [US/Can]
Therapeutic Category Antidepressant, Monoamine Oxidase Inhibitor
Use Symptomatic treatment of atypical, nonendogenous or neurotic depression
Usual Dosage Adults: Oral: 15 mg 3 times/day; may increase to 60-90 mg/day during early phase of treatment, then reduce to dose for maintenance therapy slowly after maximum benefit is obtained; takes 2-4 weeks for a significant response to occur
Dosage Forms Tablet, as sulfate: 15 mg

Phenerbel-S® *(Discontinued) see page 814*

Phenergan® [US/Can] *see promethazine on page 544*

Phenergan® VC [US] *see promethazine and phenylephrine on page 546*

Phenergan® VC With Codeine *(Discontinued) see page 814*

Phenergan® With Codeine [US] *see promethazine and codeine on page 545*

Phenergan® With Dextromethorphan *(Discontinued) see page 814*

Phenetron® *(Discontinued) see page 814*

phenindamine (fen IN dah meen)
U.S./Canadian Brand Names Nolahist® [US/Can]
Therapeutic Category Antihistamine
Use Treatment of perennial and seasonal allergic rhinitis and chronic urticaria
Usual Dosage Oral:
  Children <6 years: As directed by physician
  Children 6 to <12 years: 12.5 mg every 4-6 hours, up to 75 mg/24 hours
  Adults: 25 mg every 4-6 hours, up to 150 mg/24 hours
Dosage Forms Tablet, as tartrate: 25 mg

pheniramine and naphazoline *see naphazoline and pheniramine on page 447*

phenobarbital (fee noe BAR bi tal)
Synonyms phenobarbitone; phenylethylmalonylurea
U.S./Canadian Brand Names Luminal® Sodium [US]
Therapeutic Category Anticonvulsant; Barbiturate
Controlled Substance C-IV
  (Continued)

507

phenobarbital *(Continued)*

Use Management of generalized tonic-clonic (grand mal) and partial seizures; neonatal seizures; febrile seizures in children; sedation; may also be used for prevention and treatment of neonatal hyperbilirubinemia and lowering of bilirubin in chronic cholestasis

Usual Dosage

Children:

Sedation: Oral: 2 mg/kg 3 times/day

Hypnotic: I.M., I.V., S.C.: 3-5 mg/kg at bedtime

Hyperbilirubinemia: <12 years: Oral: 3-8 mg/kg/day in 2-3 divided doses; doses up to 12 mg/kg/day have been used

Preoperative sedation: Oral, I.M., I.V.: 1-3 mg/kg 1-1.5 hours before procedure

Adults:

Sedation: Oral, I.M., I.V.: 30-120 mg/day in 2-3 divided doses

Hypnotic: Oral, I.M., I.V., S.C.: 100-320 mg at bedtime

Hyperbilirubinemia: Oral: 90-180 mg/day in 2-3 divided doses

Preoperative sedation: I.M.: 100-200 mg 1-1$\frac{1}{2}$ hours before procedure

Anticonvulsant: Status epilepticus: **Loading dose:** I.V.:

Infants, Children, and Adults: 15-18 mg/kg in a single or divided dose; usual maximum loading dose: 20 mg/kg; in select patients may administer additional 5 mg/kg/dose every 15-30 minutes until seizure is controlled or a total dose of 30 mg/kg is reached

Anticonvulsant: Maintenance dose: Oral, I.V.:

Infants: 5-6 mg/kg/day in 1-2 divided doses

Children:

1-5 years: 6-8 mg/kg/day in 1-2 divided doses

5-12 years: 4-6 mg/kg/day in 1-2 divided doses

Children >12 years and Adults: 1-3 mg/kg/day in divided doses

Dosage Forms

Elixir: 20 mg/5 mL (5 mL, 7.5 mL, 15 mL, 120 mL, 473 mL, 946 mL, 4000 mL)

Injection, as sodium: 30 mg/mL (1 mL); 60 mg/mL (1 mL); 65 mg/mL (1 mL); 130 mg/mL (1 mL)

Luminal®: 60 mg/mL (1 mL); 130 mg/mL (1 mL)

Tablet: 15 mg, 16 mg, 30 mg, 32 mg, 60 mg, 65 mg, 100 mg

phenobarbital, belladonna, and ergotamine tartrate *see* belladonna, phenobarbital, and ergotamine tartrate *on page 74*

phenobarbital, hyoscyamine, atropine, and scopolamine *see* hyoscyamine, atropine, scopolamine, and phenobarbital *on page 340*

phenobarbitone *see* phenobarbital *on previous page*

phenol *(FEE nol)*

Synonyms carbolic acid

U.S./Canadian Brand Names Baker's P & S [US/Can]; Cēpastat® [US-OTC]; Chloraseptic® [US-OTC]; Ulcerease® [US-OTC]

Therapeutic Category Pharmaceutical Aid

Use Relief of sore throat pain, mouth, gum, and throat irritations

Usual Dosage Oral: Allow to dissolve slowly in mouth; may be repeated every 2 hours as needed

Dosage Forms

Liquid, oral (Ulcerease®): 6% with glycerin (180 mL) [sugar free]

Liquid, topical (Baker's P & S): 1% with sodium chloride, liquid paraffin oil, and water (120 mL, 240 mL)

Lozenge:

Cēpastat®: 1.45% with menthol and eucalyptus oil

Cēpastat® Cherry: 0.72% with menthol and eucalyptus oil

Chloraseptic®: 32.5 mg total phenol, sugar, corn syrup

Mouthwash (Chloraseptic®): 1.4% with thymol, sodium borate, menthol, and glycerin (180 mL)

Solution (liquified phenol): 88% [880 mg/mL]
Solution, aqueous: 6% [60 mg/mL]

phenolsulfonphthalein *(Discontinued)* *see page 814*

Phenoxine® *(Discontinued)* *see page 814*

phenoxybenzamine (fen oks ee BEN za meen)

U.S./Canadian Brand Names Dibenzyline® [US/Can]

Therapeutic Category Alpha-Adrenergic Blocking Agent

Use Symptomatic management of hypertension and sweating in patients with pheochromocytoma

Usual Dosage Oral:

Children: Initial: 0.2 mg/kg (maximum: 10 mg) once daily, increase by 0.2 mg/kg increments; usual maintenance dose: 0.4-1.2 mg/kg/day every 6-8 hours, maximum single dose: 10 mg

Adults: 10-40 mg every 8-12 hours

Dosage Forms Capsule, as hydrochloride: 10 mg

phenoxymethyl penicillin *see* penicillin V potassium *on page 499*

phentermine (FEN ter meen)

U.S./Canadian Brand Names Adipex-P® [US]; Ionamin® [US/Can]

Therapeutic Category Anorexiant

Controlled Substance C-IV

Use Short-term adjunct in exogenous obesity

Usual Dosage Oral: Adults: Obesity: 8 mg 3 times/day 30 minutes before meals or food or 15-37.5 mg/day before breakfast or 10-14 hours before retiring

Dosage Forms

Capsule, as hydrochloride: 15 mg, 18.75 mg, 30 mg, 37.5 mg
  Adipex-P®: 37.5 mg
Capsule, resin complex, as hydrochloride (Ionamin®): 15 mg, 30 mg
Tablet, as hydrochloride: 8 mg, 37.5 mg
  Adipex-P®: 37.5 mg

phentolamine (fen TOLE a meen)

U.S./Canadian Brand Names Rogitine® [Can]

Therapeutic Category Alpha-Adrenergic Blocking Agent; Diagnostic Agent

Use Diagnosis of pheochromocytoma; treatment of hypertension associated with pheochromocytoma or other causes of excess sympathomimetic amines; local treatment of dermal necrosis after extravasation of drugs with alpha-adrenergic effects (dobutamine, dopamine, epinephrine, metaraminol, norepinephrine, phenylephrine)

Usual Dosage

Treatment of extravasation: Infiltrate area S.C. with small amount of solution made by diluting 5-10 mg in 10 mL 0.9% NaCl within 12 hours of extravasation; for children, use 0.1-0.2 mg/kg up to a maximum of 10 mg

Children: I.M., I.V.:
Diagnosis of pheochromocytoma: 0.05-0.1 mg/kg/dose, maximum single dose: 5 mg
Hypertension: 0.05-0.1 mg/kg/dose administered 1-2 hours before procedure; repeat as needed until hypertension is controlled; maximum single dose: 5 mg
Adults: I.M., I.V.:
Diagnosis of pheochromocytoma: 5 mg
Hypertension: 5 mg administered 1-2 hours before procedure

Dosage Forms Injection, as mesylate: 5 mg/mL (1 mL)

Phenurone® *(Discontinued)* *see page 814*

phenylalanine mustard *see* melphalan *on page 406*

phenylazo diamino pyridine hydrochloride *see* phenazopyridine *on page 506*

Phenyldrine® *(Discontinued) see page 814*

phenylephrine (fen il EF rin)

U.S./Canadian Brand Names AK-Dilate® Ophthalmic [US]; AK-Nefrin® Ophthalmic [US]; Children's Nostril® [US]; Dionephrine® [Can]; Mydfrin® Ophthalmic [US/Can]; Neo-Synephrine® Injection [US/Can]; Neo-Synephrine® Nasal [US-OTC]; Neo-Synephrine® Ophthalmic [US]; Nostril® Nasal [US-OTC]; Prefrin™ Ophthalmic [US]; Rhinall® Nasal [US-OTC]; Vicks Sinex® Nasal [US-OTC]

Therapeutic Category Adrenergic Agonist Agent

Use Treatment of hypotension and vascular failure in shock; supraventricular tachycardia; as a vasoconstrictor in regional analgesia; symptomatic relief of nasal and nasopharyngeal mucosal congestion; as a mydriatic in ophthalmic procedures and treatment of wide-angle glaucoma

Usual Dosage

Ophthalmic procedures:

Infants <1 year: Instill 1 drop of 2.5% 15-30 minutes before procedures

Children and Adults: Instill 1 drop of 2.5% or 10% solution, may repeat in 10-60 minutes as needed

Nasal decongestant:

Children:

2-6 years: Instill 1 drop every 2-4 hours of 0.125% solution as needed

6-12 years: Instill 1-2 sprays or instill 1-2 drops every 4 hours of 0.25% solution as needed

Children >12 years and Adults: Instill 1-2 sprays or instill 1-2 drops every 4 hours of 0.25% to 0.5% solution as needed; 1% solution may be used in adult in cases of extreme nasal congestion; do not use nasal solutions more than 3 days

Hypotension/shock:

Children:

I.M., S.C.: 0.1 mg/kg/dose every 1-2 hours as needed (maximum: 5 mg)

I.V. bolus: 5-20 mcg/kg/dose every 10-15 minutes as needed

I.V. infusion: 0.1-0.5 mcg/kg/minute; the concentration and rate of infusion can be calculated using the following formulas: Dilute 0.6 mg x weight (kg) to 100 mL; then the dose in mcg/kg/minute = 0.1 x the infusion rate in mL/hour

Adults:

I.M., S.C.: 2-5 mg/dose every 1-2 hours as needed (initial dose should not exceed 5 mg)

I.V. bolus: 0.1-0.5 mg/dose every 10-15 minutes as needed (initial dose should not exceed 0.5 mg)

I.V. infusion: 10 mg in 250 mL D_5W or NS (1:25,000 dilution) (40 mcg/mL); start at 100-180 mcg/minute (2-5 mL/minute; 50-90 drops/minute) initially. When blood pressure is stabilized, maintenance rate: 40-60 mcg/minute (20-30 drops/minute)

Paroxysmal supraventricular tachycardia: I.V.:

Children: 5-10 mcg/kg/dose over 20-30 seconds

Adults: 0.25-0.5 mg/dose over 20-30 seconds

Dosage Forms

Injection, as hydrochloride (Neo-Synephrine®): 1% [10 mg/mL] (1 mL)

Solution, intranasal drops, as hydrochloride:

Neo-Synephrine®: 0.5% (15 mL, 30 mL)

Neo-Synephrine®, Children's Nostril®, Rhinall®: 0.25% (15 mL, 30 mL, 40 mL)

Neo-Synephrine®: 0.125% (15 mL)

Nasal spray, as hydrochloride:

Neo-Synephrine®, Rhinall®: 0.25% (15 mL, 30 mL, 40 mL)

Neo-Synephrine®: 1% (15 mL)

Neo-Synephrine®, Nostril®, Vicks Sinex®: 0.5% (15 mL, 30 mL)

Solution, ophthalmic, as hydrochloride:

AK-Dilate®, Mydfrin®, Neo-Synephrine®, Phenoptic®: 2.5% (2 mL, 3 mL, 5 mL, 15 mL)

AK-Dilate®, Neo-Synephrine®, Neo-Synephrine® Viscous: 10% (1 mL, 2 mL, 5 mL, 15 mL)

AK-Nefrin®, Prefrin™ Liquifilm®: 0.12% (0.3 mL, 15 mL, 20 mL)

phenylephrine and chlorpheniramine *see* chlorpheniramine and phenylephrine *on page 138*

phenylephrine and cyclopentolate *see* cyclopentolate and phenylephrine *on page 168*

phenylephrine and guaifenesin *see* guaifenesin and phenylephrine *on page 310*

phenylephrine and promethazine *see* promethazine and phenylephrine *on page 546*

phenylephrine and scopolamine (fen il EF rin & skoe POL a meen)

Synonyms scopolamine and phenylephrine

U.S./Canadian Brand Names Murocoll-2® [US]

Therapeutic Category Anticholinergic/Adrenergic Agonist

Use Mydriasis, cycloplegia and to break posterior synechiae in iritis

Usual Dosage Ophthalmic: Instill 1-2 drops into eye(s); repeat in 5 minutes

Dosage Forms Solution, ophthalmic: Phenylephrine hydrochloride 10% and scopolamine hydrobromide 0.3% (7.5 mL)

phenylephrine and zinc sulfate (fen il EF rin & zingk SUL fate)

U.S./Canadian Brand Names Zincfrin® [US/Can]

Therapeutic Category Adrenergic Agonist Agent

Use Soothe, moisturize, and remove redness due to minor eye irritation

Usual Dosage Ophthalmic: Instill 1-2 drops in eye(s) 2-4 times/day as needed

Dosage Forms Solution, ophthalmic: Phenylephrine hydrochloride 0.12% and zinc sulfate 0.25% (15 mL)

phenylephrine, hydrocodone, chlorpheniramine, acetaminophen, and caffeine *see* hydrocodone, chlorpheniramine, phenylephrine, acetaminophen, and caffeine *on page 332*

phenylephrine, promethazine, and codeine *see* promethazine, phenylephrine, and codeine *on page 546*

phenylethylmalonylurea *see* phenobarbital *on page 507*

Phenylfenesin® L.A. (Discontinued) *see page 814*

Phenylgesic® [US-OTC] *see* acetaminophen and phenyltoloxamine *on page 6*

phenylisohydantoin *see* pemoline *on page 496*

Phenytek™ [US] *see* phenytoin *on this page*

phenytoin (FEN i toyn)

Synonyms diphenylhydantoin; DPH

U.S./Canadian Brand Names Dilantin® [US/Can]; Phenytek™ [US]

Therapeutic Category Antiarrhythmic Agent, Class I-B; Hydantoin

Use Management of generalized tonic-clonic (grand mal), simple partial and complex partial seizures; prevention of seizures following head trauma/neurosurgery; ventricular arrhythmias, including those associated with digitalis intoxication, prolonged Q-T interval and surgical repair of congenital heart diseases in children; epidermolysis bullosa

Usual Dosage

Status epilepticus: I.V.:

Infants and Children: Loading dose: 15-18 mg/kg in a single or divided dose; maintenance, anticonvulsant: Initial: 5 mg/kg/day in 2 divided doses, usual doses:

6 months to 3 years: 8-10 mg/kg/day

(Continued)

phenytoin *(Continued)*

4-6 years: 7.5-9 mg/kg/day

7-9 years: 7-8 mg/kg/day

10-16 years: 6-7 mg/kg/day, some patients may require every 8 hours dosing

Adults: Loading dose: 15-18 mg/kg in a single or divided dose; maintenance, anticonvulsant: usual: 300 mg/day or 5-6 mg/kg/day in 3 divided doses or 1-2 divided doses using extended release

Anticonvulsant: Children and Adults: Oral: Loading dose: 15-20 mg/kg; based on phenytoin serum concentrations and recent dosing history; administer oral loading dose in 3 divided doses administered every 2-4 hours to decrease GI adverse effects and to ensure complete oral absorption; maintenance dose: same as I.V.

Arrhythmias:

Children and Adults: Loading dose: I.V.: 1.25 mg/kg IVP every 5 minutes may repeat up to total loading dose: 15 mg/kg

Children: Maintenance dose: Oral, I.V.: 5-10 mg/kg/day in 2 divided doses

Adults: Maintenance dose: Oral: 250 mg 4 times/day for 1 day, 250 mg twice daily for 2 days, then maintenance at 300-400 mg/day in divided doses 1-4 times/day

Dosage Forms

Capsule, extended release, as sodium:

Dilantin®: 30 mg [contains sodium benzoate], 100 mg

Phenytek™: 200 mg, 300 mg

Capsule, prompt release, as sodium: 100 mg

Injection, solution, as sodium: 50 mg/mL (2 mL, 5 mL) [contains alcohol]

Suspension, oral (Dilantin®): 125 mg/5 mL (240 mL) [contains alcohol <0.6%, sodium benzoate; orange-vanilla flavor]

Tablet, chewable (Dilantin®): 50 mg

Pherazine® VC With Codeine *(Discontinued)* see page 814

Pherazine® With Codeine *(Discontinued)* see page 814

Pherazine® With DM *(Discontinued)* see page 814

Phicon® [US-OTC] see pramoxine on page 534

Phillips'® Milk of Magnesia [US-OTC] see magnesium hydroxide on page 397

pHisoHex® [US/Can] see hexachlorophene on page 321

Phos-Ex® 62.5 *(Discontinued)* see page 814

Phos-Ex® 125 *(Discontinued)* see page 814

Phos-Ex® 167 *(Discontinued)* see page 814

Phos-Ex® 250 *(Discontinued)* see page 814

Phos-Flur® [US] see fluoride on page 278

PhosLo® [US] see calcium acetate on page 104

pHos-pHaid® *(Discontinued)* see page 814

Phosphaljel® *(Discontinued)* see page 814

Phospholine Iodide® [US] see echothiophate iodide on page 221

phosphonoformic acid see foscarnet on page 288

phosphorated carbohydrate solution

(FOS for ate ed kar boe HYE drate soe LOO shun)

Synonyms dextrose, levulose and phosphoric acid; levulose, dextrose and phosphoric acid; phosphoric acid, levulose and dextrose

U.S./Canadian Brand Names Emetrol® [US-OTC]; Nausetrol® [US-OTC]

Therapeutic Category Antiemetic

Use Relief of nausea associated with upset stomach that occurs with intestinal flu, pregnancy, food indiscretions, and emotional upsets

Usual Dosage Oral:
Morning sickness: 15-30 mL on arising; repeat every 3 hours or when nausea threatens
Motion sickness and vomiting due to drug therapy: 5 mL doses for young children; 15 mL doses for older children and adults
Regurgitation in infants: 5 or 10 mL, 10-15 minutes before each feeding; in refractory cases: 10-15 mL, 30 minutes before each feeding
Vomiting due to psychogenic factors:
Children: 5-10 mL; repeat dose every 15 minutes until distress subsides; do not take for more than 1 hour
Adults: 15-30 mL; repeat dose every 15 minutes until distress subsides; do not take for more than 1 hour

Dosage Forms
Liquid, oral:
Emetrol®: Dextrose, fructose, and phosphoric acid (118 mL, 236 mL, 473 mL)
Nausetrol®: Dextrose, fructose, and orthophosphoric acid (118 mL, 473 mL, 3785 mL)

phosphoric acid, levulose and dextrose *see* phosphorated carbohydrate solution *on previous page*

Photofrin® [US/Can] *see* porfimer *on page 527*

Phoxal-timolol [Can] *see* timolol *on page 639*

Phrenilin® [US] *see* butalbital, acetaminophen, and caffeine *on page 99*

Phrenilin Forte® [US] *see* butalbital, acetaminophen, and caffeine *on page 99*

p-hydroxyampicillin *see* amoxicillin *on page 37*

Phyllocontin® [Can] *see* aminophylline *on page 33*

Phyllocontin®-350 [Can] *see* aminophylline *on page 33*

phylloquinone *see* phytonadione *on this page*

physostigmine (fye zoe STIG meen)
Therapeutic Category Cholinesterase Inhibitor
Use Reverse toxic CNS and cardiac effects caused by anticholinergics and tricyclic antidepressants; ophthalmic solution is used to treat open-angle glaucoma
Usual Dosage
Children: Reserve for life-threatening situations only: I.V.: 0.01-0.03 mg/kg/dose; may repeat after 15-20 minutes to a maximum total dose of 2 mg
Adults:
I.M., I.V., S.C.: 0.5-2 mg to start, repeat every 20 minutes until response occurs or adverse effect occurs
I.M., I.V. to reverse the anticholinergic effects of atropine or scopolamine administered as preanesthetic medications: Administer twice the dose, on a weight basis of the anticholinergic drug
Ophthalmic: 1-2 drops of 0.25% or 0.5% solution every 4-8 hours (up to 4 times/day); the ointment can be instilled at night
Dosage Forms
Injection, as salicylate: 1 mg/mL (2 mL)
Ointment, ophthalmic, as sulfate: 0.25% (3.5 g, 3.75 g)

phytomenadione *see* phytonadione *on this page*

phytonadione (fye toe na DYE one)
Synonyms methylphytyl napthoquinone; phylloquinone; phytomenadione; vitamin K_1
U.S./Canadian Brand Names AquaMEPHYTON® [US/Can]; Mephyton® [US/Can]
Therapeutic Category Vitamin, Fat Soluble
Use Prevention and treatment of hypoprothrombinemia caused by vitamin K deficiency or anticoagulant-induced hypoprothrombinemia; hemorrhagic disease of the newborn
Usual Dosage I.V. route should be restricted for emergency use only
(Continued)

phytonadione *(Continued)*

Hemorrhagic disease of the newborn:
Prophylaxis: I.M., S.C.: 0.5-1 mg within 1 hour of birth
Treatment: I.M., S.C.: 1-2 mg/dose/day
Oral anticoagulant overdose:
Infants: I.M., I.V., S.C.: 1-2 mg/dose every 4-8 hours
Children and Adults: Oral, I.M., I.V., S.C.: 2.5-10 mg/dose; rarely up to 25-50 mg has
been used; may repeat in 6-8 hours if administered by I.M., I.V., S.C. route; may
repeat 12-48 hours after oral route
Vitamin K deficiency: Due to drugs, malabsorption or decreased synthesis of vitamin K
Infants and Children:
Oral: 2.5-5 mg/24 hours
I.M., I.V.: 1-2 mg/dose as a single dose
Adults:
Oral: 5-25 mg/24 hours
I.M., I.V.: 10 mg
Minimum daily requirement: Not well established
Infants: 1-5 mcg/kg/day
Adults: 0.03 mcg/kg/day

Dosage Forms
Injection, aqueous, colloidal: 2 mg/mL (0.5 mL)
Injection, aqueous: 10 mg/mL (1 mL)
Tablet: 5 mg

Pilagan® **Ophthalmic** *(Discontinued)* see page 814

Pilocar® **[US]** see pilocarpine on this page

pilocarpine (pye loe KAR peen)

U.S./Canadian Brand Names Diocarpine [Can]; Isopto® Carpine [US/Can]; Miocar-
pine® [Can]; Pilocar® [US]; Pilopine HS® [US/Can]; Piloptic® [US]; Salagen® [US/Can]
Therapeutic Category Cholinergic Agent
Use
Ophthalmic: Management of chronic simple glaucoma, chronic and acute angle-closure
glaucoma; counter effects of cycloplegics
Oral: Symptomatic treatment of xerostomia caused by salivary gland hypofunction
resulting from radiotherapy for cancer of the head and neck
Usual Dosage Adults:
Oral: 5 mg 3 times/day, titration up to 10 mg 3 times/day may be considered for patients
who have not responded adequately
Ophthalmic:
Nitrate solution: Shake well before using; instill 1-2 drops 2-4 times/day
Hydrochloride solution:
Instill 1-2 drops up to 6 times/day; adjust the concentration and frequency as required
to control elevated intraocular pressure
To counteract the mydriatic effects of sympathomimetic agents: Instill 1 drop of a 1%
solution in the affected eye
Gel: Instill 0.5" ribbon into lower conjunctival sac once daily at bedtime
Ocular systems: Systems are labeled in terms of mean rate of release of pilocarpine
over 7 days; begin with 20 mcg/hour at night and adjust based on response
Dosage Forms
Gel, ophthalmic, as hydrochloride (Pilopine HS®): 4% (3.5 g) [contains benzalkonium
chloride]
Solution, ophthalmic, as hydrochloride: 1% (15 mL), 2% (15 mL), 4% (15 mL), 6% (15
mL) [may contain benzalkonium chloride]
Isopto® Carpine: 1% (15 mL); 2% (15 mL, 30 mL); 4% (15 mL, 30 mL); 6% (15 mL); 8%
(15 mL) [contains benzalkonium chloride]
Pilocar®: 0.5% (15 mL); 1% (1 mL, 15 mL); 2% (1 mL, 15 mL); 3% (15 mL); 4% (1 mL,
15 mL); 6% (15 mL) [contains benzalkonium chloride]

Piloptic®: 0.5% (15 mL); 1% (15 mL); 2% (15 mL); 3% (15 mL); 4% (15 mL); 6% (15 mL) [contains benzalkonium chloride]

Tablet, as hydrochloride (Salagen®): 5 mg

pilocarpine and epinephrine (pye loe KAR peen & ep i NEF rin)

Synonyms epinephrine and pilocarpine

U.S./Canadian Brand Names P_6E_1® [US]

Therapeutic Category Cholinergic Agent

Use Treatment of glaucoma; counter effect of cycloplegics

Usual Dosage Ophthalmic: Instill 1-2 drops up to 6 times/day

Dosage Forms Solution, ophthalmic: Epinephrine bitartrate 1% and pilocarpine hydrochloride 6% (15 mL)

Pilopine HS® [US/Can] *see* pilocarpine *on previous page*

Piloptic® [US] *see* pilocarpine *on previous page*

Pilostat® Ophthalmic *(Discontinued)* *see page 814*

Pima® [US] *see* potassium iodide *on page 531*

pimaricin *see* natamycin *on page 449*

pimecrolimus (pim e KROE li mus)

U.S./Canadian Brand Names Elidel® [US]

Therapeutic Category Immunosuppressant Agent; Topical Skin Product

Use Short-term and intermittent long-term treatment of mild to moderate atopic dermatitis in patients not responsive to conventional therapy or when conventional therapy is not appropriate

Usual Dosage Children ≥2 years and Adults: Topical: Apply thin layer of 1% cream to affected area twice daily; rub in gently and completely. **Note:** Continue as long as signs and symptoms persist; discontinue if resolution occurs; re-evaluate if symptoms persist >6 weeks.

Dosage Forms Cream, topical: 1% (15 g, 30 g, 100 g)

pimozide (PI moe zide)

U.S./Canadian Brand Names Orap™ [US/Can]

Therapeutic Category Neuroleptic Agent

Use Suppression of severe motor and phonic tics in patients with Tourette's disorder

Usual Dosage Children >12 years and Adults: Oral: Initial: 1-2 mg/day, then increase dosage as needed every other day; range: 7-16 mg/day, maximum dose: 20 mg/day or 0.3 mg/kg/day should not be exceeded

Dosage Forms Tablet: 1 mg, 2 mg

pinaverium *(Canada only)* (pin ah VEER ee um)

U.S./Canadian Brand Names Dicetel® [Can]

Therapeutic Category Calcium Antagonist; Gastrointestinal Agent, Miscellaneous

Use For the treatment and relief of symptoms associated with irritable bowel syndrome (IBS): abdominal pain, bowel disturbances and intestinal discomfort; treatment of symptoms related to functional disorders of the biliary tract

Usual Dosage Adults: Oral: Three 50 mg tablets (1 tablet 3 times a day). In exceptional cases, the dosage may be increased up to 6 tablets a day (2 tablets 3 times/day). It is recommended that the tablet be taken with a glass of water during meals or snacks. The tablet should not be swallowed when in the lying position or just before bedtime.

Dosage Forms Tablet, as bromide: 50 mg, 100 mg

Pindac® *(Discontinued)* *see page 814*

pindolol (PIN doe lole)
U.S./Canadian Brand Names Apo®-Pindol [Can]; Gen-Pindolol [Can]; Novo-Pindol [Can]; Nu-Pindol [Can]; PMS-Pindolol [Can]; Visken® [US/Can]
Therapeutic Category Beta-Adrenergic Blocker
Use Management of hypertension
Usual Dosage Oral: 5 mg twice daily
Dosage Forms Tablet: 5 mg, 10 mg

pink bismuth *see* bismuth subsalicylate *on page 87*

Pin-Rid® *(Discontinued) see page 814*

Pin-X® [US-OTC] *see* pyrantel pamoate *on page 555*

PIO *see* pemoline *on page 496*

pioglitazone (pye oh GLI ta zone)
U.S./Canadian Brand Names Actos® [US/Can]
Therapeutic Category Antidiabetic Agent; Thiazolidinedione Derivative
Use
Type 2 diabetes, monotherapy: Adjunct to diet and exercise, to improve glycemic control
Type 2 diabetes, combination therapy with sulfonylurea, metformin, or insulin: When diet, exercise, and a single agent alone does not result in adequate glycemic control
Usual Dosage Adults: Oral:
Monotherapy: Initial: 15-30 mg once daily; if response is inadequate, the dosage may be increased in increments up to 45 mg once daily; maximum recommended dose: 45 mg once daily
Combination therapy:
With sulfonylureas: Initial: 15-30 mg once daily; dose of sulfonylurea should be reduced if the patient reports hypoglycemia
With metformin: Initial: 15-30 mg once daily; it is unlikely that the dose of metformin will need to be reduced due to hypoglycemia
With insulin: Initial: 15-30 mg once daily; dose of insulin should be reduced by 10% to 25% if the patient reports hypoglycemia or if the plasma glucose falls to below 100 mg/dL. Doses greater than 30 mg/day have not been evaluated in combination regimens.
A 1-week washout period is recommended in patients with normal liver enzymes who are changed from troglitazone to pioglitazone therapy.
Dosage Forms Tablet: 15 mg, 30 mg, 45 mg

pipecuronium (pi pe kur OH nee um)
U.S./Canadian Brand Names Arduan® [US/Can]
Therapeutic Category Skeletal Muscle Relaxant
Use Adjunct to general anesthesia, to provide skeletal muscle relaxation during surgery and to provide skeletal muscle relaxation for endotracheal intubation; recommended only for procedures anticipated to last 90 minutes or longer
Usual Dosage I.V.:
Children:
3 months to 1 year: Adult dosage
1-14 years: May be less sensitive to effects
Adults: Dose is individualized based on ideal body weight, ranges are 85-100 mcg/kg initially to a maintenance dose of 5-25 mcg/kg
Dosage Forms Injection, as bromide: 10 mg (10 mL)

piperacillin (pi PER a sil in)
U.S./Canadian Brand Names Pipracil® [US/Can]
Therapeutic Category Penicillin

Use Treatment of serious infections caused by susceptible strains of gram-positive, gram-negative, and anaerobic bacilli; mixed aerobic-anaerobic bacterial infections or empiric antibiotic therapy in granulocytopenic patients. Its primary use is in the treatment of serious carbenicillin-resistant or ticarcillin-resistant *Pseudomonas aeruginosa* infections susceptible to piperacillin.

Usual Dosage
Infants and Children: I.M., I.V.: 200-300 mg/kg/day in divided doses every 4-6 hours; maximum dose: 24 g/day
Higher doses have been used in cystic fibrosis: 350-500 mg/kg/day in divided doses every 4 hours
Adults:
I.M.: 2-3 g/dose every 6-12 hours I.M.; maximum 24 g/24 hours
I.V.: 3-4 g/dose every 4-6 hours; maximum 24 g/24 hours

Dosage Forms Injection, powder for reconstitution, as sodium: 2 g, 3 g, 4 g, 40 g

piperacillin and tazobactam sodium
(pi PER a sil in & ta zoe BAK tam SOW dee um)

Synonyms tazobactam and piperacillin

U.S./Canadian Brand Names Tazocin® [Can]; Zosyn® [US]

Therapeutic Category Penicillin

Use Treatment of infections caused by piperacillin-resistant, beta-lactamase-producing strains that are piperacillin/tazobactam susceptible involving the lower respiratory tract, urinary tract, skin and skin structures, gynecologic, intra-abdominal, and septicemia. Tazobactam expands activity of piperacillin to include beta-lactamase-producing strains of *S. aureus*, *H. influenzae*, *B. fragilis*, *Klebsiella*, *E. coli*, and *Acinetobacter*.

Usual Dosage Adults: I.V.: 3.375 g (3 g piperacillin/0.375 g tazobactam) every 6 hours

Dosage Forms Vials at an 8:1 ratio of piperacillin sodium/tazobactam sodium:
Injection:
Piperacillin sodium 2 g and tazobactam sodium 0.25 g
Piperacillin sodium 3 g and tazobactam sodium 0.375 g
Piperacillin sodium 4 g and tazobactam sodium 0.5 g

piperazine estrone sulfate *see* estropipate *on page 242*

piperonyl butoxide and pyrethrins *see* pyrethrins *on page 555*

Pipracil® [US/Can] *see* piperacillin *on previous page*

pirbuterol (peer BYOO ter ole)

U.S./Canadian Brand Names Maxair™ Autohaler™ [US]; Maxair™ [US]

Therapeutic Category Adrenergic Agonist Agent

Use Prevention and treatment of reversible bronchospasm including asthma

Usual Dosage Children >12 years and Adults: 2 inhalations every 4-6 hours for prevention; 2 inhalations at an interval of at least 1-3 minutes, followed by a third inhalation in treatment of bronchospasm, not to exceed 12 inhalations/day

Dosage Forms Aerosol for oral inhalation, as acetate:
Maxair™ Autohaler™: 0.2 mg per actuation (2.8 g - 80 inhalations, 14 g - 400 inhalations)
Maxair™: 0.2 mg per actuation (25.6 g - 300 inhalations)

piroxicam (peer OKS i kam)

U.S./Canadian Brand Names Alti-Piroxicam [Can]; Apo®-Piroxicam [Can]; Feldene® [US/Can]; Gen-Piroxicam [Can]; Novo-Pirocam® [Can]; Nu-Pirox [Can]; Pexicam® [Can]

Therapeutic Category Analgesic, Non-narcotic; Nonsteroidal Anti-inflammatory Drug (NSAID)

Use Management of inflammatory disorders; symptomatic treatment of acute and chronic rheumatoid arthritis, osteoarthritis, and ankylosing spondylitis; also used to treat sunburn; dysmenorrhea
(Continued)

piroxicam *(Continued)*

Usual Dosage Oral:

Children: 0.2-0.3 mg/kg/day once daily; maximum dose: 15 mg/day

Adults: 10-20 mg/day once daily; although associated with increases in GI adverse effects, doses >20 mg/day have been used (ie, 30-40 mg/day)

Therapeutic efficacy of the drug should not be assessed for at least 2 weeks after initiation of therapy or adjustment of dosage

Dosage Forms Capsule: 10 mg, 20 mg

piroxicam and cyclodextrin *(Canada only)*

(peer OKS i kam & sye kloe DEKS trin)

U.S./Canadian Brand Names Brexidol® 20 [Can]

Therapeutic Category Analgesic, Non-narcotic; Nonsteroidal Anti-inflammatory Drug (NSAID)

Use For the short-term relief of mild to moderately severe acute pain. Complexation with cyclodextrin allows faster absorption of piroxicam

Dosage Forms Tablet: Piroxicam-cyclodextrin 191.2 mg, equivalent to piroxicam 20 mg and beta-cyclodextrin 171.2 mg

p-isobutylhydratropic acid *see* ibuprofen *on page 342*

PIT *see* oxytocin *on page 487*

Pitocin® [US/Can] *see* oxytocin *on page 487*

Pitressin® [US] *see* vasopressin *on page 674*

Pitrex [Can] *see* tolnaftate *on page 644*

pit vipers antivenin *see* antivenin *(Crotalidae)* polyvalent *on page 48*

pivampicillin *(Canada only)* (piv am pi SIL in)

U.S./Canadian Brand Names Pondocillin® [Can]

Therapeutic Category Antibiotic, Penicillin

Use For the treatment of respiratory tract infections (including acute bronchitis, acute exacerbations of chronic bronchitis and pneumonia); ear, nose and throat infections; gynecological infections; urinary tract infections (including acute uncomplicated gonococcal urethritis) when caused by nonpenicillinase-producing susceptible strains of the following organisms: gram-positive organisms, ie, streptococci, pneumococci and staphylococci; gram-negative organisms, ie, *H. influenzae, N. gonorrhoeae, E. coli, P. mirabilis.*

Usual Dosage Oral

Suspension:

Infants 3 to 12 months: 40-60 mg/kg body weight daily divided into 2 equal doses

Children:

1 to 3 years: 5 mL (175 mg) twice daily

4 to 6 years: 7.5 mL (262.5 mg) twice daily

7 to 10 years: 10 mL (350 mg) twice daily

In children 10 years of age or less the dosage range is 25 to 35 mg/kg/day and should not exceed the recommended adult dose of 500 mg twice daily

Children over 10 years and adults: 15 mL (525 mg) twice daily. For severe infections: Dosage may be doubled.

Tablet: Adults and children over 10 years: 500 mg twice daily; double in severe infections

In gonococcal urethritis: 1.5 g as a single dose with 1 g probenecid concurrently

Dosage Forms

Suspension, oral: 35 mg/5 mL (100 mL, 150 mL, 200 mL)

Tablet: 500 mg (equivalent to ampicillin 377 mg)

pix carbonis *see* coal tar *on page 158*

pizotifen *(Canada only)* (pi ZOE ti fen)
U.S./Canadian Brand Names Sandomigran® [Can]; Sandomigran DS® [Can]
Therapeutic Category Antimigraine Agent
Use Migraine prophylaxis; also used for cyclical vomiting
Usual Dosage
  Migraine prophylaxis:
   Children: Up to 1.5 mg/day in divided doses
   Adult: Initial: 0.5 mg; usual adult daily dose: ~1.5 mg; maximum daily dose: 4.5 mg
  Cyclical vomiting: Children: 1.5 mg nightly
Dosage Forms
  Tablet (Sandomigran®): 0.5 mg [pizotifen malate 0.73 mg]
  Tablet, double strength (Sandomigran® DS): 1 mg [pizotifen malate 1.46 mg]

Placidyl® **[US]** *see* ethchlorvynol *on page 244*

plague vaccine (plaig vak SEEN)
Therapeutic Category Vaccine, Inactivated Bacteria
Use Vaccination of persons at high risk exposure to plaque
Usual Dosage Three I.M. doses: First dose 1 mL, second dose (0.2 mL) 1 month later, third dose (0.2 mL) 5 months after the second dose; booster doses (0.2 mL) at 1- to 2-year intervals if exposure continues
Dosage Forms Injection: 2 mL, 20 mL

Plan B™ **[US/Can]** *see* levonorgestrel *on page 381*

plantago seed *see* psyllium *on page 554*

plantain seed *see* psyllium *on page 554*

Plaquase® **[US]** *see* collagenase *on page 161*

Plaquenil® **[US/Can]** *see* hydroxychloroquine *on page 336*

Plasbumin® **[US/Can]** *see* albumin *on page 18*

Plasmanate® **[US]** *see* plasma protein fraction *on this page*

plasma protein fraction (PLAS mah PROE teen FRAK shun)
U.S./Canadian Brand Names Plasmanate® [US]
Therapeutic Category Blood Product Derivative
Use Plasma volume expansion and maintenance of cardiac output in the treatment of certain types of shock or impending shock
Usual Dosage I.V.: 250-1500 mL/day
Dosage Forms Injection: 5% (50 mL, 250 mL, 500 mL)

Plasmatein® *(Discontinued) see page 814*

Platinol® **[US]** *see* cisplatin *on page 148*

Platinol®**-AQ [US]** *see* cisplatin *on page 148*

Plavix® **[US/Can]** *see* clopidogrel *on page 155*

Plegine® *(Discontinued) see page 814*

Plendil® **[US/Can]** *see* felodipine *on page 264*

Pletal® **[US/Can]** *see* cilostazol *on page 146*

plicamycin (plye kay MYE sin)
Synonyms mithramycin
U.S./Canadian Brand Names Mithracin® [US/Can]
Therapeutic Category Antidote; Antineoplastic Agent
Use Malignant testicular tumors; treatment of hypercalcemia and hypercalciuria of malignancy not responsive to conventional treatment; chronic myelogenous leukemia in blast phase; Paget's disease
(Continued)

plicamycin *(Continued)*

Usual Dosage Refer to individual protocols. Adults: I.V. (dose based on ideal body weight):

Testicular cancer: 25-50 mcg/kg/day or every other day for 5-10 days

Blastic chronic granulocytic leukemia: 25 mcg/kg over 2-4 hours every other day for 3 weeks

Paget's disease: 15 mcg/kg/day once daily for 10 days

Hypercalcemia:

25 mcg/kg single dose which may be repeated in 48 hours if no response occurs

or 25 mcg/kg/day for 3-4 days

or 25-50 mcg/kg/dose every other day for 3-8 doses

Dosage Forms Injection, powder for reconstitution: 2.5 mg

PMPA *see* tenofovir *on page 622*

PMS-Amantadine [Can] *see* amantadine *on page 30*

PMS-Atenolol [Can] *see* atenolol *on page 60*

PMS-Baclofen [Can] *see* baclofen *on page 70*

PMS-Benzydamine [Can] *see* benzydamine *(Canada only) on page 81*

PMS-Bezafibrate [Can] *see* bezafibrate *(Canada only) on page 85*

PMS-Bromocriptine [Can] *see* bromocriptine *on page 93*

PMS-Buspirone [Can] *see* buspirone *on page 98*

PMS-Captopril® [Can] *see* captopril *on page 112*

PMS-Carbamazepine [Can] *see* carbamazepine *on page 113*

PMS-Cefaclor [Can] *see* cefaclor *on page 120*

PMS-Chloral Hydrate [Can] *see* chloral hydrate *on page 132*

PMS-Cholestyramine [Can] *see* cholestyramine resin *on page 143*

PMS-Cimetidine [Can] *see* cimetidine *on page 146*

PMS-Clonazepam [Can] *see* clonazepam *on page 154*

PMS-Conjugated Estrogens [Can] *see* estrogens (conjugated/equine) *on page 242*

PMS-Desipramine *see* desipramine *on page 181*

PMS-Dexamethasone [Can] *see* dexamethasone (systemic) *on page 184*

PMS-Diclofenac [Can] *see* diclofenac *on page 193*

PMS-Diclofenac SR [Can] *see* diclofenac *on page 193*

PMS-Diphenhydramine [Can] *see* diphenhydramine *on page 202*

PMS-Dipivefrin [Can] *see* dipivefrin *on page 205*

PMS-Docusate Calcium [Can] *see* docusate *on page 208*

PMS-Docusate Sodium [Can] *see* docusate *on page 208*

PMS-Domperidone [Can] *see* domperidone *(Canada only) on page 211*

PMS-Erythromycin [Can] *see* erythromycin (systemic) *on page 235*

PMS-Fenofibrate Micro [Can] *see* fenofibrate *on page 265*

PMS-Fluoxetine [Can] *see* fluoxetine *on page 279*

PMS-Fluphenazine Decanoate [Can] *see* fluphenazine *on page 281*

PMS-Flutamide [Can] *see* flutamide *on page 282*

PMS-Fluvoxamine [Can] *see* fluvoxamine *on page 285*

PMS-Gemfibrozil [Can] *see* gemfibrozil *on page 295*

PMS-Glyburide [Can] *see* glyburide *on page 301*

PMS-Haloperidol LA [Can] *see* haloperidol *on page 316*

PMS-Hydromorphone [Can] *see* hydromorphone *on page 335*

PMS-Hydroxyzine [Can] *see* hydroxyzine *on page 339*

PMS-Indapamide [Can] *see* indapamide *on page 348*

PMS-Ipratropium [Can] *see* ipratropium *on page 358*

PMS-Isoniazid [Can] *see* isoniazid *on page 361*

PMS-Lactulose [Can] *see* lactulose *on page 372*

PMS-Levobunolol [Can] *see* levobunolol *on page 379*

PMS-Lindane [Can] *see* lindane *on page 385*

PMS-Lithium Carbonate [Can] *see* lithium *on page 388*

PMS-Lithium Citrate [Can] *see* lithium *on page 388*

PMS-Loperamine [Can] *see* loperamide *on page 390*

PMS-Loxapine [Can] *see* loxapine *on page 394*

PMS-Mefenamic Acid [Can] *see* mefenamic acid *on page 405*

PMS-Methylphenidate [Can] *see* methylphenidate *on page 422*

PMS-Metoprolol [Can] *see* metoprolol *on page 425*

PMS-Nortriptyline [Can] *see* nortriptyline *on page 466*

PMS-Nystatin [Can] *see* nystatin *on page 473*

PMS-Oxybutynin [Can] *see* oxybutynin *on page 484*

PMS-Pindolol [Can] *see* pindolol *on page 516*

PMS-Polytrimethoprim [Can] *see* trimethoprim and polymyxin B *on page 657*

PMS-Pseudoephedrine [Can] *see* pseudoephedrine *on page 552*

PMS-Sodium Polystyrene Sulfonate [Can] *see* sodium polystyrene sulfonate *on page 600*

PMS-Sotalol [Can] *see* sotalol *on page 602*

PMS-Sucralate [Can] *see* sucralfate *on page 609*

PMS-Tamoxifen [Can] *see* tamoxifen *on page 618*

PMS-Temazepam [Can] *see* temazepam *on page 621*

PMS-Tiaprofenic [Can] *see* tiaprofenic acid *(Canada only) on page 638*

PMS-Timolol [Can] *see* timolol *on page 639*

PMS-Tobramycin [Can] *see* tobramycin *on page 641*

PMS-Trazodone [Can] *see* trazodone *on page 649*

PMS-Valproic Acid [Can] *see* valproic acid and derivatives *on page 670*

PMS-Valproic Acid E.C. [Can] *see* valproic acid and derivatives *on page 670*

PMS-Yohimbine [Can] *see* yohimbine *on page 687*

Pneumo 23™ [Can] *see* pneumococcal vaccine *on page 523*

pneumococcal 7-valent conjugate vaccine *see* pneumococcal conjugate vaccine (7-valent) *on this page*

pneumococcal conjugate vaccine (7-valent)
(noo moe KOK al KON ju gate vak SEEN seven-vay lent)
Synonyms diphtheria CRM_{197} protein; PCV7; pneumococcal 7-valent conjugate vaccine
U.S./Canadian Brand Names Prevnar™ [US]
Therapeutic Category Vaccine
Use Immunization of infants and toddlers against *Streptococcus pneumoniae* infection caused by serotypes included in the vaccine
American Academy of Pediatrics policy statement: Recommended for all children ≤23 months of age; it is administered concurrently with other recommended vaccines at 2-, (Continued)

pneumococcal conjugate vaccine (7-valent) *(Continued)*

4-, 6-, and 12-15 months. The number of doses required depends upon the age of initiation. All children 24-59 months of age who are at high risk should receive the vaccine (see Usual Dosage).

High Risk (attack rate of invasive pneumococcal disease >150/100,000 cases per year): Sickle cell disease, congenital or acquired asplenia, or splenic dysfunction, HIV infection

Presumed high Risk (attack rate not calculated):

Congenital immune deficiency; Some B- (humoral) or T-lymphocyte deficiencies, complement deficiencies (particularly C1, C2, C3, and C4 deficiencies), or phagocytic disorders (excluding chronic granulomatous disease)

Chronic cardiac disease (particularly cyanotic congenital heart disease and cardiac failure)

Chronic pulmonary disease (including asthma treated with high-dose oral corticosteroid therapy)

Cerebrospinal fluid leaks

Chronic renal insufficiency (including nephrotic syndrome)

Diseases associated with immunosuppressive therapy or radiation therapy (including malignant neoplasms, leukemias, lymphomas, and Hodgkin's disease) and solid organ transplant (guidelines for use of pneumococcal vaccines for children who have undergone bone marrow transplants are currently under revision)

Diabetes mellitus

Moderate Risk (attack rate of invasive pneumococcal disease >20/100,000 per year):

All children 24-35 months of age

Children 36-59 months of age attending "out of home" care

Children 36-59 months of age who are Native American (American Indian or Alaska Native) or are of African American descent

Usual Dosage I.M.:

Infants: 2-6 months: 0.5 mL at approximately 2-month intervals for 3 consecutive doses, followed by a fourth dose of 0.5 mL at 12-15 months of age; first dose may be given as young as 6 weeks of age, but is typically given at 2 months of age. In case of a moderate shortage of vaccine, defer the fourth dose until shortage is resolved; in case of a severe shortage of vaccine, defer third and fourth doses until shortage is resolved.

Previously Unvaccinated Infants and Children:

7-11 months: 0.5 mL for a total of 3 doses; 2 doses at least 4 weeks apart, followed by a third dose after the 1-year birthday (12-15 months), separated from the second dose by at least 2 months. In case of a severe shortage of vaccine, defer the third dose until shortage is resolved.

12-23 months: 0.5 mL for a total of 2 doses, separated by at least 2 months. In case of a severe shortage of vaccine, defer the second dose until shortage is resolved.

24-59 months:

Healthy Children: 0.5 mL as a single dose. In case of a severe shortage of vaccine, defer dosing until shortage is resolved.

Children with sickle cell disease, asplenia, HIV infection, chronic illness or immunocompromising conditions (not including bone marrow transplants - results pending; use PPV23 [pneumococcal polysaccharide vaccine, polyvalent] at 12- and 24-months until studies are complete): 0.5 mL for a total of 2 doses, separated by 2 months

Previously Vaccinated Children with a lapse in vaccine administration:

7-11 months: Previously received 1 or 2 doses PCV7: 0.5 mL dose at 7-11 months of age, followed by a second dose ≥2 months later at 12-15 months of age

12-23 months:

Previously received 1 dose before 12 months of age: 0.5 mL dose, followed by a second dose ≥2 months later

Previously received 2 doses before age 12 months: 0.5 mL dose ≥2 months after the most recent dose

24-59 months: Any incomplete schedule: 0.5 mL as a single dose; **Note:** Patients with chronic diseases or immunosuppressing conditions should receive 2 doses ≥2 months apart

Dosage Forms Injection: 2 mcg of each saccharide for each of six serotypes and 4 mcg of a seventh serotype; also 20 mcg of CRM197 carrier protein and 0.125 mg of aluminum phosphate adjuvant per 0.5 mL dose

pneumococcal polysaccharide vaccine *see* pneumococcal vaccine *on this page*

pneumococcal vaccine (noo moe KOK al vak SEEN)

Synonyms pneumococcal polysaccharide vaccine

U.S./Canadian Brand Names Pneumo 23™ [Can]; Pneumovax® 23 [US/Can]; Pnu-Imune® 23 [US]

Therapeutic Category Vaccine, Inactivated Bacteria

Use Immunity to pneumococcal lobar pneumonia and bacteremia in individuals ≥2 years of age who are at high risk of morbidity and mortality from pneumococcal infection

Usual Dosage Children >2 years and Adults: I.M., S.C.: 0.5 mL
Revaccination should be considered if ≥6 years since initial vaccination; revaccination is recommended in patients who received 14-valent pneumococcal vaccine and are at highest risk (asplenic) for fatal infection, or at ≥6 years in patients with nephrotic syndrome, renal failure, or transplant recipients, or 3-5 years in children with nephrotic syndrome, asplenia, or sickle cell disease

Dosage Forms Injection: 25 mcg each of 23 polysaccharide isolates/0.5 mL dose (0.5 mL, 1 mL, 5 mL)

Pneumomist® *(Discontinued) see page 814*

Pneumovax® 23 [US/Can] *see* pneumococcal vaccine *on this page*

Pnu-Imune® 23 [US] *see* pneumococcal vaccine *on this page*

Pod-Ben-25® *(Discontinued) see page 814*

Podocon-25™ [US] *see* podophyllum resin *on this page*

Podofilm® [Can] *see* podophyllum resin *on this page*

podofilox (po do FIL oks)

U.S./Canadian Brand Names Condyline™ [Can]; Condylox® [US]; Wartec® [Can]

Therapeutic Category Keratolytic Agent

Use Treatment of external genital warts

Usual Dosage Adults: Topical: Apply twice daily (morning and evening) for 3 consecutive days, then withhold use for 4 consecutive days; cycle may be repeated up to 4 times until there is no visible wart tissue

Dosage Forms
Gel: 0.5%
Solution, topical: 0.5% (3.5 mL)

Podofin® *(Discontinued) see page 814*

podophyllum resin (po DOF fil um REZ in)

Synonyms mandrake; may apple

U.S./Canadian Brand Names Podocon-25™ [US]; Podofilm® [Can]

Therapeutic Category Keratolytic Agent

Use Topical treatment of benign growths including external genital and perianal warts (condylomata acuminata), papillomas, fibroids

Usual Dosage Topical:
Children and Adults: 10% to 25% solution in compound benzoin tincture; apply drug to dry surface, use 1 drop at a time allowing drying between drops until area is covered; total volume should be limited to <0.5 mL per treatment session
(Continued)

podophyllum resin *(Continued)*

Condylomata acuminatum: 25% solution is applied daily; use a 10% solution when applied to or near mucous membranes

Verrucae: 25% solution is applied 3-5 times/day directly to the wart

Dosage Forms Liquid, topical: 25% (15 mL) [in benzoin tincture]

Point-Two® *(Discontinued)* *see page 814*

Poladex® *(Discontinued)* *see page 814*

Polaramine® **[US]** *see dexchlorpheniramine on page 185*

Polargen® *(Discontinued)* *see page 814*

poliomyelitis vaccine *see poliovirus vaccine (inactivated) on this page*

Poliovax® Injection *(Discontinued)* *see page 814*

poliovirus vaccine (inactivated)

(POE lee oh VYE rus vak SEEN in ak ti VAY ted)

Synonyms IPV; poliomyelitis vaccine; Salk vaccine

U.S./Canadian Brand Names IPOL™ [US/Can]

Therapeutic Category Vaccine, Live Virus and Inactivated Virus

Use Active immunization for the prevention of poliomyelitis

Usual Dosage

S.C.: 3 doses of 0.5 mL; the first 2 doses should be administered at an interval of 8 weeks; the third dose should be administered at least 6 and preferably 12 months after the second dose

Booster dose: All children who have received the 3 dose primary series in infancy and early childhood should receive a booster dose of 0.5 mL before entering school. However, if the third dose of the primary series is administered on or after the fourth birthday, a fourth (booster) dose is not required at school entry.

Dosage Forms Injection, suspension (E-IPV, Enhanced-Potency Inactivated Poliovirus Vaccine, IPOL™, Poliomyelitis Vaccine, Salk): 3 types of poliovirus (Types 1, 2, and 3) (0.5 mL) [grown in human diploid cell cultures]

poliovirus vaccine, live, trivalent, oral

(POE lee oh VYE rus vak SEEN, live, try VAY lent, OR al)

Synonyms OPV; Sabin vaccine; TOPV

U.S./Canadian Brand Names Orimune® [US]

Therapeutic Category Vaccine, Live Virus

Use Poliovirus immunization

Usual Dosage Oral:

Infants: 0.5 mL dose at age 2 months, 4 months, and 18 months; optional dose may be administered at 6 months in areas where poliomyelitis is endemic

Older Children, Adolescents and Adults: Two 0.5 mL doses 8 weeks apart; third dose of 0.5 mL 6-12 months after second dose; a reinforcing dose of 0.5 mL should be administered before entry to school, in children who received the third primary dose before their fourth birthday

Dosage Forms Solution, oral (Orimune®): Mixture of type 1, 2, and 3 viruses in monkey kidney tissue (0.5 mL)

Polocaine® **[US/Can]** *see mepivacaine on page 409*

Polycidin® **Ophthalmic** *see bacitracin and polymyxin B on page 68*

Polycillin-N® Injection *(Discontinued)* *see page 814*

Polycillin® Oral *(Discontinued)* *see page 814*

Polycillin-PRB® *(Discontinued)* *see page 814*

Polycitra® **[US]** *see sodium citrate and potassium citrate mixture on page 596*

Polycitra®-K **[US]** *see potassium citrate and citric acid on page 531*

Polycose® **[US-OTC]** *see* glucose polymers *on page 301*

Polydine® **[US-OTC]** *see* povidone-iodine *on page 533*

Polydryl® **[US-OTC]** *see* diphenhydramine *on page 202*

polyethylene glycol-electrolyte solution

(pol i ETH i leen GLY kol-EE lec tro e lyte soe LOO shun)

Synonyms electrolyte lavage solution; PEG-ES

U.S./Canadian Brand Names Colyte® [US/Can]; GoLYTELY® [US]; Klean-Prep® [Can]; Lyteprep™ [Can]; MiraLax™ [US]; NuLytely® [US]; OCL® [US]; PegLyte® [Can]

Therapeutic Category Laxative

Use For bowel cleansing prior to GI examination

Usual Dosage The recommended dose for adults is 4 L of solution prior to gastrointestinal examination, as ingestion of this dose produces a satisfactory preparation in >95% of patients. The solution is usually administered orally, but may be administered via nasogastric tube to patients who are unwilling or unable to drink the solution.

Children: Oral: 25-40 mL/kg/hour for 4-10 hours

Adults:

Oral: At a rate of 240 mL (8 oz) every 10 minutes, until 4 liters are consumed or the rectal effluent is clear; rapid drinking of each portion is preferred to drinking small amounts continuously

Nasogastric tube: At the rate of 20-30 mL/minute (1.2-1.8 L/hour); the first bowel movement should occur approximately one hour after the start of administration

Dosage Forms

Powder for oral solution:

Colyte®:

PEG 3350 240 g, sodium sulfate 22.72 g, sodium bicarbonate 6.72 g, sodium chloride 5.84 g, and potassium chloride 2.98 g (to make 4000 mL) [cherry, citrus berry, lemon-lime, and pineapple flavors]

PEG 3350 227.1 g, sodium sulfate 21.5 g, sodium bicarbonate 6.36 g, sodium chloride 5.53 g, and potassium chloride 2.82 g (to make 4000 mL) [pineapple and regular flavors]

GoLYTELY®:

Disposable jug: PEG 3350 236 g, sodium sulfate 22.74 g, sodium bicarbonate 6.74 g, sodium chloride 5.86 g, and potassium chloride 2.97 g (to make 4000 mL) [pineapple and regular flavors]

Packets: PEG 3350 227.1 g, sodium sulfate 21.5 g, sodium bicarbonate 6.36 g, sodium chloride 5.53 g, and potassium chloride 2.82 g (to make 4000 mL) [regular flavor]

MiraLax™: PEG 3350 255 g (to make 14 oz); PEG 3350 527 g (to make 26 oz)

NuLytely®: PEG 3350 420 g, sodium bicarbonate 5.72 g, sodium chloride 11.2 g, and potassium chloride 1.48 (to make 4000 mL) [cherry, lemon-lime, and orange flavors]

Solution, oral (OCL®): PEG 3350 6 g, sodium sulfate decahydrate 1.29 g, sodium bicarbonate 168 mg, potassium chloride 75 mg, and polysorbate 80 30 mg per 100 mL (1500 mL)

Polyflex® **Tablet** *(Discontinued) see page 814*

Polygam® **Injection** *(Discontinued) see page 814*

Polygam® **S/D [US]** *see* immune globulin (intravenous) *on page 347*

Poly-Histine CS® *(Discontinued) see page 814*

Poly-Histine-D® **Capsule** *(Discontinued) see page 814*

Polymox® *(Discontinued) see page 814*

polymyxin B (pol i MIKS in bee)

Therapeutic Category Antibiotic, Irrigation; Antibiotic, Miscellaneous

Use Parenteral use of polymyxin B has mainly been replaced by less toxic antibiotics; it is reserved for life-threatening infections caused by organisms resistant to the preferred drugs (eg, pseudomonal meningitis - intrathecal administration)

Usual Dosage

Otic: 1-2 drops, 3-4 times/day; should be used sparingly to avoid accumulation of excess debris

Infants <2 years:

I.M.: Up to 40,000 units/kg/day divided every 6 hours (not routinely recommended due to pain at injection sites)

I.V.: Up to 40,000 units/kg/day by continuous I.V. infusion

Intrathecal: 20,000 units/day for 3-4 days, then 25,000 units every other day for at least 2 weeks after CSF cultures are negative and CSF (glucose) has returned to within normal limits

Children ≥2 years and Adults:

I.M.: 25,000-30,000 units/kg/day divided every 4-6 hours (not routinely recommended due to pain at injection sites)

I.V.: 15,000-25,000 units/kg/day divided every 12 hours or by continuous infusion

Intrathecal: 50,000 units/day for 3-4 days, then every other day for at least 2 weeks after CSF cultures are negative and CSF (glucose) has returned to within normal limits

Total daily dose should not exceed 2,000,000 units/day

Bladder irrigation: Continuous irrigant or rinse in the urinary bladder for up to 10 days using 20 mg (equal to 200,000 units) added to 1 L of normal saline; usually no more than 1 L of irrigant is used per day unless urine flow rate is high; administration rate is adjusted to patient's urine output

Topical irrigation or topical solution: 500,000 units/L of normal saline; topical irrigation should not exceed 2 million units/day in adults

Gut sterilization: Oral: 15,000-25,000 units/kg/day in divided doses every 6 hours

Clostridium difficile enteritis: Oral: 25,000 units every 6 hours for 10 days

Ophthalmic: A concentration of 0.1% to 0.25% is administered as 1-3 drops every hour, then increasing the interval as response indicates to 1-2 drops 4-6 times/day

Dosage Forms Powder: 500,000 units/vial

polymyxin B and bacitracin *see* bacitracin and polymyxin B *on page 68*

polymyxin B and neomycin *see* neomycin and polymyxin B *on page 452*

polymyxin B and oxytetracycline *see* oxytetracycline and polymyxin B *on page 487*

polymyxin B and trimethoprim *see* trimethoprim and polymyxin B *on page 657*

polymyxin B, bacitracin, and neomycin *see* bacitracin, neomycin, and polymyxin B *on page 69*

polymyxin B, bacitracin, neomycin, and hydrocortisone *see* bacitracin, neomycin, polymyxin B, and hydrocortisone *on page 69*

polymyxin B, neomycin, and dexamethasone *see* neomycin, polymyxin B, and dexamethasone *on page 452*

polymyxin B, neomycin, and gramicidin *see* neomycin, polymyxin B, and gramicidin *on page 453*

polymyxin B, neomycin, and hydrocortisone *see* neomycin, polymyxin B, and hydrocortisone *on page 453*

polymyxin B, neomycin, and prednisolone *see* neomycin, polymyxin B, and prednisolone *on page 454*

Poly-Pred® [US] *see* neomycin, polymyxin B, and prednisolone *on page 454*

polysaccharide-iron complex (pol i SAK a ride-EYE ern KOM pleks)
U.S./Canadian Brand Names Hytinic® [US-OTC]; Niferex® [US-OTC]; Nu-Iron® [US-OTC]
Therapeutic Category Electrolyte Supplement, Oral
Use Prevention and treatment of iron deficiency anemias
Usual Dosage Oral:
Children: 3 mg/kg 3 times/day
Adults: 200 mg 3-4 times/day
Dosage Forms
Capsule: Elemental iron 150 mg
Elixir: Elemental iron 100 mg/5 mL (240 mL)
Tablet: Elemental iron 50 mg

Polysporin® Ophthalmic [US] see bacitracin and polymyxin B on page 68

Polysporin® Topical [US-OTC] see bacitracin and polymyxin B on page 68

Polytapp® Allergy Dye-Free Medication [US-OTC] see brompheniramine on page 93

Polytar® [US-OTC] see coal tar on page 158

polythiazide (pol i THYE a zide)
U.S./Canadian Brand Names Renese® [US]
Therapeutic Category Diuretic, Thiazide
Use Adjunctive therapy in treatment of edema and hypertension
Usual Dosage Adults: Oral: 1-4 mg/day
Dosage Forms Tablet: 1 mg, 2 mg, 4 mg

polythiazide and prazosin see prazosin and polythiazide on page 536

Polytrim® [US/Can] see trimethoprim and polymyxin B on page 657

Poly-Vi-Flor® [US] see vitamin (multiple/pediatric) on page 683

polyvinyl alcohol see artificial tears on page 56

Poly-Vi-Sol® [US-OTC] see vitamin (multiple/pediatric) on page 683

Pondimin® (Discontinued) see page 814

Pondocillin® [Can] see pivampicillin (Canada only) on page 518

Ponstan® [Can] see mefenamic acid on page 405

Ponstel® [US/Can] see mefenamic acid on page 405

Pontocaine® [US/Can] see tetracaine on page 627

Pontocaine® With Dextrose [US] see tetracaine and dextrose on page 628

poractant alfa (por AKT ant AL fa)
U.S./Canadian Brand Names Curosurf® [US/Can]
Therapeutic Category Lung Surfactant
Use Treatment of respiratory distress syndrome (RDS) in premature infants
Usual Dosage Intratracheal use only: Premature infant with RDS: Initial dose is 2.5 mL/kg of birth weight. Up to 2 subsequent doses of 1.25 mL/kg birth weight can be administered at 12-hour intervals if needed in infants who continue to require mechanical ventilation and supplemental oxygen.
Dosage Forms Suspension for intratracheal instillation: 80 mg/mL (1.5 mL, 3 mL)

Porcelana® Sunscreen (Discontinued) see page 814

porfimer (POR fi mer)
U.S./Canadian Brand Names Photofrin® [US/Can]
Therapeutic Category Antineoplastic Agent
(Continued)

porfimer *(Continued)*

Use Esophageal cancer: Photodynamic therapy (PDT) with porfimer for palliation of patients with completely obstructing esophageal cancer, or of patients with partially obstructing esophageal cancer who cannot be satisfactorily treated with Nd:YAG laser therapy; early-stage lung cancer (endobronchial microinvasive nonsmall cell)

Usual Dosage I.V. (refer to individual protocols):
Children: Safety and efficacy have not been established
Adults: I.V.: 2 mg/kg over 3-5 minutes
Photodynamic therapy is a two-stage process requiring administration of both drug and light. The first stage of PDT is the I.V. injection of porfimer. Illumination with laser light 40-50 hours following the injection with porfimer constitutes the second stage of therapy. A second laser light application may be administered 90-120 hours after injection, preceded by gentle debridement of residual tumor.
Patients may receive a second course of PDT a minimum of 30 days after the initial therapy; up to three courses of PDT (each separated by a minimum of 30 days) can be given. Before each course of treatment, evaluate patients for the presence of a tracheoesophageal or bronchoesophageal fistula.

Dosage Forms Injection, powder for reconstitution, as sodium: 75 mg

Portagen® [US-OTC] *see* nutritional formula, enteral/oral *on page 472*

Portia™ [US] *see* ethinyl estradiol and levonorgestrel *on page 248*

Posicor® *(Discontinued)* *see page 814*

Posture® [US-OTC] *see* calcium phosphate (dibasic) *on page 108*

Potasalan® *(Discontinued)* *see page 814*

potassium acetate *(poe TASS ee um AS e tate)*

Therapeutic Category Electrolyte Supplement, Oral

Use Potassium deficiency, treatment of hypokalemia, correction of metabolic acidosis through conversion of acetate to bicarbonate

Usual Dosage I.V. infusion:
Children: Not to exceed 3 mEq/kg/day
Adults: Up to 150 mEq/day administered at a rate up to 20 mEq/hour; maximum concentration: 40 mEq/L

Dosage Forms Injection: 2 mEq/mL (20 mL, 50 mL, 100 mL); 4 mEq/mL (50 mL)

potassium acetate, potassium bicarbonate, and potassium citrate

(poe TASS ee um AS e tate, poe TASS ee um bye KAR bun ate, & poe TASS ee um SIT rate)

U.S./Canadian Brand Names Tri-K® [US]

Therapeutic Category Electrolyte Supplement, Oral

Use Treatment or prevention of hypokalemia

Usual Dosage Oral:
Children: 1-4 mEq/kg/24 hours in divided doses as required to maintain normal serum potassium
Adults:
Prevention: 16-24 mEq/day in 2-4 divided doses
Treatment: 40-100 mEq/day in 2-4 divided doses

Dosage Forms Solution, oral: 45 mEq/15 mL from potassium acetate 1500 mg, potassium bicarbonate 1500 mg, and potassium citrate 1500 mg per 15 mL

potassium acid phosphate *(poe TASS ee um AS id FOS fate)*

U.S./Canadian Brand Names K-Phos® Original [US]

Therapeutic Category Urinary Acidifying Agent

Use Acidify the urine and lower urinary calcium concentration; reduces odor and rash caused by ammoniacal urine

Usual Dosage Adults: Oral: 1000 mg dissolved in 6-8 oz of water 4 times/day with meals and at bedtime

Dosage Forms Tablet: 500 mg [potassium 3.67 mEq] [sodium free]

potassium bicarbonate (poe TASS ee um bye KAR bun ate)

U.S./Canadian Brand Names K+ Care® ET [US]

Therapeutic Category Electrolyte Supplement, Oral

Use Potassium deficiency, hypokalemia

Usual Dosage Oral:

Normal daily requirements:
Children: 2-3 mEq/kg/day
Adults: 40-80 mEq/day

Prevention during diuretic therapy:
Children: 1-2 mEq/kg/day in 1-2 divided doses
Adults: 20-40 mEq/day in 1-2 divided doses

Treatment of hypokalemia: Children: 1-2 mEq/kg initially, then as needed based on frequently obtained lab values. If deficits are severe or ongoing losses are great, I.V. route should be considered.

Treatment of hypokalemia: Adults:
Potassium >2.5 mEq/L: 60-80 mEq/day plus additional amounts if needed
Potassium <2.5 mEq/L: Up to 40-60 mEq initial dose, followed by further doses based on lab values; deficits at a plasma level of 2 mEq/L may be as high as 400-800 mEq of potassium

Dosage Forms

Tablet for oral solution, effervescent: 6.5 mEq, 20 mEq, 25 mEq
K+ Care® ET: 25 mEq

potassium bicarbonate and potassium chloride, effervescent

(poe TASS ee um bye KAR bun ate & poe TASS ee um KLOR ide, ef er VES ent)

U.S./Canadian Brand Names K-Lyte/Cl® [US/Can]

Therapeutic Category Electrolyte Supplement, Oral

Use Treatment or prevention of hypokalemia

Usual Dosage Oral:

Children: 1-4 mEq/kg/24 hours in divided doses as required to maintain normal serum potassium

Adults:
Prevention: 16-24 mEq/day in 2-4 divided doses
Treatment: 40-100 mEq/day in 2-4 divided doses

Dosage Forms

Tablet for oral solution, effervescent:
Klorvess®: 20 mEq per packet
K-Lyte/Cl®: 25 mEq, 50 mEq per packet

potassium bicarbonate and potassium citrate, effervescent

(poe TASS ee um bye KAR bun ate & poe TASS ee um SIT rate, ef er VES ent)

Synonyms potassium citrate and potassium bicarbonate, effervescent

U.S./Canadian Brand Names Effer-K™ [US]; Klor-Con®/EF [US]; K-Lyte® [US/Can]

Therapeutic Category Electrolyte Supplement, Oral

Use Treatment or prevention of hypokalemia

Usual Dosage Oral:

Children: 1-4 mEq/kg/24 hours as required to maintain normal serum potassium
Adults:
Prevention: 16-24 mEq/day in 2-4 divided doses
Treatment: 40-100 mEq/day in 2-4 divided doses

Dosage Forms Tablet, effervescent: 25 mEq

potassium chloride (poe TASS ee um KLOR ide)

Synonyms KCl

U.S./Canadian Brand Names Apo®-K [Can]; Cena-K® [US]; K+ 10® [US]; Kaochlor® [US]; Kaon-Cl® [US]; Kaon-Cl-10® [US]; Kay Ciel® [US]; K+ Care® [US]; K-Dur® 10 [US/Can]; K-Dur® 20 [US/Can]; K-Lor™ [US/Can]; Klor-Con® [US]; Klor-Con® 8 [US]; Klor-Con® 10 [US]; Klor-Con®/25 [US]; Klorvess® [US]; Klotrix® [US]; K-Tab® [US]; Micro-K® 10 Extencaps® [US]; Micro-K® Extencaps [US/Can]; Roychlor® [Can]; Rum-K® [US]; Slow-K® [Can]

Therapeutic Category Electrolyte Supplement, Oral

Use Potassium deficiency, treatment or prevention of hypokalemia

Usual Dosage I.V. doses should be incorporated into the patient's maintenance I.V. fluids, intermittent I.V. potassium administration should be reserved for severe depletion situations in patients undergoing EKG monitoring.

Normal daily requirement: Oral, I.V.:
Newborns: 2-6 mEq/kg/day
Children: 2-3 mEq/kg/day
Adults: 40-80 mEq/day
Prevention during diuretic therapy: Oral:
Children: 1-2 mEq/kg/day in 1-2 divided doses
Adults: 20-40 mEq/day in 1-2 divided doses
Treatment: Oral, I.V.:
Children: 2-3 mEq/kg/day
Adults: 40-100 mEq/day
I.V. intermittent infusion:
Children: Dose should not exceed 0.5 mEq/kg/hour, not to exceed 20 mEq/hour
Adults: 10-20 mEq/hour, not to exceed 40 mEq/hour and 150 mEq/day

Dosage Forms

Capsule, controlled release, microencapsulated: 600 mg [8 mEq]; 750 mg [10 mEq]
Micro-K® 10 Extencaps®: 750 mg [10 mEq]
Micro-K® Extencaps®: 600 mg [8 mEq]
Liquid: 10% [20 mEq/15 mL] (480 mL, 4000 mL); 20% [40 mEq/15 mL] (480 mL, 4000 mL)
Cena-K®, Kaochlor®, Kay Ciel®, Klorvess®, Potasalan®: 10% [20 mEq/15 mL] (480 mL, 4000 mL)
Cena-K®, Kaon-Cl 20%: 20% [40 mEq/15 mL] (480 mL, 4000 mL)
Rum-K®: 15% [30 mEq/15 mL] (480 mL, 4000 mL)
Infusion: 0.1 mEq/mL (100 mL); 0.2 mEq/mL (50 mL, 100 mL); 0.3 mEq/mL (100 mL); 0.4 mEq/mL (50 mL, 100 mL); 0.6 mEq/mL (50 mL); 0.8 mEq/mL (50 mL)
Injection, concentrate: 2 mEq/mL
Powder:
K+ Care®, Kay Ciel®, K-Lor™, Klor-Con®: 20 mEq per packet (30s, 100s)
K+ Care®: 15 mEq per packet (30s, 100s)
K+ Care®, Klor-Con®/25: 25 mEq per packet (30s, 100s)
Tablet, controlled release, microencapsulated:
K-Dur® 10: 750 mg [10 mEq]
K-Dur® 20: 1500 mg [20 mEq]
Tablet, controlled release, wax matrix: 600 mg [8 mEq]; 750 mg [10 mEq]
K+ 10®, Kaon-Cl-10®, Klor-Con® 10, Klotrix®, K-Tab®: 750 mg [10 mEq]
Kaon-Cl®: 500 mg [6.7 mEq]
Klor-Con® 8, Slow-K®: 600 mg [8 mEq]

potassium citrate (poe TASS ee um SIT rate)

U.S./Canadian Brand Names Urocit®-K [US]

Therapeutic Category Alkalinizing Agent

Use Prevention of uric acid nephrolithiasis; prevention of calcium renal stones in patients with hypocitraturia; urinary alkalinizer when sodium citrate is contraindicated

Usual Dosage Adults: Oral: 10-20 mEq 3 times/day with meals, up to 100 mEq/day

Dosage Forms Tablet: 540 mg [5 mEq]; 1080 mg [10 mEq]

potassium citrate and citric acid
(poe TASS ee um SIT rate & SI trik AS id)

Synonyms citric acid and potassium citrate

U.S./Canadian Brand Names Polycitra®-K [US]

Therapeutic Category Alkalinizing Agent

Use Treatment of metabolic acidosis; alkalinizing agent in conditions where long-term maintenance of an alkaline urine is desirable

Usual Dosage Oral:
Mild to moderate hypocitraturia: 10 mEq 3 times/day with meals
Severe hypocitraturia: Initial: 20 mEq 3 times/day or 15 mEq 4 times/day with meals or within 30 minutes after meals; do not exceed 100 mEq/day

Dosage Forms
Crystals for reconstitution: Potassium citrate 3300 mg and citric acid 1002 mg per packet
Solution, oral: Potassium citrate 1100 mg and citric acid 334 mg per 5 mL

potassium citrate and potassium bicarbonate, effervescent *see* potassium
bicarbonate and potassium citrate, effervescent *on page 529*

potassium citrate and potassium gluconate
(poe TASS ee um SIT rate & poe TASS ee um GLOO coe nate)

U.S./Canadian Brand Names Twin-K® [US]

Therapeutic Category Electrolyte Supplement, Oral

Use Treatment or prevention of hypokalemia

Usual Dosage Oral:
Children: 1-4 mEq/kg/24 hours in divided doses as required to maintain normal serum potassium
Adults:
Prevention: 16-24 mEq/day in 2-4 divided doses
Treatment: 40-100 mEq/day in 2-4 divided doses

Dosage Forms Solution, oral: 20 mEq/5 mL from potassium citrate 170 mg and potassium gluconate 170 mg per 5 mL

potassium gluconate (poe TASS ee um GLOO coe nate)

U.S./Canadian Brand Names Glu-K® [US-OTC]; Kaon® [US/Can]

Therapeutic Category Electrolyte Supplement, Oral

Use Treatment or prevention of hypokalemia

Usual Dosage Oral:
Normal daily requirement:
Children: 2-3 mEq/kg/day
Adults: 40-80 mEq/day
Prevention during diuretic therapy:
Children: 1-2 mEq/kg/day in 1-2 divided doses
Adults: 20-40 mEq/day in 1-2 divided doses
Treatment of hypokalemia:
Children: 2-3 mEq/kg/day in 2-4 divided doses
Adults: 40-100 mEq/day in 2-4 divided doses

Dosage Forms
Elixir (Kaon®): 20 mEq/15 mL
Tablet (Glu-K®): 2 mEq

potassium iodide (poe TASS ee um EYE oh dide)

Synonyms KI; Lugol's solution; strong iodine solution

U.S./Canadian Brand Names Pima® [US]; SSKI® [US]; Thyro-Block® [Can]

Therapeutic Category Antithyroid Agent; Expectorant

Use Expectorant for the symptomatic treatment of chronic pulmonary diseases complicated by mucous; reduce thyroid vascularity prior to thyroidectomy and management of
(Continued)

potassium iodide (Continued)

thyrotoxic crisis; block thyroidal uptake of radioactive isotopes of iodine in a radiation emergency or other exposure to radioactive iodine

Usual Dosage Oral:

Adults RDA: 130 mcg

Expectorant:

Children: 60-250 mg every 6-8 hours; maximum single dose: 500 mg

Adults: 300-1000 mg 2-3 times/day, may increase to 1-1.5 g 3 times/day

Preoperative thyroidectomy: Children and Adults: 50-250 mg 3 times/day (2-6 drops strong iodine solution); administer for 10 days before surgery

Thyrotoxic crisis:

Infants <1 year: $\frac{1}{2}$ adult dosage

Children and Adults: 300 mg = 6 drops SSKI® every 8 hours

Graves' disease in neonates: 1 drop of Lugol's solution every 8 hours

Sporotrichosis:

Initial:

Preschool: 50 mg/dose 3 times/day

Children: 250 mg/dose 3 times/day

Adults: 500 mg/dose 3 times/day

Oral increase 50 mg/dose daily

Maximum dose:

Preschool: 500 mg/dose 3 times/day

Children and Adults: 1-2 g/dose 3 times/day

Continue treatment for 4-6 weeks after lesions have completely healed

Dosage Forms

Solution, oral:

SSKI®: 1 g/mL (30 mL, 240 mL) [contains sodium thiosulfate]

Lugol's solution, strong iodine: Potassium iodide 100 mg/mL with iodine 50 mg/mL

Syrup (Pima®): 325 mg/5 mL [equivalent to iodide 249 mg/5 mL] (473 mL) [black raspberry flavor]

potassium phosphate (poe TASS ee um FOS fate)

U.S./Canadian Brand Names Neutra-Phos®-K [US]

Therapeutic Category Electrolyte Supplement, Oral

Use Treatment and prevention of hypophosphatemia

Usual Dosage I.V. doses should be incorporated into the patient's maintenance I.V. fluids; intermittent I.V. infusion should be reserved for severe depletion situations and requires continuous cardiac monitoring. It is difficult to determine total body phosphorus deficit, the following dosages are empiric guidelines: **Note:** Doses listed as mmol of **phosphate**:

Replacement intermittent infusion: I.V.:

Children:

Low dose: 0.08 mmol/kg over 6 hours; use if recent losses and uncomplicated

Intermediate dose: 0.16-0.24 mmol/kg over 4-6 hours; use if serum phosphorus level 0.5-1 mg/dL

High dose: 0.36 mmol/kg over 6 hours; use if serum phosphorus <0.5 mg/dL

Adults: Varying dosages: 0.15-0.3 mmol/kg/dose over 12 hours; may repeat as needed to achieve desired serum level **or**

15 mmol/dose over 2 hours; use if serum phosphorus <2 mg/dL **or**

Low dose: 0.16 mmol/kg over 4-6 hours; use if serum phosphorus level 2.3-3 mg/dL

Intermediate dose: 0.32 mmol/kg over 4-6 hours; use if serum phosphorus level 1.6-2.2 mg/dL

High dose: 0.64 mmol/kg over 8-12 hours; use if serum phosphorus <1.5 mg/dL

Maintenance:

Children: 0.5-1.5 mmol/kg/24 hours I.V. or 2-3 mmol/kg/24 hours orally in divided doses

Adults: 50-70 mmol/24 hours I.V. or 50-150 mmol/24 hours orally in divided doses

Dosage Forms
  Injection (per mL): Phosphate 3 mmol, potassium 4.4 mEq
  Powder [capsule] (Neutra-Phos®-K): Elemental phosphorus 250 mg, phosphate 8 mmol, potassium 14.2 mEq

potassium phosphate and sodium phosphate
(poe TASS ee um FOS fate & SOW dee um FOS fate)

Synonyms sodium phosphate and potassium phosphate

U.S./Canadian Brand Names K-Phos® MF [US]; K-Phos® Neutral [US]; K-Phos® No. 2 [US]; Neutra-Phos® Powder [US]; Uro-KP-Neutral® [US]

Therapeutic Category Electrolyte Supplement, Oral

Use Treatment of conditions associated with excessive renal phosphate loss or inadequate GI absorption of phosphate

Usual Dosage All dosage forms to be mixed in 6-8 oz of water prior to administration
  Children: 2-3 mmol phosphate/kg/24 hours administered 4 times/day
  Adults: 100-150 mmol phosphate/24 hours in divided doses after meals and at bedtime; 1-8 tablets or capsules/day, administered 4 times/day

Dosage Forms
  Liquid: Whole cow's milk (per mL): Phosphate 0.29 mmol, sodium 0.025 mEq, potassium 0.035 mEq
  Powder, concentrated [capsule] (Neutra-Phos®): Elemental phosphorus 250 mg, phosphate 8 mmol, sodium 7.1 mEq, potassium 7.1 mEq
  Tablet:
    K-Phos® MF: Elemental phosphorus 125.6 mg, phosphate 4 mmol, sodium 2.9 mEq, potassium 1.1 mEq
    K-Phos® Neutral: Elemental phosphorus 250 mg, phosphate 8 mmol, sodium 13 mEq, potassium 1.1 mEq
    K-Phos® No. 2: Elemental phosphorus 250 mg, phosphate 8 mmol, sodium 5.8 mEq, potassium 2.3 mEq
    Uro-KP-Neutral®: Elemental phosphorus 250 mg, phosphate 8 mmol, sodium 10.8 mEq, potassium 1.3 mEq

Povidex® [US-OTC] *see povidone-iodine on this page*

povidone-iodine (POE vi done-EYE oh dyne)
U.S./Canadian Brand Names Acu-Dyne® Skin [US-OTC]; Aplicare® [US-OTC]; Betadine® [US/Can]; Minidyne® [US-OTC]; Operand® [US-OTC]; Polydine® [US-OTC]; Povidex® [US-OTC]; Proviodine [Can]; PVP-Duoswab® [US-OTC]; Summer's Eve® Special Care [US-OTC]; Vagi-Gard® Douche [US-OTC]

Therapeutic Category Antibacterial, Topical

Use External antiseptic with broad microbicidal spectrum against bacteria, fungi, viruses, protozoa, and yeasts

Usual Dosage Apply as needed for treatment and prevention of susceptible microbial infections

Dosage Forms
  Aerosol, topical: 5% (88.7 mL, 90 mL)
  Antiseptic gauze pads, topical: 10% (3" x 9")
  Cleanser: 60 mL, 240 mL
  Cleanser, skin: 7.5% (30 mL, 118 mL)
  Cleanser, skin, foam: 7.5% (170 g)
  Cream: 5% (14 g)
  Foam, topical: 10% (250 g)
  Gel, lubricating, topical: 5% (5 g)
  Gel, vaginal: 10% (18 g, 90 g)
  Liquid, concentrate [whirlpool]: 3840 mL
  Liquid, topical: 473 mL
  Ointment, topical: 1% (30 g, 454 g); 10% (0.94 g, 3.8 g, 28 g, 30 g, 454 g); 1 g, 1.2 g, 2.7 g packets
  (Continued)

povidone-iodine *(Continued)*

Shampoo: 7.5% (118 mL)
Solution, douche: 10% (240 mL) [0.5 oz/packet] (6/box)
Solution, douche, concentrate: 10% (240 mL); 20% (120 mL, 240 mL)
Solution, douche, diluted: 0.3% (135 mL, 180 mL)
Solution, mouthwash: 0.5% (177 mL)
Solution, ophthalmic, sterile prep: 5% (50 mL)
Solution, prep: 10% (30 mL, 60 mL, 240 mL, 473 mL, 1000 mL, 4000 mL)
Solution, swab aid: 1%
Solution, swabsticks: 10%
Solution, topical: 1% (480 mL, 4000 mL); 10% (15 mL, 30 mL, 120 mL, 237 mL, 473 mL, 480 mL, 1000 mL, 4000 mL)
Solution, topical concentrate [perineal wash]: 1% (240 mL); 10% (236 mL)
Solution, topical [surgical scrub]: 7.5% (15 mL, 473 mL, 946 mL)
Suppositories, vaginal: 10% (7s)

PPD *see* tuberculin tests *on page 662*

PPL *see* benzylpenicilloyl-polylysine *on page 81*

PPS *see* pentosan polysulfate sodium *on page 502*

pralidoxime (pra li DOKS eem)

Synonyms 2-PAM; 2-pyridine aldoxime methochloride
U.S./Canadian Brand Names Protopam® Injection [US/Can]
Therapeutic Category Antidote
Use Reverse muscle paralysis associated with toxic exposure to organophosphate anticholinesterase pesticides and chemicals; control of overdosage by anticholinesterase drugs used to treat myasthenia gravis
Usual Dosage Poisoning: I.V.:
Children: 20-50 mg/kg/dose; repeat in 1-2 hours if muscle weakness has not been relieved, then at 10- to 12-hour intervals if cholinergic signs recur
Adults: 1-2 g; repeat in 1-2 hours if muscle weakness has not been relieved, then at 10- to 12-hour intervals if cholinergic signs recur
Dosage Forms
Injection: 20 mL vial containing 1 g each pralidoxime chloride with one 20 mL ampul diluent, disposable syringe, needle, and alcohol swab
Injection, as chloride: 300 mg/mL (2 mL)

PrameGel® [US-OTC] *see* pramoxine *on this page*

Pramet® FA *(Discontinued)* *see page 814*

Pramilet® FA *(Discontinued)* *see page 814*

pramipexole (pra mi PEX ole)

U.S./Canadian Brand Names Mirapex® [US/Can]
Therapeutic Category Dopaminergic Agent (Anti-Parkinson's)
Use Treatment of the signs and symptoms of idiopathic Parkinson's Disease
Usual Dosage Adults: Oral: Initial: 0.375 mg/day given in 3 divided doses, increase gradually by 0.125 mg/dose every 5-7 days; range: 1.5-4.5 mg/day
Dosage Forms Tablet: 0.125 mg, 0.25 mg, 0.5 mg, 1 mg, 1.5 mg

Pramosone® [US] *see* pramoxine and hydrocortisone *on next page*

Pramox® HC [Can] *see* pramoxine and hydrocortisone *on next page*

pramoxine (pra MOKS een)

U.S./Canadian Brand Names Anusol® [US-OTC]; Fleet® Pain Relief [US-OTC]; Itch-X® [US-OTC]; Phicon® [US-OTC]; PrameGel® [US-OTC]; Prax® [US-OTC]; ProctoFoam® NS [US-OTC]; Tronolane® [US-OTC]; Tronothane® [US-OTC]

Therapeutic Category Local Anesthetic
Use Temporary relief of pain and itching associated with anogenital pruritus or irritation; dermatosis, minor burns or hemorrhoids
Usual Dosage Apply as directed, usually every 3-4 hours
Dosage Forms
 Aerosol, foam, as hydrochloride (ProctoFoam® NS): 1% (15 g)
 Cream, as hydrochloride:
  Prax®: 1% (30 g, 113.4 g, 454 g)
  Tronolane®: 1% (30 g, 60 g)
 Gel, topical, as hydrochloride:
  Itch-X®: 1% (35.4 g)
  PrameGel®: 1% (118 g)
 Lotion, as hydrochloride (Prax®): 1% (15 mL, 120 mL, 240 mL)
 Ointment, as hydrochloride (Anusol®): 1% (30 g)
 Pads, as hydrochloride (Fleet® Pain Relief): 1% (100s)
 Solution, topical, as hydrochloride [spray] (Itch-X®): 1% (60 mL)

pramoxine and hydrocortisone (pra MOKS een & hye droe KOR ti sone)
Synonyms hydrocortisone and pramoxine
U.S./Canadian Brand Names Analpram-HC® [US]; Enzone® [US]; Epifoam® [US]; Pramosone® [US]; Pramox® HC [Can]; ProctoFoam®-HC [US/Can]; Zone-A Forte® [US]
Therapeutic Category Anesthetic/Corticosteroid
Use Treatment of severe anorectal or perianal inflammation
Usual Dosage Apply to affected areas 3-4 times/day
Dosage Forms
 Cream: Pramoxine hydrochloride 1% and hydrocortisone acetate 1%; pramoxine hydrochloride 1% and hydrocortisone acetate 2.5%
 Foam, rectal: Pramoxine hydrochloride 1% and hydrocortisone acetate 1% (10 g)
 Lotion: Pramoxine hydrochloride 1% and hydrocortisone 1%; pramoxine hydrochloride 2.5% and hydrocortisone 1% (37.5 mL, 120 mL, 240 mL)

Prandin™ [US/Can] see repaglinide on page 567

Pravachol® [US/Can] see pravastatin on this page

pravastatin (PRA va stat in)
U.S./Canadian Brand Names Lin-Pravastatin [Can]; Pravachol® [US/Can]
Therapeutic Category HMG-CoA Reductase Inhibitor
Use Adjunct to diet for the reduction of elevated total and LDL-cholesterol levels in patients with hypercholesterolemia (Type IIa and IIb)
Usual Dosage Adults: Oral: 10-20 mg once daily at bedtime
Dosage Forms Tablet, as sodium: 10 mg, 20 mg, 40 mg, 80 mg

Prax® [US-OTC] see pramoxine on previous page

praziquantel (pray zi KWON tel)
U.S./Canadian Brand Names Biltricide® [US/Can]
Therapeutic Category Anthelmintic
Use All stages of schistosomiasis caused by all *Schistosoma* species pathogenic to humans; clonorchiasis and opisthorchiasis
Usual Dosage Children >4 years and Adults: Oral:
 Schistosomiasis: 20 mg/kg/dose 2-3 times/day for 1 day at 4- to 6-hour intervals
 Flukes: 25 mg/kg/dose every 8 hours for 1-2 days
 Cysticercosis: 50 mg/kg/day divided every 8 hours for 14 days
 Tapeworms: 10-20 mg/kg as a single dose (25 mg/kg for *Hymenolepis nana*)
 Clonorchiasis/opisthorchiasis: 3 doses of 25 mg/kg as a 1-day treatment
Dosage Forms Tablet, tri-scored: 600 mg

prazosin (PRA zoe sin)

Synonyms furazosin

U.S./Canadian Brand Names Alti-Prazosin [Can]; Apo®-Prazo [Can]; Minipress® [US/Can]; Novo-Prazin [Can]; Nu-Prazo [Can]

Therapeutic Category Alpha-Adrenergic Blocking Agent

Use Hypertension, severe congestive heart failure (in conjunction with diuretics and cardiac glycosides)

Unlabeled use: Symptoms of benign prostatic hyperplasia

Usual Dosage Oral:

Children: Initial: 5 mcg/kg/dose (to assess hypotensive effects); usual dosing interval every 6 hours; increase dosage gradually up to maintenance of 25-150 mcg/kg/day divided every 6 hours

Adults: Initial: 1 mg/dose 2-3 times/day; usual maintenance dose: 3-15 mg/day in divided doses 2-4 times/day; maximum daily dose: 20 mg

Dosage Forms Capsule, as hydrochloride: 1 mg, 2 mg, 5 mg

prazosin and polythiazide (PRA zoe sin & pol i THYE a zide)

Synonyms polythiazide and prazosin

U.S./Canadian Brand Names Minizide® [US]

Therapeutic Category Antihypertensive Agent, Combination

Use Management of mild to moderate hypertension

Usual Dosage Adults: Oral: 1 capsule 2-3 times/day

Dosage Forms Capsule:

1: Prazosin 1 mg and polythiazide 0.5 mg
2: Prazosin 2 mg and polythiazide 0.5 mg
5: Prazosin 5 mg and polythiazide 0.5 mg

Precedex™ [US/Can] see dexmedetomidine on page 186

Precose® [US/Can] see acarbose on page 3

Predair® *(Discontinued)* see page 814

Predaject-50® *(Discontinued)* see page 814

Predalone® *(Discontinued)* see page 814

Predcor® *(Discontinued)* see page 814

Predcor-TBA® *(Discontinued)* see page 814

Pred Forte® [US/Can] see prednisolone (ophthalmic) on next page

Pred-G® [US] see prednisolone and gentamicin on next page

Predicort-50® *(Discontinued)* see page 814

Pred Mild® [US/Can] see prednisolone (ophthalmic) on next page

prednicarbate (PRED ni kar bate)

U.S./Canadian Brand Names Dermatop® [US]

Therapeutic Category Corticosteroid, Topical

Use Relief of the inflammatory and pruritic manifestations of corticosteroid-responsive dermatoses

Usual Dosage Adults: Topical: Apply a thin film to affected area twice daily. Therapy should be discontinued when control is achieved. If no improvement is seen, reassessment of diagnosis may be necessary.

Dosage Forms

Cream: 0.1% (15 g, 60 g)
Ointment: 0.1% (15 g, 60 g)

Prednicen-M® *(Discontinued)* see page 814

Prednicot® [US] see prednisone on page 538

prednisolone and gentamicin (pred NIS oh lone & jen ta MYE sin)

Synonyms gentamicin and prednisolone

U.S./Canadian Brand Names Pred-G® [US]

Therapeutic Category Antibiotic/Corticosteroid, Ophthalmic

Use Treatment of steroid responsive inflammatory conditions and superficial ocular infections due to strains of microorganisms susceptible to gentamicin such as *Staphylococcus*, *E. coli*, *H. influenzae*, *Klebsiella*, *Neisseria*, *Pseudomonas*, *Proteus*, and *Serratia* species

Usual Dosage Children and Adults: Ophthalmic: 1 drop 2-4 times/day; during the initial 24-48 hours, the dosing frequency may be increased if necessary

Dosage Forms

Ointment, ophthalmic: Prednisolone acetate 0.6% and gentamicin sulfate 0.3% (3.5 g)

Suspension, ophthalmic: Prednisolone acetate 1% and gentamicin sulfate 0.3% (2 mL, 5 mL, 10 mL)

prednisolone and sulfacetamide see sulfacetamide and prednisolone *on page 611*

prednisolone, neomycin, and polymyxin B see neomycin, polymyxin B, and prednisolone *on page 454*

prednisolone (ophthalmic) (pred NIS oh lone op THAL mik)

Tall-Man predniso**LONE** (ophthalmic)

U.S./Canadian Brand Names AK-Pred® [US]; Diopred® [Can]; Econopred® Plus [US]; Econopred® [US]; Inflamase® Forte [US/Can]; Inflamase® Mild [US/Can]; Metreton® [US]; Ophtho-Tate® [Can]; Pred Forte® [US/Can]; Pred Mild® [US/Can]

Therapeutic Category Adrenal Corticosteroid

Use Treatment of palpebral and bulbar conjunctivitis; corneal injury from chemical, radiation, thermal burns, or foreign body penetration

Usual Dosage Adults: Ophthalmic: 1-2 drops into conjunctival sac every hour during day, every 2 hours at night until favorable response is obtained, then use 1 drop every 4 hours

Dosage Forms

Solution, ophthalmic, as sodium phosphate: 0.125% (5 mL, 10 mL, 15 mL); 1% (5 mL, 10 mL, 15 mL)

Suspension, ophthalmic, as acetate: 0.12% (5 mL, 10 mL); 0.125% (5 mL, 10 mL, 15 mL); 1% (1 mL, 5 mL, 10 mL, 15 mL)

prednisolone (systemic) (pred NIS oh lone sis TEM ik)

Synonyms deltahydrocortisone; metacortandralone

Tall-Man predniso**LONE** (systemic)

U.S./Canadian Brand Names Delta-Cortef® [US]; Key-Pred-SP® [US]; Key-Pred® [US]; Orapred™ [US]; Pediapred® [US/Can]; Prednisol® TBA [US]; Prelone® [US]

Therapeutic Category Adrenal Corticosteroid

Use Treatment of endocrine disorders, rheumatic disorders, collagen diseases, dermatologic diseases, allergic states, ophthalmic diseases, respiratory diseases, hematologic disorders, neoplastic diseases, edematous states, and gastrointestinal diseases

Usual Dosage Dose depends upon condition being treated and response of patient; dosage for infants and children should be based on severity of the disease and response of the patient rather than on strict adherence to dosage indicated by age, weight, or body surface area. Consider alternate day therapy for long-term therapy. Discontinuation of long-term therapy requires gradual withdrawal by tapering the dose.

Children:

Acute asthma:

Oral: 1-2 mg/kg/day in divided doses 1-2 times/day for 3-5 days

I.V.: 2-4 mg/kg/day divided 3-4 times/day

Anti-inflammatory or immunosuppressive dose: Oral, I.V.: 0.1-2 mg/kg/day in divided doses 1-4 times/day

(Continued)

prednisolone (systemic) *(Continued)*

Nephrotic syndrome: Oral: Initial: 2 mg/kg/day (maximum: 80 mg/day) in divided doses 3-4 times/day until urine is protein free for 5 days (maximum: 28 days); if proteinuria persists, use 4 mg/kg/dose every other day for an additional 28 days (maximum: 120 mg/day); maintenance: 2 mg/kg/dose every other day for 28 days (maximum: 80 mg/dose); then taper over 4-6 weeks

Adults:

Oral, I.V.: 5-60 mg/day

Dosage Forms

Injection, as acetate (for I.M., intralesional, intra-articular, or soft tissue administration only): 25 mg/mL (10 mL, 30 mL); 50 mg/mL (30 mL)

Injection, as sodium phosphate (for I.M., I.V., intra-articular, intralesional, or soft tissue administration): 20 mg/mL (2 mL, 5 mL, 10 mL)

Injection, as tebutate (for intra-articular, intralesional, soft tissue administration only): 20 mg/mL (1 mL, 5 mL, 10 mL)

Liquid, oral, as sodium phosphate: 5 mg/5 mL (120 mL)

Solution, oral, as sodium phosphate: 15 mg/5 mL (240 mL)

Syrup: 15 mg/5 mL (240 mL)

Tablet: 5 mg

Prednisol® TBA [US] *see* prednisolone (systemic) *on previous page*

prednisone (PRED ni sone)

Synonyms deltacortisone; deltadehydrocortisone

Tall-Man predniSONE

U.S./Canadian Brand Names Apo®-Prednisone [Can]; Deltasone® [US]; Meticorten® [US]; Prednicot® [US]; Sterapred® DS [US]; Sterapred® [US]; Winpred™ [Can]

Therapeutic Category Adrenal Corticosteroid

Use Management of adrenocortical insufficiency; used for its anti-inflammatory or immunosuppressant effects

Usual Dosage Dose depends upon condition being treated and response of patient; dosage for infants and children should be based on severity of the disease and response of the patient rather than on strict adherence to dosage indicated by age, weight, or body surface area. Consider alternate day therapy for long-term therapy. Discontinuation of long-term therapy requires gradual withdrawal by tapering the dose.

Children: Oral: 0.05-2 mg/kg/day (anti-inflammatory or immunosuppressive dose) divided 1-4 times/day

Acute asthma: Oral: 1-2 mg/kg/day in divided doses 1-2 times/day for 3-5 days

Nephrotic syndrome: Oral: Initial: 2 mg/kg/day (maximum: of 80 mg/day) in divided doses 3-4 times/day until urine is protein free for 5 days (maximum: 28 days); if proteinuria persists, use 4 mg/kg/dose every other day (maximum: 120 mg/day) for an additional 28 days; maintenance: 2 mg/kg/dose every other day for 28 days (maximum: 80 mg/day); then taper over 4-6 weeks

Children and Adults: Physiologic replacement: 4-5 mg/m^2/day

Adults: Oral: 5-60 mg/day in divided doses 1-4 times/day

Dosage Forms

Solution, oral: 1 mg/mL (5 mL, 120 mL, 500 mL) [contains alcohol 5%]

Solution, oral concentrate: 5 mg/mL (30 mL) [contains alcohol 30%]

Syrup: 1 mg/mL (120 mL, 240 mL)

Tablet: 1 mg, 2.5 mg, 5 mg, 10 mg, 20 mg, 50 mg

Prefrin™ Ophthalmic [US] *see* phenylephrine *on page 510*

Pregestimil® [US-OTC] *see* nutritional formula, enteral/oral *on page 472*

pregnenedione *see* progesterone *on page 543*

Pregnyl® [US/Can] *see* chorionic gonadotropin (human) *on page 144*

Prelone® [US] *see* prednisolone (systemic) *on previous page*

Prelu-2® **[US]** *see* phendimetrazine *on page 507*

Preludin® *(Discontinued) see page 814*

Premarin® **[US/Can]** *see* estrogens (conjugated/equine) *on page 242*

Premarin® **With Methyltestosterone** *(Discontinued) see page 814*

Premphase® **[US/Can]** *see* estrogens and medroxyprogesterone *on page 241*

Prempro™ **[US/Can]** *see* estrogens and medroxyprogesterone *on page 241*

prenatal vitamins *see* vitamin (multiple/prenatal) *on page 683*

Prenavite® **[US-OTC]** *see* vitamin (multiple/prenatal) *on page 683*

Preparation H® **Cleansing Pads [Can]** *see* witch hazel *on page 686*

Prepcat® **[US]** *see* radiological/contrast media (ionic) *on page 561*

Pre-Pen® **[US]** *see* benzylpenicilloyl-polylysine *on page 81*

Prepidil® **Vaginal Gel [US/Can]** *see* dinoprostone *on page 201*

Prescription Strength Desenex® *(Discontinued) see page 814*

Pressyn® **[Can]** *see* vasopressin *on page 674*

PreSun® **29 [US-OTC]** *see* methoxycinnamate and oxybenzone *on page 419*

Pretz-D® **[US-OTC]** *see* ephedrine *on page 228*

Pretz® **[US-OTC]** *see* sodium chloride *on page 595*

Prevacid® **[US/Can]** *see* lansoprazole *on page 374*

Prevalite® **[US]** *see* cholestyramine resin *on page 143*

PREVEN™ **[US]** *see* ethinyl estradiol and levonorgestrel *on page 248*

Prevex® **[Can]** *see* betamethasone (topical) *on page 83*

Prevex® **HC [Can]** *see* hydrocortisone (topical) *on page 334*

PreviDent® **[US]** *see* fluoride *on page 278*

PreviDent® **5000 Plus**™ **[US]** *see* fluoride *on page 278*

Prevnar™ **[US]** *see* pneumococcal conjugate vaccine (7-valent) *on page 521*

Prevpac™ **[US/Can]** *see* lansoprazole, amoxicillin, and clarithromycin *on page 375*

Priftin® **[US/Can]** *see* rifapentine *on page 573*

prilocaine (PRIL oh kane)
    U.S./Canadian Brand Names Citanest® Forte [Can]; Citanest® Plain [US/Can]
    Therapeutic Category Local Anesthetic
    Use In dentistry for infiltration anesthesia and for nerve block anesthesia
    Usual Dosage Dose varies with procedure, desired depth, and duration of anesthesia, desired muscle relaxation, vascularity of tissues, physical condition, and age of patient
    Dosage Forms Injection: 4% (1.8 mL)

prilocaine and lidocaine *see* lidocaine and prilocaine *on page 384*

Prilosec® **[US/Can]** *see* omeprazole *on page 476*

primaclone *see* primidone *on next page*

Primacor® **[US/Can]** *see* milrinone *on page 431*

primaquine (PRIM a kween)
    Synonyms prymaccone
    Therapeutic Category Aminoquinoline (Antimalarial)
    Use In conjunction with a blood schizonticidal agent to provide radical cure of *P. vivax* or *P. ovale* malaria after a clinical attack has been confirmed by blood smear or serologic titer; prevention of relapse of *P. ovale* or *P. vivax* malaria; malaria postexposure prophylaxis
    (Continued)

primaquine *(Continued)*

Usual Dosage Oral:

Children: 0.3 mg base/kg/day once daily for 14 days not to exceed 15 mg/day or 0.9 mg base/kg once weekly for 8 weeks not to exceed 45 mg base/week

Adults: 15 mg/day (base) once daily for 14 days or 45 mg base once weekly for 8 weeks

Dosage Forms Tablet, as phosphate: 26.3 mg [15 mg base]

Primatene® Mist [US-OTC] *see* epinephrine *on page 228*

Primaxin® [US/Can] *see* imipenem and cilastatin *on page 345*

primidone (PRI mi done)

Synonyms desoxyphenobarbital; primaclone

U.S./Canadian Brand Names Apo®-Primidone [Can]; Mysoline® [US/Can]

Therapeutic Category Anticonvulsant; Barbiturate

Use Management of generalized tonic-clonic (grand mal), complex partial and simple partial (focal) seizures

Usual Dosage Oral:

Children <8 years: Initial: 50-125 mg/day given at bedtime; increase by 50-125 mg/day increments every 3-7 days; usual dose: 10-25 mg/kg/day in divided doses 3-4 times/day

Children >8 years and Adults: Initial: 125-250 mg/day at bedtime; increase by 125-250 mg/day every 3-7 days; usual dose: 750-1500 mg/day in divided doses 3-4 times/day with maximum dosage of 2 g/day

Dosage Forms

Suspension, oral: 250 mg/5 mL (240 mL)

Tablet: 50 mg, 250 mg

Primsol® [US] *see* trimethoprim *on page 657*

Principen® [US] *see* ampicillin *on page 40*

Prinivil® [US/Can] *see* lisinopril *on page 388*

Prinzide® [US/Can] *see* lisinopril and hydrochlorothiazide *on page 388*

Priorix™ [Can] *see* measles, mumps, and rubella vaccines, combined *on page 402*

Priscoline® [US] *see* tolazoline *on page 643*

pristinamycin *see* quinupristin and dalfopristin *on page 560*

Privine® [US-OTC] *see* naphazoline *on page 446*

ProAmatine [US] *see* midodrine *on page 430*

Proampacin® *(Discontinued) see page 814*

Pro-Banthine® *(Discontinued) see page 814*

probenecid (proe BEN e sid)

U.S./Canadian Brand Names Benuryl™ [Can]

Therapeutic Category Uricosuric Agent

Use Prevention of gouty arthritis; hyperuricemia; prolong serum levels of penicillin/cephalosporin

Usual Dosage Oral:

Children:

<2 years: Not recommended

2-14 years: Prolong penicillin serum levels: 25 mg/kg starting dose, then 40 mg/kg/day administered 4 times/day

Gonorrhea: <45 kg: 25 mg/kg x 1 (maximum: 1 g/dose) 30 minutes before penicillin, ampicillin or amoxicillin

Adults:

Hyperuricemia with gout: 250 mg twice daily for one week; increase to 500 mg 2 times/ day; may increase by 500 mg/month, if needed, to maximum of 2-3 g/day (dosages may be decreased by 500 mg every 6 months if serum urate concentrations are controlled)

Prolong penicillin serum levels: 500 mg 4 times/day

Gonorrhea: 1 g 30 minutes before penicillin, ampicillin or amoxicillin

Dosage Forms Tablet: 500 mg

probenecid and colchicine *see* colchicine and probenecid *on page 160*

Pro-Bionate® [US-OTC] *see* Lactobacillus *on page 372*

Probiotica® [US-OTC] *see* Lactobacillus *on page 372*

procainamide (proe kane A mide)

Synonyms procaine amide hydrochloride

U.S./Canadian Brand Names Apo®-Procainamide [Can]; Procanbid® [US]; Procan™ SR [Can]; Pronestyl® [US/Can]; Pronestyl-SR® [US/Can]

Therapeutic Category Antiarrhythmic Agent, Class I-A

Use Ventricular tachycardia, premature ventricular contractions, paroxysmal atrial tachycardia, and atrial fibrillation; to prevent recurrence of ventricular tachycardia, paroxysmal supraventricular tachycardia, atrial fibrillation or flutter

Usual Dosage Must be titrated to patient's response

Children:

Oral: 15-50 mg/kg/24 hours divided every 3-6 hours; maximum 4 g/24 hours

I.M.: 20-30 mg/kg/24 hours divided every 4-6 hours in divided doses; maximum 4 g/24 hours

I.V.: Load: 3-6 mg/kg/dose over 5 minutes not to exceed 100 mg/dose; may repeat every 5-10 minutes to maximum of 15 mg/kg/load; maintenance as continuous I.V. infusion: 20-80 mcg/kg/minute; maximum: 2 g/24 hours

Adults:

Oral: 250-500 mg/dose every 3-6 hours or 500 mg to 1 g every 6 hours sustained release; usual dose: 50 mg/kg/24 hours or 2-4 g/24 hours

I.V.: Load: 50-100 mg/dose, repeated every 5-10 minutes until patient controlled; or load with 15-18 mg/kg, maximum loading dose: 1-1.5 g; maintenance: 2-6 mg/minute continuous I.V. infusion, usual maintenance: 3-4 mg/minute

Dosage Forms

Capsule, as hydrochloride: 250 mg, 375 mg, 500 mg

Injection, as hydrochloride: 100 mg/mL (10 mL); 500 mg/mL (2 mL)

Tablet, as hydrochloride: 250 mg, 375 mg, 500 mg

Tablet, sustained release, as hydrochloride: 250 mg, 500 mg, 750 mg, 1000 mg

Procanbid®: 500 mg, 1000 mg

procaine (PROE kane)

U.S./Canadian Brand Names Novocain® [US/Can]

Therapeutic Category Local Anesthetic

Use Produce spinal anesthesia and epidural and peripheral nerve block by injection and infiltration methods

Usual Dosage Dose varies with procedure, desired depth and duration of anesthesia, desired muscle relaxation, vascularity of tissues, physical condition, and age of patient

Dosage Forms Injection, as hydrochloride: 1% [10 mg/mL] (2 mL, 6 mL, 30 mL, 100 mL); 2% [20 mg/mL] (30 mL, 100 mL); 10% (2 mL)

procaine amide hydrochloride *see* procainamide *on this page*

procaine benzylpenicillin *see* penicillin G procaine *on page 499*

procaine penicillin G *see* penicillin G procaine *on page 499*

Pro-Cal-Sof® *(Discontinued)* *see page 814*

Procanbid® **[US]** *see* procainamide *on previous page*

Procan™ **SR** *(Discontinued) see page 814*

Procan™ **SR [Can]** *see* procainamide *on previous page*

procarbazine (proe KAR ba zeen)

Synonyms ibenzmethyzin; MIH; n-methylhydrazine

U.S./Canadian Brand Names Matulane® [US/Can]; Natulan® [Can]

Therapeutic Category Antineoplastic Agent

Use Treatment of Hodgkin's disease, non-Hodgkin's lymphoma, brain tumor, bronchogenic carcinoma

Usual Dosage Refer to individual protocols. Oral:

Children: 50-100 mg/m^2/day in a single dose; doses as high as 100-200 mg/m^2/day once daily have been used for neuroblastoma and medulloblastoma

Adults: Initial: 2-4 mg/kg/day in single or divided doses for 7 days then increase dose to 4-6 mg/kg/day until response is obtained or leukocyte count decreased <4000/mm^3 or the platelet count decreased <100,000/mm^3; maintenance: 1-2 mg/kg/day

Dosage Forms Capsule, as hydrochloride: 50 mg

Procardia® **[US/Can]** *see* nifedipine *on page 459*

Procardia XL® **[US]** *see* nifedipine *on page 459*

procetofene *see* fenofibrate *on page 265*

prochlorperazine (proe klor PER a zeen)

U.S./Canadian Brand Names Compazine® [US/Can]; Compro™ [US]; Nu-Prochlor [Can]; Stemetil® [Can]

Therapeutic Category Phenothiazine Derivative

Use Management of nausea and vomiting; acute and chronic psychoses

Usual Dosage

Children: Oral, rectal:

>10 kg: 0.4 mg/kg/24 hours in 3-4 divided doses; **or**

9-14 kg: 2.5 mg every 12-24 hours as needed; maximum: 7.5 mg/day

14-18 kg: 2.5 mg every 8-12 hours as needed; maximum: 10 mg/day

18-39 kg: 2.5 mg every 8 hours or 5 mg every 12 hours as needed; maximum: 15 mg/day

I.M.: 0.1-0.15 mg/kg/dose; usual: 0.13 mg/kg/dose; change to oral as soon as possible

I.V.: Not recommended

Adults:

Oral: 5-10 mg 3-4 times/day; usual maximum: 40 mg/day; doses up to 150 mg/day may be required in some patients

I.M.: 5-10 mg every 3-4 hours; usual maximum: 40 mg/day; doses up to 10-20 mg every 4-6 hours may be required in some patients

I.V.: 2.5-10 mg; maximum 10 mg/dose or 40 mg/day; may repeat dose every 3-4 hours as needed

Rectal: 25 mg twice daily

Dosage Forms

Capsule, sustained action, as maleate: 10 mg, 15 mg, 30 mg

Injection, as edisylate: 5 mg/mL (2 mL, 10 mL)

Suppository, rectal: 2.5 mg, 5 mg, 25 mg (12/box)

Syrup, as edisylate: 5 mg/5 mL (120 mL)

Tablet, as maleate: 5 mg, 10 mg, 25 mg

Procrit® **[US]** *see* epoetin alfa *on page 230*

Proctocort™ **Rectal [US]** *see* hydrocortisone (rectal) *on page 333*

ProctoCream ® **HC Cream [US]** *see* hydrocortisone (rectal) *on page 333*

proctofene *see* fenofibrate *on page 265*

ProctoFoam®**-HC [US/Can]** *see* pramoxine and hydrocortisone *on page 535*

ProctoFoam® **NS [US-OTC]** *see* pramoxine *on page 534*

Procyclid™ **[Can]** *see* procyclidine *on this page*

procyclidine (proe SYE kli deen)

U.S./Canadian Brand Names Kemadrin® [US/Can]; Procyclid™ [Can]

Therapeutic Category Anticholinergic Agent; Anti-Parkinson's Agent

Use Relief of symptoms of Parkinsonian syndrome and drug-induced extrapyramidal symptoms

Usual Dosage Adults: Oral: 2-2.5 mg 3 times/day after meals; if tolerated, gradually increase dose to 4-5 mg 3 times/day

Dosage Forms Tablet, as hydrochloride: 5 mg

Procytox® **[Can]** *see* cyclophosphamide *on page 169*

Prodium™ **[US-OTC]** *see* phenazopyridine *on page 506*

Prodrox® **[US]** *see* hydroxyprogesterone caproate *on page 337*

Profasi® **[US]** *see* chorionic gonadotropin (human) *on page 144*

Profasi® **HP [Can]** *see* chorionic gonadotropin (human) *on page 144*

Profenal® ***(Discontinued)*** *see page 814*

Profen II DM® ***(Discontinued)*** *see page 814*

Profen® **II [US-OTC]** *see* guaifenesin and pseudoephedrine *on page 310*

Profen LA® ***(Discontinued)*** *see page 814*

Profilate-HP® ***(Discontinued)*** *see page 814*

Profilnine® **SD [US]** *see* factor IX complex (human) *on page 261*

Proflavanol C™ **[Can]** *see* ascorbic acid *on page 57*

Progestaject® **Injection *(Discontinued)*** *see page 814*

Progestasert® **[US]** *see* progesterone *on this page*

progesterone (proe JES ter one)

Synonyms pregnenedione; progestin

U.S./Canadian Brand Names Crinone® [US/Can]; Progestasert® [US]; Prometrium® [US/Can]

Therapeutic Category Progestin

Use Intrauterine contraception in women who have had at least 1 child, are in a stable, mutually monogamous relationship, and have no history of pelvic inflammatory disease; amenorrhea; functional uterine bleeding; replacement therapy

Oral: Prevention of endometrial hyperplasia in nonhysterectomized postmenopausal women who are receiving conjugated estrogen tablets; secondary amenorrhea

Intravaginal gel: Part of assisted reproductive technology for infertile women with progesterone deficiency; secondary amenorrhea (8% gel is used in those who fail to respond to 4%)

Usual Dosage

I.M.: Adults: Female:

Amenorrhea: 5-10 mg/day for 6-8 consecutive days

Functional uterine bleeding: 5-10 mg/day for 6 doses

IUD: Adults: Female: Contraception: Insert a single system into the uterine cavity; contraceptive effectiveness is retained for 1 year and system must be replaced 1 year after insertion

Oral: Adults: Female:

Prevention of endometrial hyperplasia (in postmenopausal women with a uterus who are receiving daily conjugated estrogen tablets): 200 mg as a single daily dose every evening for 12 days sequentially per 28-day cycle

Amenorrhea: 400 mg every evening for 10 days

(Continued)

543

progesterone *(Continued)*

Intravaginal gel: Adults: Female:
ART in women who require progesterone supplementation: 90 mg (8% gel) once daily; if pregnancy occurs, may continue treatment for up to 10-12 weeks
ART in women with partial or complete ovarian failure: 90 mg (8% gel) intravaginally twice daily; if pregnancy occurs, may continue up to 10-12 weeks
Secondary amenorrhea: 45 mg (4% gel) intravaginally every other day for up to 6 doses; women who fail to respond may be increased to 90 mg (8% gel) every other day for up to 6 doses

Dosage Forms
Capsule (Prometrium®): 100 mg, 200 mg [contains peanut oil]
Gel, vaginal (Crinone®): 4% (45 mg); 8% (90 mg)
Injection [in oil]: 50 mg/mL (10 mL) [may contain benzyl alcohol, sesame oil]
Intrauterine system, reservoir [in silicone fluid] (Progestasert®): 38 mg [delivers progesterone 65 mcg/day over 1 year]

progestin *see* progesterone *on previous page*

Proglycem® [US/Can] *see* diazoxide *on page 192*

Prograf® [US/Can] *see* tacrolimus *on page 617*

ProHance® [US] *see* radiological/contrast media (non-ionic) *on page 563*

ProHIBiT® *(Discontinued)* *see page 814*

Prokine™ Injection *(Discontinued)* *see page 814*

Prolamine® *(Discontinued)* *see page 814*

Prolapa® [Can] *see* benserazide and levodopa *(Canada only) on page 75*

Prolastin® [US/Can] *see* alpha₁-proteinase inhibitor *on page 24*

Proleukin® [US/Can] *see* aldesleukin *on page 20*

Prolex-D [US] *see* guaifenesin and phenylephrine *on page 310*

Prolixin® [US] *see* fluphenazine *on page 281*

Prolixin Decanoate® [US] *see* fluphenazine *on page 281*

Prolixin Enanthate® [US] *see* fluphenazine *on page 281*

Proloid® *(Discontinued)* *see page 814*

Proloprim® [US/Can] *see* trimethoprim *on page 657*

Promacet® [US] *see* butalbital, acetaminophen, and caffeine *on page 99*

Promatussin® DM [Can] *see* promethazine and dextromethorphan *on next page*

promazine *(PROE ma zeen)*

Therapeutic Category Phenothiazine Derivative
Use Treatment of psychoses
Usual Dosage I.M.:
Children >12 years: Antipsychotic: 10-25 mg every 4-6 hours
Adults:
Psychosis: 10-200 mg every 4-6 hours not to exceed 1000 mg/day
Antiemetic: 25-50 mg every 4-6 hours as needed
Dosage Forms Injection, as hydrochloride: 25 mg/mL (10 mL); 50 mg/mL (1 mL, 2 mL, 10 mL)

Prometa® *(Discontinued)* *see page 814*

Prometh® *(Discontinued)* *see page 814*

promethazine *(proe METH a zeen)*

U.S./Canadian Brand Names Anergan® [US]; Phenergan® [US/Can]
Therapeutic Category Antiemetic; Phenothiazine Derivative

Use Symptomatic treatment of various allergic conditions and motion sickness; sedative and an antiemetic

Usual Dosage
Children:
Antihistamine: Oral: 0.1 mg/kg/dose every 6 hours during the day and 0.5 mg/kg/dose at bedtime as needed
Antiemetic: Oral, I.M., I.V., rectal: 0.25-1 mg/kg 4-6 times/day as needed
Motion sickness: Oral: 0.5 mg/kg 30 minutes to 1 hour before departure, then every 12 hours as needed
Sedation: Oral, I.M., I.V., rectal: 0.5-1 mg/kg/dose every 6 hours as needed
Adults:
Antihistamine:
Oral: 25 mg at bedtime or 12.5 mg 3 times/day
I.M., I.V., rectal: 25 mg, may repeat in 2 hours
Antiemetic: Oral, I.M., I.V., rectal: 12.5-25 mg every 4 hours as needed
Motion sickness: Oral: 25 mg 30 minutes to 1 hour before departure, then every 12 hours as needed
Sedation: Oral, I.M., I.V., rectal: 25-50 mg/dose

Dosage Forms
Injection, as hydrochloride: 25 mg/mL (1 mL, 10 mL); 50 mg/mL (1 mL, 10 mL)
Suppository, rectal, as hydrochloride: 12.5 mg, 25 mg, 50 mg
Syrup, as hydrochloride: 6.25 mg/5 mL (5 mL, 120 mL, 480 mL, 4000 mL); 25 mg/5 mL (120 mL, 480 mL, 4000 mL)
Tablet, as hydrochloride: 12.5 mg, 25 mg, 50 mg

promethazine and codeine (proe METH a zeen & KOE deen)
Synonyms codeine and promethazine
U.S./Canadian Brand Names Phenergan® With Codeine [US]
Therapeutic Category Antihistamine/Antitussive
Controlled Substance C-V
Use Temporary relief of coughs and upper respiratory symptoms associated with allergy or the common cold
Usual Dosage Oral (in terms of codeine):
Children: 1-1.5 mg/kg/day every 4 hours as needed; maximum: 30 mg/day **or**
2-6 years: 1.25-2.5 mL every 4-6 hours or 2.5-5 mg/dose every 4-6 hours as needed; maximum: 30 mg codeine/day
6-12 years: 2.5-5 mL every 4-6 hours as needed or 5-10 mg/dose every 4-6 hours as needed; maximum: 60 mg codeine/day
Adults: 10-20 mg/dose every 4-6 hours as needed; maximum: 120 mg codeine/day; or 5-10 mL every 4-6 hours as needed
Dosage Forms Syrup: Promethazine hydrochloride 6.25 mg and codeine phosphate 10 mg per 5 mL (120 mL, 180 mL, 473 mL)

promethazine and dextromethorphan
(proe METH a zeen & deks troe meth OR fan)
Synonyms dextromethorphan and promethazine
U.S./Canadian Brand Names Promatussin® DM [Can]
Therapeutic Category Antihistamine/Antitussive
Use Temporary relief of coughs and upper respiratory symptoms associated with allergy or the common cold
Usual Dosage Oral:
Children:
2-6 years: 1.25-2.5 mL every 4-6 hours up to 10 mL in 24 hours
6-12 years: 2.5-5 mL every 4-6 hours up to 20 mL in 24 hours
Adults: 5 mL every 4-6 hours up to 30 mL in 24 hours
Dosage Forms Syrup: Promethazine hydrochloride 6.25 mg and dextromethorphan hydrobromide 15 mg per 5 mL (120 mL, 480 mL, 4000 mL) [contains alcohol 7%]

promethazine and meperidine *see* meperidine and promethazine *on page 408*

promethazine and phenylephrine (proe METH a zeen & fen il EF rin)

Synonyms phenylephrine and promethazine

U.S./Canadian Brand Names Phenergan® VC [US]; Promethazine VC Plain [US]; Promethazine VC [US]

Therapeutic Category Antihistamine/Decongestant Combination

Use Temporary relief of upper respiratory symptoms associated with allergy or the common cold

Usual Dosage Oral:
Children:
2-6 years: 1.25 mL every 4-6 hours, not to exceed 7.5 mL in 24 hours
6-12 years: 2.5 mL every 4-6 hours, not to exceed 15 mL in 24 hours
Children >12 years and Adults: 5 mL every 4-6 hours, not to exceed 30 mL in 24 hours

Dosage Forms Liquid: Promethazine hydrochloride 6.25 mg and phenylephrine hydrochloride 5 mg per 5 mL (120 mL, 240 mL, 473 mL)

promethazine, phenylephrine, and codeine

(proe METH a zeen, fen il EF rin, & KOE deen)

Synonyms codeine, promethazine, and phenylephrine; phenylephrine, promethazine, and codeine

Therapeutic Category Antihistamine/Decongestant/Antitussive

Controlled Substance C-V

Use Temporary relief of coughs and upper respiratory symptoms including nasal congestion

Usual Dosage Oral:
Children (expressed in terms of codeine dosage): 1-1.5 mg/kg/day every 4 hours, maximum: 30 mg/day **or**
<2 years: Not recommended
2 to 6 years:
Weight 25 lb: 1.25-2.5 mL every 4-6 hours, not to exceed 6 mL/24 hours
Weight 30 lb: 1.25-2.5 mL every 4-6 hours, not to exceed 7 mL/24 hours
Weight 35 lb: 1.25-2.5 mL every 4-6 hours, not to exceed 8 mL/24 hours
Weight 40 lb: 1.25-2.5 mL every 4-6 hours, not to exceed 9 mL/24 hours
6 to <12 years: 2.5-5 mL every 4-6 hours, not to exceed 15 mL/24 hours
Adults: 5 mL every 4-6 hours, not to exceed 30 mL/24 hours

Dosage Forms Liquid: Promethazine hydrochloride 6.25 mg, phenylephrine hydrochloride 5 mg, and codeine phosphate 10 mg per 5 mL (120 mL, 240 mL, 480 mL, 4000 mL) [contains alcohol 7%]

Promethazine VC [US] *see* promethazine and phenylephrine *on this page*

Promethazine VC Plain [US] *see* promethazine and phenylephrine *on this page*

Promethist® With Codeine *(Discontinued)* *see page 814*

Prometh® VC Plain Liquid *(Discontinued)* *see page 814*

Prometh® VC With Codeine *(Discontinued)* *see page 814*

Prometrium® [US/Can] *see* progesterone *on page 543*

Promit® [US] *see* dextran 1 *on page 187*

Pronap-100® [US] *see* propoxyphene and acetaminophen *on page 548*

Pronestyl® [US/Can] *see* procainamide *on page 541*

Pronestyl-SR® [US/Can] *see* procainamide *on page 541*

Pronto® [US-OTC] *see* pyrethrins *on page 555*

Propacet® *(Discontinued)* *see page 814*

Propac™ [US-OTC] *see* nutritional formula, enteral/oral *on page 472*

Propaderm® **[Can]** *see* beclomethasone *on page 73*

propafenone (proe pa FEEN one)
U.S./Canadian Brand Names Rythmol® [US/Can]
Therapeutic Category Antiarrhythmic Agent, Class I-C
Use Life-threatening ventricular arrhythmias; an oral sodium channel blocker similar to encainide and flecainide; in clinical trials was used effectively to treat atrial flutter, atrial fibrillation and other arrhythmias, but are not labeled indications; can worsen or even cause new ventricular arrhythmias (proarrhythmic effect)
Usual Dosage Adults: Oral: 150 mg every 8 hours, up to 300 mg every 8 hours
Dosage Forms Tablet, as hydrochloride: 150 mg, 225 mg, 300 mg

Propagest® *(Discontinued)* see page 814

Propanthel™ **[Can]** *see* propantheline *on this page*

propantheline (proe PAN the leen)
U.S./Canadian Brand Names Propanthel™ [Can]
Therapeutic Category Anticholinergic Agent
Use Adjunctive treatment of peptic ulcer, irritable bowel syndrome, pancreatitis, ureteral and urinary bladder spasm; to reduce duodenal motility during diagnostic radiologic procedures
Usual Dosage Oral:
  Antisecretory:
    Children: 1-2 mg/kg/day in 3-4 divided doses
    Elderly patients: 7.5 mg 3 times/day before meals and at bedtime
  Antispasmodic:
    Children: 2-3 mg/kg/day in divided doses every 4-6 hours and at bedtime
    Adults: 15 mg 3 times/day before meals or food and 30 mg at bedtime
Dosage Forms Tablet, as bromide: 15 mg

proparacaine (proe PAR a kane)
Synonyms proxymetacaine
U.S./Canadian Brand Names Alcaine® [US/Can]; Diocaine® [Can]; Ophthetic® [US]; Parcaine® [US]
Therapeutic Category Local Anesthetic
Use Local anesthesia for tonometry, gonioscopy; suture removal from cornea; removal of corneal foreign body; cataract extraction, glaucoma surgery; short operative procedure involving the cornea and conjunctiva
Usual Dosage Children and Adults:
  Ophthalmic surgery: Instill 1 drop of 0.5% solution in eye every 5-10 minutes for 5-7 doses
  Tonometry, gonioscopy, suture removal: Instill 1-2 drops 0.5% solution in eye just prior to procedure
Dosage Forms Solution, ophthalmic, as hydrochloride: 0.5% (2 mL, 15 mL) [contains benzalkonium chloride]

proparacaine and fluorescein (proe PAR a kane & FLURE e seen)
U.S./Canadian Brand Names Fluoracaine® [US]
Therapeutic Category Diagnostic Agent; Local Anesthetic
Use Anesthesia for tonometry, gonioscopy; suture removal from cornea; removal of corneal foreign body; cataract extraction, glaucoma surgery
Usual Dosage
  Tonometry, gonioscopy, suture removal: Adults: Instill 1-2 drops 0.5% solution in eye just prior to procedure
  Ophthalmic surgery: Children and Adults: Instill 1 drop of 0.5% solution in eye every 5-10 minutes for 5-7 doses
(Continued)

proparacaine and fluorescein *(Continued)*

Dosage Forms Solution: Proparacaine hydrochloride 0.5% and fluorescein sodium 0.25% (5 mL)

Propecia® **[US/Can]** *see* finasteride *on page 272*

Propine® **[US/Can]** *see* dipivefrin *on page 205*

Proplex® **SX-T Injection** *(Discontinued) see page 814*

Proplex® **T [US]** *see* factor IX complex (human) *on page 261*

propofol (PROE po fole)

U.S./Canadian Brand Names Diprivan® [US/Can]

Therapeutic Category General Anesthetic

Use Induction or maintenance of anesthesia; sedation

Usual Dosage Dosage must be individualized and titrated to the desired clinical effect; however, as a general guideline:

No pediatric dose has been established

Induction: I.V.:

Adults ≤55 years, and/or ASA I or II patients: 2-2.5 mg/kg of body weight (approximately 40 mg every 10 seconds until onset of induction)

Elderly, debilitated, hypovolemic, and/or ASA III or IV patients: 1-1.5 mg/kg of body weight (approximately 20 mg every 10 seconds until onset of induction)

Maintenance: I.V. infusion:

Adults ≤55 years, and/or ASA I or II patients: 0.1-0.2 mg/kg of body weight/minute (6-12 mg/kg of body weight/hour)

Elderly, debilitated, hypovolemic, and/or ASA III or IV patients: 0.05-0.1 mg/kg of body weight/minute (3-6 mg/kg of body weight/hour)

I.V. intermittent: 25-50 mg increments, as needed

Dosage Forms Injection [with EDTA preservative]: 10 mg/mL (20 mL, 50 mL, 100 mL)

Propoxacet-N® *(Discontinued) see page 814*

propoxyphene (proe POKS i feen)

Synonyms dextropropoxyphene

U.S./Canadian Brand Names Darvon® [US]; Darvon-N® Tablet [US/Can]; 642® Tablet [Can]

Therapeutic Category Analgesic, Narcotic

Controlled Substance C-IV

Use Management of mild to moderate pain

Usual Dosage Adults: Oral:

Hydrochloride: 65 mg every 3-4 hours as needed for pain; maximum: 390 mg/day

Napsylate: 100 mg every 4 hours as needed for pain; maximum: 600 mg/day

Dosage Forms

Capsule, as hydrochloride: 65 mg

Tablet, as napsylate: 100 mg

propoxyphene and acetaminophen

(proe POKS i feen & a seet a MIN oh fen)

Synonyms acetaminophen and propoxyphene

U.S./Canadian Brand Names Darvocet-N® 50 [US/Can]; Darvocet-N® 100 [US/Can]; Pronap-100® [US]

Therapeutic Category Analgesic, Narcotic

Controlled Substance C-IV

Use Management of mild to moderate pain

Usual Dosage Adults: Oral:

Darvocet-N®: 1-2 tablets every 4 hours as needed; maximum: 600 mg propoxyphene napsylate/day

Darvocet-N® 100: 1 tablet every 4 hours as needed; maximum: 600 mg propoxyphene napsylate/day
Dosage Forms
Tablet:
Darvocet-N® 50: Propoxyphene napsylate 50 mg and acetaminophen 325 mg
Darvocet-N® 100, Pronap-100®: Propoxyphene napsylate 100 mg and acetaminophen 650 mg

propoxyphene and aspirin (proe POKS i feen & AS pir in)

Synonyms aspirin and propoxyphene
U.S./Canadian Brand Names Darvon® Compound-65 [US]; PC-Cap® [US]
Therapeutic Category Analgesic, Narcotic
Controlled Substance C-IV
Use Management of mild to moderate pain
Usual Dosage Oral: 1-2 capsules every 4 hours as needed
Dosage Forms Capsule: Propoxyphene hydrochloride 65 mg and aspirin 389 mg with caffeine 32.4 mg

propranolol (proe PRAN oh lole)

U.S./Canadian Brand Names Apo®-Propranolol [Can]; Inderal® LA [US/Can]; Inderal® [US/Can]; Nu-Propranolol [Can]
Therapeutic Category Antiarrhythmic Agent, Class II; Beta-Adrenergic Blocker
Use Management of hypertension, angina pectoris, pheochromocytoma, essential tremor, tetralogy of Fallot cyanotic spells, and arrhythmias (such as atrial fibrillation and flutter, A-V nodal re-entrant tachycardias, and catecholamine-induced arrhythmias); prevention of myocardial infarction, migraine headache; symptomatic treatment of hypertrophic subaortic stenosis; short-term adjunctive therapy of thyrotoxicosis
Usual Dosage
Tachyarrhythmias:
Oral:
Children: Initial: 0.5-1 mg/kg/day in divided doses every 6-8 hours; titrate dosage upward every 3-7 days; usual dose: 2-4 mg/kg/day; higher doses may be needed; do not exceed 16 mg/kg/day or 60 mg/day
Adults: 10-80 mg/dose every 6-8 hours
I.V.:
Children: 0.01-0.1 mg/kg slow IVP over 10 minutes; maximum dose: 1 mg
Adults: 1 mg/dose slow IVP; repeat every 5 minutes up to a total of 5 mg
Hypertension: Oral:
Children: Initial: 0.5-1 mg/kg/day in divided doses every 6-12 hours; increase gradually every 3-7 days; maximum: 2 mg/kg/24 hours
Adults: Initial: 40 mg twice daily or 60-80 mg once daily as sustained release capsules; increase dosage every 3-7 days; usual dose: ≤320 mg divided in 2-3 doses/day or once daily as sustained release; maximum daily dose: 640 mg
Migraine headache prophylaxis: Oral:
Children: 0.6-1.5 mg/kg/day **or**
≤35 kg: 10-20 mg 3 times/day
>35 kg: 20-40 mg 3 times/day
Adults: Initial: 80 mg/day divided every 6-8 hours; increase by 20-40 mg/dose every 3-4 weeks to a maximum of 160-240 mg/day administered in divided doses every 6-8 hours; if satisfactory response not achieved within 6 weeks of starting therapy, drug should be withdrawn gradually over several weeks
Tetralogy spells: Children: Oral: 1-2 mg/kg/day every 6 hours as needed, may increase by 1 mg/kg/day to a maximum of 5 mg/kg/day, or if refractory may increase slowly to a maximum of 10-15 mg/kg/day
Thyrotoxicosis:
Adolescents and Adults: Oral: 10-40 mg/dose every 6 hours
Adults: I.V.: 1-3 mg/dose slow IVP as a single dose
(Continued)

propranolol *(Continued)*

Adults: Oral:
Angina: 80-320 mg/day in doses divided 2-4 times/day or 80-160 mg of sustained release once daily
Pheochromocytoma: 30-60 mg/day in divided doses
Myocardial infarction prophylaxis: 180-240 mg/day in 3-4divided doses
Hypertrophic subaortic stenosis: 20-40 mg 3-4 times/day
Essential tremor: 40 mg twice daily initially; maintenance doses: usually 120-320 mg/day

Dosage Forms
Capsule, long-acting, as hydrochloride: 60 mg, 80 mg, 120 mg, 160 mg
Injection, as hydrochloride: 1 mg/mL (1 mL)
Solution, oral, as hydrochloride: 4 mg/mL (5 mL, 500 mL); 8 mg/mL (5 mL, 500 mL) [strawberry-mint flavor]
Solution, oral concentrate, as hydrochloride: 80 mg/mL (30 mL)
Tablet, as hydrochloride: 10 mg, 20 mg, 40 mg, 60 mg, 80 mg, 90 mg

propranolol and hydrochlorothiazide

(proe PRAN oh lole & hye droe klor oh THYE a zide)
Synonyms hydrochlorothiazide and propranolol
U.S./Canadian Brand Names Inderide® LA [US]; Inderide® [US]
Therapeutic Category Antihypertensive Agent, Combination
Use Management of hypertension
Usual Dosage Dose is individualized
Dosage Forms
Capsule, long-acting (Inderide® LA):
80/50: Propranolol hydrochloride 80 mg and hydrochlorothiazide 50 mg
120/50: Propranolol hydrochloride 120 mg and hydrochlorothiazide 50 mg
160/50: Propranolol hydrochloride 160 mg and hydrochlorothiazide 50 mg
Tablet (Inderide®):
40/25: Propranolol hydrochloride 40 mg and hydrochlorothiazide 25 mg
80/25: Propranolol hydrochloride 80 mg and hydrochlorothiazide 25 mg

Propulsid® [US] *see* cisapride *on page 147*

propylene glycol and salicylic acid *see* salicylic acid and propylene glycol *on page 581*

propylhexedrine

(proe pil HEKS e dreen)
U.S./Canadian Brand Names Benzedrex® [US-OTC]
Therapeutic Category Adrenergic Agonist Agent
Use Topical nasal decongestant
Usual Dosage Inhale through each nostril while blocking the other
Dosage Forms Solution, intranasal [spray]: 250 mg (0.42 mL)

2-propylpentanoic acid *see* valproic acid and derivatives *on page 670*

propylthiouracil

(proe pil thye oh YOOR a sil)
Synonyms PTU
U.S./Canadian Brand Names Propyl-Thyracil® [Can]
Therapeutic Category Antithyroid Agent
Use Palliative treatment of hyperthyroidism, adjunct to ameliorate hyperthyroidism in preparation for surgical treatment or radioactive iodine therapy, management of thyrotoxic crisis
Usual Dosage Oral:
Children: Initial: 5-7 mg/kg/day in divided doses every 8 hours or
6-10 years: 50-150 mg/day
>10 years: 150-300 mg/day

Maintenance: 1/3 to 2/3 of the initial dose in divided doses every 8-12 hours
Adults: Initial: 300-450 mg/day in divided doses every 8 hours; maintenance: 100-150 mg/day in divided doses every 8-12 hours
Dosage Forms Tablet: 50 mg

Propyl-Thyracil® **[Can]** *see* propylthiouracil *on previous page*

2-propylvaleric acid *see* valproic acid and derivatives *on page 670*

Proscar® **[US/Can]** *see* finasteride *on page 272*

Pro-Sof® *(Discontinued) see page 814*

Pro-Sof® **Plus** *(Discontinued) see page 814*

ProSom™ **[US]** *see* estazolam *on page 238*

prostaglandin E₁ *see* alprostadil *on page 25*

prostaglandin E₂ *see* dinoprostone *on page 201*

Prostaphlin® *(Discontinued) see page 814*

ProStep® **Patch** *(Discontinued) see page 814*

Prostigmin® **[US/Can]** *see* neostigmine *on page 454*

Prostin E₂® **Vaginal Suppository [US/Can]** *see* dinoprostone *on page 201*

Prostin F₂ Alpha® *(Discontinued) see page 814*

Prostin VR Pediatric® **[US/Can]** *see* alprostadil *on page 25*

protamine sulfate (PROE ta meen SUL fate)
Therapeutic Category Antidote
Use Treatment of heparin overdosage; neutralize heparin during surgery or dialysis procedures
Usual Dosage Children and Adults: I.V.: 1 mg of protamine neutralizes 90 USP units of heparin (lung) and 115 USP units of heparin (intestinal); heparin neutralization occurs within 5 minutes following I.V. injection; administer 1 mg for each 100 units of heparin administered in preceding 3-4 hours up to a maximum dose of 50 mg
Dosage Forms Injection: 10 mg/mL (5 mL, 25 mL)

protein C (activated), human, recombinant *see* drotrecogin alfa *on page 218*

Protenate® *(Discontinued) see page 814*

Prothazine-DC® *(Discontinued) see page 814*

Protilase® *(Discontinued) see page 814*

protirelin (proe TYE re lin)
Synonyms lopremone
U.S./Canadian Brand Names Thyrel® TRH [US/Can]
Therapeutic Category Diagnostic Agent
Use Adjunct in the diagnostic assessment of thyroid function, and an adjunct to other diagnostic procedures in assessment of patients with pituitary or hypothalamic dysfunction; also causes release of prolactin from the pituitary and is used to detect defective control of prolactin secretion.
Usual Dosage I.V.:
Children: 7 mcg/kg to a maximum dose of 500 mcg
Adults: 500 mcg (range: 200-500 mcg)
Dosage Forms Injection: 500 mcg/mL (1 mL)

Protonix® **[US/Can]** *see* pantoprazole *on page 491*

Protopam® **Injection [US/Can]** *see* pralidoxime *on page 534*

Protopam® **Tablet** *(Discontinued) see page 814*

Protopic™ **[US]** *see* tacrolimus *on page 617*

Protostat® Oral *(Discontinued)* see page 814

protriptyline (proe TRIP ti leen)
   U.S./Canadian Brand Names Vivactil® [US]
   Therapeutic Category Antidepressant, Tricyclic (Secondary Amine)
   Use Treatment of various forms of depression, often in conjunction with psychotherapy
   Usual Dosage Oral:
     Adolescents: 15-20 mg/day
     Adults: 15-60 mg in 3-4 divided doses
   Dosage Forms Tablet, as hydrochloride: 5 mg, 10 mg

Protropin® [US/Can] see human growth hormone on page 324

Provatene® *(Discontinued)* see page 814

Proventil® [US] see albuterol on page 18

Proventil® HFA [US] see albuterol on page 18

Proventil® Repetabs® [US] see albuterol on page 18

Provera® [US/Can] see medroxyprogesterone acetate on page 404

Provigil® [US/Can] see modafinil on page 434

Proviodine [Can] see povidone-iodine on page 533

Provisc® [US] see sodium hyaluronate on page 597

Provocholine® [US/Can] see methacholine on page 414

Proxigel® Oral [US-OTC] see carbamide peroxide on page 113

proxymetacaine see proparacaine on page 547

Prozac® [US/Can] see fluoxetine on page 279

Prozac® Weekly™ [US] see fluoxetine on page 279

PRP-D see *Haemophilus* B conjugate vaccine on page 314

prymaccone see primaquine on page 539

Pseudocot-T® [US-OTC] see triprolidine and pseudoephedrine on page 659

pseudoephedrine (soo doe e FED rin)
   Synonyms *d*-isoephedrine
   U.S./Canadian Brand Names Balminil® Decongestant [Can]; Cenafed® [US-OTC];
     Children's Silfedrine® [US-OTC]; Children's Sudafed® Nasal Decongestant [US-OTC];
     Contac® Cold 12 Hour Relief Non Drowsy; Decofed® [US-OTC]; Dimetapp® Deconges-
     tant Liqui-Gels® [US-OTC]; Efidac/24® [US-OTC]; Eltor® [Can]; Genaphed® [US-OTC];
     PediaCare® Decongestant Infants [US-OTC]; PMS-Pseudoephedrine [Can]; Pseudofrin
     [Can]; Robidrine® [Can]; Sudafed® 12 Hour [US-OTC]; Sudafed® Children's [US-OTC];
     Sudafed® Decongestant [Can]; Sudafed® [US-OTC]; Triaminic® AM Decongestant
     Formula [US-OTC]; Triaminic® Infant Decongestant [US/Can]
   Therapeutic Category Adrenergic Agonist Agent
   Use Temporary symptomatic relief of nasal congestion due to common cold, upper
     respiratory allergies, and sinusitis; also promotes nasal or sinus drainage
   Usual Dosage Oral:
     Children:
       <2 years: 4 mg/kg/day in divided doses every 6 hours
       2-5 years: 15 mg every 6 hours; maximum: 60 mg/24 hours
       6-12 years: 30 mg every 6 hours; maximum: 120 mg/24 hours
     Adults: 60 mg every 6 hours; maximum: 240 mg/24 hours
   Dosage Forms
     Gelcap, as hydrochloride: 30 mg
     Liquid, as hydrochloride: 15 mg/5 mL (120 mL); 30 mg/5 mL (120 mL, 240 mL, 473 mL)
     Solution, oral drops, as hydrochloride: 7.5 mg/0.8 mL (15 mL)
     Syrup, as hydrochloride: 15 mg/5 mL (118 mL); 30 mg/mL (480 mL, 4000 mL)

Tablet, as hydrochloride: 30 mg, 60 mg
Tablet, chewable: 15 mg
Tablet, extended release, as sulfate: 120 mg, 240 mg

pseudoephedrine, acetaminophen, and dextromethorphan *see* acetaminophen, dextromethorphan, and pseudoephedrine *on page 8*

pseudoephedrine and acetaminophen *see* acetaminophen and pseudoephedrine *on page 6*

pseudoephedrine and acrivastine *see* acrivastine and pseudoephedrine *on page 12*

pseudoephedrine and azatadine *see* azatadine and pseudoephedrine *on page 65*

pseudoephedrine and carbinoxamine *see* carbinoxamine and pseudoephedrine *on page 115*

pseudoephedrine and chlorpheniramine *see* chlorpheniramine and pseudoephedrine *on page 138*

pseudoephedrine and dexbrompheniramine *see* dexbrompheniramine and pseudoephedrine *on page 185*

pseudoephedrine and dextromethorphan
(soo doe e FED rin & deks troe meth OR fan)
U.S./Canadian Brand Names Balminil DM D [Can]; Benylin® DM-D [Can]; Children's Sudafed® Cough & Cold [US-OTC]; Koffex DM-D [Can]; Novahistex® DM Decongestant [Can]; Novahistine® DM Decongestant [Can]; Robitussin® Childrens Cough & Cold [Can]; Robitussin® Maximum Strength Cough & Cold [US-OTC]; Robitussin® Pediatric Cough & Cold [US-OTC]; Vicks® 44D Cough & Head Congestion [US-OTC]
Therapeutic Category Antitussive/Decongestant
Use Temporary symptomatic relief of nasal congestion due to common cold, upper respiratory allergies, and sinusitis; also promotes nasal or sinus drainage; symptomatic relief of coughs caused by minor viral upper respiratory tract infections or inhaled irritants; most effective for a chronic nonproductive cough
Usual Dosage Adults: Oral: 1 capsule every 6 hours
Dosage Forms Liquid:
Children's Sudafed® Cold & Cough: Pseudoephedrine hydrochloride 15 mg and dextromethorphan hydrobromide 5 mg per 5 mL
Robitussin® Maximum Strength Cough & Cold: Pseudoephedrine hydrochloride 30 mg and dextromethorphan hydrobromide 15 mg per 5 mL
Robitussin® Pediatric Cough & Cold: Pseudoephedrine hydrochloride 15 mg and dextromethorphan hydrobromide 7.5 mg per 5 mL
Vicks® 44D Cough & Head Congestion: Pseudoephedrine hydrochloride 20 mg and dextromethorphan hydrobromide 10 mg per 5 mL

pseudoephedrine and guaifenesin *see* guaifenesin and pseudoephedrine *on page 310*

pseudoephedrine and ibuprofen
(soo doe e FED rin & eye byoo PROE fen)
U.S./Canadian Brand Names Advil® Cold & Sinus Caplets [US-OTC]; Advil® Cold & Sinus Tablet [Can]; Dristan® Sinus Caplets [US]; Dristan® Sinus Tablet [Can]
Therapeutic Category Decongestant/Analgesic
Use Temporary symptomatic relief of nasal congestion due to common cold, upper respiratory allergies, and sinusitis; also promotes nasal or sinus drainage; sinus headaches and pains
Usual Dosage Adults: Oral: 1-2 caplets every 4-6 hours
Dosage Forms
Caplet: Pseudoephedrine hydrochloride 30 mg and ibuprofen 200 mg
Tablet: Pseudoephedrine hydrochloride 30 mg and ibuprofen 200 mg

pseudoephedrine and loratadine *see* loratadine and pseudoephedrine *on page 391*

pseudoephedrine and triprolidine *see* triprolidine and pseudoephedrine *on page 659*

pseudoephedrine, dextromethorphan, and acetaminophen *see* acetaminophen, dextromethorphan, and pseudoephedrine *on page 8*

pseudoephedrine, dextromethorphan, and guaifenesin *see* guaifenesin, pseudoephedrine, and dextromethorphan *on page 312*

pseudoephedrine, guaifenesin, and codeine *see* guaifenesin, pseudoephedrine, and codeine *on page 311*

pseudoephedrine, hydrocodone, and guaifenesin *see* hydrocodone, pseudoephedrine, and guaifenesin *on page 332*

Pseudofrin [Can] *see* pseudoephedrine *on page 552*

Pseudo-Gest Plus® Tablet *(Discontinued)* *see page 814*

Pseudo GG TR [US] *see* guaifenesin and pseudoephedrine *on page 310*

pseudomonic acid A *see* mupirocin *on page 440*

Pseudovent™ [US] *see* guaifenesin and pseudoephedrine *on page 310*

Pseudovent™-Ped [US] *see* guaifenesin and pseudoephedrine *on page 310*

Psor-a-set® Soap [US-OTC] *see* salicylic acid *on page 581*

Psorcon™ [US/Can] *see* diflorasone *on page 196*

Psorcon™ E [US] *see* diflorasone *on page 196*

psoriGel® [US-OTC] *see* coal tar *on page 158*

Psorion® Topical *(Discontinued)* *see page 814*

P & S Plus® [US-OTC] *see* coal tar and salicylic acid *on page 158*

psyllium (SIL i yum)
   Synonyms plantago seed; plantain seed
   U.S./Canadian Brand Names Fiberall® Powder [US-OTC]; Fiberall® Wafer [US-OTC]; Hydrocil® [US-OTC]; Konsyl-D® [US-OTC]; Konsyl® [US-OTC]; Metamucil® Smooth Texture [US-OTC]; Metamucil® [US/Can]; Modane® Bulk [US-OTC]; Novo-Mucilax [Can]; Perdiem® Plain [US-OTC]; Reguloid® [US-OTC]; Serutan® [US-OTC]; Syllact® [US-OTC]
   Therapeutic Category Laxative
   Use Treatment of chronic atonic or spastic constipation and in constipation associated with rectal disorders; management of irritable bowel syndrome
   Usual Dosage Oral:
      Children 6-11 years: $^1/_2$ to 1 rounded teaspoonful 1-3 times/day
      Adults: 1-2 rounded teaspoonfuls or 1-2 packets 1-4 times/day
   Dosage Forms
      Granules for oral solution: 4.03 g per rounded teaspoon (100 g, 250 g); 2.5 g per rounded teaspoon
      Powder for oral solution, psyllium hydrophilic: 3.4 g per rounded teaspoon (210 g, 300 g, 420 g, 630 g)
      Wafers: 3.4 g

P.T.E.-4® [US] *see* trace metals *on page 646*

P.T.E.-5® [US] *see* trace metals *on page 646*

pteroylglutamic acid *see* folic acid *on page 285*

PTU *see* propylthiouracil *on page 550*

Pulmicort® Nebuamp® *see* budesonide *on page 95*

Pulmicort Respules™ [US] *see* budesonide *on page 95*

Pulmicort Turbuhaler® **[US/Can]** *see* budesonide *on page 95*

Pulmozyme® **[US/Can]** *see* dornase alfa *on page 212*

Puralube® Tears [US-OTC] *see* artificial tears *on page 56*

Purge® [US-OTC] *see* castor oil *on page 119*

Puri-Clens™ [US-OTC] *see* methylbenzethonium chloride *on page 420*

purified protein derivative *see* tuberculin tests *on page 662*

Purinethol® **[US/Can]** *see* mercaptopurine *on page 410*

PVF® K [Can] *see* penicillin V potassium *on page 499*

PVP-Duoswab® [US-OTC] *see* povidone-iodine *on page 533*

pyrantel pamoate (pi RAN tel PAM oh ate)
U.S./Canadian Brand Names Ascarel® [US-OTC]; Combantrin™ [Can]; Pamix® [US-OTC]; Pin-X® [US-OTC]; Reese's® Pinworm Medicine [US-OTC]
Therapeutic Category Anthelmintic
Use Roundworm (*Ascaris lumbricoides*), pinworm (*Enterobius vermicularis*), and hookworm (*Ancylostoma duodenale* and *Necator americanus*) infestations, and trichostrongyliasis
Usual Dosage Children and Adults: Oral:
Roundworm, pinworm, or trichostrongyliasis: 11 mg/kg administered as a single dose; maximum dose is 1 g; dosage should be repeated in 2 weeks for pinworm infection
Hookworm: 11 mg/kg/day once daily for 3 days
Dosage Forms
Capsule: 180 mg
Liquid: 50 mg/mL (30 mL)
Suspension, oral: 50 mg/mL (60 mL) [caramel-currant flavor]

pyrazinamide (peer a ZIN a mide)
Synonyms pyrazinoic acid amide
U.S./Canadian Brand Names Tebrazid™ [Can]
Therapeutic Category Antitubercular Agent
Use In combination with other antituberculosis agents in the treatment of *Mycobacterium tuberculosis* infection (especially useful in disseminated and meningeal tuberculosis); CDC currently recommends a 3 or 4 multidrug regimen which includes pyrazinamide, rifampin, INH, and at times ethambutol or streptomycin for the treatment of tuberculosis
Usual Dosage Oral:
Children: 15-30 mg/kg/day in divided doses every 12-24 hours; daily dose not to exceed 2 g
Adults: 15-30 mg/kg/day in 3-4 divided doses; maximum daily dose: 2 g/day
Dosage Forms Tablet: 500 mg

pyrazinamide, rifampin, and isoniazid *see* rifampin, isoniazid, and pyrazinamide *on page 573*

pyrazinoic acid amide *see* pyrazinamide *on this page*

pyrethrins (pye RE thrins)
Synonyms piperonyl butoxide and pyrethrins
U.S./Canadian Brand Names A-200™ [US-OTC]; End Lice® [US-OTC]; Pronto® [US-OTC]; Pyrinex® Pediculicide [US-OTC]; Pyrinyl Plus® [US-OTC]; Pyrinyl® [US-OTC]; R & C™ II [Can]; R & C™ Shampoo/Conditioner [Can]; R & C® [US-OTC]; RID® Mousse [Can]; RID® [US-OTC]; Tisit® Blue Gel [US-OTC]; Tisit® [US-OTC]
Therapeutic Category Scabicides/Pediculicides
Use Treatment of *Pediculus humanus* infestations
Usual Dosage Application of pyrethrins: Topical:
Apply enough solution to completely wet infested area, including hair
Allow to remain on area for 10 minutes
(Continued)

pyrethrins *(Continued)*

Wash and rinse with large amounts of warm water
Use fine-toothed comb to remove lice and eggs from hair
Shampoo hair to restore body and luster
Treatment may be repeated if necessary once in a 24-hours period
Repeat treatment in 7-10 days to kill newly hatched lice

Dosage Forms All in combination with piperonyl butoxide:
Gel: 0.3% (30 g)
Liquid, topical: 0.2% (60 mL, 120 mL); 0.3% (60 mL, 118 mL, 120 mL, 177 mL, 237 mL, 240 mL)
Shampoo: 0.3% (59 mL, 60 mL, 118 mL, 120 mL, 240 mL); 0.33% (120 mL)

Pyridiate® [US] *see* phenazopyridine *on page 506*

2-pyridine aldoxime methochloride *see* pralidoxime *on page 534*

Pyridium® [US/Can] *see* phenazopyridine *on page 506*

Pyridium Plus® *(Discontinued)* *see page 814*

pyridostigmine (peer id oh STIG meen)

U.S./Canadian Brand Names Mestinon®-SR [Can]; Mestinon® Timespan® [US]; Mestinon® [US/Can]; Regonol® [US]
Therapeutic Category Cholinergic Agent
Use Symptomatic treatment of myasthenia gravis by improving muscle strength; reversal of effects of nondepolarizing neuromuscular blocking agents
Usual Dosage Normally, sustained-release dosage form is used at bedtime for patients who complain of morning weakness

Myasthenia gravis:
Oral:
Children: 7 mg/kg/day in 5-6 divided doses
Adults: Initial: 60 mg 3 times/day with maintenance dose ranging from 60 mg to 1.5 g/day; sustained-release formulation should be dosed at least every 6 hours (usually 12-24 hours)
I.M., I.V.:
Children: 0.05-0.15 mg/kg/dose (maximum single dose: 10 mg)
Adults: 2 mg every 2-3 hours or 1/30th of oral dose
Reversal of nondepolarizing neuromuscular blocker: I.M., I.V.:
Children: 0.1-0.25 mg/kg/dose preceded by atropine
Adults: 10-20 mg preceded by atropine
Dosage Forms
Injection, as bromide:
Mestinon®: 5 mg/mL (2 mL)
Regonol®: 5 mg/mL (2 mL, 5 mL) [contains benzyl alcohol 1%]
Syrup, as bromide (Mestinon®): 60 mg/5 mL (480 mL) [contains alcohol 5%; raspberry flavor]
Tablet, as bromide (Mestinon®): 60 mg
Tablet, sustained release, as bromide (Mestinon® Timespan®): 180 mg

pyridoxine (peer i DOKS een)

Synonyms vitamin B_6
U.S./Canadian Brand Names Aminoxin® [US-OTC]
Therapeutic Category Vitamin, Water Soluble
Use Prevent and treat vitamin B_6 deficiency, pyridoxine-dependent seizures in infants, treatment of drug-induced deficiency (eg, isoniazid or hydralazine)
Usual Dosage
Pyridoxine-dependent Infants:
Oral: 2-100 mg/day
I.M., I.V.: 10-100 mg

Dietary deficiency: Oral:
  Children: 5-10 mg/24 hours for 3 weeks
  Adults: 10-20 mg/day for 3 weeks
Drug-induced neuritis (eg, isoniazid, hydralazine, penicillamine, cycloserine): Oral treatment:
  Children: 10-50 mg/24 hours; prophylaxis: 1-2 mg/kg/24 hours
  Adults: 100-200 mg/24 hours; prophylaxis: 10-100 mg/24 hours

For the treatment of seizures and/or coma from acute isoniazid toxicity, a dose of pyridoxine hydrochloride equal to the amount of INH ingested can be administered I.M./I.V. in divided doses together with other anticonvulsants

Dosage Forms
  Injection, as hydrochloride: 100 mg/mL (10 mL, 30 mL)
  Tablet, as hydrochloride: 25 mg, 50 mg, 100 mg, 250 mg, 500 mg
  Tablet, enteric coated, as hydrochloride: 20 mg

pyridoxine, folic acid, and cyanocobalamin *see* folic acid, cyanocobalamin, and pyridoxine *on page 286*

pyrimethamine (peer i METH a meen)

U.S./Canadian Brand Names Daraprim® [US/Can]
Therapeutic Category Folic Acid Antagonist (Antimalarial)
Use Prophylaxis of malaria due to susceptible strains of plasmodia; used in conjunction with quinine and sulfadoxine for the treatment of uncomplicated attacks of chloroquine-resistant *P. falciparum* malaria; used in conjunction with fast-acting schizonticide to initiate transmission control and suppression cure; synergistic combination with sulfadiazine in treatment of toxoplasmosis
Usual Dosage Oral:
  Malaria chemoprophylaxis:
    Children: 0.5 mg/kg once weekly; not to exceed 25 mg/dose **or**
    Children:
      <4 years: 6.25 mg once weekly
      4-10 years: 12.5 mg once weekly
    Children >10 years and Adults: 25 mg once weekly
    Dosage should be continued for all age groups for at least 6-10 weeks after leaving endemic areas
  Chloroquine-resistant *P. falciparum* malaria (when used in conjunction with quinine and sulfadiazine):
    Children:
      <10 kg: 6.25 mg/day once daily for 3 days
      10-20 kg: 12.5 mg/day once daily for 3 days
      20-40 kg: 25 mg/day once daily for 3 days
    Adults: 25 mg twice daily for 3 days
  Toxoplasmosis (with sulfadiazine or trisulfapyrimidines):
    Children: 1 mg/kg/day divided into 2 equal daily doses; decrease dose after 2-4 days by 50%, continue for about 1 month; used with 100 mg sulfadiazine/kg/day divided every 6 hours; **or** 2 mg/kg/day divided every 12 hours for 3 days followed by 1 mg/kg/day once daily for 4 weeks
    Adults: 50-75 mg/day together with 1-4 g of a sulfonamide for 1-3 weeks depending on patient's tolerance and response
Dosage Forms Tablet: 25 mg

Pyrinex® Pediculicide [US-OTC] *see* pyrethrins *on page 555*
Pyrinyl Plus® [US-OTC] *see* pyrethrins *on page 555*
Pyrinyl® [US-OTC] *see* pyrethrins *on page 555*

pyrithione zinc (peer i THYE one zingk)

U.S./Canadian Brand Names DHS Zinc® [US-OTC]; Head & Shoulders® [US-OTC]; Theraplex Z® [US-OTC]; Zincon® [US-OTC]; ZNP® Bar [US-OTC]
(Continued)

pyrithione zinc *(Continued)*

Therapeutic Category Antiseborrheic Agent, Topical

Use Relieves the itching, irritation and scalp flaking associated with dandruff and/or seborrheal dermatitis of the scalp

Usual Dosage Topical: Shampoo hair twice weekly, wet hair, apply to scalp and massage vigorously, rinse and repeat

Dosage Forms
Bar, topical: 2% (119 g)
Shampoo, topical: 1% (120 mL, 240 mL); 2% (120 mL, 180 mL, 240 mL, 360 mL)

Q-Dryl® [US-OTC] *see* diphenhydramine *on page 202*

Qualisone® [US] *see* betamethasone (topical) *on page 83*

quazepam *(KWAY ze pam)*

U.S./Canadian Brand Names Doral® [US/Can]

Therapeutic Category Benzodiazepine

Controlled Substance C-IV

Use Short-term treatment of insomnia

Usual Dosage Adults: Oral: Initial: 15 mg at bedtime; in some patients the dose may be reduced to 7.5 mg after a few nights

Dosage Forms Tablet: 7.5 mg, 15 mg

Quelicin® [US/Can] *see* succinylcholine *on page 608*

Queltuss® *(Discontinued)* *see page 814*

Quenalin® [US-OTC] *see* diphenhydramine *on page 202*

Questran® Light [US/Can] *see* cholestyramine resin *on page 143*

Questran® Powder [US/Can] *see* cholestyramine resin *on page 143*

Questran® Tablet *(Discontinued)* *see page 814*

quetiapine *(kwe TYE a peen)*

U.S./Canadian Brand Names Seroquel® [US/Can]

Therapeutic Category Antipsychotic Agent

Use Management of psychotic disorders; this antipsychotic drug belongs to a new chemical class, the dibenzothiazepine derivatives

Usual Dosage Adults: Oral: 25-100 mg 2-3 times/day

Dosage Forms Tablet, as fumarate: 25 mg, 100 mg, 200 mg, 300 mg

Quibron® [US] *see* theophylline and guaifenesin *on page 631*

Quibron®-T [US] *see* theophylline *on page 630*

Quibron®-T/SR [US/Can] *see* theophylline *on page 630*

Quiess® Injection *(Discontinued)* *see page 814*

Quinaglute® Dura-Tabs® [US] *see* quinidine *on next page*

Quinalan® *(Discontinued)* *see page 814*

quinalbarbitone *see* secobarbital *on page 586*

Quinamm® *(Discontinued)* *see page 814*

quinapril *(KWIN a pril)*

U.S./Canadian Brand Names Accupril® [US/Can]

Therapeutic Category Angiotensin-Converting Enzyme (ACE) Inhibitor

Use Treatment of hypertension, either alone or in combination with other antihypertensive agents

Usual Dosage Adults: Oral: Initial: 10 mg once daily, adjust according to blood pressure response at peak and trough blood levels; in general, the normal dosage range is 40-80 mg/day

Dosage Forms Tablet, as hydrochloride: 5 mg, 10 mg, 20 mg, 40 mg

quinapril and hydrochlorothiazide
(KWIN a pril & hye droe klor oh THYE a zide)
U.S./Canadian Brand Names Accuretic™ [US/Can]
Therapeutic Category Antihypertensive Agent, Combination
Use Treatment of hypertension (not for initial therapy)
Usual Dosage Oral:
Children: Safety and efficacy have not been established.
Adults: Initial:
Patients who have failed quinapril monotherapy:
Quinapril 10 mg/hydrochlorothiazide 12.5 mg **or**
Quinapril 20 mg/hydrochlorothiazide 12.5 mg once daily
Patients with adequate blood pressure control on hydrochlorothiazide 25 mg/day, but significant potassium loss:
Quinapril 10 mg/hydrochlorothiazide 12.5 mg **or**
Quinapril 20 mg/hydrochlorothiazide 12.5 mg once daily
Note: Clinical trials of quinapril/hydrochlorothiazide combinations used quinapril doses of 2.5-40 mg/day and hydrochlorothiazide doses of 6.25-25 mg/day.
Dosage Forms Tablet:
10/25: Quinapril hydrochloride 10 mg and hydrochlorothiazide 12.5 mg
20/12.5: Quinapril hydrochloride 20 mg and hydrochlorothiazide 12.5 mg
20/25: Quinapril hydrochloride 20 mg and hydrochlorothiazide 25 mg

Quinidex® Extentabs® [US] see quinidine on this page

quinidine (KWIN i deen)
U.S./Canadian Brand Names Apo®-Quinidine [Can]; Quinaglute® Dura-Tabs® [US]; Quinidex® Extentabs® [US]
Therapeutic Category Antiarrhythmic Agent, Class I-A
Use Prophylaxis after cardioversion of atrial fibrillation and/or flutter to maintain normal sinus rhythm; also used to prevent reoccurrence of paroxysmal supraventricular tachycardia, paroxysmal A-V junctional rhythm, paroxysmal ventricular tachycardia, paroxysmal atrial fibrillation, and atrial or ventricular premature contractions; also has activity against *Plasmodium falciparum* malaria
Usual Dosage Dosage expressed in terms of the salt: 267 mg of quinidine gluconate = 200 mg of quinidine sulfate.
Oral (quinidine sulfate): 15-60 mg/kg/day in 4-5 divided doses or 6 mg/kg every 4-6 hours; usual 30 mg/kg/day or 900 mg/m^2/day given in 5 daily doses at a rate ≤10 mg/minute every 3-6 hours as needed
Oral (for malaria):
Sulfate: 100-600 mg/dose every 4-6 hours; begin at 200 mg/dose and titrate to desired effect (maximum daily dose: 3-4 g)
Gluconate: 324-972 mg every 8-12 hours
Dosage Forms
Injection, solution, as gluconate: 80 mg/mL (10 mL) [equivalent to quinidine base 50 mg]
Tablet, as sulfate: 200 mg, 300 mg
Tablet, extended release, as gluconate (Quinaglute® Dura-Tabs®): 324 mg [equivalent to quinidine base 202 mg]
Tablet, extended release, as sulfate (Quinidex® Extentabs®): 300 mg [equivalent to quinidine base 249 mg]

quinine (KWYE nine)
U.S./Canadian Brand Names Quinine-Odan™ [Can]
Therapeutic Category Antimalarial Agent
(Continued)

quinine *(Continued)*

Use Suppression or treatment of chloroquine-resistant *P. falciparum* malaria (inactive against sporozoites, pre-erythrocytic or exoerythrocytic forms of plasmodia); treatment of *Babesia microti* infection

Usual Dosage Oral (parenteral dosage form may be obtained from Centers for Disease Control if needed):

Children: Chloroquine-resistant malaria and babesiosis: 25 mg/kg/day in divided doses every 8 hours for 7 days; maximum: 650 mg/dose

Adults:

Chloroquine-resistant malaria: 650 mg every 8 hours for 7 days in conjunction with another agent

Babesiosis: 650 mg every 6-8 hours for 7 days

Dosage Forms

Capsule, as sulfate: 200 mg, 325 mg

Tablet, as sulfate: 260 mg

Quinine-Odan™ [Can] *see quinine on previous page*

quinol *see hydroquinone on page 336*

Quinora® *(Discontinued)* *see page 814*

Quinsana Plus® [US-OTC] *see tolnaftate on page 644*

Quintasa® [Can] *see mesalamine on page 411*

quinupristin and dalfopristin (kwi NYOO pris tin & dal FOE pris tin)

Synonyms pristinamycin; RP59500

U.S./Canadian Brand Names Synercid® [US/Can]

Therapeutic Category Antibiotic, Streptogramin

Use Treatment of serious or life-threatening infections associated with vancomycin-resistant *Enterococcus faecium* bacteremia; treatment of complicated skin and skin structure infections caused by methcillin-susceptible *Staphylococcus aureus* or *Streptococcus pyogenes*

Investigational use: Has been studied in the treatment of a variety of infections caused by *Enterococcus faecium* (not *E. fecalis*) including vancomycin-resistant strains. May also be effective in the treatment of serious infections caused by *Staphylococcus* species including those resistant to methicillin.

Usual Dosage Adults: I.V.:

Vancomycin-resistant *Enterococcus faecium:* 7.5 mg/kg every 8 hours

Complicated skin and skin structure infection: 7.5 mg/kg every 12 hours

Dosage Forms Injection, powder for reconstitution: 500 mg (dalfopristin 350 mg and quinupristin 150 mg)

Quiphile® *(Discontinued)* *see page 814*

Quixin™ Ophthalmic [US] *see levofloxacin on page 380*

QVAR™ [US/Can] *see beclomethasone on page 73*

Q-vel® *(Discontinued)* *see page 814*

rabeprazole (ra BE pray zole)

Synonyms pariprazole

U.S./Canadian Brand Names Aciphex™ [US/Can]

Therapeutic Category Gastric Acid Secretion Inhibitor

Use Short-term (4-8 weeks) treatment and maintenance of erosive or ulcerative gastroesophageal reflux disease (GERD); symptomatic GERD; short-term (up to 4 weeks) treatment of duodenal ulcers; long-term treatment of pathological hypersecretory conditions, including Zollinger-Ellison syndrome

Usual Dosage Adults and Elderly:

GERD: 20 mg once daily for 4-8 weeks; maintenance: 20 mg once daily

Duodenal ulcer: 20 mg/day after breakfast for 4 weeks

Hypersecretory conditions: 60 mg once daily; dose may need to be adjusted as necessary. Doses as high as 100 mg and 60 mg twice daily have been used.

Dosage Forms Tablet, delayed release, enteric coated: 20 mg

rabies immune globulin (human)
(RAY beez i MYUN GLOB yoo lin HYU man)

Synonyms RIG

U.S./Canadian Brand Names BayRab® [US/Can]; Imogam® Rabies Pasteurized [Can]; Imogam® [US]

Therapeutic Category Immune Globulin

Use Passive immunity to rabies for postexposure prophylaxis of individuals exposed to the virus

Usual Dosage Children and Adults: I.M.: 20 units/kg in a single dose (RIG should always be administered in conjunction with rabies vaccine (HDCV)) (infiltrate ½ of the dose locally around the wound; administer the remainder I.M.)

Dosage Forms Injection, solution: 150 units/mL (2 mL, 10 mL)

rabies virus vaccine (RAY beez VYE rus vak SEEN)

Synonyms HDCV; HDRS

U.S./Canadian Brand Names Imovax® Rabies [US/Can]

Therapeutic Category Vaccine, Inactivated Virus

Use Pre-exposure rabies immunization for high risk persons; postexposure antirabies immunization along with local treatment and immune globulin

Usual Dosage

Pre-exposure prophylaxis: Two 1 mL doses I.M. or I.D. one week apart, third dose 3 weeks after second dose. If exposure continues, booster doses can be administered every 2 years, or an antibody titer determined and a booster dose administered if the titer is inadequate.

Postexposure prophylaxis: All postexposure treatment should begin with immediate cleansing of the wound with soap and water. Persons not previously immunized as above: Rabies immune globulin 20 units/kg body weight, half infiltrated at bite site if possible, remainder I.M.; and 5 doses of rabies vaccine, 1 mL I.M., one each on days 0, 3, 7, 14, 28.

Persons who have previously received postexposure prophylaxis with rabies vaccine, received a recommended I.M. or I.D. pre-exposure series of rabies vaccine or have a previously documented rabies antibody titer considered adequate: Two doses of rabies vaccine, 1 mL I.M., one each on days 0 and 3

Dosage Forms Injection, powder for reconstitution: 2.5 int. units [freeze dried suspension grown in human diploid cell culture; contains albumin <100 mg, neomycin <150 mcg]

radiological/contrast media (ionic)

U.S./Canadian Brand Names Anatrast® [US]; Angio Conray® [US]; Angiovist® [US]; Baricon® [US]; Barobag® [US]; Baro-CAT® [US]; Baroflave® [US]; Barosperse® [US]; Bar-Test® [US]; Bilopaque® [US]; Cholebrine® [US]; Cholografin® Meglumine [US]; Conray® [US]; Cystografin® [US]; Dionosil Oily® [US]; Enecat® [US]; Entrobar® [US]; Epi-C® [US]; Ethiodol® [US]; Flo-Coat® [US]; Gastrografin® [US]; HD 85® [US]; HD 200 Plus® [US]; Hexabrix™ [US]; Hypaque-Cysto® [US]; Hypaque® Meglumine [US]; Hypaque® Sodium [US]; Liquid Barosperse® [US]; Liquipake® [US]; Lymphazurin® [US]; Magnevist® [US]; MD-Gastroview® [US]; Oragrafin® Calcium [US]; Oragrafin® Sodium [US]; Perchloracap® [US]; Prepcat® [US]; Reno-M-30® [US]; Reno-M-60® [US]; Reno-M-DIP® [US]; Renovue®-65 [US]; Renovue®-DIP [US]; Sinografin® [US]; Telepaque® [US]; Tomocat® [US]; Tonopaque® [US]; Urovist Cysto® [US]; Urovist® Meglumine [US]; Urovist® Sodium 300 [US]; Vascoray® [US]

Therapeutic Category Radiopaque Agents

(Continued)

radiological/contrast media (ionic) *(Continued)*

Dosage Forms

Oral cholecystographic agents:
Iocetamic acid: Tablet (Cholebrine®): 750 mg
Iopanoic acid: Tablet (Telepaque®): 500 mg
Ipodate calcium: Granules for oral suspension (Oragrafin® Calcium): 3 g
Ipodate sodium: Capsule (Bilivist®, Oragrafin® Sodium): 500 mg
Tyropanoate sodium: Capsule (Bilopaque®): 750 mg

GI contrast agents: Barium sulfate:
Paste (Anatrast®): 100% (500 g)
Powder:
 Baroflave®: 100%
 Baricon®, HD 200 Plus®: 98%
 Barosperse®, Tonopaque®: 95%
Suspension:
 Baro-CAT®, Prepcat®: 1.5%
 Enecat®, Tomocat®: 5%
 Entrobar®: 50%
 Liquid Barasperse®: 60%
 HD 85®: 85%
 Barobag®: 97%
 Flo-Coat®, Liquipake®: 100%
 Epi-C®: 150%
Tablet (Bar-Test®): 650 mg

Parenteral agents: Injection:
Diatrizoate meglumine:
 Hypaque® Meglumine
 Reno-M-DIP®
 Urovist® Meglumine
 Angiovist® 282
 Hypaque® Meglumine
 Reno-M-60®
Diatrizoate sodium:
 Hypaque® Sodium
 Urovist® Sodium 300
Gadopentetate dimeglumine: Magnevist®
Iodamide meglumine:
 Renovue®-DIP
 Renovue®-65
Iodipamide meglumine: Cholografin® meglumine
Iothalamate meglumine:
 Conray® 30
 Conray® 43
 Conray®
Iothalamate sodium:
 Angio Conray®
 Conray® 325
 Conray® 400
Diatrizoate meglumine and diatrizoate sodium:
 Angiovist® 292
 Angiovist® 370
 Hypaque-76®
 Hypaque-M®, 75%
 Hypaque-M®, 90%
 MD-60®
 MD-76®
 Renografin-60®
 Renografin-76®

Renovist® II
Renovist®
Iothalamate meglumine and iothalamate sodium:
Vascoray®
Hexabrix™

Miscellaneous agents (NOT for intravascular use, for instillation into various cavities):
Diatrizoate meglumine: Urogenital solution, sterile:
Crystografin®
Crystografin® Dilute
Hypaque-Cysto®
Reno-M-30®
Urovist Cysto®
Diatrizoate meglumine and diatrizoate sodium: Solution, oral or rectal:
Gastrografin®
MD-Gastroview®
Diatrizoate sodium:
Solution, oral or rectal (Hypaque® sodium oral)
Solution, urogenital (Hypaque® sodium 20%)
Iothalamate meglumine: Solution, urogenital:
Cysto-Conray®
Cysto-Conray® II

Diatrizoate meglumine and iodipamide meglumine:
Injection, urogenital for intrauterine instillation (Sinografin®)
Ethiodized oil: Injection (Ethiodol®)
Propyliodone: Suspension (Dionosil Oily®)
Isosulfan blue: Injection (Lymphazurin® 1%)
Potassium perchlorate: Capsule (Perchloracap®): 200 mg

radiological/contrast media (non-ionic)

U.S./Canadian Brand Names Amipaque® [US]; Isovue® [US]; Omnipaque® [US]; Optiray® [US]; ProHance® [US]
Therapeutic Category Radiopaque Agents
Dosage Forms
Injection, solution:
Gadoteridol (ProHance®): 279.3 mg/mL (15 mL, 30 mL, 50 mL) [single use vial]; 279.3 mg/mL (20 mL) [prefilled syringe]
Iohexol (Omnipaque®): 140 mg/mL, 180 mg/mL, 210 mg/mL, 240 mg/mL, 300 mg/mL, 350 mg/mL
Iopamidol:
Isovue-128®
Isovue-200®
Isovue-300®
Isovue-370®
Isovue-M 200®
Isovue-M 300®
Ioversol:
Optiray® 160
Optiray® 240
Optiray® 320
Metrizamide: Amipaque®

R-albuterol *see* levalbuterol *on page 378*

raloxifene (ral OX i feen)

U.S./Canadian Brand Names Evista® [US/Can]
Therapeutic Category Selective Estrogen Receptor Modulator (SERM)
Use Prevention and treatment of osteoporosis in postmenopausal women
(Continued)

raloxifene *(Continued)*

Usual Dosage Adults: Oral: 1 tablet daily, may be administered any time of the day without regard to meals

Dosage Forms Tablet, as hydrochloride: 60 mg

raltitrexed *(Canada only)* (ral ti TREX ed)

U.S./Canadian Brand Names Tomudex® [Can]

Therapeutic Category Antineoplastic Agent

Use Undergoing clinical trials for a variety of neoplasms, including breast, colorectal nonsmall cell lung, ovarian, and pancreatic cancers

Usual Dosage Refer to individual protocols.
I.V.: 3 mg/m^2 every 3 weeks

Dosage Forms Powder for injection, lyophilized: 2 mg

ramipril (ra MI pril)

U.S./Canadian Brand Names Altace™ [US/Can]

Therapeutic Category Angiotensin-Converting Enzyme (ACE) Inhibitor

Use Treatment of hypertension, alone or in combination with thiazide diuretics; congestive heart failure immediately after myocardial infarction

Usual Dosage Adults: Oral: 2.5-5 mg once daily

Dosage Forms Capsule: 1.25 mg, 2.5 mg, 5 mg, 10 mg

ranitidine bismuth citrate (ra NI ti deen BIZ muth SIT rate)

Synonyms RBC

U.S./Canadian Brand Names Tritec® [US]

Therapeutic Category Gastrointestinal Agent, Gastric or Duodenal Ulcer Treatment

Use In combination with clarithromycin for the treatment of active duodenal ulcer associated with *H. pylori* infection; not to be used alone for the treatment of active duodenal ulcer

Usual Dosage Adults: Oral: 400 mg twice daily for 4 weeks (28 days) in conjunction with clarithromycin 500 mg 3 times/day for first 2 weeks

Dosage Forms Tablet: 400 mg (ranitidine 162 mg, trivalent bismuth 128 mg, and citrate 110 mg)

ranitidine hydrochloride (ra NI ti deen hye droe KLOR ide)

U.S./Canadian Brand Names Alti-Ranitidine [Can]; Apo®-Ranitidine [Can]; Gen-Ranitidine [Can]; Novo-Ranidine [Can]; Nu-Ranit [Can]; Zanta [Can]; Zantac® [US/Can]; Zantac® 75 [US-OTC]

Therapeutic Category Histamine H$_2$ Antagonist

Use Short-term treatment of active duodenal ulcers and benign gastric ulcers; long-term prophylaxis of duodenal ulcer and gastric hypersecretory states; gastroesophageal reflux (GER)

Usual Dosage
Children:
Oral: 1.5-2 mg/kg/dose every 12 hours
I.M., I.V.: 0.75-1.5 mg/kg/dose every 6-8 hours, maximum daily dose: 400 mg
Continuous infusion: 0.1-0.25 mg/kg/hour (preferred for stress ulcer prophylaxis in patients with concurrent maintenance I.V.s or TPNs)
Adults:
Short-term treatment of ulceration: 150 mg/dose twice daily or 300 mg at bedtime
Prophylaxis of recurrent duodenal ulcer: 150 mg at bedtime
Gastric hypersecretory conditions: Oral: 150 mg twice daily, up to 600 mg /day
I.M., I.V.: 50 mg/dose every 6-8 hours (dose not to exceed 400 mg/day)

Dosage Forms
Capsule, as hydrochloride: 150 mg, 300 mg

Granules, effervescent, as hydrochloride (Zantac® EFFERdose®): 150 mg (60s) [contains sodium 7.55 mEq/packet, phenylalanine 16.84 mg/packet, and sodium benzoate]

Infusion, as hydrochloride [premixed in NaCl 0.45%; preservative free] (Zantac®): 50 mg (50 mL)

Injection, solution, as hydrochloride (Zantac®): 25 mg/mL (2 mL, 6 mL, 40 mL) [contains phenol 0.5% as preservative]

Syrup, as hydrochloride: 15 mg/mL (10 mL) [contains alcohol 7.5%; peppermint flavor]
Zantac®: 15 mg/mL (473 mL) [contains alcohol 7.5%; peppermint flavor]

Tablet, as hydrochloride: 75 mg [OTC], 150 mg, 300 mg
Zantac®: 150 mg, 300 mg
Zantac® 75: 75 mg

Tablet, effervescent, as hydrochloride (Zantac® EFFERdose®): 150 mg [contains sodium 7.96 mEq/tablet, phenylalanine 16.84 mg/tablet, and sodium benzoate]

rapacuronium (ra pa kyoo ROE nee um)
U.S./Canadian Brand Names Raplon™ [US/Can]

Therapeutic Category Neuromuscular Blocker Agent, Nondepolarizing

Use Adjunct to general anesthesia to facilitate tracheal intubation; to provide skeletal muscle relaxation during surgical procedures; does not relieve pain

Usual Dosage I.V. (do not administer I.M.):

Children 1 month to 12 years: Initial: 2 mg/kg. Repeat dosing is not recommended in pediatric patients.

Children 13-17 years: Clinicians should consider the physical maturity, height and weight of the patient in determining the dose. Adults (1.5 mg/kg), pediatric (2 mg/kg) and Cesarean section (2.5 mg/kg) dosing recommendations may serve as a general guideline in determining an intubating dose in this age group.

Adults: Tracheal Intubation:

Initial: Short surgical procedures: 1.5 mg/kg; Cesarean section: 2.5 mg/kg

Repeat dosing: Up to three maintenance doses of 0.5 mg/kg, administered at 25% recovery of control T1 may be administered. **Note:** The duration of neuromuscular blockade increases with each additional dose.

Dosage Forms Powder for injection: 100 mg (5 mL); 200 mg (10 mL)

Rapamune® [US/Can] *see* sirolimus *on page 592*

Raplon™ [US/Can] *see* rapacuronium *on this page*

rasburicase (ras BYOOR i kayse)
U.S./Canadian Brand Names Elitek™ [US]

Therapeutic Category Enzyme

Use Initial management of uric acid levels in pediatric patients with leukemia, lymphoma, and solid tumor malignancies receiving anticancer therapy expected to result in tumor lysis and elevation of plasma uric acid

Usual Dosage I.V.: Children: Management of uric acid levels: 0.15 mg/kg or 0.2 mg/kg once daily for 5 days; begin chemotherapy 4-24 hours after the first dose

Dosage Forms Injection, powder for reconstitution: 1.5 mg [packaged with three 1 mL ampules of diluent]

Raudixin® *(Discontinued)* *see page 814*

Rauverid® *(Discontinued)* *see page 814*

Raxar® *(Discontinued)* *see page 814*

RBC *see* ranitidine bismuth citrate *on previous page*

R & C™ II [Can] *see* pyrethrins *on page 555*

R & C® Lice [US] *see* permethrin *on page 505*

R & C™ Shampoo/Conditioner [Can] *see* pyrethrins *on page 555*

R & C® [US-OTC] *see* pyrethrins *on page 555*

Reactine™ [Can] *see* cetirizine *on page 129*

Rea-Lo® [US-OTC] *see* urea *on page 666*

Rebetol® [US] *see* ribavirin *on page 570*

Rebetron™ [US/Can] *see* interferon alfa-2b and ribavirin combination pack *on page 355*

Rebif® [US/Can] *see* interferon beta-1a *on page 356*

recombinant human deoxyribonuclease *see* dornase alfa *on page 212*

recombinant human interleukin-11 *see* oprelvekin *on page 478*

recombinant interleukin-11 *see* oprelvekin *on page 478*

recombinant plasminogen activator *see* reteplase *on page 568*

Recombinate™ [US/Can] *see* antihemophilic factor (recombinant) *on page 46*

Recombivax HB® [US/Can] *see* hepatitis B vaccine *on page 320*

Rectacort® Suppository *(Discontinued)* *see page 814*

Redisol® *(Discontinued)* *see page 814*

Redutemp® [US-OTC] *see* acetaminophen *on page 3*

Redux® *(Discontinued)* *see page 814*

Reese's® Pinworm Medicine [US-OTC] *see* pyrantel pamoate *on page 555*

Refludan® [US/Can] *see* lepirudin *on page 376*

Refresh® Plus [US/Can] *see* artificial tears *on page 56*

Refresh® Tears [US/Can] *see* artificial tears *on page 56*

Refresh® [US-OTC] *see* artificial tears *on page 56*

Regitine® *(Discontinued)* *see page 814*

Reglan® [US] *see* metoclopramide *on page 424*

Regonol® [US] *see* pyridostigmine *on page 556*

Regranex® [US/Can] *see* becaplermin *on page 72*

Regulace® *(Discontinued)* *see page 814*

Regular Iletin® II [US] *see* insulin preparations *on page 352*

Regulax SS® *(Discontinued)* *see page 814*

Regulex® [Can] *see* docusate *on page 208*

Reguloid® [US-OTC] *see* psyllium *on page 554*

Regutol® *(Discontinued)* *see page 814*

Rejuva-A® [Can] *see* tretinoin (topical) *on page 650*

Relafen® [US/Can] *see* nabumetone *on page 443*

Relefact® TRH *(Discontinued)* *see page 814*

Relenza® [US/Can] *see* zanamivir *on page 688*

Relief® Ophthalmic Solution *(Discontinued)* *see page 814*

Remeron® [US] *see* mirtazapine *on page 432*

Remeron® SolTab™ [US] *see* mirtazapine *on page 432*

Remicade® [US] *see* infliximab *on page 350*

remifentanil (rem i FEN ta nil)
   U.S./Canadian Brand Names Ultiva™ [US/Can]
   Therapeutic Category Analgesic, Narcotic
   Use Analgesic for use during general anesthesia for continued analgesia
   Usual Dosage Adults: I.V. continuous infusion:
      During induction: 0.5-1 mcg/kg/minute

During maintenance:
  With nitrous oxide (66%): 0.4 mcg/kg/minute (range: 0.1-2 mcg/kg/min)
  With isoflurane: 0.25 mcg/kg/minute (range: 0.05-2 mcg/kg/min)
  With propofol: 0.25 mcg/kg/minute (range: 0.05-2 mcg/kg/min)
  Continuation as an analgesic in immediate postoperative period: 0.1 mcg/kg/minute (range: 0.025-0.2 mcg/kg/min)
Dosage Forms Injection, powder for reconstitution: 1 mg, 2 mg, 5 mg

Reminyl® **[US]** *see* galantamine *on page 292*

Remodulin™ **[US]** *see* treprostinil *on page 649*

Renacidin® **[US]** *see* citric acid bladder mixture *on page 149*

Renagel® **[US/Can]** *see* sevelamer *on page 589*

Renedil® **[Can]** *see* felodipine *on page 264*

Renese® **[US]** *see* polythiazide *on page 527*

Reno-M-30® **[US]** *see* radiological/contrast media (ionic) *on page 561*

Reno-M-60® **[US]** *see* radiological/contrast media (ionic) *on page 561*

Reno-M-DIP® **[US]** *see* radiological/contrast media (ionic) *on page 561*

Renoquid® *(Discontinued) see page 814*

Renormax® **[US]** *see* spirapril *on page 604*

Renova® **[US]** *see* tretinoin (topical) *on page 650*

Renovue®**-65 [US]** *see* radiological/contrast media (ionic) *on page 561*

Renovue®**-DIP [US]** *see* radiological/contrast media (ionic) *on page 561*

Rentamine® **[US-OTC]** *see* chlorpheniramine, ephedrine, phenylephrine, and carbetapentane *on page 139*

ReoPro® **[US/Can]** *see* abciximab *on page 2*

repaglinide (re PAG li nide)

U.S./Canadian Brand Names GlucoNorm® [Can]; Prandin™ [US/Can]
Therapeutic Category Hypoglycemic Agent, Oral
Use As an adjunct to diet and exercise to lower blood glucose on noninsulin-dependent (Type II) diabetes patients
Usual Dosage Oral: Adults: 0.5-4 mg before each meal
  Oral hypoglycemic-naive individuals or those with HbA1c levels <8%: Initial: 0.5 mg before each meal; for other patients, the starting dose is 1-2 mg before each meal
  Dose can be adjusted (by prescribers) up to 4 mg before each meal. If a meal is skipped, the patient should also skip the repaglinide dose.
Dosage Forms Tablet: 0.5 mg, 1 mg, 2 mg

Repan® **[US]** *see* butalbital, acetaminophen, and caffeine *on page 99*

Repan CF® **[US]** *see* butalbital, acetaminophen, and caffeine *on page 99*

Reposans-10® **Oral** *(Discontinued) see page 814*

Rep-Pred® *(Discontinued) see page 814*

Repronex® **[US]** *see* menotropins *on page 407*

ReQuip® **[US/Can]** *see* ropinirole *on page 578*

Resa® *(Discontinued) see page 814*

Resaid® *(Discontinued) see page 814*

Rescaps-D® **S.R. Capsule** *(Discontinued) see page 814*

Rescon® **Liquid** *(Discontinued) see page 814*

Rescriptor® **[US/Can]** *see* delavirdine *on page 178*

Rescula® **[US]** *see* unoprostone *on page 666*

Resectisol® Irrigation Solution [US] *see* mannitol *on page 400*

reserpine (re SER peen)
Therapeutic Category Rauwolfia Alkaloid
Use Management of mild to moderate hypertension
Usual Dosage Adults: Oral: 0.1-0.5 mg/day in 1-2 doses
Dosage Forms Tablet: 0.1 mg, 0.25 mg

reserpine, hydralazine, and hydrochlorothiazide *see* hydralazine, hydrochloro-thiazide, and reserpine *on page 328*

Respa-1st® [US] *see* guaifenesin and pseudoephedrine *on page 310*

Respa® DM [US] *see* guaifenesin and dextromethorphan *on page 308*

Respa-GF® [US] *see* guaifenesin *on page 307*

Respaire®-60 SR [US] *see* guaifenesin and pseudoephedrine *on page 310*

Respaire®-120 SR [US] *see* guaifenesin and pseudoephedrine *on page 310*

Respbid® *(Discontinued)* *see page 814*

RespiGam™ [US] *see* respiratory syncytial virus immune globulin (intravenous) *on this page*

respiratory syncytial virus immune globulin (intravenous)
(RES peer rah tor ee sin SISH al VYE rus i MYUN GLOB yoo lin in tra VEE nus)
Synonyms RSV-IGIV
U.S./Canadian Brand Names RespiGam™ [US]
Therapeutic Category Immune Globulin
Use Prevention of serious lower respiratory infection caused by respiratory syncytial virus (RSV) in children <24 months of age with bronchopulmonary dysplasia (BPD) or a history of premature birth (≤35 weeks gestation)
Usual Dosage I.V.: 750 mg/kg/month according to the following infusion schedule: 1.5 mL/kg/hour for 15 minutes, then at 3 mL/kg/hour for the next 15 minutes if the clinical condition does not contraindicate a higher rate, and finally, administer at 6 mL/kg/hour until completion of dose
Dosage Forms Injection, solution [preservative free]: 50 mg/mL (50 mL)

Resporal® [US] *see* dexbrompheniramine and pseudoephedrine *on page 185*

Restall® [US] *see* hydroxyzine *on page 339*

Restoril® [US/Can] *see* temazepam *on page 621*

Retavase® [US/Can] *see* reteplase *on this page*

reteplase (RE ta plase)
Synonyms recombinant plasminogen activator; r-PA
U.S./Canadian Brand Names Retavase® [US/Can]
Therapeutic Category Fibrinolytic Agent
Use Management of acute myocardial infarction
Usual Dosage Adults: I.V.: Given as two (2) bolus doses of 10 units each over a period of 2 minutes (second dose given 30 minutes after the initiation of the first dose)
Dosage Forms Injection, powder for reconstitution [preservative free]: 10.4 units [equivalent to reteplase 18.1 mg; packaged with sterile water for injection]

Retin-A® [US/Can] *see* tretinoin (topical) *on page 650*

Retin-A® Micro [US] *see* tretinoin (topical) *on page 650*

retinoic acid *see* tretinoin (topical) *on page 650*

Retinova® [Can] *see* tretinoin (topical) *on page 650*

Retrovir® [US/Can] *see* zidovudine *on page 689*

Reversol® [US] *see* edrophonium *on page 223*

Revex® [US] *see* nalmefene *on page 445*

Rēv-Eyes™ [US] *see* dapiprazole *on page 175*

ReVia® [US/Can] *see* naltrexone *on page 446*

Revitalose C-1000® [Can] *see* ascorbic acid *on page 57*

Rexigen Forte® *(Discontinued) see page 814*

Rezulin® *(Discontinued) see page 814*

rFVIIa *see* factor VIIa (recombinant) *on page 262*

R-Gel® *(Discontinued) see page 814*

R-Gen® *(Discontinued) see page 814*

R-Gene® [US] *see* arginine *on page 55*

RGM-CSF *see* sargramostim *on page 583*

r-hCG *see* chorionic gonadotropin (recombinant) *on page 145*

Rheaban® *(Discontinued) see page 814*

Rheomacrodex® [US] *see* dextran *on page 187*

Rhesonativ® Injection *(Discontinued) see page 814*

Rheumatrex® [US] *see* methotrexate *on page 417*

rhIL-11 *see* oprelvekin *on page 478*

Rhinalar® [Can] *see* flunisolide *on page 276*

Rhinall® Nasal [US-OTC] *see* phenylephrine *on page 510*

Rhinatate® [US] *see* chlorpheniramine, pyrilamine, and phenylephrine *on page 141*

Rhinatate® Tablet *(Discontinued) see page 814*

Rhindecon® *(Discontinued) see page 814*

Rhinocort® [US/Can] *see* budesonide *on page 95*

Rhinocort® Aqua™ [US/Can] *see* budesonide *on page 95*

Rhinolar® *(Discontinued) see page 814*

Rhinosyn-PD® [US-OTC] *see* chlorpheniramine and pseudoephedrine *on page 138*

Rhinosyn® [US-OTC] *see* chlorpheniramine and pseudoephedrine *on page 138*

Rho-Clonazepam [Can] *see* clonazepam *on page 154*

Rhodacine® [Can] *see* indomethacin *on page 349*

Rh$_o$(D) immune globulin
(ar aych oh (dee) i MYUN GLOB yoo lin IN tra MUS kyoo ler)

U.S./Canadian Brand Names BayRho-D® Full-Dose [US]; BayRho-D® Mini-Dose [US]; RhoGAM® [US]; WinRho SDF® [US]

Therapeutic Category Immune Globulin

Use Prevent isoimmunization in Rh-negative individuals exposed to Rh-positive blood during delivery of an Rh-positive infant, as a result of an abortion, following amniocentesis or abdominal trauma, or following a transfusion accident; to prevent hemolytic disease of the newborn if there is a subsequent pregnancy with an Rh-positive fetus

Usual Dosage
Prevention of Rh isoimmunization: I.V.: 1500 int. units (300 mcg) at 28 weeks gestation or immediately after amniocentesis if before 34 weeks gestation or after chorionic villus sampling; repeat this dose every 12 weeks during the pregnancy. Administer 600 int. units (120 mcg) at delivery (within 72 hours) and after invasive intrauterine procedures such as abortion, amniocentesis, or any other manipulation if at >34 weeks gestation. **Note:** If the Rh status of the baby is not known at 72 hours, administer Rh$_o$(D) immune
(Continued)

Rh₀(D) immune globulin *(Continued)*

globulin to the mother at 72 hours after delivery. If >72 hours have elapsed, do not withhold Rh₀(D) immune globulin, but administer as soon as possible, up to 28 days after delivery.

I.M.: Reconstitute vial with 1.25 mL and administer as above

Transfusion: Administer within 72 hours after exposure for treatment of incompatible blood transfusions or massive fetal hemorrhage as follows:

I.V.: 3000 int. units (600 mcg) every 8 hours until the total dose is administered (45 int. units [9 mcg] of Rh-positive blood/mL blood; 90 int. units [18 mcg] Rh-positive red cells/mL cells)

I.M.: 6000 int. units [1200 mcg] every 12 hours until the total dose is administered (60 int. units [12 mcg] of Rh-positive blood/mL blood; 120 int. units [24 mcg] Rh-positive red cells/mL cells)

Treatment of ITP: I.V.: Initial: 25-50 mcg/kg depending on the patient's Hgb concentration; maintenance: 25-60 mcg/kg depending on the clinical response

Dosage Forms

Injection, solution [preservative free]:

BayRho-D® Full-Dose, RhoGAM®, WinRho SDF®: 300 mcg

BayRho-D® Mini-Dose: 50 mcg

Rhodis™ [Can] *see* ketoprofen *on page 368*

Rhodis-EC™ [Can] *see* ketoprofen *on page 368*

Rhodis SR™ [Can] *see* ketoprofen *on page 368*

Rho®-Fluphenazin Decanoate [Can] *see* fluphenazine *on page 281*

RhoGAM® [US] *see* Rh₀(D) immune globulin *on previous page*

Rho®-Haloperidol Decanoate [Can] *see* haloperidol *on page 316*

Rho®-Metformin [Can] *see* metformin *on page 414*

Rho®-Sotalol [Can] *see* sotalol *on page 602*

Rhotral [Can] *see* acebutolol *on page 3*

Rhotrimine® [Can] *see* trimipramine *on page 658*

Rhovane® [Can] *see* zopiclone *(Canada only) on page 693*

Rhoxal-atenolol [Can] *see* atenolol *on page 60*

Rhoxal-diltiazem SR [Can] *see* diltiazem *on page 199*

Rhoxal-famotidine [Can] *see* famotidine *on page 262*

Rhoxal-fluoxetine [Can] *see* fluoxetine *on page 279*

Rhoxal-loperamine [Can] *see* loperamide *on page 390*

Rhoxal-Minocycline [Can] *see* minocycline *on page 431*

Rhoxal-orphendrine [Can] *see* orphenadrine *on page 480*

Rhoxal-ticlopidine [Can] *see* ticlopidine *on page 639*

Rhoxal-valproic [Can] *see* valproic acid and derivatives *on page 670*

RHUEPO-α *see* epoetin alfa *on page 230*

Rhulicaine® *(Discontinued)* *see page 814*

Rhuli® Cream *(Discontinued)* *see page 814*

ribavirin (rye ba VYE rin)

Synonyms RTCA; tribavirin

U.S./Canadian Brand Names Rebetol® [US]; Virazole® [US/Can]

Therapeutic Category Antiviral Agent

Use

Inhalation: Treatment of patients with respiratory syncytial virus (RSV) infections; may also be used in other viral infections including influenza A and B and adenovirus;

specially indicated for treatment of severe lower respiratory tract RSV infections in patients with an underlying compromising condition (prematurity, bronchopulmonary dysplasia and other chronic lung conditions, congenital heart disease, immunodeficiency, immunosuppression), and recent transplant recipients

Oral capsules: The combination therapy of oral ribavirin with interferon alfa-2b, recombinant (Intron® A) injection is indicated for the treatment of chronic hepatitis C in patients with compensated liver disease who have relapsed after alpha interferon therapy or were previously untreated with alpha interferons

Usual Dosage

Aerosol inhalation: Infants and children: Use with Viratek® small particle aerosol generator (SPAG-2) at a concentration of 20 mg/mL (6 g reconstituted with 300 mL of sterile water without preservatives). Continuous aerosol administration: 12-18 hours/day for 3 days, up to 7 days in length

Oral: Adults:

Chronic hepatitis C (in combination with interferon alfa-2b):

≤75 kg: 400 mg in the morning, then 600 mg in the evening

>75 kg: 600 mg in the morning, then 600 mg in the evening

Note: If HCV-RNA is undetectable at 24 weeks, duration of therapy is 48 weeks. In patients who relapse following interferon therapy, duration of dual therapy is 24 weeks.

Chronic hepatitis C (in combination with peginterferon alfa-2b): 400 mg twice daily; duration of therapy is 1 year; after 24 weeks of treatment, if serum HCV-RNA is not below the limit of detection of the assay, consider discontinuation.

Dosage Forms

Capsule (Rebetol®): 200 mg

Powder for aerosol (Virazole®): 6 g

riboflavin (RYE boe flay vin)

Synonyms lactoflavin; vitamin B_2; vitamin G

Therapeutic Category Vitamin, Water Soluble

Use Prevent riboflavin deficiency and treat ariboflavinosis

Usual Dosage Oral:

Riboflavin deficiency:

Children: 2.5-10 mg/day in divided doses

Adults: 5-30 mg/day in divided doses

Recommended daily allowance: Adults:

Male: 1.4-4.8 mg

Female: 1.2-1.3 mg

Dosage Forms

Capsule: 100 mg

Tablet: 25 mg, 50 mg, 100 mg

Ridactate® [US] see calcium lactate on page 108

Rid-A-Pain® [US] see capsaicin on page 111

Rid-A-Pain-HP® [US] see capsaicin on page 111

Ridaura® [US/Can] see auranofin on page 64

Ridifed® [US-OTC] see triprolidine and pseudoephedrine on page 659

RID® Mousse [Can] see pyrethrins on page 555

RID® Spray [US-OTC] see permethrin on page 505

RID® [US-OTC] see pyrethrins on page 555

rifabutin (rif a BYOO tin)

Synonyms ansamycin

U.S./Canadian Brand Names Mycobutin® [US/Can]

Therapeutic Category Antibiotic, Miscellaneous

(Continued)

rifabutin *(Continued)*

Use Prevention of disseminated *Mycobacterium avium* complex (MAC) in patients with advanced HIV infection; utilized in multiple drug regimens for treatment of MAC

Usual Dosage Oral:

Children: Efficacy and safety of rifabutin have not been established in children; a limited number of HIV-positive children with MAC (n=22) have been given rifabutin for MAC prophylaxis; doses of 5 mg/kg/day have been useful

Adults: 300 mg once daily; for patients who experience gastrointestinal upset, rifabutin can be administered 150 mg twice daily with food

Dosage Forms Capsule: 150 mg

Rifadin® **[US/Can]** *see* rifampin *on this page*

Rifamate® **[US/Can]** *see* rifampin and isoniazid *on this page*

rifampicin *see* rifampin *on this page*

rifampin *(RIF am pin)*

Synonyms rifampicin

U.S./Canadian Brand Names Rifadin® [US/Can]; Rimactane® [US]; Rofact™ [Can]

Therapeutic Category Antibiotic, Miscellaneous

Use In combination with other antitubercular drugs for the treatment of active tuberculosis; eliminate meningococci from asymptomatic carriers; prophylaxis in contacts of patients with *Haemophilus influenzae* type B infection; used in combination with other anti-infectives in the treatment of staphylococcal infections

Usual Dosage Oral (I.V. infusion dose is the same as for the oral route):

Tuberculosis:

Children: 10-20 mg/kg/day in divided doses every 12-24 hours

Adults: 10 mg/kg/day; maximum: 600 mg/day

American Thoracic Society and CDC currently recommend twice weekly therapy as part of a short-course regimen which follows 1-2 months of daily treatment of uncomplicated pulmonary tuberculosis in the compliant patient

Children: 10-20 mg/kg/dose (up to 600 mg) twice weekly under supervision to ensure compliance

Adults: 10 mg/kg (up to 600 mg) twice weekly

H. influenzae prophylaxis:

Infants and Children: 20 mg/kg/day every 24 hours for 4 days

Adults: 600 mg every 24 hours for 4 days

Meningococcal prophylaxis:

<1 month: 10 mg/kg/day in divided doses every 12 hours

Infants and Children: 20 mg/kg/day in divided doses every 12 hours for 2 days

Adults: 600 mg every 12 hours for 2 days

Nasal carriers of *Staphylococcus aureus*: Adults: 600 mg/day for 5-10 days in combination with other antibiotics

Dosage Forms

Capsule: 150 mg, 300 mg

Rifadin®: 150 mg, 300 mg

Rimactane®: 300 mg

Injection, powder for reconstitution (Rifadin®): 600 mg

rifampin and isoniazid *(RIF am pin & eye soe NYE a zid)*

Synonyms isoniazid and rifampin

U.S./Canadian Brand Names Rifamate® [US/Can]

Therapeutic Category Antibiotic, Miscellaneous

Use Management of active tuberculosis; see individual monographs for additional information

Usual Dosage Oral: 2 capsules/day

Dosage Forms Capsule: Rifampin 300 mg and isoniazid 150 mg

rifampin, isoniazid, and pyrazinamide
(RIF am pin, eye soe NYE a zid, & peer a ZIN a mide)
Synonyms isoniazid, rifampin, and pyrazinamide; pyrazinamide, rifampin, and isoniazid
U.S./Canadian Brand Names Rifater® [US/Can]
Therapeutic Category Antibiotic, Miscellaneous
Use Management of active tuberculosis
Usual Dosage Adults: Oral: Patients weighing:
  ≤44 kg: 4 tablets
  45-54 kg: 5 tablets
  ≥55 kg: 6 tablets
  Doses should be administered in a single daily dose
Dosage Forms Tablet: Rifampin 120 mg, isoniazid 50 mg, and pyrazinamide 300 mg

rifapentine (RIF a pen teen)
U.S./Canadian Brand Names Priftin® [US/Can]
Therapeutic Category Antitubercular Agent
Use Treatment of pulmonary tuberculosis (indication is based on the 6-month follow-up treatment outcome observed in controlled clinical trial). Rifapentine must always be used in conjunction with at least one other antituberculosis drug to which the isolate is susceptible; it may also be necessary to add a third agent (either streptomycin or ethambutol) until susceptibility is known.
Usual Dosage
  Children: No dosing information available
  Adults: **Rifapentine should not be used alone**; initial phase should include a 3- to 4-drug regimen
    Intensive phase of short-term therapy: 600 mg (four 150 mg tablets) given weekly (every 72 hours); following the intensive phase, treatment should continue with rifapentine 600 mg once weekly for 4 months in combination with INH or appropriate agent for susceptible organisms
Dosage Forms Tablet, film coated: 150 mg

Rifater® [US/Can] *see* rifampin, isoniazid, and pyrazinamide *on this page*

rIFN-A *see* interferon alfa-2a *on page 353*

RIG *see* rabies immune globulin (human) *on page 561*

rIL-11 *see* oprelvekin *on page 478*

Rilutek® [US] *see* riluzole *on this page*

riluzole (RIL yoo zole)
Synonyms 2-amino-6-trifluoromethoxy-benzothiazole; RP54274
U.S./Canadian Brand Names Rilutek® [US]
Therapeutic Category Miscellaneous Product
Use Treatment of amyotrophic lateral sclerosis (ALS), also known as Lou Gehrig's disease
Usual Dosage Adults: Oral: 50 mg twice daily
Dosage Forms Tablet: 50 mg

Rimactane® [US] *see* rifampin *on previous page*

rimantadine (ri MAN ta deen)
U.S./Canadian Brand Names Flumadine® [US/Can]
Therapeutic Category Antiviral Agent
Use Prophylaxis (adults and children) and treatment (adults) of influenza A viral infection
Usual Dosage Oral:
  Prophylaxis:
    Children <10 years: 5 mg/kg administered once daily
    Children >10 years and Adults: 100 mg twice daily
  (Continued)

rimantadine *(Continued)*

Treatment: Adults: 100 mg twice daily

Dosage Forms
Syrup, as hydrochloride: 50 mg/5 mL (240 mL) [raspberry flavor]
Tablet, as hydrochloride: 100 mg

rimexolone (ri MEKS oh lone)

U.S./Canadian Brand Names Vexol® [US/Can]
Therapeutic Category Adrenal Corticosteroid
Use Treatment of inflammation after ocular surgery and the treatment of anterior uveitis
Usual Dosage Children >2 years and Adults: Ophthalmic: Instill 1-2 drops into conjunctival sac every hour during day, every 2 hours at night until favorable response is obtained, then use 1 drop every 4 hours; for mild to moderate inflammation, instill 1-2 drops into conjunctival sac 2-4 times/day
Dosage Forms Suspension, ophthalmic: 1% (5 mL, 10 mL) [contains benzalkonium chloride]

Rimso®-50 [US/Can] *see* dimethyl sulfoxide *on page 201*

Riobin® *(Discontinued)* *see page 814*

Riopan Plus® Double Strength [US-OTC] *see* magaldrate and simethicone *on page 396*

Riopan Plus® [US-OTC] *see* magaldrate and simethicone *on page 396*

Riopan® [US-OTC] *see* magaldrate *on page 396*

Riphenidate [Can] *see* methylphenidate *on page 422*

risedronate (ris ED roe nate)

U.S./Canadian Brand Names Actonel™ [US/Can]
Therapeutic Category Bisphosphonate Derivative
Use Treatment of hypercalcemia associated with malignancy, osteolytic bone lesions of multiple myeloma; also used in postmenopausal osteoporosis; primary hyperparathyroidism and Paget's disease (moderate to severe)
Usual Dosage Adults: Oral: 30 mg once daily for 2 months
Dosage Forms Tablet, as sodium: 5 mg, 30 mg, 35 mg

Risperdal® [US/Can] *see* risperidone *on this page*

Risperdal Consta™ [Investigational] [US] *see* risperidone *on this page*

risperidone (ris PER i done)

U.S./Canadian Brand Names Risperdal Consta™ [Investigational] [US]; Risperdal® [US/Can]
Therapeutic Category Antipsychotic Agent, Benzisoxazole
Use Management of psychotic disorders (eg, schizophrenia)
Usual Dosage Oral: Recommended starting dose: 1 mg twice daily; slowly increase to the optimum range of 4-8 mg/day; daily dosages >10 mg does not appear to confer any additional benefit, and the incidence of extrapyramidal reactions is higher than with lower doses
Dosage Forms
Injection, microspheres for reconstitution, extended release (Risperdal Consta™): 25 mg, 37.5 mg, 50 mg [currently investigational, not commercially available]
Solution, oral: 1 mg/mL (30 mL) [contains benzoic acid]
Tablet: 0.25 mg, 0.5 mg, 1 mg, 2 mg, 3 mg, 4 mg

Ritalin® [US/Can] *see* methylphenidate *on page 422*

Ritalin® LA [US] *see* methylphenidate *on page 422*

Ritalin-SR® [US/Can] *see* methylphenidate *on page 422*

Ritifed® **[US-OTC]** see triprolidine and pseudoephedrine on page 659

ritonavir (rye TON a veer)
U.S./Canadian Brand Names Norvir® SEC [Can]; Norvir® [US/Can]
Therapeutic Category Antiviral Agent
Use Treatment of HIV, especially advanced cases; usually is used as part of triple or double therapy with other nucleoside and protease inhibitors
Usual Dosage Adults: Oral: 600 mg twice daily with meals
Dosage Forms
Capsule: 100 mg [contains ethanol and polyoxyl 35 castor oil]
Solution: 80 mg/mL (240 mL) [contains ethanol and polyoxyl 35 castor oil]

Rituxan® **[US/Can]** see rituximab on this page

rituximab (ri TUK si mab)
Synonyms anti-CD20 monoclonal antibodies; C2B8 monoclonal antibody; Pan-B antibodies
U.S./Canadian Brand Names Rituxan® [US/Can]
Therapeutic Category Antineoplastic Agent
Use Treatment of patients with relapsed or refractory low-grade or follicular, CD20 positive, B-cell non-Hodgkin's lymphoma
Usual Dosage Adults: I.V.: 375 mg/m^2 given as an I.V. infusion once weekly for 4 doses (days 1, 8, 15, and 22); may be administered in an outpatient setting; **do not administer as an intravenous push or bolus**
Dosage Forms Injection, solution [preservative free]: 10 mg/mL (10 mL, 50 mL)

Riva-Diclofenac [Can] see diclofenac on page 193
Riva-Diclofenac-K [Can] see diclofenac on page 193
Riva-Loperamine [Can] see loperamide on page 390
Riva-Lorazepam [Can] see lorazepam on page 391
Riva-Naproxen [Can] see naproxen on page 447
Rivanase AQ [Can] see beclomethasone on page 73
Riva-Norfloxacin [Can] see norfloxacin on page 465
Rivasol [Can] see zinc sulfate on page 691

rivastigmine (ri va STIG meen)
Synonyms ENA 713; SDZ ENA 713
U.S./Canadian Brand Names Exelon® [US/Can]
Therapeutic Category Acetylcholinesterase Inhibitor; Cholinergic Agent
Use Mild to moderate dementia from Alzheimer's disease
Usual Dosage Adults: Oral: Initial: 1.5 mg twice daily to start; if dose is tolerated for at least 2 weeks then it may be increased to 3 mg twice daily; increases to 4.5 mg twice daily and 6 mg twice daily should only be attempted after at least 2 weeks at the previous dose; maximum dose: 6 mg twice daily. If adverse events such as nausea, vomiting, abdominal pain, or loss of appetite occur, the patient should be instructed to discontinue treatment for several doses then restart at the same or next lower dosage level; antiemetics have been used to control GI symptoms.
Dosage Forms
Capsule, as tartrate: 1.5 mg, 3 mg, 4.5 mg, 6 mg
Solution, oral, as tartrate: 2 mg/mL (120 mL) [contains sodium benzoate]

Rivotril® **[Can]** see clonazepam on page 154

rizatriptan (rye za TRIP tan)
U.S./Canadian Brand Names Maxalt-MLT™ [US]; Maxalt RPD™ [Can]; Maxalt® [US/Can]
(Continued)

rizatriptan *(Continued)*

Therapeutic Category Antimigraine Agent; Serotonin Agonist

Use Acute treatment of migraine with or without aura

Usual Dosage Oral: 10-20 mg, repeat after 2 hours if significant relief is not attained

Dosage Forms

Tablet, as benzoate (Maxalt®): 5 mg, 10 mg

Tablet, orally-disintegrating, as benzoate (Maxalt-MLT®): 5 mg [contains phenylalanine 1.05 mg/tablet; peppermint flavor]; 10 mg [contains phenylalanine 2.1 mg/tablet; peppermint flavor]

rLFN-α2 *see* interferon alfa-2b *on page 354*

RMS® [US] *see* morphine sulfate *on page 437*

Ro 11-1163 *see* moclobemide *(Canada only) on page 434*

Robafen® AC [US] *see* guaifenesin and codeine *on page 308*

Robafen® CF *(Discontinued)* *see page 814*

Robaxin® [US/Can] *see* methocarbamol *on page 417*

Robaxisal® [US/Can] *see* methocarbamol and aspirin *on page 417*

Robaxisal® Extra Strength [Can] *see* methocarbamol and aspirin *on page 417*

Robicillin® Tablet *(Discontinued)* *see page 814*

Robidrine® [Can] *see* pseudoephedrine *on page 552*

Robinul® [US] *see* glycopyrrolate *on page 303*

Robinul® Forte [US] *see* glycopyrrolate *on page 303*

Robitet® *(Discontinued)* *see page 814*

Robitussin® [US/Can] *see* guaifenesin *on page 307*

Robitussin® A-C *(Discontinued)* *see page 814*

Robitussin-CF® *(Discontinued)* *see page 814*

Robitussin® Childrens Cough & Cold [Can] *see* pseudoephedrine and dextromethorphan *on page 553*

Robitussin® Cold and Congestion [US-OTC] *see* guaifenesin, pseudoephedrine, and dextromethorphan *on page 312*

Robitussin® Cough and Cold Infant [US-OTC] *see* guaifenesin, pseudoephedrine, and dextromethorphan *on page 312*

Robitussin® Cough Calmers [US-OTC] *see* dextromethorphan *on page 189*

Robitussin®-DAC *(Discontinued)* *see page 814*

Robitussin® DM [US/Can] *see* guaifenesin and dextromethorphan *on page 308*

Robitussin® Maximum Strength Cough & Cold [US-OTC] *see* pseudoephedrine and dextromethorphan *on page 553*

Robitussin® Pediatric Cough & Cold [US-OTC] *see* pseudoephedrine and dextromethorphan *on page 553*

Robitussin® Pediatric [US-OTC] *see* dextromethorphan *on page 189*

Robitussin-PE® [US-OTC] *see* guaifenesin and pseudoephedrine *on page 310*

Robitussin® Severe Congestion [US-OTC] *see* guaifenesin and pseudoephedrine *on page 310*

Robitussin® Sugar Free Cough [US-OTC] *see* guaifenesin and dextromethorphan *on page 308*

Rocaltrol® [US/Can] *see* calcitriol *on page 104*

Rocephin® [US/Can] *see* ceftriaxone *on page 126*

rocuronium (roe kyoor OH nee um)
U.S./Canadian Brand Names Zemuron® [US/Can]
Therapeutic Category Skeletal Muscle Relaxant
Use Produces skeletal muscle relaxation during surgery after induction of general anesthesia, increases pulmonary compliance during assisted mechanical respiration, facilitates endotracheal intubation
Usual Dosage I.V.:
Children:
Initial: 0.6 mg/kg under halothane anesthesia produce excellent to good intubating conditions within 1 minute and will provide a median time of 41 minutes of clinical relaxation in children 3 months to 1 year of age, and 27 minutes in children 1-12 years
Maintenance: 0.075-0.125 mg/kg administered upon return of T_1 to 25% of control provides clinical relaxation for 7-10 minutes
Adults:
Tracheal intubation:
Initial: 0.6 mg/kg is expected to provide approximately 31 minutes of clinical relaxation under opioid/nitrous oxide/oxygen anesthesia with neuromuscular block sufficient for intubation attained in 1-2 minutes; lower doses (0.45 mg/kg) may be used to provide 22 minutes of clinical relaxation with median time to neuromuscular block of 1-3 minutes; maximum blockade is achieved in <4 minutes
Maximum: 0.9-1.2 mg/kg may be administered during surgery under opioid/nitrous oxide/oxygen anesthesia without adverse cardiovascular effects and is expected to provide 58-67 minutes of clinical relaxation; neuromuscular blockade sufficient for intubation is achieved in <2 minutes with maximum blockade in <3 minutes
Maintenance: 0.1, 0.15, and 0.2 mg/kg administered at 25% recovery of control T_1 (defined as 3 twitches of train-of-four) provides a median of 12, 17, and 24 minutes of clinical duration under anesthesia
Rapid sequence intubation: 0.6-1.2 mg/kg in appropriately premedicated and anesthetized patients with excellent or good intubating conditions within 2 minutes
Continuous infusion: Initial: 0.01-0.012 mg/kg/minute only after early evidence of spontaneous recovery of neuromuscular function is evident
Dosage Forms Injection, solution, as bromide: 10 mg/mL (5 mL, 10 mL)

Rofact™ **[Can]** *see* rifampin *on page 572*

rofecoxib (roe fe COX ib)
U.S./Canadian Brand Names Vioxx® [US/Can]
Therapeutic Category Nonsteroidal Anti-inflammatory Drug (NSAID), COX-2 Selective
Use Relief of the signs and symptoms of osteoarthritis; management of acute pain in adults; treatment of primary dysmenorrhea
Usual Dosage Adult: Oral:
Osteoarthritis: 12.5 mg once daily; may be increased to a maximum of 25 mg once daily
Acute pain and management of dysmenorrhea: 50 mg once daily as needed (use for longer than 5 days has not been studied)
Dosage Forms
Suspension, oral: 12.5 mg/5 mL (150 mL); 25 mg/5 mL (150 mL) [strawberry flavor]
Tablet: 12.5 mg, 25 mg, 50 mg

Roferon-A® **[US/Can]** *see* interferon alfa-2a *on page 353*
Rogaine® **[Can]** *see* minoxidil *on page 432*
Rogaine® **Extra Strength for Men [US-OTC]** *see* minoxidil *on page 432*
Rogaine® **for Men [US-OTC]** *see* minoxidil *on page 432*
Rogaine® **for Women [US-OTC]** *see* minoxidil *on page 432*
Rogitine® **[Can]** *see* phentolamine *on page 509*
Rolaids® **Calcium Rich [US-OTC]** *see* calcium carbonate *on page 104*
Rolatuss® **Plain Liquid** *(Discontinued)* *see page 814*

Romazicon® **[US/Can]** *see* flumazenil *on page 275*

Romilar® **AC [US]** *see* guaifenesin and codeine *on page 308*

Romycin® **[US]** *see* erythromycin (ophthalmic/topical) *on page 235*

Rondec®-DM Drops [US] *see* carbinoxamine, pseudoephedrine, and dextromethorphan *on page 115*

Rondec® Drops [US] *see* carbinoxamine and pseudoephedrine *on page 115*

Rondec® Syrup [US] *see* brompheniramine and pseudoephedrine *on page 94*

Rondec® Tablets [US] *see* carbinoxamine and pseudoephedrine *on page 115*

Rondec-TR® [US] *see* carbinoxamine and pseudoephedrine *on page 115*

Rondomycin® Capsule *(Discontinued) see page 814*

ropinirole (roe PIN i role)

U.S./Canadian Brand Names ReQuip® [US/Can]

Therapeutic Category Anti-Parkinson's Agent

Use Treatment of idiopathic Parkinson's disease; in patients with early Parkinson's disease who were not receiving concomitant levodopa therapy as well as in patients with advanced disease on concomitant levodopa

Usual Dosage Adults: Oral: Dosage should be increased to achieve a maximum therapeutic effect, balanced against the principal side effects of nausea, dizziness, somnolence, and dyskinesia

Recommended starting dose: 0.25 mg 3 times/day; based on individual patient response, the dosage should be titrated with weekly increments
Week 1: 0.25 mg 3 times/day; total daily dose: 0.75 mg
Week 2: 0.5 mg 3 times/day; total daily dose: 1.5 mg
Week 3: 0.75 mg 3 times/day; total daily dose: 2.25 mg
Week 4: 1 mg 3 times/day; total daily dose: 3 mg
After week 4, if necessary, daily dosage may be increased by 1.5 mg/day on a weekly basis up to a dose of 9 mg/day, and then by up to 3 mg/day weekly to a total of 24 mg/day

Dosage Forms Tablet, as hydrochloride: 0.25 mg, 0.5 mg, 1 mg, 2 mg, 4 mg, 5 mg

ropivacaine (roe PIV a kane)

U.S./Canadian Brand Names Naropin™ [US/Can]

Therapeutic Category Local Anesthetic

Use Production of local or regional anesthesia for surgery, postoperative pain management and obstetrical procedures by infiltration anesthesia and nerve block anesthesia

Usual Dosage Administer the smallest dose and concentration required to produce the desired result

Dosage Forms
Infusion, as hydrochloride: 2 mg/mL (100 mL, 200 mL)
Injection, solution, as hydrochloride [single dose]: 2 mg/mL (10 mL, 20 mL); 5 mg/mL (10 mL, 20 mL, 30 mL); 7.5 mg/mL (10 mL, 20 mL); 10 mg/mL (10 mL, 20 mL)

rosiglitazone (roe si GLI ta zone)

U.S./Canadian Brand Names Avandia® [US/Can]

Therapeutic Category Hypoglycemic Agent, Oral; Thiazolidinedione Derivative

Use

Type II diabetes, monotherapy: Improve glycemic control as an adjunct to diet and exercise

Type II diabetes, combination therapy: In combination with metformin when diet, exercise and metformin alone or diet, exercise and rosiglitazone alone do not result in adequate glycemic control.

Usual Dosage Adults: Oral: Initial: 4 mg daily as a single daily dose or in divided doses twice daily. If response is inadequate after 12 weeks of treatment, the dosage may be increased to 8 mg daily as a single daily dose or in divided doses twice daily.

Dosage Forms Tablet: 2 mg, 4 mg, 8 mg

RotaShield® *(Discontinued)* *see page 814*

Rovamycine® [Can] *see* spiramycin *(Canada only)* *on page 604*

Rowasa® [US/Can] *see* mesalamine *on page 411*

Roxanol® [US] *see* morphine sulfate *on page 437*

Roxanol 100® [US] *see* morphine sulfate *on page 437*

Roxanol SR™ Oral *(Discontinued)* *see page 814*

Roxanol®-T [US] *see* morphine sulfate *on page 437*

Roxicet® [US] *see* oxycodone and acetaminophen *on page 485*

Roxicet® 5/500 [US] *see* oxycodone and acetaminophen *on page 485*

Roxicodone™ [US] *see* oxycodone *on page 484*

Roxicodone™ Intensol™ [US] *see* oxycodone *on page 484*

Roxiprin® *(Discontinued)* *see page 814*

Roychlor® [Can] *see* potassium chloride *on page 530*

RP54274 *see* riluzole *on page 573*

RP59500 *see* quinupristin and dalfopristin *on page 560*

r-PA *see* reteplase *on page 568*

RSV-IGIV *see* respiratory syncytial virus immune globulin (intravenous) *on page 568*

R-Tannamine® [US] *see* chlorpheniramine, pyrilamine, and phenylephrine *on page 141*

R-Tannate® [US] *see* chlorpheniramine, pyrilamine, and phenylephrine *on page 141*

RTCA *see* ribavirin *on page 570*

RU-486 *see* mifepristone *on page 430*

RU-38486 *see* mifepristone *on page 430*

rubella and measles vaccines, combined *see* measles and rubella vaccines, combined *on page 402*

rubella and mumps vaccines, combined
(rue BEL a & mumpz vak SEENS, kom BINED)
U.S./Canadian Brand Names Biavax® II [US]
Therapeutic Category Vaccine, Live Virus
Use Promote active immunity to rubella and mumps by inducing production of antibodies
Usual Dosage Children >12 months and Adults: 1 vial in outer aspect of the upper arm
Dosage Forms Injection (mixture of 2 viruses):
1. Wistar RA 27/3 strain of rubella virus
2. Jeryl Lynn (B level) mumps strain grown cell cultures of chick embryo

rubella virus vaccine (live) (rue BEL a VYE rus vak SEEN live)
Synonyms German measles vaccine
U.S./Canadian Brand Names Meruvax® II [US]
Therapeutic Category Vaccine, Live Virus
Use Provide vaccine-induced immunity to rubella
Usual Dosage S.C.: 1000 $TCID_{50}$ of rubella
Dosage Forms Injection, powder for reconstitution [single dose]: 1000 $TCID_{50}$ (Wistar RA 27/3 Strain) [contains gelatin, human albumin, and neomycin]

rubeola vaccine *see* measles virus vaccine (live) *on page 402*

Rubex® [US] *see* doxorubicin *on page 214*

rubidomycin *see* daunorubicin hydrochloride *on page 176*

Rubramin-PC® *(Discontinued) see page 814*

Rufen® *(Discontinued) see page 814*

Rum-K® [US] *see* potassium chloride *on page 530*

Ru-Tuss® Liquid *(Discontinued) see page 814*

Ru-Tuss® Tablet *(Discontinued) see page 814*

Ru-Vert-M® *(Discontinued) see page 814*

Rx-Otic® Drops [US] *see* antipyrine and benzocaine *on page 47*

Rymed® *(Discontinued) see page 814*

Rymed-TR® *(Discontinued) see page 814*

Ryna-C® [US] *see* chlorpheniramine, pseudoephedrine, and codeine *on page 140*

Rynatan® [US] *see* azatadine and pseudoephedrine *on page 65*

Rynatan® Pediatric Suspension [US] *see* chlorpheniramine, pyrilamine, and phenylephrine *on page 141*

Rynatuss® Pediatric Suspension [US-OTC] *see* chlorpheniramine, ephedrine, phenylephrine, and carbetapentane *on page 139*

Rynatuss® [US-OTC] *see* chlorpheniramine, ephedrine, phenylephrine, and carbetapentane *on page 139*

Ryna® [US-OTC] *see* chlorpheniramine and pseudoephedrine *on page 138*

Rythmodan® [Can] *see* disopyramide *on page 207*

Rythmodan®-LA [Can] *see* disopyramide *on page 207*

Rythmol® [US/Can] *see* propafenone *on page 547*

Sabin vaccine *see* poliovirus vaccine, live, trivalent, oral *on page 524*

Sabril® [US/Can] *see* vigabatrin *(Canada only) on page 678*

sacrosidase (sak RO se dase)

U.S./Canadian Brand Names Sucraid™ [US/Can]
Therapeutic Category Enzyme
Use An enzyme replacement therapy for the treatment of the genetically determined sucrase deficiency, which is part of congenital sucrase-isomaltase deficiency (CSID)
Usual Dosage Oral:
<15 kg: 1 mL [8500 int. units] (one full measuring scoop or 22 drops) per meal or snack
>15 kg: 2 mL [17,000 int. units] (two full measuring scoops or 44 drops) per meal or snack

It is recommended that approximately half of the dosage be taken at the beginning of each meal or snack, and the remainder be taken at the end of each meal or snack.

The beverage or infant formula should be served cold or at room temperature; the beverage or infant formula should not be warmed or heated before or after addition of sacrosidase

Dosage Forms Solution, oral: 8500 int. units per mL (118 mL)

Safe Tussin® 30 [US-OTC] *see* guaifenesin and dextromethorphan *on page 308*

Saizen® [US/Can] *see* human growth hormone *on page 324*

Salacid® Ointment *(Discontinued) see page 814*

Sal-Acid® Plaster [US-OTC] *see* salicylic acid *on next page*

Salactic® Film [US-OTC] *see* salicylic acid *on next page*

Salagen® [US/Can] *see* pilocarpine *on page 514*

Salazopyrin® [Can] *see* sulfasalazine *on page 613*

Salazopyrin En-Tabs® **[Can]** *see* sulfasalazine *on page 613*

salbutamol *see* albuterol *on page 18*

Saleto-200® *(Discontinued) see page 814*

Saleto-400® *(Discontinued) see page 814*

Salflex® **[US/Can]** *see* salsalate *on page 583*

Salgesic® *(Discontinued) see page 814*

salicylazosulfapyridine *see* sulfasalazine *on page 613*

salicylic acid (sal i SIL ik AS id)

U.S./Canadian Brand Names Compound W® [US-OTC]; Dr Scholl's® Disk [US-OTC]; Dr Scholl's® Wart Remover [US-OTC]; DuoFilm® [US-OTC]; Duoforte® 27 [Can]; DuoPlant® [US-OTC]; Freezone® [US-OTC]; Gordofilm® [US-OTC]; Mediplast® Plaster [US-OTC]; Mosco® [US-OTC]; Occlusal™ [Can]; Occlusal®-HP [US/Can]; Off-Ezy® Wart Remover [US-OTC]; Psor-a-set® Soap [US-OTC]; Sal-Acid® Plaster [US-OTC]; Salactic® Film [US-OTC]; Sal-Plant® [US-OTC]; Sebcur® [Can]; Soluver® [Can]; Soluver® Plus [Can]; Trans-Ver-Sal® [Can]; Trans-Ver-Sal® AdultPatch [US-OTC]; Trans-Ver-Sal® PediaPatch [US-OTC]; Trans-Ver-Sal® PlantarPatch [US-OTC]; Wart-Off® [US-OTC]

Therapeutic Category Keratolytic Agent

Use Topically for its keratolytic effect in controlling seborrheic dermatitis or psoriasis of body and scalp, dandruff, and other scaling dermatoses; to remove warts, corns, calluses; also used in the treatment of acne

Usual Dosage

Shampoo: Apply to scalp and allow to remain for a few minutes, then rinse, initially use every day or every other day; 2 treatments/week are usually sufficient to maintain control

Topical: Apply to affected area and place under occlusion at night; hydrate skin for at least 5 minutes before use

Dosage Forms

Cream: 2% (30 g, 120 g)

Disk: 40%

Gel: 5% (60 g); 6% (30 g); 17% (7.5 g, 14.2 g)

Liquid: 13.6% (9.3 mL); 17% (9.3 mL, 10 mL, 13.5 mL, 15 mL); 16.7% (15 mL)

Lotion: 3% (120 mL)

Ointment: 3% (90 g)

Patch, transdermal: 15% (20 mm); 40% (20 mm)

Plaster: 40%

Soap: 2% (97.5 g)

Strip: 40%

salicylic acid and lactic acid (sal i SIL ik AS id & LAK tik AS id)

Synonyms lactic acid and salicylic acid

U.S./Canadian Brand Names Duofilm® Solution [US]

Therapeutic Category Keratolytic Agent

Use Treatment of benign epithelial tumors such as warts

Usual Dosage Topical: Apply a thin layer directly to wart once daily (may be useful to apply at bedtime and wash off in morning)

Dosage Forms Solution, topical: Salicylic acid 16.7% and lactic acid 16.7% in flexible collodion (15 mL)

salicylic acid and propylene glycol

(sal i SIL ik AS id & PROE pi leen GLYE cole)

Synonyms propylene glycol and salicylic acid

U.S./Canadian Brand Names Keralyt® Gel [US-OTC]

Therapeutic Category Keratolytic Agent

(Continued)

salicylic acid and propylene glycol *(Continued)*

Use Removal of excessive keratin in hyperkeratotic skin disorders, including various ichthyosis, keratosis palmaris and plantaris and psoriasis; may be used to remove excessive keratin in dorsal and plantar hyperkeratotic lesions

Usual Dosage Topical: Apply to area at night after soaking region for at least 5 minutes to hydrate area, and place under occlusion; medication is washed off in morning

Dosage Forms Gel, topical: Salicylic acid 6% and propylene glycol 60% in ethyl alcohol 19.4% with hydroxypropyl methylcellulose and water (30 g)

salicylic acid and sulfur *see* sulfur and salicylic acid *on page 614*

Salinex® [US-OTC] *see* sodium chloride *on page 595*

Salivart® [US-OTC] *see* saliva substitute *on this page*

saliva substitute *(sa LYE va SUB stee tute)*

U.S./Canadian Brand Names Entertainer's Secret® [US-OTC]; Moi-Stir® [US-OTC]; MouthKote® [US-OTC]; Salivart® [US-OTC]; Salix® Lozenge [US-OTC]

Therapeutic Category Gastrointestinal Agent, Miscellaneous

Use Relief of dry mouth and throat in xerostomia

Usual Dosage Use as needed

Dosage Forms Product may contain additional ingredients; refer to package labeling for additional information.

Lozenge: 100s

Solution: 50 mL, 60 mL, 120 mL, 240 mL, 555 mL

Swabstix: 3s

Salix® Lozenge [US-OTC] *see* saliva substitute *on this page*

Salk vaccine *see* poliovirus vaccine (inactivated) *on page 524*

salmeterol *(sal ME te role)*

U.S./Canadian Brand Names Serevent® Diskus® [US]; Serevent® [US/Can]

Therapeutic Category Adrenergic Agonist Agent

Use Maintenance treatment of asthma; prevention of bronchospasm in patients >12 years of age with reversible obstructive airway disease, including patients with symptoms of nocturnal asthma who require regular treatment with inhaled, short-acting beta$_2$ agonists; prevention of exercise-induced bronchospasm

Usual Dosage

Inhalation: 42 mcg (2 puffs) twice daily (12 hours apart) for maintenance and prevention of symptoms of asthma

Prevention of exercise-induced asthma: 42 mcg (2 puffs) 30-60 minutes prior to exercise; additional doses should not be used for 12 hours

Dosage Forms

Aerosol for oral inhalation, as xinafoate (Serevent®): 21 mcg/spray [60 inhalations] (6.5 g), [120 inhalations] (13 g)

Powder for oral inhalation (Serevent® Diskus®): 50 mcg [46 mcg/inhalation] (60 doses)

salmeterol and fluticasone *see* fluticasone and salmeterol *on page 282*

Salmonella typhi Vi capsular polysaccharide vaccine *(Canada only)* *(sal mo NEL la TI fi vi CAP su lar po le SAK ar ide VAK seen)*

U.S./Canadian Brand Names Typherix™ [Can]

Therapeutic Category Vaccine

Use For active immunization against typhoid fever in persons 2 years of age and older.

Usual Dosage One dose administered I.M. ensures protection for at least 3 years. The vaccine must be given at least 2 weeks prior to travel to endemic areas.

Dosage Forms Injection: Vi polysaccharide vaccine of *S. typhi* 25 mcg (0.5 mL)

Salmonine® *(Discontinued)* *see* page 814

Salofalk® **[Can]** *see* mesalamine *on page 411*

Sal-Plant® **[US-OTC]** *see* salicylic acid *on page 581*

salsalate (SAL sa late)

Synonyms disalicylic acid

U.S./Canadian Brand Names Amigesic® [US/Can]; Argesic®-SA [US]; Disalcid® [US]; Mono-Gesic® [US]; Salflex® [US/Can]

Therapeutic Category Analgesic, Non-narcotic; Antipyretic; Nonsteroidal Anti-inflammatory Drug (NSAID)

Use Treatment of minor pain or fever; rheumatoid arthritis, osteoarthritis, and related inflammatory conditions

Usual Dosage Adults: Oral: 1 g 2-4 times/day

Dosage Forms
Capsule: 500 mg
Tablet: 500 mg, 750 mg

Salsitab® *(Discontinued) see page 814*

salt *see* sodium chloride *on page 595*

Sal-Tropine™ **[US]** *see* atropine *on page 62*

Saluron® *(Discontinued) see page 814*

Salutensin® *(Discontinued) see page 814*

Salutensin-Demi® *(Discontinued) see page 814*

Sandimmune® **[US/Can]** *see* cyclosporine *on page 169*

Sandomigran® **[Can]** *see* pizotifen *(Canada only) on page 519*

Sandomigran DS® **[Can]** *see* pizotifen *(Canada only) on page 519*

Sandostatin® **[US/Can]** *see* octreotide *on page 474*

Sandostatin LAR® **[US/Can]** *see* octreotide *on page 474*

SangCya™ *(Discontinued) see page 814*

Sani-Supp® **[US-OTC]** *see* glycerin *on page 302*

Sanorex® *(Discontinued) see page 814*

Sansert® **[US/Can]** *see* methysergide *on page 424*

Santyl® **[US/Can]** *see* collagenase *on page 161*

saquinavir (sa KWIN a veer)

U.S./Canadian Brand Names Fortovase® [US/Can]; Invirase® [US/Can]

Therapeutic Category Antiviral Agent

Use Treatment of advanced HIV infection, used in combination with older nucleoside analog medications

Usual Dosage Adults: Oral:
Fortovase®: Six 200 mg (1200 mg) capsules 3 times/day within 2 hours after a meal
Invirase®: Three 200 mg (600 mg) capsules 3 times/day within 2 hours after a full meal

Dosage Forms
Capsule, as mesylate (Invirase®): 200 mg
Capsule, soft gelatin (Fortovase®): 200 mg

Sarafem™ **[US]** *see* fluoxetine *on page 279*

sargramostim (sar GRAM oh stim)

Synonyms GM-CSF; granulocyte-macrophage colony-stimulating factor; RGM-CSF

U.S./Canadian Brand Names Leukine™ [US/Can]

Therapeutic Category Colony-Stimulating Factor

Use Myeloid reconstitution after autologous bone marrow transplantation; to accelerate myeloid recovery in patients with non-Hodgkin's lymphoma, Hodgkin's lymphoma, and
(Continued)

sargramostim *(Continued)*

acute lymphoblastic leukemia undergoing autologous BMT; following induction chemotherapy in patients with acute myelogenous leukemia to shorten time to neutrophil
recovery

Usual Dosage

Children and Adults: I.V. infusion over ≥2 hours or S.C.

Existing clinical data suggest that starting GM-CSF between 24 and 72 hours
subsequent to chemotherapy may provide optimal neutrophil recover; continue
therapy until the occurrence of an absolute neutrophil count of 10,000/μL after the
neutrophil nadir

**The available data suggest that rounding the dose to the nearest vial size may
enhance patient convenience and reduce costs without clinical detriment**

**Myeloid reconstitution after peripheral stem cell, allogeneic or autologous bone
marrow transplant:** I.V.: 250 mcg/m^2/day for 21 days to begin 2-4 hours after the
marrow infusion on day 0 of autologous bone marrow transplant or ≥24 hours after
chemotherapy or 12 hours after last dose of radiotherapy

If a severe adverse reaction occurs, reduce or temporarily discontinue the dose until
the reaction abates

If blast cells appear or progression of the underlying disease occurs, disrupt treatment

Interrupt or reduce the dose by half if ANC is >20,000 cells/mm^3

Patients should not receive sargramostim until the postmarrow infusion ANC is <500
cells/mm^3

Neutrophil recovery following chemotherapy in AML: I.V.: 250 mcg/m^2/day over a 4-
hour period starting ~day 11 or 4 days following the completion of induction chemotherapy, if day 10 bone marrow is hypoblastic with <5% blasts

If a second cycle of chemotherapy is necessary, administer ~4 days after the completion of chemotherapy if the bone marrow is hypoblastic with <5% blasts

Continue sargramostim until ANC is >1500 cells/mm^3 for consecutive days or a
maximum of 42 days

Discontinue sargramostim immediately if leukemic regrowth occurs

If a severe adverse reaction occurs, reduce the dose by 50% or temporarily discontinue the dose until the reaction abates

Mobilization of peripheral blood progenitor cells: I.V.: 250 mcg/m^2/day over 24
hours or S.C. once daily

Continue the same dose through the period of PBPC collection

The optimal schedule for PBPC collection has not been established (usually begun by
day 5 and performed daily until protocol specified targets are achieved)

If WBC >50,000 cells/mm^3, reduce the dose by 50%

If adequate numbers of progenitor cells are not collected, consider other mobilization
therapy

Postperipheral blood progenitor cell transplantation: I.V.: 250 mcg/m^2/day over 24
hours or S.C. once daily beginning immediately following infusion of progenitor cells
and continuing until ANC is >1500 for 3 consecutive days is attained

BMT failure or engraftment delay: I.V.: 250 mcg/m^2/day for 14 days as a 2-hour
infusion

The dose can be repeated after 7 days off therapy if engraftment has not occurred

If engraftment still has not occurred, a third course of 500 mcg/m^2/day for 14 days may
be tried after another 7 days off therapy; if there is still no improvement, it is unlikely
that further dose escalation will be beneficial

If a severe adverse reaction occurs, reduce or temporarily discontinue the dose until
the reaction abates

If blast cells appear or disease progression occurs, discontinue treatment

Dosage Forms Injection: 250 mcg, 500 mcg

Sarna® HC [Can] *see* hydrocortisone (topical) *on page 334*

Sarna® [US-OTC] *see* camphor, menthol, and phenol *on page 109*

S.A.S.™ [Can] *see* sulfasalazine *on page 613*

Sastid® Plain Therapeutic Shampoo and Acne Wash [US-OTC] *see* sulfur and salicylic acid *on page 614*

Scabene® *(Discontinued)* *see page 814*

Scalpicin® [US] *see* hydrocortisone (topical) *on page 334*

S-Citalopram *see* escitalopram *on page 236*

Sclavo Test - PPD® *(Discontinued)* *see page 814*

Scleromate™ [US] *see* morrhuate sodium *on page 438*

Scopace® [US] *see* scopolamine *on this page*

scopolamine (skoe POL a meen)

Synonyms hyoscine

U.S./Canadian Brand Names Isopto® Hyoscine [US]; Scopace® [US]; Transderm Scōp® [US]; Transderm-V® [Can]

Therapeutic Category Anticholinergic Agent

Use Preoperative medication to produce amnesia and decrease salivary and respiratory secretions; to produce cycloplegia and mydriasis; treatment of iridocyclitis; prevention of motion sickness; prevention of nausea/vomiting associated with anesthesia or opiate analgesia (patch)

Usual Dosage

Preoperatively:

Children: I.M., S.C.: 6 mcg/kg/dose (maximum: 0.3 mg/dose) or 0.2 mg/m^2 may be repeated every 6-8 hours **or** alternatively:

4-7 months: 0.1 mg

7 months to 3 years: 0.15 mg

3-8 years: 0.2 mg

8-12 years: 0.3 mg

Adults: I.M., I.V., S.C.: 0.3-0.65 mg; may be repeated every 4-6 hours

Motion sickness: Transdermal: Children >12 years and Adults: Apply 1 disc behind the ear at least 4 hours prior to exposure and every 3 days as needed

Ophthalmic:

Refraction:

Children: Instill 1 drop of 0.25% to eye(s) twice daily for 2 days before procedure

Adults: Instill 1-2 drops of 0.25% to eye(s) 1 hour before procedure

Iridocyclitis:

Children: Instill 1 drop of 0.25% to eye(s) up to 3 times/day

Adults: Instill 1-2 drops of 0.25% to eye(s) up to 4 times/day

Dosage Forms

Injection, as hydrobromide: 0.4 mg/mL (0.5 mL, 1 mL)

Solution, ophthalmic, as hydrobromide (Isopto® Hyoscine, Scopace®): 0.25% (5 mL, 15 mL)

Tablet, as hydrobromide: 0.4 mg

Transdermal system (Transderm Scōp®): 0.33 mg/24 hours [2.5 cm^2] total scopolamine 1.5 mg per patch [releases ~1 mg over 72 hours]

scopolamine and phenylephrine *see* phenylephrine and scopolamine *on page 511*

scopolamine, hyoscyamine, atropine, and phenobarbital *see* hyoscyamine, atropine, scopolamine, and phenobarbital *on page 340*

Scot-Tussin DM® Cough Chasers [US-OTC] *see* dextromethorphan *on page 189*

Scot-Tussin® Sugar Free Expectorant [US-OTC] *see* guaifenesin *on page 307*

SDZ ENA 713 *see* rivastigmine *on page 575*

SeaMist® [US-OTC] *see* sodium chloride *on page 595*

Seba-Gel™ [US] *see* benzoyl peroxide *on page 79*

Sebcur® **[Can]** *see* salicylic acid *on page 581*

Sebcur/T® **[Can]** *see* coal tar and salicylic acid *on page 158*

Sebizon® **[US]** *see* sulfacetamide *on page 610*

secobarbital (see koe BAR bi tal)
Synonyms quinalbarbitone
U.S./Canadian Brand Names Seconal™ [US]
Therapeutic Category Barbiturate
Controlled Substance C-II
Use Short-term treatment of insomnia and as preanesthetic agent
Usual Dosage Oral:
Children: Preoperative sedation: 2-6 mg/kg (maximum 100 mg)
Adults:
Hypnotic: 100 mg
Preoperative sedation: 200-300 mg 1-2 hours before surgery
Dosage Forms Capsule, as sodium: 100 mg

secobarbital and amobarbital *see* amobarbital and secobarbital *on page 36*

Seconal™ [US] *see* secobarbital *on this page*

Secran® *(Discontinued) see page 814*

SecreFlo™ [US] *see* secretin *on this page*

secretin (SEE kre tin)
U.S./Canadian Brand Names SecreFlo™ [US]
Therapeutic Category Diagnostic Agent
Use Diagnosis of Zollinger-Ellison syndrome, chronic pancreatic dysfunction, and some
hepatobiliary diseases such as obstructive jaundice resulting from cancer or stones in
the biliary tract
Usual Dosage I.V.:
Pancreatic function: 1 CU/kg slow I.V. injection over 1 minute
Zollinger-Ellison: 2 CU/kg slow I.V. injection over 1 minute
Dosage Forms Injection, powder for reconstitution: 16 mcg

Sectral® **[US/Can]** *see* acebutolol *on page 3*

Sedapap® **[US]** *see* butalbital, acetaminophen, and caffeine *on page 99*

Selax® **[Can]** *see* docusate *on page 208*

Seldane® *(Discontinued) see page 814*

Seldane-D® *(Discontinued) see page 814*

Selecor® *(Discontinued) see page 814*

Select™ 1/35 [Can] *see* ethinyl estradiol and norethindrone *on page 251*

Selectol® *(Discontinued) see page 814*

selegiline (seh LEDGE ah leen)
Synonyms deprenyl; *l*-deprenyl
U.S./Canadian Brand Names Apo®-Selegiline [Can]; Atapryl® [US]; Eldepryl® [US/
Can]; Gen-Selegiline [Can]; Novo-Selegiline [Can]; Nu-Selegiline [Can]; Selpak® [US]
Therapeutic Category Anti-Parkinson's Agent; Dopaminergic Agent (Anti-Parkinson's)
Use Adjunct in the management of parkinsonian patients in which levodopa/carbidopa
therapy is deteriorating
Unlabeled uses: Early Parkinson's disease, Alzheimer's disease
Usual Dosage Adults: Oral: 5 mg twice daily
Dosage Forms
Capsule, as hydrochloride (Eldepryl®): 5 mg
Tablet, as hydrochloride: 5 mg

selenium sulfide (se LEE nee um SUL fide)

U.S./Canadian Brand Names Exsel® [US]; Head & Shoulders® Intensive Treatment [US-OTC]; Selsun Blue® [US-OTC]; Selsun Gold® for Women [US-OTC]; Selsun® [US]; Versel® [Can]

Therapeutic Category Antiseborrheic Agent, Topical

Use Treat itching and flaking of the scalp associated with dandruff; to control scalp seborrheic dermatitis; treatment of tinea versicolor

Usual Dosage Topical:

Dandruff, seborrhea: Massage 5-10 mL into wet scalp, leave on scalp 2-3 minutes, rinse thoroughly and repeat application; shampoo twice weekly for 2 weeks initially, then use once every 1-4 weeks as indicated depending upon control

Tinea versicolor: Apply the 2.5% lotion to affected area and lather with small amounts of water; leave on skin for 10 minutes, then rinse thoroughly; apply every day for 7 days

Dosage Forms

Lotion: 1% (120 mL, 210 mL, 240 mL); 2.5% (120 mL)

Shampoo: 1% (120 mL, 210 mL, 330 mL)

Sele-Pak® [US] *see* trace metals *on page 646*

Selepen® [US] *see* trace metals *on page 646*

Selestoject® (Discontinued) *see page 814*

Selpak® [US] *see* selegiline *on previous page*

Selsun® [US] *see* selenium sulfide *on this page*

Selsun Blue® [US-OTC] *see* selenium sulfide *on this page*

Selsun Gold® for Women [US-OTC] *see* selenium sulfide *on this page*

Semicid® [US-OTC] *see* nonoxynol 9 *on page 464*

Semprex®-D [US] *see* acrivastine and pseudoephedrine *on page 12*

Senexon® [US-OTC] *see* senna *on this page*

senna (SEN na)

U.S./Canadian Brand Names Black Draught® [US-OTC]; Ex-Lax® [US]; Ex-Lax® Maximum Relief [US]; Senexon® [US-OTC]; Senna-Gen® [US-OTC]; Senokot® [US-OTC]; X-Prep® [US-OTC]

Therapeutic Category Laxative

Use Short-term treatment of constipation; evacuate the colon for bowel or rectal examinations

Usual Dosage

Children:

Oral:

>6 years: 10-20 mg/kg/dose at bedtime; maximum daily dose: 872 mg

6-12 years, >27 kg: 1 tablet at bedtime, up to 4 tablets/day **or** 1/2 teaspoonful of granules (326 mg/tsp) at bedtime (up to 2 teaspoonfuls/day)

Liquid:

2-5 years: 5-10 mL at bedtime

6-15 years: 10-15 mL at bedtime

Suppository: 1/2 at bedtime

Syrup:

1 month to 1 year: 1.25-2.5 mL at bedtime up to 5 mL/day

1-5 years: 2.5-5 mL at bedtime up to 10 mL/day

5-10 years: 5-10 mL at bedtime up to 20 mL/day

Adults:

Granules (326 mg/teaspoon): 1 teaspoonful at bedtime, not to exceed 2 teaspoonfuls twice daily

Liquid: 15-30 mL with meals and at bedtime

Suppository: 1 at bedtime, may repeat once in 2 hours

Syrup: 2-3 teaspoonfuls at bedtime, not to exceed 30 mL/day

(Continued)

senna *(Continued)*

Tablet: 187 mg: 2 tablets at bedtime, not to exceed 8 tablets/day
Tablet: 374 mg: 1 at bedtime, up to 4/day; 600 mg: 2 tablets at bedtime, up to 3 tablets/day

Dosage Forms
Granules: 326 mg/teaspoonful
Liquid: 6.5% [65 mg/mL] (75 mL, 150 mL); 7% [70 mg/mL] (130 mL, 360 mL)
Suppository, rectal: 652 mg
Syrup: 218 mg/5 mL (60 mL, 240 mL)
Tablet: 187 mg, 217 mg, 600 mg

Senna-Gen® [US-OTC] *see* senna *on previous page*

Senokot® [US-OTC] *see* senna *on previous page*

Senolax® *(Discontinued)* *see page 814*

Sensorcaine® [US/Can] *see* bupivacaine *on page 97*

Sensorcaine®-MPF [US] *see* bupivacaine *on page 97*

Septa® Topical Ointment *(Discontinued)* *see page 814*

Septisol® *(Discontinued)* *see page 814*

Septra® [US/Can] *see* sulfamethoxazole and trimethoprim *on page 612*

Septra® DS [US/Can] *see* sulfamethoxazole and trimethoprim *on page 612*

Ser-A-Gen® *(Discontinued)* *see page 814*

Ser-Ap-Es® *(Discontinued)* *see page 814*

Serax® [US] *see* oxazepam *on page 482*

Serc® [Can] *see* betahistine *(Canada only) on page 82*

Serentil® [US/Can] *see* mesoridazine *on page 411*

Serevent® [US/Can] *see* salmeterol *on page 582*

Serevent® Diskus® [US] *see* salmeterol *on page 582*

sermorelin acetate (ser moe REL in AS e tate)

U.S./Canadian Brand Names Geref® Diagnostic [US]; Geref® [US]
Therapeutic Category Diagnostic Agent
Use Evaluate ability of the somatotroph of the pituitary gland to secrete growth hormone
Usual Dosage I.V. (in a single dose in the morning following an overnight fast):
Children or subjects <50 kg: Draw venous blood samples for GH determinations 15 minutes before and immediately prior to administration, then administer 1 mcg/kg followed by a 3 mL normal saline flush, draw blood samples again for GH determinations
Adults or subjects >50 kg: Determine the number of ampules needed based on a dose of 1 mcg/kg, draw venous blood samples for GH determinations 15 minutes before and immediately prior to administration, then administer 1 mcg/kg followed by a 3 mL normal saline flush, draw blood samples again for GH determinations
Dosage Forms
Injection, powder for reconstitution:
Geref®: 0.5 mg, 1 mg
Geref® Diagnostic: 50 mcg

Seromycin® Pulvules® [US] *see* cycloserine *on page 169*

Serophene® [US/Can] *see* clomiphene *on page 154*

Seroquel® [US/Can] *see* quetiapine *on page 558*

Serostim® [US/Can] *see* human growth hormone *on page 324*

Serpalan® *(Discontinued)* *see page 814*

Serpasil® *(Discontinued)* *see page 814*

Serpatabs® *(Discontinued)* see page 814

sertraline (SER tra leen)
U.S./Canadian Brand Names Apo®-Sertraline [Can]; Novo-Sertraline [Can]; Zoloft® [US/Can]
Therapeutic Category Antidepressant, Selective Serotonin Reuptake Inhibitor
Use Treatment of major depression; pediatric obsessive-compulsive disorder; also being studied for use in obesity
Usual Dosage Oral: Initial: 50 mg/day as a single dose, dosage may be increased at intervals of at least 1 week to a maximum recommended dosage of 200 mg/day
Dosage Forms
Solution, oral concentrate: 20 mg/mL (60 mL)
Tablet, as hydrochloride: 25 mg, 50 mg, 100 mg

Serutan® **[US-OTC]** see psyllium on page 554

Serzone® **[US/Can]** see nefazodone on page 450

sevelamer (se VEL a mer)
U.S./Canadian Brand Names Renagel® [US/Can]
Therapeutic Category Phosphate Binder
Use Reduction of serum phosphorous in patients with end-stage renal disease
Usual Dosage Adults: Oral: 2-4 capsules 3 times/day with meals; the initial dose may be based on serum phosphorous:
(Phosphorous: Initial dose)
>6.0 and <7.5: 2 capsules 3 times/day
>7.5 and <9.0: 3 capsules 3 times/day
≥9.0: 4 capsules 3 times/day
Dosage should be adjusted based on serum phosphorous concentration, with a goal of lowering to <6.0 mg/dL; maximum daily dose studied was 30 capsules/day
Dosage Forms
Capsule: 403 mg
Tablet: 400 mg, 800 mg

sevoflurane (see voe FLOO rane)
U.S./Canadian Brand Names Sevorane AF™ [Can]; Ultane® [US]
Therapeutic Category General Anesthetic
Use General induction and maintenance of anesthesia (inhalation)
Usual Dosage Surgical levels of anesthesia can usually be obtained with concentrations of 0.5% to 3%
Dosage Forms Liquid for inhalation: 250 mL

Sevorane AF™ [Can] see sevoflurane on this page

Shur-Seal® **[US-OTC]** see nonoxynol 9 on page 464

Sibelium® **[Can]** see flunarizine *(Canada only)* on page 275

Siblin® *(Discontinued)* see page 814

sibutramine (si BYOO tra meen)
U.S./Canadian Brand Names Meridia™ [US/Can]
Therapeutic Category Anorexiant
Use Management of obesity, including weight loss and maintenance of weight loss, and should be used in conjunction with a reduced calorie diet
Usual Dosage Adults ≥16 years: Initial: 10 mg once daily; after 4 weeks may titrate up to 15 mg once daily as needed and tolerated
Dosage Forms Capsule, as hydrochloride: 5 mg, 10 mg, 15 mg

Silace-C® **[US-OTC]** see docusate and casanthranol on page 209

Siladryl® **Allerfy**® **[US-OTC]** *see* diphenhydramine *on page 202*

Silafed® **[US-OTC]** *see* triprolidine and pseudoephedrine *on page 659*

Silain® *(Discontinued) see page 814*

Silaminic® **Cold Syrup** *(Discontinued) see page 814*

Silaminic® **Expectorant** *(Discontinued) see page 814*

Silapap® **Children's [US-OTC]** *see* acetaminophen *on page 3*

Silapap® **Infants [US-OTC]** *see* acetaminophen *on page 3*

sildenafil (sil DEN a fil)

Synonyms UK 92480

U.S./Canadian Brand Names Viagra® [US/Can]

Therapeutic Category Phosphodiesterase (Type 5) Enzyme Inhibitor

Use Effective in most men with erectile dysfunction (ED), the medical term for impotence, which is associated with a broad range of physical or psychological medical conditions.

Usual Dosage Oral: Adults: 50 mg taken one hour before sexual activity; individuals may need more (100 mg) or less (25 mg) and dosing should be determined by a physician depending on effectiveness and side effects. The drug should not be used more than once daily.

Dosage Forms Tablet, as citrate: 25 mg, 50 mg, 100 mg

Sildicon-E® *(Discontinued) see page 814*

Silexin® **[US-OTC]** *see* guaifenesin and dextromethorphan *on page 308*

Silphen DM® **[US-OTC]** *see* dextromethorphan *on page 189*

Silphen® **[US-OTC]** *see* diphenhydramine *on page 202*

Siltussin-CF® *(Discontinued) see page 814*

Silvadene® **[US]** *see* silver sulfadiazine *on this page*

silver nitrate (SIL ver NYE trate)

Synonyms AgNO$_3$

Therapeutic Category Topical Skin Product

Use Prevention of gonococcal ophthalmia neonatorum; cauterization of wounds and sluggish ulcers, removal of granulation tissue and warts

Usual Dosage

Neonates: Ophthalmic: Instill 2 drops immediately after birth into conjunctival sac of each eye as a single dose; do not irrigate eyes following instillation of eye drops

Children and Adults:

Sticks: Apply to mucous membranes and other moist skin surfaces only on area to be treated 2-3 times/week for 2-3 weeks

Topical solution: Apply a cotton applicator dipped in solution on the affected area 2-3 times/week for 2-3 weeks

Dosage Forms

Applicator sticks: 75% (6") [with potassium nitrate 25%]

Ointment: 10% (30 g)

Solution, ophthalmic [wax ampuls]: 1%

Solution, topical: 10% (30 mL); 25% (30 mL); 50% (30 mL)

silver sulfadiazine (SIL ver sul fa DYE a zeen)

U.S./Canadian Brand Names Dermazin™ [Can]; Flamazine® [Can]; Silvadene® [US]; SSD® AF [US]; SSD® Cream [US/Can]; Thermazene® [US]

Therapeutic Category Antibacterial, Topical

Use Adjunct in the prevention and treatment of infection in second and third degree burns

Usual Dosage Children and Adults: Topical: Apply once or twice daily with a sterile gloved hand; apply to a thickness of $^1/_{16}$"; burned area should be covered with cream at all times

Dosage Forms Cream: 1% [10 mg/g] (20 g, 50 g, 85 g, 100 g, 400 g, 1000 g)

simethicone (sye METH i kone)
Synonyms activated dimethicone; activated methylpolysiloxane
U.S./Canadian Brand Names Flatulex® [US-OTC]; Gas-X® [US-OTC]; Maalox® Anti-Gas [US-OTC]; Mylanta® Gas [US-OTC]; Mylicon® [US-OTC]; Ovol® [Can]; Phazyme® [Can]
Therapeutic Category Antiflatulent
Use Relieve flatulence, functional gastric bloating, and postoperative gas pains
Usual Dosage Oral:
Infants: 20 mg 4 times/day
Children <12 years: 40 mg 4 times/day
Children >12 years and Adults: 40-120 mg after meals and at bedtime as needed, not to exceed 500 mg/day
Dosage Forms
Capsule: 125 mg
Suspension, oral [drops]: 40 mg/0.6 mL (30 mL)
Tablet: 60 mg, 95 mg
Tablet, chewable: 40 mg, 80 mg, 125 mg

simethicone and calcium carbonate see calcium carbonate and simethicone on page 105

simethicone and magaldrate see magaldrate and simethicone on page 396

Simply Sleep® [US-OTC] see diphenhydramine on page 202

Simulect® [US/Can] see basiliximab on page 71

simvastatin (SIM va stat in)
U.S./Canadian Brand Names Zocor® [US/Can]
Therapeutic Category HMG-CoA Reductase Inhibitor
Use Adjunct to dietary therapy to decrease elevated serum total and LDL cholesterol concentrations in primary hypercholesterolemia; lowering elevated triglyceride levels
Usual Dosage Adults: Oral: Start with 5-10 mg/day as a single bedtime dose; starting dose of 5 mg/day should be considered for patients with LDL-C of ≤190 mg/dL and for the elderly; patients with LDL-C levels >190 mg/dL should be started on 10 mg/day; adjustments of dosage should be made at intervals of 4 weeks or more; maximum recommended dose: 40 mg/day
Dosage Forms Tablet: 5 mg, 10 mg, 20 mg, 40 mg, 80 mg

sincalide (SIN ka lide)
Synonyms C8-CCK; OP-CCK
U.S./Canadian Brand Names Kinevac® [US]
Therapeutic Category Diagnostic Agent
Use Postevacuation cholecystography; gallbladder bile sampling; stimulate pancreatic secretion for analysis
Usual Dosage Adults: I.V.:
Contraction of gallbladder: 0.02 mcg/kg over 30 seconds to 1 minute, may repeat in 15 minutes a 0.04 mcg/kg dose
Pancreatic function: 0.02 mcg/kg over 30 minutes
Dosage Forms Injection: 5 mcg

Sine-Aid® IB (Discontinued) see page 814

Sinemet® [US/Can] see levodopa and carbidopa on page 380

Sinemet® CR [US/Can] see levodopa and carbidopa on page 380

Sinequan® [US/Can] see doxepin on page 213

Singulair® [US/Can] see montelukast on page 437

Sinografin® [US] see radiological/contrast media (ionic) on page 561

Sinubid® *(Discontinued)* see page 814

Sinufed® **Timecelles**® *(Discontinued)* see page 814

Sinumed® *(Discontinued)* see page 814

Sinumist®**-SR Capsulets**® *(Discontinued)* see page 814

Sinus-Relief® **[US-OTC]** see acetaminophen and pseudoephedrine on page 6

Sinutab® **Non Drowsy [Can]** see acetaminophen and pseudoephedrine on page 6

Sinutab® **Sinus & Allergy [Can]** see acetaminophen, chlorpheniramine, and pseudoephedrine on page 7

Sinutab® **Sinus Allergy Maximum Strength [US-OTC]** see acetaminophen, chlorpheniramine, and pseudoephedrine on page 7

Sinutab® **Sinus Maximum Strength Without Drowsiness [US-OTC]** see acetaminophen and pseudoephedrine on page 6

sirolimus (sir OH li mus)

U.S./Canadian Brand Names Rapamune® [US/Can]

Therapeutic Category Immunosuppressant Agent

Use Prophylaxis of organ rejection in patients receiving renal transplants, in combination with cyclosporin and corticosteroids

Unlabeled use: Prophylaxis of organ rejection in solid organ transplant patients in combination with tacrolimus and corticosteroids

Usual Dosage Oral:

Adults ≥40 kg: Loading dose: For *de novo* transplant recipients, a loading dose of 3 times the daily maintenance dose should be administered on day 1 of dosing. Maintenance dose: 2 mg/day. Doses should be taken 4 hours after cyclosporine, and should be taken consistently either with or without food.

Children ≥13 years or Adults <40 kg: Loading dose: 3 mg/m^2 (day 1); followed by a maintenance of 1 mg/m^2/day.

Dosage Forms

Solution, oral: 1 mg/mL (1 mL, 2 mL, 5 mL, 60 mL, 150 mL)

Tablet: 1 mg

SK see streptokinase on page 606

Skelaxin® **[US/Can]** see metaxalone on page 414

Skelex® *(Discontinued)* see page 814

Skelid® **[US]** see tiludronate on page 639

SKF 104864 see topotecan on page 645

skin test antigens, multiple (skin test AN tee gens, MUL ti pul)

U.S./Canadian Brand Names Multitest CMI® [US]

Therapeutic Category Diagnostic Agent

Use Detection of nonresponsiveness to antigens by means of delayed hypersensitivity skin testing

Usual Dosage Select only test sites that permit sufficient surface area and subcutaneous tissue to allow adequate penetration of all 8 points, avoid hairy areas

Press loaded unit into the skin with sufficient pressure to puncture the skin and allow adequate penetration of all points, maintain firm contact for at least five seconds, during application the device should not be "rocked" back and forth and side to side without removing any of the test heads from the skin sites

If adequate pressure is applied it will be possible to observe:

1. The puncture marks of the nine tines on each of the eight test heads
2. An imprint of the circular platform surrounding each test head
3. Residual antigen and glycerin at each of the eight sites

If any of the above three criteria are not fully followed, the test results may not be reliable

Reading should be done in good light, read the test sites at both 24 and 48 hours, the largest reaction recorded from the two readings at each test site should be used; if two readings are not possible, a single 48 hour is recommended

A positive reaction from any of the seven delayed hypersensitivity skin test antigens is **induration of ≥2 mm** providing there is no induration at the negative control site; the size of the induration reactions with this test may be smaller than those obtained with other intradermal procedures

Dosage Forms Applicator, skin test [carton; preloaded]: 7 antigens and a glycerin control

Sleep-Aid® **[US-OTC]** *see* doxylamine *on page 216*

Sleep-eze 3® **Oral** *(Discontinued) see page 814*

Sleepinal® **[US-OTC]** *see* diphenhydramine *on page 202*

Sleep® **Tabs [US-OTC]** *see* diphenhydramine *on page 202*

Sleepwell 2-nite® *(Discontinued) see page 814*

Slim-Mint® *(Discontinued) see page 814*

Sloan's Liniment® **[US]** *see* capsaicin *on page 111*

Slo-bid™ *(Discontinued) see page 814*

Slo-Niacin® **[US-OTC]** *see* niacin *on page 456*

Slo-Phyllin® **[US]** *see* theophylline *on page 630*

Slo-Phyllin® **GG** *(Discontinued) see page 814*

Slo-Salt® *(Discontinued) see page 814*

Slow FE® **[US-OTC]** *see* ferrous sulfate *on page 269*

Slow-K® *(Discontinued) see page 814*

Slow-K® **[Can]** *see* potassium chloride *on page 530*

Slow-Mag® **[US/Can]** *see* magnesium chloride *on page 397*

Slow-Trasicor® **[Can]** *see* oxprenolol *(Canada only) on page 483*

smelling salts *see* ammonia spirit (aromatic) *on page 36*

SMX-TMP *see* sulfamethoxazole and trimethoprim *on page 612*

snake (pit vipers) antivenin *see* antivenin *(Crotalidae) polyvalent on page 48*

Snaplets-EX® *(Discontinued) see page 814*

sodium 2-mercaptoethane sulfonate *see* mesna *on page 411*

sodium acetate (SOW dee um AS e tate)

Therapeutic Category Alkalinizing Agent; Electrolyte Supplement, Oral

Use Sodium salt replacement; correction of acidosis through conversion of acetate to bicarbonate

Usual Dosage Sodium acetate is metabolized to bicarbonate on an equimolar basis outside the liver; administer in large volume I.V. fluids as a sodium source. Refer to sodium bicarbonate monograph.

Maintenance electrolyte requirements of sodium in parenteral nutrition solutions:
Daily requirements: 3-4 mEq/kg/24 hours or 25-40 mEq/1000 kcal/24 hours
Maximum: 100-150 mEq/24 hours

Dosage Forms Injection: 2 mEq/mL (20 mL, 50 mL, 100 mL); 4 mEq/mL (50 mL, 100 mL)

sodium acid carbonate *see* sodium bicarbonate *on next page*

sodium ascorbate (SOW dee um a SKOR bate)
U.S./Canadian Brand Names Cenolate® [US]
Therapeutic Category Vitamin, Water Soluble
Use Prevention and treatment of scurvy and to acidify the urine; large doses may decrease the severity of "colds"
Usual Dosage Oral, I.V.:
Children:
Scurvy: 100-300 mg/day in divided doses for at least 2 weeks
Urinary acidification: 500 mg every 6-8 hours
Dietary supplement: 35-45 mg/day
Adults:
Scurvy: 100-250 mg 1-2 times/day for at least 2 weeks
Urinary acidification: 4-12 g/day in divided doses
Dietary supplement: 50-60 mg/day
Prevention and treatment of cold: 1-3 g/day
Dosage Forms Injection: 562.5 mg/mL [ascorbic acid 500 mg/mL] (1 mL, 2 mL)

sodium benzoate and caffeine *see* caffeine and sodium benzoate *on page 102*

sodium bicarbonate (SOW dee um bye KAR bun ate)
Synonyms baking soda; NaHCO$_3$; sodium acid carbonate; sodium hydrogen carbonate
U.S./Canadian Brand Names Neut® [US]
Therapeutic Category Alkalinizing Agent; Antacid; Electrolyte Supplement, Oral
Use Management of metabolic acidosis; antacid; alkalinize urine; stabilization of acid base status in cardiac arrest, and treatment of life-threatening hyperkalemia
Usual Dosage
Cardiac arrest (patient should be adequately ventilated before administering NaHCO$_3$):
Infants: Use 1:1 dilution of 1 mEq/mL NaHCO$_3$ or use 0.5 mEq/mL NaHCO$_3$ at a dose of 1 mEq/kg slow IVP initially; may repeat with 0.5 mEq/kg in 10 minutes one time or as indicated by the patient's acid-base status. Rate of administration should not exceed 10 mEq/minute.
Children and Adults: IVP: 1 mEq/kg initially; may repeat with 0.5 mEq/kg in 10 minutes one time or as indicated by the patient's acid-base status
Metabolic acidosis: Dosage should be based on the following formula if blood gases and pH measurements are available:
Infants and Children: HCO$_3$-(mEq) = 0.3 x weight (kg) x base deficit (mEq/L) **or** HCO$_3$-(mEq) = 0.5 x weight (kg) x (24 - serum HCO$_3$-) (mEq/L)
Adults: HCO$_3$-(mEq) = 0.2 x weight (kg) x base deficit (mEq/L) **or** HCO$_3$-(mEq) = 0.5 x weight (kg) x (24 - serum HCO$_3$-) (mEq/L)
If acid-base status is not available: Dose for older Children and Adults: 2-5 mEq/kg I.V. infusion over 4-8 hours; subsequent doses should be based on patient's acid-base status
Chronic renal failure: Oral: Children: 1-3 mEq/kg/day
Renal tubular acidosis: Oral:
Distal:
Children: 2-3 mEq/kg/day
Adults: 1 mEq/kg/day
Proximal: Children: Initial: 5-10 mEq/kg/day; maintenance: Increase as required to maintain serum bicarbonate in the normal range
Urine alkalinization: Oral:
Children: 1-10 mEq (84-840 mg)/kg/day in divided doses; dose should be titrated to desired urinary pH
Adults: Initial: 48 mEq (4 g), then 12-24 mEq (1-2 g) every 4 hours; dose should be titrated to desired urinary pH; doses up to 16 g/day have been used
Dosage Forms
Injection:
4% [40 mg/mL = 2.4 mEq/5 mL] (5 mL)

4.2% [42 mg/mL = 5 mEq/10 mL] (10 mL)
5% [50 mg/mL = 5.95 mEq/10 mL] (500 mL)
7.5% [75 mg/mL = 8.92 mEq/10 mL] (10 mL, 50 mL)
8.4% [84 mg/mL = 10 mEq/10 mL] (10 mL, 50 mL)
Powder: 120 g, 480 g
Tablet: 325 mg [3.8 mEq]; 520 mg [6.3 mEq]; 650 mg [7.6 mEq]

sodium cellulose phosphate *see* cellulose sodium phosphate *on page 127*

sodium chloride (SOW dee um KLOR ide)

Synonyms NaCl; normal saline; salt

U.S./Canadian Brand Names Altamist [US-OTC]; Ayr® Baby Saline [US-OTC]; Ayr® Saline [US-OTC]; Breathe Free® [US-OTC]; Breathe Right® Saline [US-OTC]; Broncho Saline® [US]; Entsol® Mist [US-OTC]; Entsol® Single Use [US-OTC]; Entsol® [US-OTC]; Muro 128® [US-OTC]; Nasal Moist® [US-OTC]; NāSal™ [US-OTC]; Na-Zone® [US-OTC]; Ocean® [US-OTC]; Pediamist® [US-OTC]; Pretz® [US-OTC]; Salinex® [US-OTC]; SeaMist® [US-OTC]; Wound Wash Saline™ [US-OTC]

Therapeutic Category Electrolyte Supplement, Oral; Lubricant, Ocular

Use Prevention of muscle cramps and heat prostration; restoration of sodium ion in hyponatremia; restore moisture to nasal membranes; reduction of corneal edema

Usual Dosage

Newborn electrolyte requirement:

Premature: 2-8 mEq/kg/24 hours

Term:

0-48 hours: 0-2 mEq/kg/24 hours

>48 hours: 1-4 mEq/kg/24 hours

Children: I.V.: Hypertonic solutions (>0.9%) should only be used for the initial treatment of acute serious symptomatic hyponatremia; maintenance: 3-4 mEq/kg/day; maximum: 100-150 mEq/day; dosage varies widely depending on clinical condition

Replacement: Determined by laboratory determinations mEq

Sodium deficiency (mEq/kg) = [% dehydration (L/kg)/100 x 70 (mEq/L) = [0.6 (L/kg) x (140 - serum sodium) (mEq/L)]

Nasal: Use as often as needed

Adults:

GI irrigant: 1-3 L/day by intermittent irrigation

Heat cramps: Oral: 0.5-1 g with full glass of water, up to 4.8 g/day

Replacement I.V.: Determined by laboratory determinations mEq

Sodium deficiency (mEq/kg) = [% dehydration (L/kg)/100 x 70 (mEq/L)] + [0.6 (L/kg) x (140 - serum sodium) (mEq/L)]

To correct acute, serious hyponatremia: mEq sodium = (desired sodium (mEq/L) - actual sodium (mEq/L) x 0.6 x wt (kg)); for acute correction use 125 mEq/L as the desired serum sodium; acutely correct serum sodium in 5 mEq/L/dose increments; more gradual correction in increments of 10 mEq/L/day is indicated in the asymptomatic patient

Chloride maintenance electrolyte requirement in parenteral nutrition: 2-4 mEq/kg/24 hours or 25-40 mEq/1000 kcals/24 hours; maximum: 100-150 mEq/24 hours

Sodium maintenance electrolyte requirement in parenteral nutrition: 3-4 mEq/kg/24 hours or 25-40 mEq/1000 kcals/24 hours; maximum: 100-150 mEq/24 hours.

Nasal: Use as often as needed

Ophthalmic:

Ointment: Apply once daily or more often

Solution: Instill 1-2 drops into affected eye(s) every 3-4 hours

Abortifacient: 20% (250 mL) administered by transabdominal intra-amniotic instillation

Dosage Forms

Aero, intranasal, buffered (Entsol®): 3% (100 mL)

Gel, intranasal (Nasal Moist®): 0.65% (30 g)

(Continued)

sodium chloride *(Continued)*

Injection, solution: 0.45% (25 mL, 50 mL, 100 mL, 250 mL, 500 mL, 1000 mL, 1500 mL, 2000 mL); 0.9% (2 mL, 3 mL, 5 mL, 10 mL, 20 mL, 25 mL, 30 mL, 50 mL, 100 mL, 150 mL, 250 mL, 500 mL, 1000 mL); 2.5 % (250 mL); 3% (500 mL); 5% (500 mL)

Solution for injection [preservative free]: 0.9% (2mL, 5 mL, 10 mL, 20 mL, 50 mL, 100 mL)

Injection, solution, bacteriostatic: 0.9% (10 mL, 20 mL, 30 mL)

Injection, concentrated solution: 14.6% (20 mL, 40 mL, 250 mL); 23.4% (30 mL 50 mL, 100 mL, 200 mL, 250 mL)

Ointment, ophthalmic: 5% (3.5 g)
Muro-128®: 5% (3.5g)

Powder, solution (Entsol®) 3% (10.5 g)

Solution, inhalation: 0.45% (3 mL, 5 mL); 0.9% (3 mL, 5 mL); 3% (15 mL); 10% (15 mL)
Broncho Saline®: 0.9% (90 mL, 240 mL)

Solution, intranasal: 0.65% (45 mL, 90 mL)
Salinex®: 0.4% (15 mL, 50 mL)
Pediamist®: 0.5% (15 mL)
Altamist: 0.65% (60 mL)
Ayr® Baby Saline: 0.65% (30 mL)
Ayr® Saline, Ayr® Saline Mist: 0.65% (50 mL)
Breathe Free®, Breathe Right® Saline: 0.65% (44 mL)
NaSal™: 0.65% (15 mL, 30 mL)
Nasal Moist®: 0.65% (15 mL, 45 mL)
Ocean®: 0.65% (45 mL)
Sea Mist®: 0.65% (15 mL)
Pretz® Irrigation: 0.75% (240 mL)
Na-Zone®: 0.75% (60 mL)
Entsol® Mist: 3% (30 mL)
Enstol® Single Use [buffered; prefilled; preservative free nasal wash]: 3% (240 mL)

Solution, irrigation: 0.45% (2000 mL); 0.9% (250 mL, 500 mL, 1000 mL, 2000 mL, 3000 mL, 4000 mL)
Wound Wash Saline™: 0.9% (90 mL, 210 mL)

Solution, ophthalmic: 5% (15 mL)
Muro-128®: 2% (15 mL), 5% (15 mL, 30 mL)

Tablet: 1 g

sodium citrate and potassium citrate mixture

(SOW dee um SIT rate & poe TASS ee um SIT rate MIKS chur)

U.S./Canadian Brand Names Polycitra® [US]

Therapeutic Category Alkalinizing Agent

Use Conditions where long-term maintenance of an alkaline urine is desirable as in control and dissolution of uric acid and cystine calculi of the urinary tract

Usual Dosage Oral:

Children: 5-15 mL diluted in water after meals and at bedtime

Adults: 15-30 mL diluted in water after meals and at bedtime

Dosage Forms

Solution, oral (Polycitra®-LC): Sodium citrate 500 mg and citric acid 334 mg with potassium citrate 550 mg per 5 mL [sugar free]

Syrup, oral (Polycitra®): Sodium citrate 500 mg and citric acid 334 mg with potassium citrate 550 mg per 5 mL

sodium edetate *see* edetate disodium *on page 222*

sodium ethacrynate *see* ethacrynic acid *on page 243*

sodium etidronate *see* etidronate disodium *on page 258*

sodium fusidate *see* fusidic acid *(Canada only) on page 291*

sodium hyaluronate (SOW dee um hye al yoor ON nate)
Synonyms hyaluronic acid
U.S./Canadian Brand Names Biolon® [US/Can]; Cystistat® [Can]; Eyestil [Can]; Healon® [Can]; Healon® GV [Can]; Hyalgan® [US]; Provisc® [US]; Supartz® [US]; Suplasyn® [Can]; Vitrax® [US]
Therapeutic Category Ophthalmic Agent, Viscoelastic
Use Surgical aid in cataract extraction, intraocular implantation, corneal transplant, glaucoma filtration, and retinal attachment surgery

Intra-articular injection (Hyalgan®, Suppartz®): Treatment of pain in osteoarthritis in knee in patients who have failed nonpharmacologic treatment and simple analgesics
Usual Dosage Depends upon procedure
Dosage Forms
Injection (Hyalgan®, Supartz®): 10 mg/mL (2 mL, 2.5 mL)
Liquid:
Biolon®: 10 mg/mL (0.5 mL, 1 mL)
Provisc®: 10 mg/mL (0.4 mL, 0.55 mL, 0.85 mL)
Vitrax®: 30 mg/mL (0.65 mL)

sodium hyaluronate-chrondroitin sulfate *see* chondroitin sulfate-sodium hyaluronate *on page 144*

sodium hyaluronate/hylan G-F 20
(SOW dee um hye al yoor ON ate/HYE lan gee-eff TWEN tee)
U.S./Canadian Brand Names Synvisc® [US/Can]
Therapeutic Category Miscellaneous Product
Use Treatment of pain in osteoarthritis of the knee in patients who have failed to respond adequately to conservative nonpharmacologic therapy and simple analgesics
Usual Dosage The recommended treatment regimen is 3 injections in the knee, 1 week apart. To achieve maximum effect, it is essential to administer all 3 injections. The maximum recommended dosage is 6 injections within 6 months, with a minimum of 4 weeks between treatment regimens. The duration of effect for those patients who respond to treatment is generally 12 to 26 weeks, although shorter and longer periods have also been observed. Synvisc® does not produce a general systemic effect.
Dosage Forms Injection: Hylan polymers 16 mg/2 mL; Each mL contains: hylan 8 mg, sodium chloride 8.5 mg, disodium hydrogen phosphate 0.16 mg, sodium dihydrogen phosphate hydrate 0.04 mg, sterile water for injection USP q.s.

sodium hydrogen carbonate *see* sodium bicarbonate *on page 594*

sodium hypochlorite solution
(SOW dee um hye poe KLOR ite soe LOO shun)
Synonyms Dakin's solution; modified Dakin's solution
Therapeutic Category Disinfectant
Use Treatment of athlete's foot (0.5%); wound irrigation (0.5%); to disinfect utensils and equipment (5%)
Usual Dosage Topical irrigation
Dosage Forms
Solution, topical: 5% (4000 mL)
Solution, topical (Dakin's):
Full strength: 0.5% (1000 mL)
Half strength: 0.25% (1000 mL)
Quarter strength: 0.125% (1000 mL)

sodium lactate (SOW dee um LAK tate)
Therapeutic Category Alkalinizing Agent
Use Source of bicarbonate for prevention and treatment of mild to moderate metabolic acidosis
(Continued)

sodium lactate *(Continued)*

Usual Dosage Dosage depends on degree of acidosis

Dosage Forms

Injection:

560 mg/mL [sodium 5 mEq sodium and lactate 5 mEq per mL] (10 mL, 500 mL)

1.87 g/100 mL [sodium 16.7 mEq and lactate 16.7 mEq per 100 mL] (1000 mL)

sodium nitroferricyanide *see* nitroprusside *on page 463*

Sodium P.A.S.® *(Discontinued) see page 814*

sodium-pca and lactic acid *see* lactic acid and sodium-PCA *on page 371*

sodium phenylacetate and sodium benzoate

(SOW dee um fen il AS e tate & SOW dee um BENZ oh ate)

U.S./Canadian Brand Names Ucephan® [US]

Therapeutic Category Ammonium Detoxicant

Use Adjunctive therapy to prevent/treat hyperammonemia in patients with urea cycle enzymopathy involving partial or complete deficiencies of carbamoyl-phosphate synthetase, ornithine transcarbamoylase or argininosuccinate synthetase

Usual Dosage Infants and Children: Oral: 2.5 mL (250 mg sodium benzoate and 250 mg sodium phenylacetate)/kg/day divided 3-6 times/day; total daily dose should not exceed 100 mL

Dosage Forms Solution: Sodium phenylacetate 100 mg and sodium benzoate 100 mg per mL (100 mL)

sodium phenylbutyrate (SOW dee um fen il BYOO ti rate)

Synonyms ammonapse

U.S./Canadian Brand Names Buphenyl® [US]

Therapeutic Category Miscellaneous Product

Use Adjunctive therapy in the chronic management of patients with urea cycle disorder involving deficiencies of carbamoylphosphate synthetase, ornithine transcarbamylase, or argininosuccinic acid synthetase

Usual Dosage

Powder: Patients weighing <20 kg: 450-600 mg/kg/day or 9.9-13 g/m^2/day, administered in equally divided amounts with each meal or feeding, 4-6 times/day; safety and efficacy of doses >20 g/day have not been established

Tablet: Children >20 kg and Adults: 450-600 mg/kg/day or 9.9-13 g/m^2/day, administered in equally divided amounts with each meal; safety and efficacy of doses >20 g/day have not been established

Dosage Forms

Powder: 3.2 g [sodium phenylbutyrate 3 g] per **teaspoon** (500 mL, 950 mL)

Tablet: 500 mg

sodium phosphate and potassium phosphate *see* potassium phosphate and sodium phosphate *on page 533*

sodium phosphates (SOW dee um FOS fates)

U.S./Canadian Brand Names Fleet® Enema [US/Can]; Fleet® Phospho®-Soda [US/Can]; Visicol™ [US]

Therapeutic Category Electrolyte Supplement, Oral; Laxative

Use Source of phosphate in large volume I.V. fluids; short-term treatment of constipation (oral/rectal) and to evacuate the colon for rectal and bowel exams; treatment and prevention of hypophosphatemia

Usual Dosage

Normal requirements elemental phosphorus: Oral:

0-6 months: Adequate intake: 100 mg/day

6-12 months: Adequate intake: 275 mg/day

1-3 years: RDA: 460 mg

4-8 years: RDA: 500 mg
9-18 years: RDA: 1250 mg
≥19 years: RDA: 700 mg

Hypophosphatemia: It is difficult to provide concrete guidelines for the treatment of severe hypophosphatemia because the extent of total body deficits and response to therapy are difficult to predict. Aggressive doses of phosphate may result in a transient serum elevation followed by redistribution into intracellular compartments or bone tissue. Intermittent I.V. infusion should be reserved for severe depletion situations (<1 mg/dL in adults); large doses of oral phosphate may cause diarrhea and intestinal absorption may be unreliable. I.V. solutions should be infused slowly. Use caution when mixing with calcium and magnesium, precipitate may form. The following dosages are empiric guidelines. **Note:** 1 mmol phosphate = 31 mg phosphorus; 1 mg phosphorus = 0.032 mmol phosphate

Hypophosphatemia treatment: Doses listed as mmol of phosphate:
Intermittent I.V. infusion: Acute repletion or replacement:
Children:
Low dose: 0.08 mmol/kg over 6 hours; use if losses are recent and uncomplicated
Intermediate dose: 0.16-0.24 mmol/kg over 4-6 hours; use if serum phosphorus level 0.5-1 mg/dL
High dose: 0.36 mmol/kg over 6 hours; use if serum phosphorus <0.5 mg/dL
Adults: Varying dosages: 0.15-0.3 mmol/kg/dose over 12 hours; may repeat as needed to achieve desired serum level **or**
15 mmol/dose over 2 hours; use if serum phosphorus <2 mg/dL **or**
Low dose: 0.16 mmol/kg over 4-6 hours; use if serum phosphorus level 2.3-3 mg/dL
Intermediate dose: 0.32 mmol/kg over 4-6 hours; use if serum phosphorus level 1.6-2.2 mg/dL
High dose: 0.64 mmol/kg over 8-12 hours; use if serum phosphorus <1.5 mg/dL
Oral: Adults: 0.5-1 g elemental phosphorus 2-3 times/day may be used when serum phosphorus level is 1-2.5 mg/dL
Maintenance: Doses listed as mmol of phosphate:
Children:
Oral: 2-3 mmol/kg/day in divided doses
I.V.: 0.5-1.5 mmol/kg/day
Adults:
Oral: 50-150 mmol/day in divided doses
I.V.: 50-70 mmol/day

Laxative (Fleet®): Rectal:
Children 2-<5 years: One-half contents of one 2.25 oz pediatric enema
Children 5-12 years: Contents of one 2.25 oz pediatric enema, may repeat
Children ≥12 years and Adults: Contents of one 4.5 oz enema as a single dose, may repeat

Laxative (Fleet® Phospho®-Soda): Oral: Take on an empty stomach; dilute dose with 4 ounces cool water, then follow dose with 8 ounces water; **do not repeat dose within 24 hours**
Children 5-9 years: 5-10 mL as a single dose
Children 10-12 years: 10-20 mL as a single dose
Children ≥12 years and Adults: 20-45 mL as a single dose

Bowel cleansing prior to colonoscopy (Visicol™): Oral: Adults: A total of 40 tablets divided as follows:
Evening before colonoscopy: 3 tablets every 15 minutes for 6 doses, then 2 additional tablets in 15 minutes (total of 20 tablets)
3-5 hours prior to colonoscopy: 3 tablets every 15 minutes for 6 doses, then 2 additional tablets in 15 minutes (total of 20 tablets)
Note: Each dose should be taken with a minimum of 8 ounces of clear liquids. Do not repeat treatment within 7 days. Do not use additional agents, especially sodium phosphate products.
(Continued)

sodium phosphates *(Continued)*

Dosage Forms
Enema:
Fleet®: Monobasic sodium phosphate 19 g and dibasic sodium phosphate 7 g per 118 mL
Fleet® for Children: Monobasic sodium phosphate 9.5 g and dibasic sodium phosphate 3.5 g per 59 mL
Injection: Phosphate 3 mmol and sodium 4 mEq per mL (5 mL, 15 mL, 50 mL)
Solution, oral (Fleet® Phospho®-Soda): Monobasic sodium phosphate monohydrate 2.4 g and dibasic sodium phosphate heptahydrate 0.9 g per 5 mL (45 mL, 90 mL)
Tablet, oral (Visicol™): Sodium phosphate monobasic monohydrate 1.102 g and sodium phosphate dibasic anhydrous 0.398 g (1.5 g total sodium phosphate per tablet)

sodium polystyrene sulfonate

(SOW dee um pol ee STYE reen SUL fon ate)
U.S./Canadian Brand Names Kayexalate® [US/Can]; Kionex™ [US]; PMS-Sodium Polystyrene Sulfonate [Can]; SPS® [US]
Therapeutic Category Antidote
Use Treatment of hyperkalemia
Usual Dosage
Children:
Oral: 1 g/kg/dose every 6 hours
Rectal: 1 g/kg/dose every 2-6 hours (In small children and infants employ lower doses by using the practical exchange ratio of 1 mEq potassium/g of resin as the basis for calculation)
Adults:
Oral: 15 g (60 mL) 1-4 times/day
Rectal: 30-50 g every 6 hours
Dosage Forms
Powder for suspension, oral/rectal: 454 g
Suspension, oral/rectal: 1.25 g/5 mL (60 mL, 120 mL, 200 mL, 500 mL) [contains alcohol 0.3% and sorbitol 33%]

sodium salicylate (SOW dee um sa LIS i late)

Therapeutic Category Analgesic, Non-narcotic; Antipyretic
Use Treatment of minor pain or fever; arthritis
Usual Dosage Adults: Oral: 325-650 mg every 4 hours
Dosage Forms Tablet, enteric coated: 325 mg, 650 mg

Sodium Sulamyd® [US/Can] *see* sulfacetamide *on page 610*

sodium tetradecyl (SOW dee um tetra DEK il)

U.S./Canadian Brand Names Sotradecol® [US]; Trombovar® [Can]
Therapeutic Category Sclerosing Agent
Use Treatment of small, uncomplicated varicose veins of the lower extremities; endoscopic sclerotherapy in the management of bleeding esophageal varices
Usual Dosage I.V.: 0.5-2 mL of 1% (5-20 mg) for small veins; 0.5-2 mL of 3% (15-60 mg) for medium or large veins
Dosage Forms Injection, as sulfate: 1% [10 mg/mL] (2 mL); 3% [30 mg/mL] (2 mL)

sodium thiosulfate (SOW dee um thye oh SUL fate)

Therapeutic Category Antidote; Antifungal Agent
Use
Parenteral: Used alone or with sodium nitrite or amyl nitrite in cyanide poisoning or arsenic poisoning; reduce the risk of nephrotoxicity associated with cisplatin therapy; local infiltration (in diluted form) of selected chemotherapy extravasation
Topical: Treatment of tinea versicolor

Usual Dosage I.V.:
Cyanide and nitroprusside antidote:
Children <25 kg: 50 mg/kg after receiving 4.5-10 mg/kg sodium nitrite; a half dose of each may be repeated if necessary
Children >25 kg and Adults: 12.5 g after 300 mg of sodium nitrite; a half dose of each may be repeated if necessary
Cyanide poisoning: Dose should be based on determination as with nitrite, at rate of 2.5-5 mL/minute to maximum of 50 mL
Dosage Forms
Injection: 100 mg/mL (10 mL); 250 mg/mL (50 mL)
Lotion: 25% (120 mL, 180 mL) [contains isopropyl alcohol 10% and salicylic acid 1%]

Sofarin® *(Discontinued)* see page 814

Soflax™ **[Can]** see docusate on page 208

Sofra-Tulle® **[Can]** see framycetin *(Canada only)* on page 289

Solagé™ **[US/Can]** see mequinol and tretinoin on page 409

Solaquin® **[US/Can]** see hydroquinone on page 336

Solaquin Forte® **[US/Can]** see hydroquinone on page 336

Solaraze™ **[US]** see diclofenac on page 193

Solarcaine® **Aloe Extra Burn Relief [US-OTC]** see lidocaine on page 383

Solarcaine® **[US-OTC]** see benzocaine on page 77

Solatene® *(Discontinued)* see page 814

Solfoton® *(Discontinued)* see page 814

Solganal® **[US/Can]** see aurothioglucose on page 64

soluble fluorescein see fluorescein sodium on page 277

Solu-Cortef® **[US/Can]** see hydrocortisone (systemic) on page 333

Solugel® **[Can]** see benzoyl peroxide on page 79

Solu-Medrol® **[US/Can]** see methylprednisolone on page 423

Solurex L.A.® **[US]** see dexamethasone (systemic) on page 184

Soluver® **[Can]** see salicylic acid on page 581

Soluver® **Plus [Can]** see salicylic acid on page 581

Soma® **[US/Can]** see carisoprodol on page 117

Soma® **Compound [US]** see carisoprodol and aspirin on page 117

Soma® **Compound w/Codeine [US]** see carisoprodol, aspirin, and codeine on page 117

somatostatin *(Canada only)* (soe mat oh STA tin)
U.S./Canadian Brand Names Stilamin® [Can]
Therapeutic Category Variceal Bleeding (Acute) Agent
Use For the symptomatic treatment of acute bleeding from esophageal varices. Other treatment options for long-term management of the condition may be considered if necessary, once initial control has been established.
Usual Dosage Slow 250 mcg I.V. bolus injection over 3 to 5 minutes, followed by a continuous infusion at a rate of 250 mcg/hour until bleeding from the varices has stopped (usually within 12 to 24 hours). Once bleeding has been controlled, it is recommended that the infusion be continued for at least another 48 to 72 hours, or out to a maximum of 120 hours to prevent recurrent bleeding.
Dosage Forms Injection: 250 mcg, 3 mg

somatrem see human growth hormone on page 324

somatropin see human growth hormone on page 324

Sominex® **[US-OTC]** *see* diphenhydramine *on page 202*

Somnote® **[US]** *see* chloral hydrate *on page 132*

Sonata® **[US/Can]** *see* zaleplon *on page 688*

sorbitol (SOR bi tole)

U.S./Canadian Brand Names Arlex® [US]

Therapeutic Category Genitourinary Irrigant; Laxative

Use Humectant; sweetening agent; hyperosmotic laxative; facilitate the passage of sodium polystyrene sulfonate or a charcoal-toxin complex through the intestinal tract

Usual Dosage Hyperosmotic laxative (as single dose, at infrequent intervals):

Children 2-11 years:

Oral: 2 mL/kg (as 70% solution)

Rectal enema: 30-60 mL as 25% to 30% solution

Children >12 years and Adults:

Oral: 30-150 mL (as 70% solution)

Rectal enema: 120 mL as 25% to 30% solution

Adjunct to sodium polystyrene sulfonate: 15 mL as 70% solution orally until diarrhea occurs (10-20 mL/2 hours) or 20-100 mL as an oral vehicle for the sodium polystyrene sulfonate resin

When administered with charcoal: Oral:

Children: 4.3 mL/kg of 35% sorbitol with 1 g/kg of activated charcoal

Adults: 4.3 mL/kg of 70% sorbitol with 1 g/kg of activated charcoal

Dosage Forms

Solution: 70% (480 mL, 3840 mL)

Solution, genitourinary irrigation: 3% (1500 mL, 3000 mL); 3.3% (2000 mL)

Soriatane® **[US/Can]** *see* acitretin *on page 12*

Sorine™ **[US]** *see* sotalol *on this page*

Sotacor® *see* sotalol *on this page*

sotalol (SOE ta lole)

U.S./Canadian Brand Names Alti-Sotalol [Can]; Apo®-Sotalol [Can]; Betapace AF™ [US/Can]; Betapace® [US]; Gen-Sotalol [Can]; Novo-Sotalol [Can]; Nu-Sotalol [Can]; PMS-Sotalol [Can]; Rho®-Sotalol [Can]; Sorine™ [US]; Sotacor®

Therapeutic Category Antiarrhythmic Agent, Class II; Antiarrhythmic Agent, Class III; Beta-Adrenergic Blocker, Nonselective

Use Treatment of ventricular arrhythmias

Usual Dosage Sotalol should be initiated and doses increased in a hospital with facilities for cardiac rhythm monitoring and assessment. Proarrhythmic events can occur after initiation of therapy and with each upward dosage adjustment.

Children: Oral: The safety and efficacy of sotalol in children have not been established

Note: Dosing per manufacturer, based on pediatric pharmacokinetic data; wait at least 36 hours between dosage adjustments to allow monitoring of QT intervals

≤2 years: Dosage should be adjusted (deceased) by plotting of the child's age on a logarithmic scale provided by the manufacturer (refer to package labeling)

>2 years: Initial: 90 mg/m^2/day in 3 divided doses; may be incrementally increased to a maximum of 180 mg/m^2/day

Adults: Oral:

Ventricular arrhythmias (Betapace®, Sorine™):

Initial: 80 mg twice daily

Dose may be increased gradually to 240-320 mg/day; allow 3 days between dosing increments in order to attain steady-state plasma concentrations and to allow monitoring of QT intervals

Most patients respond to a total daily dose of 160-320 mg/day in 2-3 divided doses.

Some patients, with life-threatening refractory ventricular arrhythmias, may require doses as high as 480-640 mg/day; however, these doses should only be prescribed when the potential benefit outweighs the increased of adverse events.

Atrial fibrillation or atrial flutter (Betapace AF™): Initial: 80 mg twice daily

If the initial dose does not reduce the frequency of relapses of atrial fibrillation/flutter and is tolerated without excessive QT prolongation (not >520 msec) after 3 days, the dose may be increased to 120 mg twice daily This may be further increased to 160 mg twice daily if response is inadequate and QT prolongation is not excessive.

Dosage Forms Tablet, as hydrochloride:
Betapace® [light blue]: 80 mg, 120 mg, 160 mg, 240 mg
Betapace AF™ [white]: 80 mg, 120 mg, 160 mg
Sorine™ [white]: 80 mg, 120 mg, 160 mg, 240 mg

Sotradecol® [US] *see* sodium tetradecyl *on page 600*

Soyacal® [US] *see* fat emulsion *on page 263*

Soyalac® [US-OTC] *see* nutritional formula, enteral/oral *on page 472*

Spacol [US] *see* hyoscyamine *on page 339*

Spacol T/S [US] *see* hyoscyamine *on page 339*

Span-FF® *(Discontinued)* *see page 814*

sparfloxacin (spar FLOKS a sin)

U.S./Canadian Brand Names Zagam® [US]

Therapeutic Category Quinolone

Use Treatment of adult patients with community acquired pneumonia caused by susceptible strains of *Chlamydia pneumoniae*, *Haemophilus influenzae*, *Haemophilus parainfluenzae*, *Moraxella catarrhalis*, *Mycoplasma pneumoniae*, or *Streptococcus pneumoniae* and acute bacterial exacerbations of acute bronchitis caused by susceptible strains of *Chlamydia pneumoniae*, *Enterobacter cloacae*, *Haemophilus influenzae*, *Haemophilus parainfluenzae*, *Klebsiella pneumoniae*, *Moraxella catarrhalis*, *Staphylococcus aureus*, or *Streptococcus pneumoniae*

Usual Dosage Adults: Oral: 400 mg on day 1, then 200 mg/day for the next 9 days (11 tablets total). In patients with creatinine clearance <50 mL/minute, administer 400 mg on day 1, then begin 200 mg every 48 hours on day 3 for a total of 9 days (6 tablets total).

Dosage Forms Tablet: 200 mg

Sparine® *(Discontinued)* *see page 814*

Spasmoject® *(Discontinued)* *see page 814*

Spasmolin® *(Discontinued)* *see page 814*

Spec-T® *(Discontinued)* *see page 814*

Spectazole™ [US/Can] *see* econazole *on page 221*

spectinomycin (spek ti noe MYE sin)

U.S./Canadian Brand Names Trobicin® [US]

Therapeutic Category Antibiotic, Miscellaneous

Use Treatment of uncomplicated gonorrhea (ineffective against syphilis)

Usual Dosage I.M.:
Children:
<45 kg: 40 mg/kg/dose 1 time
≥45 kg: See adult dose
Children >8 years who are allergic to penicillins/cephalosporins may be treated with oral tetracycline
Adults: 2 g deep I.M. or 4 g where antibiotic resistance is prevalent 1 time; 4 g (10 mL) dose should be administered as 2-5 mL injections

Dosage Forms Injection, powder for reconstitution, as hydrochloride: 2 g

Spectracef™ **[US]** *see* cefditoren *on page 122*

Spectrobid® **Tablet** *(Discontinued) see page 814*

Spectrocin Plus® **[US-OTC]** *see* bacitracin, neomycin, polymyxin B, and lidocaine *on page 69*

Spherulin® *(Discontinued) see page 814*

spiramycin *(Canada only)* (speer a MYE sin)

U.S./Canadian Brand Names Rovamycine® [Can]

Therapeutic Category Antibiotic, Macrolide

Use Treatment of infections of the respiratory tract, buccal cavity, skin and soft tissues due to susceptible organisms. *N. gonorrheae*: as an alternate choice of treatment for gonorrhea in patients allergic to the penicillins. Before treatment of gonorrhea, the possibility of concomitant infection due to *T. pallidum* should be excluded.

Usual Dosage Oral:

Children: The usual daily dosage is based on 150,000 units/kg body weight in 2 or 3 divided doses

Adults: 6,000,000-9,000,000 units per 24 hours, in 2 divided doses; in severe infections, the daily dosage may be increased to 12,000,000-15,000,000 units per day

Gonorrhea: 12,000,000-13,500000 units in a single dose.

Dosage Forms Capsule:

Rovamycine® "250": 750,000 int. units

Rovamycine® "500": 1,500,000 int. units

spirapril (SPYE ra pril)

U.S./Canadian Brand Names Renormax® [US]

Therapeutic Category Angiotensin-Converting Enzyme (ACE) Inhibitor

Use Management of mild to severe hypertension

Usual Dosage Adults: Oral: 12 mg/day in 1-2 divided doses

Dosage Forms Tablet: 3 mg, 6 mg, 12 mg, 24 mg

Spironazide® *(Discontinued) see page 814*

spironolactone (speer on oh LAK tone)

U.S./Canadian Brand Names Aldactone® [US/Can]; Novo-Spiroton [Can]

Therapeutic Category Diuretic, Potassium Sparing

Use Management of edema associated with excessive aldosterone excretion; hypertension; primary hyperaldosteronism; hypokalemia; treatment of hirsutism

Usual Dosage Oral:

Children: 1.5-3.5 mg/kg/day in divided doses every 6-24 hours

Diagnosis of primary aldosteronism: 125-375 mg/m^2/day in divided doses

Vaso-occlusive disease: 7.5 mg/kg/day in divided doses twice daily (non-FDA approved dose)

Adults:

Edema, hypertension, hypokalemia: 25-200 mg/day in 1-2 divided doses

Diagnosis of primary aldosteronism: 100-400 mg/day in 1-2 divided doses

Dosage Forms Tablet: 25 mg, 50 mg, 100 mg

spironolactone and hydrochlorothiazide *see* hydrochlorothiazide and spironolactone *on page 329*

Spirozide® *(Discontinued) see page 814*

Sporanox® **[US/Can]** *see* itraconazole *on page 364*

Sportscreme® **[US-OTC]** *see* triethanolamine salicylate *on page 654*

Sportsmed® **[US]** *see* capsaicin *on page 111*

SPS® **[US]** *see* sodium polystyrene sulfonate *on page 600*

SRC® **Expectorant** *(Discontinued) see page 814*

SSD® AF [US] *see* silver sulfadiazine *on page 590*

SSD® Cream [US/Can] *see* silver sulfadiazine *on page 590*

SSKI® [US] *see* potassium iodide *on page 531*

ST1571 *see* imatinib *on page 345*

Stadol® [US] *see* butorphanol *on page 101*

Stadol® NS [US/Can] *see* butorphanol *on page 101*

Stagesic® [US] *see* hydrocodone and acetaminophen *on page 329*

Stahist® *(Discontinued)* *see page 814*

stanozolol (stan OH zoe lole)
  U.S./Canadian Brand Names Winstrol® [US]
  Therapeutic Category Anabolic Steroid
  Controlled Substance C-III
  Use Prophylactic use against angioedema
  Usual Dosage
    Children: Acute attacks:
    <6 years: 1 mg/day
    6-12 years: 2 mg/day
    Adults: Oral: Initial: 2 mg 3 times/day, may then reduce to a maintenance dose of 2 mg/day or 2 mg every other day after 1-3 months
  Dosage Forms Tablet: 2 mg

Staphcillin® *(Discontinued)* *see page 814*

Starlix® [US] *see* nateglinide *on page 449*

Starnoc® [Can] *see* zaleplon *on page 688*

Statex® [Can] *see* morphine sulfate *on page 437*

Staticin® [US] *see* erythromycin (ophthalmic/topical) *on page 235*

Statobex® *(Discontinued)* *see page 814*

stavudine (STAV yoo deen)
  Synonyms d4T
  U.S./Canadian Brand Names Zerit® [US/Can]
  Therapeutic Category Antiviral Agent
  Use Treatment of advanced HIV infection in patients who experience intolerance, toxicity, resistance, or HIV disease progression with either zidovudine or didanosine therapy; active against most zidovudine-resistant strains; in adults, stavudine used alone in patients with 50-500 CD4 cells/mm^3 and at least 6 months previous treatment with zidovudine was more effective than continued zidovudine in preventing disease progression and death
  Usual Dosage Oral:
    Children 7 months to 15 years: 1-2 mg/kg/day divided twice daily
    Adults: 0.5-1 mg/kg/day **or**
    <60 kg: 30 mg every 12 hours
    ≥60 kg: 40 mg every 12 hours
    If peripheral neuropathy or elevations in liver enzymes occur, stavudine should be discontinued; once adverse effects resolve, reinitiate therapy at a lower dose of 20 mg every 12 hours (for ≥60 kg patients) or 15 mg every 12 hours (for <60 kg patients)
  Dosage Forms
    Capsule: 15 mg, 20 mg, 30 mg, 40 mg
    Powder, oral solution: 1 mg/mL (200 mL)

S-T Cort® [US] *see* hydrocortisone (topical) *on page 334*

Stelazine® [US] *see* trifluoperazine *on page 655*

Stemetil® [Can] *see* prochlorperazine *on page 542*

Stemex® *(Discontinued)* see page 814

Sterapred® [US] see prednisone on page 538

Sterapred® DS [US] see prednisone on page 538

Stilamin® [Can] see somatostatin *(Canada only)* on page 601

stilbestrol see diethylstilbestrol on page 196

Stilphostrol® [US] see diethylstilbestrol on page 196

Stimate™ [US] see desmopressin acetate on page 182

St. Joseph® Cough Suppressant [US-OTC] see dextromethorphan on page 189

St. Joseph® Measured Dose Nasal Solution *(Discontinued)* see page 814

St. Joseph® Pain Reliever [US-OTC] see aspirin on page 58

Stop® [US-OTC] see fluoride on page 278

Streptase® [US/Can] see streptokinase on this page

streptokinase (strep toe KYE nase)

Synonyms SK

U.S./Canadian Brand Names Streptase® [US/Can]

Therapeutic Category Fibrinolytic Agent

Use Thrombolytic agent used in treatment of recent severe or massive deep vein thrombosis, pulmonary emboli, myocardial infarction, and occluded arteriovenous cannulas

Usual Dosage I.V.:

Children: Safety and efficacy not established; limited studies have used: 3500-4000 units/kg over 30 minutes followed by 1000-1500 units/kg/hour; clotted catheter: 25,000 units, clamp for 2 hours then aspirate contents and flush with normal saline

Adults (best results are realized if used within 5-6 hours of myocardial infarction; antibodies to streptokinase remain for 3-6 months after initial dose, use another thrombolytic enzyme, ie, urokinase, if thrombolytic therapy is indicated):

Guidelines for Acute Myocardial Infarction (AMI):

1.5 million units infused over 60 minutes. Monitor for the first few hours for signs of anaphylaxis or allergic reaction. **Infusion should be slowed if lowering of 25 mm Hg in blood pressure or terminated if asthmatic symptoms appear.** Begin heparin 5000-10,000 unit bolus followed by 1000 units/hour approximately 3-4 hours after completion of streptokinase infusion or when PTT is <100 seconds.

Guidelines for Acute Pulmonary Embolism (APE):

3 million unit dose; administer 250,000 units over 30 minutes followed by 100,000 units/hour for 24 hours. Monitor for the first few hours for signs of anaphylaxis or allergic reaction. **Infusion should be slowed if blood pressure is lowered by 25 mm Hg or if asthmatic symptoms appear.** Begin heparin 1000 units/hour approximately 3-4 hours after completion of streptokinase infusion or when PTT is <100 seconds.

Thromboses: 250,000 units to start, then 100,000 units/hour for 24-72 hours depending on location

Cannula occlusion: 250,000 units into cannula, clamp for 2 hours, then aspirate contents and flush with normal saline. **Not recommended**

Dosage Forms Injection, powder for reconstitution: 250,000 units, 750,000 units, 1,500,000 units

streptomycin (strep toe MYE sin)

Therapeutic Category Antibiotic, Aminoglycoside; Antitubercular Agent

Use Combination therapy of active tuberculosis; used in combination with other agents for treatment of streptococcal or enterococcal endocarditis, mycobacterial infections, plague, tularemia, and brucellosis. Streptomycin is indicated for persons from endemic areas of drug-resistant *Mycobacterium tuberculosis* or who are HIV infected.

Usual Dosage Intramuscular (may also be given intravenous piggyback):

Tuberculosis therapy: **Note:** A four-drug regimen (isoniazid, rifampin, pyrazinamide and either streptomycin or ethambutol) is preferred for the initial, empiric treatment of TB. When the drug susceptibility results are available, the regimen should be altered as appropriate.

Patients with TB and without HIV infection:

OPTION 1:

Isoniazid resistance rate <4%: Administer daily isoniazid, rifampin, and pyrazinamide for 8 weeks followed by isoniazid and rifampin daily or directly observed therapy (DOT) 2-3 times/week for 16 weeks

If isoniazid resistance rate is not documented, ethambutol or streptomycin should also be administered until susceptibility to isoniazid or rifampin is demonstrated. Continue treatment for at least 6 months or 3 months beyond culture conversion.

OPTION 2: Administer daily isoniazid, rifampin, pyrazinamide, and either streptomycin or ethambutol for 2 weeks followed by DOT 2 times/week administration of the same drugs for 6 weeks, and subsequently, with isoniazid and rifampin DOT 2 times/week administration for 16 weeks

OPTION 3: Administer isoniazid, rifampin, pyrazinamide, and either ethambutol or streptomycin by DOT 3 times/week for 6 months

Patients with TB and with HIV infection: Administer any of the above OPTIONS 1, 2 or 3, however, treatment should be continued for a total of 9 months and at least 6 months beyond culture conversion

Note: Some experts recommend that the duration of therapy should be extended to 9 months for patients with disseminated disease, miliary disease, disease involving the bones or joints, or tuberculosis lymphadenitis

Children:

Daily therapy: 20-30 mg/kg/day (maximum: 1 g/day)

Directly observed therapy (DOT): Twice weekly: 25-30 mg/kg (maximum: 1.5 g)

DOT: 3 times/week: 25-30 mg/kg (maximum: 1 g)

Adults:

Daily therapy: 15 mg/kg/day (maximum: 1 g)

Directly observed therapy (DOT): Twice weekly: 25-30 mg/kg (maximum: 1.5 g)

DOT: 3 times/week: 25-30 mg/kg (maximum: 1 g)

Enterococcal endocarditis: 1 g every 12 hours for 2 weeks, 500 mg every 12 hours for 4 weeks in combination with penicillin

Streptococcal endocarditis: 1 g every 12 hours for 1 week, 500 mg every 12 hours for 1 week

Tularemia: 1-2 g/day in divided doses for 7-10 days or until patient is afebrile for 5-7 days

Plague: 2-4 g/day in divided doses until the patient is afebrile for at least 3 days

Dosage Forms Injection, as sulfate: 400 mg/mL (2.5 mL) [1 g vial]

streptozocin (strep toe ZOE sin)

U.S./Canadian Brand Names Zanosar® [US/Can]

Therapeutic Category Antineoplastic Agent

Use Treat metastatic islet cell carcinoma of the pancreas, carcinoid tumor and syndrome, Hodgkin's disease, palliative treatment of colorectal cancer

Usual Dosage Children and Adults: I.V.: 500 mg/m^2 for 5 days every 6 weeks until optimal benefit or toxicity occurs; or may be administered in single dose 1000 mg/m^2 at weekly intervals for 2 doses, then increased to 1500 mg/m^2 weekly; the median total dose to onset of response is about 2000 mg/m^2 and the median total dose to maximum response is about 4000 mg/m^2

Dosage Forms Injection: 1 g

Stresstabs® 600 Advanced Formula [US-OTC] *see* vitamin (multiple/oral) *on page 683*

Strifon Forte® [Can] *see* chlorzoxazone *on page 142*

Stromectol® [US] *see* ivermectin *on page 364*

strong iodine solution *see* potassium iodide *on page 531*

strontium-89 (STRON shee um-atey nine)
U.S./Canadian Brand Names Metastron® [US/Can]
Therapeutic Category Radiopharmaceutical
Use Relief of bone pain in patients with skeletal metastases
Usual Dosage Adults: I.V.: 148 megabecquerel (4 millicurie) administered by slow I.V. injection over 1-2 minutes or 1.5-2.2 megabecquerel (40-60 microcurie)/kg; repeated doses are generally not recommended at intervals <90 days
Dosage Forms Injection, as chloride: 10.9-22.6 mg/mL [148 megabecquerel, 4 millicurie] (10 mL)

Stuartnatal® Plus 3™ [US-OTC] *see* vitamin (multiple/prenatal) *on page 683*

Stuart Prenatal® [US-OTC] *see* vitamin (multiple/prenatal) *on page 683*

Sublimaze® [US] *see* fentanyl *on page 266*

succimer (SUKS i mer)
U.S./Canadian Brand Names Chemet® [US/Can]
Therapeutic Category Chelating Agent
Use Treatment of lead poisoning in children with blood levels >45 mcg/dL. It is not indicated for prophylaxis of lead poisoning in a lead-containing environment.
Usual Dosage Children and Adults: Oral: 30 mg/kg/day in divided doses every 8 hours for an additional 5 days followed by 20 mg/kg/day for 14 days
Dosage Forms Capsule: 100 mg

succinate mafenide acetate *see* mafenide *on page 396*

succinylcholine (suks in il KOE leen)
Synonyms suxamethonium
U.S./Canadian Brand Names Anectine® Chloride [US]; Anectine® Flo-Pack® [US]; Quelicin® [US/Can]
Therapeutic Category Skeletal Muscle Relaxant
Use Produces skeletal muscle relaxation in procedures of short duration such as endotracheal intubation or endoscopic exams
Usual Dosage I.M., I.V.:
Children: 1-2 mg/kg
Intermittent: Initial: 1 mg/kg/dose one time; maintenance: 0.3-0.6 mg/kg every 5-10 minutes as needed
Adults: 0.6 mg/kg (range: 0.3-1.1 mg/kg) over 10-30 seconds, up to 150 mg total dose
Maintenance: 0.04-0.07 mg/kg every 5-10 minutes as needed
Continuous infusion: 2.5 mg/minute (or 0.5-10 mg/minute); dilute to concentration of 1-2 mg/mL in D_5W or NS
Note: Pretreatment with atropine may reduce occurrence of bradycardia
Dosage Forms
Injection, as chloride: 20 mg/mL (10 mL); 50 mg/mL (10 mL); 100 mg/mL (5 mL, 10 mL, 20 mL)
Injection, powder for reconstitution, as chloride: 500 mg, 1 g

Sucostrin® *(Discontinued)* *see page 814*

Sucraid™ [US/Can] *see* sacrosidase *on page 580*

sucralfate (soo KRAL fate)

Synonyms aluminum sucrose sulfate, basic

U.S./Canadian Brand Names Apo®-Sucralate [Can]; Carafate® [US]; Novo-Sucralate [Can]; Nu-Sucralate [Can]; PMS-Sucralate [Can]; Sulcrate® [Can]; Sulcrate® Suspension Plus [Can]

Therapeutic Category Gastrointestinal Agent, Gastric or Duodenal Ulcer Treatment

Use Short-term management of duodenal ulcers; gastric ulcers; suspension may be used topically for treatment of stomatitis due to cancer chemotherapy or other causes of esophageal and gastric erosions

Usual Dosage

Children: Dose not established, doses of 40-80 mg/kg/day divided every 6 hours have been used

Stomatitis: Oral: 2.5-5 mL (1 g/10 mL suspension), swish and spit or swish and swallow 4 times/day

Adults:

Duodenal ulcer treatment: Oral: 1 g 4 times/day, 1 hour before meals or food and at bedtime for 4-8 weeks, or alternatively 2 g twice daily

Duodenal ulcer maintenance therapy: Oral: 1 g twice daily

Stomatitis: Oral: 1 g/10 mL suspension, swish and spit or swish and swallow 4 times/day

Dosage Forms

Suspension, oral: 1 g/10 mL (10 mL, 420 mL)

Tablet: 1 g

Sucrets® Cough Calmers *(Discontinued)* see page 814

Sucrets® Sore Throat [US-OTC] see hexylresorcinol on page 321

Sucrets® [US-OTC] see dyclonine on page 220

Sudafed® 12 Hour [US-OTC] see pseudoephedrine on page 552

Sudafed® Children's [US-OTC] see pseudoephedrine on page 552

Sudafed® Cold & Allergy [US-OTC] see chlorpheniramine and pseudoephedrine on page 138

Sudafed® Cold and Sinus [US-OTC] see acetaminophen and pseudoephedrine on page 6

Sudafed® Cold & Cough Extra Strength [Can] see acetaminophen, dextromethorphan, and pseudoephedrine on page 8

Sudafed® Cough *(Discontinued)* see page 814

Sudafed® Decongestant [Can] see pseudoephedrine on page 552

Sudafed® Head Cold and Sinus Extra Strength [Can] see acetaminophen and pseudoephedrine on page 6

Sudafed Plus® Liquid *(Discontinued)* see page 814

Sudafed® Severe Cold [US-OTC] see acetaminophen, dextromethorphan, and pseudoephedrine on page 8

Sudafed® Sinus Headache [US-OTC] see acetaminophen and pseudoephedrine on page 6

Sudafed® [US-OTC] see pseudoephedrine on page 552

Sudex® *(Discontinued)* see page 814

Sufedrin® *(Discontinued)* see page 814

Sufenta® [US/Can] see sufentanil on this page

sufentanil (soo FEN ta nil)

U.S./Canadian Brand Names Sufenta® [US/Can]

Therapeutic Category Analgesic, Narcotic; General Anesthetic

Controlled Substance C-II

(Continued)

sufentanil *(Continued)*

Use Analgesia; analgesia adjunct; anesthetic agent

Usual Dosage I.V.:

Children <12 years: 10-25 mcg/kg with 100% O_2, maintenance: 25-50 mcg as needed (total dose of up to 1-2 mcg/kg)

Adults: Dose should be based on body weight. **Note:** In obese patients (ie, >20% above ideal body weight), use lean body weight to determine dosage

1-2 mcg/kg with N_2O/O_2 for endotracheal intubation; maintenance: 10-25 mcg as needed

2-8 mcg/kg with N_2O/O_2 more complicated major surgical procedures; maintenance: 10-50 mcg as needed

8-30 mcg/kg with 100% O_2 and muscle relaxant produces sleep; at doses of ≥8 mcg/kg maintains a deep level of anesthesia; maintenance: 10-50 mcg as needed

Dosage Forms Injection, as citrate: 50 mcg/mL (1 mL, 2 mL, 5 mL)

Sular® **[US]** *see* nisoldipine *on page 460*

sulbactam and ampicillin *see* ampicillin and sulbactam *on page 41*

sulconazole *(sul KON a zole)*

U.S./Canadian Brand Names Exelderm® [US/Can]

Therapeutic Category Antifungal Agent

Use Treatment of superficial fungal infections of the skin, including tinea cruris, tinea corporis, tinea versicolor and possibly tinea pedis

Usual Dosage Topical: Apply once or twice daily for 4-6 weeks

Dosage Forms

Cream, as nitrate: 1% (15 g, 30 g, 60 g)

Solution, topical, as nitrate: 1% (30 mL)

Sulcrate® **[Can]** *see* sucralfate *on previous page*

Sulcrate® Suspension Plus [Can] *see* sucralfate *on previous page*

Sulf-10® **[US]** *see* sulfacetamide *on this page*

sulfabenzamide, sulfacetamide, and sulfathiazole

(sul fa BENZ a mide, sul fa SEE ta mide, & sul fa THYE a zole)

Synonyms sulfacetamide, sulfabenzamide, and sulfathiazole; sulfathiazole, sulfacetamide, and sulfabenzamide; triple sulfa

U.S./Canadian Brand Names V.V.S.® [US]

Therapeutic Category Antibiotic, Vaginal

Use Treatment of *Haemophilus vaginalis* vaginitis

Usual Dosage Adults: Vaginal:

Cream: Insert 1 applicatorful in vagina twice daily for 4-6 days; dosage may then be decreased to $1/2$ to $1/4$ of an applicatorful twice daily

Tablet: Insert 1 intravaginally twice daily for 10 days

Dosage Forms

Cream, vaginal: Sulfabenzamide 3.7%, sulfacetamide 2.86%, and sulfathiazole 3.42% (78 g [with applicator], 90 g, 120 g)

Tablet, vaginal: Sulfabenzamide 184 mg, sulfacetamide 143.75 mg, and sulfathiazole 172.5 mg [with applicator] (20 tablets/box)

sulfacetamide *(sul fa SEE ta mide)*

U.S./Canadian Brand Names AK-Sulf® [US]; Bleph®-10 [US]; Carmol® Scalp [US]; Cetamide® [US/Can]; Diosulf™ [Can]; Klaron® [US]; Ocu-Sul® [US]; Sebizon® [US]; Sodium Sulamyd® [US/Can]; Sulf-10® [US]

Therapeutic Category Antibiotic, Ophthalmic

Use Treatment and prophylaxis of conjunctivitis, corneal ulcers, and other superficial ocular infections due to susceptible organisms; adjunctive treatment with systemic sulfonamides for therapy of trachoma

Usual Dosage Children >2 months and Adults: Ophthalmic:
Ointment: Apply to lower conjunctival sac 1-4 times/day and at bedtime
Solution: 1-2 drops every 2-3 hours in the lower conjunctival sac during the waking hours and less frequently at night
Dosage Forms
Lotion, as sodium: 10% (59 mL, 85 g)
Ointment, ophthalmic, as sodium: 10% (3.5 g)
Solution, ophthalmic, as sodium: 10% (1 mL, 2 mL, 2.5 mL, 5 mL, 15 mL); 15% (5 mL, 15 mL); 30% (15 mL)

sulfacetamide and prednisolone (sul fa SEE ta mide & pred NIS oh lone)
Synonyms prednisolone and sulfacetamide
U.S./Canadian Brand Names AK-Cide® [US]; Blephamide® [US/Can]; Dioptimyd® [Can]; Metimyd® [US]; Vasocidin® [US/Can]
Therapeutic Category Antibiotic/Corticosteroid, Ophthalmic
Use Steroid-responsive inflammatory ocular conditions where infection is present or there is a risk of infection; ophthalmic suspension may be used as an otic preparation
Usual Dosage Children >2 and Adults: Ophthalmic:
Ointment: Apply to lower conjunctival sac 1-4 times/day
Solution: Instill 1-3 drops every 2-3 hours while awake
Dosage Forms
Ointment, ophthalmic:
AK-Cide®, Metimyd®, Vasocidin®: Sulfacetamide sodium 10% and prednisolone acetate 0.5% (3.5 g)
Blephamide®: Sulfacetamide sodium 10% and prednisolone acetate 0.2% (3.5 g)
Suspension, ophthalmic: Sulfacetamide sodium 10% and prednisolone sodium phosphate 0.25% (5 mL)
AK-Cide®, Metimyd®: Sulfacetamide sodium 10% and prednisolone acetate 0.5% (5 mL)
Blephamide®: Sulfacetamide sodium 10% and prednisolone acetate 0.2% (2.5 mL, 5 mL, 10 mL)
Vasocidin®: Sulfacetamide sodium 10% and prednisolone sodium phosphate: 0.25% (5 mL, 10 mL)

sulfacetamide and sulfur *see* sulfur and sulfacetamide *on page 615*

sulfacetamide sodium and fluorometholone
(sul fa SEE ta mide SOW dee um & flure oh METH oh lone)
Synonyms fluorometholone and sulfacetamide
U.S./Canadian Brand Names FML-S® [US]
Therapeutic Category Antibiotic/Corticosteroid, Ophthalmic
Use Steroid-responsive inflammatory ocular conditions where infection is present or there is a risk of infection
Usual Dosage Children >2 months and Adults: Ophthalmic: Instill 1-3 drops every 2-3 hours while awake
Dosage Forms Suspension, ophthalmic: Sulfacetamide sodium 10% and fluorometholone 0.1% (5 mL, 10 mL)

sulfacetamide, sulfabenzamide, and sulfathiazole *see* sulfabenzamide, sulfacetamide, and sulfathiazole *on previous page*

Sulfacet-R® [US] *see* sulfur and sulfacetamide *on page 615*

sulfadiazine (sul fa DYE a zeen)
Tall-Man sulfaDIAZINE
Therapeutic Category Sulfonamide
Use Adjunctive treatment in toxoplasmosis; treatment of urinary tract infections and nocardiosis; rheumatic fever prophylaxis in penicillin-allergic patient; uncomplicated attack of malaria
(Continued)

sulfadiazine *(Continued)*

Usual Dosage Oral:

Congenital toxoplasmosis:

Newborns and Children <2 months: 100 mg/kg/day divided every 6 hours in conjunction with pyrimethamine 1 mg/kg/day once daily and supplemental folinic acid 5 mg every 3 days for 6 months

Children >2 months: 25-50 mg/kg/dose 4 times/day

Toxoplasmosis:

Children: 120-150 mg/kg/day, maximum dose: 6 g/day; divided every 6 hours in conjunction with pyrimethamine 2 mg/kg/day divided every 12 hours for 3 days followed by 1 mg/kg/day once daily (maximum: 25 mg/day) with supplemental folinic acid

Adults: 2-8 g/day divided every 6 hours in conjunction with pyrimethamine 25 mg/day and with supplemental folinic acid

Dosage Forms Tablet: 500 mg

sulfadoxine and pyrimethamine (sul fa DOKS een & peer i METH a meen)

U.S./Canadian Brand Names Fansidar® [US]

Therapeutic Category Antimalarial Agent

Use Treatment of *Plasmodium falciparum* malaria in patients in whom chloroquine resistance is suspected; malaria prophylaxis for travelers to areas where chloroquine-resistant malaria is endemic

Usual Dosage Children and Adults: Oral:

Treatment of acute attack of malaria: A single dose of the following number of Fansidar® tablets is used in sequence with quinine or alone:

2-11 months: 1/4 tablet

1-3 years: 1/2 tablet

4-8 years: 1 tablet

9-14 years: 2 tablets

>14 years: 3 tablets

Malaria prophylaxis: A single dose should be carried for self-treatment in the event of febrile illness when medical attention is not immediately available:

2-11 months: 1/4 tablet

1-3 years: 1/2 tablet

4-8 years: 1 tablet

9-14 years: 2 tablets

>14 years and Adults: 3 tablets

Dosage Forms Tablet: Sulfadoxine 500 mg and pyrimethamine 25 mg

Sulfa-Gyn® *(Discontinued)* see page 814

Sulfamethoprim® *(Discontinued)* see page 814

sulfamethoxazole and trimethoprim

(sul fa meth OKS a zole & trye METH oh prim)

Synonyms co-trimoxazole; SMX-TMP; TMP-SMX; trimethoprim and sulfamethoxazole

U.S./Canadian Brand Names Apo®-Sulfatrim [Can]; Bactrim™ DS [US]; Bactrim™ [US]; Novo-Trimel [Can]; Novo-Trimel D.S. [Can]; Nu-Cotrimox® [Can]; Septra® DS [US/Can]; Septra® [US/Can]; Sulfatrim® DS [US]; Sulfatrim® [US]

Therapeutic Category Sulfonamide

Use Treatment of urinary tract infections caused by susceptible *E. coli, Klebsiella, Enterobacter, Proteus mirabilis, Proteus* (indole positive); acute otitis media due to amoxicillin-resistant *H. influenzae, S. pneumoniae,* and *M. catarrhalis*; acute exacerbations of chronic bronchitis; prophylaxis and treatment of *Pneumocystis carinii* pneumonitis (PCP); treatment of susceptible shigellosis, typhoid fever, *Nocardia asteroides* infection, and *Xanthomonas maltophilia* infection; the I.V. preparation is used for treatment of *Pneumocystis carinii* pneumonitis, *Shigella,* and severe urinary tract infections

Usual Dosage Oral, I.V. (dosage recommendations are based on the trimethoprim component):

Children >2 months:

Mild to moderate infections: 6-12 mg TMP/kg/day in divided doses every 12 hours

Serious infection/*Pneumocystis*: 15-20 mg TMP/kg/day in divided doses every 6 hours

Urinary tract infection prophylaxis: 2 mg TMP/kg/dose daily

Prophylaxis of *Pneumocystis*: 5-10 mg TMP/kg/day or 150 mg TMP/m^2/day in divided doses every 12 hours 3 days/week; dose should not exceed 320 mg trimethoprim and 1600 mg sulfamethoxazole 3 days/week; Mon, Tue, Wed

Adults: Urinary tract infection/chronic bronchitis: 1 double strength tablet every 12 hours for 10-14 days

Dosage Forms The 5:1 ratio (SMX:TMP) remains constant in all dosage forms:

Injection: Sulfamethoxazole 80 mg and trimethoprim 16 mg per mL (5 mL, 10 mL, 20 mL, 30 mL, 50 mL)

Suspension, oral: Sulfamethoxazole 200 mg and trimethoprim 40 mg per 5 mL (20 mL, 100 mL, 150 mL, 200 mL, 480 mL)

Tablet: Sulfamethoxazole 400 mg and trimethoprim 80 mg

Tablet, double strength: Sulfamethoxazole 800 mg and trimethoprim 160 mg

Sulfamylon® [US] *see* mafenide *on page 396*

sulfanilamide (sul fa NIL a mide)

U.S./Canadian Brand Names AVC™ [US/Can]

Therapeutic Category Antifungal Agent

Use Treatment of vulvovaginitis caused by *Candida albicans*

Usual Dosage Vaginal: 1 applicatorful once or twice daily continued through 1 complete menstrual cycle

Dosage Forms

Cream, vaginal [with applicator]: 15% [150 mg/g] (120 g)

Suppository, vaginal: 1.05 g (16s)

sulfasalazine (sul fa SAL a zeen)

Synonyms salicylazosulfapyridine

U.S./Canadian Brand Names Alti-Sulfasalazine® [Can]; Azulfidine® EN-tabs® [US]; Azulfidine® Tablet [US]; Salazopyrin® [Can]; Salazopyrin En-Tabs® [Can]; S.A.S.™ [Can]

Therapeutic Category 5-Aminosalicylic Acid Derivative

Use Management of ulcerative colitis; treatment of active Crohn's disease

Usual Dosage Oral:

Children >2 years:

Initial: 40-60 mg/kg/day divided every 4-6 hour

Maintenance dose: 20-30 mg/kg/day divided every 6 hours, up to a maximum of 2 g/day

Adults:

Initial: 3-4 g/day divided every 4-6 hours

Maintenance dose: 2 g/day divided every 6 hours

Dosage Forms

Tablet: 500 mg

Tablet, enteric coated: 500 mg

sulfathiazole, sulfacetamide, and sulfabenzamide *see* sulfabenzamide, sulfacetamide, and sulfathiazole *on page 610*

Sulfatrim® [US] *see* sulfamethoxazole and trimethoprim *on previous page*

Sulfatrim® DS [US] *see* sulfamethoxazole and trimethoprim *on previous page*

Sulfa-Trip® *(Discontinued)* *see page 814*

sulfinpyrazone (sul fin PEER a zone)

U.S./Canadian Brand Names Anturane® [US]; Apo®-Sulfinpyrazone [Can]; Nu-Sulfin-pyrazone [Can]

Therapeutic Category Uricosuric Agent

Use Treatment of chronic gouty arthritis and intermittent gouty arthritis

Usual Dosage Oral: 200 mg twice daily

Dosage Forms
Capsule: 200 mg
Tablet: 100 mg

sulfisoxazole (sul fi SOKS a zole)

Synonyms sulphafurazole

Tall-Man sulfiSOXAZOLE

U.S./Canadian Brand Names Gantrisin® Pediatric Suspension [US]; Sulfizole® [Can]; Truxazole® [US]

Therapeutic Category Sulfonamide

Use Treatment of uncomplicated urinary tract infections, otitis media, *Chlamydia*; nocardiosis; treatment of acute pelvic inflammatory disease in prepubertal children

Usual Dosage
Children >2 months: Oral: 75 mg/kg stat, 120-150 mg/kg/day in divided doses every 4-6 hours; not to exceed 6 g/day
Pelvic inflammatory disease: 100 mg/kg/day in divided doses every 6 hours; used in combination with ceftriaxone
Chlamydia trachomatis: 100 mg/kg/day divided every 6 hours
Adults: Oral: 2-4 g stat, 4-8 g/day in divided doses every 4-6 hours

Dosage Forms
Suspension, oral, pediatric, as acetyl: 500 mg/5 mL (480 mL) [raspberry flavor]
Tablet: 500 mg

sulfisoxazole and erythromycin *see* erythromycin and sulfisoxazole *on page 235*

sulfisoxazole and phenazopyridine

(sul fi SOKS a zole & fen az oh PEER i deen)

Synonyms phenazopyridine and sulfisoxazole

Therapeutic Category Sulfonamide

Use Treatment of urinary tract infections and nocardiosis

Usual Dosage Oral: 4-6 tablets to start, then 2 tablets 4 times/day for 2 days, then continue with sulfisoxazole only

Dosage Forms Tablet: Sulfisoxazole 500 mg and phenazopyridine 50 mg

Sulfizole® [Can] *see* sulfisoxazole *on this page*

sulfur and salicylic acid (SUL fur & sal i SIL ik AS id)

Synonyms salicylic acid and sulfur

U.S./Canadian Brand Names Aveeno® Cleansing Bar [US-OTC]; Fostex® [US-OTC]; Pernox® [US-OTC]; Sastid® Plain Therapeutic Shampoo and Acne Wash [US-OTC]

Therapeutic Category Antiseborrheic Agent, Topical

Use Therapeutic shampoo for dandruff and seborrheal dermatitis; acne skin cleanser

Usual Dosage Children and Adults: Topical:
Shampoo: Initial: Use daily or every other day; 1-2 treatments/week will usually maintain control
Soap: Use daily or every other day

Dosage Forms
Cake: Sulfur 2% and salicylic acid 2% (123 g)
Cleanser: Sulfur 2% and salicylic acid 1.5% (60 mL, 120 mL)
Shampoo: Micropulverized sulfur 2% and salicylic acid 2% (120 mL, 240 mL)
Soap: Micropulverized sulfur 2% and salicylic acid 2% (113 g)

Wash: Sulfur 1.6% and salicylic acid 1.6% (75 mL)

sulfur and sulfacetamide (SUL fur & sul fa SEE ta mide)
Synonyms sulfacetamide and sulfur
U.S./Canadian Brand Names Novacet® [US]; Sulfacet-R® [US]
Therapeutic Category Antiseborrheic Agent, Topical
Use Aid in the treatment of acne vulgaris, acne rosacea and seborrheic dermatitis
Usual Dosage Topical: Apply in a thin film 1-3 times/day
Dosage Forms Lotion, topical: Sulfur colloid 5% and sulfacetamide sodium 10% (30 mL)

sulindac (sul IN dak)
U.S./Canadian Brand Names Apo®-Sulin [Can]; Clinoril® [US]; Novo-Sundac [Can]; Nu-Sundac [Can]
Therapeutic Category Analgesic, Non-narcotic; Nonsteroidal Anti-inflammatory Drug (NSAID)
Use Management of inflammatory disease, rheumatoid disorders; acute gouty arthritis
Usual Dosage Oral:
Children: Dose not established
Adults: 150-200 mg twice daily; not to exceed 400 mg/day
Dosage Forms Tablet: 150 mg, 200 mg

sulphafurazole *see* sulfisoxazole *on previous page*

Sultrin™ *(Discontinued) see page 814*

sumatriptan succinate (SOO ma trip tan SUKS i nate)
U.S./Canadian Brand Names Imitrex® [US/Can]
Therapeutic Category Antimigraine Agent
Use Acute treatment of migraine with or without aura
Unlabeled use: Cluster headaches
Usual Dosage Adults:
Oral: 25 mg (taken with fluids); maximum recommended dose is 100 mg. If a satisfactory response has not been obtained at 2 hours, a second dose of up to 100 mg may be given. Efficacy of this second dose has not been examined. If a headache returns, additional doses may be taken at intervals of at least 2 hours up to a daily maximum of 300 mg. There is no evidence that an initial dose of 100 mg provides substantially greater relief than 25 mg.
Intranasal: Single dose of 5, 10, or 20 mg administered in one nostril; a 10 mg dose may be achieved by administration of a single 5 mg dose in each nostril; if headache returns, the dose may be repeated once after 2 hours, not to exceed a total daily dose of 40 mg
S.C.: 6 mg; a second injection may be administered at least 1 hour after the initial dose, but not more than two injections in a 24-hour period
Dosage Forms
Injection: 12 mg/mL (0.5 mL, 2 mL)
Nasal spray [100 μL unit dose spray device]: 5 mg, 20 mg
Tablet: 25 mg, 50 mg, 100 mg

Summer's Eve® Special Care [US-OTC] *see* povidone-iodine *on page 533*

Sumycin® [US] *see* tetracycline *on page 628*

Sun-Benz [Can] *see* benzydamine *(Canada only) on page 81*

sunscreen (paba-free) *see* methoxycinnamate and oxybenzone *on page 419*

Supartz® [US] *see* sodium hyaluronate *on page 597*

Superchar® *(Discontinued) see page 814*

Superchar® With Sorbitol *(Discontinued) see page 814*

Superdophilus® [US-OTC] *see* Lactobacillus *on page 372*

Supeudol® **[Can]** *see* oxycodone *on page 484*

Suplasyn® **[Can]** *see* sodium hyaluronate *on page 597*

Supprelin™ **[US]** *see* histrelin *on page 323*

Suppress® *(Discontinued) see page 814*

Suprane® **[US/Can]** *see* desflurane *on page 181*

Suprax® **[US/Can]** *see* cefixime *on page 122*

Surbex-T® **Filmtabs**® **[US-OTC]** *see* vitamin B complex with vitamin C *on page 681*

Surbex® **With C Filmtabs**® **[US-OTC]** *see* vitamin B complex with vitamin C *on page 681*

Sureprin 81™ **[US-OTC]** *see* aspirin *on page 58*

Surfak® **[US-OTC]** *see* docusate *on page 208*

Surgam® **[Can]** *see* tiaprofenic acid *(Canada only) on page 638*

Surgam® **SR [Can]** *see* tiaprofenic acid *(Canada only) on page 638*

Surgicel® **[US]** *see* cellulose, oxidized *on page 127*

Surital® *(Discontinued) see page 814*

Surmontil® **[US/Can]** *see* trimipramine *on page 658*

Survanta® **[US/Can]** *see* beractant *on page 81*

Suspen® **[US]** *see* penicillin V potassium *on page 499*

Sus-Phrine® *(Discontinued) see page 814*

Sustaire® *(Discontinued) see page 814*

Sustiva® **[US/Can]** *see* efavirenz *on page 223*

Su-Tuss®**-HD [US]** *see* hydrocodone, pseudoephedrine, and guaifenesin *on page 332*

suxamethonium *see* succinylcholine *on page 608*

Sween Cream® **[US-OTC]** *see* methylbenzethonium chloride *on page 420*

Swim-Ear® **Otic [US-OTC]** *see* boric acid *on page 90*

Syllact® **[US-OTC]** *see* psyllium *on page 554*

Symadine® *(Discontinued) see page 814*

Symax SL [US] *see* hyoscyamine *on page 339*

Symax SR [US] *see* hyoscyamine *on page 339*

Symmetrel® **[US/Can]** *see* amantadine *on page 30*

Symmetrel® **Capsule** *(Discontinued) see page 814*

Synacort® **[US]** *see* hydrocortisone (topical) *on page 334*

synacthen *see* cosyntropin *on page 165*

Synagis® **[US]** *see* palivizumab *on page 488*

Synalar® **[US/Can]** *see* fluocinolone *on page 276*

Synalar-HP® **Topical** *(Discontinued) see page 814*

Synalgos®**-DC [US]** *see* dihydrocodeine compound *on page 198*

Synarel® **[US/Can]** *see* nafarelin *on page 443*

Syn-Diltiazem® **[Can]** *see* diltiazem *on page 199*

Synemol® **Topical** *(Discontinued) see page 814*

Synercid® **[US/Can]** *see* quinupristin and dalfopristin *on page 560*

Synflex® **[Can]** *see* naproxen *on page 447*

Synflex® **DS [Can]** *see* naproxen *on page 447*

Synkayvite® *(Discontinued)* see page 814

Synphasic® **[Can]** see ethinyl estradiol and norethindrone on page 251

synthetic lung surfactant see colfosceril palmitate on page 161

Synthroid® **[US/Can]** see levothyroxine on page 382

Syntocinon® **Nasal** *(Discontinued)* see page 814

Synvisc® **[US/Can]** see sodium hyaluronate/hylan G-F 20 on page 597

Syprine® **[US/Can]** see trientine on page 654

Sytobex® *(Discontinued)* see page 814

t₃/t₄ liotrix see liotrix on page 387

t₃ thyronine see liothyronine on page 386

t₄ thyroxine see levothyroxine on page 382

642® **Tablet [Can]** see propoxyphene on page 548

Tabron® *(Discontinued)* see page 814

Tac™-3 Injection [US] see triamcinolone (systemic) on page 651

Tac™-40 Injection *(Discontinued)* see page 814

Tacaryl® *(Discontinued)* see page 814

TACE® *(Discontinued)* see page 814

tacrine (TAK reen)
Synonyms tetrahydroaminoacrine; THA
U.S./Canadian Brand Names Cognex® [US]
Therapeutic Category Acetylcholinesterase Inhibitor; Cholinergic Agent
Use Treatment of Alzheimer's disease
Usual Dosage Adults: Oral: 40 mg/day
Dosage Forms Capsule, as hydrochloride: 10 mg, 20 mg, 30 mg, 40 mg

tacrolimus (ta KROE li mus)
Synonyms FK506
U.S./Canadian Brand Names Prograf® [US/Can]; Protopic® [US]
Therapeutic Category Immunosuppressant Agent
Use
  Oral/injection: Potent immunosuppressive drug used in liver or kidney transplant recipients
  Topical: Moderate to severe atopic dermatitis in patients not responsive to conventional therapy or when conventional therapy is not appropriate
  Unlabeled uses: Potent immunosuppressive drug used in heart, lung, small bowel transplant recipients; immunosuppressive drug for peripheral stem cell/bone marrow transplantation
Usual Dosage
  Initial: I.V. continuous infusion: 0.1 mg/kg/day until the tolerance of oral intake
  Oral: Usually 3-4 times the I.V. dose, or 0.3 mg/kg/day in divided doses every 12 hours
Dosage Forms
  Capsule: 0.5 mg, 1 mg, 5 mg
  Injection: 5 mg/mL (1 mL) [contains alcohol and surfactant]
  Ointment, topical: 0.03% (30 g, 60 g); 0.1% (30 g, 60g)

Tagamet® **[US/Can]** see cimetidine on page 146

Tagamet® **HB [US/Can]** see cimetidine on page 146

Talacen® **[US]** see pentazocine compound on page 501

Talwin® **[US/Can]** see pentazocine on page 501

Talwin® **Compound [US]** see pentazocine compound on page 501

Talwin® NX **[US]** *see* pentazocine *on page 501*

Tambocor™ [US/Can] *see* flecainide *on page 273*

Tamiflu™ [US/Can] *see* oseltamivir *on page 481*

Tamine® *(Discontinued) see page 814*

Tamofen® [Can] *see* tamoxifen *on this page*

tamoxifen (ta MOKS i fen)

U.S./Canadian Brand Names Apo®-Tamox [Can]; Gen-Tamoxifen [Can]; Nolvadex® [US/Can]; Nolvadex®-D [Can]; Novo-Tamoxifen [Can]; PMS-Tamoxifen [Can]; Tamofen® [Can]

Therapeutic Category Antineoplastic Agent

Use Palliative or adjunctive treatment of advanced breast cancer in postmenopausal women

Usual Dosage Oral: 10-20 mg twice daily

Dosage Forms Tablet, as citrate: 10 mg, 20 mg

tamsulosin (tam SOO loe sin)

U.S./Canadian Brand Names Flomax® [US/Can]

Therapeutic Category Alpha-Adrenergic Blocking Agent

Use Treatment of signs and symptoms of benign prostatic hyperplasia (BPH)

Usual Dosage Oral: Adults: 0.4 mg once daily approximately 30 minutes after the same meal each day

Dosage Forms Capsule, as hydrochloride: 0.4 mg

Tanac® *(Discontinued) see page 814*

Tanoral® Tablet *(Discontinued) see page 814*

Tantum™ [Can] *see* benzydamine *(Canada only) on page 81*

Tao® [US] *see* troleandomycin *on page 660*

Tapazole® [US/Can] *see* methimazole *on page 416*

Tarabine® PFS *(Discontinued) see page 814*

Taractan® *(Discontinued) see page 814*

Targel® [Can] *see* coal tar *on page 158*

Targretin® [US/Can] *see* bexarotene *on page 85*

Tarka® [US] *see* trandolapril and verapamil *on page 647*

Taro-Carbamazepin [Can] *see* carbamazepine *on page 113*

Taro-Desoximetasone [Can] *see* desoximetasone *on page 183*

Taro-Sone® [Can] *see* betamethasone (topical) *on page 83*

Taro-Warfarin [Can] *see* warfarin *on page 685*

Tasmar® [US] *see* tolcapone *on page 643*

TAT *see* tetanus antitoxin *on page 626*

Tavist® [US] *see* clemastine *on page 150*

Tavist®-1 [US-OTC] *see* clemastine *on page 150*

Tavist-D® *(Discontinued) see page 814*

Taxol® [US/Can] *see* paclitaxel *on page 488*

Taxotere® [US/Can] *see* docetaxel *on page 208*

tazarotene (taz AR oh teen)

U.S./Canadian Brand Names Tazorac® [US/Can]

Therapeutic Category Keratolytic Agent

Use Topical treatment of facial acne vulgaris; topical treatment of stable plaque psoriasis of up to 20% body surface area involvement

Usual Dosage Children >12 years and Adults: Topical:

Acne: Cleanse the face gently. After the skin is dry, apply a thin film of tazarotene (2 mg/ cm^2) once daily, in the evening, to the skin where the acne lesions appear. Use enough to cover the entire affected area. Tazarotene was investigated ≤12 weeks during clinical trials for acne.

Psoriasis: Apply tazarotene once daily, in the evening, to psoriatic lesions using enough (2 mg/cm^2) to cover only the lesion with a thin film to no more than 20% of body surface area. If a bath or shower is taken prior to application, dry the skin before applying the gel. Because unaffected skin may be more susceptible to irritation, avoid application of tazarotene to these areas. Tazarotene was investigated for up to 12 months during clinical trials for psoriasis.

Dosage Forms

Cream: 0.05% (15 g, 30 g, 60 g); 0.1% (15 g, 30 g, 60 g)
Gel: 0.05% (30 g, 100 g); 0.1% (30 g, 100 g)

Tazicef® **[US]** *see* ceftazidime *on page 125*

Tazidime® **[US/Can]** *see* ceftazidime *on page 125*

tazobactam and piperacillin *see* piperacillin and tazobactam sodium *on page 517*

Tazocin® **[Can]** *see* piperacillin and tazobactam sodium *on page 517*

Tazorac® **[US/Can]** *see* tazarotene *on previous page*

3TC® **[Can]** *see* lamivudine *on page 373*

T-Caine® **Lozenge** *(Discontinued)* *see page 814*

TCN *see* tetracycline *on page 628*

Td *see* diphtheria and tetanus toxoid *on page 203*

TDF *see* tenofovir *on page 622*

Teardrops® **[Can]** *see* artificial tears *on page 56*

Tear Drop® **Solution** *(Discontinued)* *see page 814*

TearGard® **Ophthalmic Solution** *(Discontinued)* *see page 814*

Teargen® **II [US-OTC]** *see* artificial tears *on page 56*

Teargen® **[US-OTC]** *see* artificial tears *on page 56*

Tearisol® **[US-OTC]** *see* artificial tears *on page 56*

Tears Again® **[US-OTC]** *see* artificial tears *on page 56*

Tears Naturale® **Free [US-OTC]** *see* artificial tears *on page 56*

Tears Naturale® **II [US-OTC]** *see* artificial tears *on page 56*

Tears Naturale® **[US-OTC]** *see* artificial tears *on page 56*

Tears Plus® **[US-OTC]** *see* artificial tears *on page 56*

Tears Renewed® **[US-OTC]** *see* artificial tears *on page 56*

Tebamide® *(Discontinued)* *see page 814*

Tebrazid™ **[Can]** *see* pyrazinamide *on page 555*

Tecnal® **[Can]** *see* butalbital, aspirin, and caffeine *on page 100*

Tecnal C 1/2 [Can] *see* butalbital compound and codeine *on page 100*

Tecnal C 1/4 [Can] *see* butalbital compound and codeine *on page 100*

Teczem® **[US/Can]** *see* enalapril and diltiazem *on page 226*

Tedral® *(Discontinued)* *see page 814*

Teejel® **[Can]** *see* choline salicylate *on page 144*

tegaserod (teg a SER od)
Synonyms HTF919
U.S./Canadian Brand Names Zelnorm™ [US]
Therapeutic Category Serotonin 5-HT$_4$ Receptor Agonist
Use Short-term treatment of constipation-predominate irritable bowel syndrome (IBS) in women
Usual Dosage Oral:
Adults: Female: IBS with constipation: 6 mg twice daily, before meals, for 4-6 weeks; may consider continuing treatment for an additional 4-6 weeks in patients who respond initially.
Dosage Forms Tablet, as maleate: 2 mg, 6 mg

Tega-Vert® **Oral** *(Discontinued)* *see page 814*

Tegison® **[US]** *see etretinate on page 259*

Tegopen® *(Discontinued)* *see page 814*

Tegretol® **[US/Can]** *see carbamazepine on page 113*

Tegretol®**-XR [US]** *see carbamazepine on page 113*

Tegrin® **Dandruff Shampoo [US-OTC]** *see coal tar on page 158*

Tegrin®**-HC [US-OTC]** *see hydrocortisone (topical) on page 334*

Telachlor® **Oral** *(Discontinued)* *see page 814*

Teladar® **Topical** *(Discontinued)* *see page 814*

Teldrin® **Oral** *(Discontinued)* *see page 814*

Telepaque® **[US]** *see radiological/contrast media (ionic) on page 561*

Teline® *(Discontinued)* *see page 814*

telmisartan (tel mi SAR tan)
U.S./Canadian Brand Names Micardis® [US/Can]
Therapeutic Category Angiotensin II Receptor Antagonist
Use Treatment of hypertension alone or in combination with other antihypertensives
Usual Dosage Adults: Oral: The usual starting dose is 40 mg once daily. Blood pressure response is dose-related over the range of 20 mg-80 mg/day; when additional antihypertensive effects are needed beyond that achieved with 80 mg/day, a diuretic may be added.
Dosage Forms Tablet: 20 mg, 40 mg, 80 mg

telmisartan and hydrochlorothiazide
(tel mi SAR tan & hye droe klor oh THYE a zide)
U.S./Canadian Brand Names Micardis® HCT [US]
Therapeutic Category Antihypertensive Agent, Combination
Use Treatment of hypertension; combination product should not be used for initial therapy
Usual Dosage Adults: Oral: Replacement therapy: Combination product can be substituted for individual titrated agents. Initiation of combination therapy when monotherapy has failed to achieve desired effects:
Patients currently on telmisartan: Initial dose if blood pressure is not currently controlled on monotherapy of 80 mg telmisartan: Telmisartan 80 mg/hydrochlorothiazide 12.5 mg once daily; may titrate up to telmisartan 160 mg/hydrochlorothiazide 25 mg if needed
Patients currently on HCTZ: Initial dose if blood pressure is not currently controlled on monotherapy of 25 mg once daily, or is controlled and experiencing hypokalemia: Telmisartan 80 mg/hydrochlorothiazide 12.5 mg once daily; may titrate up to telmisartan 160 mg/hydrochlorothiazide 25 mg if blood pressure remains uncontrolled after 2-4 weeks of therapy

Dosage Forms
Tablet:
Telmisartan 40 mg and hydrochlorothiazide 12.5 mg
Telmisartan 80 mg and hydrochlorothiazide 12.5 mg

Temaril® *(Discontinued)* *see page 814*

temazepam (te MAZ e pam)

U.S./Canadian Brand Names Apo®-Temazepam [Can]; Gen-Temazepam [Can]; Novo-Temazepam [Can]; Nu-Temazepam [Can]; PMS-Temazepam [Can]; Restoril® [US/Can]
Therapeutic Category Benzodiazepine
Controlled Substance C-IV
Use Treatment of anxiety and as an adjunct in the treatment of depression; also may be used in the management of panic attacks; transient insomnia and sleep latency
Usual Dosage Adults: Oral: 15-30 mg at bedtime
Dosage Forms Capsule: 7.5 mg, 15 mg, 30 mg

Temazin® Cold Syrup *(Discontinued)* *see page 814*

Temodal™ [Can] *see temozolomide on this page*

Temodar® [US/Can] *see temozolomide on this page*

Temovate® [US] *see clobetasol on page 152*

temozolomide (te mo ZOLE oh mide)

U.S./Canadian Brand Names Temodal™ [Can]; Temodar® [US/Can]
Therapeutic Category Antineoplastic Agent, Alkylating Agent
Use Treatment of adult patients with refractory (first relapse) anaplastic astrocytoma who have experienced disease progression on nitrosourea and procarbazine
Unlabeled use: Glioma, first relapse/advanced metastatic malignant melanoma
Usual Dosage The dosage is adjusted according to nadir neutrophil and platelet counts of previous cycle and counts at the time of the next cycle.
Adults: Initial dose: 150 mg/m^2 once daily for 5 consecutive days per 28-day treatment cycle
Measure day 22 ANC and platelets. Measure day 29 ANC and platelets. Based on lowest counts at either day 22 or day 29:
On day 22 or day 29, if ANC <1,000/µL or the platelet count is <50,000/µL, postpone therapy until ANC >1,500/µL and platelet count >100,000/µL. Reduce dose by 50 mg/m^2 for subsequent cycle.
If ANC 1,000-1,500/µL or platelets 50,000-100,000/µL, postpone therapy until ANC >1,500/µL and platelet count >100,000/µL; maintain initial dose.
If ANC >1,500/µL (on day 22 and day 29) and platelet count >100,000/µL, increase dose to, or maintain dose at 200 mg/m^2/day for 5 for subsequent cycle.
Dosage Forms Capsule: 5 mg, 20 mg, 100 mg, 250 mg

Tempra® [Can] *see acetaminophen on page 3*

Tenake® [US] *see butalbital, acetaminophen, and caffeine on page 99*

Tencon® [US] *see butalbital, acetaminophen, and caffeine on page 99*

tenecteplase (ten EK te plase)

U.S./Canadian Brand Names TNKase™ [US]
Therapeutic Category Thrombolytic Agent
Use Reduce mortality associated with acute myocardial infarction
Usual Dosage I.V.:
Adult: Recommended total dose should not exceed 50 mg and is based on patient's weight; administer as a bolus over 5 seconds
If patient's weight:
<60 kg, dose: 30 mg
(Continued)

tenecteplase *(Continued)*

≥60 to <70 kg, dose: 35 mg
≥70 to <80 kg, dose: 40 mg
≥80 to <90 kg, dose: 45 mg
≥90 kg, dose: 50 mg

All patients received 150-325 mg of aspirin as soon as possible and then daily. Intravenous heparin was initiated as soon as possible and PTT was maintained between 50-70 seconds.

Dosage Forms Injection, powder for reconstitution, recombinant: 50 mg

Tenex® **[US/Can]** *see* guanfacine *on page 313*

teniposide (ten i POE side)

Synonyms EPT; VM-26
U.S./Canadian Brand Names Vumon® [US/Can]
Therapeutic Category Antineoplastic Agent
Use Treatment of Hodgkin's and non-Hodgkin's lymphomas, acute lymphocytic leukemia, bladder carcinoma and neuroblastoma
Usual Dosage I.V.:
Children: 130 mg/m^2/week, increasing to 150 mg/m^2 after 3 weeks and to 180 mg/m^2 after 6 weeks
Adults: 50-180 mg/m^2 once or twice weekly for 4-6 weeks
Dosage Forms Injection: 10 mg/mL (5 mL)

Ten-K® *(Discontinued)* *see page 814*

tenofovir (te NOE fo veer)

Synonyms PMPA; TDF; tenofovir disoproxil fumarate
U.S./Canadian Brand Names Viread™ [US]
Therapeutic Category Antiretroviral Agent, Reverse Transcriptase Inhibitor (Nucleotide)
Use Management of HIV infections in combination with at least two other antiretroviral agents
Usual Dosage Oral: Adults: HIV infection: 300 mg once daily
Dosage Forms Tablet, as disoproxil fumarate: 300 mg [equivalent to 245 mg tenofovir disoproxil]

tenofovir disoproxil fumarate *see* tenofovir *on this page*

Tenolin [Can] *see* atenolol *on page 60*

Tenoretic® **[US/Can]** *see* atenolol and chlorthalidone *on page 60*

Tenormin® **[US/Can]** *see* atenolol *on page 60*

Tensilon® **[US]** *see* edrophonium *on page 223*

Tenuate® **[US/Can]** *see* diethylpropion *on page 195*

Tenuate® **Dospan®** **[US/Can]** *see* diethylpropion *on page 195*

Tepanil® *(Discontinued)* *see page 814*

Tepanil® **TenTabs®** *(Discontinued)* *see page 814*

Tequin® **[US/Can]** *see* gatifloxacin *on page 293*

Terazol® **3 [US/Can]** *see* terconazole *on page 624*

Terazol® **7 [US/Can]** *see* terconazole *on page 624*

terazosin (ter AY zoe sin)

U.S./Canadian Brand Names Alti-Terazosin [Can]; Apo®-Terazosin [Can]; Hytrin® [US/Can]; Novo-Terazosin [Can]; Nu-Terazosin [Can]
Therapeutic Category Alpha-Adrenergic Blocking Agent

Use Management of mild to moderate hypertension; considered a step 2 drug in stepped approach to hypertension; benign prostate hypertrophy

Usual Dosage Adults: Oral: 1 mg; slowly increase dose to achieve desired blood pressure, up to 20 mg/day

Dosage Forms
Capsule: 1 mg, 2 mg, 5 mg, 10 mg
Tablet: 1 mg, 2 mg, 5 mg, 10 mg

terbinafine (oral) (TER bin a feen OR al)

U.S./Canadian Brand Names Lamisil® Oral [US/Can]

Therapeutic Category Antifungal Agent

Use Treatment of onychomycosis infections of the toenail or fingernail

Usual Dosage Adults: Oral:
Fingernail onychomycosis: 250 mg once daily for 6 weeks
Toenail onychomycosis: 250 mg once daily for 12 weeks

Dosage Forms Tablet: 250 mg

terbinafine (topical) (TER bin a feen TOP i kal)

U.S./Canadian Brand Names Lamisil® Cream [US]

Therapeutic Category Antifungal Agent

Use Topical antifungal for the treatment of tinea pedis (athlete's foot), tinea cruris (jock itch), and tinea corporis (ring worm); tinea versicolor (lotion)

Unlabeled use: Cutaneous candidiasis

Usual Dosage Adults: Topical:
Athlete's foot: Apply to affected area twice daily for at least 1 week, not to exceed 4 weeks
Ringworm and jock itch: Apply to affected area once or twice daily for at least 1 week, not to exceed 4 weeks

Dosage Forms
Cream: 1% (15 g, 30 g)
Lotion: 1%

terbutaline (ter BYOO ta leen)

U.S./Canadian Brand Names Brethine® [US]; Bricanyl® [Can]

Therapeutic Category Adrenergic Agonist Agent

Use Bronchodilator in reversible airway obstruction and bronchial asthma

Usual Dosage
Children <6 years:
Oral: Initial: 0.05 mg/kg/dose 3 times/day, increased gradually as required; maximum: 0.15 mg/kg/dose 3-4 times/day or a total of 5 mg/24 hours
S.C.: 0.005-0.01 mg/kg/dose to a maximum of 0.3 mg/dose every 15-20 minutes for 3 doses
Inhalation nebulization dose: 0.06 mg/kg; maximum: 8 mg
Inhalation: 0.3 mg/kg/dose up to maximum of 10 mg/dose every 4-6 hours
Children >6 years and Adults:
Oral:
6-15 years: 2.5 mg every 6 hours 3 times/day; not to exceed 7.5 mg in 24 hours
>15 years: 5 mg/dose every 6 hours 3 times/day; if side effects occur, reduce dose to 2.5 mg every 6 hours; not to exceed 15 mg in 24 hours
S.C.: 0.25 mg/dose repeated in 15-30 minutes for one time only; a total dose of 0.5 mg should not be exceeded within a 4-hour period

Dosage Forms
Injection, as sulfate: 1 mg/mL (1 mL)
Tablet, as sulfate: 2.5 mg, 5 mg

terconazole (ter KONE a zole)

Synonyms triaconazole

U.S./Canadian Brand Names Terazol® 3 [US/Can]; Terazol® 7 [US/Can]

Therapeutic Category Antifungal Agent

Use Local treatment of vulvovaginal candidiasis

Usual Dosage Vaginal: 1 applicatorful in vagina at bedtime for 7 consecutive days

Dosage Forms

Cream, vaginal:

Terazol® 7: 0.4% (45 g)

Terazol® 3: 0.8% (20 g)

Suppository, vaginal (Terazol® 3): 80 mg (3s)

teriparatide (ter i PAR a tide)

U.S./Canadian Brand Names Parathar™ [US]

Therapeutic Category Diagnostic Agent

Use Diagnosis of hypocalcemia in either hypoparathyroidism or pseudohypoparathyroidism

Usual Dosage I.V.:

Children ≥3 years: 3 units/kg up to 200 units

Adults: 200 units over 10 minutes

Dosage Forms Powder for injection: 200 units hPTH activity (10 mL)

terpin hydrate *(Discontinued)* *see page 814*

terpin hydrate and codeine *(Discontinued)* *see page 814*

Terra-Cortril® Ophthalmic Suspension *(Discontinued)* *see page 814*

Terramycin® I.M. [US/Can] *see* oxytetracycline *on page 487*

Terramycin® Oral *(Discontinued)* *see page 814*

Terramycin® w/Polymyxin B Ophthalmic [US] *see* oxytetracycline and polymyxin B *on page 487*

Tesamone® Injection *(Discontinued)* *see page 814*

Teslac® [US/Can] *see* testolactone *on this page*

TESPA *see* thiotepa *on page 635*

Tessalon® Perles [US/Can] *see* benzonatate *on page 79*

Tes-Tape® *(Discontinued)* *see page 814*

Testoderm® [US] *see* testosterone *on next page*

Testoderm® TTS [US] *see* testosterone *on next page*

Testoderm® with Adhesive [US] *see* testosterone *on next page*

testolactone (tes toe LAK tone)

U.S./Canadian Brand Names Teslac® [US/Can]

Therapeutic Category Androgen

Use Palliative treatment of advanced disseminated breast carcinoma

Usual Dosage Adults: Females: Oral: 250 mg 4 times/day for at least 3 months; desired response may take as long as 3 months

Dosage Forms Tablet: 50 mg

Testomar® *(Discontinued)* *see page 814*

Testopel® Pellet *(Discontinued)* *see page 814*

testosterone (tes TOS ter one)

Synonyms aqueous testosterone

U.S./Canadian Brand Names Andriol® [Can]; Androderm® [US]; AndroGel® [US]; Delatestryl® [US/Can]; Depo®-Testosterone [US]; Testoderm® [US]; Testoderm® TTS [US]; Testoderm® with Adhesive [US]; Testro® AQ [US]; Testro® LA [US]

Therapeutic Category Androgen

Controlled Substance C-III

Use Androgen replacement therapy in the treatment of delayed male puberty; male hypogonadism

Usual Dosage

Children: I.M.:

Male hypogonadism:

Initiation of pubertal growth: 40-50 mg/m^2/dose (cypionate or enanthate ester) monthly until the growth rate falls to prepubertal levels

Terminal growth phase: 100 mg/m^2/dose (cypionate or enanthate ester) monthly until growth ceases

Maintenance virilizing dose: 100 mg/m^2/dose (cypionate or enanthate ester) twice monthly

Delayed puberty: 40-50 mg/m^2/dose monthly (cypionate or enanthate ester) for 6 months

Adults: Inoperable breast cancer: I.M.: 200-400 mg every 2-4 weeks

Male: Short-acting formulations: Testosterone Aqueous/Testosterone Propionate (in oil): I.M.:

Androgen replacement therapy: 10-50 mg 2-3 times/week

Male hypogonadism: 40-50 mg/m^2/dose monthly until the growth rate falls to prepubertal levels (~5 cm/year); during terminal growth phase: 100 mg/m^2/dose monthly until growth ceases; maintenance virilizing dose: 100 mg/m^2/dose twice monthly or 50-400 mg/dose every 2-4 weeks

Male: Long-acting formulations: Testosterone enanthate (in oil)/testosterone cypionate (in oil): I.M.:

Male hypogonadism: 50-400 mg every 2-4 weeks

Male with delayed puberty: 50-200 mg every 2-4 weeks for a limited duration

Male ≥18 years: Transdermal: Primary hypogonadism **or** hypogonadotropic hypogonadism:

Testoderm®: Apply 6 mg patch daily to scrotum (if scrotum is inadequate, use a 4 mg daily system)

Testoderm-TTS®: Apply 5 mg patch daily to clean, dry area of skin on the arm, back or upper buttocks. **Do not apply Testoderm-TTS® to the scrotum.**

Androderm®: Apply 2 systems nightly to clean, dry area on the back, abdomen, upper arms, or thighs for 24 hours for a total of 5 mg/day

AndroGel®: Males >18 years of age: 5 g (to deliver 50 mg of testosterone) applied once daily (preferably in the morning) to clean, dry, intact skin of the shoulder and upper arms and/or abdomen. Upon opening the packet(s), the entire contents should be squeezed into the palm of the hand and immediately applied to the application site(s). Application sites should be allowed to dry for a few minutes prior to dressing. Hands should be washed with soap and water after application. **Do not apply AndroGel® to the genitals.**

Dosage Forms

Gel, transdermal (AndroGel®): 1%: 50 mg (5 g gel); 75 mg (7.5 g gel)

Injection, aqueous suspension (Testro® AQ): 25 mg/mL (10 mL, 30 mL); 50 mg/mL (10 mL, 30 mL); 100 mg/mL (10 mL, 30 mL)

Injection, as cypionate [in oil] (Depo® Testosterone): 100 mg/mL (1 mL, 10 mL); 200 mg/mL (1 mL, 10 mL)

Injection, as enanthate [in oil] (Delatestryl®, Testro® LA): 200 mg/mL (1 mL, 5 mL, 10 mL)

Injection, as propionate [in oil]: 100 mg/mL (10 mL)

Transdermal system:

Androderm®: 2.5 mg/day; 5 mg/day

(Continued)

testosterone *(Continued)*
Testoderm®: 4 mg/day; 6 mg/day
Testoderm® TTS: 5 mg/day

Testred® [US] *see* methyltestosterone *on page 423*

Testro® AQ [US] *see* testosterone *on previous page*

Testro® LA [US] *see* testosterone *on previous page*

tetanus and diphtheria toxoid *see* diphtheria and tetanus toxoid *on page 203*

tetanus antitoxin (TET a nus an tee TOKS in)
Synonyms TAT
Therapeutic Category Antitoxin
Use Tetanus prophylaxis or treatment of active tetanus only when tetanus immune globulin (TIG) is not available
Usual Dosage
Prophylaxis: I.M., S.C.:
Children <30 kg: 1500 units
Children and Adults >30 kg: 3000-5000 units
Treatment: Children and Adults: Inject 10,000-40,000 units into wound; administer 40,000-100,000 units I.V.
Dosage Forms Injection, equine: Not less than 400 units/mL (12.5 mL, 50 mL)

tetanus immune globulin (human)
(TET a nus i MYUN GLOB yoo lin HYU man)
Synonyms TIG
U.S./Canadian Brand Names BayTet™ [US/Can]
Therapeutic Category Immune Globulin
Use Passive immunization against tetanus; tetanus immune globulin is preferred over tetanus antitoxin for treatment of active tetanus; part of the management of an unclean, nonminor wound in a person whose history of previous receipt of tetanus toxoid is unknown or who has received less than three doses of tetanus toxoid
Usual Dosage I.M.:
Prophylaxis of tetanus:
Children: 4 units/kg; some recommend administering 250 units to small children
Adults: 250 units
Treatment of tetanus:
Children: 500-3000 units; some should infiltrate locally around the wound
Adults: 3000-6000 units
Dosage Forms Injection: 250 units/mL

tetanus toxoid (adsorbed) (TET a nus TOKS oyd ad SORBED)
Therapeutic Category Toxoid
Use Active immunization against tetanus
Usual Dosage Adults: I.M.:
Primary immunization: 0.5 mL; repeat 0.5 mL at 4-8 weeks after first dose and at 6-12 months after second dose
Routine booster doses are recommended only every 5-10 years
Dosage Forms
Injection, adsorbed:
Tetanus 5 Lf units per 0.5 mL dose (0.5 mL, 5 mL)
Tetanus 10 Lf units per 0.5 mL dose (0.5 mL, 5 mL)

tetanus toxoid (fluid) (TET a nus TOKS oyd FLOO id)
Synonyms tetanus toxoid plain
Therapeutic Category Toxoid
Use Active immunization against tetanus in adults and children

Usual Dosage Inject 3 doses of 0.5 mL I.M. or S.C. at 4- to 8-week intervals with fourth dose administered only 6-12 months after third dose

Dosage Forms
Injection, fluid:
Tetanus 4 Lf units per 0.5 mL dose (7.5 mL)
Tetanus 5 Lf units per 0.5 mL dose (0.5 mL, 7.5 mL)

tetanus toxoid plain *see* tetanus toxoid (fluid) *on previous page*

tetrabenazine *(Canada only)* (tet ra BENZ a zeen)

U.S./Canadian Brand Names Nitoman® [Can]

Therapeutic Category Monoamine Depleting Agent

Use Treatment of hyperkinetic movement disorders such as Huntington's chorea, hemiballismus, senile chorea, tic and Gilles de la Tourette syndrome and tardive dyskinesia; not indicated for the treatment of levodopa-induced dyskinetic/choreiform movements; should only be used by (or in consultation with) physicians who are experienced in the treatment of hyperkinetic movement disorders.

Usual Dosage Oral:
Children: No adequately controlled clinical studies have been performed in children. Limited clinical experience suggests that treatment should be started at approximately half the adult dose, and titrated slowly and carefully according to tolerance and individual response.
Adults: Initial starting dose: 12.5 mg 2-3 times/day is recommended. This can be increased by 12.5 mg/day every 3-5 days until the maximal tolerated and effective dose is reached for the individual, and may have to be up/down titrated depending on individual tolerance. In most cases the maximal tolerated dose will be 25 mg 3 times/day. In very rare cases, a 200 mg dose has been reached (the maximum recommended dose in some publications). If there is no improvement at the maximal tolerated dose in 7 days, it is unlikely that Nitoman® will be of benefit to the patient, either by increasing the dose or by extending the duration of treatment.

Dosage Forms Tablet: 25 mg

tetracaine (TET ra kane)

Synonyms amethocaine

U.S./Canadian Brand Names Ametop™ [Can]; Pontocaine® [US/Can]

Therapeutic Category Local Anesthetic

Use Local anesthesia in the eye for various diagnostic and examination purposes; spinal anesthesia; topical anesthesia for local skin disorders; local anesthesia for mucous membranes

Usual Dosage
Children: Safety and efficacy have not been established
Adults:
Ophthalmic (not for prolonged use):
Ointment: Apply ½" to 1" to lower conjunctival fornix
Solution: Instill 1-2 drops
Spinal anesthesia 1% solution:
Subarachnoid injection: 5-20 mg
Saddle block: 2-5 mg; a 1% solution should be diluted with equal volume of CSF before administration
Topical mucous membranes (2% solution): Apply as needed; dose should not exceed 20 mg
Topical for skin: Apply to affected areas as needed

Dosage Forms
Cream, as hydrochloride: 1% (28 g)
Injection, as hydrochloride: 1% [10 mg/mL] (2 mL)
Injection, powder for reconstitution, as hydrochloride: 20 mg
Injection, as hydrochloride [contains dextrose 6%]: 0.2% [2 mg/mL] (2 mL); 0.3% [3 mg/mL] (5 mL)
(Continued)

tetracaine *(Continued)*

Ointment, as hydrochloride: 0.5% [5 mg/mL] (28 g)
Ointment, ophthalmic, as hydrochloride: 0.5% [5 mg/mL] (3.75 g)
Solution, ophthalmic, as hydrochloride: 0.5% [5 mg/mL] (1 mL, 2 mL, 15 mL, 59 mL)
Solution, topical, as hydrochloride: 2% [20 mg/mL] (30 mL, 118 mL)

tetracaine and dextrose (TET ra kane & DEKS trose)

U.S./Canadian Brand Names Pontocaine® With Dextrose [US]
Therapeutic Category Local Anesthetic
Use Spinal anesthesia (saddle block)
Usual Dosage Dose varies with procedure, depth of anesthesia, duration desired, and physical condition of patient
Dosage Forms
Injection:
Tetracaine hydrochloride 0.2% and dextrose 6% (2 mL)
Tetracaine hydrochloride 0.3% and dextrose 6% (5 mL)

tetracaine hydrochloride, benzocaine, butyl aminobenzoate, and benzalkonium chloride *see* benzocaine, butyl aminobenzoate, tetracaine, and benzalkonium chloride *on page 78*

TetraCap® *(Discontinued) see page 814*

tetracosactide *see* cosyntropin *on page 165*

tetracycline (tet ra SYE kleen)

Synonyms TCN
U.S./Canadian Brand Names Apo®-Tetra [Can]; Brodspec® [US]; EmTet® [US]; Novo-Tetra [Can]; Nu-Tetra [Can]; Sumycin® [US]; Wesmycin® [US]
Therapeutic Category Antibiotic, Ophthalmic; Antibiotic, Topical; Tetracycline Derivative
Use
Children, Adolescents, and Adults: Treatment of Rocky Mountain spotted fever caused by susceptible Rickettsia or brucellosis
Adolescents and Adults: Presumptive treatment of chlamydial infection in patients with gonorrhea
Older Children, Adolescents, and Adults: Treatment of Lyme disease, mycoplasmal disease or *Legionella*
Usual Dosage
Children >8 years:
Oral: 25-50 mg/kg/day in divided doses every 6 hours; not to exceed 3 g/day
Ophthalmic:
Suspension: Instill 1-2 drops 2-4 times/day or more often as needed
Ointment: Instill every 2-12 hours
Adults:
Oral: 250-500 mg/dose every 6 hours
Ophthalmic:
Suspension: Instill 1-2 drops 2-4 times/day or more often as needed
Ointment: Instill every 2-12 hours
Topical: Apply to affected areas 1-4 times/day
Dosage Forms
Capsule, as hydrochloride: 250 mg, 500 mg
Ointment, as hydrochloride: 3% [30 mg/mL] (14.2 g, 30 g)
Ointment, ophthalmic: 1% [10 mg/mL] (3.5 g)
Solution, topical: 2.2 mg/mL (70 mL)
Suspension, ophthalmic: 1% [10 mg/mL] (0.5 mL, 1 mL, 4 mL)
Suspension, oral, as hydrochloride: 125 mg/5 mL (60 mL, 480 mL)
Tablet, as hydrochloride: 250 mg, 500 mg

tetrahydroaminoacrine *see* tacrine *on page 617*

tetrahydrocannabinol *see* dronabinol *on page 217*

tetrahydrozoline (tet ra hye DROZ a leen)

Synonyms tetryzoline

U.S./Canadian Brand Names Collyrium Fresh® [US-OTC]; Eyesine® [US-OTC]; Geneye® [US-OTC]; Mallazine® Eye Drops [US-OTC]; Murine® Plus Ophthalmic [US-OTC]; Optigene® [US-OTC]; Tetrasine® Extra [US-OTC]; Tetrasine® [US-OTC]; Tyzine® [US]; Visine® Extra [US-OTC]

Therapeutic Category Adrenergic Agonist Agent

Use Symptomatic relief of nasal congestion and conjunctival congestion

Usual Dosage

Nasal congestion:

Children 2-6 years: Instill 2-3 drops of 0.05% solution every 4-6 hours as needed

Children >6 years and Adults: Instill 2-4 drops or 0.1% spray nasal mucosa every 4-6 hours as needed

Conjunctival congestion: Adults: Instill 1-2 drops in each eye 2-3 times/day

Dosage Forms

Solution, intranasal, as hydrochloride [spray]: 0.05% (15 mL); 0.1% (30 mL, 473 mL)

Solution, ophthalmic, as hydrochloride: 0.05% (15 mL)

Tetralan® *(Discontinued) see page 814*

Tetram® *(Discontinued) see page 814*

Tetramune® *(Discontinued) see page 814*

Tetrasine® Extra Ophthalmic *(Discontinued) see page 814*

Tetrasine® Extra [US-OTC] *see* tetrahydrozoline *on this page*

Tetrasine® Ophthalmic *(Discontinued) see page 814*

Tetrasine® [US-OTC] *see* tetrahydrozoline *on this page*

tetryzoline *see* tetrahydrozoline *on this page*

Teveten® [US] *see* eprosartan *on page 231*

Texacort® [US] *see* hydrocortisone (topical) *on page 334*

TG *see* thioguanine *on page 633*

6-TG *see* thioguanine *on page 633*

T/Gel® [US-OTC] *see* coal tar *on page 158*

T-Gen® *(Discontinued) see page 814*

T-Gesic® [US] *see* hydrocodone and acetaminophen *on page 329*

THA *see* tacrine *on page 617*

thalidomide (tha LI doe mide)

U.S./Canadian Brand Names Thalomid® [US/Can]

Therapeutic Category Immunosuppressant Agent

Use Treatment or prevention of graft-versus-host reactions after bone marrow transplantation; in aphthous ulceration in HIV-positive patients; reactional lepromatous or erythema nodosum leprosy; Langerhans cell histiocytosis, Behçet's syndrome; hypnotic agent; also may be effective in rheumatoid arthritis, discoid lupus, and erythema multiforme; useful in type 2 lepra reactions, but not type 1; can assist in healing mouth ulcers in AIDS patients

Usual Dosage

Leprosy: Up to 400 mg/day; usual maintenance dose: 50-100 mg/day

Behçet's syndrome: 100-400 mg/day

Graft-vs-host reactions:

Children: 3 mg/kg 4 times/day

Adults: 100-1600 mg/day; usual initial dose: 200 mg 4 times/day for use up to 700 days

(Continued)

thalidomide *(Continued)*

AIDS-related aphthous stomatitis: 200 mg twice daily for 5 days, then 200 mg/day for up to 8 weeks

Discoid lupus erythematosus: 100-400 mg/day; maintenance dose: 25-50 mg

Dosage Forms Capsule: 50 mg

Thalitone® **[US]** *see* chlorthalidone *on page 142*

Thalomid® **[US/Can]** *see* thalidomide *on previous page*

THAM® **[US]** *see* tromethamine *on page 661*

THC *see* dronabinol *on page 217*

Theelin® **Aqueous Injection** *(Discontinued)* *see page 814*

Theo-24® **[US]** *see* theophylline *on this page*

Theobid® *(Discontinued)* *see page 814*

Theobid® **Jr Duracaps®** *(Discontinued)* *see page 814*

Theochron® **[US]** *see* theophylline *on this page*

Theoclear-80® *(Discontinued)* *see page 814*

Theoclear®-L.A. *(Discontinued)* *see page 814*

Theocon® **[US]** *see* theophylline and guaifenesin *on next page*

Theo-Dur® **[US/Can]** *see* theophylline *on this page*

Theo-Dur® **Sprinkle®** *(Discontinued)* *see page 814*

Theolair™ **[US/Can]** *see* theophylline *on this page*

Theolair™-SR *(Discontinued)* *see page 814*

Theolate® **[US]** *see* theophylline and guaifenesin *on next page*

Theomar® **GG [US]** *see* theophylline and guaifenesin *on next page*

Theo-Organidin® *(Discontinued)* *see page 814*

theophylline (thee OF i lin)

U.S./Canadian Brand Names Aerolate III® [US]; Aerolate JR® [US]; Aerolate SR® [US]; Apo®-Theo LA [Can]; Elixophyllin® [US]; Novo-Theophyl SR [Can]; Quibron®-T/SR [US/Can]; Quibron®-T [US]; Slo-Phyllin® [US]; Theo-24® [US]; Theochron® [US]; Theo-Dur® [US/Can]; Theolair™ [US/Can]; T-Phyl® [US]; Uniphyl® [US/Can]

Therapeutic Category Theophylline Derivative

Use Treatment of symptoms and reversible airway obstruction due to chronic asthma, chronic bronchitis, or COPD; for treatment of idiopathic apnea of prematurity in neonates

Usual Dosage

Apnea: Dosage should be determined by plasma level monitoring; each 0.5 mg/kg of theophylline administered as a loading dose will result in a 1 mcg/mL increase in serum theophylline concentration

Loading dose: 5 mg/kg; dilute dose in 1-hour I.V. fluid via syringe pump over 1 hour

Maintenance: 2 mg/kg every 8-12 hours or 1-3 mg/kg/dose every 8-12 hours; administer I.V. push 1 mL/minute (2 mg/minute)

Treatment of acute bronchospasm in older patients: (>6 months of age): Loading dose (in patients not currently receiving theophylline): 6 mg/kg (based on aminophylline) administered I.V. over 20-30 minutes; 4.7 mg/kg (based on theophylline) administered I.V. over 20-30 minutes; administration rate should not exceed 20 mg (1 mL)/minute (theophylline) or 25 mg (1 mL)/minute (aminophylline)

Approximate maintenance dosage for treatment of acute bronchospasm:

Children:

6 months to 9 years: 1.2 mg/kg/hour (aminophylline); 0.95 mg/kg/hour (theophylline)

9-16 years and young adult smokers: 1 mg/kg/hour (aminophylline); 0.79 mg/kg/hour (theophylline)

Adults (healthy, nonsmoking): 0.7 mg/kg/hour (aminophylline); 0.55 mg/kg/hour (theophylline)

Older patients and patients with cor pulmonale: 0.6 mg/kg/hour (aminophylline); 0.47 mg/kg/hour (theophylline)

Patients with CHF or liver failure: 0.5 mg/kg/hour (aminophylline); 0.39 mg/kg/hour (theophylline)

Chronic therapy: Slow clinical titration is generally preferred

Initial dose: 16 mg/kg/24 hours or 400 mg/24 hours, whichever is less

Increasing dose: The above dosage may be increased in ~25% increments at 2- to 3-day intervals so long as the drug is tolerated or until the maximum dose is reached; monitor serum levels

Exercise caution in younger children who cannot complain of minor side effects, older adults, and those with cor pulmonale; CHF or liver disease may have unusually low dosage requirements

Dosage Forms

Capsule, immediate release: 100 mg, 200 mg

Capsule, timed release:
8-12 hours (Aerolate®): 65 mg [III], 130 mg [JR], 260 mg [SR]
8-12 hours (Slo-Phyllin® Gyrocaps®): 60 mg, 125 mg, 250 mg
24 hours (Theo-24®): 100 mg, 200 mg, 300 mg

Elixir (Elixophyllin®): 80 mg/15 mL (15 mL, 30 mL, 480 mL, 4000 mL)

Infusion [in D$_5$W]: 0.4 mg/mL (1000 mL); 0.8 mg/mL (500 mL, 1000 mL); 1.6 mg/mL (250 mL, 500 mL); 2 mg/mL (100 mL); 3.2 mg/mL (250 mL); 4 mg/mL (50 mL, 100 mL);

Solution, oral (Theolair™): 80 mg/15 mL (15 mL, 18.75 mL, 30 mL, 480 mL)

Syrup (Slo-Phyllin®): 80 mg/15 mL (15 mL, 30 mL, 500 mL)

Tablet, immediate release:
Quibron®-T: 300 mg
Slo-Phyllin®: 100 mg, 200 mg
Theolair™: 125 mg, 250 mg

Tablet, controlled release (Theo-X®): 100 mg, 200 mg, 300 mg

Tablet, timed release:
8-12 hours (Quibron®-T/SR): 300 mg
8-12 hours (Respbid®): 250 mg, 500 mg
8-12 hours (T-Phyl®): 200 mg
8-24 hours (Theo-Dur®): 100 mg, 200 mg, 300 mg, 450 mg
12-24 hours: 100 mg, 200 mg, 300 mg, 450 mg
12-24 hours (Theochron®): 100 mg, 200 mg, 300 mg
24 hours (Theolair™-SR): 200 mg, 300 mg, 500 mg
24 hours (Uni-Dur®, Uniphyl®): 400 mg, 600 mg

theophylline and guaifenesin (thee OF i lin & gwye FEN e sin)

Synonyms guaifenesin and theophylline

U.S./Canadian Brand Names Elixophyllin® GG [US]; Neoasma® [US]; Quibron® [US]; Theocon® [US]; Theolate® [US]; Theomar® GG [US]

Therapeutic Category Theophylline Derivative

Use Symptomatic treatment of bronchospasm associated with bronchial asthma, chronic bronchitis and pulmonary emphysema

Usual Dosage Adults: Oral: 1-2 capsules every 6-8 hours

Dosage Forms

Capsule: Theophylline 150 mg and guaifenesin 90 mg

Elixir: Theophylline 150 mg and guaifenesin 90 mg per 15 mL (480 mL)

Liquid: Theophylline 100 mg and guaifenesin 100 mg per 15 mL (480 mL)

Syrup: Theophylline 150 mg and guaifenesin 90 mg per 15 mL (480 mL)

Tablet: Theophylline 125 mg and guaifenesin 100 mg

theophylline ethylenediamine see aminophylline on page 33

Theo-Sav® (Discontinued) see page 814

Theospan®-SR (Discontinued) see page 814

Theostat-80® *(Discontinued)* *see page 814*

Theovent® *(Discontinued)* *see page 814*

Theo-X® *(Discontinued)* *see page 814*

Therabid® *(Discontinued)* *see page 814*

TheraCys® **[US]** *see* BCG vaccine *on page 72*

Thera-Flu® **Flu and Cold [US]** *see* acetaminophen, chlorpheniramine, and pseudoephedrine *on page 7*

Thera-Flu® **Non-Drowsy Flu, Cold and Cough [US-OTC]** *see* acetaminophen, dextromethorphan, and pseudoephedrine *on page 8*

Thera-Flur® *(Discontinued)* *see page 814*

Thera-Flur-N® **[US]** *see* fluoride *on page 278*

Theragen® **[US]** *see* capsaicin *on page 111*

Theragen HP® **[US]** *see* capsaicin *on page 111*

Theragran® **Hematinic®** **[US]** *see* vitamin (multiple/oral) *on page 683*

Theragran® **Liquid [US-OTC]** *see* vitamin (multiple/oral) *on page 683*

Theragran-M® **[US-OTC]** *see* vitamin (multiple/oral) *on page 683*

Theragran® **[US-OTC]** *see* vitamin (multiple/oral) *on page 683*

Thera-Hist® **Syrup** *(Discontinued)* *see page 814*

Theramine® **Expectorant** *(Discontinued)* *see page 814*

Theramycin Z® **[US]** *see* erythromycin (ophthalmic/topical) *on page 235*

Therapatch Warm® **[US]** *see* capsaicin *on page 111*

Theraplex Z® **[US-OTC]** *see* pyrithione zinc *on page 557*

Thermazene® **[US]** *see* silver sulfadiazine *on page 590*

thiabendazole (thye a BEN da zole)

Synonyms tiabendazole
U.S./Canadian Brand Names Mintezol® [US]
Therapeutic Category Anthelmintic
Use Treatment of strongyloidiasis, cutaneous larva migrans, visceral larva migrans, dracunculosis, trichinosis, and mixed helminthic infections
Usual Dosage Children and Adults: Oral: 50 mg/kg/day divided every 12 hours (maximum dose: 3 g/day)
  Strongyloidiasis: For 2 consecutive days
  Cutaneous larva migrans: For 2-5 consecutive days
  Visceral larva migrans: For 5-7 consecutive days
  Trichinosis: For 2-4 consecutive days
  Dracunculosis: 50-75 mg/kg/day divided every 12 hours for 3 days
Dosage Forms
  Suspension, oral: 500 mg/5 mL (120 mL)
  Tablet, chewable: 500 mg [orange flavor]

Thiacide® *(Discontinued)* *see page 814*

thiamazole *see* methimazole *on page 416*

Thiamilate® **[US]** *see* thiamine *on this page*

thiamine (THYE a min)

Synonyms aneurine; thiaminium; vitamin B_1
U.S./Canadian Brand Names Betaxin® [Can]; Thiamilate® [US]
Therapeutic Category Vitamin, Water Soluble

Use Treatment of thiamine deficiency including beriberi, Wernicke's encephalopathy syndrome, and peripheral neuritis associated with pellagra; alcoholic patients with altered sensorium; various genetic metabolic disorders

Usual Dosage Dietary supplement (depends on caloric or carbohydrate content of the diet):

Infants: 0.3-0.5 mg/day

Children: 0.5-1 mg/day

Adults: 1-2 mg/day

Note: The above doses can be found as a combination in multivitamin preparations

Children:

Noncritically ill thiamine deficiency: Oral: 10-50 mg/day in divided doses every day for 2 weeks followed by 5-10 mg/day for one month

Beriberi: I.M.: 10-25 mg/day for 2 weeks, then 5-10 mg orally every day for one month (oral as therapeutic multivitamin)

Adults:

Wernicke's encephalopathy: I.M., I.V.: 50 mg as a single dose, then 50 mg I.M. every day until normal diet resumed

Noncritically ill thiamine deficiency: Oral: 10-50 mg/day in divided doses

Beriberi: I.M., I.V.: 10-30 mg 3 times/day for 2 weeks, then switch to 5-10 mg orally every day for one month (oral as therapeutic multivitamin)

Dosage Forms

Injection, as hydrochloride: 100 mg/mL (1 mL, 2 mL, 10 mL, 30 mL); 200 mg/mL (30 mL)

Tablet, as hydrochloride: 50 mg, 100 mg, 250 mg, 500 mg

Tablet, enteric coated, as hydrochloride (Thiamilate®): 20 mg

thiaminium *see thiamine on previous page*

thiethylperazine (thye eth il PER a zeen)

U.S./Canadian Brand Names Torecan® [US]

Therapeutic Category Phenothiazine Derivative

Use Relief of nausea and vomiting

Usual Dosage Children >12 years and Adults: Oral: 10 mg 1-3 times/day as needed

Dosage Forms Tablet, as maleate: 10 mg [contains sodium benzoate and tartrazine]

thimerosal (thye MER oh sal)

U.S./Canadian Brand Names Mersol® [US-OTC]; Merthiolate® [US-OTC]

Therapeutic Category Antibacterial, Topical

Use Organomercurial antiseptic with sustained bacteriostatic and fungistatic activity

Usual Dosage Apply 1-3 times/day

Dosage Forms

Ointment, ophthalmic, topical: 0.02% [0.2 mg/mL] (3.5 g)

Solution, topical: 0.1% [1 mg/mL = 1:1000] (120 mL, 480 mL, 4000 mL)

Solution, topical [spray]: 0.1% [1 mg/mL = 1:1000] with alcohol 2% (90 mL)

Tincture, topical: 0.1% [1 mg/mL = 1:1000] with alcohol 50% (120 mL, 480 mL, 4000 mL)

thioguanine (thye oh GWAH neen)

Synonyms 2-amino-6-mercaptopurine; TG; 6-TG; 6-thioguanine; tioguanine

U.S./Canadian Brand Names Lanvis® [Can]

Therapeutic Category Antineoplastic Agent

Use Remission induction in acute myelogenous (nonlymphocytic) leukemia; treatment of chronic myelogenous leukemia and acute lymphocytic leukemia

Usual Dosage Refer to individual protocols. Oral:

Infants <3 years: Combination drug therapy for acute nonlymphocytic leukemia: 3.3 mg/kg/day in divided doses twice daily for 4 days

Children and Adults: 2-3 mg/kg/day calculated to nearest 20 mg or 75-200 mg/m^2/day in 1-2 divided doses for 5-7 days or until remission is attained

(Continued)

thioguanine *(Continued)*
Dosage Forms Tablet, scored: 40 mg

6-thioguanine *see* thioguanine *on previous page*

Thiola™ [US/Can] *see* tiopronin *on page 640*

thiopental (thye oh PEN tal)
U.S./Canadian Brand Names Pentothal® Sodium [US/Can]
Therapeutic Category Barbiturate
Controlled Substance C-III
Use Induction of anesthesia; adjunct for intubation in head injury patients; control of convulsive states; treatment of elevated intracranial pressure
Usual Dosage I.V.:
Induction anesthesia:
  Infants: 5-8 mg/kg
  Children 1-12 years: 5-6 mg/kg
  Adults: 3-5 mg/kg
Maintenance anesthesia:
  Children: 1 mg/kg as needed
  Adults: 25-100 mg as needed
Increased intracranial pressure: Children and Adults: 1.5-5 mg/kg/dose; repeat as needed to control intracranial pressure
Seizures:
  Children: 2-3 mg/kg/dose, repeat as needed
  Adults: 75-250 mg/dose, repeat as needed
Rectal administration: (Patient should be NPO for no less than 3 hours prior to administration)
Suggested initial doses of thiopental rectal suspension are:
  <3 months: 15 mg/kg/dose
  >3 months: 25 mg/kg/dose
Note: The age of a premature infant should be adjusted to reflect the age that the infant would have been if full-term (eg, an infant, now age 4 months, who was 2 months premature should be considered to be a 2-month old infant).
Doses should be rounded downward to the nearest 50 mg increment to allow for accurate measurement of the dose
Inactive or debilitated patients and patients recently medicated with other sedatives, (eg, chloral hydrate, meperidine, chlorpromazine, and promethazine), may require smaller doses than usual
If the patient is not sedated within 15-20 minutes, a single repeat dose of thiopental can be administered; the single repeat doses are:
  <3 months of age: <7.5 mg/kg/dose
  >3 months of age: 15 mg/kg/dose
Adults weighing >90 kg should not receive >3 g as a total dose (initial plus repeat doses)
Children weighing >34 kg should not receive >1 g as a total dose (initial plus repeat doses)
Neither adults nor children should receive more than one course of thiopental rectal suspension (initial dose plus repeat dose) per 24-hour period
Dosage Forms
Injection, as sodium: 250 mg, 400 mg, 500 mg, 1 g, 2.5 g, 5 g
Suspension, rectal, as sodium: 400 mg/g (2 g)

Thioplex® [US] *see* thiotepa *on next page*

thioproperazine *(Canada only)* (thye oh pro PER a zeen)
U.S./Canadian Brand Names Majeptil® [Can]
Therapeutic Category Neuroleptic Agent

Use All types of acute and chronic schizophrenia, including those which did not respond to the usual neuroleptics; manic syndromes.

Usual Dosage Initial treatment: Adults: It is recommended to start treatment at a low dosage of about 5 mg/day in a single dose or in divided doses. This initial dosage is gradually increased by the same amount every 2-3 days until the usual effective dosage of 30-40 mg/day is reached. In some cases, higher dosages of 90 mg or more per day, are necessary to control the psychotic manifestations.

Children >10 years of age: Start treatment with a daily dosage of 1-3 mg following the method of treatment described for adults

Maintenance therapy: Adults and Children: Dosage should be reduced gradually to the lowest effective level, which may be as low as a few mg per day and maintained as long as necessary

Dosage Forms Tablet, as mesylate: 10 mg

thioridazine (thye oh RID a zeen)

U.S./Canadian Brand Names Apo®-Thioridazine [Can]; Mellaril® [US/Can]

Therapeutic Category Phenothiazine Derivative

Use Management of psychotic disorders; depressive neurosis; dementia in elderly; severe behavioral problems in children

Usual Dosage Oral:

Children >2 years: Range: 0.5-3 mg/kg/day in 2-3 divided doses; usual: 1 mg/kg/day; maximum: 3 mg/kg/day

Behavior problems: Initial: 10 mg 2-3 times/day, increase gradually

Severe psychoses: Initial: 25 mg 2-3 times/day, increase gradually

Adults:

Psychoses: Initial: 50-100 mg 3 times/day with gradual increments as needed and tolerated; maximum daily dose: 800 mg/day in 2-4 divided doses

Depressive disorders, dementia: Initial: 25 mg 3 times/day; maintenance dose: 20-200 mg/day

Dosage Forms

Solution, oral concentrate, as hydrochloride: 30 mg/mL (120 mL); 100 mg/mL (3.4 mL, 120 mL)

Tablet, as hydrochloride: 10 mg, 15 mg, 25 mg, 50 mg, 100 mg, 150 mg, 200 mg

thiotepa (thye oh TEP a)

Synonyms TESPA; triethylenethiophosphoramide; TSPA

U.S./Canadian Brand Names Thioplex® [US]

Therapeutic Category Antineoplastic Agent

Use Treatment of superficial tumors of the bladder; palliative treatment of adenocarcinoma of breast or ovary; lymphomas and sarcomas; meningeal neoplasms; control pleural, pericardial or peritoneal effusions caused by metastatic tumors; high-dose regimens with autologous bone marrow transplantation

Usual Dosage Refer to individual protocols.

Children: Sarcomas: I.V.: 25-65 mg/m^2 as a single dose every 21 days

Adults:

I.M., I.V., S.C.: 8 mg/m^2 daily for 5 days or 30-60 mg/m^2 once per week

High-dose therapy for bone marrow transplant: I.V.: 500 mg/m^2

Intracavitary: 0.6-0.8 mg/kg or 60 mg in 60 mL SWI instilled into the bladder at 1- to 4-week intervals

Intrathecal: Doses of 1-10 mg/m^2 administered 1-2 times/week

Dosage Forms Injection, powder for reconstitution: 15 mg

thiothixene (thye oh THIKS een)

Synonyms tiotixene

U.S./Canadian Brand Names Navane® [US/Can]

Therapeutic Category Thioxanthene Derivative

Use Management of psychotic disorders

(Continued)

thiothixene *(Continued)*

Usual Dosage
Children <12 years: 0.25 mg/kg/24 hours in divided doses (dose not well established)
Children >12 years and Adults: Mild to moderate psychosis: 2 mg 3 times/day, up to 20-30 mg/day; more severe psychosis: Initial: 5 mg 2 times/day, may increase gradually, if necessary; maximum: 60 mg/day
Hemodialysis: Not dialyzable (0% to 5%)

Dosage Forms
Capsule: 1 mg, 2 mg, 5 mg, 10 mg, 20 mg
Injection, powder for reconstitution, as hydrochloride: 5 mg/mL (2 mL)
Solution, oral concentrate, as hydrochloride: 5 mg/mL (30 mL, 120 mL)

Thorazine® [US] *see* chlorpromazine *on page 141*

Thrombate III™ [US/Can] *see* antithrombin III *on page 47*

Thrombinar® *(Discontinued)* *see page 814*

thrombin (topical) (THROM bin TOP i kal)

U.S./Canadian Brand Names Thrombogen® [US]; Thrombostat® [Can]
Therapeutic Category Hemostatic Agent
Use Hemostasis whenever minor bleeding from capillaries and small venules is accessible
Usual Dosage Use 1000-2000 units/mL of solution where bleeding is profuse; apply powder directly to the site of bleeding or on oozing surfaces; use 100 units/mL for bleeding from skin or mucosal surfaces
Dosage Forms Powder: 1000 units, 5000 units, 10,000 units, 20,000 units, 50,000 units

Thrombogen® [US] *see* thrombin (topical) *on this page*

Thrombostat® *(Discontinued)* *see page 814*

Thrombostat® [Can] *see* thrombin (topical) *on this page*

Thymoglobulin® [US] *see* antithymocyte globulin (rabbit) *on page 47*

Thypinone® *(Discontinued)* *see page 814*

Thyrar® *(Discontinued)* *see page 814*

Thyrel® TRH [US/Can] *see* protirelin *on page 551*

Thyro-Block® *(Discontinued)* *see page 814*

Thyro-Block® [Can] *see* potassium iodide *on page 531*

Thyrogen® [US] *see* thyrotropin alpha *on next page*

thyroid (THYE royd)

Synonyms desiccated thyroid; thyroid extract
U.S./Canadian Brand Names Armour® Thyroid [US]; Nature-Throid® NT [US]; Westhroid® [US]
Therapeutic Category Thyroid Product
Use Replacement or supplemental therapy in hypothyroidism
Usual Dosage Adults: Oral: Start at 30 mg/day and titrate by 30 mg/day in increments of 2- to 3-week intervals; usual maintenance dose: 60-120 mg/day
Dosage Forms
Capsule, pork source in soybean oil (S-P-T): 60 mg, 120 mg, 180 mg, 300 mg
Tablet:
Armour® Thyroid: 15 mg, 30 mg, 60 mg, 90 mg, 120 mg, 180 mg, 240 mg, 300 mg
Thyroid USP: 15 mg, 30 mg, 60 mg, 120 mg, 180 mg, 300 mg

thyroid extract *see* thyroid *on this page*

thyroid-stimulating hormone *see* thyrotropin *on next page*

Thyroid Strong® *(Discontinued)* *see page 814*

Thyrolar® [US/Can] *see liotrix on page 387*

thyrotropin (thye roe TROE pin)
Synonyms thyroid-stimulating hormone; TSH
U.S./Canadian Brand Names Thytropar® [US]
Therapeutic Category Diagnostic Agent
Use Diagnostic aid to determine subclinical hypothyroidism or decreased thyroid reserve, to differentiate between primary and secondary hypothyroidism and between primary hypothyroidism and euthyroidism in patients receiving thyroid replacement
Usual Dosage I.M., S.C.: 10 units/day for 1-3 days; follow by a radioiodine study 24 hours past last injection, no response in thyroid failure, substantial response in pituitary failure
Dosage Forms Injection: 10 units

thyrotropin alpha (thye roe TROE pin AL fa)
Synonyms human thyroid-stimulating hormone
U.S./Canadian Brand Names Thyrogen® [US]
Therapeutic Category Diagnostic Agent
Use As an adjunctive diagnostic tool for serum thyroglobulin (Tg) testing with or without radioiodine imaging in the follow-up of patients with well-differentiated thyroid cancer
Potential clinical uses:
  1. Patients with an undetectable Tg on thyroid hormone suppressive therapy to exclude the diagnosis of residual or recurrent thyroid cancer
  2. Patients requiring serum Tg testing and radioiodine imaging who are unwilling to undergo thyroid hormone withdrawal testing and whose treating physician believes that use of a less sensitive test is justified
  3. Patients who are either unable to mount an adequate endogenous TSH response to thyroid hormone withdrawal or in whom withdrawal is medically contraindicated
Usual Dosage Children >16 years and Adults: I.M.: 0.9 mg every 24 hours for 2 doses or every 72 hours for 3 doses. For radioiodine imaging, radioiodine administration should be given 24 hours following the final Thyrogen® injection. Scanning should be performed 48 hours after radioiodine administration (72 hours after the final injection of Thyrogen®).
Dosage Forms Injection, powder for reconstitution [kit]: 1.1 mg vials (>4 int. units) [two vials of Thyrogen® and two vials of SWFI - 10 mL]

Thytropar® [US] *see thyrotropin on this page*
tiabendazole *see thiabendazole on page 632*

tiagabine (tye AG a bene)
U.S./Canadian Brand Names Gabitril® [US/Can]
Therapeutic Category Anticonvulsant
Use Adjunctive therapy in adults and children 12 years and older in the treatment of partial seizures
Usual Dosage Children >12 years and Adults: Oral: Initial: 4 mg, once daily; the total daily dose may be increased in 4 mg increments beginning the second week of therapy; thereafter, the daily dose may be increased by 4-8 mg/day until clinical response is achieved, up to a maximum of 32 mg/day; the total daily dose at higher levels should be given in divided doses, 2-4 times/day
Dosage Forms Tablet: 2 mg, 4 mg, 12 mg, 16 mg, 20 mg

Tiamate® (Discontinued) *see page 814*
Tiamol® [Can] *see fluocinonide on page 277*

tiaprofenic acid *(Canada only)* (tye ah PRO fen ik AS id)

U.S./Canadian Brand Names Albert® Tiafen [Can]; Apo®-Tiaprofenic [Can]; Novo-Tiaprofenic [Can]; Nu-Tiaprofenic [Can]; PMS-Tiaprofenic [Can]; Surgam® [Can]; Surgam® SR [Can]

Therapeutic Category Nonsteroidal Anti-inflammatory Drug (NSAID)

Use Relief of signs and symptoms of rheumatoid arthritis and osteoarthritis (degenerative joint disease)

Usual Dosage Adults: Oral:

Tablet:

Rheumatoid arthritis: Usual initial and maintenance dose: 600 mg/day in 3 divided doses; some patients may do well on 300 mg twice daily; maximum daily dose: 600 mg

Osteoarthritis: Usual initial and maintenance dose: 600 mg/day in 2 or 3 divided doses; in rare instances patients may be maintained on 300 mg/day in divided doses; maximum daily dose: 600 mg

Extended release capsule:

Rheumatoid arthritis or osteoarthritis: Initial and maintenance dose: 2 sustained release capsules of 300 mg once daily; Surgam® SR capsules should be swallowed whole

Dosage Forms

Capsule, sustained release: 300 mg

Tablet: 200 mg, 300 mg

Tiazac® [US/Can] *see* diltiazem *on page 199*

Ticar® [US] *see* ticarcillin *on this page*

ticarcillin (tye kar SIL in)

U.S./Canadian Brand Names Ticar® [US]

Therapeutic Category Penicillin

Use Treatment of infections such as septicemia, acute and chronic respiratory tract infections, skin and soft tissue infections, and urinary tract infections due to susceptible strains of *Pseudomonas*, *Proteus*, *Escherichia coli*, and *Enterobacter*

Usual Dosage I.V. (ticarcillin is generally administered I.M. only for the treatment of uncomplicated urinary tract infections):

Infants and Children: 200-300 mg/kg/day in divided doses every 4-6 hours; maximum dose: 24 g/day

Adults: 1-4 g every 4-6 hours

Dosage Forms Injection, powder for reconstitution, as disodium: 3 g, 20 g

ticarcillin and clavulanate potassium

(tye kar SIL in & klav yoo LAN ate poe TASS ee um)

Synonyms clavulanic acid and ticarcillin; ticarcillin and clavulanic acid

U.S./Canadian Brand Names Timentin® [US/Can]

Therapeutic Category Penicillin

Use Treatment of infections caused by susceptible organisms involving the lower respiratory tract, urinary tract, skin and skin structures, bone and joint, and septicemia. Clavulanate expands activity of ticarcillin to include beta-lactamase producing strains of *S. aureus*, *H. influenzae*, *Moraxella catarrhalis*, *B. fragilis*, *Klebsiella*, and *Proteus* species

Usual Dosage I.V.:

Children: 200-300 mg of ticarcillin/kg/day in divided doses every 4-6 hours

Adults: 3.1 g (ticarcillin 3 g plus clavulanic acid 0.1 g) every 4-6 hours; maximum: 18-24 g/day; for urinary tract infections: 3.1 g every 6-8 hours

Dosage Forms

Infusion [premixed, frozen]: Ticarcillin disodium 3 g and clavulanate potassium 0.1 g (100 mL)

Injection, powder for reconstitution: Ticarcillin disodium 3 g and clavulanate potassium 0.1 g (3.1 g, 31 g)

ticarcillin and clavulanic acid *see* ticarcillin and clavulanate potassium *on previous page*

TICE® BCG [US] *see* BCG vaccine *on page 72*

Ticlid® [US/Can] *see* ticlopidine *on this page*

ticlopidine (tye KLOE pi deen)
U.S./Canadian Brand Names Alti-Ticlopidine [Can]; Apo®-Ticlopidine [Can]; Gen-Ticlopidine [Can]; Nu-Ticlopidine [Can]; Rhoxal-ticlopidine [Can]; Ticlid® [US/Can]
Therapeutic Category Antiplatelet Agent
Use Platelet aggregation inhibitor that reduces the risk of thrombotic stroke in patients who have had a stroke or stroke precursors
Usual Dosage Adults: Oral: 1 tablet twice daily with food
Dosage Forms Tablet, as hydrochloride: 250 mg

Ticon® *(Discontinued) see page 814*

TIG *see* tetanus immune globulin (human) *on page 626*

Tigan® [US/Can] *see* trimethobenzamide *on page 657*

Tiject-20® *(Discontinued) see page 814*

Tikosyn™ [US/Can] *see* dofetilide *on page 209*

Tilade® [US/Can] *see* nedocromil (inhalation) *on page 450*

tiludronate (tye LOO droe nate)
Synonyms tiludronic acid
U.S./Canadian Brand Names Skelid® [US]
Therapeutic Category Bisphosphonate Derivative
Use Paget's disease of the bone
Usual Dosage Adults: Oral: 400 mg/day (2 tablets) [tiludronic acid]
Dosage Forms Dosage expressed in terms of tiludronic acid:
  Tablet, as disodium: 240 mg [tiludronic acid 200 mg]

tiludronic acid *see* tiludronate *on this page*

Tim-AK [Can] *see* timolol *on this page*

Timecelles® *(Discontinued) see page 814*

Timentin® [US/Can] *see* ticarcillin and clavulanate potassium *on previous page*

timolol (TYE moe lole)
U.S./Canadian Brand Names Apo®-Timol [Can]; Apo®-Timop [Can]; Betimol® [US]; Blocadren® [US]; Gen-Timolol [Can]; Nu-Timolol [Can]; Phoxal-timolol [Can]; PMS-Timolol [Can]; Tim-AK [Can]; Timoptic® OcuDose® [US]; Timoptic® [US/Can]; Timoptic-XE® [US/Can]
Therapeutic Category Beta-Adrenergic Blocker
Use Ophthalmic dosage form used to treat elevated intraocular pressure such as glaucoma or ocular hypertension; orally for treatment of hypertension and angina and for prevention of myocardial infarction and migraine headaches
Usual Dosage
  Children and Adults: Ophthalmic: Initial: 0.25% solution, instill 1 drop twice daily; increase to 0.5% solution if response not adequate; decrease to 1 drop/day if controlled; do not exceed 1 drop twice daily of 0.5% solution
  Adults: Oral:
  Hypertension: Initial: 10 mg twice daily, increase gradually every 7 days, usual dosage: 20-40 mg/day in 2 divided doses; maximum: 60 mg/day
  Prevention of myocardial infarction: 10 mg twice daily initiated within 1-4 weeks after infarction
  Migraine headache: Initial: 10 mg twice daily, increase to maximum of 30 mg/day
(Continued)

timolol *(Continued)*

Dosage Forms

Gel-forming solution, ophthalmic, as maleate (Timoptic-XE®): 0.25% (2.5 mL, 5 mL); 0.5% (2.5 mL, 5 mL)

Solution, ophthalmic, as hemihydrate (Betimol®): 0.25% (5 mL, 10 mL, 15 mL); 0.5% (5 mL, 10 mL, 15 mL) [contains benzalkonium chloride]

Solution, ophthalmic, as maleate: 0.25% (5 mL, 10 mL, 15 mL); 0.5% (5 mL, 10 mL, 15 mL) [contains benzalkonium chloride]

Timoptic®: 0.25% (5 mL, 10 mL); 0.5% (5 mL, 10 mL) [contains benzalkonium chloride]

Solution, ophthalmic, as maleate [preservative free] (Timoptic® OcuDose®): 0.25% (0.2 mL);0.5% (0.2 mL) [single use]

Tablet, as maleate (Blocadren®): 5 mg, 10 mg, 20 mg

Timoptic® [US/Can] *see* timolol *on previous page*

Timoptic® OcuDose® [US] *see* timolol *on previous page*

Timoptic-XE® [US/Can] *see* timolol *on previous page*

Tinactin® for Jock Itch [US-OTC] *see* tolnaftate *on page 644*

Tinactin® [US-OTC] *see* tolnaftate *on page 644*

TinBen® [US-OTC] *see* benzoin *on page 79*

Tindal® *(Discontinued)* *see page 814*

Tine Test PPD [US] *see* tuberculin tests *on page 662*

Ting® [US-OTC] *see* tolnaftate *on page 644*

Tinver® *(Discontinued)* *see page 814*

tinzaparin (tin ZA pa rin)

U.S./Canadian Brand Names Innohep® [US/Can]

Therapeutic Category Anticoagulant (Other)

Use Treatment of acute symptomatic deep vein thrombosis, with or without pulmonary embolism, in conjunction with warfarin sodium

Usual Dosage S.C.:

Adults: 175 anti-Xa int. units/kg of body weight once daily. Warfarin sodium should be started when appropriate. Administer tinzaparin for at least 6 days and until patient is adequately anticoagulated with warfarin.

Note: To calculate the volume of solution to administer per dose: Volume to be administered (mL) = patient weight (kg) x 0.00875 mL/kg (may be rounded off to the nearest 0.05 mL)

Dosage Forms Injection: 20,000 anti-Xa int. units/mL (2 mL vial)

tioconazole (tye oh KONE a zole)

U.S./Canadian Brand Names 1-Day™ [US-OTC]; GyneCure™ [Can]; Trosyd™ AF [Can]; Trosyd™ J [Can]; Vagistat®-1 [US-OTC]

Therapeutic Category Antifungal Agent

Use Local treatment of vulvovaginal candidiasis

Usual Dosage Vaginal: Insert 1 applicatorful in vagina, just prior to bedtime, as a single dose

Dosage Forms Ointment, vaginal: 6.5% (4.6 g) [with applicator]

tioguanine *see* thioguanine *on page 633*

tiopronin (tye oh PROE nin)

U.S./Canadian Brand Names Thiola™ [US/Can]

Therapeutic Category Urinary Tract Product

Use Prevention of kidney stone (cystine) formation in patients with severe homozygous cystinuric who have urinary cystine >500 mg/day who are resistant to treatment with high fluid intake, alkali, and diet modification, or who have had adverse reactions to penicillamine

Usual Dosage Adults: Initial: 800 mg/day; average dose: 1000 mg/day

Dosage Forms Tablet: 100 mg

tiotixene *see* thiothixene *on page 635*

tirofiban (tye roe FYE ban)

U.S./Canadian Brand Names Aggrastat® [US/Can]

Therapeutic Category Antiplatelet Agent

Use In combination with heparin, is indicated for the treatment of acute coronary syndrome, including patients who are to be managed medically and those undergoing PTCA or atherectomy. In this setting, it has been shown to decrease the rate of a combined endpoint of death, new myocardial infarction or refractory ischemia/repeat cardiac procedure.

Usual Dosage Adults: I.V.: Initial rate of 0.4 mcg/kg/minute for 30 minutes and then continued at 0.1 mcg/kg/minute

Dosage Forms

Injection [premixed] 50 mcg/mL (500 mL)

Injection, solution: 250 mcg/mL (50 mL)

Ti-Screen® [US-OTC] *see* methoxycinnamate and oxybenzone *on page 419*

Tisit® Blue Gel [US-OTC] *see* pyrethrins *on page 555*

Tisit® [US-OTC] *see* pyrethrins *on page 555*

Tisseel® VH Fibrin Sealant Kit [US/Can] *see* fibrin sealant kit *on page 271*

tissue plasminogen activator, recombinant *see* alteplase *on page 26*

Titralac® Plus Liquid [US-OTC] *see* calcium carbonate and simethicone *on page 105*

Ti-U-Lac® H [Can] *see* urea and hydrocortisone *on page 667*

tizanidine (tye ZAN i deen)

U.S./Canadian Brand Names Zanaflex® [US/Can]

Therapeutic Category Alpha$_2$-Adrenergic Agonist Agent

Use Intermittent management of increased muscle tone associated with spasticity (eg, multiple sclerosis, spinal cord injury)

Usual Dosage Adults: Oral: Initial: 4 mg every 6-8 hours, not to exceed 3 doses/day or 36 mg in a 24-hour period; doses may be increased at 2 mg or 4 mg increments with single doses not exceeding 12 mg

Dosage Forms Tablet: 2 mg, 4 mg

TMP *see* trimethoprim *on page 657*

TMP-SMX *see* sulfamethoxazole and trimethoprim *on page 612*

TNKase™ [US] *see* tenecteplase *on page 621*

TOBI™ [US/Can] *see* tobramycin *on this page*

TobraDex® [US/Can] *see* tobramycin and dexamethasone *on next page*

tobramycin (toe bra MYE sin)

U.S./Canadian Brand Names AKTob® [US]; Nebcin® [US/Can]; PMS-Tobramycin [Can]; TOBI™ [US/Can]; Tobrex® [US/Can]; Tomycine™ [Can]

Therapeutic Category Aminoglycoside (Antibiotic); Antibiotic, Ophthalmic

Use Treatment of documented or suspected infections caused by susceptible gram-negative bacilli including *Pseudomonas aeruginosa*; infection with a nonpseudomonal enteric bacillus which is more sensitive to tobramycin than gentamicin based on susceptibility tests; susceptible organisms in lower respiratory tract infections, septicemia; intra-abdominal, skin, bone, and urinary tract infections; empiric therapy in cystic (Continued)

tobramycin *(Continued)*

fibrosis and immunocompromised patients; used topically to treat superficial ophthalmic infections caused by susceptible bacteria

Usual Dosage Dosage should be based on an estimate of ideal body weight

Infants and Children: I.M., I.V.: 2.5 mg/kg/dose every 8 hours

Note: Some patients may require larger or more frequent doses if serum levels document the need (ie, cystic fibrosis or febrile granulocytopenic patients)

Adults: I.M., I.V.: 3-5 mg/kg/day in 3 divided doses

Children and Adults:

Renal dysfunction: 2.5 mg/kg (2-3 serum level measurements should be obtained after the initial dose to measure the half-life in order to determine the frequency of subsequent doses)

Ophthalmic: 1-2 drops every 4 hours; apply ointment 2-3 times/day; for severe infections apply ointment every 3-4 hours, or 2 drops every 30-60 minutes initially, then reduce to less frequent intervals

Dosage Forms

Injection, as sulfate (Nebcin®): 10 mg/mL (2 mL, 6 mL, 8 mL); 40 mg/mL (1 mL, 2 mL, 30 mL, 50 mL)

Injection, powder for reconstitution (Nebcin®): 40 mg/mL (1.2 g vials)

Ointment, ophthalmic (Tobrex®): 0.3% (3.5 g)

Solution for nebulization (TOBI™): 60 mg/mL (5 mL)

Solution, ophthalmic: 0.3% (5 mL)

AKTob®, Tobrex®: 0.3% (5 mL)

tobramycin and dexamethasone (toe bra MYE sin & deks a METH a sone)

Synonyms dexamethasone and tobramycin

U.S./Canadian Brand Names TobraDex® [US/Can]

Therapeutic Category Antibiotic/Corticosteroid, Ophthalmic

Use Treatment of external ocular infection caused by susceptible gram-negative bacteria and steroid responsive inflammatory conditions of the palpebral and bulbar conjunctiva, lid, cornea, and anterior segment of the globe

Usual Dosage Ophthalmic: Adults:

Ointment: Apply 1.25 cm (½") every 3-4 hours to 2-3 times/day

Suspension: Instill 1-2 drops every 4-6 hours (first 24-48 hours may increase frequency to every 2 hours until signs of clinical improvement are seen); apply every 30-60 minutes for severe infections

Dosage Forms

Ointment, ophthalmic: Tobramycin 0.3% and dexamethasone 0.1% (3.5 g)

Suspension, ophthalmic: Tobramycin 0.3% and dexamethasone 0.1% (2.5 mL, 5 mL)

Tobrex® **[US/Can]** *see* tobramycin *on previous page*

tocainide (toe KAY nide)

U.S./Canadian Brand Names Tonocard® [US]

Therapeutic Category Antiarrhythmic Agent, Class I-B

Use Suppress and prevent symptomatic ventricular arrhythmias

Usual Dosage Adults: Oral: 1200-1800 mg/day in 3 divided doses

Dosage Forms Tablet, as hydrochloride: 400 mg, 600 mg

tocophersolan (toe kof er SOE lan)

Synonyms TPGS

U.S./Canadian Brand Names Liqui-E® [US]

Therapeutic Category Vitamin, Fat Soluble

Use Treatment of vitamin E deficiency resulting from malabsorption due to prolonged cholestatic hepatobiliary disease

Usual Dosage Dietary supplement: Oral: 15 mg (400 units) every day

Dosage Forms Liquid: 26.6 units/mL

Tofranil® **[US/Can]** *see* imipramine *on page 346*

Tofranil-PM® **[US]** *see* imipramine *on page 346*

tolazamide (tole AZ a mide)

Tall-Man **TOLAZ**amide

U.S./Canadian Brand Names Tolinase® [US/Can]

Therapeutic Category Antidiabetic Agent, Oral

Use Adjunct to diet for the management of mild to moderately severe, stable, noninsulin-dependent (type II) diabetes mellitus

Usual Dosage Adults: Oral: 100-1000 mg/day

Dosage Forms Tablet: 100 mg, 250 mg, 500 mg

tolazoline (tole AZ oh leen)

Synonyms benzazoline

U.S./Canadian Brand Names Priscoline® [US]

Therapeutic Category Alpha-Adrenergic Blocking Agent

Use Persistent pulmonary hypertension of the newborn (PPHN), also known as persistent fetal circulation (PFC); peripheral vasospastic disorders

Usual Dosage

Neonates: Initial: I.V.: 1-2 mg/kg over 10-15 minutes via scalp vein or upper extremity; maintenance: 1-2 mg/kg/hour; use lower maintenance doses in patients with decreased renal function. Also used in neonates for acute vasospasm "cath toes" at 0.25 mg/kg/hour (no load)

Adults: Peripheral vasospastic disorder: I.M., I.V., S.C.: 10-50 mg 4 times/day

Dosage Forms Injection, as hydrochloride: 25 mg/mL (4 mL)

tolbutamide (tole BYOO ta mide)

Tall-Man **TOLBUT**amide

U.S./Canadian Brand Names Apo®-Tolbutamide [Can]; Orinase® Diagnostic [US]; Tol-Tab® [US]

Therapeutic Category Antidiabetic Agent, Oral

Use Adjunct to diet for the management of mild to moderately severe, stable, noninsulin-dependent (type II) diabetes mellitus

Usual Dosage Adults:
Oral: 250-2000 mg/day
I.V. bolus: 20 mg/kg

Dosage Forms
Injection, powder for reconstitution, as sodium (Orinase Diagnostic®): 1 g
Tablet (Tol-Tab®): 500 mg

tolcapone (TOLE ka pone)

U.S./Canadian Brand Names Tasmar® [US]

Therapeutic Category Anti-Parkinson's Agent

Use Adjunct to levodopa and carbidopa for the treatment of signs and symptoms of idiopathic Parkinson's disease

Usual Dosage Adults: Oral: Initial: 100 mg 3 times/day, may increase to 200 mg 3 times/day

Dosage Forms Tablet: 100 mg, 200 mg

Tolectin® **[US/Can]** *see* tolmetin *on next page*

Tolectin® **DS [US]** *see* tolmetin *on next page*

Tolinase® **[US/Can]** *see* tolazamide *on this page*

tolmetin (TOLE met in)

U.S./Canadian Brand Names Tolectin® DS [US]; Tolectin® [US/Can]

Therapeutic Category Analgesic, Non-narcotic; Nonsteroidal Anti-inflammatory Drug (NSAID)

Use Treatment of inflammatory and rheumatoid disorders, including juvenile rheumatoid arthritis

Usual Dosage Oral:

Children ≥2 years: Anti-inflammatory: Initial: 20 mg/kg/day in 3 divided doses, then 15-30 mg/kg/day in 3 divided doses; maximum dose: 30 mg/kg/day

Adults: 400 mg 3 times/day; usual dose: 600 mg to 1.8 g/day; maximum: 2 g/day

Dosage Forms

Capsule, as sodium (Tolectin® DS): 400 mg

Tablet, as sodium (Tolectin®): 200 mg, 600 mg

tolnaftate (tole NAF tate)

U.S./Canadian Brand Names Absorbine Jr.® Antifungal [US-OTC]; Aftate® for Athlete's Foot [US-OTC]; Aftate® for Jock Itch [US-OTC]; Blis-To-Sol® [US-OTC]; Dr Scholl's Athlete's Foot [US-OTC]; Dr Scholl's Maximum Strength Tritin [US-OTC]; Genaspor® [US-OTC]; Pitrex [Can]; Quinsana Plus® [US-OTC]; Tinactin® for Jock Itch [US-OTC]; Tinactin® [US-OTC]; Ting® [US-OTC]; ZeaSorb® AF [Can]

Therapeutic Category Antifungal Agent

Use Treatment of tinea pedis, tinea cruris, tinea corporis, tinea manuum caused by *Trichophyton rubrum*, *T. mentagrophytes*, *T. tonsurans*, *M. canis*, *M. audouinii*, and *E. floccosum*; also effective in the treatment of tinea versicolor infections due to *Malassezia furfur*

Usual Dosage Children and Adults: Topical: Wash and dry affected area; apply 1-2 drops of solution or a small amount of cream or powder and rub into the affected areas twice daily for 2-4 weeks

Dosage Forms

Aerosol, topical liquid: 1% (59.2 mL, 90 mL, 120 mL)

Aerosol, topical powder: 1% (56.7 g, 100 g, 105 g, 150 g)

Cream: 1% (15 g, 30 g)

Gel: 1% (15 g)

Powder: 1% (45 g, 90 g)

Solution, topical: 1% (10 mL)

Tol-Tab® [US] *see* tolbutamide *on previous page*

tolterodine (tole TER oh dine)

U.S./Canadian Brand Names Detrol® LA [US]; Detrol® [US/Can]

Therapeutic Category Anticholinergic Agent

Use Treatment of patients with an overactive bladder with symptoms of urinary frequency, urgency, or urge incontinence

Usual Dosage

Children: Safety and efficacy in pediatric patients have not been established

Adults: Treatment of overactive bladder: Oral:

Immediate release tablet: 2 mg twice daily; the dose may be lowered to 1 mg twice daily based on individual response and tolerability

Dosing adjustment in patients concurrently taking CYP3A4 inhibitors: 1 mg twice daily

Extended release capsule: 4 mg once a day; dose may be lowered to 2 mg daily based on individual response and tolerability

Dosing adjustment in patients concurrently taking CYP3A4 inhibitors: 2 mg daily

Dosage Forms

Capsule, extended release, as tartrate: 2 mg, 4 mg

Tablet, as tartrate: 1 mg, 2 mg

Tolu-Sed® DM [US-OTC] *see* guaifenesin and dextromethorphan *on page 308*

Tomocat® [US] *see* radiological/contrast media (ionic) *on page 561*

Tomudex® **[Can]** *see* raltitrexed *(Canada only) on page 564*

Tomycine™ **[Can]** *see* tobramycin *on page 641*

Tonocard® **[US]** *see* tocainide *on page 642*

Tonopaque® **[US]** *see* radiological/contrast media (ionic) *on page 561*

Topamax® **[US/Can]** *see* topiramate *on this page*

Topicort® **[US/Can]** *see* desoximetasone *on page 183*

Topicort®-LP **[US]** *see* desoximetasone *on page 183*

Topicycline® **Topical** *(Discontinued) see page 814*

Topilene® **[Can]** *see* betamethasone (topical) *on page 83*

topiramate (toe PYE ra mate)

U.S./Canadian Brand Names Topamax® [US/Can]

Therapeutic Category Anticonvulsant

Use Adjunctive therapy for partial onset seizures in adults

Usual Dosage

Adults: Initial: 25-50 mg/day; titrate in increments of 25-50 mg per week until an effective daily dose is reached; the daily dose may be increased by 25 mg at weekly intervals for the first 4 weeks; thereafter, the daily dose may be increased by 25-50 mg weekly to an effective daily dose (usually at least 400 mg); usual maximum dose: 1600 mg/day

Note: A more rapid titration schedule has been previously recommended (ie, 50 mg/week), and may be attempted in some clinical situations; however, this may reduce the patient's ability to tolerate topiramate.

Children 2-16 years: Partial seizures (adjunctive therapy): Initial dose titration should begin at 25 mg (or less, based on a range of 1-3 mg/kg/day) nightly for the first week. Dosage may be increased in increments of 1-3 mg/kg/day (administered in two divided doses) at 1- or 2-week intervals to a total daily dose of 5-9 mg/kg/day.

Dosage Forms

Capsule, sprinkle (Topamax®): 15 mg, 25 mg

Tablet (Topamax®): 25 mg, 100 mg, 200 mg

Topisone® *see* betamethasone (topical) *on page 83*

Toposar® **[US]** *see* etoposide *on page 259*

topotecan (toe poe TEE kan)

Synonyms hycamptamine; SKF 104864

U.S./Canadian Brand Names Hycamtin™ [US/Can]

Therapeutic Category Antineoplastic Agent

Use Metastatic carcinoma of the ovary after failure of initial or subsequent chemotherapy; experimentally in childhood solid tumors and leukemia resistant to standard therapies; treatment of small cell lung cancer sensitive disease after failure of first-line chemotherapy (sensitive disease is defined as disease responding to chemotherapy but subsequently progressing at least 60 days or at least 90 days after chemotherapy)

Usual Dosage

Children: A phase I study in pediatric patients by CCSG determined the recommended phase II dose to be 5.5 mg/m^2 as a 24-hour continuous infusion

Adults: Most phase II studies currently utilize topotecan at 1.5-2.0 mg/m^2/day for 5 days, repeated every 21-28 days. Alternative dosing regimens evaluated in phase I studies have included 21-day continuous infusion (recommended phase II dose: 0.53-0.7 mg/m^2/day) and weekly 24-hour infusions (recommended phase II dose: 1.5 mg/m^2/week). Dose modifications: Dosage modification may be required for toxicity

Dosage Forms Injection, powder for reconstitution, as hydrochloride: 4 mg (base)

Toprol-XL® **[US/Can]** *see* metoprolol *on page 425*

Topsyn® **[Can]** *see* fluocinonide *on page 277*

TOPV *see* poliovirus vaccine, live, trivalent, oral *on page 524*

Toradol® **[US/Can]** *see* ketorolac *on page 368*

Torecan® **[US]** *see* thiethylperazine *on page 633*

Torecan® **Suppository** *(Discontinued)* *see page 814*

toremifene (TORE em i feen)
Synonyms FC1157a
U.S./Canadian Brand Names Fareston® [US/Can]
Therapeutic Category Antineoplastic Agent
Use Treatment of advanced breast cancer; management of desmoid tumors and endometrial carcinoma
Usual Dosage Refer to individual protocols.
  Adults: Oral: 60 mg once daily, generally continued until disease progression is observed
Dosage Forms Tablet, as citrate: 60 mg

Tornalate® **[US/Can]** *see* bitolterol *on page 88*

torsemide (TOR se mide)
U.S./Canadian Brand Names Demadex® [US]
Therapeutic Category Diuretic, Loop
Use Management of edema associated with congestive heart failure and hepatic or renal disease; used alone or in combination with antihypertensives in treatment of hypertension
Usual Dosage Adults:
  Oral: 5-10 mg once daily; if ineffective, may double dose until desired effect is achieved
  I.V.: 10-20 mg/dose repeated in 2 hours as needed with a doubling of the dose with each succeeding dose until desired diuresis is achieved
  Continues to be effective in patients with cirrhosis, no apparent change in dose is necessary
Dosage Forms
  Injection: 10 mg/mL (2 mL, 5 mL)
  Tablet: 5 mg, 10 mg, 20 mg, 100 mg

Totacillin® *(Discontinued)* *see page 814*

Totacillin-N® *(Discontinued)* *see page 814*

Touro™ **Allergy [US]** *see* brompheniramine and pseudoephedrine *on page 94*

Touro™ **CC [US]** *see* guaifenesin, pseudoephedrine, and dextromethorphan *on page 312*

Touro® **DM [US]** *see* guaifenesin and dextromethorphan *on page 308*

Touro Ex® **[US]** *see* guaifenesin *on page 307*

Touro LA® **[US]** *see* guaifenesin and pseudoephedrine *on page 310*

t-PA *see* alteplase *on page 26*

TPGS *see* tocophersolan *on page 642*

T-Phyl® **[US]** *see* theophylline *on page 630*

Trace-4® **[US]** *see* trace metals *on this page*

trace metals (trase MET als)
Synonyms chromium injection; copper injection; manganese injection; molybdenum injection; neonatal trace metals; zinc injection
U.S./Canadian Brand Names Chroma-Pak® [US]; Iodopen® [US]; Molypen® [US]; M.T.E.-4® [US]; M.T.E.-5® [US]; M.T.E.-6® [US]; MulTE-PAK-4® [US]; MulTE-PAK-5® [US]; Neotrace-4® [US]; PedTE-PAK-4® [US]; Pedtrace-4® [US]; P.T.E.-4® [US]; P.T.E.-5® [US]; Sele-Pak® [US]; Selepen® [US]; Trace-4® [US]; Zinca-Pak® [US]

Therapeutic Category Trace Element
Use Prevent and correct trace metal deficiencies
Dosage Forms
Injection:
Chromium: 4 mcg/mL, 20 mcg/mL
Copper: 0.4 mg/mL, 2 mg/mL
Manganese: 0.1 mg/mL (as chloride or sulfate salt)
Molybdenum: 25 mcg/mL
Selenium: 40 mcg/mL
Zinc: 1 mg/mL (sulfate); 1 mg/mL (chloride); 5 mg/mL (sulfate)

Tracleer™ [US] *see* bosentan *on page 90*

Tracrium® [US] *see* atracurium *on page 62*

Tral® (Discontinued) *see page 814*

tramadol (TRA ma dole)

U.S./Canadian Brand Names Ultram® [US/Can]
Therapeutic Category Analgesic, Non-narcotic
Use Relief of moderate to moderately severe pain
Usual Dosage Adults: Oral: 50-100 mg every 4-6 hours, not to exceed 400 mg/day
Dosage Forms Tablet, as hydrochloride: 50 mg

Trandate® [US/Can] *see* labetalol *on page 370*

trandolapril (tran DOE la pril)

U.S./Canadian Brand Names Mavik® [US/Can]
Therapeutic Category Angiotensin-Converting Enzyme (ACE) Inhibitor
Use Management of hypertension alone or in combination with other antihypertensive agents
Unlabeled use: As a class, ACE inhibitors are recommended in the treatment of systolic congestive heart failure
Usual Dosage Adults:
Non-Black patients: 0.5-1 mg for those not receiving diuretics; increase dose at 0.5-1 mg increments at 1- to 2-week intervals; maximum dose: 4 mg/day
Black patients: Initiate doses of 1-2 mg; maximum dose: 4 mg/day
Dosage Forms Tablet: 1 mg, 2 mg, 4 mg

trandolapril and verapamil (tran DOE la pril & ver AP a mil)

U.S./Canadian Brand Names Tarka® [US]
Therapeutic Category Antihypertensive Agent, Combination
Use Combination drug for the treatment of hypertension
Usual Dosage Dose is individualized
Dosage Forms
Tablet, combination [trandolapril component is immediate release, verapamil component is sustained release]:
Trandolapril 1 mg and verapamil hydrochloride 240 mg
Trandolapril 2 mg and verapamil hydrochloride 180 mg
Trandolapril 2 mg and verapamil hydrochloride 240 mg
Trandolapril 4 mg and verapamil hydrochloride 240 mg

tranexamic acid (tran eks AM ik AS id)

U.S./Canadian Brand Names Cyklokapron® [US/Can]
Therapeutic Category Antihemophilic Agent
Use Short-term use (2-8 days) in hemophilia patients during and following tooth extraction to reduce or prevent hemorrhage
Usual Dosage Children and Adults: I.V.: 10 mg/kg immediately before surgery, then 25 mg/kg/dose orally 3-4 times/day for 2-8 days
(Continued)

tranexamic acid *(Continued)*

Alternatively:
Oral: 25 mg/kg 3-4 times/day beginning 1 day prior to surgery
I.V.: 10 mg/kg 3-4 times/day in patients who are unable to take oral

Dosage Forms
Injection: 100 mg/mL (10 mL)
Tablet: 500 mg

transamine *see* tranylcypromine *on this page*

Transdermal-NTG® Patch *(Discontinued)* *see page 814*

Transderm-Nitro® [Can] *see* nitroglycerin *on page 462*

Transderm Scōp® [US] *see* scopolamine *on page 585*

Transderm-V® [Can] *see* scopolamine *on page 585*

Trans-Plantar® Transdermal Patch *(Discontinued)* *see page 814*

Trans-Ver-Sal® [Can] *see* salicylic acid *on page 581*

Trans-Ver-Sal® AdultPatch [US-OTC] *see* salicylic acid *on page 581*

Trans-Ver-Sal® PediaPatch [US-OTC] *see* salicylic acid *on page 581*

Trans-Ver-Sal® PlantarPatch [US-OTC] *see* salicylic acid *on page 581*

Tranxene® [US/Can] *see* clorazepate *on page 156*

tranylcypromine (tran il SIP roe meen)

Synonyms transamine
U.S./Canadian Brand Names Parnate® [US/Can]
Therapeutic Category Antidepressant, Monoamine Oxidase Inhibitor
Use Symptomatic treatment of depressed patients refractory to or intolerant to tricyclic antidepressants or electroconvulsive therapy; has a more rapid onset of therapeutic effect than other MAO inhibitors, but causes more severe hypertensive reactions
Usual Dosage Adults: Oral: 10 mg twice daily, increase by 10 mg increments at 1- to 3-week intervals; maximum: 60 mg/day
Dosage Forms Tablet, as sulfate: 10 mg

Trasicor® [Can] *see* oxprenolol *(Canada only) on page 483*

trastuzumab (tras TU zoo mab)

U.S./Canadian Brand Names Herceptin® [US/Can]
Therapeutic Category Antineoplastic Agent
Use Treatment of patients with metastatic breast cancer whose tumors overexpress the HER2 protein
Usual Dosage Adults: I.V.:
Loading dose: 4 mg/kg over 90 minutes; do not administer as an I.V. bolus or I.V. push
Maintenance dose: 2 mg/kg once weekly (may be infused over 30 minutes if prior infusions are well tolerated)
Dosage Forms Injection [vial; with vial of bacteriostatic water]: 440 mg

Trasylol® [US/Can] *see* aprotinin *on page 53*

Travase® *(Discontinued)* *see page 814*

Travatan™ [US] *see* travoprost *on this page*

travoprost (TRA voe prost)

U.S./Canadian Brand Names Travatan™ [US]
Therapeutic Category Prostaglandin, Ophthalmic

Use Reduction of elevated intraocular pressure in patients with open-angle glaucoma or ocular hypertension who are intolerant of the other IOP-lowering medications or insufficiently responsive (failed to achieve target IOP determined after multiple measurements over time) to another IOP-lowering medication

Usual Dosage Ophthalmic: Adults: Glaucoma (open angle) or ocular hypertension: Instill 1 drop into affected eye(s) once daily in the evening; do not exceed once-daily dosing (may decrease IOP-lowering effect). If used with other topical ophthalmic agents, separate administration by at least 5 minutes.

Dosage Forms Solution, ophthalmic: 0.004% (2.5 mL) [contains benzalkonium chloride]

trazodone (TRAZ oh done)

U.S./Canadian Brand Names Alti-Trazodone [Can]; Apo®-Trazodone [Can]; Apo®-Trazodone D; Desyrel® [US/Can]; Gen-Trazodone [Can]; Novo-Trazodone [Can]; Nu-Trazodone [Can]; PMS-Trazodone [Can]; Trazorel [Can]

Therapeutic Category Antidepressant, Triazolopyridine

Use Treatment of depression

Usual Dosage Oral:
Adolescents: Initial: 25-50 mg/day; increase to 100-150 mg/day in divided doses
Adults: Initial: 150 mg/day in 3 divided doses (may increase by 50 mg/day every 3-7 days); maximum: 600 mg/day

Dosage Forms Tablet, as hydrochloride: 50 mg, 100 mg, 150 mg, 300 mg

Trazorel [Can] *see* trazodone *on this page*

Trecator®-SC [US/Can] *see* ethionamide *on page 256*

Trelstar™ Depot [US/Can] *see* triptorelin *on page 659*

Trelstar™ LA [US] *see* triptorelin *on page 659*

Trendar® *(Discontinued) see page 814*

Trental® [US/Can] *see* pentoxifylline *on page 502*

treprostinil (tre PROST in il)

U.S./Canadian Brand Names Remodulin™ [US]

Therapeutic Category Vasodilator

Use Treatment of pulmonary arterial hypertension (PAH) in patients with NYHA Class II-IV symptoms to decrease exercise-associated symptoms

Usual Dosage S.C. infusion:
Adults: PAH: Initial: 1.25 ng/kg/minute continuous; if dose cannot be tolerated, reduce to 0.625 ng/kg/minute. Increase at rate not >1.25 ng/kg/minute per week for first 4 weeks, and not >2.5 ng/kg/minute per week for remainder of therapy. Limited experience with doses >40 ng/kg/minute.
Note: Dose must be carefully and individually titrated (symptom improvement with minimal adverse effects).

Dosage Forms Injection, solution; 1 mg/mL (20 mL); 2.5 mg/mL (20 mL); 5 mg/mL (20 mL); 10 mg/mL (20 mL)

tretinoin (oral) (TRET i noyn oral)

Synonyms all-*trans*-retinoic acid

U.S./Canadian Brand Names Vesanoid® [US/Can]

Therapeutic Category Antineoplastic Agent

Use Acute promyelocytic leukemia (APL): Induction of remission in patients with APL, French American British (FAB) classification M3 (including the M3 variant), characterized by the presence of the t(15;17) translocation or the presence of the PML/RARα gene who are refractory to or who have relapsed from anthracycline chemotherapy, or for whom anthracycline-based chemotherapy is contraindicated. Tretinoin is for the induction of remission only. All patients should receive an accepted form of remission consolidation or maintenance therapy for APL after completion of induction therapy with tretinoin.
(Continued)

tretinoin (oral) *(Continued)*

Usual Dosage Oral:

Children: There are limited clinical data on the pediatric use of tretinoin. Of 15 pediatric patients (age range: 1-16 years) treated with tretinoin, the incidence of complete remission was 67%. Safety and efficacy in pediatric patients <1 year of age have not been established. Some pediatric patients experience severe headache and pseudotumor cerebri, requiring analgesic treatment and lumbar puncture for relief. Increased caution is recommended. Consider dose reduction in children experiencing serious or intolerable toxicity; however, the efficacy and safety of tretinoin at doses <45 mg/m^2/ day have not been evaluated.

Adults: 45 mg/m^2/day administered as two evenly divided doses until complete remission is documented. Discontinue therapy 30 days after achievement of complete remission or after 90 days of treatment, whichever occurs first. If after initiation of treatment the presence of the t(15;17) translocation is not confirmed by cytogenetics or by polymerase chain reaction studies and the patient has not responded to tretinoin, consider alternative therapy.

Note: Tretinoin is for the induction of remission only. Optimal consolidation or maintenance regimens have not been determined. All patients should, therefore, receive a standard consolidation or maintenance chemotherapy regimen for APL after induction therapy with tretinoin unless otherwise contraindicated.

Dosage Forms Capsule: 10 mg

tretinoin (topical) (TRET i noyn TOP i kal)

Synonyms retinoic acid; vitamin A acid

U.S./Canadian Brand Names Altinac™ [US]; Avita® [US]; Rejuva-A® [Can]; Renova® [US]; Retin-A® Micro [US]; Retin-A® [US/Can]; Retinova® [Can]

Therapeutic Category Retinoic Acid Derivative

Use Treatment of acne vulgaris, photodamaged skin, and some skin cancers

Usual Dosage Children >12 years and Adults: Topical: Apply once daily before retiring; if stinging or irritation develop, decrease frequency of application

Dosage Forms

Cream, topical:

Altinac™: 0.025% (20 g, 45 g); 0.05% (20 g, 45 g); 0.1% (20 g, 45 g)

Avita®: 0.025% (20 g, 45 g)

Retin-A®: 0.025% (20 g, 45 g); 0.05% (20 g, 45 g); 0.1% (20 g, 45 g)

Cream, emollient, topical (Renova®): 0.02% (40 g); 0.05% (20 g, 40 g, 60 g)

Gel, topical:

Retin-A®: 0.01% (15 g, 45 g); 0.025% (15 g, 45 g)

Retin-A® Micro [microsphere]: 0.04% (20 g, 45 g); 0.1% (20 g, 45 g)

Liquid, topical (Retin-A®): 0.05% (28 mL)

Trexall™ [US] *see* methotrexate *on page 417*

triacetin (trye a SEE tin)

Synonyms glycerol triacetate

U.S./Canadian Brand Names Ony-Clear® Nail [US-OTC]

Therapeutic Category Antifungal Agent

Use Fungistat for athlete's foot and other superficial fungal infections

Usual Dosage Topical: Apply twice daily, cleanse areas with dilute alcohol or mild soap and water before application; continue treatment for 7 days after symptoms have disappeared

Dosage Forms

Aerosol, topical: With cetylpyridinium chloride, chloroxylenol, and benzalkonium chloride (45 mL, 60 mL)

Cream, topical: With cetylpyridinium chloride and chloroxylenol (30 g)

Liquid, topical: With cetylpyridinium chloride and chloroxylenol (30 mL)

Solution, topical: With cetylpyridinium chloride, chloroxylenol, and benzalkonium chloride in an oil base (15 mL)

Triacet™ **Topical [US] Oracort [Can]** *see* triamcinolone (topical) *on next page*
triacetyloleandomycin *see* troleandomycin *on page 660*
Triacin-C® **[US]** *see* triprolidine, pseudoephedrine, and codeine *on page 659*
Triacin® **[US-OTC]** *see* triprolidine and pseudoephedrine *on page 659*
triaconazole *see* terconazole *on page 624*
Triad® **[US]** *see* butalbital, acetaminophen, and caffeine *on page 99*
Triaderm [Can] *see* triamcinolone (topical) *on next page*
Triafed® *(Discontinued)* *see page 814*
Triam-A® **Injection [US]** *see* triamcinolone (systemic) *on this page*
triamcinolone and nystatin *see* nystatin and triamcinolone *on page 473*

triamcinolone (inhalation, nasal)
(trye am SIN oh lone in hil LA shun, NAY sal)
U.S./Canadian Brand Names Nasacort® AQ [US/Can]; Nasacort® [US/Can]; Trinasal® [Can]
Therapeutic Category Corticosteroid, Topical
Use Symptoms of seasonal and perennial allergic rhinitis
Usual Dosage Children >12 years and Adults: Intranasal: 2 sprays in each nostril once daily; may increase after 4-7 days up to 4 sprays once daily or 1 spray 4 times/day in each nostril
Dosage Forms
Aerosol, nasal: 55 mcg per actuation (15 mL)
Spray, nasal: 55 mcg per actuation in aqueous base (16.5 g)

triamcinolone (inhalation, oral) (trye am SIN oh lone in hil LA shun, OR al)
U.S./Canadian Brand Names Azmacort® [US]
Therapeutic Category Adrenal Corticosteroid
Use Asthma
Usual Dosage
Children 6-12 years: Inhalation: 1-2 inhalations 3-4 times/day, not to exceed 12 inhalations/day
Children >12 years and Adults: Oral inhalation: 2 inhalations 3-4 times/day, not to exceed 16 inhalations/day
Dosage Forms Aerosol: Oral inhalation: 100 mcg/metered spray (2 oz)

triamcinolone (systemic) (trye am SIN oh lone sis TEM ik)
U.S./Canadian Brand Names Aristocort® Forte Injection [US]; Aristocort® Intralesional Injection [US]; Aristocort® Tablet [US/Can]; Aristospan® Intra-articular Injection [US/Can]; Aristospan® Intralesional Injection [US/Can]; Kenalog® Injection [US/Can]; Tac™-3 Injection [US]; Triam-A® Injection [US]; Triam Forte® Injection [US]
Therapeutic Category Adrenal Corticosteroid
Use Severe inflammation or immunosuppression
Usual Dosage In general, single I.M. dose of 4-7 times oral dose will control patient from 4-7 days up to 3-4 weeks

Children 6-12 years:
I.M.: Acetonide or hexacetonide: 0.03-0.2 mg/kg at 1- to 7-day intervals
Children >12 years and Adults:
Oral: 4-100 mg/day
I.M.: Acetonide or hexacetonide: 60 mg (of 40 mg/mL), additional 20-100 mg doses (usual: 40-80 mg) may be administered when signs and symptoms recur, best at 6-week intervals to minimize HPA suppression
(Continued)

triamcinolone (systemic) *(Continued)*

Intra-articularly, intrasynovially, intralesionally: 2.5-40 mg as diacetate salt or acetonide salt, dose may be repeated when signs and symptoms recur

Intra-articularly: Hexacetonide: 2-20 mg every 3-4 weeks as hexacetonide salt

Intralesional (use 10 mg/mL): Diacetate or acetonide: 1 mg/injection site, may be repeated one or more times/week depending upon patients response; maximum; 30 mg at any one time; may use multiple injections if they are more than 1 cm apart

Intra-articular, intrasynovial, and soft-tissue injection (use 10 mg/mL or 40 mg/mL): Diacetate or acetonide: 2.5-40 mg depending upon location, size of joints, and degree of inflammation; repeat when signs and symptoms recur

Sublesionally (as acetonide): Up to 1 mg per injection site and may be repeated one or more times weekly; multiple sites may be injected if they are 1 cm or more apart, not to exceed 30 mg

Dosage Forms

Syrup: 2 mg/5 mL (120 mL); 4 mg/5 mL (120 mL)

Tablet: 1 mg, 2 mg, 4 mg, 8 mg

Triamcinolone acetonide:
Injection: 10 mg/mL (5 mL); 40 mg/mL (1 mL, 5 mL, 10 mL)

Triamcinolone diacetate: Injection: 25 mg/mL (5 mL); 40 mg/mL (1 mL, 5 mL, 10 mL)

Triamcinolone hexacetonide: Injection: 5 mg/mL (5 mL); 20 mg/mL (1 mL, 5 mL)

triamcinolone (topical) (trye am SIN oh lone TOP i kal)

U.S./Canadian Brand Names Aristocort® A Topical [US]; Aristocort® Topical [US/Can]; Kenalog® in Orabase® [US/Can]; Kenalog® Topical [US/Can]; Triacet™ Topical [US] Oracort [Can]; Triaderm [Can]

Therapeutic Category Corticosteroid, Topical

Use Severe inflammation or immunosuppression; nasal spray for symptoms of seasonal and perennial allergic rhinitis

Usual Dosage Children >12 years and Adults: Topical: Apply a thin film 2-3 times/day. Therapy should be discontinued when control is achieved. If no improvement is seen, reassessment of diagnosis may be necessary.

Dosage Forms

Aerosol, topical: 0.2 mg/2 second spray (23 g, 63 g)

Cream: 0.025% (15 g, 60 g, 80 g, 240 g, 454 g); 0.1% (15 g, 30 g, 60 g, 80 g, 90 g, 120 g, 240 g); 0.5% (15 g, 20 g, 30 g, 240 g)

Lotion: 0.025% (60 mL); 0.1% (15 mL, 60 mL)

Ointment, oral: 0.1% (5 g)

Ointment, topical: 0.025% (15 g, 30 g, 60 g, 80 g, 120 g, 454 g); 0.1% (15 g, 30 g, 60 g, 80 g, 120 g, 240 g, 454 g); 0.5% (15 g, 20 g, 30 g, 240 g)

Triam Forte® Injection [US] *see* triamcinolone (systemic) *on previous page*

Triaminic® Allergy Tablet *(Discontinued) see page 814*

Triaminic® AM Decongestant Formula [US-OTC] *see* pseudoephedrine *on page 552*

Triaminic® Cold Tablet *(Discontinued) see page 814*

Triaminic® Expectorant *(Discontinued) see page 814*

Triaminic® Infant Decongestant [US/Can] *see* pseudoephedrine *on page 552*

Triaminicol® Multi-Symptom Cold Syrup *(Discontinued) see page 814*

Triaminic® Oral Infant, Drops *(Discontinued) see page 814*

Triaminic® Sore Throat Formula [US-OTC] *see* acetaminophen, dextromethorphan, and pseudoephedrine *on page 8*

Triaminic® Syrup *(Discontinued) see page 814*

Triamonide® Injection *(Discontinued) see page 814*

triamterene (trye AM ter een)
U.S./Canadian Brand Names Dyrenium® [US/Can]
Therapeutic Category Diuretic, Potassium Sparing
Use Alone or in combination with other diuretics to treat edema and hypertension; decreases potassium excretion caused by kaliuretic diuretics
Usual Dosage Oral:
Children: 2-4 mg/kg/day in 1-2 divided doses; maximum: 300 mg/day
Adults: 100-300 mg/day in 1-2 divided doses; maximum: 300 mg/day
Dosage Forms Capsule: 50 mg, 100 mg

triamterene and hydrochlorothiazide *see* hydrochlorothiazide and triamterene *on page 329*

Trianal® [Can] *see* butalbital, aspirin, and caffeine *on page 100*

Triapin® (Discontinued) *see page 814*

Triatec-8 [Can] *see* acetaminophen and codeine *on page 5*

Triatec-30 [Can] *see* acetaminophen and codeine *on page 5*

Triatec-Strong [Can] *see* acetaminophen and codeine *on page 5*

Triavil® [US/Can] *see* amitriptyline and perphenazine *on page 35*

Triavil® 4-50 (Discontinued) *see page 814*

Triaz® [US] *see* benzoyl peroxide *on page 79*

Triaz® Cleanser [US] *see* benzoyl peroxide *on page 79*

triazolam (trye AY zoe lam)
U.S./Canadian Brand Names Apo®-Triazo [Can]; Gen-Triazolam [Can]; Halcion® [US/Can]
Therapeutic Category Benzodiazepine
Controlled Substance C-IV
Use Short-term treatment of insomnia
Usual Dosage Oral (onset of action is rapid, patient should be in bed when taking medication):
Children <18 years: Dosage not established
Adults: 0.125-0.25 mg at bedtime
Dosage Forms Tablet: 0.125 mg, 0.25 mg

tribavirin *see* ribavirin *on page 570*

Tri-Chlor® [US] *see* trichloroacetic acid *on this page*

Trichlorex® [Can] *see* trichlormethiazide *on this page*

trichlormethiazide (trye klor meth EYE a zide)
U.S./Canadian Brand Names Aquacot® [US]; Metatensin® [Can]; Naqua® [US/Can]; Trichlorex® [Can]
Therapeutic Category Diuretic, Thiazide
Use Management of mild to moderate hypertension; treatment of edema in congestive heart failure and nephrotic syndrome
Usual Dosage Oral:
Children >6 months: 0.07 mg/kg/24 hours or 2 mg/m^2/24 hours
Adults: 1-4 mg/day
Dosage Forms Tablet: 2 mg, 4 mg

trichloroacetaldehyde monohydrate *see* chloral hydrate *on page 132*

trichloroacetic acid (trye klor oh a SEE tik AS id)
U.S./Canadian Brand Names Tri-Chlor® [US]
Therapeutic Category Keratolytic Agent
(Continued)

trichloroacetic acid *(Continued)*

Use Debride callous tissue

Usual Dosage Apply to verruca, cover with bandage for 5-6 days, remove verruca, reapply as needed

Dosage Forms Liquid: 80% (15 mL)

Trichophyton skin test (trye koe FYE ton skin test)

U.S./Canadian Brand Names Dermatophytin® [US]

Therapeutic Category Diagnostic Agent

Use Assess cell-mediated immunity

Usual Dosage 0.1 mL intradermally, examine reaction site in 24-48 hours; induration of ≥5 mm in diameter is a positive reaction

Dosage Forms

Injection, diluted: 1:30 V/V (5 mL)

Injection, undiluted: 5 mL

Tri-Clear® Expectorant *(Discontinued)* see page 814

TriCor® [US/Can] see fenofibrate on page 265

Tricosal® [US] see choline magnesium trisalicylate on page 143

Tridesilon® [US] see desonide on page 182

Tridil® Injection *(Discontinued)* see page 814

Tridione® *(Discontinued)* see page 814

Tridione® Suppository *(Discontinued)* see page 814

trientine (TRYE en teen)

U.S./Canadian Brand Names Syprine® [US/Can]

Therapeutic Category Chelating Agent

Use Treatment of Wilson's disease in patients intolerant to penicillamine

Usual Dosage Oral (administer on an empty stomach):

Children <12 years: 500-750 mg/day in divided doses 2-4 times/day; maximum: 1.5 g/day

Adults: 750-1250 mg/day in divided doses 2-4 times/day; maximum daily dose: 2 g

Dosage Forms Capsule, as hydrochloride: 250 mg

triethanolamine polypeptide oleate-condensate

(trye eth a NOLE a meen pol i PEP tide OH lee ate-KON den sate)

U.S./Canadian Brand Names Cerumenex® [US/Can]

Therapeutic Category Otic Agent, Ceruminolytic

Use Removal of ear wax (cerumen)

Usual Dosage Children and Adults: Otic: Fill ear canal, insert cotton plug; allow to remain 15-30 minutes; flush ear with lukewarm water

Dosage Forms Solution, otic: 6 mL, 12 mL

triethanolamine salicylate (trye eth a NOLE a meen sa LIS i late)

U.S./Canadian Brand Names Antiphlogistine Rub A-535 No Odour [Can]; Myoflex® [US/Can]; Sportscreme® [US-OTC]

Therapeutic Category Analgesic, Topical

Use Relief of pain of muscular aches, rheumatism, neuralgia, sprains, arthritis on intact skin

Usual Dosage Topical: Apply to area as needed

Dosage Forms Cream: 10% in a nongreasy base

triethylenethiophosphoramide see thiotepa on page 635

Trifed-C® *(Discontinued)* see page 814

Tri-Fed® **[US-OTC]** *see* triprolidine and pseudoephedrine *on page 659*

trifluoperazine (trye floo oh PER a zeen)
   U.S./Canadian Brand Names Apo®-Trifluoperazine [Can]; Stelazine® [US]
   Therapeutic Category Phenothiazine Derivative
   Use Treatment of psychoses and management of anxiety
   Usual Dosage
      Children 6-12 years: Psychoses:
         Oral: Hospitalized or well supervised patients: Initial dose: 1 mg 1-2 times/day, gradually increase until symptoms are controlled or adverse effects become troublesome; maximum: 15 mg/day
         I.M.: 1 mg twice daily
      Adults:
         Psychoses:
            Outpatients: Oral: 1-2 mg twice daily
            Hospitalized or well supervised patients: Initial dose: 2-5 mg twice daily with optimum response in the 15-20 mg/day range; do not exceed 40 mg/day
            I.M.: 1-2 mg every 4-6 hours as needed up to 10 mg/24 hours maximum
         Nonpsychotic anxiety: Oral: 1-2 mg twice daily; maximum: 6 mg/day; therapy for anxiety should not exceed 12 weeks; do not exceed 6 mg/day for longer than 12 weeks when treating anxiety; agitation, jitteriness or insomnia may be confused with original neurotic or psychotic symptoms
   Dosage Forms
      Injection, as hydrochloride: 2 mg/mL (10 mL)
      Solution, oral concentrate, as hydrochloride: 10 mg/mL (60 mL)
      Tablet, as hydrochloride: 1 mg, 2 mg, 5 mg, 10 mg

trifluorothymidine *see* trifluridine *on this page*

triflupromazine (trye floo PROE ma zeen)
   U.S./Canadian Brand Names Vesprin® [US/Can]
   Therapeutic Category Phenothiazine Derivative
   Use Treatment of psychoses, nausea, vomiting, and intractable hiccups
   Usual Dosage
      Children: I.M.: 0.2-0.25 mg/kg
      Adults:
         I.M.: 5-15 mg every 4 hours
         I.V.: 1 mg
   Dosage Forms Injection, as hydrochloride: 10 mg/mL (10 mL) [multidose vial]; 20 mg/mL (1 mL)

trifluridine (trye FLURE i deen)
   Synonyms f_3t; trifluorothymidine
   U.S./Canadian Brand Names Viroptic® [US/Can]
   Therapeutic Category Antiviral Agent
   Use Treatment of primary keratoconjunctivitis and recurrent epithelial keratitis caused by herpes simplex virus types I and II
   Usual Dosage Adults: Ophthalmic: Instill 1 drop into affected eye every 2 hours while awake, to a maximum of 9 drops/day, until re-epithelialization of corneal ulcer occurs; then use 1 drop every 4 hours for another 7 days; do **not** exceed 21 days of treatment
   Dosage Forms Solution, ophthalmic: 1% (7.5 mL)

triglycerides, medium chain *see* medium chain triglycerides *on page 404*

trihexyphenidyl (trye heks ee FEN i dil)
   Synonyms benzhexol
   U.S./Canadian Brand Names Apo®-Trihex [Can]; Artane® [US]
   Therapeutic Category Anticholinergic Agent; Anti-Parkinson's Agent
      (Continued)

trihexyphenidyl *(Continued)*

Use Adjunctive treatment of Parkinson's disease; also used in treatment of drug-induced extrapyramidal effects and acute dystonic reactions

Usual Dosage Oral:

Parkinsonism: Initial: Administer 1-2 mg the first day; increase by 2 mg increments at intervals of 3-5 days, until a total of 6-10 mg is administered daily. Many patients derive maximum benefit from a total daily dose of 6-10 mg; however, postencephalitic patients may require a total daily dose of 12-15 mg in 3-4 divided doses

Concomitant use with levodopa: 3-6 mg/day in divided doses is usually adequate

Drug-induced extrapyramidal disorders: Start with a single 1 mg dose; daily dosage usually ranges between 5-15 mg in 3-4 divided doses

Dosage Forms

Elixir, as hydrochloride: 2 mg/5 mL (480 mL)

Tablet, as hydrochloride: 2 mg, 5 mg

TriHIBit® [US] *see* diphtheria, tetanus toxoids, and acellular pertussis vaccine and *Haemophilus* b conjugate vaccine *on page 205*

Tri-Immunol® *(Discontinued)* *see page 814*

Tri-K® [US] *see* potassium acetate, potassium bicarbonate, and potassium citrate *on page 528*

TRIKOF-D® *(Discontinued)* *see page 814*

Tri-Kort® Injection *(Discontinued)* *see page 814*

Trilafon® [US/Can] *see* perphenazine *on page 505*

Trileptal® [US/Can] *see* oxcarbazepine *on page 482*

Tri-Levlen® [US] *see* ethinyl estradiol and levonorgestrel *on page 248*

Trilisate® [US/Can] *see* choline magnesium trisalicylate *on page 143*

Trilog® Injection *(Discontinued)* *see page 814*

Trilone® Injection *(Discontinued)* *see page 814*

Tri-Luma™ [US] *see* fluocinolone, hydroquinone, and tretinoin *on page 276*

Trimazide® *(Discontinued)* *see page 814*

trimebutine *(Canada only)* (trye me BYOO teen)

U.S./Canadian Brand Names Modulon® [Can]

Therapeutic Category Antispasmodic Agent, Gastrointestinal

Use For the treatment and relief of symptoms associated with the irritable bowel syndrome (spastic colon). In postoperative paralytic ileus in order to accelerate the resumption of the intestinal transit following abdominal surgery.

Usual Dosage Adults:

Parenteral: Dosage should be individually tailored according to response, but the total parenteral daily dose should not exceed 300 mg. The usual adult dose is 50-100 mg 3 times daily, administered as an I.M. injection, as a 3-minute I.V. injection, or as a 60-minute I.V. infusion (in D_5W or NS), until resumption of intestinal motility.

Tablets: Up to 600 mg daily in divided doses. It may be administered as two 100 mg tablets 3 times daily before meals or one 200 mg tablet 3 times daily before meals.

Dosage Forms Tablet, as maleate: 100 mg, 200 mg

trimeprazine *(Canada only)* (trye MEP re zeen)

U.S./Canadian Brand Names Panectyl® [Can]

Therapeutic Category Antihistamine

Use Perennial and seasonal allergic rhinitis and other allergic symptoms including urticaria

Usual Dosage Oral:

Children:

6 months to 3 years: 1.25 mg at bedtime or 3 times/day if needed

>3 years: 2.5 mg at bedtime or 3 times/day if needed
>6 years: 5 mg/day
Adults: 2.5 mg 4 times/day
Dosage Forms Tablet, as tartrate: 2.5 mg, 5 mg

trimethobenzamide (trye meth oh BEN za mide)
U.S./Canadian Brand Names Benzacot® [US]; Tigan® [US/Can]
Therapeutic Category Anticholinergic Agent; Antiemetic
Use Control of nausea and vomiting (especially for long-term antiemetic therapy)
Usual Dosage Rectal use: Contraindicated in neonates and premature infants
Children:
Oral, rectal: 15-20 mg/kg/day or 400-500 mg/m^2/day divided into 3-4 doses
I.M.: Not recommended
Adults:
Oral: 250 mg 3-4 times/day
I.M., rectal: 200 mg 3-4 times/day
Dosage Forms
Capsule, as hydrochloride: 250 mg, 300 mg
Injection, solution, as hydrochloride: 100 mg/mL (2 mL, 20 mL)
Suppository, rectal, as hydrochloride: 100 mg, 200 mg [contains benzocaine]

trimethoprim (trye METH oh prim)
Synonyms TMP
U.S./Canadian Brand Names Primsol® [US]; Proloprim® [US/Can]
Therapeutic Category Antibiotic, Miscellaneous
Use Treatment of urinary tract infections due to susceptible strains of *E. coli, P. mirabilis, K. pneumoniae, Enterobacter* sp and coagulase-negative *Staphylococcus* including *S. saprophyticus*; acute otitis media in children; acute exacerbations of chronic bronchitis in adults; in combination with other agents for treatment of toxoplasmosis, *Pneumocystis carinii*; treatment of superficial ocular infections involving the conjunctiva and cornea
Usual Dosage Adults: Oral: 100 mg every 12 hours or 200 mg every 24 hours
Dosage Forms
Solution, oral (Primsol®): 50 mg (base)/5 mL (480 mL) [contains sodium benzoate; bubblegum flavor]
Tablet: 100 mg
Proloprim®: 100 mg, 200 mg

trimethoprim and polymyxin B (trye METH oh prim & pol i MIKS in bee)
Synonyms polymyxin B and trimethoprim
U.S./Canadian Brand Names PMS-Polytrimethoprim [Can]; Polytrim® [US/Can]
Therapeutic Category Antibiotic, Ophthalmic
Use Treatment of surface ocular bacterial conjunctivitis and blepharoconjunctivitis
Usual Dosage Ophthalmic: Instill 1-2 drops in eye(s) every 4-6 hours
Dosage Forms Solution, ophthalmic: Trimethoprim sulfate 1 mg and polymyxin B sulfate 10,000 units per mL (10 mL)

trimethoprim and sulfamethoxazole *see* sulfamethoxazole and trimethoprim *on page 612*

trimethylpsoralen *see* trioxsalen *on next page*

trimetrexate glucuronate (tri me TREKS ate gloo KYOOR oh nate)
U.S./Canadian Brand Names Neutrexin® [US]
Therapeutic Category Antibiotic, Miscellaneous
Use Alternative therapy for the treatment of moderate-to-severe *Pneumocystis carinii* pneumonia (PCP) in immunocompromised patients, including patients with acquired
(Continued)

trimetrexate glucuronate *(Continued)*

immunodeficiency syndrome (AIDS), who are intolerant of, or are refractory to, co-trimoxazole therapy or for whom co-trimoxazole is contraindicated

Usual Dosage Adults: I.V.: 45 mg/m^2 once daily over 60 minutes for 21 days; it is necessary to reduce the dose in patients with liver dysfunction, although no specific recommendations exist

Dosage Forms Injection, powder for reconstitution: 25 mg, 200 mg

trimipramine (trye MI pra meen)

U.S./Canadian Brand Names Apo®-Trimip [Can]; Novo-Tripramine [Can]; Nu-Trimipramine [Can]; Rhotrimine® [Can]; Surmontil® [US/Can]

Therapeutic Category Antidepressant, Tricyclic (Tertiary Amine)

Use Treatment of various forms of depression, often in conjunction with psychotherapy

Usual Dosage Oral: 50-150 mg/day as a single bedtime dose

Dosage Forms Capsule, as maleate: 25 mg, 50 mg, 100 mg

Trimox® [US] *see* amoxicillin *on page 37*

Trimox® 500 mg *(Discontinued)* *see page 814*

Trinalin® Repetabs® [US/Can] *see* azatadine and pseudoephedrine *on page 65*

Trinasal® [Can] *see* triamcinolone (inhalation, nasal) *on page 651*

Tri-Nefrin® Extra Strength Tablet *(Discontinued)* *see page 814*

Tri-Norinyl® [US] *see* ethinyl estradiol and norethindrone *on page 251*

Triofed® Syrup *(Discontinued)* *see page 814*

Triostat™ [US] *see* liothyronine *on page 386*

Triotann® [US] *see* chlorpheniramine, pyrilamine, and phenylephrine *on page 141*

trioxsalen (trye OKS a len)

Synonyms trimethylpsoralen

U.S./Canadian Brand Names Trisoralen® [US]

Therapeutic Category Psoralen

Use In conjunction with controlled exposure to ultraviolet light or sunlight for repigmentation of idiopathic vitiligo; increasing tolerance to sunlight with albinism; enhance pigmentation

Usual Dosage Children >12 years and Adults: Oral: 10 mg/day as a single dose, 2-4 hours before controlled exposure to UVA or sunlight

Dosage Forms Tablet: 5 mg

Tripedia® [US] *see* diphtheria, tetanus toxoids, and acellular pertussis vaccine *on page 204*

Triphasil® [US/Can] *see* ethinyl estradiol and levonorgestrel *on page 248*

Triphed® [US-OTC] *see* triprolidine and pseudoephedrine *on next page*

Tri-Phen-Chlor® *(Discontinued)* *see page 814*

Triphenyl® Expectorant *(Discontinued)* *see page 814*

Triphenyl® Syrup *(Discontinued)* *see page 814*

Triple Antibiotic® [US] *see* bacitracin, neomycin, and polymyxin B *on page 69*

triple sulfa *see* sulfabenzamide, sulfacetamide, and sulfathiazole *on page 610*

Tri-P® Oral Infant Drops *(Discontinued)* *see page 814*

Triposed® Syrup *(Discontinued)* *see page 814*

Triposed® Tablet [US-OTC] *see* triprolidine and pseudoephedrine *on next page*

triprolidine and pseudoephedrine
(trye PROE li deen & soo doe e FED rin)

Synonyms pseudoephedrine and triprolidine

U.S./Canadian Brand Names Actanol® [US-OTC]; Actedril® [US-OTC]; Actifed® [US/Can]; Allerfed® [US-OTC]; Allerfrim® [US-OTC]; Allerphed® [US-OTC]; Altafed® [US-OTC]; Aphedrid™ [US-OTC]; Aprodine® [US-OTC]; Biofed-PE® [US-OTC]; Cenafed® Plus Tablet [US-OTC]; Genac® Tablet [US-OTC]; Histafed® [US-OTC]; Hista-Tabs® [US-OTC]; Pseudocot-T® [US-OTC]; Ridifed® [US-OTC]; Ritifed® [US-OTC]; Silafed® [US-OTC]; Triacin® [US-OTC]; Tri-Fed® [US-OTC]; Triphed® [US-OTC]; Triposed® Tablet [US-OTC]; Tri-Pseudafed® [US-OTC]; Tri-Sofed® [US-OTC]; Tri-Sudo® [US-OTC]; Uni-Fed® [US-OTC]; Vi-Sudo® [US-OTC]

Therapeutic Category Antihistamine/Decongestant Combination

Use Temporary relief of nasal congestion, running nose, sneezing, itching of nose or throat and itchy, watery eyes due to common cold, hay fever or other upper respiratory allergies

Usual Dosage May dose according to **pseudoephedrine** component (4 mg/kg/day in divided doses 3-4 times/day) Oral:

Children:
4 months to 2 years: 1.25 mL 3-4 times/day
2-4 years: 2.5 mL 3-4 times/day
4-6 years: 3.75 mL 3-4 times/day
6-12 years: 5 mL or ½ tablet 3-4 times/day, not to exceed 2 tablets/day
Children >12 years and Adults: 10 mL or 1 tablet 3-4 times/day, not to exceed 4 tablets/day

Dosage Forms
Capsule: Triprolidine hydrochloride 2.5 mg and pseudoephedrine hydrochloride 60 mg
Capsule, extended release: Triprolidine hydrochloride 5 mg and pseudoephedrine hydrochloride 120 mg
Syrup: Triprolidine hydrochloride 1.25 mg and pseudoephedrine hydrochloride 30 mg per 5 mL
Tablet: Triprolidine hydrochloride 2.5 mg and pseudoephedrine hydrochloride 60 mg

triprolidine, pseudoephedrine, and codeine
(trye PROE li deen, soo doe e FED rin, & KOE deen)

U.S./Canadian Brand Names Aprodine® w/C [US]; CoActifed® [Can]; Triacin-C® [US]

Therapeutic Category Antihistamine/Decongestant/Antitussive

Controlled Substance C-V

Use Symptomatic relief of cough

Usual Dosage Oral:
Children:
2-6 years: 2.5 mL 4 times/day
7-12 years: 5 mL 4 times/day
Children >12 years and Adults: 10 mL 4 times/day

Dosage Forms Syrup: Triprolidine hydrochloride 1.25 mg, pseudoephedrine hydrochloride 30 mg, and codeine phosphate 10 mg per 5 mL [contains alcohol 4.3%]

Tri-Pseudafed® [US-OTC] *see* triprolidine and pseudoephedrine *on this page*

Tri-Pseudo® (Discontinued) *see page 814*

TripTone® Caplets® [US-OTC] *see* dimenhydrinate *on page 200*

triptorelin (trip toe REL in)

Synonyms triptorelin pamoate

U.S./Canadian Brand Names Trelstar™ Depot [US/Can]; Trelstar™ LA [US]

Therapeutic Category Luteinizing Hormone-Releasing Hormone Analog

Use Palliative treatment of advanced prostate cancer as an alternative to orchiectomy or estrogen administration

Usual Dosage I.M.: Adults: Prostate cancer:
(Continued)

659

triptorelin *(Continued)*

Trelstar™ Depot: 3.75 mg once every 28 days
Trelstar™ LA: 11.25 mg once every 84 days
Dosage Forms Injection, powder for reconstitution, as pamoate [also available packaged with Debioclip™ (prefilled syringe containing sterile water)]:
Trelstar™ Depot: 3.75 mg
Trelstar™ LA: 11.25 mg

triptorelin pamoate *see triptorelin on previous page*

Triquilar® **[Can]** *see ethinyl estradiol and levonorgestrel on page 248*

tris buffer *see tromethamine on next page*

Trisenox™ **[US]** *see arsenic trioxide on page 56*

tris(hydroxymethyl)aminomethane *see tromethamine on next page*

Tri-Sofed® **[US-OTC]** *see triprolidine and pseudoephedrine on previous page*

Trisoject® **Injection** *(Discontinued)* *see page 814*

Trisoralen® **[US]** *see trioxsalen on page 658*

Tri-Statin® **II Topical** *(Discontinued)* *see page 814*

Trisudex® *(Discontinued)* *see page 814*

Tri-Sudo® **[US-OTC]** *see triprolidine and pseudoephedrine on previous page*

Tri-Tannate® **[US]** *see chlorpheniramine, pyrilamine, and phenylephrine on page 141*

Tri-Tannate Plus® *(Discontinued)* *see page 814*

Tritec® **[US]** *see ranitidine bismuth citrate on page 564*

Trivagizole 3™ *(Discontinued)* *see page 814*

Tri-Vi-Flor® **[US]** *see vitamin (multiple/pediatric) on page 683*

Tri-Vi-Sol® **[US-OTC]** *see vitamin (multiple/pediatric) on page 683*

Trivora® **[US]** *see ethinyl estradiol and levonorgestrel on page 248*

Trixaicin® **[US]** *see capsaicin on page 111*

Trixaicin HP® **[US]** *see capsaicin on page 111*

Trizivir® **[US/Can]** *see abacavir, lamivudine, and zidovudine on page 2*

Trobicin® **[US]** *see spectinomycin on page 603*

Trocaine® **[US-OTC]** *see benzocaine on page 77*

Trocal® **[US-OTC]** *see dextromethorphan on page 189*

Trofan® *(Discontinued)* *see page 814*

Trofan DS® *(Discontinued)* *see page 814*

troleandomycin (troe lee an doe MYE sin)

Synonyms triacetyloleandomycin
U.S./Canadian Brand Names Tao® [US]
Therapeutic Category Macrolide (Antibiotic)
Use Adjunct in the treatment of severe corticosteroid-dependent asthma due to its steroid-sparing properties; obsolete antibiotic with spectrum of activity similar to erythromycin
Usual Dosage Oral:
Children: 25-40 mg/kg/day divided every 6 hours
Adjunct in corticosteroid-dependent asthma: 14 mg/kg/day in divided doses every 6-12 hours not to exceed 250 mg every 6 hours; dose is tapered to once daily then alternate day dosing
Adults: 250-500 mg 4 times/day
Dosage Forms Capsule: 250 mg

Trombovar® **[Can]** *see* sodium tetradecyl *on page 600*

tromethamine (troe METH a meen)

Synonyms tris buffer; tris(hydroxymethyl)aminomethane

U.S./Canadian Brand Names THAM® [US]

Therapeutic Category Alkalinizing Agent

Use Correction of metabolic acidosis associated with cardiac bypass surgery or cardiac arrest; to correct excess acidity of stored blood that is preserved with acid citrate dextrose (ACD); to prime the pump-oxygenator during cardiac bypass surgery; indicated in severe metabolic acidosis in patients in whom sodium or carbon dioxide elimination is restricted [eg, infants needing alkalinization after receiving maximum sodium bicarbonate (8-10 mEq/kg/24 hours)]

Usual Dosage Dose depends on buffer base deficit; when deficit is known: tromethamine mL of 0.3 M solution = body weight (kg) x base deficit (mEq/L); when base deficit is not known: 3-6 mL/kg/dose I.V. (1-2 mEq/kg/dose)

Metabolic acidosis with cardiac arrest:

I.V.: 3.5-6 mL/kg (1-2 mEq/kg/dose) into large peripheral vein; 500-1000 mL if needed in adults

I.V. continuous drip: Infuse slowly by syringe pump over 3-6 hours

Excess acidity of ACD priming blood: 14-70 mL of 0.3 molar solution added to each 500 mL of blood

Dosage Forms Injection (THAM®): 18 g [0.3 molar] (500 mL)

Tronolane® **[US-OTC]** *see* pramoxine *on page 534*

Tronothane® **[US-OTC]** *see* pramoxine *on page 534*

tropicamide (troe PIK a mide)

Synonyms bistropamide

U.S./Canadian Brand Names Diotrope® [Can]; Mydriacyl® [US/Can]

Therapeutic Category Anticholinergic Agent

Use Short-acting mydriatic used in diagnostic procedures; as well as preoperatively and postoperatively; treatment of some cases of acute iritis, iridocyclitis, and keratitis

Usual Dosage Children and Adults: Ophthalmic:

Cycloplegia: 1-2 drops (1%); may repeat in 5 minutes

Mydriasis: 1-2 drops (0.5%) 15-20 minutes before exam; may repeat every 30 minutes as needed

Dosage Forms Solution, ophthalmic: 0.5% (2 mL, 15 mL); 1% (2 mL, 3 mL, 15 mL)

Trosyd™ **AF [Can]** *see* tioconazole *on page 640*

Trosyd™ **J [Can]** *see* tioconazole *on page 640*

trovafloxacin (TROE va flox a sin)

Synonyms alatrofloxacin; CP-99,219-27

U.S./Canadian Brand Names Trovan® [US/Can]

Therapeutic Category Antibiotic, Quinolone

Use Should be used only in life- or limb-threatening infections

Treatment of nosocomial pneumonia, community-acquired pneumonia, complicated intra-abdominal infections, gynecologic/pelvic infections, complicated skin and skin structure infections

Usual Dosage Adults:

Nosocomial pneumonia: I.V.: 300 mg single dose followed by 200 mg/day orally for a total duration of 10-14 days

Community-acquired pneumonia: Oral, I.V.: 200 mg/day for 7-14 days

Complicated intra-abdominal infections, including postsurgical infections/gynecologic and pelvic infections: I.V.: 300 mg as a single dose followed by 200 mg/day orally for a total duration of 7-14 days

(Continued)

trovafloxacin *(Continued)*

Skin and skin structure infections, complicated, including diabetic foot infections: Oral, I.V.: 200 mg/day for 10-14 days

Dosage Forms
Injection, as mesylate (alatrofloxacin): 5 mg/mL (40 mL, 60 mL)
Tablet, as mesylate (trovafloxacin): 100 mg, 200 mg

Trovan® **[US/Can]** *see* trovafloxacin *on previous page*

Truphylline® *(Discontinued) see page 814*

Trusopt® **[US/Can]** *see* dorzolamide *on page 212*

Truxadryl® **[US-OTC]** *see* diphenhydramine *on page 202*

Truxazole® **[US]** *see* sulfisoxazole *on page 614*

Truxcillin® **[US]** *see* penicillin V potassium *on page 499*

trypsin, balsam Peru, and castor oil

(TRIP sin, BAL sam pe RUE, & KAS tor oyl)
U.S./Canadian Brand Names Granulex [US]
Therapeutic Category Protectant, Topical
Use Treatment of decubitus ulcers, varicose ulcers, debridement of eschar, dehiscent wounds and sunburn
Usual Dosage Topical: Apply a minimum of twice daily or as often as necessary
Dosage Forms Aerosol, topical: Trypsin 0.1 mg, balsam Peru 72.5 mg, and castor oil 650 mg per 0.82 mL (60 g, 120 g)

Tryptacin® *(Discontinued) see page 814*

Trysul® *(Discontinued) see page 814*

TSH *see* thyrotropin *on page 637*

TSPA *see* thiotepa *on page 635*

T-Stat® **[US]** *see* erythromycin (ophthalmic/topical) *on page 235*

tuberculin tests (too BER kyoo lin tests)

Synonyms Mantoux; old tuberculin; PPD; purified protein derivative
U.S./Canadian Brand Names Aplisol® [US]; Tine Test PPD [US]; Tubersol® [US]
Therapeutic Category Diagnostic Agent
Use Skin test in diagnosis of tuberculosis, to aid in assessment of cell-mediated immunity; routine tuberculin testing is recommended at 12 months of age and at every 1-2 years thereafter, before the measles vaccination
Usual Dosage Children and Adults: Intradermally: 0.1 mL approximately 4" below elbow; use $1/4$" to $1/2$" or 26- or 27-gauge needle; significant reactions are ≥5 mm in diameter
Dosage Forms
Injection:
First test strength: 1 TU/0.1 mL (1 mL)
Intermediate test strength: 5 TU/0.1 mL (1 mL, 5 mL, 10 mL)
Second test strength: 250 TU/0.1 mL (1 mL)
Tine: 5 TU each test

Tubersol® **[US]** *see* tuberculin tests *on this page*

tubocurarine (too boe kyoor AR een)

Synonyms *d*-tubocurarine
Therapeutic Category Skeletal Muscle Relaxant
Use Adjunct to anesthesia to induce skeletal muscle relaxation
Usual Dosage Children and Adults: I.V.: 0.2-0.4 mg/kg as a single dose; maintenance: 0.04-0.2 mg/kg/dose as needed to maintain paralysis

Alternative adult dose: 6-9 mg once daily, then 3-4.5 mg as needed to maintain paralysis

Dosage Forms Injection, as chloride: 3 mg/mL [3 units/mL] (5 mL, 10 mL, 20 mL)

Tucks® **Cream** *(Discontinued)* *see page 814*

Tucks® **[US-OTC]** *see* witch hazel *on page 686*

Tuinal® **[US]** *see* amobarbital and secobarbital *on page 36*

Tums® **E-X Extra Strength Tablet [US-OTC]** *see* calcium carbonate *on page 104*

Tums® **Ultra [US-OTC]** *see* calcium carbonate *on page 104*

Tums® **[US-OTC]** *see* calcium carbonate *on page 104*

Tusal® *(Discontinued)* *see page 814*

Tusibron® *(Discontinued)* *see page 814*

Tusibron-DM® *(Discontinued)* *see page 814*

Tussafin® **Expectorant** *(Discontinued)* *see page 814*

Tuss-Allergine® **Modified T.D. Capsule** *(Discontinued)* *see page 814*

Tussend® **Expectorant [US]** *see* hydrocodone, pseudoephedrine, and guaifenesin *on page 332*

Tussigon® **[US]** *see* hydrocodone and homatropine *on page 331*

Tussionex® **[US]** *see* hydrocodone and chlorpheniramine *on page 330*

Tussi-Organidin® *(Discontinued)* *see page 814*

Tussi-Organidin® **DM** *(Discontinued)* *see page 814*

Tussi-Organidin® **DM NR [US]** *see* guaifenesin and dextromethorphan *on page 308*

Tussi-Organidin® **NR [US]** *see* guaifenesin and codeine *on page 308*

Tussi-Organidin® **S-NR [US]** *see* guaifenesin and codeine *on page 308*

Tuss-LA® *(Discontinued)* *see page 814*

Tusso-DM® *(Discontinued)* *see page 814*

Tussogest® **Extended Release Capsule** *(Discontinued)* *see page 814*

Tuss-Ornade® *(Discontinued)* *see page 814*

Tusstat® **[US-OTC]** *see* diphenhydramine *on page 202*

Twelve Resin-K® **[US]** *see* cyanocobalamin *on page 167*

Twice-A-Day® **[US-OTC]** *see* oxymetazoline *on page 486*

Twilite® **[US-OTC]** *see* diphenhydramine *on page 202*

Twin-K® **[US]** *see* potassium citrate and potassium gluconate *on page 531*

Twinrix® **[US/Can]** *see* hepatitis A inactivated and hepatitis B (recombinant) vaccine *on page 319*

Two-Dyne® *(Discontinued)* *see page 814*

Tylenol® **[US/Can]** *see* acetaminophen *on page 3*

Tylenol® **Allergy Sinus [US/Can]** *see* acetaminophen, chlorpheniramine, and pseudoephedrine *on page 7*

Tylenol® **Arthritis Pain [US-OTC]** *see* acetaminophen *on page 3*

Tylenol® **Children's [US-OTC]** *see* acetaminophen *on page 3*

Tylenol® **Cold [Can]** *see* acetaminophen, dextromethorphan, and pseudoephedrine *on page 8*

Tylenol® **Cold Effervescent Medication Tablet** *(Discontinued)* *see page 814*

Tylenol® Cold Non-Drowsy [US-OTC] *see* acetaminophen, dextromethorphan, and pseudoephedrine *on page 8*

Tylenol® Decongestant [Can] *see* acetaminophen and pseudoephedrine *on page 6*

Tylenol® Extra Strength [US-OTC] *see* acetaminophen *on page 3*

Tylenol® Flu Non-Drowsy Maximum Strength [US-OTC] *see* acetaminophen, dextromethorphan, and pseudoephedrine *on page 8*

Tylenol® Infants [US-OTC] *see* acetaminophen *on page 3*

Tylenol® Junior Strength [US-OTC] *see* acetaminophen *on page 3*

Tylenol® PM Extra Strength [US-OTC] *see* acetaminophen and diphenhydramine *on page 5*

Tylenol® Severe Allergy [US-OTC] *see* acetaminophen and diphenhydramine *on page 5*

Tylenol® Sinus [Can] *see* acetaminophen and pseudoephedrine *on page 6*

Tylenol® Sinus Non-Drowsy [US-OTC] *see* acetaminophen and pseudoephedrine *on page 6*

Tylenol® Sore Throat [US-OTC] *see* acetaminophen *on page 3*

Tylenol® with Codeine [US/Can] *see* acetaminophen and codeine *on page 5*

Tylox® [US] *see* oxycodone and acetaminophen *on page 485*

Typherix™ [Can] *see* Salmonella typhi Vi capsular polysaccharide vaccine *(Canada only) on page 582*

Typhim Vi® [US] *see* typhoid vaccine *on this page*

typhoid vaccine (TYE foid vak SEEN)

Synonyms typhoid vaccine live oral Ty21a

U.S./Canadian Brand Names Typhim Vi® [US]; Vivotif Berna™ [US/Can]

Therapeutic Category Vaccine, Inactivated Bacteria

Use Promotes active immunity to typhoid fever for patients exposed to typhoid carrier or foreign travel to typhoid fever endemic area

Usual Dosage

Oral: Adults:

Primary immunization: 1 capsule on alternate days (day 1, 3, 5, and 7)

Booster immunization: Repeat full course of primary immunization every 5 years

S.C.:

Children 6 months to 10 years: 0.25 mL; repeat in ≥4 weeks (total immunization is 2 doses)

Children >10 years and Adults: 0.5 mL; repeat dose in ≥4 weeks (total immunization is 2 doses)

Booster: 0.25 mL every 3 years for children 6 months to 10 years and 0.5 mL every 3 years for adults and children >10 years

Dosage Forms

Capsule, enteric coated (Vivotif Berna™): Viable *S. typhi* Ty21a colony-forming units 2-6 x 10^9 and nonviable *S. typhi* Ty21a colony-forming units 50 x 10^9 with sucrose, ascorbic acid, amino acid mixture, lactose, and magnesium stearate

Injection (Typhim Vi®): Purified Vi capsular polysaccharide 25 mcg/0.5 mL (0.5 mL)

Injection, suspension (H-P): Heat- and phenol-inactivated, killed Ty-2 strain of *S. typhi* organisms; provides 8 units/mL, ≤1 billion/mL and ≤35 mcg nitrogen/mL (5 mL, 10 mL)

Powder for suspension (AKD): 8 units/mL ≤1 billion/mL, acetone inactivated dried (50 doses)

typhoid vaccine live oral Ty21a *see* typhoid vaccine *on this page*

Tyrodone® Liquid *(Discontinued)* *see page 814*

Tyzine® [US] *see* tetrahydrozoline *on page 629*

U-90152S *see* delavirdine *on page 178*

UAA® **[US]** *see* methenamine, phenyl salicylate, atropine, hyoscyamine, benzoic acid, and methylene blue *on page 416*

UAD Otic® *(Discontinued) see page 814*

UCB-P071 *see* cetirizine *on page 129*

Ucephan® **[US]** *see* sodium phenylacetate and sodium benzoate *on page 598*

U-Cort™ **[US]** *see* hydrocortisone (topical) *on page 334*

UK *see* urokinase *on page 668*

UK-68-798 *see* dofetilide *on page 209*

UK 92480 *see* sildenafil *on page 590*

UK109496 *see* voriconazole *on page 685*

Ulcerease® **[US-OTC]** *see* phenol *on page 508*

Ulcidine® **[Can]** *see* famotidine *on page 262*

ULR-LA® *(Discontinued) see page 814*

Ultane® **[US]** *see* sevoflurane *on page 589*

Ultiva™ **[US/Can]** *see* remifentanil *on page 566*

Ultracet™ **[US]** *see* acetaminophen and tramadol *on page 7*

Ultralente® **U** *(Discontinued) see page 814*

Ultram® **[US/Can]** *see* tramadol *on page 647*

Ultra Mide® **[US/Can]** *see* urea *on next page*

Ultramop™ **[Can]** *see* methoxsalen *on page 418*

Ultraquin™ **[Can]** *see* hydroquinone *on page 336*

Ultrase® **[US/Can]** *see* pancrelipase *on page 489*

Ultrase® **MT12 [US/Can]** *see* pancrelipase *on page 489*

Ultrase® **MT18 [US/Can]** *see* pancrelipase *on page 489*

Ultrase® **MT20 [US/Can]** *see* pancrelipase *on page 489*

Ultrase® **MT24** *(Discontinued) see page 814*

Ultra Tears® **[US-OTC]** *see* artificial tears *on page 56*

Ultravate™ **[US/Can]** *see* halobetasol *on page 315*

Unasyn® **[US/Can]** *see* ampicillin and sulbactam *on page 41*

undecylenic acid and derivatives (un de sil EN ik AS id & dah RIV ah tivs)

Synonyms zinc undecylenate

U.S./Canadian Brand Names Fungi-Nail® [US-OTC]

Therapeutic Category Antifungal Agent

Use Treatment of athlete's foot (tinea pedis), ringworm (except nails and scalp), prickly heat, jock itch (tinea cruris), diaper rash and other minor skin irritations due to superficial dermatophytes

Usual Dosage Children and Adults: Topical: Apply as needed twice daily after cleansing the affected area for 2-4 weeks

Dosage Forms Solution, topical: Undecylenic acid 25% (29.57 mL)

Unguentine® *(Discontinued) see page 814*

Uni-Bent® **Cough Syrup** *(Discontinued) see page 814*

Unicap® **[US-OTC]** *see* vitamin (multiple/oral) *on page 683*

Uni-Decon® *(Discontinued) see page 814*

Uni-Dur® *(Discontinued) see page 814*

Uni-Fed® **[US-OTC]** *see* triprolidine and pseudoephedrine *on page 659*

Unipen® *(Discontinued)* see page 814

Uniphyl® [US/Can] see theophylline on page 630

Unipres® *(Discontinued)* see page 814

Uni-Pro® *(Discontinued)* see page 814

Uniretic™ [US/Can] see moexipril and hydrochlorothiazide on page 435

Unisom® [US-OTC] see doxylamine on page 216

Unison® Sleepgels® Maximum Strength [US-OTC] see diphenhydramine on page 202

Unithroid™ [US] see levothyroxine on page 382

Unitrol® *(Discontinued)* see page 814

Uni-tussin® *(Discontinued)* see page 814

Uni-tussin® DM *(Discontinued)* see page 814

Univasc® [US] see moexipril on page 435

Univol® [Can] see aluminum hydroxide and magnesium hydroxide on page 29

Unna's boot see zinc gelatin on page 690

Unna's paste see zinc gelatin on page 690

unoprostone (yoo noe PROS tone)

Synonyms unoprostone isopropyl
U.S./Canadian Brand Names Rescula® [US]
Therapeutic Category Ophthalmic Agent, Miscellaneous
Use To lower intraocular pressure (IOP) in patients with open-angle glaucoma or ocular hypertension; should be used in patients who are not tolerant of, or failed treatment with other IOP-lowering medications
Usual Dosage Ophthalmic: Adults: Instill 1 drop into affected eye(s) twice daily
Dosage Forms Solution, ophthalmic: 0.15% (5 mL) [contains benzalkonium chloride]

unoprostone isopropyl see unoprostone on this page

Urabeth® *(Discontinued)* see page 814

Uracel® *(Discontinued)* see page 814

Urasal® [Can] see methenamine on page 416

urea (yoor EE a)

Synonyms carbamide
U.S./Canadian Brand Names Amino-Cerv™ [US]; Aquacare® [US-OTC]; Aquaphilic® With Carbamide [US-OTC]; Carmol® 10 [US-OTC]; Carmol® 20 [US-OTC]; Carmol® 40 [US]; Carmol® Deep Cleaning [US]; Carmol® Scalp Treatment [US]; Gormel® [US-OTC]; Lanaphilic® [US-OTC]; Nutraplus® [US-OTC]; Rea-Lo® [US-OTC]; Ultra Mide® [US/Can]; Ureacin® [US-OTC]; Ureaphil® [US]; Uremol® [Can]; Urisec® [Can]
Therapeutic Category Diuretic, Osmotic; Topical Skin Product
Use Reduce intracranial pressure and intraocular pressure (30%); promotes hydration and removal of excess keratin in hyperkeratotic conditions and dry skin; mild cervicitis
Usual Dosage
Children: I.V. slow infusion:
<2 years: 0.1-0.5 g/kg
>2 years: 0.5-1.5 g/kg
Adults:
I.V. infusion: 1-1.5 g/kg by slow infusion (1-2$\frac{1}{2}$ hours); maximum: 120 g/24 hours
Topical: Apply 1-3 times/day
Vaginal: 1 applicatorful in vagina at bedtime for 2-4 weeks
Dosage Forms
Cream:
Aquacare®: 10% (75 g)

Carmol® 20: 20% (90 g)
Carmol® 40: 40% (30 g, 90 g, 210 g)
Gormel®: 20% (75 g, 120 g, 454 g, 2270 g)
Nutraplus®: 10% (90 g, 454 g)
Rea-Lo®: 30% (60 g, 240 g)
Ureacin®-20: 20% (120 g)
Cream, vaginal (Amino-Cerv™): 8.34% [83.4 mg/g] (82.5 g)
Injection, powder for reconstitution (Ureaphil®): 40 g
Lotion:
Aquacare®: 10% (240 mL)
Carmol® 10: 10% (180 mL)
Carmol® 40: 40% (240 mL)
Carmol® Scalp Treatment: 10% (90 mL)
Nutraplus®: 10% (240 mL, 480 mL)
Rea-Lo®: 15% (120 mL)
Ultra Mide®: 25% (120 mL, 240 mL)
Ureacin®-10: 10% (240 mL)
Ointment:
Aquaphilic® with Carbamide: 10% (180 g, 480 g); 20% (480 g)
Lanaphilic®: 10% (454 g); 20% (454 g)
Shampoo: Carmol® Deep Cleaning: 10% (240 mL)

urea and hydrocortisone (yoor EE a & hye droe KOR ti sone)

Synonyms hydrocortisone and urea
U.S./Canadian Brand Names Carmol-HC® [US]; Ti-U-Lac® H [Can]; Uremol® HC [Can]
Therapeutic Category Corticosteroid, Topical
Use Inflammation of corticosteroid-responsive dermatoses
Usual Dosage Topical: Apply thin film and rub in well 1-4 times/day. Therapy should be discontinued when control is achieved. If no improvement is seen, reassessment of diagnosis may be necessary.
Dosage Forms Cream: Urea 10% and hydrocortisone acetate 1% (30 g) [in water soluble vanishing cream base]

Ureacin®-40 Topical *(Discontinued)* see page 814

Ureacin® [US-OTC] see urea on previous page

urea peroxide see carbamide peroxide on page 113

Ureaphil® [US] see urea on previous page

Urecholine® [US] see bethanechol on page 84

Uremol® [Can] see urea on previous page

Uremol® HC [Can] see urea and hydrocortisone on this page

Urex® [US/Can] see methenamine on page 416

Uridon Modified® [US] see methenamine, phenyl salicylate, atropine, hyoscyamine, benzoic acid, and methylene blue on page 416

Urisec® [Can] see urea on previous page

Urised® [US] see methenamine, phenyl salicylate, atropine, hyoscyamine, benzoic acid, and methylene blue on page 416

Urispas® [US/Can] see flavoxate on page 272

Uristat® [US-OTC] see phenazopyridine on page 506

Uri-Tet® *(Discontinued)* see page 814

Uritin® [US] see methenamine, phenyl salicylate, atropine, hyoscyamine, benzoic acid, and methylene blue on page 416

Urobak® *(Discontinued)* see page 814

Urobiotic-25® *(Discontinued)* see page 814

Urocit®-K [US] *see* potassium citrate *on page 530*

Urodine® *(Discontinued) see page 814*

Urodol® [US-OTC] *see* phenazopyridine *on page 506*

Urofemme® [US-OTC] *see* phenazopyridine *on page 506*

urofollitropin (yoor oh fol li TROE pin)
  U.S./Canadian Brand Names Fertinex® [US]; Fertinorm® H.P. [Can]; Metrodin® [US]
  Therapeutic Category Ovulation Stimulator
  Use Induction of ovulation in patients with polycystic ovarian disease and to stimulate the development of multiple oocytes
  Usual Dosage Adults: Female: S.C.: 75 units/day for 7-12 days, used with hCG may repeat course of treatment 2 more times
  Dosage Forms Injection: 0.83 mg [75 units FSH activity] (2 mL); 1.66 mg [150 units FSH activity]

Urogesic® [US] *see* phenazopyridine *on page 506*

urokinase (yoor oh KIN ase)
  Synonyms UK
  U.S./Canadian Brand Names Abbokinase® [US]
  Therapeutic Category Fibrinolytic Agent
  Use Treatment of recent severe or massive deep vein or arterial thrombosis, pulmonary emboli, and occluded arteriovenous cannulas
  Usual Dosage
    Children and Adults: Deep vein thrombosis: I.V.: Loading: 4400 units/kg over 10 minutes, then 4400 units/kg/hour for 12 hours
    Adults:
      Myocardial infarction: Intracoronary: 750,000 units over 2 hours (6000 units/minute over up to 2 hours)
      Occluded I.V. catheters:
        5000 units (use only Abbokinase® Open Cath) in each lumen over 1-2 minutes, leave in lumen for 1-4 hours, then aspirate; may repeat with 10,000 units in each lumen if 5000 units fails to clear the catheter; **do not infuse into the patient**; volume to instill into catheter is equal to the volume of the catheter
        I.V. infusion: 200 units/kg/hour in each lumen for 12-48 hours at a rate of at least 20 mL/hour
      Dialysis patients: 5000 units is administered in each lumen over 1-2 minutes; leave urokinase in lumen for 1-2 days, then aspirate
      Clot lysis (large vessel thrombi): Loading: I.V.: 4400 units/kg over 10 minutes, increase to 6000 units/kg/hour; maintenance: 4400-6000 units/kg/hour adjusted to achieve clot lysis or patency of affected vessel; doses up to 50,000 units/kg/hour have been used. **Note:** Therapy should be initiated as soon as possible after diagnosis of thrombi and continued until clot is dissolved (usually 24-72 hours).

    Acute pulmonary embolism: Three treatment alternatives: 3 million unit dosage
      Alternative 1: 12-hour infusion: 4400 units/kg (2000 units/lb) bolus over 10 minutes followed by 4400 units/kg/hour (2000 units/lb); begin heparin 1000 units/hour approximately 3-4 hours after completion of urokinase infusion or when PTT is <100 seconds
      Alternative 2: 2-hour infusion: 1 million unit bolus over 10 minutes followed by 2 million units over 110 minutes; begin heparin 1000 units/hour approximately 3-4 hours after completion of urokinase infusion or when PTT is <100 seconds
      Alternative 3: Bolus dose only: 15,000 units/kg over 10 minutes; begin heparin 1000 units/hour approximately 3-4 hours after completion of urokinase infusion or when PTT is <100 seconds
  Dosage Forms
    Injection, powder for reconstitution: 250,000 units
    Injection, powder for reconstitution [catheter clear]: 5000 units, 9000 units

Uro-KP-Neutral® [US] *see* potassium phosphate and sodium phosphate *on page 533*

Urolene Blue® [US] *see* methylene blue *on page 421*

Uro-Mag® [US-OTC] *see* magnesium oxide *on page 398*

Uromitexan™ [Can] *see* mesna *on page 411*

Uroplus® DS *(Discontinued)* *see page 814*

Uroplus® SS *(Discontinued)* *see page 814*

Urovist Cysto® [US] *see* radiological/contrast media (ionic) *on page 561*

Urovist® Meglumine [US] *see* radiological/contrast media (ionic) *on page 561*

Urovist® Sodium 300 [US] *see* radiological/contrast media (ionic) *on page 561*

Urso® [US/Can] *see* ursodiol *on this page*

ursodeoxycholic acid *see* ursodiol *on this page*

ursodiol (ER soe dye ole)
Synonyms ursodeoxycholic acid
U.S./Canadian Brand Names Actigall™ [US]; Urso® [US/Can]
Therapeutic Category Gallstone Dissolution Agent
Use Gallbladder stone dissolution
Usual Dosage Oral: 8-10 mg/kg/day in 2-3 divided doses
Dosage Forms
  Capsule (Actigall®): 300 mg
  Tablet, film coated (Urso®): 250 mg

Uticort® *(Discontinued)* *see page 814*

Utradol™ [Can] *see* etodolac *on page 258*

Uvadex® [US/Can] *see* methoxsalen *on page 418*

Vagifem® [US/Can] *see* estradiol *on page 238*

Vagi-Gard® Douche [US-OTC] *see* povidone-iodine *on page 533*

Vagistat®-1 [US-OTC] *see* tioconazole *on page 640*

Vagitrol® *(Discontinued)* *see page 814*

valacyclovir (val ay SYE kloe veer)
U.S./Canadian Brand Names Valtrex® [US/Can]
Therapeutic Category Antiviral Agent
Use Treatment of herpes zoster (shingles) in immunocompetent patients; episodic treatment or prophylaxis of recurrent genital herpes in immunocompetent patients; for first episode genital herpes; treatment of herpes labialis (cold sores)
Usual Dosage Oral: Adults:
  Herpes zoster (shingles): 1 g 3 times/day for 7 days
  Genital herpes:
   Initial episode: 1 g 2 times/day for 10 days
   Episodic treatment: 500 mg twice daily for 3 days
   Prophylaxis: 500-1000 mg once daily
  Herpes labialis (cold sores): 2 g twice daily for one day (separate doses by ~12 hours)
Dosage Forms Caplet: 500 mg, 1000 mg

Valadol® *(Discontinued)* *see page 814*

Valcyte™ [US] *see* valganciclovir *on next page*

valdecoxib (val de KOX ib)
U.S./Canadian Brand Names Bextra™ [US]
Therapeutic Category Nonsteroidal Anti-inflammatory Drug (NSAID), COX-2 Selective
(Continued)

valdecoxib *(Continued)*

Use Relief of signs and symptoms of osteoarthritis and adult rheumatoid arthritis; treatment of primary dysmenorrhea

Usual Dosage Oral: Adults:

Osteoarthritis and rheumatoid arthritis: 10 mg once daily; **Note:** No additional benefits seen with 20 mg/day

Primary dysmenorrhea: 20 mg twice daily as needed

Dosage Forms Tablet: 10 mg, 20 mg

Valergen® Injection *(Discontinued)* see page 814

Valertest No.1® [US] *see* estradiol and testosterone on page 240

valganciclovir (val gan SYE kloh veer)

U.S./Canadian Brand Names Valcyte™ [US]

Therapeutic Category Antiviral Agent

Use Treatment of cytomegalovirus (CMV) retinitis in patients with acquired immunodeficiency syndrome (AIDS)

Usual Dosage Oral: Adults: CMV retinitis:

Induction: 900 mg twice daily for 21 days (with food)

Maintenance: Following induction treatment, or for patients with inactive CMV retinitis who require maintenance therapy: Recommended dose: 900 mg once daily (with food)

Dosage Forms Tablet, as hydrochloride: 450 mg [496.3 mg valganciclovir hydrochloride equivalent to 450 mg valganciclovir]

Valisone® Scalp Lotion [Can] *see* betamethasone (topical) on page 83

Valisone® Topical *(Discontinued)* see page 814

Valium® [US/Can] *see* diazepam on page 191

Valmid® Capsule *(Discontinued)* see page 814

Valorin Extra [US-OTC] *see* acetaminophen on page 3

Valorin [US-OTC] *see* acetaminophen on page 3

Valpin® 50 *(Discontinued)* see page 814

valproic acid and derivatives (val PROE ik AS id & dah RIV ah tives)

Synonyms dipropylacetic acid; DPA; 2-propylpentanoic acid; 2-propylvaleric acid

U.S./Canadian Brand Names Alti-Divalproex [Can]; Apo®-Divalproex [Can]; Depacon® [US]; Depakene® [US/Can]; Depakote® Delayed Release [US]; Depakote® ER [US]; Depakote® Sprinkle® [US]; Epival® I.V. [Can]; Gen-Divalproex [Can]; Novo-Divalproex [Can]; Nu-Divalproex [Can]; PMS-Valproic Acid [Can]; PMS-Valproic Acid E.C. [Can]; Rhoxal-valproic [Can]

Therapeutic Category Anticonvulsant

Use

Mania associated with bipolar disorder (Depakote®)

Migraine prophylaxis (Depakote®, Depakote® ER)

Monotherapy and adjunctive therapy in the treatment of patients with complex partial seizures that occur either in isolation or in association with other types of seizures (Depacon™, Depakote®)

Sole and adjunctive therapy of simple and complex absence seizures (Depacon™, Depakene®, Depakote®)

Adjunctively in patients with multiple seizure types that include absence seizures (Depacon™, Depakene®)

Unlabeled use: Behavior disorders in Alzheimer's disease

Usual Dosage
Seizures:

Children >10 years and Adults:

Oral: Initial: 10-15 mg/kg/day in 1-3 divided doses; increase by 5-10 mg/kg/day at weekly intervals until therapeutic levels are achieved; maintenance: 30-60 mg/kg/day in 2-3 divided doses. Adult usual dose: 1000-2500 mg/day

Children receiving more than one anticonvulsant (ie, polytherapy) may require doses up to 100 mg/kg/day in 3-4 divided doses

I.V.: Administer as a 60-minute infusion (≤20 mg/minute) with the same frequency as oral products; switch patient to oral products as soon as possible

Rectal: Dilute syrup 1:1 with water for use as a retention enema; loading dose: 17-20 mg/kg one time; maintenance: 10-15 mg/kg/dose every 8 hours

Mania: Adults: Oral: 750 mg/day in divided doses; dose should be adjusted as rapidly as possible to desired clinical effect; a loading dose of 20 mg/kg may be used; maximum recommended dosage: 60 mg/kg/day

Migraine prophylaxis: Adults: Oral:

Extended release tablets: 500 mg once daily for 7 days, then increase to 1000 mg once daily; adjust dose based on patient response; usual dosage range 500-1000 mg/day

Delayed release tablets: 250 mg twice daily; adjust dose based on patient response, up to 1000 mg/day

Dosage Forms
Capsule, as valproic acid (Depakene®): 250 mg

Capsule, sprinkles, as divalproex sodium (Depakote® Sprinkle®): 125 mg

Injection, solution, as sodium valproate (Depacon®): 100 mg/mL (5 mL)

Syrup, as sodium valproate: 250 mg/5 mL (5 mL, 480 mL)

Depakene®: 250 mg/mL (480 mL)

Tablet, delayed release, as divalproex sodium (Depakote®): 125 mg, 250 mg, 500 mg

Tablet, extended release, as divalproex sodium (Depakote® ER): 500 mg

Valrelease® *(Discontinued)* see page 814

valrubicin (val ru BYE cin)
U.S./Canadian Brand Names Valstar™ [US/Can]

Therapeutic Category Antineoplastic Agent, Anthracycline

Use Intravesical therapy of BCG-refractory carcinoma *in situ* of the urinary bladder

Usual Dosage Adults: Intravesical: 800 mg once weekly for 6 weeks

Dosage Forms Injection: 40 mg/mL (5 mL)

valsartan (val SAR tan)
U.S./Canadian Brand Names Diovan™ [US/Can]

Therapeutic Category Angiotensin II Receptor Antagonist

Use Treatment of hypertension alone or in combination with other antihypertensives

Usual Dosage Adults: Oral: 80 mg/day; may be increased to 160 mg if needed (maximal effects observed in 4-6 weeks)

Dosage Forms Tablet: 80 mg, 160 mg, 320 mg""

Capsule: 80 mg, 160 mg, 320 mg [Note: This form to be discontinued]

Tablet: 40 mg, 80 mg, 160 mg, 320 mg

valsartan and hydrochlorothiazide
(val SAR tan & hye droe klor oh THYE a zide)

U.S./Canadian Brand Names Diovan HCT™ [US/Can]

Therapeutic Category Antihypertensive Agent, Combination

Use Treatment of hypertension

Usual Dosage Adults: Oral: Dose is individualized

Dosage Forms Tablet:

Valsartan 80 mg and hydrochlorothiazide 12.5 mg

Valsartan 160 mg and hydrochlorothiazide 12.5 mg

(Continued)

valsartan and hydrochlorothiazide *(Continued)*
Valsartan 160 mg and hydrochlorothiazide 25 mg

Valstar™ [US/Can] *see* valrubicin *on previous page*

Valtrex® [US/Can] *see* valacyclovir *on page 669*

Vamate® Oral *(Discontinued)* *see page 814*

Vanatrip® [US] *see* amitriptyline *on page 34*

Vancenase® AQ 84 mcg [US] *see* beclomethasone *on page 73*

Vancenase® Pockethaler® [US] *see* beclomethasone *on page 73*

Vanceril® [US/Can] *see* beclomethasone *on page 73*

Vancocin® [US/Can] *see* vancomycin *on this page*

Vancoled® [US] *see* vancomycin *on this page*

vancomycin (van koe MYE sin)
U.S./Canadian Brand Names Vancocin® [US/Can]; Vancoled® [US]
Therapeutic Category Antibiotic, Miscellaneous
Use Treatment of patients with the following infections or conditions: treatment of infections due to documented or suspected methicillin-resistant *S. aureus* or beta-lactam resistant coagulase-negative *Staphylococcus*; treatment of serious or life-threatening infections (ie, endocarditis, meningitis, osteomyelitis) due to documented or suspected staphylococcal or streptococcal infections in patients who are allergic to penicillins and/or cephalosporins; empiric therapy of infections associated with central lines, VP shunts, hemodialysis shunts, vascular grafts, prosthetic heart valves; used orally for staphylococcal enterocolitis or for antibiotic-associated pseudomembranous colitis produced by *C. difficile*
Usual Dosage I.V. (initial dosage recommendation):
Infants >1 month and Children: 40 mg/kg/day in divided doses every 6 hours
Infants >1 month and Children with staphylococcal central nervous system infection: 60 mg/kg/day in divided doses every 6 hours
Adults: With normal renal function: 0.5 g every 6 hours or 1 g every 12 hours

Intrathecal:
 Children: 5-20 mg/day
 Adults: 20 mg/day
Oral:
 Children: 10-50 mg/kg/day in divided doses every 6-8 hours; not to exceed 2 g/day
 Adults: 0.5-2 g/day in divided doses every 6-8 hours
Pseudomembranous colitis produced by *C. difficile*:
 Children: 40 mg/kg/day in divided doses, added to fluids
 Adults: 500 mg to 2 g/day administered in 3 or 4 divided doses for 7-10 days
Dosage Forms
Capsule, as hydrochloride: 125 mg, 250 mg
Injection, powder for reconstitution, as hydrochloride: 500 mg, 1 g, 2 g, 5 g, 10 g
Powder for oral solution, as hydrochloride: 1 g, 10 g

Vanex-LA® *(Discontinued)* *see page 814*

Vaniqa™ [US] *see* eflornithine *on page 224*

Vanoxide® *(Discontinued)* *see page 814*

Vanoxide-HC® [US/Can] *see* benzoyl peroxide and hydrocortisone *on page 80*

Vanquish® Extra Strength Pain Reliever [US-OTC] *see* acetaminophen, aspirin, and caffeine *on page 7*

Vanseb-T® Shampoo *(Discontinued)* *see page 814*

Vansil™ *(Discontinued)* *see page 814*

Vantin® [US/Can] *see* cefpodoxime *on page 124*

Vaponefrin® *(Discontinued)* see page 814

Vaponefrin® **[Can]** see epinephrine on page 228

VAQTA® **[US/Can]** see hepatitis A vaccine on page 319

varicella virus vaccine (var i SEL a VYE rus vak SEEN)

Synonyms chickenpox vaccine; varicella-zoster virus (VZV) vaccine

U.S./Canadian Brand Names Varivax® [US/Can]

Therapeutic Category Vaccine, Live Virus

Use The American Association of Pediatrics recommends that the chickenpox vaccine should be given to all healthy children between 12 months and 18 years; children between 12 months and 13 years who have not been immunized or who have not had chickenpox should receive 1 vaccination while children 13-18 years of age require 2 vaccinations 4-8 weeks apart; the vaccine has been added to the childhood immunization schedule for infants 12-28 months of age and children 11-12 years of age who have not been vaccinated previously or who have not had the disease; it is recommended to be given with the measles, mumps, and rubella (MMR) vaccine

Usual Dosage S.C.:

Children 12 months to 12 years: 0.5 mL

Children 12 years to Adults: 2 doses of 0.5 mL separated by 4-8 weeks

Dosage Forms Injection, powder for reconstitution [preservative free; single-dose vial]: 1350 plaque-forming units (PFU)/0.5 mL [contains gelatin and trace amounts of neomycin]

varicella-zoster immune globulin (human)

(var i SEL a-ZOS ter i MYUN GLOB yoo lin HYU man)

Synonyms VZIG

Therapeutic Category Immune Globulin

Use Passive immunization of susceptible immunodeficient patients after exposure to varicella; most effective if begun within 96 hours of exposure

VZIG supplies are limited, restrict administration to those meeting the following criteria:

One of the following underlying illnesses or conditions:

Neoplastic disease (eg, leukemia or lymphoma)

Congenital or acquired immunodeficiency

Immunosuppressive therapy with steroids, antimetabolites or other immunosuppressive treatment regimens

Newborn of mother who had onset of chickenpox within 5 days before delivery or within 48 hours after delivery

Premature (≥28 weeks gestation) whose mother has no history of chickenpox

Premature (<28 weeks gestation or ≤1000 g VZIG) regardless of maternal history

One of the following types of exposure to chickenpox or zoster patient(s):

Continuous household contact

Playmate contact (>1 hour play indoors)

Hospital contact (in same 2-4 bedroom or adjacent beds in a large ward or prolonged face-to-face contact with an infectious staff member or patient)

Susceptible to varicella-zoster

Age of <15 years; administer to immunocompromised adolescents and adults and to other older patients on an individual basis

An acceptable alternative to VZIG prophylaxis is to treat varicella, if it occurs, with high-dose I.V. acyclovir

Usual Dosage High-risk susceptible patients who are exposed again more than 3 weeks after a prior dose of VZIG should receive another full dose; there is no evidence VZIG modifies established varicella-zoster infections.

I.M.: Administer by deep injection in the gluteal muscle or in another large muscle mass. Inject 125 units/10 kg (22 lb); maximum dose: 625 units (5 vials); minimum dose: 125 units; do not administer fractional doses. Do not inject I.V.

(Continued)

673

varicella-zoster immune globulin (human) *(Continued)*

Dosage Forms Injection: 125 units of antibody in single dose vials; 625 units of antibody

varicella-zoster virus (VZV) vaccine *see* varicella virus vaccine *on previous page*

Varivax® **[US/Can]** *see* varicella virus vaccine *on previous page*

Vascor® **[US/Can]** *see* bepridil *on page 81*

Vascoray® **[US]** *see* radiological/contrast media (ionic) *on page 561*

Vaseretic® **[US/Can]** *see* enalapril and hydrochlorothiazide *on page 226*

Vasocidin® **[US/Can]** *see* sulfacetamide and prednisolone *on page 611*

VasoClear® **[US-OTC]** *see* naphazoline *on page 446*

Vasocon® **[Can]** *see* naphazoline *on page 446*

Vasocon-A® **[US/Can]** *see* naphazoline and antazoline *on page 447*

Vasocon Regular® **Ophthalmic** *(Discontinued)* *see page 814*

Vasodilan® **[US]** *see* isoxsuprine *on page 363*

vasopressin (vay soe PRES in)

Synonyms antidiuretic hormone (ADH); 8-arginine vasopressin
U.S./Canadian Brand Names Pitressin® [US]; Pressyn® [Can]
Therapeutic Category Hormone, Posterior Pituitary
Use Treatment of diabetes insipidus; prevention and treatment of postoperative abdominal distention; differential diagnosis of diabetes insipidus; adjunct in the treatment of acute massive hemorrhage of GI tract or esophageal varices
Usual Dosage
Diabetes insipidus:
I.M., S.C.:
Children: 2.5-5 units 2-4 times/day as needed
Adults: 5-10 units 2-4 times/day as needed (dosage range 5-60 units/day)
Intranasal: Administer on cotton pledget or nasal spray
Abdominal distention Adults: I.M.: 5 mg stat, 10 mg every 3-4 hours
GI hemorrhage: I.V.: Administer in a peripheral vein; dilute aqueous in NS or D_5W to 0.1-1 unit/mL and infuse at 0.2-0.4 unit/minute and progressively increase to 0.9 unit/minute if necessary; I.V. infusion administration requires the use of an infusion pump and should be administered in a peripheral line to minimize adverse reactions on coronary arteries
Dosage Forms Injection, aqueous: 20 vasopressor units/mL (0.5 mL, 1 mL, 10 mL)

Vasosulf® **Ophthalmic** *(Discontinued)* *see page 814*

Vasotec® **[US/Can]** *see* enalapril *on page 225*

Vasotec® **I.V.** **[US/Can]** *see* enalapril *on page 225*

Vasoxyl® *(Discontinued)* *see page 814*

Vaxigrip® **[Can]** *see* influenza virus vaccine *on page 350*

VCF™ **[US-OTC]** *see* nonoxynol 9 *on page 464*

V-Cillin K® *(Discontinued)* *see page 814*

VCR *see* vincristine *on page 678*

V-Dec-M® **[US]** *see* guaifenesin and pseudoephedrine *on page 310*

Vectrin® *(Discontinued)* *see page 814*

vecuronium (ve KYOO roe nee um)

Synonyms ORG NC 45
U.S./Canadian Brand Names Norcuron® [US/Can]
Therapeutic Category Skeletal Muscle Relaxant

Use Adjunct to anesthesia, to facilitate endotracheal intubation, and provide skeletal muscle relaxation during surgery or mechanical ventilation

Usual Dosage I.V.:

Infants >7 weeks to 1 year: Initial: 0.08-0.1 mg/kg/dose; maintenance: 0.05-0.1 mg/kg/ every hour as needed

Children >1 year and Adults: Initial: 0.08-0.1 mg/kg/dose; maintenance: 0.05-0.1 mg/kg/ every hour as needed; may be administered as a continuous infusion at 0.1 mg/kg/hour

Note: Children may require slightly higher initial doses and slightly more frequent supplementation

Dosage Forms Injection, powder for reconstitution: 10 mg (5 mL, 10 mL)

Veetids® **[US]** *see* penicillin V potassium *on page 499*

Velban® **[US/Can]** *see* vinblastine *on page 678*

Velosef® **[US]** *see* cephradine *on page 129*

Velosulin® **BR (Buffered) [US]** *see* insulin preparations *on page 352*

Velsar® **Injection** *(Discontinued)* *see page 814*

venlafaxine (VEN la faks een)

U.S./Canadian Brand Names Effexor® [US/Can]; Effexor® XR [US/Can]

Therapeutic Category Antidepressant, Phenethylamine

Use Treatment of depression

Usual Dosage Adults: Oral:

Capsule: One capsule daily

Tablet: 75 mg/day, administered in 2 or 3 divided doses, taken with food; dose may be increased in 75 mg/day increments at intervals of at least 4 days, up to 225-375 mg/ day

Dosage Forms

Capsule, extended release (Effexor® XR): 37.5 mg, 75 mg, 150 mg

Tablet (Effexor®): 25 mg, 37.5 mg, 50 mg, 75 mg, 100 mg

Venofer® **[US]** *see* iron sucrose *on page 360*

Venoglobulin®-I *(Discontinued)* *see page 814*

Venoglobulin®-S [US] *see* immune globulin (intravenous) *on page 347*

Ventolin® **[US]** *see* albuterol *on page 18*

Ventolin® **HFA [US]** *see* albuterol *on page 18*

VePesid® **[US/Can]** *see* etoposide *on page 259*

verapamil (ver AP a mil)

Synonyms iproveratril

U.S./Canadian Brand Names Alti-Verapamil [Can]; Apo®-Verap [Can]; Calan® SR [US]; Calan® [US/Can]; Chronovera® [Can]; Covera® [Can]; Covera-HS® [US]; Gen-Verapamil [Can]; Gen-Verapamil SR [Can]; Isoptin® SR [US/Can]; Isoptin® [US/Can]; Novo-Veramil [Can]; Novo-Veramil SR [Can]; Nu-Verap [Can]; Verelan® PM [US]; Verelan® [US]

Therapeutic Category Antiarrhythmic Agent, Class IV; Calcium Channel Blocker

Use Angina, hypertension; I.V. for supraventricular tachyarrhythmias (PSVT, atrial fibrillation, atrial flutter)

Usual Dosage

Children: I.V.:

0-1 year: 0.1-0.2 mg/kg/dose, repeated after 30 minutes as needed

1-16 years: 0.1-0.3 mg/kg over 2-3 minutes; maximum: 5 mg/dose, may repeat dose once in 30 minutes if adequate response not achieved; maximum for second dose: 10 mg/dose

Children: Oral (dose not well established):

4-8 mg/kg/day in 3 divided doses **or** 1-5 years: 40-80 mg every 8 hours

(Continued)

verapamil *(Continued)*

>5 years: 80 mg every 6-8 hours
Adults:
Oral: 240-480 mg/24 hours divided 3-4 times/day
I.V.: 5-10 mg (0.075-0.15 mg/kg); may repeat 10 mg (0.15 mg/kg) 15-30 minutes after the initial dose if needed and if patient tolerated initial dose

Dosage Forms
Capsule, sustained release, as hydrochloride: 120 mg, 180 mg, 240 mg, 360 mg
Verelan®: 120 mg, 180 mg, 240 mg, 360 mg
Verelan® PM: 100 mg, 200 mg, 300 mg
Injection, as hydrochloride: 2.5 mg/mL (2 mL, 4 mL)
Isoptin®: 2.5 mg/mL (2 mL, 4 mL)
Tablet, as hydrochloride: 40 mg, 80 mg, 120 mg
Calan®, Isoptin®: 40 mg, 80 mg, 120 mg
Tablet, sustained release, as hydrochloride: 180 mg, 240 mg
Calan® SR, Isoptin® SR: 120 mg, 180 mg, 240 mg
Covera-HS®: 180 mg, 240 mg

Verazinc® Oral *(Discontinued)* see page 814

Vercyte® *(Discontinued)* see page 814

Verelan® [US] see verapamil on previous page

Verelan® PM [US] see verapamil on previous page

Vergogel® Gel *(Discontinued)* see page 814

Vergon® *(Discontinued)* see page 814

Vermizine® *(Discontinued)* see page 814

Vermox® [US/Can] see mebendazole on page 403

Verr-Canth™ *(Discontinued)* see page 814

Verrex-C&M® *(Discontinued)* see page 814

Verrusol® *(Discontinued)* see page 814

Versacaps® [US] see guaifenesin and pseudoephedrine on page 310

Versed® *(Discontinued)* see page 814

Versed® [Can] see midazolam on page 429

Versel® [Can] see selenium sulfide on page 587

Versiclear™ *(Discontinued)* see page 814

verteporfin (ver te POR fin)

U.S./Canadian Brand Names Visudyne™ [US/Can]
Therapeutic Category Ophthalmic Agent
Use Treatment of age-related macular degeneration in patients with classic subfoveal choroidal neovascularization
Usual Dosage Therapy is a two-step process; first the infusion of verteporfin, then the activation of verteporfin with a nonthermal diode laser
Adults: I.V.: 6 mg/m^2 body surface area
Dosage Forms Powder for injection: 2 mg/mL (7.5 mL)

Verukan® Solution *(Discontinued)* see page 814

Vesanoid® [US/Can] see tretinoin (oral) on page 649

Vesprin® [US/Can] see triflupromazine on page 655

Vexol® [US/Can] see rimexolone on page 574

VFEND® [US] see voriconazole on page 685

V-Gan® Injection *(Discontinued)* see page 814

Viadur® **[US/Can]** *see* leuprolide acetate *on page 377*

Viagra® **[US/Can]** *see* sildenafil *on page 590*

Vibazine® *(Discontinued) see page 814*

Vibramycin® **[US]** *see* doxycycline *on page 215*

Vibra-Tabs® **[US/Can]** *see* doxycycline *on page 215*

Vicks® **44D Cough & Head Congestion [US-OTC]** *see* pseudoephedrine and dextromethorphan *on page 553*

Vicks® **44E [US-OTC]** *see* guaifenesin and dextromethorphan *on page 308*

Vicks® **44 Non-Drowsy Cold & Cough Liqui-Caps** *(Discontinued) see page 814*

Vicks® **Children's Chloraseptic**® *(Discontinued) see page 814*

Vicks® **Chloraseptic**® **Sore Throat** *(Discontinued) see page 814*

Vicks® **DayQuil**® **Allergy Relief 4 Hour Tablet** *(Discontinued) see page 814*

Vicks® **DayQuil**® **Cold and Flu Non-Drowsy [US-OTC]** *see* acetaminophen, dextromethorphan, and pseudoephedrine *on page 8*

Vicks® **DayQuil**® **Sinus Pressure & Congestion Relief** *(Discontinued) see page 814*

Vicks Formula 44® **Pediatric Formula [US-OTC]** *see* dextromethorphan *on page 189*

Vicks Formula 44® **[US-OTC]** *see* dextromethorphan *on page 189*

Vicks® **Pediatric Formula 44E [US-OTC]** *see* guaifenesin and dextromethorphan *on page 308*

Vicks Sinex® **12 Hour Ultrafine Mist [US-OTC]** *see* oxymetazoline *on page 486*

Vicks Sinex® **Nasal [US-OTC]** *see* phenylephrine *on page 510*

Vicks® **Vatronol**® *(Discontinued) see page 814*

Vicodin® **[US]** *see* hydrocodone and acetaminophen *on page 329*

Vicodin® **ES [US]** *see* hydrocodone and acetaminophen *on page 329*

Vicodin® **HP [US]** *see* hydrocodone and acetaminophen *on page 329*

Vicodin Tuss™ **[US]** *see* hydrocodone and guaifenesin *on page 331*

Vicon-C® **[US-OTC]** *see* vitamin B complex with vitamin C *on page 681*

Vicon Forte® **[US]** *see* vitamin (multiple/oral) *on page 683*

Vicon® **Plus [US-OTC]** *see* vitamin (multiple/oral) *on page 683*

Vicoprofen® **[US/Can]** *see* hydrocodone and ibuprofen *on page 331*

vidarabine (vye DARE a been)

Synonyms adenine arabinoside; ARA-A; arabinofuranosyladenine

U.S./Canadian Brand Names Vira-A® [US]

Therapeutic Category Antiviral Agent

Use Treatment of acute keratoconjunctivitis and epithelial keratitis due to herpes simplex virus; herpes simplex encephalitis; neonatal herpes simplex virus infections; disseminated varicella-zoster in immunosuppressed patients

Usual Dosage Children and Adults: Ophthalmic: Keratoconjunctivitis: ½" of ointment in lower conjunctival sac 5 times/day every 3 hours while awake until complete re-epithelialization has occurred, then twice daily for an additional 7 days

Dosage Forms Ointment, ophthalmic, as monohydrate: 3% [30 mg/mL = 28 mg/mL base] (3.5 g)

ViDaylin® **[US]** *see* vitamin (multiple/oral) *on page 683*

Vi-Daylin/F® **[US]** *see* vitamin (multiple/pediatric) *on page 683*

Vi-Daylin® **[US-OTC]** *see* vitamin (multiple/pediatric) *on page 683*

Videx® **[US/Can]** *see* didanosine *on page 195*

Videx® **EC** **[US]** *see* didanosine *on page 195*

vigabatrin *(Canada only)* (vye GA ba trin)

Synonyms GVG; MDL-71754

U.S./Canadian Brand Names Sabril® [US/Can]

Therapeutic Category Anticonvulsant

Use Partial/secondary generalized seizures; useful for spasticity or tardive dyskinesia

Usual Dosage
Initial dose: 1-2 g/day then titrate to maintenance dose of 2-4 g/day in 1-2 divided doses (lower initial doses in the elderly, patients with renal insufficiency, or patients with psychiatric illnesses)
Infantile spasm: 50-200 mg/kg/day
Spasticity: 2-3 g/day
Tardive dyskinesia: 2-8 g/day

Dosage Forms
Powder for oral suspension [sachets]: 0.5 g [contains povidone]
Tablet: 500 mg

vinblastine (vin BLAS teen)

Synonyms vincaleukoblastine; VLB

Tall-Man vinBLAStine

U.S./Canadian Brand Names Velban® [US/Can]

Therapeutic Category Antineoplastic Agent

Use Palliative treatment of Hodgkin's disease; advanced testicular germinal-cell cancers; non-Hodgkin's lymphoma, histiocytosis, and choriocarcinoma

Usual Dosage Refer to individual protocol. Varies depending upon clinical and hematological response. Administer at intervals of at least 7 days and only after leukocyte count has returned to at least 4000/mm^3; maintenance therapy should be titrated according to leukocyte count. Dosage should be reduced in patients with recent exposure to radiation therapy or chemotherapy; single doses in these patients should not exceed 5.5 mg/m^2.

Children and Adults: I.V.: 4-12 mg/m^2 every 7-10 days **or** 5-day continuous infusion of 1.4-1.8 mg/m^2/day **or** 0.1-0.5 mg/kg/week

Dosage Forms
Injection, as sulfate: 1 mg/mL (10 mL)
Injection, powder for reconstitution, as sulfate: 10 mg

vincaleukoblastine *see* vinblastine *on this page*

Vincasar® PFS® **[US/Can]** *see* vincristine *on this page*

vincristine (vin KRIS teen)

Synonyms LCR; leurocristine; VCR

Tall-Man vinCRIStine

U.S./Canadian Brand Names Oncovin® [US/Can]; Vincasar® PFS® [US/Can]

Therapeutic Category Antineoplastic Agent

Use Treatment of leukemias, Hodgkin's disease, neuroblastoma, malignant lymphomas, Wilms' tumor, and rhabdomyosarcoma

Usual Dosage Refer to individual protocol as dosages vary with protocol used. Adjustments are made depending upon clinical and hematological response and upon adverse reactions.

Children: I.V.:
≤10 kg or BSA <1 m^2: 0.05 mg/kg once weekly
2 mg/m^2; may repeat every week

Adults: I.V.: 0.4-1.4 mg/m^2, up to 2 mg maximum; may repeat every week
Dosage Forms Injection, as sulfate: 1 mg/mL (1 mL, 2 mL, 5 mL)

vinorelbine (vi NOR el been)

Synonyms vinorelbine tartrate hydrochloride
U.S./Canadian Brand Names Navelbine® [US/Can]
Therapeutic Category Antineoplastic Agent
Use Treatment of nonsmall cell lung cancer (as a single agent or in combination with cisplatin)
    Unlabeled uses: Breast cancer, ovarian carcinoma (cisplatin-resistant), Hodgkin's disease
Usual Dosage Varies depending upon clinical and hematological response (refer to individual protocols).

Adults: I.V.: 30 mg/m^2 every 7 days
Dosage adjustment in hematological toxicity (based on granulocyte counts):
Granulocytes ≥1500 cells/mm^3 on day of treatment: Administer 30 mg/m^2
Granulocytes 1000-1499 cells/mm^3 on day of treatment: Administer 15 mg/m^2
Granulocytes <1000 cells/mm^3 on day of treatment: Do not administer. Repeat granulocyte count in one week; if 3 consecutive doses are held because granulocyte count is <1000 cells/mm^3, discontinue vinorelbine

For patients who, during treatment, have experienced fever or sepsis while granulocytopenic or had 2 consecutive weekly doses held due to granulocytopenia, subsequent doses of vinorelbine should be:
22.5 mg/m^2 for granulocytes ≥1,500 cells/mm^3
11.25 mg/m^2 for granulocytes 1000-1499 cells/mm^3
Dosage Forms Injection, as tartrate: 10 mg/mL (1 mL, 5 mL)

vinorelbine tartrate hydrochloride *see* vinorelbine *on this page*
Vioform® *(Discontinued)* *see page 814*
Vioform®-Hydrocortisone Topical *(Discontinued)* *see page 814*
Viokase® [US/Can] *see* pancrelipase *on page 489*
viosterol *see* ergocalciferol *on page 232*
Vioxx® [US/Can] *see* rofecoxib *on page 577*
Vira-A® [US] *see* vidarabine *on page 677*
Viracept® [US/Can] *see* nelfinavir *on page 450*
Viramune® [US/Can] *see* nevirapine *on page 456*
Virazole® [US/Can] *see* ribavirin *on page 570*
Viread™ [US] *see* tenofovir *on page 622*
Virilon® [US] *see* methyltestosterone *on page 423*
Viroptic® [US/Can] *see* trifluridine *on page 655*
Viscoat® [US] *see* chondroitin sulfate-sodium hyaluronate *on page 144*
Visicol™ [US] *see* sodium phosphates *on page 598*
Visine-A™ [US-OTC] *see* naphazoline and pheniramine *on page 447*
Visine® Extra [US-OTC] *see* tetrahydrozoline *on page 629*
Visine® L.R. [US-OTC] *see* oxymetazoline *on page 486*
Visken® [US/Can] *see* pindolol *on page 516*
Vistacon-50® Injection *(Discontinued)* *see page 814*
Vistacot® [US] *see* hydroxyzine *on page 339*
Vistaject-25® *(Discontinued)* *see page 814*
Vistaject-50® *(Discontinued)* *see page 814*

Vistaquel® Injection *(Discontinued)* *see page 814*

Vistaril® [US/Can] *see* hydroxyzine *on page 339*

Vistazine® Injection *(Discontinued)* *see page 814*

Vistide® [US] *see* cidofovir *on page 145*

Vi-Sudo® [US-OTC] *see* triprolidine and pseudoephedrine *on page 659*

Visudyne™ [US/Can] *see* verteporfin *on page 676*

Vita 3B [Can] *see* vitamin B complex *on next page*

Vita 3B+C [Can] *see* vitamin B complex with vitamin C *on next page*

Vita® #12 [US] *see* cyanocobalamin *on page 167*

Vitabee® 12 [US] *see* cyanocobalamin *on page 167*

VitaCarn® Oral *(Discontinued)* *see page 814*

Vita-C® [US-OTC] *see* ascorbic acid *on page 57*

Vital HN® [US-OTC] *see* nutritional formula, enteral/oral *on page 472*

vitamin A (VYE ta min aye)

Synonyms oleovitamin A

U.S./Canadian Brand Names Aquasol A® [US]; Palmitate-A® [US-OTC]

Therapeutic Category Vitamin, Fat Soluble

Use Treatment and prevention of vitamin A deficiency; supplementation in patients with measles

Usual Dosage

RDA:

0-3 years: 400 mcg*

4-6 years: 500 mcg*

7-10 years: 700 mcg*

>10 years: 800-1000 mcg*

*mcg retinol equivalent (0.3 mcg retinol = 1 unit vitamin A)

Supplementation in measles: Children: Oral:

<1 year: 100,000 units/day for 2 days

>1 year: 200,000 units/day for 2 days

Severe deficiency with xerophthalmia:

Children 1-8 years:

Oral: 5000-10,000 units/kg/day for 5 days or until recovery occurs

I.M.: 5000-15,000 units/day for 10 days

Children >8 years and Adults:

Oral: 500,000 units/day for 3 days, then 50,000 units/day for 14 days, then 10,000-20,000 units/day for 2 months

I.M.: 50,000-100,000 units/day for 3 days, 50,000 units/day for 14 days

Deficiency (without corneal changes): Oral:

Infants <1 year: 10,000 units/kg/day for 5 days, then 7500-15,000 units/day for 10 days

Children 1-8 years: 5000-10,000 units/kg/day for 5 days, then 17,000-35,000 units/day for 10 days

Children >8 years and Adults: 100,000 units/day for 3 days then 50,000 units/day for 14 days

Malabsorption syndrome (prophylaxis): Children >8 years and Adults: Oral: 10,000-50,000 units/day of water miscible product

Dietary supplement: Oral:

Infants up to 6 months: 1500 units/day

Children:

6 months to 3 years: 1500-2000 units/day

4-6 years: 2500 units/day

7-10 years: 3300-3500 units/day

Children >10 years and Adults: 4000-5000 units/day

Dosage Forms
Capsule: 8000 units, 10,000 units [OTC], 25,000 units, 50,000 units
Injection (Aquasol®-A): 50,000 units/mL (2 mL)
Tablet [OTC]: 5000 units, 10,000 units, 15,000 units
Palmitate-A®: 5000 units, 15,000 units

vitamin A acid *see* tretinoin (topical) *on page 650*

vitamin A and vitamin D (VYE ta min aye & VYE ta min dee)
Synonyms cod liver oil
U.S./Canadian Brand Names A and D™ Ointment [US-OTC]
Therapeutic Category Protectant, Topical
Use Temporary relief of discomfort due to chapped skin, diaper rash, minor burns, abrasions, as well as irritations associated with ostomy skin care
Usual Dosage
Oral, oil: Dietary supplement: 2.5 mL/day
Topical: Apply locally with gentle massage as needed
Dosage Forms Ointment: (60 g) [in lanolin-petrolatum base]

vitamin B₁ *see* thiamine *on page 632*

vitamin B₂ *see* riboflavin *on page 571*

vitamin B₃ *see* niacin *on page 456*

vitamin B₅ *see* pantothenic acid *on page 491*

vitamin B₆ *see* pyridoxine *on page 556*

vitamin B₁₂ *see* cyanocobalamin *on page 167*

vitamin B complex (VYE ta min bee KOM pleks)
U.S./Canadian Brand Names Apatate® [US-OTC]; Gevrabon® [US-OTC]; Mega B® [US-OTC]; Orexin® [US-OTC]; Penta/3B® [Can]; Vita 3B [Can]
Therapeutic Category Vitamin, Water Soluble
Usual Dosage Dosage is usually 1 tablet or capsule/day; please refer to package insert
Dosage Forms Content may vary slightly depending on product used
Capsule/Tablet: Vitamin B₁ 10-15 mg, vitamin B₂ 10 mg, vitamin B₃ 100 mg, vitamin B₅ 20 mg, vitamin B₆ 2-5 mg, vitamin B₁₂ 6-10 mg
Solution: 5 mL, 360 mL

vitamin B complex with vitamin C
(VYE ta min bee KOM pleks with VYE ta min see)
U.S./Canadian Brand Names Allbee® With C [US-OTC]; Penta/3B®+C [Can]; Surbex-T® Filmtabs® [US-OTC]; Surbex® With C Filmtabs® [US-OTC]; Vicon-C® [US-OTC]; Vita 3B+C [Can]
Therapeutic Category Vitamin, Water Soluble
Use Supportive nutritional supplementation in conditions in which water-soluble vitamins are required like GI disorders, chronic alcoholism, pregnancy, severe burns, and recovery from surgery
Usual Dosage Adults: Oral: 1 tablet/capsule daily
Dosage Forms Content may vary slightly depending on product used
Capsule/Tablet: Vitamin B₁ 6-25 mg, vitamin B₂ 6-50 mg, vitamin B₃ 30-150 mg, vitamin B₅ 10-50 mg, vitamin B₆ 2-50 mg, vitamin B₁₂ 5-25 mg, vitamin C 250-600 mg

vitamin B complex with vitamin C and folic acid
(VYE ta min bee KOM pleks with VYE ta min see & FOE lik AS id)
U.S./Canadian Brand Names Berocca® [US]; Nephrocaps® [US]
Therapeutic Category Vitamin, Water Soluble
(Continued)

vitamin B complex with vitamin C and folic acid *(Continued)*

Use Supportive nutritional supplementation in conditions in which water-soluble vitamins are required like GI disorders, chronic alcoholism, pregnancy, severe burns, and recovery from surgery

Usual Dosage Adults: Oral: 1 capsule/day

Dosage Forms Content may vary slightly depending on product used:

Capsule/Tablet: Folic acid 0.1-0.4 mg, vitamin B_1 10-15 mg, vitamin B_2 10 mg, vitamin B_3 100 mg, vitamin B_5 20 mg, vitamin B_6 2-5 mg, vitamin B_{12} 6-10 mg, vitamin C 300-500 mg

vitamin C *see* ascorbic acid *on page 57*

vitamin D_2 *see* ergocalciferol *on page 232*

vitamin E (VYE ta min ee)

Synonyms *d*-alpha tocopherol; *dl*-alpha tocopherol

U.S./Canadian Brand Names Amino-Opti-E® [US-OTC]; Aquasol E® [US-OTC]; E-Complex-600® [US-OTC]; E-Vitamin® [US-OTC]; Vita-Plus® E Softgels® [US-OTC]; Vitec® [US-OTC]; Vite E® Creme [US-OTC]

Therapeutic Category Vitamin, Fat Soluble; Vitamin, Topical

Use Prevention and treatment of vitamin E deficiency

Usual Dosage

RDA: Oral:

Premature Infants ≤3 months: 25 units/day

Infants:

≤6 months: 4.5 units/day

6-12 months: 6 units/day

Children:

1-3 years: 9 units/day

4-10 years: 10.5 units/day

Adults >11 years:

Female: 12 units/day

Male: 15 units/day

Prevention of vitamin E deficiency: Neonates, premature, low birthweight (results in normal levels within 1 week): Oral: 25-50 units/24 hours until 6-10 weeks of age or 125-150 units/kg total in 4 doses on days 1, 2, 7, and 8 of life

Vitamin E deficiency treatment: Adults: Oral: 50-200 units/24 hours for 2 weeks

Topical: Apply a thin layer over affected areas as needed

Dosage Forms

Capsule: 100 units, 200 units, 400 units, 500 units, 600 units, 1000 units

Capsule, water miscible: 73.5 mg, 147 mg, 165 mg, 330 mg, 400 units

Cream: 50 mg/g (15 g, 30 g, 60 g, 75 g, 120 g, 454 g)

Liquid, oral drops: 50 mg/mL (12 mL, 30 mL)

Liquid, topical: 10 mL, 15 mL, 30 mL, 60 mL

Lotion: 120 mL

Oil: 15 mL, 30 mL, 60 mL

Ointment: 30 mg/g (45 g, 60 g)

Tablet: 200 units, 400 units

vitamin G *see* riboflavin *on page 571*

vitamin K_1 *see* phytonadione *on page 513*

vitamin (multiple/injectable) (VYE ta min, MUL ti pul/in JEC ta bul)

U.S./Canadian Brand Names M.V.C.® 9 + 3 [US]; M.V.I.®-12 [US]; M.V.I.® Concentrate [US]; M.V.I.® Pediatric [US]

Therapeutic Category Vitamin

Usual Dosage I.V.:
Children:
≤5 kg: 10 mL/1000 mL TPN (M.V.I.® Pediatric)
5.1 kg to 11 years: 5 mL/one TPN bag/day (M.V.I.® Pediatric)
Children >11 years and Adults: 5 mL of vials 1 and 2 (M.V.I.®-12)/one TPN bag/day
Dosage Forms See multiple vitamin table

vitamin (multiple/oral) (VYE ta mins MUL ti pul/OR al)
U.S./Canadian Brand Names Cefol® Filmtab® [US]; Eldercaps® [US-OTC]; Niferex®-PN [US]; Stresstabs® 600 Advanced Formula [US-OTC]; Theragran® Hematinic® [US]; Theragran® Liquid [US-OTC]; Theragran-M® [US-OTC]; Theragran® [US-OTC]; Unicap® [US-OTC]; Vicon Forte® [US]; Vicon® Plus [US-OTC]; ViDaylin® [US]
Therapeutic Category Vitamin
Use Dietary supplement
Usual Dosage Adults: Oral: 1 tablet/day or 5 mL/day liquid
Dosage Forms See multiple vitamin table

vitamin (multiple/pediatric) (VYE ta min, MUL ti pul/pee dee AT rik)
Synonyms children's vitamins; multivitamins/fluoride
U.S./Canadian Brand Names Adeflor® [US]; ADEKs® Pediatric Drops [US]; LKV-Drops® [US-OTC]; Multi Vit® Drops [US-OTC]; Poly-Vi-Flor® [US]; Poly-Vi-Sol® [US-OTC]; Tri-Vi-Flor® [US]; Tri-Vi-Sol® [US-OTC]; Vi-Daylin/F® [US]; Vi-Daylin® [US-OTC]
Therapeutic Category Vitamin
Use Nutritional supplement, vitamin deficiency
Usual Dosage Oral: 0.6 mL or 1 mL/day; please refer to package insert
Dosage Forms See multiple vitamin table

vitamin (multiple/prenatal) (VYE ta mins MUL ti pul/pre NAY tal)
Synonyms prenatal vitamins
U.S./Canadian Brand Names Chromagen® OB [US-OTC]; Natalins® [US-OTC]; Prenavite® [US-OTC]; Stuartnatal® Plus 3™ [US-OTC]; Stuart Prenatal® [US-OTC]
Therapeutic Category Vitamin
Use Nutritional supplement, vitamin deficiency
Usual Dosage Oral: 1 tablet or capsule daily; please refer to package insert
Dosage Forms See multiple vitamin table

Vitaneed™ [US-OTC] *see* nutritional formula, enteral/oral *on page 472*

Vita-Plus® E Softgels® [US-OTC] *see* vitamin E *on previous page*

Vitec® [US-OTC] *see* vitamin E *on previous page*

Vite E® Creme [US-OTC] *see* vitamin E *on previous page*

Vitrasert® [US/Can] *see* ganciclovir *on page 293*

Vitravene™ [US/Can] *see* fomivirsen *on page 287*

Vitrax® [US] *see* sodium hyaluronate *on page 597*

Vivactil® [US] *see* protriptyline *on page 552*

Viva-Drops® [US-OTC] *see* artificial tears *on page 56*

Vivelle® [US/Can] *see* estradiol *on page 238*

Vivelle-Dot® [US] *see* estradiol *on page 238*

Vivonex® T.E.N. [US-OTC] *see* nutritional formula, enteral/oral *on page 472*

Vivonex® [US-OTC] *see* nutritional formula, enteral/oral *on page 472*

Vivotif Berna™ [US/Can] *see* typhoid vaccine *on page 664*

VLB *see* vinblastine *on page 678*

VM-26 *see* teniposide *on page 622*

Volmax® [US] *see* albuterol *on page 18*

Multivitamin Products Available

Product	Content Given Per	A IU	D IU	E IU	C mg	FA mg	B_1 mg	B_2 mg	B_3 mg	B_6 mg	B_{12} mcg	Other
Theragran®	5 mL liquid	10,000	400		200		10	10	100	4.1	5	B_5 21.4 mg
Vi-Daylin®	1 mL drops	1500	400	4.1	35		0.5	0.6	8	0.4	1.5	Alcohol <0.5%
Vi-Daylin® Iron	1 mL	1500	400	4.1	35		0.5	0.6	8	0.4		Fe 10 mg
Albee® with C	tablet				300		15	10.2		5		Niacinamide 50 mg, pantothenic acid 10 mg
Vitamin B complex	tablet					400 mcg	1.5	1.7		2	6	Niacinamide 20 mg
Hexavitamin	cap/tab	5000	400		75		2	3	20			
Iberet-Folic-500®	tablet				500	0.8	6	6	30	5	25	B_5 10 mg, Fe 105 mg
Stuartnatal® 1+1	tablet	4000	400	11	120	1	1.5	3	20	10	12	Cu, Zn 25 mg, Fe 65 mg, Ca 200 mg
Theragran-M®	tablet	5000	400	30	90	0.4	3	3.4	30	3	9	Cl, Cr, I, K, B_5, 10 mg, Mg, Mn, Mo, P, Se, Zn 15 mg, Fe 27 mg, biotin 30 mcg, beta-carotene 1250 IU
Vi-Daylin®	tablet	2500	400	15	60	0.3	1.05	1.2	13.5	1.05	4.5	
M.V.I.®-12 injection	5 mL	3300	200	10	100	0.4	3	3.6	40	4	5	B_5 15 mg, biotin 60 mcg
M.V.I.®-12 unit vial	20 mL											
M.V.I.® pediatric powder	5 mL	2300	400	7	80	0.14	1.2	1.4	17	1	1	B_5 5 mg, biotin 20 mcg, vitamin K 200 mcg

Voltaren® **[US/Can]** *see* diclofenac *on page 193*

Voltaren Rapide® **[Can]** *see* diclofenac *on page 193*

Voltaren®**-XR [US]** *see* diclofenac *on page 193*

Voltare Ophtha® **[Can]** *see* diclofenac *on page 193*

Vontrol® *(Discontinued) see page 814*

voriconazole (vor i KOE na zole)
Synonyms UK109496
U.S./Canadian Brand Names VFEND® [US]
Therapeutic Category Antifungal Agent
Use Treatment of invasive aspergillosis; treatment of serious fungal infections caused by *Scedosporium apiospermum* and *Fusarium* spp (including *Fusarium solani*) in patients intolerant of, or refractory to, other therapy
Usual Dosage Children >12 years and Adults: I.V.: Initial: Loading dose: 6 mg/kg every 12 hours for 2 doses; followed by maintenance dose of 4 mg/kg every 12 hours
Conversion to oral dosing:
Patients >40 kg: 200 mg every 12 hours
Patients ≤40 kg: 100 mg every 12 hours
Note: Dosage may be increased by 100 mg/dose in patients who fail to respond adequately (50 mg/dose in patients ≤40 kg)
Dosage Forms
Injection, powder for reconstitution: 200 mg [contains SBECD 3200 mg]
Tablet: 50 mg, 200 mg [contains lactose]

VōSol® **[US]** *see* acetic acid *on page 10*

VōSol® **HC [US/Can]** *see* acetic acid, propylene glycol diacetate, and hydrocortisone *on page 10*

VP-16 *see* etoposide *on page 259*

Vumon® **[US/Can]** *see* teniposide *on page 622*

V.V.S.® **[US]** *see* sulfabenzamide, sulfacetamide, and sulfathiazole *on page 610*

Vytone® **[US]** *see* iodoquinol and hydrocortisone *on page 358*

VZIG *see* varicella-zoster immune globulin (human) *on page 673*

warfarin (WAR far in)
U.S./Canadian Brand Names Coumadin® [US/Can]; Taro-Warfarin [Can]
Therapeutic Category Anticoagulant (Other)
Use Prophylaxis and treatment of venous thromboembolic disorders; prevention of arterial thromboembolism in patients with prosthetic heart valves or atrial fibrillation; prevention of death, venous thromboembolism, and recurrent MI after acute MI
Usual Dosage
Oral:
Infants and Children: 0.05-0.34 mg/kg/day; infants <12 months of age may require doses at or near the high end of this range; consistent anticoagulation may be difficult to maintain in children <5 years of age
Adults: 5-15 mg/day for 2-5 days, then adjust dose according to results of prothrombin time; usual maintenance dose ranges from 2-10 mg/day
I.V. (administer as a slow bolus injection): 2-5 mg/day
Dosage Forms
Injection, powder for reconstitution, as sodium: 5 mg
Tablet, as sodium: 1 mg, 2 mg, 2.5 mg, 3 mg, 4 mg, 5 mg, 6 mg, 7.5 mg, 10 mg

Wartec® **[Can]** *see* podofilox *on page 523*

Wart-Off® **[US-OTC]** *see* salicylic acid *on page 581*

4-Way® **Long Acting [US-OTC]** *see* oxymetazoline *on page 486*

Wehamine® Injection *(Discontinued)* *see page 814*

Wehdryl® *(Discontinued)* *see page 814*

WelChol™ **[US/Can]** *see* colesevelam *on page 161*

Wellbutrin® **[US/Can]** *see* bupropion *on page 97*

Wellbutrin® **SR [US]** *see* bupropion *on page 97*

Wellcovorin® **[US]** *see* leucovorin *on page 377*

Wesmycin® **[US]** *see* tetracycline *on page 628*

Wesprin® **Buffered** *(Discontinued)* *see page 814*

Westcort® **[US/Can]** *see* hydrocortisone (topical) *on page 334*

Westhroid® **[US]** *see* thyroid *on page 636*

Wigraine® **[US]** *see* ergotamine *on page 233*

40 Winks® *(Discontinued)* *see page 814*

Winpred™ **[Can]** *see* prednisone *on page 538*

WinRho SD® *(Discontinued)* *see page 814*

WinRho SDF® **[US]** *see* Rh₀(D) immune globulin *on page 569*

Winstrol® **[US]** *see* stanozolol *on page 605*

witch hazel (witch HAY zel)
  Synonyms hamamelis water
  U.S./Canadian Brand Names Preparation H® Cleansing Pads [Can]; Tucks® [US-OTC]
  Therapeutic Category Astringent
  Use After-stool wipe to remove most causes of local irritation; temporary management of vulvitis, pruritus ani and vulva; help relieve the discomfort of simple hemorrhoids, anorectal surgical wounds, and episiotomies
  Usual Dosage Apply to anorectal area as needed
  Dosage Forms
    Liquid, topical: 100% (60 mL, 120 mL, 240 mL, 480 mL)
    Pads: 50% (20s, 50s)
    Tucks®: 50% (12s, 40s, 100s)

Wolfina® *(Discontinued)* *see page 814*

wood sugar *see* d-xylose *on page 220*

Wound Wash Saline™ **[US-OTC]** *see* sodium chloride *on page 595*

Wyamine® **Sulfate [US]** *see* mephentermine *on page 408*

Wyamycin S® *(Discontinued)* *see page 814*

Wycillin® **[US/Can]** *see* penicillin G procaine *on page 499*

Wydase® *(Discontinued)* *see page 814*

Wygesic® *(Discontinued)* *see page 814*

Wymox® **[US]** *see* amoxicillin *on page 37*

Wytensin® *(Discontinued)* *see page 814*

Xalatan® **[US/Can]** *see* latanoprost *on page 375*

Xana TS™ **[Can]** *see* alprazolam *on page 24*

Xanax® **[US/Can]** *see* alprazolam *on page 24*

Xeloda® **[US/Can]** *see* capecitabine *on page 111*

Xenical® **[US/Can]** *see* orlistat *on page 479*

Xigris™ **[US]** *see* drotrecogin alfa *on page 218*

Xiral® **[US]** *see* chlorpheniramine, pseudoephedrine, and methscopolamine *on page 140*

Xopenex™ **[US/Can]** *see* levalbuterol *on page 378*

X-Prep® **[US-OTC]** *see* senna *on page 587*

X-Seb™ **T [US-OTC]** *see* coal tar and salicylic acid *on page 158*

Xylocaine® **[US/Can]** *see* lidocaine *on page 383*

Xylocaine® **With Epinephrine [US/Can]** *see* lidocaine and epinephrine *on page 384*

Xylocard® **[Can]** *see* lidocaine *on page 383*

xylometazoline (zye loe met AZ oh leen)
U.S./Canadian Brand Names Decongest [Can]
Therapeutic Category Adrenergic Agonist Agent
Use Symptomatic relief of nasal and nasopharyngeal mucosal congestion
Usual Dosage
Children <12 years: 2-3 drops (0.05%) in each nostril every 8-10 hours
Children >12 years and Adults: 2-3 drops or sprays (0.1%) in each nostril every 8-10 hours
Dosage Forms Solution, intranasal drops, as hydrochloride:

Xylo-Pfan® **[US-OTC]** *see* d-xylose *on page 220*

Y-90 zevalin *see* ibritumomab *on page 342*

Yasmin® **[US]** *see* ethinyl estradiol and drospirenone *on page 245*

yellow fever vaccine (YEL oh FEE ver vak SEEN)
U.S./Canadian Brand Names YF-VAX® [US/Can]
Therapeutic Category Vaccine, Live Virus
Use Induction of active immunity against yellow fever virus, primarily among persons traveling or living in areas where yellow fever infection exists. (Some countries require a valid international Certification of Vaccination showing receipt of vaccine; if a pregnant woman is to be vaccinated only to satisfy an international requirement, efforts should be made to obtain a waiver letter.) The WHO requires revaccination every 10 years to maintain traveler's vaccination certificate.
Usual Dosage Single-dose S.C.: 0.5 mL
Dosage Forms Injection, powder for reconstitution [preservative free; diluent provided]: Not less than 5.04 Log_{10} plaque-forming units (PFU) [single-dose vial]; Not less than 25.2 Log_{10} plaque-forming units (PFU) [5-dose vial]

yellow mercuric oxide *see* mercuric oxide *on page 410*

YF-VAX® **[US/Can]** *see* yellow fever vaccine *on this page*

Yocon® **[US/Can]** *see* yohimbine *on this page*

Yodoxin® **[US]** *see* iodoquinol *on page 357*

yohimbine (yo HIM bine)
U.S./Canadian Brand Names Aphrodyne® [US]; PMS-Yohimbine [Can]; Yocon® [US/Can]
Therapeutic Category Miscellaneous Product
Use No FDA sanctioned indications
Usual Dosage Adults: Oral: 1 tablet 3 times/day
Dosage Forms Tablet, as hydrochloride: 5.4 mg

Yohimex™ *(Discontinued)* *see page 814*

Yutopar® *(Discontinued)* *see page 814*

Zaditen® **[Can]** *see* ketotifen *on page 368*

Zaditor™ **[US/Can]** *see* ketotifen *on page 368*

zafirlukast (za FIR loo kast)
Synonyms ICI 204, 219
U.S./Canadian Brand Names Accolate® [US/Can]
Therapeutic Category Leukotriene Receptor Antagonist
Use Prophylaxis and chronic treatment of asthma in adults and children ≥7 years of age
Usual Dosage
  Children <7 years: Safety and effectiveness has not been established
  Children 7-11 years: 10 mg twice daily
  Adults: Oral: 20 mg twice daily; administer 1 hour before food or 2 hours after food
Dosage Forms Tablet: 10 mg, 20 mg

Zagam® [US] see sparfloxacin on page 603

zalcitabine (zal SITE a been)
Synonyms ddC; dideoxycytidine
U.S./Canadian Brand Names Hivid® [US/Can]
Therapeutic Category Antiviral Agent
Use Treatment of HIV infections as monotherapy (in patients intolerant to zidovudine or with disease progression while on zidovudine) or in combination with zidovudine in patients with advanced HIV disease (adult CD4 cell count of 150-300 cells/mm^3)
Usual Dosage Oral:
  Safety and efficacy in children <13 years of age have not been established
  Adults (dosed in combination with zidovudine): Daily dose: 0.750 mg every 8 hours, administered together with 200 mg of zidovudine (ie, total daily dose: 2.25 mg of zalcitabine and 600 mg of zidovudine)
Dosage Forms Tablet: 0.375 mg, 0.75 mg

zaleplon (ZAL e plon)
U.S./Canadian Brand Names Sonata® [US/Can]; Starnoc® [Can]
Therapeutic Category Hypnotic, Nonbenzodiazepine (Pyrazolopyrimidine)
Use Short-term treatment of insomnia
Usual Dosage
  Adults: Oral: 10 mg at bedtime (range: 5-20 mg)
Dosage Forms Capsule: 5 mg, 10 mg [contains tartrazine]

Zanaflex® [US/Can] see tizanidine on page 641

zanamivir (za NA mi veer)
U.S./Canadian Brand Names Relenza® [US/Can]
Therapeutic Category Antiviral Agent, Inhalation Therapy
Use Treatment of uncomplicated acute illness due to influenza virus in adults and adolescents 12 years of age or older. Treatment should only be initiated in patients who have been symptomatic for no more than 2 days.
Usual Dosage Adolescents ≥12 years and Adults: 2 Inhalations: (10 mg total) twice daily for 5 days. Two doses should be taken on the first day of dosing, regardless of interval, while doses should be spaced by approximately 12 hours on subsequent days.
Dosage Forms Powder for oral inhalation: 5 mg/blister (20s) [4 blisters per Rotadisk®, 5 Rotadisk® per package]

Zanosar® [US/Can] see streptozocin on page 607

Zanta [Can] see ranitidine hydrochloride on page 564

Zantac® [US/Can] see ranitidine hydrochloride on page 564

Zantac® 75 [US-OTC] see ranitidine hydrochloride on page 564

Zantryl® *(Discontinued)* see page 814

Zapzyt® [US-OTC] see benzoyl peroxide on page 79

Zarontin® [US/Can] see ethosuximide on page 257

Zaroxolyn® **[US/Can]** *see* metolazone *on page 425*

Zartan® *(Discontinued) see page 814*

Z-Chlopenthixol *see* zuclopenthixol *(Canada only) on page 693*

ZeaSorb® **AF [Can]** *see* tolnaftate *on page 644*

Zeasorb®-AF [US-OTC] *see* miconazole *on page 427*

Zebeta® **[US/Can]** *see* bisoprolol *on page 88*

Zebrax® *(Discontinued) see page 814*

Zebutal® **[US]** *see* butalbital, acetaminophen, and caffeine *on page 99*

Zefazone® *(Discontinued) see page 814*

Zelnorm™ [US] *see* tegaserod *on page 620*

Zemplar™ [US/Can] *see* paricalcitol *on page 493*

Zemuron® **[US/Can]** *see* rocuronium *on page 577*

Zenapax® **[US/Can]** *see* daclizumab *on page 173*

Zephiran® **[US-OTC]** *see* benzalkonium chloride *on page 76*

Zephrex® **[US]** *see* guaifenesin and pseudoephedrine *on page 310*

Zephrex LA® **[US]** *see* guaifenesin and pseudoephedrine *on page 310*

Zerit® **[US/Can]** *see* stavudine *on page 605*

Zestoretic® **[US/Can]** *see* lisinopril and hydrochlorothiazide *on page 388*

Zestril® **[US/Can]** *see* lisinopril *on page 388*

Zetar® **[US/Can]** *see* coal tar *on page 158*

Zetran® *(Discontinued) see page 814*

Zevalin™ [US] *see* ibritumomab *on page 342*

Ziac® **[US/Can]** *see* bisoprolol and hydrochlorothiazide *on page 88*

Ziagen® **[US/Can]** *see* abacavir *on page 2*

Zide® **[US]** *see* hydrochlorothiazide *on page 328*

zidovudine (zye DOE vyoo deen)

Synonyms azidothymidine; AZT; compound S

U.S./Canadian Brand Names Apo®-Zidovudine [Can]; AZT™ [Can]; Novo-AZT [Can]; Retrovir® [US/Can]

Therapeutic Category Antiviral Agent

Use Management of patients with HIV infections who have had at least one episode of *Pneumocystis carinii* pneumonia or who have CD4 cell counts (cells/mm^3) of ≤500 in children >6 years and adults, <750 in children 2-6 years, <1000 in children 1-2 years, and <1750 for children <1 year; patients who have HIV-related symptoms or who are asymptomatic with abnormal laboratory values indicating HIV-related immunosuppression; prevention of maternal-fetal HIV transmission

Usual Dosage

Children 3 months to 12 years:
 Oral: 90-180 mg/m^2/dose every 6 hours; maximum: 200 mg every 6 hours
 I.V. continuous infusion: 0.5-1.8 mg/kg/hour
 I.V. intermittent infusion: 100 mg/m^2/dose every 6 hours
Adults:
 Oral:
  Asymptomatic infection: 100 mg every 4 hours while awake (500 mg/day)
  Symptomatic HIV infection: Initial: 200 mg every 4 hours (1200 mg/day), then after 1 month, 100 mg every 4 hours (600 mg/day)
 I.V.: 1-2 mg/kg/dose every 4 hours

Dosage Forms

Capsule: 100 mg

(Continued)

zidovudine *(Continued)*

Injection, solution: 10 mg/mL (20 mL)
Syrup: 50 mg/5 mL (240 mL) [contains sodium benzoate; strawberry flavor]
Tablet: 300 mg

zidovudine and lamivudine (zye DOE vyoo deen & la MI vyoo deen)

Synonyms AZT + 3TC
U.S./Canadian Brand Names Combivir® [US/Can]
Therapeutic Category Antiviral Agent
Use Combivir® given twice a day, provides an alternative regimen to lamivudine 150 mg twice a day plus zidovudine 600 mg per day in divided doses; this drug form reduces capsule/tablet intake for these two drugs to two per day instead of up to eight
Usual Dosage Children >12 years and Adults: Oral: One tablet twice daily
Dosage Forms Tablet: Zidovudine 300 mg and lamivudine 150 mg

Zilactin® [Can] *see* lidocaine *on page 383*

Zilactin®-B [US/Can] *see* benzocaine *on page 77*

Zilactin® Baby [US/Can] *see* benzocaine *on page 77*

Zilactin-L® [US-OTC] *see* lidocaine *on page 383*

zileuton (zye LOO ton)

U.S./Canadian Brand Names Zyflo™ [US]
Therapeutic Category 5-Lipoxygenase Inhibitor
Use Prophylaxis and chronic treatment of asthma in adults and children ≥12 years of age
Usual Dosage Children ≥12 years and Adults: Oral: 1 tablet 4 times/day, may be taken with meals and at bedtime
Dosage Forms Tablet: 600 mg

Zinacef® [US/Can] *see* cefuroxime *on page 126*

Zinca-Pak® [US] *see* trace metals *on page 646*

Zincate® [US] *see* zinc sulfate *on next page*

zinc chloride (zingk KLOR ide)

Therapeutic Category Trace Element
Use Cofactor for replacement therapy to different enzymes helps maintain normal growth rates, normal skin hydration and senses of taste and smell
Usual Dosage Clinical response may not occur for up to 6-8 weeks
Supplemental to I.V. solutions:
Premature Infants <1500 g, up to 3 kg: 300 mcg/kg/day
Full-term Infants and Children ≤5 years: 100 mcg/kg/day
Adults:
Stable with fluid loss from small bowel: 12.2 mg zinc/liter TPN or 17.1 mg zinc/kg (added to 1000 mL I.V. fluids) of stool or ileostomy output
Metabolically stable: 2.5-4 mg/day, add 2 mg/day for acute catabolic states
Dosage Forms Injection, solution: 1 mg/mL (10 mL, 50 mL)

Zincfrin® [US/Can] *see* phenylephrine and zinc sulfate *on page 511*

zinc gelatin (zingk JEL ah tin)

Synonyms Unna's boot; Unna's paste
U.S./Canadian Brand Names Gelucast® [US]
Therapeutic Category Protectant, Topical
Use Protectant and to support varicosities and similar lesions of the lower limbs
Usual Dosage Apply externally as an occlusive boot
Dosage Forms Bandage: 3" x 10 yards; 4" x 10 yards

zinc injection *see* trace metals *on page 646*

Zincofax® [Can] *see* zinc oxide *on this page*

Zincon® [US-OTC] *see* pyrithione zinc *on page 557*

zinc oxide (zingk OKS ide)

Synonyms Lassar's zinc paste

U.S./Canadian Brand Names Ammens® Medicated Deodorant [US-OTC]; Balmex® [US-OTC]; Boudreaux's® Butt Paste [US-OTC]; Critic-Aid Skin Care® [US-OTC]; Desitin® Creamy [US-OTC]; Zincofax® [Can]

Therapeutic Category Topical Skin Product

Use Protective coating for mild skin irritations and abrasions; soothing and protective ointment to promote healing of chapped skin, diaper rash

Usual Dosage Infants, Children, and Adults: Topical: Apply several times daily to affected area

Dosage Forms

Ointment, topical: 20% (30 g, 60 g, 480 g)

Balmex®: 11.3% (60 g, 120 g, 480 g)

Desitin® Creamy: 10% (60 g, 120 g)

Paste, topical:

Boudreaux's® Butt Paste: 16% (30 g, 60 g, 120 g, 480 g) [contains castor oil, boric acid, mineral oil, and Peruvian balsam]

Critic-Aid Skin Care®: 20% (71 g, 170 g)

Powder, topical (Ammens® Medicated Deodorant): 9.1% (187.5 g, 330 g) [original and shower fresh scent]

zinc oxide, cod liver oil, and talc (zingk OKS ide, kod LIV er oyl, & talk)

U.S./Canadian Brand Names Desitin® [US-OTC]

Therapeutic Category Protectant, Topical

Use Relief of diaper rash, superficial wounds and burns, and other minor skin irritations

Usual Dosage Topical: Apply thin layer as needed

Dosage Forms Ointment, topical: Zinc oxide, cod liver oil and talc in a petrolatum and lanolin base (30 g, 60 g, 120 g, 240 g, 270 g)

zinc sulfate (zingk SUL fate)

U.S./Canadian Brand Names Orazinc® [US-OTC]; Rivasol [Can]; Zincate® [US]

Therapeutic Category Electrolyte Supplement, Oral

Use Zinc supplement (oral and parenteral); may improve wound healing in those who are deficient

Usual Dosage

RDA: Oral:

Birth to 6 months: 3 mg elemental zinc/day

6-12 months: 5 mg elemental zinc/day

1-10 years: 10 mg elemental zinc/day

≥11 years: 15 mg elemental zinc/day

Zinc deficiency: Oral:

Infants and Children: 0.5-1 mg elemental zinc/kg/day divided 1-3 times/day; somewhat larger quantities may be needed if there is impaired intestinal absorption or an excessive loss of zinc

Adults: 110-220 mg zinc sulfate (25-50 mg elemental zinc)/dose 3 times/day

Dosage Forms

Capsule (Orazinc®, Zincate®): 220 mg [elemental zinc 50 mg]

Injection, solution [preservative free]: 1 mg elemental zinc/mL (10 mL); 5 mg elemental zinc/mL (5 mL)

Tablet (Orazinc®): 110 mg [elemental zinc 25 mg]

zinc undecylenate *see* undecylenic acid and derivatives *on page 665*

Zinecard® **[US/Can]** *see* dexrazoxane *on page 187*

ziprasidone (zi PRAY si done)

U.S./Canadian Brand Names Geodon® [US]
Therapeutic Category Antipsychotic Agent
Use Treatment of schizophrenia
Usual Dosage
Adults: Psychosis: Oral: Initial: 20 mg twice daily (with food)
Maintenance: Range 20-100 mg twice daily; however, dosages >80 mg twice daily are generally not recommended
Dosage Forms
Capsule, as hydrochloride: 20 mg, 40 mg, 60 mg, 80 mg
Injection, powder for reconstitution, as mesylate: 20 mg

Zithromax® **[US/Can]** *see* azithromycin *on page 66*

ZNP® **Bar [US-OTC]** *see* pyrithione zinc *on page 557*

Zocor® **[US/Can]** *see* simvastatin *on page 591*

Zofran® **[US/Can]** *see* ondansetron *on page 477*

Zofran® **ODT [US/Can]** *see* ondansetron *on page 477*

Zoladex® **[US/Can]** *see* goserelin *on page 305*

Zoladex® **LA [Can]** *see* goserelin *on page 305*

Zoledronate *see* zoledronic acid *on this page*

zoledronic acid (ZOE le dron ik AS id)

Synonyms CGP-42446; Zoledronate
U.S./Canadian Brand Names Zometa® [US/Can]
Therapeutic Category Bisphosphonate Derivative
Use Treatment of hypercalcemia of malignancy
Usual Dosage I.V.: Adults: Hypercalcemia of malignancy (albumin-corrected serum calcium ≥12 mg/dL): 4 mg (maximum) given as a single dose infused over **no less than 15 minutes**; patients should be adequately hydrated prior to treatment (restoring urine output to ~2 L/day). Monitor serum calcium and wait at least 7 days before considering retreatment.
Dosage Forms Injection, powder for reconstitution: 4 mg [as monohydrate 4.264 mg]

Zolicef® *(Discontinued)* *see page 814*

zolmitriptan (zohl mi TRIP tan)

Synonyms 311C90
U.S./Canadian Brand Names Zomig® [US/Can]; Zomig-ZMT™ [US]
Therapeutic Category Antimigraine Agent; Serotonin Agonist
Use Acute treatment of adult migraine, with or without auras.
Usual Dosage Oral:
Children: Safety and efficacy have not been established
Adults: Migraine:
Tablet: Initial: ≤2.5 mg at the onset of migraine headache; may break 2.5 mg tablet in half
Orally-disintegrating tablet: Initial: 2.5 mg at the onset of migraine headache
Note: Use the lowest possible dose to minimize adverse events. If the headache returns, the dose may be repeated after 2 hours; do not exceed 10 mg within a 24-hour period. Controlled trials have not established the effectiveness of a second dose if the initial one was ineffective
Dosage Forms
Tablet (Zomig®): 2.5 mg, 5 mg
Tablet, orally-disintegrating (Zomig-ZMT™): 2.5 mg [contains phenylalanine 2.81 mg/tablet; orange flavor]; 5 mg [contains phenylalanine 5.62 mg/tablet; orange flavor]

Zoloft® **[US/Can]** *see* sertraline *on page 589*

zolpidem (zole PI dem)
U.S./Canadian Brand Names Ambien® [US/Can]
Therapeutic Category Hypnotic, Nonbarbiturate
Use Short-term treatment of insomnia
Usual Dosage Adults: Oral: 10 mg immediately before bedtime
Dosage Forms Tablet, as tartrate: 5 mg, 10 mg

Zolyse® *(Discontinued) see page 814*

Zometa® **[US/Can]** *see* zoledronic acid *on previous page*

Zomig® **[US/Can]** *see* zolmitriptan *on previous page*

Zomig-ZMT™ **[US]** *see* zolmitriptan *on previous page*

Zonalon® Cream [US/Can] *see* doxepin *on page 213*

Zone-A Forte® [US] *see* pramoxine and hydrocortisone *on page 535*

Zonegran™ [US/Can] *see* zonisamide *on this page*

zonisamide (zoe NIS a mide)
U.S./Canadian Brand Names Zonegran™ [US/Can]
Therapeutic Category Anticonvulsant, Sulfonamide
Use Adjunct treatment of partial seizures in adults with epilepsy
Usual Dosage
 Children >16 years and Adults: Oral: For the adjunctive treatment of partial seizures, initial dose is 100 mg/day. Dose may be increased to 200 mg/day after 2 weeks. Further dosage increases to 300 mg and 400 mg/day can then be made with a minimum of 2 weeks between adjustments, in order to reach steady state at each dosage level. Doses of up to 600 mg/day have been studied, however, there is no evidence of increased response with doses above 400 mg/day.
Dosage Forms Capsule: 100 mg

zopiclone *(Canada only)* (ZOE pi clone)
U.S./Canadian Brand Names Apo®-Zopiclone [Can]; Gen-Zopiclone [Can]; Imovane® [Can]; Nu-Zopiclone [Can]; Rhovane® [Can]
Therapeutic Category Hypnotic
Use Treatment of insomnia (to be used <28-day duration)
Usual Dosage Oral: 7.5 mg 30-60 minutes before bedtime
Dosage Forms Tablet: 5 mg, 7.5 mg

ZORprin® **[US]** *see* aspirin *on page 58*

Zostrix® **[US/Can]** *see* capsaicin *on page 111*

Zostrix High Potency® **[US]** *see* capsaicin *on page 111*

Zostrix®-HP [US/Can] *see* capsaicin *on page 111*

Zostrix Sports® **[US]** *see* capsaicin *on page 111*

Zosyn® **[US]** *see* piperacillin and tazobactam sodium *on page 517*

Zovia™ [US] *see* ethinyl estradiol and ethynodiol diacetate *on page 246*

Zovirax® **[US/Can]** *see* acyclovir *on page 13*

Z-PAK® **[US/Can]** *see* azithromycin *on page 66*

zuclopenthixol *(Canada only)* (zoo kloe pen THIX ol)
Synonyms Z-Chlopenthixol
U.S./Canadian Brand Names Clopixol-Acuphase® [Can]; Clopixol® [Can]; Clopixol® Depot [Can]
Therapeutic Category Antipsychotic Agent
 (Continued)

zuclopenthixol *(Canada only)* *(Continued)*

Use Schizophrenia, bipolar disorder, psychoses; usually useful in agitated states

Usual Dosage

Oral: Zuclopenthixol hydrochloride: Initial: 20-30 mg/day in divided doses; usual maintenance dose: 20-75 mg/day; maximum daily dose: 150 mg

I.M.:

Zuclopenthixol acetate: 50-150 mg; may be repeated in 2-3 days; no more than 4 injections should be given in the course of treatment; maximum dose during course of treatment: 400 mg

Zuclopenthixol decanoate: 100 mg by deep I.M. injection; additional doses of 100-200 mg (I.M.) may be given over the following 1-4 weeks; maximum weekly dose: 600 mg

Dosage Forms

Injection:

Clopixol-Acuphase®, as acetate: 50 mg/mL [zuclopenthixol 42.5 mg/mL] (1 mL, 2 mL)

Clopixol® Depot, as decanoate: 200 mg/mL [zuclopenthixol 144.4 mg/mL] (10 mL)

Tablet, as dihydrochloride (Clopixol®): 10 mg, 25 mg, 40 mg

Zyban® **[US/Can]** *see* bupropion *on page 97*

Zyban™ 100 mg *(Discontinued) see page 814*

Zydone® **[US]** *see* hydrocodone and acetaminophen *on page 329*

Zyflo™ [US] *see* zileuton *on page 690*

Zyloprim® **[US/Can]** *see* allopurinol *on page 23*

Zymase® *(Discontinued) see page 814*

Zyprexa® **[US/Can]** *see* olanzapine *on page 475*

Zyprexa® Zydis® **[US]** *see* olanzapine *on page 475*

Zyrtec® **[US]** *see* cetirizine *on page 129*

Zyrtec-D 12 Hour™ [US] *see* cetirizine and pseudoephedrine *on page 130*

Zyvox™ [US] *see* linezolid *on page 386*

APPENDIX

ABBREVIATIONS & SYMBOLS COMMONLY USED IN MEDICAL ORDERS

Abbreviation	From	Meaning
μg		microgram
μmol		micromole
°C		degrees Celsius (Centigrade)
<		less than
>		greater than
≤		less than or equal to
≥		greater than or equal to
aa, aa	ana	of each
AA		Alcoholics Anonymous
ABG		arterial blood gas
ac	ante cibum	before meals or food
ACE		angiotensin-converting enzyme
ACLS		adult cardiac life support
ad	ad	to, up to
a.d.	aurio dextra	right ear
ADH		antidiuretic hormone
ADHD		attention-deficit/hyperactivity disorder
ADLs		activities of daily living
ad lib	ad libitum	at pleasure
AED		antiepileptic drug
AIMS		Abnormal Involuntary Movement Scale
a.l.	aurio laeva	left ear
ALL		acute lymphoblastic leukemia
ALT		alanine aminotransferase (was SGPT)
AM	ante meridiem	morning
AML		acute myeloblastic leukemia
amp		ampul
amt		amount
ANA		antinuclear antibodies
ANC		absolute neutrophil count
ANL		acute nonlymphoblastic leukemia
aq	aqua	water
aq. dest.	aqua destillata	distilled water
APTT		activated partial thromboplastin time
a.s.	aurio sinister	left ear
ASA (class I-IV)		classification of surgical patients according to their baseline health (eg, healthy ASA and II or increased severity of illness ASA III or IV)
ASAP		as soon as possible
AST		aspartate aminotransferase (was SGOT)
a.u.	aures utrae	each ear
AUC		area under the curve
A-V		atrial-ventricular
BDI		Beck Depression Inventory
bid	bis in die	twice daily
bm		bowel movement
BMT		bone marrow transplant
bp		blood pressure
BPRS		Brief Psychiatric Rating Scale
BSA		body surface area
BUN		blood urea nitrogen
c	cong	a gallon
c̄	cum	with
cal		calorie
cAMP		cyclic adenosine monophosphate
cap	capsula	capsule
CBC		complete blood count
CBT		cognitive behavioral therapy

(continued)

Abbreviation	From	Meaning
cc		cubic centimeter
CGI		Clinical Global Impression
CHF		congestive heart failure
CI		cardiac index
CIV		continuous I.V. infusion
Cl_{cr}		creatinine clearance
cm		centimeter
CNS		central nervous system
comp	compositus	compound
cont		continue
COPD		chronic obstructive pulmonary disease
CSF		cerebral spinal fluid
CT		computed tomography
CVA		cerebral vascular accident
CVP		central venous pressure
d	dies	day
D_5W		dextrose 5% in water
$D_{10}W$		dextrose 10% in water
d/c		discontinue
DIC		disseminated intravascular coagulation
dil	dilue	dilute
disp	dispensa	dispense
div	divide	divide
DNA		deoxyribonucleic acid
DSM-IV		Diagnostic and Statistical Manual
DTs		delirium tremens
dtd	dentur tales doses	give of such a dose
DVT		deep vein thrombosis
ECT		electroconvulsive therapy
EEG		electroencephalogram
EKG		electrocardiogram
elix, el	elixir	elixir
emp		as directed
EPS		extrapyramidal side effects
ESR		erythrocyte sedimentation rate
E.T.		endotracheal
et	et	and
ex aq		in water
f, ft	fac, fiat, fiant	make, let be made
FDA		Food and Drug Administration
FEV_11		forced expiratory volume
FVC		forced vital capacity
g	gramma	gram
G-6-PD		glucose-6-phosphate dehydrogenase
GA		gestational age
GABA		gamma-aminobutyric acid
GAD		generalized anxiety disorder
GAF		Global Assessment of Functioning Scale
GE		gastroesophageal
GI		gastrointestinal
GITS		gastrointestinal therapeutic system
gr	granum	grain
gtt	gutta	a drop
GU		genitourinary
h	hora	hour
HAM-A		Hamilton Anxiety Scale
HAM-D		Hamilton Depression Scale
HIV		human immunodeficiency virus
HPLC		high performance liquid chromatography
hs	hora somni	at bedtime
IBW		ideal body weight

APPENDIX

Abbreviation	From	Meaning
ICP		intracranial pressure
IgG		immune globulin G
I.M.		intramuscular
INR		international normalized ratio
I.O.		intraosseous
I & O		input and output
IOP		intraocular pressure
I.T.		intrathecal
IU		international unit
I.V.		intravenous
IVH		intraventricular hemorrhage
IVP		intravenous push
JRA		juvenile rheumatoid arthritis
kcal		kilocalorie
kg		kilogram
KIU		kallikrein inhibitor unit
L		liter
LAMM		L-α-acetyl methadol
LDH		lactate dehydrogenase
LE		lupus erythematosus
liq	liquor	a liquor, solution
LP		lumbar puncture
M	misce	mix
MADRS		Montgomery Asbery Depression Rating Scale
MAOIs		monoamine oxidase inhibitors
MAP		mean arterial pressure
mcg		microgram
MDEA		3,4-methylene-dioxy amphetamine
m. dict	more dictor	as directed
MDMA		3,4-methylene-dioxy methamphetamine
mEq		milliequivalent
mg		milligram
MI		myocardial infarction
min		minute
mixt	mixtura	a mixture
mL		milliliter
mm		millimeter
MMSE		Mini-Mental State Examination
mo		month
mOsm		milliosmols
MPPP		l-methyl-4-proprionoxy-4-phenyl pyridine
MR		mental retardation
MRI		magnetic resonance image
ND		nasoduodenal
NF		National Formulary
ng		nanogram
NMS		neuroleptic malignant syndrome
no.	numerus	number
noc	nocturnal	in the night
non rep	non repetatur	do not repeat, no refills
NPO		nothing by mouth
NSAID		nonsteroidal anti-inflammatory drug
O, Oct	octarius	a pint
OCD		obsessive-compulsive disorder
o.d.	oculus dexter	right eye
o.l.	oculus laevus	left eye
O.R.		operating room
o.s.	oculus sinister	left eye
OTC		over-the-counter (nonprescription)
o.u.	oculo uterque	each eye
PALS		pediatric advanced life support

(continued)

Abbreviation	From	Meaning
PANSS		Positive and Negative Symptom Scale
pc, post cib	post cibos	after meals
PCA		postconceptional age
PCP		*Pneumocystis carinii* pneumonia
PCWP		pulmonary capillary wedge pressure
PDA		patent ductus arteriosus
per		through or by
PM	post meridiem	afternoon or evening
PNA		postnatal age
P.O.	per os	by mouth
P.R.	per rectum	rectally
prn	pro re nata	as needed
PSVT		paroxysmal supraventricular tachycardia
PT		prothrombin time
PTT		partial thromboplastin time
PTSD		post-traumatic stress disorder
PUD		peptic ulcer disease
pulv	pulvis	a powder
PVC		premature ventricular contraction
q		every
qad	quoque alternis die	every other day
qd		every day
qh	quiaque hora	every hour
qid	quater in die	four times a day
qod		every other day
qs	quantum sufficiat	a sufficient quantity
qs ad		a sufficient quantity to make
qty		quantity
qv	quam volueris	as much as you wish
Rx	recipe	take, a recipe
RAP		right atrial pressure
REM		rapid eye movement
rep	repetatur	let it be repeated
$\bar{s}$	sine	without
S-A		sino-atrial
sa	secundum artem	according to art
sat	sataratus	saturated
S.C.		subcutaneous
S_{cr}		serum creatinine
SIADH		syndrome of inappropriate antidiuretic hormone
sig	signa	label, or let it be printed
S.L.		sublingual
SLE		systemic lupus erythematosus
sol	solutio	solution
solv		dissolve
$\overline{ss}$, ss	semis	one-half
sos	si opus sit	if there is need
SSRIs		selective serotonin reuptake inhibitors
stat	statim	at once, immediately
supp	suppositorium	suppository
SVR		systemic vascular resistance
SVT		supraventricular tachycardia
SWI		sterile water for injection
syr	syrupus	syrup
tab	tabella	tablet
tal		such
TCA		tricyclic antidepressant
TD		tardive dyskinesia
tid	ter in die	three times a day
tr, tinct	tincture	tincture
trit		triturate

(continued)

Abbreviation	From	Meaning
tsp		teaspoonful
TT		thrombin time
u.d., ut dict	ut dictum	as directed
ULN		upper limits of normal
ung	unguentum	ointment
USAN		United States Adopted Names
USP		United States Pharmacopeia
UTI		urinary tract infection
V_d		volume of distribution
V_{dss}		volume of distribution at steady-state
v.o.		verbal order
w.a.		while awake
x3		3 times
x4		4 times
y		year
YBOC		Yale Brown Obsessive-Compulsive Scale
YMRS		Young Mania Rating Scale

NORMAL LABORATORY VALUES FOR ADULTS

Automated Chemistry (CHEMISTRY A)

Test	Values	Remarks
SERUM PLASMA		
Acetone	Negative	
Albumin	3.2-5 g/dL	
Alcohol, ethyl	Negative	
Aldolase	1.2-7.6 IU/L	
Ammonia	20-70 mcg/dL	Specimen to be placed on ice as soon as collected
Amylase	30-110 units/L	
Bilirubin, direct	0-0.3 mg/dL	
Bilirubin, total	0.1-1.2 mg/dL	
Calcium	8.6-10.3 mg/dL	
Calcium, ionized	2.24-2.46 mEq/L	
Chloride	95-108 mEq/L	
Cholesterol, total	≤220 mg/dL	Fasted blood required --- normal value affected by dietary habits This reference range is for a general adult population
HDL cholesterol	40-60 mg/dL	Fasted blood required --- normal value affected by dietary habits
LDL cholesterol	65-170 mg/dL	LDLC calculated by Friewald formula... which has certain inaccuracies and is invalid at trig levels >300 mg/dL
CO_2	23-30 mEq/L	
Creatine kinase (CK) isoenzymes		
CK-BB	0%	
CK-MB (cardiac)	0%-3.9%	
CK-MM (muscle)	96%-100%	

CK-MB levels must be both ≥4% and 10 IU/L to meet diagnostic criteria for CK-MB positive result consistent with myocardial injury.

Test	Values	Remarks
Creatine phosphokinase (CPK)	8-150 IU/L	
Creatinine	0.5-1.4 mg/dL	
Ferritin	13-300 ng/mL	
Folate	3.6-20 ng/dL	
GGT (gamma-glutamyltranspeptidase)		
male	11-63 IU/L	
female	8-35 IU/L	
GLDH	To be determined	
Glucose (2-h postprandial)	Up to 140 mg/dL	
Glucose, fasting	60-110 mg/dL	
Glucose, nonfasting (2-h postprandial)	60-140 mg/dL	
Hemoglobin A_{1c}	8	
Hemoglobin, plasma free	<2.5 mg/100 mL	
Hemoglobin, total glycosolated (Hb A_1)	4%-8%	
Iron	65-150 mcg/dL	
Iron binding capacity, total (TIBC)	250-420 mcg/dL	
Lactic acid	0.7-2.1 mEq/L	Specimen to be kept on ice and sent to lab as soon as possible
Lactate dehydrogenase (LDH)	56-194 IU/L	
Lactate dehydrogenase (LDH) isoenzymes		
LD_1	20%-34%	
LD_2	29%-41%	
LD_3	15%-25%	
LD_4	1%-12%	
LD_5	1%-15%	

APPENDIX

Test	Values	Remarks
Flipped LD_1/LD_2 ratios (>1 may be consistent with myocardial injury) particularly when considered in combination with a recent CK-MB positive result		
Lipase	23-208 units/L	
Magnesium	1.6-2.5 mg/dL	Increased by slight hemolysis
Osmolality	289-308 mOsm/kg	
Phosphatase, alkaline		
adults 25-60 y	33-131 IU/L	
adults 61 y or older	51-153 IU/L	
infancy-adolescence	Values range up to 3-5 times higher than adults	
Phosphate, inorganic	2.8-4.2 mg/dL	
Potassium	3.5-5.2 mEq/L	Increased by slight hemolysis
Prealbumin	>15 mg/dL	
Protein, total	6.5-7.9 g/dL	
SGOT (AST)	<35 IU/L (20-48)	
SGPT (ALT) (10-35)	<35 IU/L	
Sodium	134-149 mEq/L	
Transferrin	>200 mg/dL	
Triglycerides	45-155 mg/dL	Fasted blood required
Urea nitrogen (BUN)	7-20 mg/dL	
Uric acid		
male	2.0-8.0 mg/dL	
female	2.0-7.5 mg/dL	

Test	Values	Remarks
CEREBROSPINAL FLUID		
Glucose	50-70 mg/dL	
Protein		
adults and children	15-45 mg/dL	CSF obtained by lumbar puncture
newborn infants	60-90 mg/dL	

On CSF obtained by cisternal puncture: About 25 mg/dL

On CSF obtained by ventricular puncture: About 10 mg/dL

Note: Bloody specimen gives erroneously high value due to contamination with blood proteins

Test	Values	Remarks
URINE		
(24-hour specimen is required for all these tests unless specified)		
Amylase	32-641 units/L	The value is in units/L and **not** calculated for total volume
Amylase, fluid (random samples)		Interpretation of value left for physician, depends on the nature of fluid
Calcium	Depends upon dietary intake	
Creatine		
male	150 mg/24 h	Higher value on children and during pregnancy
female	250 mg/24 h	
Creatinine	1000-2000 mg/24 h	
Creatinine clearance (endogenous)		
male	85-125 mL/min	A blood sample must
female	75-115 mL/min	accompany urine specimen
Glucose	1 g/24 h	
5-hydroxyindoleacetic acid	2-8 mg/24 h	
Iron	0.15 mg/24 h	Acid washed container required
Magnesium	146-209 mg/24 h	
Osmolality	500-800 mOsm/kg	With normal fluid intake
Oxalate	10-40 mg/24 h	
Phosphate	400-1300 mg/24 h	
Potassium	25-120 mEq/24 h	Varies with diet; the interpretation of urine electrolytes and osmolality should be left for the physician
Sodium	40-220 mEq/24 h	
Porphobilinogen, qualitative	Negative	
Porphyrins, qualitative	Negative	
Proteins	0.05-0.1 g/24 h	
Salicylate	Negative	
Urea clearance	60-95 mL/min	A blood sample must accompany specimen
Urea N	10-40 g/24 h	Dependent on protein intake
Uric acid	250-750 mg/24 h	Dependent on diet and therapy
Urobilinogen	0.5-3.5 mg/24 h	For qualitative determination on random urine, send sample to urinalysis section in Hematology Lab
Xylose absorption test		
children	16%-33% of ingested xylose	
adults	>4 g in 5 h	
FECES		
Fat, 3-day collection	<5 g/d	Value depends on fat intake of 100 g/d for 3 days preceding and during collection
GASTRIC ACIDITY		
Acidity, total, 12 h	10-60 mEq/L	Titrated at pH 7

BLOOD GASES

	Arterial	Capillary	Venous
pH	7.35-7.45	7.35-7.45	7.32-7.42
pCO_2 (mm Hg)	35-45	35-45	38-52
pO_2 (mm Hg)	70-100	60-80	24-48
HCO_3 (mEq/L)	19-25	19-25	19-25
TCO_2 (mEq/L)	19-29	19-29	23-33
O_2 saturation (%)	90-95	90-95	40-70
Base excess (mEq/L)	-5 to +5	-5 to +5	-5 to +5

HEMATOLOGY

Complete Blood Count

Age	Hgb (g/dL)	Hct (%)	MCV (fL)	MCH (pg)	MCHC (%)	RBC (mill/mm^3)	RDW	PLTS (x 10^3/mm^3)
0-3 d	15.0-20.0	45-61	95-115	31-37	29-37	4.0-5.9	<18.0	250-450
1-2 wk	12.5-18.5	39-57	86-110	28-36	28-38	3.6-5.5	<17.0	250-450
1-6 mo	10.0-13.0	29-42	74-96	25-35	30-36	3.1-4.3	<16.5	300-700
7 mo - 2 y	10.5-13.0	33-38	70-84	23-30	31-37	3.7-4.9	<16.0	250-600
2-5 y	11.5-13.0	34-39	75-87	24-30	31-37	3.9-5.0	<15.0	250-550
5-8 y	11.5-14.5	35-42	77-95	25-33	31-37	4.0-4.9	<15.0	250-550
13-18 y	12.0-15.2	36-47	78-96	25-35	31-37	4.5-5.1	<14.5	150-450
Adult male	13.5-16.5	41-50	80-100	26-34	31-37	4.5-5.5	<14.5	150-450
Adult female	12.0-15.0	36-44	80-100	26-34	31-37	4.0-4.9	<14.5	150-450

WBC and Diff

Age	WBC (x 10^3/mm^3)	Segs	Bands	Eos	Basos	Lymphs	Atypical Lymphs	Monos	# of NRBCs
0-3 d	9.0-35.0	32-62	10-18	0-2	0-1	19-29	0-8	5-7	0-2
1-2 wk	5.0-20.0	14-34	6-14	0-2	0-1	36-45	0-8	6-10	0
1-6 mo	6.0-17.5	13-33	4-12	0-3	0-1	41-71	0-8	4-7	0
7 mo - 2 y	6.0-17.0	15-35	5-11	0-3	0-1	45-76	0-8	3-6	0
2-5 y	5.5-15.5	23-45	5-11	0-3	0-1	35-65	0-8	3-6	0
5-8 y	5.0-14.5	32-54	5-11	0-3	0-1	28-48	0-8	3-6	0
13-18 y	4.5-13.0	34-64	5-11	0-3	0-1	25-45	0-8	3-6	0
Adults	4.5-11.0	35-66	5-11	0-3	0-1	24-44	0-8	3-6	0

Erythrocyte Sedimentation Rates and Reticulocyte Counts

Sedimentation rate, Westergren

    Children   0-20 mm/hour

    Adult male   0-15 mm/hour

    Adult female   0-20 mm/hour

Sedimentation rate, Wintrobe

    Children   0-13 mm/hour

    Adult male   0-10 mm/hour

    Adult female   0-15 mm/hour

Reticulocyte count

    Newborns   2%-6%

    1-6 mo   0%-2.8%

    Adults   0.5%-1.5%

NORMAL LABORATORY VALUES FOR CHILDREN

CHEMISTRY		Normal Values
Albumin	0-1 y	2.0-4.0 g/dL
	1 y - adult	3.5-5.5 g/dL
Ammonia	Newborns	90-150 µg/dL
	Children	40-120 µg/dL
	Adults	18-54 µg/dL
Amylase	Newborns	0-60 units/L
	Adults	30-110 units/L
Bilirubin, conjugated, direct	Newborns	<1.5 mg/dL
	1 mo - adult	0-0.5 mg/dL
Bilirubin, total	0-3 d	2.0-10.0 mg/dL
	1 mo - adult	0-1.5 mg/dL
Bilirubin, unconjugated, indirect		0.6-10.5 mg/dL
Calcium	Newborns	7.0-12.0 mg/dL
	0-2 y	8.8-11.2 mg/dL
	2 y - adult	9.0-11.0 mg/dL
Calcium, ionized, whole blood		4.4-5.4 mg/dL
Carbon dioxide, total		23-33 mEq/L
Chloride		95-105 mEq/L
Cholesterol	Newborns	45-170 mg/dL
	0-1 y	65-175 mg/dL
	1-20 y	120-230 mg/dL
Creatinine	0-1 y	≤0.6 mg/dL
	1 y - adult	0.5-1.5 mg/dL
Glucose	Newborns	30-90 mg/dL
	0-2 y	60-105 mg/dL
	Children - Adults	70-110 mg/dL
Iron	Newborns	110-270 µg/dL
	Infants	30-70 µg/dL
	Children	55-120 µg/dL
	Adults	70-180 µg/dL
Iron binding	Newborns	59-175 µg/dL
	Infants	100-400 µg/dL
	Adults	250-400 µg/dL
Lactic acid, lactate		2-20 mg/dL
Lead, whole blood		<10 µg/dL
Lipase	Children	20-140 units/L
	Adults	0-190 units/L
Magnesium		1.5-2.5 mEq/L
Osmolality, serum		275-296 mOsm/kg

CHEMISTRY		Normal Values
Osmolality, urine		50-1400 mOsm/kg
Phosphorus	Newborns	4.2-9.0 mg/dL
	6 wk - 19 mo	3.8-6.7 mg/dL
	19 mo - 3 y	2.9-5.9 mg/dL
	3-15 y	3.6-5.6 mg/dL
	>15 y	2.5-5.0 mg/dL
Potassium, plasma	Newborns	4.5-7.2 mEq/L
	2 d - 3 mo	4.0-6.2 mEq/L
	3 mo - 1 y	3.7-5.6 mEq/L
	1-16 y	3.5-5.0 mEq/L
Protein, total	0-2 y	4.2-7.4 g/dL
	>2 y	6.0-8.0 g/dL
Sodium		136-145 mEq/L
Triglycerides	Infants	0-171 mg/dL
	Children	20-130 mg/dL
	Adults	30-200 mg/dL
Urea nitrogen, blood	0-2 y	4-15 mg/dL
	2 y - adult	5-20 mg/dL
Uric acid	Male	3.0-7.0 mg/dL
	Female	2.0-6.0 mg/dL

ENZYMES

Alanine aminotransferase (ALT) (SGPT)	0-2 mo	8-78 units/L
	>2 mo	8-36 units/L
Alkaline phosphatase (ALKP)	Newborns	60-130 units/L
	0-16 y	85-400 units/L
	>16 y	30-115 units/L
Aspartate aminotransferase (AST) (SGOT)	Infants	18-74 units/L
	Children	15-46 units/L
	Adults	5-35 units/L
Creatine kinase (CK)	Infants	20-200 units/L
	Children	10-90 units/L
	Adult Male	0-206 units/L
	Adult Female	0-175 units/L
Lactate dehydrogenase (LDH)	Newborns	290-501 units/L
	1 mo - 2 y	110-144 units/L
	>16 y	60-170 units/L

THYROID FUNCTION TESTS

T_4 (thyroxine)	1-7 d	10.1-20.9 µg/dL
	8-14 d	9.8-16.6 µg/dL
	1 mo - 1 y	5.5-16.0 µg/dL
	>1 y	4.0-12.0 µg/dL
FTI	1-3 d	9.3-26.6
	1-4 wk	7.6-20.8
	1-4 mo	7.4-17.9
	4-12 mo	5.1-14.5
	1-6 y	5.7-13.3
	>6 y	4.8-14.0
T_3	Newborns	100-470 ng/dL
	1-5 y	100-260 ng/dL
	5-10 y	90-240 ng/dL
	10 y - adult	70-210 ng/dL
T_3 uptake		35%-45%
TSH	Cord	3-22 µU/mL
	1-3 d	<40 µU/mL
	3-7 d	<25 µU/mL
	>7 d	0-10 µU/mL

APOTHECARY/METRIC CONVERSIONS

Approximate Liquid Measures

Basic equivalent: 1 fluid ounce = 30 mL

Examples:

1 gallon	3800 mL	4 fluid oz	120 mL
1 quart	960 mL	15 minims	1 mL
1 pint	480 mL	10 minims	0.6 mL
8 fluid oz	240 mL		

1 gallon	128 fluid ounces
1 quart	32 fluid ounces
1 pint	16 fluid ounces

Approximate Household Equivalents

1 teaspoonful . . . . 5 mL   1 tablespoonful . . . 15 mL

Weights

Basic equivalents:

1 oz = 30 g   15 gr = 1 g

Examples:

4 oz	120 g	1 gr	60 mg
2 oz	60 g	$\frac{1}{100}$ gr	600 mcg
10 gr	600 mg	$\frac{1}{150}$ gr	400 mcg
7 $\frac{1}{2}$ gr	500 mg	$\frac{1}{200}$ gr	300 mcg
16 oz	1 pound		

Metric Conversions

Basic equivalents:

1 g . . . . 1000 mg   1 mg . . . . 1000 mcg

Examples:

5 g	5000 mg	5 mg	5000 mcg
0.5 g	500 mg	0.5 mg	500 mcg
0.05 g	50 mg	0.05 mg	50 mcg

Exact Equivalents

1 g = 15.43 grains	0.1 mg = $\frac{1}{600}$ gr
1 milliliter (mL) = 16.23 minims	0.12 mg = $\frac{1}{500}$ gr
1 minim = 0.06 milliliter	0.15 mg = $\frac{1}{400}$ gr
1 gr = 64.8 milligrams	0.2 mg = $\frac{1}{300}$ gr
1 pint (pt) = 473.2 milliliters	0.3 mg = $\frac{1}{200}$ gr
1 oz = 28.35 grams	0.4 mg = $\frac{1}{150}$ gr
1 lb = 453.6 grams	0.5 mg = $\frac{1}{120}$ gr
1 kg = 2.2 pounds	0.6 mg = $\frac{1}{100}$ gr
1 qt = 946.4 milliliters	0.8 mg = $\frac{1}{80}$ gr
	1 mg = $\frac{1}{65}$ gr

Solids*

$\frac{1}{4}$ grain = 15 mg
$\frac{1}{2}$ grain = 30 mg
1 grain = 60 mg
$1\frac{1}{2}$ grains = 90 mg
5 grains = 300 mg
10 grains = 600 mg

*Use exact equivalents for compounding and calculations requiring a high degree of accuracy.

POUNDS/KILOGRAMS CONVERSION

1 pound = 0.45359 kilograms
1 kilogram = 2.2 pounds

lb	=	kg	lb	=	kg	lb	=	kg
1		0.45	70		31.75	140		63.50
5		2.27	75		34.02	145		65.77
10		4.54	80		36.29	150		68.04
15		6.80	85		38.56	155		70.31
20		9.07	90		40.82	160		72.58
25		11.34	95		43.09	165		74.84
30		13.61	100		45.36	170		77.11
35		15.88	105		47.63	175		79.38
40		18.14	110		49.90	180		81.65
45		20.41	115		52.16	185		83.92
50		22.68	120		54.43	190		86.18
55		24.95	125		56.70	195		88.45
60		27.22	130		58.91	200		90.72
65		29.48	135		61.24			

TEMPERATURE CONVERSION

Centigrade to Fahrenheit = (°C x 9/5) + 32 = °F
Fahrenheit to Centigrade = (°F - 32) x 5/9 = °C

°C	=	°F	°C	=	°F	°C	=	°F
100.0		212.0	39.0		102.2	36.8		98.2
50.0		122.0	38.8		101.8	36.6		97.9
41.0		105.8	38.6		101.5	36.4		97.5
40.8		105.4	38.4		101.1	36.2		97.2
40.6		105.1	38.2		100.8	36.0		96.8
40.4		104.7	38.0		100.4	35.8		96.4
40.2		104.4	37.8		100.1	35.6		96.1
40.0		104.0	37.6		99.7	35.4		95.7
39.8		103.6	37.4		99.3	35.2		95.4
39.6		103.3	37.2		99.0	35.0		95.0
39.4		102.9	37.0		98.6	0		32.0
39.2		102.6						

ACQUIRED IMMUNODEFICIENCY SYNDROME (AIDS) — LAB TESTS AND APPROVED DRUGS FOR HIV INFECTION AND AIDS-RELATED CONDITIONS

This list of tests is not intended in any way to suggest patterns of physician's orders, nor is it complete. These tests may support possible clinical diagnoses or rule out other diagnostic possibilities. Each laboratory test relevant to AIDS is listed and weighted. Two symbols (**) indicate that the test is diagnostic, that is, documents the diagnosis if the expected is found. A single symbol (*) indicates a test frequently used in the diagnosis or management of the disease. The other listed tests are useful on a selective basis with consideration of clinical factors and specific aspects of the case.

Acid-Fast Stain
Acid-Fast Stain, Modified, *Nocardia* Species
Antimicrobial Susceptibility Testing, Fungi
Antimicrobial Susceptibility Testing, Mycobacteria
Arthropod Identification
Babesiosis Serological Test
Bacteremia Detection, Buffy Coat Micromethod
Bacterial Culture, Blood
Bacterial Culture, Bronchoscopy Specimen
Bacterial Culture, Sputum
Bacterial Culture, Stool
Bacterial Culture, Throat
Bacterial Culture, Urine, Clean Catch
Beta$_2$-Microglobulin
Blood and Fluid Precautions, Specimen Collection
Bronchial Washings Cytology
Bronchoalveolar Lavage Cytology
Brushings Cytology
Candida Antigen
Candidiasis Serologic Test
Cat Scratch Disease Serology
CD4/CD8 Enumeration
Cerebrospinal Fluid Cytology
Cryptococcal Antigen Titer
Cryptosporidium Diagnostic Procedures
Cytomegalic Inclusion Disease Cytology
Cytomegalovirus Antibody
Cytomegalovirus Antigen Detection
Cytomegalovirus Culture
Cytomegalovirus DNA Detection
Darkfield Examination, Syphilis
Electron Microscopy
Folic Acid, Serum
Fungal Culture, Biopsy or Body Fluid
Fungal Culture, Blood
Fungal Culture, Cerebrospinal Fluid
Fungal Culture, Sputum
Fungal Culture, Stool
Fungal Culture, Urine
Hemoglobin A$_2$
Hepatitis B Surface Antigen
Herpes Cytology
Herpes Simplex Virus Antigen Detection
Herpes Simplex Virus Culture
Histopathology
Histoplasmosis Antibody

Histoplasmosis Antigen
**HIV-1/HIV-2 Serology
HTLV-I/II Antibody
*Human Immunodeficiency Virus Culture
*Human Immunodeficiency Virus DNA Amplification
India Ink Preparation
Inhibitor, Lupus, Phospholipid Type
KOH Preparation
Leishmaniasis Serological Test
Leukocyte Immunophenotyping
Lymphocyte Transformation Test
Microsporidia Diagnostic Procedures
Mycobacteria by DNA Probe
Mycobacterial Culture, Biopsy or Body Fluid
Mycobacterial Culture, Cerebrospinal Fluid
Mycobacterial Culture, Cutaneous and Subcutaneous Tissue
Mycobacterial Culture, Sputum
Mycobacterial Culture, Stool
Neisseria gonorrhoeae Culture and Smear
Nocardia Culture
Ova and Parasites, Stool
*p24 Antigen
Platelet Count
Pneumocystis carinii Preparation
Pneumocystis Immunofluorescence
Polymerase Chain Reaction
Red Blood Cell Indices
Risks of Transfusion
Skin Biopsy
Sputum Cytology
Toxoplasmosis Serology
VDRL, Serum
Viral Culture
Viral Culture, Blood
Viral Culture, Body Fluid
Viral Culture, Central Nervous System Symptoms
Viral Culture, Dermatological Symptoms
Viral Culture, Tissue
Virus, Direct Detection by Fluorescent Antibody
White Blood Count

CURRENTLY APPROVED DRUGS FOR HIV

Protease Inhibitors

amprenavir (Agenerase®)
indinavir (Crixivan®)
lopinavir and ritonavir (Kaletra®)
nelfinavir (Viracept®)
ritonavir (Norvir®)
saquinavir (Fortovase®)

Nucleoside/Nucleotide Reverse Transcriptase Inhibitors (NTRIs)
abacavir (Ziagen®)
didanosine (Videx®)
lamivudine (Epivir®)
stavudine (Zerit®)
tenofovir (Viread®)

zalcitabine (Hivid®)
zidovudine, lamivudine, and abacavir (Trizivir®)
zidovudine (Retrovir®)
zidovudine and lamivudine (Combivir®)

Non-Nucleoside Reverse Transcriptase Inhibitors (NNRTIs)
delavirdine (Rescriptor®)
efavirenz (Sustiva®)
nevirapine (Viramune®)

Drugs Being Studied in HIV/AIDS Clinical Trials

A-007 [antineoplastic]
ABT-378 (new name: lopinavir) [protease inhibitor]
acetaminophen (Tylenol®, Panadol®) [analgesic, antipyretic]
acetylcysteine (Mucomyst®, Respaire®) [antiretroviral, mycolytic]
acitretin (Soriatane®) [antipsoriatic]
ACT (activated cellular therapy) [other/HIV]
acyclovir (Zovirax®) [antiviral]
aldesleukin (Proleukin®) [immunomodulator, antineoplastic]
alitretinoin (Panretin®) [retinoic acid]
AL 721 [antiviral]
ALVAC-HIV gp 160 MN (vCP125) [vaccine]
ALVAC-HIV MN120TMG (vCP205) [vaccine]
ALVAC-HIV MN120TMGNP (vCP300) [vaccine]
ALVAC-RG rabies glycoprotein (vCP65) [vaccine]
allopurinol (Zyloprim®) [xanthine oxidase inhibitor]
aluminum hydroxide (Amphogel®) [adjuvant, immunostimulant]
alvircept sudotox (CD4-*Pseudomonas* exotoxin) [immunomodulator, antiretroviral]
amikacin sulfate (Kanamycin®) [antibacterial]
amikacin (MiKasome) [no data]
aminosalicylic acid [antibacterial]
amitriptyline hydrochloride (Elavil®) [antidepressant, analgesic]
amoxicillin (Amoxil®) [antimicrobial]
amphotericin B (Fungizone®) [antifungal]
ampligen (Atvogen®) [antiretroviral, immunomodulator]
anti-HIV immune serum globulin (HIVIG®) [immunomodulator]
anti-Rh antibodies (Anti-D) [immunomodulator]
APL 400-003 [vaccine]
AS-101 (ammonium trichlorotellurate) [immunomodulator]
atevirdine mesylate (U-87201E) [antiretroviral]
azidodideoxyuridine (AzdU) [antiretroviral]
BCH 10652 [reverse transcriptase inhibitor/HIV]
beclomethasone dipropionate (Beclovent®) [anti-inflammatory]
benzimidavir (1263W94) [CMV-DNA inhibitor/CMV]
benztropine mesylate (Cogentin®) [anticholinergic, antiparkinsonian]
bis-POM PMEA [antiretroviral]
bleomycin (Blenoxane®) [antineoplastic]
BMS 232 [protease inhibitor]
BMS 232632 [protease azapeptide inhibitor/HIV]
BMS 234475 [second generation protease inhibitor/HIV]
BMS 234475/CGP-61755 [other/HIV]
butyldeoxynojirimicin (SC-48334) [antiretroviral]
calanolide A [antiviral]
capreomycin sulfate (Caprocin®) [antibacterial]
CD4 antigen [antiretroviral]
CD4-IgG [antiretroviral, immunomodulator]
ceftriaxone sodium (Rocephin®) [antimicrobial]

cefuroxime axetil (Ceftin®) [antibiotic]
chimeric anti-TNF monoclonal antibody (Chimeric A2) [immunomodulator]
chlorhexidine gluconate (Peridex®, Hibiclens®) [topical antibacterial, antimicrobial]
cidofovir gel (Forvade®) [antiviral/genital herpes]
cimetidine (Tagamet®) [immunomodulator, histamine receptor antagonist]
ciprofloxacin (Cipro®) [antibacterial]
CI-0694 (Sulfasim®) [immunomodulator]
clavulanate potassium [antibacterial]
clindamycin (Cleocin®) [antibacterial]
clofazimine (Lamprene®) [antimicrobial, antileprotic]
clotrimazole (Lotrimin®, Mycelex®, FemCare®) [antifungal]
Cryptosporidium immune whey protein (bovine anticryptosporidium immunoglobulin)
    [antidiarrheal]
CS-92 [nucleoside reverse transcriptase inhibitor/HIV]
CTL [gene therapy/HIV]
curdlan sulfate [antiviral]
cyclophosphamide (Cytoxan®) [antineoplastic, immunosuppressant]
cycloserine (Seromycin®) [antibacterial]
cysteamine (MEA; mercaptoethylamine) [antiretroviral, antiurolithic]
cytarabine (Cytosar-U®) [antimetabolite, antineoplastic, antiviral,
    immunosuppressant]
cytolin [nontoxic AIDS monoclonal antibody/HIV]
cytomegalovirus immune globulin intravenous (human) (CytoGam®)
    [immunomodulator]
dacarbazine [antineoplastic]
DAPD [purine dioxolane nucleoside/HIV]
dapsone [antibacterial]
delavirdine mesylate (U-90152) [antiretroviral]
deoxy-fluorothymidine (FDT) [antiretroviral]
dexamethasone (Decadron®) [anti-inflammatory, immunomodulator, antineoplastic]
dextran sulfate [antiretroviral]
diclazuril [antiprotozoal]
dideoxyadenosine (ddA) [antiretroviral]
diethylhomospermine (DEHSPM) [antidiarrheal]
dinitrochlorobenzene (DNCB) [contact allergen, immunomodulator]
disulfiram (Antabuse®) [alcohol abuse deterrent, immunomodulator, antiretroviral]
ditiocarb sodium (Imuthiol®) [immunomodulator, chelator]
DMP-266 [non-nucleoside reverse transcriptase inhibitor/HIV]
DMP-450 [second generation protease inhibitor/HIV]
doxorubicin (Adriamycin®, Rubex®) [antineoplastic]
emtricitabine (Coviracil) [nucleoside analog]
env 2-3 [vaccine]
ethambutol hydrochloride (Myambutol®) [antibacterial]
ethionamide [antibacterial]
etoposide (VePesid®) [antineoplastic]
F105 human monoclonal antibody [immunomodulator]
fiacitabine (FIAC) [antiviral]
fialuridine (FIAU) [antiviral]
flucytosine (Ancobon®) [antifungal]
fluorouracil (5-FU) [antineoplastic]
G3139 [antisense compound/nonhodgkin's lymphoma]
GEM 132 [hybrid antisense oligonucleotide/CMV retinitis]
glutamic acid (Feracid®) [gastric acidifier]
gp-160 (MicroGeneSys®, VaxSyn®) [vaccine]
gp-160 vaccine (Immuno-AG) [vaccine]
guaifenesin (Robitussin®) [expectorant]
GW275175 [CMV-DNA maturation inhibitor/CMV retinitis]
HBY 097 [antiretroviral]

hepatitis B vaccine (Engerix-B®, Recombivax HB®) [vaccine]
heptavalent pneumococcal conjugate vaccine [vaccine]
HIV p17/p24: Ty-VLP [vaccine]
HIV-1 C4-V3 polyvalent peptide vaccine [vaccine]
HIVAC-1e [vaccine]
hydroxyurea (Hydrea®) [anticancer drug]
hypericin (VIMRyxn®) [antiretroviral]
ibuprofen (Advil®; Motrin®; Nuprin®) [nonsteroidal anti-inflammatory]
ifosfamide [antineoplastic]
imipramine hydrochloride (Tofranil®) [antidepressant]
inosine pranobex (Isoprinosine®) [antiviral, immunostimulant, antiretroviral]
insulin-like growth factor (Somatomedin C®) [immunomodulator]
interferon alfa-n1 (Wellferon®) [antineoplastic, antiviral, immunomodulator]
interferon alfa-n3 (Alferon N®) [antineoplastic, antiviral, immunomodulator]
interferon beta (Betaseron®) [antineoplastic, antiviral, immunomodulator, antiretroviral]
interferon gamma (Actimmune®) [antineoplastic, antiviral, immunomodulator]
interleukin-3 (IL-3) [immunomodulator, hematopoietic]
interleukin-4 (IL-4) [immunomodulator, antineoplastic]
interleukin-10 (IL-10) [immunomodulator]
interleukin-12 (IL-12) [antiviral]
iodenosine (f-dda) [purine-based reverse transcriptase inhibitor/HIV]
ISIS 13312 [second generation antisense compound/CMV retinitis]
ISIS 2922 [antiviral]
isoniazid (INH) [antibacterial]
isotretinoin (Accutane®) [keratolytic]
ketoconazole (Nizoral®) [antifungal, antineoplastic, antiadrenal]
keyhole-limpet hemocyanin [immunomodulator]
kynostatin 272 (KNI-272®) [protease inhibitor, antiretroviral]
L-756,423 [protease inhibitor]
lentinan [immunomodulator, antineoplastic]
letrazuril [antiprotozoal]
leucovorin calcium (Wellcovorin®) [antianemic, antidote for folic acid antagonists]
levamisole [immunomodulator]
levocarnitine [antihyperlipoproteinemic]
levofloxacin [antimicrobial, antiretroviral]
liposome - encapsulated monophosphoryl lipid A [adjuvant, immunostimulant]
Liposyn® III (I.V. fat emulsion 2%) [nutritional support]
Liposyn® II (I.V. fat emulsion 20%) [nutritional support]
lobucavir [antiviral]
lodenosine (F-ddA) [nucleoside analog type drug similar to ddI]
lymphocytes, activated [immunomodulator]
L-697, 639 [antiretroviral]
L-697, 661 [antiretroviral]
magnesium sulfate [electrolyte replenisher, anticonvulsant, laxative]
MDL 28574 [antiretroviral]
MDX-240 [virus-specific bispecific antibody/HIV]
memantine [NMDA receptor antagonist/neuroprotective agent/dementia]
methadone hydrochloride (Dolophine®) [detoxification maintenance, narcotic analgesic]
methotrexate (MTX) [antineoplastic, folic acid antagonist, anti-inflammatory]
methoxsalen (Oxsoralen-ultra®) [photochemotherapeutic]
methylprednisolone (Medrol®) [anti-inflammatory, immunosuppressant]
mexiletine hydrochloride (Mexitil®) [analgesic, antiarrhythmic]
MF59 [adjuvant, immunostimulant]
microparticulate monovalent HIV-1 peptide vaccine [vaccine]
mitoguazone dihydrochloride (MGBG) [antineoplastic]
mitoxantrone hydrochloride (Novantrone®) [antineoplastic]

MKC-442 [antiviral-NNRTI]
monophosphoryl lipid A [adjuvant, immunostimulant]
MTP-PE/MF59 [immunostimulant, adjuvant emulsion]
multikine [immunotherapeutic agent/HIV]
multivalent HIV-1 peptide immunogen [vaccine]
n-docosanol (Lidakol®) [antiviral]
nimodipine (Nimotop®) [calcium channel blocker, vasodilator]
nitazoxanide (NTZ) [antiparasitic]
nystatin (Mycostatin®) [antifungal]
octreotide acetate (Sandostatin®) [antidiarrheal]
OPC 14117 [antioxidant]
oxandrolone (Oxandrin®) [steroid]
oxazepam (Serax®) [anxiolytic, minor tranquilizer]
P3C541b lipopeptide [vaccine]
paclitaxel (Taxol®) [antineoplastic]
paromomycin sulfate (Humatin®) [antibiotic, amebicidal, anthelmintic]
PCLUS [vaccine]
penicillin G [antibacterial]
pentosan polysulfate sodium [antineoplastic, antiviral, anticoagulant, anti-inflammatory, antiretroviral]
pentoxifylline (Trental®) [vasodilator, hemorrheologic]
peptide T [antiretroviral, immunomodulator]
phenylhydrazone [antiviral/HIV]
piritrexim isethionate [antifolate, antineoplastic, antiproliferative, antiprotozoal]
PMEA [antiretroviral]
pneumococcal vaccine polyvalent [vaccine]
polyethylene glycolated IL-2 (PEG IL-2) [immunomodulator]
polymyxin B sulfate/bacitracin zinc ointment (Bacitracin®, Polysporin®) [antibacterial]
prednisone [glucocorticoid]
primaquine [antimalarial]
probenecid (Benemid®) [renal tubular blocker, uricosuric]
probucol (Panavir®) [antiviral]
pseudoephedrine (Sudafed®) [decongestant, sympathomimetic]
pyrazinamide [antibacterial]
pyridoxine hydrochloride (vitamin B_6) [vitamin (coenzyme)]
QS-21 [adjuvant, immunostimulant]
quinine [antimalarial, neuromuscular]
ranitidine hydrochloride (Zantac®) [histamine receptor antagonist, immunomodulator]
recombinant p24 vaccine [vaccine]
rgp 120/HIV-1IIIB [vaccine]
rgp 120/HIV-1MN [vaccine]
rgp 120/HIV 1MN monovalent octameric V3 peptide (SynVac®) [vaccine]
rgp 120/HIV-1SF2 [vaccine]
ribavirin (Virazole®) [antiviral, antiretroviral]
rifalazil (PA-1648) [rifampin derivative]
rifampin (Rifadin®, Rimactane®) [antibacterial]
RMP-7 [antifungal]
RO 24-7429 [antiretroviral, *tat* inhibitor]
Saccharomyces boulardii [antidiarrheal]
SC-49483 [antiretroviral]
SC-52151 [protease inhibitor, antiretroviral]
SCH 39304 [antifungal]
selegiline hydrochloride (Deprenyl®) [MAO inhibitor, antidyskinetic, antiparkinsonian]
sevirumab (human monoclonal antibody to cytomegalovirus) [antiviral, immunomodulator]
smallpox vaccine (Dryvax®) [vaccine]
sorivudine (Brovavir®) [antiviral]

SP-303T [antiviral]
sparfloxacin (Zagam®) [antibacterial]
spiramycin [antibacterial, antiprotozoal]
streptomycin sulfate [antibacterial]
SU5416 [angiogenesis inhibitor/HIV]
sulfadiazine [antibacterial]
sulfadoxine (Fansidar® when combined with pyrimethamine) [antibacterial]
syntex adjuvant formulation [adjuvant, immunostimulant]
T1249 [fusion inhibitor]
T20 [fusion inhibitor]
TAT antagonist [antiviral]
TBC-3B [vaccine]
tecogalan sodium (SP-PG) [angiogenesis inhibitor]
tenofovir dipivoxil (PMPA) [nucleotide inhibitor]
thalidomide (Synovir®) [immunomodulator, sedative, hypnotic]
thioctic acid [antioxidant]
threonyl muramyl dipeptide [adjuvant, immunostimulant]
thymic humoral factor (THF) [immunomodulator]
thymosin alpha 1 [immunomodulator]
thymopentin (Timunox®) [immunomodulator]
tipranavir [protease inhibitor]
TNP-470 [antineoplastic]
tretinoin (Atragen®) [liposomal all-transretinoic acid]
trichosanthin (GLQ 223) [antiretroviral, immunosuppressant]
trifluridine (ophthalmic) [antiviral]
tuberculin purified protein derivative (PPD) [diagnostic aid]
tumor necrosis factor (TNF) [antineoplastic, antiretroviral]
tumor necrosis factor soluble receptor - immunoadhesion complex
    [immunomodulator]
valacyclovir hydrochloride (Valtrex®) [antiviral]
valganciclovir (Cymeval®) [antiviral/CMV retinitis]
valproic acid (Depakene®) [anticonvulsant]
varicella virus vaccine live (Varivax®) [vaccine]
vesnarinone (OPC-8212) [antiretroviral, cardiotonic]
vidarabine [antiviral]
vinblastine sulfate (Velban®) [antineoplastic]
vincristine (Oncovin®) [antineoplastic]
virulizin [macrophage activator/HIV and lymphomas]
WF10 [antiretroviral]
wobenzym [immunomodulator]
WR 6026 [antiprotozoal]
zidovudine/didanosine (Sciptene®) [heterodimer/HIV]
524W91 [antiretroviral]
882C87 [antiviral]
935U83 [antiretroviral]

CANCER CHEMOTHERAPY ACRONYMS

Acronyms	Used for
7 + 3	Leukemia — acute myeloid leukemia, induction
ABP	Lymphoma — non-Hodgkin's
ABC-P	Multiple myeloma
ABDIC	Lymphoma — Hodgkin's
ABVD	Lymphoma — Hodgkin's
AC	Sarcoma — bony sarcoma
AC	Breast cancer
AC (DC)	Multiple myeloma
ACE	Lung cancer — small cell
ACe	Breast cancer
ACMF	Breast cancer
ACOMLA	Lymphoma — non-Hodgkin's
ADOC	Thymoma (malignant)
AVM	Breast cancer
m-BACOD	Lymphoma — non-Hodgkin's
BACOP	Lymphoma — non-Hodgkin's
BAP	Multiple myeloma
BAPP	Thymoma (malignant)
BCDT	Malignant melanoma
BCNU-DAG	Brain tumors
B-CMF	Head and neck cancer
BCVM	Cervical cancer
BCP	Multiple myeloma
BEP	Genitourinary cancer — testicular, induction, good risk
BHD	Malignant melanoma
	Breast cancer
BMC	Head and neck cancer
B-MOPP	Lymphoma — Hodgkin's
BMVL	Head and neck cancer
BOMP	Cervical cancer
BVCPP	Lymphoma — Hodgkin's
CAF	Breast cancer
CAFVP	Breast cancer
CAM	Genitourinary cancer — prostate
CAMP	Lung cancer — non-small cell
CAP	Genitourinary cancer — bladder
	Head and neck cancer
	Lung cancer — non-small cell
	Adrenal cortical cancer
	Endometrial cancer
CAP-BOP	Lymphoma — non-Hodgkin's
CAP-M	Genitourinary cancer — bladder
CBM	Head and neck cancer
CC	Ovarian cancer — epithelial
CCCP	Multiple myeloma
CCNU-VP	Lymphoma — Hodgkin's
CCVPP	Lymphoma — Hodgkin's
CD	Leukemia — acute nonlymphoblastic, consolidation
	Ewing's sarcoma
	Genitourinary cancer — prostate
CDC	Ovarian cancer — epithelial
CDF	Genitourinary cancer — prostate
CE	Adrenal cortical cancer
CF	Head and neck cancer
CFM	Breast cancer
CFPT	Breast cancer
CHAP	Ovarian cancer — epithelial
CHL + PRED	Leukemia — chronic lymphocytic leukemia

APPENDIX

Acronyms	Used for
CHOP	Lymphoma — non-Hodgkin's
CHOP-B (Yale)	Lymphoma — non-Hodgkin's
CHOP-Bleo	Lymphoma — non-Hodgkin's
CHOP (P)	Lymphoma — non-Hodgkin's
CHOR	Lung cancer — small cell
CISCA	Gastric cancer Genitourinary cancer — bladder
Cladribine (2-CdA)	Leukemia — chronic lymphocytic leukemia
CMB	Cervical cancer
CMC-High Dose	Lung cancer — small cell
CMF	Breast cancer
CMFP	Breast cancer
CMFVP (Cooper's)	Breast cancer
C-MOPP	Lymphoma — non-Hodgkin's
CMV	Genitourinary cancer — bladder
COB	Head and neck cancer
CODE	Lung cancer — small cell
COPE	Lung cancer — small cell
COLP	Thymoma (malignant)
COM	Colon cancer
COMF	Colon cancer
COP-BLAM	Lymphoma — non-Hodgkin's
COP-BLAM III	Lymphoma — non-Hodgkin's
COP-BLAM IV	Lymphoma — non-Hodgkin's
COP	Lymphoma — non-Hodgkin's
COP-BLAM	Lymphoma — non-Hodgkin's
COPP (or "C" MOPP)	Lymphoma — non-Hodgkin's
CP	Ovarian cancer — epithelial
CV	Lung cancer — non-small cell
CVB	Esophageal cancer
CVI	Lung cancer — non-small cell
CVM	Gestational trophoblastic disease
CVP	Leukemia — chronic lymphocytic leukemia Lymphoma — non-Hodgkin's
CYADIC	Sarcoma — soft tissue
CYVADIC	Sarcoma — bony sarcoma Sarcoma — soft tissue
DAFS	Carcinoid (malignant)
DAT	Leukemia — acute myeloid leukemia, induction Breast cancer
DC	Multiple myeloma
DHAP	Lymphoma — non-Hodgkin's
DMC	Gestational trophoblastic cancer
DS	Genitourinary cancer — prostate
DTIC-ACTD	Malignant melanoma
DVP	Leukemia — acute lymphoblastic, induction
DVPA	Leukemia — acute lymphoblastic, induction
ELF	Gastric cancer
EMA-CO	Gestational trophoblastic disease
FAC	Breast cancer
FAC-S	Carcinoid (malignant)
FAM	Gastric cancer Lung cancer — non-small cell Pancreatic cancer
FAME	Gastric cancer
FAMTX	Gastric cancer
FAP	Gastric cancer
FAP-2	Pancreatic cancer
FCE	Gastric cancer
F-CL	Colon cancer

Acronyms	Used for
FDC	Gastric cancer
FL	Genitourinary cancer — prostate
FLe	Colon cancer
Fludarabine	Leukemia — chronic lymphocytic leukemia
FMS (SMF)	Pancreatic cancer
FMV	Colon cancer
FOAM	Breast cancer
FOMi	Lung cancer — non-small cell
FOMi/CAP	Lung cancer — non-small cell
5FU/LDLF	Colon cancer
FU/HU	Colon cancer
FU/LV	Colon cancer
5FU Hurt	Head and neck cancer
5FU/LV (weekly)	Colon cancer
FL	Genitourinary cancer — prostate
HDAC	Leukemia — acute myeloid leukemia, induction
HDMTX	Sarcoma — bony sarcoma
IC	Leukemia — acute myeloid leukemia, induction
ID	Sarcoma — soft tissue
IMAC	Sarcoma — bony sarcoma
IMF	Breast cancer
IMVP-16	Lymphoma — non-Hodgkin's
LDAC	Leukemia — acute myeloid leukemia, induction
L-VAM	Genitourinary cancer — prostate
M-2	Multiple myeloma
MAC	Genitourinary cancer — bladder Endometrial cancer
MACC	Lung cancer — non-small cell
MACOP-B	Lymphoma — non-Hodgkin's
MAID	Sarcoma — soft tissue
MAP	Head and neck cancer
MBC (MBD)	Head and neck cancer Cervical cancer Esophageal cancer
MBD	Head and neck cancer
MC	Leukemia — acute myeloid leukemia, induction
MeCP	Multiple myeloma
MF	Head and neck cancer Esophageal cancer
MICE (ICE)	Lung cancer — small cell
MINE	Lymphoma — non-Hodgkin's
MM	Leukemia — acute lymphoblastic, maintenance
MMC (MTX + MP + CTX)	Leukemia — acute lymphoblastic, maintenance
MOF-STREP	Colon cancer
MOP-BAP	Lymphoma — Hodgkin's
MOPP	Lymphoma — Hodgkin's
MOPP/ABV Hybrid	Lymphoma — Hodgkin's
MP	Multiple myeloma
m-PFL	Genitourinary cancer — bladder
MS	Adrenal cortical cancer
MV	Leukemia — acute myeloid leukemia, induction
MVAC	Genitourinary cancer — bladder
MVPP	Lymphoma — Hodgkin's
NFL	Breast cancer
PAC (CAP)	Ovarian cancer — epithelial Endometrial cancer
PE	Genitourinary cancer — testicular, induction, good risk Lung cancer — small cell
PFL	Gastric cancer Head and neck cancer
PFL + IFN	Head and neck cancer

APPENDIX

Acronyms	Used for
Pt-FU	Head and neck cancer
POCC	Lung cancer — small cell
Pro-MACE	Lymphoma — non-Hodgkin's
Pro-MACE-CytaBOM	Lymphoma — non-Hodgkin's
Pro-MACE-MOPP	Lymphoma — non-Hodgkin's
PT	Ovarian cancer — epithelial
SC	Carcinoid (malignant)
SCAB	Lymphoma — Hodgkin's
SD	Pancreatic cancer
SF	Carcinoid (malignant)
SMF	Pancreatic cancer
T-9	Ewing's sarcoma
VAB VI	Genitourinary cancer — testicular, induction, salvage
VAC	Ovarian cancer — germ cell Sarcoma — soft tissue Ewing's sarcoma
VAC (CAV) (Induction)	Lung cancer — small cell
VAD	Leukemia — acute lymphoblastic, induction Multiple myeloma
VADRIAC — High Dose	Sarcoma — bony sarcoma
VAIE	Sarcoma — bony sarcoma
VAM	Breast cancer
VAP	Multiple myeloma
VATH	Breast cancer
VBAP	Multiple myeloma
VBC	Malignant melanoma
VBP (PVB)	Genitourinary cancer — testicular, induction, salvage
VC	Lung cancer — small cell
VCAP	Multiple myeloma
VDCP	Endometrial cancer
VDP	Malignant melanoma
VIP	Genitourinary cancer — testicular, induction, poor risk
VIP (Einhorn)	Genitourinary cancer — testicular, induction, poor risk
VP	Leukemia — acute lymphoblastic, induction
VP-L-Asparaginase	Leukemia — acute lymphoblastic, induction
Wayne State	Head and neck cancer

CANCER CHEMOTHERAPY REGIMENS

ADULT REGIMENS

Adenocarcinoma – Unknown Primary

Carbo-Tax
Paclitaxel, I.V., 135 mg/m^2 over 24 hours, day 1, followed by
Carboplatin dose targeted by Calvert equation to AUC 7.5 I.V.

Repeat cycle every 21 days

EP
Cisplatin, I.V., 60-100 mg/m^2, day 1
Etoposide, I.V., 80-100 mg/m^2, days 1-3

Repeat cycle every 21 days

FAM
Fluorouracil, I.V., 600 mg/m^2, days 1, 8, 29, 36
Doxorubicin, I.V., 30 mg/m^2, days 1, 29
Mitomycin, I.V., 10 mg/m^2, day 1

Repeat cycle every 8 weeks

Paclitaxel/Carboplatin/Etoposide
Paclitaxel, I.V., 200 mg/m^2 over 1 hour, day 1, followed by
Carboplatin dose targeted by Calvert equation to AUC 6 I.V.
Etoposide, P.O., 50 mg/day alternated with 100 mg/day, days 1-10

Repeat cycle every 21 days

Breast Cancer

Standard adjuvant chemotherapy includes 4 cycles of AC or 6 cycles of CMF (d_1/d_8 variety)

AC
Doxorubicin, I.V., 60 mg/m^2, day 1
Cyclophosphamide, I.V., 400-600 mg/m^2, day 1

Repeat cycle every 21 days

ACe
Doxorubicin, I.V., 40 mg/m^2, day 1
Cyclophosphamide, P.O., 200 mg/m^2/day, days 1-3 or 3-6

Repeat cycle every 21-28 days

CAF
Cyclophosphamide, P.O., 100 mg/m^2, days 1-14 or 600 mg/m^2 I.V., day 1
Doxorubicin, I.V., 25 mg/m^2, days 1, 8 or 60 mg/m^2 I.V., day 1
Fluorouracil, I.V., 500-600 mg/m^2, days 1, 8

Repeat cycle every 28 days

or

Cyclophosphamide, I.V., 500 mg/m^2, day 1
Doxorubicin, I.V., 50 mg/m^2, day 1
Fluorouracil, I.V., 500 mg/m^2, day 1

Repeat cycle every 21 days

CFM
Cyclophosphamide, I.V., 500-600 mg/m^2, day 1
Fluorouracil, I.V., 500-600 mg/m^2, day 1
Mitoxantrone, I.V., 10-12 mg/m^2, day 1

Repeat cycle every 21 days

Breast Cancer *(continued)*

CFPT

Cyclophosphamide, I.V., 150 mg/m^2, days 1-5
Fluorouracil, I.V., 300 mg/m^2, days 1-5
Prednisone, P.O., 10 mg tid, days 1-7
Tamoxifen, P.O., 10 mg bid, days 1-42

Repeat cycle every 42 days

CMF

Cyclophosphamide, P.O., 100 mg/m^2, days 1-14 or 600 mg/m^2 I.V., days 1, 8
Methotrexate, I.V., 40 mg/m^2, days 1, 8
Fluorouracil, I.V., 600 mg/m^2, days 1, 8

Repeat cycle every 28 days

or

Cyclophosphamide, I.V., 600 mg/m^2, day 1
Methotrexate, I.V., 40 mg/m^2, day 1
Fluorouracil, I.V., 400-600 mg/m^2, day 1

Repeat cycle every 21 days

CMFP

Cyclophosphamide, P.O., 100 mg/m^2, days 1-14
Methotrexate, I.V., 40-60 mg/m^2, days 1, 8
Fluorouracil, I.V., 600-700 mg/m^2, days 1, 8
Prednisone, P.O., 40 mg (first 3 cycles only), days 1-14

Repeat cycle every 28 days

FAC

Fluorouracil, I.V., 500 mg/m^2, days 1, 8
Doxorubicin, I.V., 50 mg/m^2, day 1
Cyclophosphamide, I.V., 500 mg/m^2, day 1

Repeat cycle every 21 days

IMF

Ifosfamide, I.V., 1.5 g/m^2, days 1, 8
Mesna, I.V., 20% of ifosfamide dose, give immediately before and 4 and 8 hours after ifosfamide
    infusion, days 1, 8
Methotrexate, I.V., 40 mg/m^2, days 1, 8
Fluorouracil, I.V., 600 mg/m^2, days 1, 8

Repeat cycle every 28 days

NFL

Mitoxantrone, I.V., 12 mg/m^2, day 1
Fluorouracil, I.V., 350 mg/m^2, days 1-3, given after leucovorin calcium
Leucovorin calcium, I.V., 300 mg/m^2, days 1-3

or

Mitoxantrone, I.V., 10 mg/m^2, day 1
Fluorouracil, I.V., 1000 mg/m^2 continuous infusion, given after leucovorin calcium, days 1-3
Leucovorin calcium, I.V., 100 mg/m^2, days 1-3

Repeat cycle every 21 days

Sequential Dox-CMF

Doxorubicin, I.V., 75 mg/m^2, every 21 days for 4 cycles followed by 21- or 28-day CMF for 8
    cycles

Vinorelbine/Doxorubicin

Vinorelbine, I.V., 25 mg/m^2, days 1, 8
Doxorubicin, I.V., 50 mg/m^2, day 1

Repeat cycle every 21 days

VATH

Vinblastine, I.V., 4.5 mg/m^2, day 1
Doxorubicin, I.V., 45 mg/m^2, day 1
Thiotepa, I.V., 12 mg/m^2, day 1
Fluoxymesterone, P.O., 10 mg tid, days 1-21

Repeat cycle every 21 days

Breast Cancer *(continued)*

Single-Agent Regimens

Anastrozole, P.O., 1 mg qd

Capecitabine, P.O., 2500 mg/m^2/day, bid regimen, days 1-14, repeat cycle every 21 days

Docetaxel, I.V., 60-100 mg/m^2 over 1 hour; patient must be premedicated with dexamethasone 8 mg bid P.O. for 5 days, start 1 day before docetaxel; repeat cycle every 3 weeks

Gemcitabine, I.V., 725 mg/m^2 over 30 minutes, weekly for 3 weeks, followed by 1-week rest, repeat cycle every 28 days

Letrozole, P.O., 2.5 mg qd

Megestrol, P.O., 40 mg qid

Paclitaxel, I.V., 175 mg/m^2 over 3 hours, every 21 days or 250 mg/m^2 over 3-24 hours, every 21 days
Patient must be premedicated with:
Dexamethasone 20 mg P.O., 12 and 6 hours prior
Diphenhydramine 50 mg I.V., 30 minutes prior
Cimetidine 300 mg I.V., or ranitidine 50 mg I.V., 30 minutes prior

Tamoxifen, P.O., 20 mg qd

Toremifene citrate, P.O., 60 mg qd

Vinorelbine, I.V., 30 mg/m^2, every 7 days

Cervical Cancer

CLD-BOMP
Bleomycin, I.V., 5 mg continuous infusion, days 1-7
Cisplatin, I.V., 10 mg/m^2, day 1, 22
Vincristine, I.V., 0.7 mg/m^2, day 7
Mitomycin-C. I.V., 7 mg/m^2, day 7

Repeat cycle every 21 days

MOBP
Bleomycin, I.V., 30 units/day continuous infusion, days 1, 4
Vincristine, I.V., 0.5 mg/m^2, days 1, 4
Mitomycin-C. I.V., 10 mg/m^2, day 1
Cisplatin, I.V., 50 mg/m^2, days 1, 22

Repeat cycle every 28 days

Single-Agent Regimen

Cisplatin, I.V., 50-100 mg/m^2, every 21 days

Colon Cancer

F-CL
Fluorouracil, I.V., 375 mg/m^2, days 1-5
Leucovorin calcium, I.V., 200 mg/m^2, days 1-5

Repeat cycle every 28 days
or
Fluorouracil, I.V., 500 mg/m^2/week 1 hour after initiating the calcium leucovorin infusion for 6 weeks
Leucovorin calcium, I.V., 500 mg/m^2, over 2 hours, weekly for 6 weeks
2-week break, then repeat cycle

FLe
Fluorouracil, I.V., 450 mg/m^2 for 5 days, then, after a pause of 4 weeks, 450 mg/m^2/week for 48 weeks
Levamisole, P.O., 50 mg tid for 3 days, repeated every 2 weeks for 1 year

Colon Cancer *(continued)*

FMV

Fluorouracil, I.V., 10 mg/kg/day, days 1-5
Methyl-CCNU, P.O., 175 mg/m^2, day 1
Vincristine, I.V., 1 mg/m^2 (max: 2 mg), day 1

Repeat cycle every 35 days

FU/LV

Fluorouracil, I.V., 370-400 mg/m^2/day, days 1-5
Leucovorin calcium, I.V., 200 mg/m^2/day, commence infusion 15 minutes prior to fluorouracil
infusion, days 1-5

Repeat cycle every 21 days

or

Fluorouracil, I.V., 1000 mg/m^2/day by continuous infusion, days 1-4
Leucovorin calcium, I.V., 200 mg/m^2/day, days 1-4

Repeat cycle every 28 days

Weekly 5FU/LV

Fluorouracil, I.V., 600 mg/m^2 over 1 hour given after leucovorin, repeat weekly x 6 then 2-week
rest period = 1 cycle, days 1, 8, 15, 22, 29, 36
Leucovorin calcium, I.V., 500 mg/m^2 over 2 hours, days 1, 8, 15, 22, 29, 36

Repeat cycle every 56 days

5FU/LDLF

Fluorouracil, I.V., 425 mg/m^2/day, days 1-5
Leucovorin calcium, I.V., 20-25 mg/m^2/day, days 1-5

Repeat cycle every 28 days

Single-Agent Regimens

5-FU, I.V., 1000 mg/m^2/day, continuous infusion, days 1-5

Repeat cycle every 21-28 days

Irinotecan, I.V., 125 mg/m^2 over 90 minutes every 7 days for 4 cycles or 350 mg/m^2 over 30
minutes

Repeat cycle every 21 days

Endometrial Cancer

AP

Doxorubicin, I.V., 60 mg/m^2, day 1
Cisplatin, I.V., 60 mg/m^2, day 1

Repeat cycle every 21 days

Single-Agent Regimens

Doxorubicin, I.V., 40-60 mg/m^2, day 1

Repeat cycle every 21-28 days

Medroxyprogesterone, P.O., 200 mg/day

Gastric Cancer

EAP

Etoposide, I.V., 120 mg/m^2, days 4, 5, 6
Doxorubicin, I.V., 20 mg/m^2, days 1, 7
Cisplatin, I.V., 40 mg/m^2, days 2, 8

Repeat cycle every 28 days

ELF

Leucovorin calcium, I.V., 300 mg/m^2, days 1-3 followed by
Etoposide, I.V., 120 mg/m^2, days 1-3 followed by
Fluorouracil, I.V., 500 mg/m^2, days 1-3

Repeat cycle every 21-28 days

Gastric Cancer *(continued)*

FAM

Fluorouracil, I.V., 600 mg/m^2, days 1, 8, 29, 36
Doxorubicin, I.V., 30 mg/m^2, days 1, 29
Mitomycin C, I.V., 10 mg/m^2, day 1

Repeat cycle every 8 weeks

FAME

Fluorouracil, I.V., 350 mg/m^2, days 1-5, 36-40
Doxorubicin, I.V., 40 mg/m^2, days 1, 36
Methyl-CCNU, P.O., 150 mg/m^2, day 1

Repeat cycle every 70 days

FAMTX

Methotrexate, IVPB, 1500 mg/m^2, day 1
Fluorouracil, IVPB, 1500 mg/m^2 1 hour after methotrexate, day 1
Leucovorin calcium, P.O., 15 mg/m^2 q6h x 48 hours, 24 hours after methotrexate, day 2
Doxorubicin, IVPB, 30 mg/m^2, day 15

Repeat cycle every 28 days

FCE

Fluorouracil, I.V., 900 mg/m^2/day continuous infusion, days 1-5
Cisplatin, I.V., 20 mg/m^2, days 1-5
Etoposide, I.V., 90 mg/m^2, days 1, 3, 5

Repeat cycle every 21 days

PFL

Cisplatin, I.V., 25 mg/m^2 continuous infusion, days 1-5
Fluorouracil, I.V., 800 mg/m^2 continuous infusion, days 2-5
Leucovorin calcium, I.V., 500 mg/m^2 continuous infusion, days 1-5

Repeat cycle every 28 days

Single-Agent Regimens

Irinotecan, I.V., over 90 minutes: 125 mg/m^2/week; repeat weekly for 4 weeks, then 2-week rest period

or

Irinotecan, I.V. over 30-90 minutes: 350 mg/m^2; repeat every 21 days

Genitourinary Cancer

Bladder

CAP

Cyclophosphamide, I.V., 400 mg/m^2, day 1
Doxorubicin, I.V., 40 mg/m^2, day 1
Cisplatin, I.V., 60 mg/m^2, day 1

Repeat cycle every 21 days

CISCA

Cisplatin, I.V., 70-100 mg/m^2, day 2
Cyclophosphamide, I.V., 650 mg/m^2, day 1
Doxorubicin, I.V., 50 mg/m^2, day 1

Repeat cycle every 21-28 days

CMV

Cisplatin, I.V., 100 mg/m^2 over 4 hours, start 12 hours after MTX, day 2
Methotrexate, I.V., 30 mg/m^2, days 1, 8
Vinblastine, I.V., 4 mg/m^2, days 1, 8

Repeat cycle every 21 days

Genitourinary Cancer — Bladder *(continued)*

m-PFL

    Methotrexate, I.V., 60 mg/m^2, day 1
    Cisplatin, I.V., 25 mg/m^2 continuous infusion, days 2-6
    Fluorouracil, I.V., 800 mg/m^2 continuous infusion, days 2-6
    Leucovorin calcium, I.V., 500 mg/m^2 continuous infusion, days 2-6

        Repeat cycle every 28 days for 4 cycles

MVAC

    Methotrexate, I.V., 30 mg/m^2, days 1, 15, 22
    Vinblastine, I.V., 3 mg/m^2, days 2, 15, 22
    Doxorubicin, I.V., 30 mg/m^2, day 2
    Cisplatin, I.V., 70 mg/m^2, day 2

        Repeat cycle every 28 days

PC

    Paclitaxel, I.V., 200 mg/m^2 or 225 mg/m^2 over 3 hours, day 1
    Carboplatin, I.V., dose targeted by Calvert equation to AUC 5 or 6 after paclitaxel, day 1

        Repeat cycle every 21 days

Single-Agent Regimens

    Gemcitabine, I.V., 1200 mg/m^2, days 1, 8, 15

        Repeat cycle every 28 days

    Paclitaxel, I.V., 250 mg/m^2 over 24 hours, day 1

        Repeat cycle every 21 days

Ovarian, Epithelial

Carbo-Tax

    Paclitaxel, I.V., 135 mg/m^2 over 24 hours, day 1
        or
    175 mg/m^2 over 3 hours, day 1, followed by
    Carboplatin dose targeted by Calvert equation to AUC 7.5 I.V.

        Repeat cycle every 21 days

CC

    Carboplatin, I.V., dose targeted by Calvert equation to AUC 6-7
    Cyclophosphamide, I.V., 600 mg/m^2, day 1

        Repeat cycle every 28 days

CP

    Cyclophosphamide, I.V., 750 mg/m^2, day 1
    Cisplatin, I.V., 75 mg/m^2, day 1

        Repeat cycle every 21 days

CT

    Paclitaxel, I.V., 135 mg/m^2 over 24 hours, day 1
        or
    175 mg/m^2 over 3 hours, day 1, followed by
    Cisplatin, I.V., 75 mg/m^2

        Repeat cycle every 21 days

PAC (CAP)

    Cisplatin, I.V., 50 mg/m^2, day 1
    Doxorubicin, I.V., 50 mg/m^2, day 1
    Cyclophosphamide, I.V., 1000 mg/m^2, day 1

        Repeat cycle every 21 days x 8 cycles

Genitourinary Cancer — Ovarian, Epithelial *(continued)*

Single-Agent Regimens

Altretamine, P.O., 260 mg/m^2/day, qid for 1-15 days

Repeat cycle every 28 days for 2 cycles, then reassess

Etoposide, I.V., 50-60 mg/m^2/day, days 1-21

Repeat cycle every 28 days

Liposomal doxorubicin, I.V., 50 mg/m^2, 1-hour infusion, day 1

Repeat cycle every 21 days

Paclitaxel, I.V., 135 mg/m^2, over 3 or 24 hours, day 1

Repeat cycle every 21 days for 2 cycles, then reassess

Topotecan, I.V., 1.5 mg/m^2, over 30 minutes, days 1-5

Repeat cycle every 21 days for 2 cycles, then reassess

Ovarian, Germ Cell

BEP

Bleomycin, I.V., 30 units, days 2, 9, 16
Etoposide, I.V., 100 mg/m^2, days 1-5
Cisplatin, I.V., 20 mg/m^2, days 1-5

Repeat cycle every 21 days

VAC

Vincristine, I.V., 1.2-1.5 mg/m^2 (max: 2 mg) weekly for 10-12 weeks, or every 2 weeks for 12 doses
Dactinomycin, I.V., 0.3-0.4 mg/m^2, days 1-5
Cyclophosphamide, I.V., 150 mg/m^2, days 1-5

Repeat every 28 days

Prostate

EV

Estramustine, P.O., 200 mg tid, days 1-42
Vinblastine, I.V., 4 mg/m^2/week, begin day 1

Repeat cycle every 6 weeks

FL

Flutamide, P.O., 250 mg tid, days 1-28
Leuprolide acetate, S.C., 1 mg qd, days 1-28

Repeat cycle every 28 days

or

Flutamide, P.O., 250 mg tid, days 1-28
Leuprolide acetate depot, I.M., 7.5 mg, day 1

Repeat cycle every 28 days

FZ

Flutamide, P.O., 250 mg tid
Goserelin acetate, S.C., 3.6 mg implant, every 28 days or goserelin S.C., 10.8 mg depot every 12 weeks

L-VAM

Leuprolide acetate, S.C., 1 mg qd, days 1-28
Vinblastine, I.V., 1.5 mg/m^2/day continuous infusion, days 2-7
Doxorubicin, I.V., 50 mg/m^2 continuous infusion, day 1
Mitomycin C, I.V., 10 mg/m^2, day 2

Repeat cycle every 28 days

Mitoxantrone/Prednisone

Mitoxantrone, I.V., 12 mg/m^2, day 1
Prednisone, P.O., 5 mg bid

Repeat cycle every 21 days

Genitourinary Cancer — Prostate *(continued)*

No Known Acronym

    Bicalutamide, P.O., 50 mg/day

    Leuprolide acetate depot, I.M., 7.5 mg or goserelin S.C. 3.6 mg implant every 28 days

PE

    Paclitaxel, I.V., 120 mg/m^2, days 1-4

    Estramustine, P.O., 600 mg qd, 24 hours before paclitaxel

Repeat cycle every 21 days

Single-Agent Regimens

    Estramustine, P.O., 14 mg/kg/day, tid or qid

    Goserelin acetate implant, S.C., 3.6 mg every 28 days or 10.8 mg every 12 weeks

    Nilutamide, P.O., 300 mg qd, days 1-30, then 150 mg qd in combination with surgical castration; begin on same day or day after castration

    Prednisone, P.O., 5 mg bid

Renal

Interleukin-2 (rIL-2), S.C.
    20 million units/m^2, days 3-5, weeks 1, 4
    5 million units/m^2, days 1, 3, 5, weeks 2, 3, 5, 6

or

Interferon alfa (rIFNα2), S.C.
    6 million units/m^2, day 1, weeks 1, 4;
    6 million units/m^2, days 1, 3, 5, weeks 2, 3, 5, 6

Repeat cycle every 8 weeks

Single-Agent Regimen

Interleukin-2:
    High dose: I.V. bolus over 15 minutes, 600,000-720,000 units/kg q8h until toxicity or 14 days; administer 2 courses separated by 7-10 days
    Low dose: S.C., 18 million units/day for 5 days, then 9 million units/day for 2 days, then 18 million units/day 3 days/week for 6 weeks

or

3 million units/m^2/day for 5 days/week, every 2 weeks for 1 month, then every 4 weeks

Testicular

EP

    Etoposide, I.V., 100 mg/m^2, days 1-5

    Cisplatin, I.V., 20 mg/m^2, days 1-5

Repeat cycle every 21 days

Testicular, Induction, Good Risk

BEP

    Bleomycin, I.V., 30 units, days 2, 9, 16

    Etoposide, I.V., 100 mg/m^2, days 1-5

    Cisplatin, I.V., 20 mg/m^2, days 1-5

Repeat cycle every 21 days

PVB

    Cisplatin, I.V., 20 mg/m^2, days 1-5

    Vinblastine, I.V., 0.15 mg/kg, days 1, 2

    Bleomycin, I.V., 30 units, days 2, 9, 16

Repeat cycle every 21 days

Testicular, Induction, Poor Risk

VIP

    Etoposide, I.V., 75 mg/m^2, days 1-5
    Ifosfamide, I.V., 1.2 g/m^2, days 1-5
    Cisplatin, I.V., 20 mg/m^2, days 1-5
    Mesna, I.V., 400 mg/m^2, then 1200 mg/m^2/day continuous infusion, days 1-5

                        Repeat cycle every 21 days

VIP (Einhorn)

    Vinblastine, I.V., 0.11 mg/kg, days 1-2
    Ifosfamide, I.V., 1200 mg/m^2, days 1-5
    Cisplatin, I.V., 20 mg/m^2, days 1-5
    Mesna, I.V., 400 mg/m^2, then 1200 mg/m^2/day continuous infusion, days 1-5

                        Repeat cycle every 21 days

Testicular, Induction, Salvage

VAB VI

    Vinblastine, I.V., 4 mg/m^2, day 1
    Dactinomycin, I.V., 1 mg/m^2, day 1
    Bleomycin, I.V., 30 units push day 1, then 20 units/m^2/day continuous infusion, days 1-3
    Cisplatin, I.V., 120 mg/m^2, day 4
    Cyclophosphamide, I.V., 600 mg/m^2, day 1

                        Repeat cycle every 21 days

VBP (PVB)

    Vinblastine, I.V., 6 mg/m^2, days 1, 2
    Bleomycin, I.V., 30 units, days 1, 8, 15, (22)
    Cisplatin, I.V., 20 mg/m^2, days 1-5

                        Repeat cycle every 21-28 days

Gestational Trophoblastic Cancer

DMC

    Dactinomycin, I.V., 0.37 mg/m^2, days 1-5
    Methotrexate, I.V., 11 mg/m^2, days 1-5
    Cyclophosphamide, I.V., 110 mg/m^2, days 1-5

                        Repeat cycle every 21 days

Head and Neck Cancer

CAP

    Cyclophosphamide, I.V., 500 mg/m^2, day 1
    Doxorubicin, I.V., 50 mg/m^2, day 1
    Cisplatin, I.V., 50 mg/m^2, day 1

                        Repeat cycle every 28 days

CF

    Carboplatin, I.V., 400 mg/m^2, day 1
    Fluorouracil, I.V., 1000 mg/m^2/day continuous infusion, days 1-5

                        Repeat cycle every 21-28 days

COB

    Cisplatin, I.V., 100 mg/m^2, day 1
    Vincristine, I.V., 1 mg, days 2, 5
    Bleomycin, I.V., 30 units/day continuous infusion, days 2-5

                        Repeat cycle every 21 days

Head and Neck Cancer *(continued)*

5-FU HURT

Hydroxyurea, P.O., 1000 mg q12h x 11 doses; start PM of admission, give 2 hours prior to radiation therapy, days 0-5

Fluorouracil, I.V., 800 mg/m^2/day continuous infusion, start AM after admission, days 1-5

Paclitaxel, I.V., 5-25 mg/m^2/day continuous infusion, start AM after admission; dose escalation study – refer to protocol, days 1-5

G-CSF, S.C., 5 mcg/kg/day, days 6-12, start ≥12 hours after completion of 5-FU infusion

5-7 cycles may be administered

PFL

Cisplatin, I.V., 100 mg/m^2, day 1

Fluorouracil, I.V., 600-800 mg/m^2/day continuous infusion, days 1-5

Leucovorin calcium, I.V., 200-300 mg/m^2/day, days 1-5

Repeat cycle every 21 days

PFL+IFN

Cisplatin, I.V., 100 mg/m^2, day 1

Fluorouracil, I.V., 640 mg/m^2/day continuous infusion, days 1-5

Leucovorin calcium, P.O., 100 mg q4h, days 1-5

Interferon alfa-2b, S.C., 2 x 10^6 units/m^2, days 1-6

Pt-FU

Cisplatin, I.V., 100 mg/m^2, day 1

Fluorouracil, I.V., 1000 mg/m^2/day continuous infusion, days 1-5

Repeat cycle every 21 days for 2 cycles

TIP

Paclitaxel, I.V., 175 mg/m^2 3-hour infusion, day 1

Ifosfamide, I.V., 1000 mg/m^2 2-hour infusion, days 1-3

Mesna, I.V., 400 mg/m^2 before ifosfamide and 200 mg/m^2 I.V., 4 hours after ifosfamide

Cisplatin, I.V., 60 mg/m^2, day 1

Repeat cycle every 21-28 days

Single-Agent Regimens

Carboplatin, I.V., 300-400 mg/m^2, over 2 hours every 21-28 days

Methotrexate, I.V., I.M., 40 mg/m^2, bolus day 1; cycle repeated every 7 days for 6 cycles

Cisplatin I.V., 100 mg/m^2, every 28 days divided into 1, 2, or 4 equal doses per month

Vinorelbine, I.V., 25-30 mg/m^2, repeat weekly

Leukemia

Acute Lymphoblastic, Induction

VAD

Vincristine, I.V., 0.4 mg/day continuous infusion, days 1-4

Doxorubicin, I.V., 12 mg/m^2/day continuous infusion, days 1-4

Dexamethasone, P.O., 40 mg, days 1-4, 9-12, 17-20

VP

Vincristine, I.V., 2 mg/m^2/week for 4-6 weeks (max: 2 mg)

Prednisone, P.O., 60 mg/m^2/day in divided doses for 4 weeks, taper weeks 5-7

No Known Acronym

Cyclophosphamide, I.V., 1200 mg/m^2, day 1

Daunorubicin, I.V., 45 mg/m^2, days 1-3

Prednisone, P.O., 60 mg/m^2, days 1-21

Vincristine, I.V., 2 mg/m^2/week

L-asparaginase, I.V., 6000 units/m^2, 3 times/week

or

Pegaspargase, I.M./I.V., 2500 units/m^2, every 14 days if patient develops hypersensitivity to native L-asparaginase

Acute Lymphoblastic, Maintenance

MM
Mercaptopurine, P.O., 50-75 mg/m^2, days 1-7
Methotrexate, P.O./I.V., 20 mg/m^2, day 1

Repeat cycle every 7 days

MMC (MTX + MP + CTX)*
Methotrexate, I.V., 20 mg/m^2/week
Mercaptopurine, P.O., 50 mg/m^2/day
Cyclophosphamide, I.V., 200 mg/m^2/week
*Continue all 3 drugs until relapse of disease or after 3 years of remission.

Acute Lymphoblastic, Relapse

AVDP
Asparaginase, I.V., 15,000 units/m^2, days 1-5, 8-12, 15-19, 22-26
Vincristine, I.V., 2 mg/m^2 (max: 2 mg), days 8, 15, 22
Daunorubicin, I.V., 30-60 mg/m^2, days 8, 15, 22
Prednisone, P.O., 40 mg/m^2, days 8-12, 15-19, 22-26

Acute Myeloid Leukemia, Induction

7+3
Cytarabine, I.V., 100-200 mg/m^2/day continuous infusion, days 1-7
with
Daunorubicin, I.V., 45 mg/m^2, days 1-3
or
Idarubicin, I.V., 12 mg/m^2, days 1-3
or
Mitoxantrone, I.V., 12 mg/m^2, days 1-3

5+2*
Cytarabine, I.V., 100-200 mg/m^2/day continuous infusion, days 1-5
with
Daunorubicin, I.V., 45 mg/m^2, days 1-2
or
Mitoxantrone, I.V., 12 mg/m^2, days 1-2
*For reinduction

DAT/DCT
Daunorubicin, I.V., 60 mg/m^2/day, days 1-3
Cytarabine, I.V., 200 mg/m^2/day continuous infusion, days 1-5
Thioguanine, P.O., 100 mg/m^2 q12h, days 1-5

Modified DAT (considerations in elderly patients)
Daunorubicin, I.V., 50 mg/m^2, day 1
Cytarabine, S.C., 100 mg/m^2/day q12h, days 1-5
Thioguanine, P.O., 100 mg/m^2 q12h, days 1-5

EMA-86
Etoposide, I.V., 200 mg/m^2/day continuous infusion, days 8-10
Mitoxantrone, I.V., 12 mg/m^2, days 1-3
Cytarabine, I.V., 500 mg/m^2/day continuous infusion, days 1-3, 8-10

LDAC
Considerations in Elderly Patients
Cytarabine, S.C., 10 mg/m^2 bid, days 10-21

MC
Mitoxantrone, I.V., 12 mg/m^2/day, days 1-3
Cytarabine, I.V., 100-200 mg/m^2/day continuous infusion, days 1-7

Consolidation
Mitoxantrone, I.V., 12 mg/m^2, days 1-2
Cytarabine, I.V., 100 mg/m^2 continuous infusion, days 1-5

Repeat cycle every 28 days

Leukemia — Acute Myeloid Leukemia, Induction *(continued)*

MV

Mitoxantrone, I.V., 10 mg/m^2/day, days 1-5
Etoposide, I.V., 100 mg/m^2/day, days 1-3

Single-Agent Regimen

All transrelincic acid (ATRA), P.O., 45 mg/m^2/day (1 or 2 divided doses) with or without 7+3 induction regimen

Acute Myeloid Leukemia, Postremission

Single-Agent Regimens

Cytarabine, I.V., 100 mg/m^2/day continuous infusion, days 1-5*; repeat cycle every 28 days
*For patients >60 years of age

Cytarabine (HiDAC), I.V. 3000 mg/m^2 over 1-3 hours, every 12 hours, days 1-6
or
3000 mg/m^2 over 1-3 hours, every 12 hours, days 1, 3, 5. Administer with saline, methylcellulose, or steroid eyedrops OU, every 2-4 hours, beginning with cytarabine and continuing 48-72 hours after last cytarabine dose

Repeat cycle every 28 days

Acute Nonlymphoblastic, Consolidation

CD

Cytarabine, I.V., 3000 mg/m^2 q12h, days 1-6
Daunorubicin, I.V., 30 mg/m^2/day, days 7-9

Chronic Lymphocytic Leukemia

CHL + PRED

Chlorambucil, P.O., 0.4 mg/kg/day for 1 day every other week
Prednisone, P.O., 100 mg/day for 2 days every other week; adjust dosage according to blood counts every 2 weeks prior to therapy; increase initial dose of 0.4 mg/kg by 0.1 mg/kg every 2 weeks until toxicity or disease control is achieved

CVP

Cyclophosphamide, P.O., 400 mg/m^2/day, days 1-5
Vincristine, I.V., 1.4 mg/m^2 (max: 2 mg), day 1
Prednisone, P.O., 100 mg/m^2, days 1-5

Repeat cycle every 21 days

Single-Agent Regimens

Chlorambucil, P.O., 0.1-0.2 mg/kg/day for 3-6 weeks
or
Chlorambucil, P.O., 20-30 mg/m^2, day 1

Repeat cycle every 14-28 days

or

Chlorambucil, P.O., 0.4 mg/kg/day, for 1 day every other week
or
Chlorambucil, P.O., 0.4 mg/kg/day, for 1 day every other day

Cladribine, I.V., 0.1 mg/kg/day continuous infusion, days 1-5 or 1-7

Repeat cycle every 28-35 days

Cyclophosphamide, P.O., 2-4 mg/kg, days 1-10

Repeat cycle every 21-28 days

Fludarabine, I.V., 25-30 mg/m^2, days 1-5

Repeat cycle every 28 days

Prednisone,* P.O., 30-60 mg/m^2, days 1-5 or 1-7

*Use if patient symptomatic with autoimmune thrombocytopenia or hemolytic anemia.

Chronic Myelogenous Leukemia

Single-Agent Regimens

Busulfan, P.O., 4-8 mg/day for 5-10 weeks (until WBC reduced to 20 x 10^3/µL)

Hydroxyurea, P.O., 2-5 g/day; decrease dose by 1/2 as counts decrease (stop when WBC = 20 x 10^3/µL)

Interferon alfa-2a, S.C., 3-9 million units/day; dose may be adjusted as per response and adverse events.

Hairy-Cell Leukemia

Single-Agent Regimens

Cladribine, I.V., 0.1 mg/kg/day continuous infusion, days 1-7

Administer one cycle

Interferon alfa-2a, S.C., 3 million units, 3 times/week

Pentostatin, I.V., 4 mg/m^2, day 1

Repeat cycle every 14 days

Lung Cancer

Small Cell

CAV/VAC
Cyclophosphamide, I.V., 750-1000 mg/m^2, day 1
Doxorubicin, I.V., 50 mg/m^2, day 1
Vincristine, I.V., 1.4 mg/m^2 (max: 2 mg), day 1

Repeat cycle every 3 weeks

CAVE
Cyclophosphamide, I.V., 750 mg/m^2, day 1
Doxorubicin, I.V., 50 mg/m^2, day 1
Vincristine, I.V., 1.4 mg/m^2 (max: 2 mg), day 1
Etoposide, I.V., 60-100 mg/m^2, days 1-3

Repeat cycle every 21 days

EC
Etoposide, I.V., 100-120 mg/m^2, days 1-3
Carboplatin, I.V., 325-400 mg/m^2, day 1

Repeat cycle every 28 days

EP/PE
Etoposide, I.V., 120 mg/m^2, days 1-3
Cisplatin, I.V., 60-120 mg/m^2, day 1

Repeat cycle every 21-28 days

Single-Agent Regimen

Etoposide, P.O., 50 mg/m^2, days 1-21

Repeat cycle every 28 days

Topotecan, I.V., 1.5 mg/m^2/day, over 30 minutes, days 1-5

Repeat cycle every 21 days

Non-small Cell

Carbo-Tax
Paclitaxel, I.V., 135 mg/m^2 over 24 hours, day 1 **or**
175 mg/m^2 over 3 hours, day 1, followed by
Carboplatin dose targeted by Calvert equation to AUC 7.5 I.V.

Repeat cycle every 21 days

Lung Cancer — Non-small Cell *(continued)*

EC

Etoposide, I.V., 100-120 mg/m^2, days 1-3

with

Carboplatin, I.V., 300-325 mg/m^2, day 1

Repeat cycle every 21-28 days

EP

Etoposide, I.V., 80 mg/m^2, days 1-3
Cisplatin, I.V., 60-100 mg/m^2, day 1

Repeat cycle every 21-28 days

Gemcitabine-Cis

Gemcitabine, I.V., 1000 mg/m^2, days 1, 8, 15
Cisplatin, I.V., 100 mg/m^2, day 2 or 15

Repeat cycle every 28 days

PC

Paclitaxel, I.V., 175 mg/m^2, 3-hour infusion, day 1
Cisplatin, I.V., 80 mg/m^2, day 1

Repeat cycle every 21 days

Vinorelbine-Cis

Vinorelbine, I.V., 30 mg/m^2, every 7 days
Cisplatin, I.V., 120 mg/m^2, day 1, 29, then every 6 weeks

Single-Agent Regimens

Topotecan, I.V., 1.5 mg/m^2/day, over 30 minutes, days 1-5

Repeat cycle every 21 days

Vinorelbine, I.V., 30 mg/m^2, every 7 days

Lymphoma

Hodgkin's

ABVD

Doxorubicin, I.V., 25 mg/m^2, days 1, 15
Bleomycin, I.V., 10 units/m^2, days 1, 15
Vinblastine, I.V., 6 mg/m^2, days 1, 15
Dacarbazine, I.V., 350-375 mg/m^2, days 1, 15

Repeat cycle every 28 days

ChlVPP

Chlorambucil, P.O., 6 mg/m^2 (max: 10 mg/day), days 1-14
Vinblastine, I.V., 6 mg/m^2 (max: 10 mg dose), days 1, 8
Procarbazine, P.O., 100 mg/m^2 (max: 150 mg/day), days 1-14
Prednisone, P.O., 40 mg/day, days 1-14

Repeat cycle every 28 days

CVPP

Lomustine, P.O., 75 mg/m^2, day 1
Vinblastine, I.V., 4 mg/m^2, days 1, 8
Procarbazine, P.O., 100 mg/m^2, days 1-14
Prednisone, P.O., 30 mg/m^2, days 1-14 (cycles 1 and 4 only)

Repeat cycle every 28 days

EVA

Etoposide, I.V., 100 mg/m^2, days 1-3
Vinblastine, I.V., 6 mg/m^2, day 1
Doxorubicin, I.V., 50 mg/m^2, day 1

Repeat cycle every 28 days

Lymphoma — Hodgkin's *(continued)*
MOPP
    Mechlorethamine, I.V., 6 mg/m^2, days 1, 8
    Vincristine, I.V., 1.4 mg/m^2 (max: 2.5 mg), days 1, 8
    Procarbazine, P.O., 100 mg/m^2, days 1-14
    Prednisone, P.O., 40 mg/m^2, days 1-14

                Repeat cycle every 28 days

MOPP/ABV Hybrid
    Mechlorethamine, I.V., 6 mg/m^2, day 1
    Vincristine, I.V., 1.4 mg/m^2, day 1
    Procarbazine, P.O., 100 mg/m^2, days 1-7
    Prednisone, P.O., 40 mg/m^2, days 1-14
    Doxorubicin, I.V., 35 mg/m^2, day 8
    Bleomycin, I.V., 10 units/m^2, day 8
    Vinblastine, I.V., 6 mg/m^2, day 8

                Repeat cycle every 28 days

MVPP
    Mechlorethamine, I.V., 6 mg/m^2, days 1, 8
    Vinblastine, I.V., 6 mg/m^2, days 1, 8
    Procarbazine, P.O., 100 mg/m^2, days 1-14
    Prednisone, P.O., 40 mg/m^2, days 1-14

                Repeat cycle every 42 days

NOVP
    Mitoxantrone, I.V., 10 mg/m^2, day 1
    Vincristine, I.V., 2 mg, day 8
    Vinblastine, I.V., 6 mg/m^2, day 1
    Prednisone, P.O., 100 mg/m^2, days 1-5

                Repeat cycle every 21 days

Stanford V*
    Mechlorethamine, I.V., 6 mg/m^2, day 1
    Doxorubicin, I.V., 25 mg/m^2, days 1, 15
    Vinblastine, I.V., 6 mg/m^2, days 1, 15
    Vincristine, I.V., 1.4 mg/m^2, days 8, 22
    Bleomycin, I.V., 5 units/m^2, days 8, 22
    Etoposide, I.V., 60 mg/m^2, days 15, 16
    Prednisone, P.O., 40 mg/m^2/day, dose tapered over the last 15 days

                Repeat cycle every 28 days

*In patients older than 50 years of age, vinblastine dose decreased to 4 mg/m^2 and vincristine dose decreased to 1 mg/m^2 on weeks 9-12. Concomitant trimethoprim/sulfamethoxazole DS P.O. bid; acyclovir 200 mg P.O. tid; ketoconazole 200 mg P.O. qd; and stool softeners used.

Non-Hodgkin's

BACOP
    Bleomycin, I.V., 5 units/m^2, days 15, 22
    Doxorubicin, I.V., 25 mg/m^2, days 1, 8
    Cyclophosphamide, I.V., 650 mg/m^2, days 1, 8
    Vincristine, I.V., 1.4 mg/m^2 (max: 2 mg), days 1, 8
    Prednisone, P.O., 60 mg/m^2, days 15-28

                Repeat cycle every 28 days

CHOP
    Cyclophosphamide, I.V., 750 mg/m^2, day 1
    Doxorubicin, I.V., 50 mg/m^2, day 1
    Vincristine, I.V., 1.4 mg/m^2 (max: 2 mg), day 1
    Prednisone, P.O., 100 mg/m^2, days 1-5

                Repeat cycle every 21 days

Lymphoma — Non-Hodgkin's *(continued)*

CHOP-Bleo

Cyclophosphamide, I.V., 750 mg/m^2, day 1
Doxorubicin, I.V., 50 mg/m^2, day 1
Vincristine, I.V., 2 mg, days 1, 5
Prednisone, P.O., 100 mg, days 1-5
Bleomycin, I.V., 15 units, days 1, 5

Repeat cycle every 21-28 days

CNOP

Cyclophosphamide, I.V., 750 mg/m^2, day 1
Mitoxantrone, I.V., 10 mg/m^2, day 1
Vincristine, I.V., 1.4 mg/m^2, day 1
Prednisone, P.O., 50 mg/m^2, days 1-5

Repeat cycle every 21 days

COMLA

Cyclophosphamide, I.V., 1500 mg/m^2, day 1
Vincristine, I.V., 1.4 mg/m^2 (max: 2.5 mg), days 1, 8, 15
Methotrexate, I.V., 120 mg/m^2, days 22, 29, 36, 43, 50, 57, 64, 71
Leucovorin calcium rescue, P.O., 25 mg/m^2, q6h for 4 doses, beginning 24 hours after each
    methotrexate dose
Cytarabine, I.V., 300 mg/m^2, days 22, 29, 36, 43, 50, 57, 64, 71

Repeat cycle every 21 days

COP

Cyclophosphamide, I.V., 800 mg/m^2, day 1
Vincristine, I.V., 1.4 mg/m^2 (max: 2 mg), day 1
Prednisone, P.O., 60 mg/m^2, days 1-5

Repeat cycle every 21 days

COP-BLAM

Cyclophosphamide, I.V., 400 mg/m^2, day 1
Vincristine, I.V., 1 mg/m^2, day 1
Prednisone, P.O., 40 mg/m^2, days 1-10
Bleomycin, I.V., 15 mg, day 14
Doxorubicin, I.V., 40 mg/m^2, day 1
Procarbazine, P.O., 100 mg/m^2, days 1-10

COPP (or "C" MOPP)

Cyclophosphamide, I.V., 400-650 mg/m^2, days 1, 8
Vincristine, I.V., 1.4-1.5 mg/m^2 (max: 2 mg), days 1, 8
Procarbazine, P.O., 100 mg/m^2, days 1-14
Prednisone, P.O., 40 mg/m^2, days 1-14

Repeat cycle every 28 days

CVP

Cyclophosphamide, P.O., 400 mg/m^2, days 1-5
Vincristine, I.V., 1.4 mg/m^2 (max: 2 mg), day 1
Prednisone, P.O., 100 mg/m^2, days 1-5

Repeat cycle every 21 days

DHAP*

Dexamethasone, I.V., 10 mg q6h, days 1-4
Cytarabine, I.V., 2 g/m^2 q12h x 2 doses, day 2
Cisplatin, I.V., 100 mg/m^2 continuous infusion, day 1

Repeat cycle every 21-28 days

*Administer with saline, methylcellulose, or steroid eyedrops OU, every 2-4 hours, beginning with
cytarabine and continuing 48-72 hours after last cytarabine dose.

Lymphoma — Non-Hodgkin's *(continued)*
ESHAP*
Etoposide, I.V., 60 mg/m^2, days 1-4
Cisplatin, I.V., 25 mg/m^2/day continuous infusion, days 1-4
Cytarabine, I.V., 2 g/m^2, immediately following completion of etoposide and cisplatin therapy
Methylprednisolone, I.V., 500 mg/day, days 1-4

Repeat cycle every 21-28 days

*Administer with saline, methylcellulose, or steroid eyedrops OU, every 2-4 hours, beginning with cytarabine and continuing 48-72 hours after last cytarabine dose.

IMVP-16
Ifosfamide, I.V., 4 g/m^2 continuous infusion over 24 hours, day 1
Mesna, I.V., 800 mg/m^2 bolus prior to ifosfamide, then 4 g/m^2 continuous infusion over 12 hours
   concurrent w/ifosfamide; then 2.4 g/m^2 continuous infusion over 12 hours after ifosfamide
   infusion, day 1
Methotrexate, I.V., 30 mg/m^2, days 3, 10
Etoposide, I.V., 100 mg/m^2, days 1-3

Repeat cycle every 21-28 days

MACOP-B
Methotrexate, I.V., 400 mg/m^2, weeks 2, 6, 10
Doxorubicin, I.V., 50 mg/m^2, weeks 1, 3, 5, 7, 9, 11
Cyclophosphamide, I.V., 350 mg/m^2, weeks 1, 3, 5, 7, 9, 11
Vincristine, I.V., 1.4 mg/m^2 (max: 2 mg), weeks 2, 4, 8, 10, 12
Bleomycin, I.V., 10 units/m^2, weeks 4, 8, 12
Prednisone, P.O., 75 mg/day tapered over 15 d, days 1-15
Leucovorin calcium, P.O., 15 mg/m^2, q6h x 6 doses 24 hours after methotrexate, weeks 2, 6, 10
Trimethoprim/sulfamethoxazole DS, P.O., tablet, bid, for 12 weeks
Ketoconazole, P.O., 200 mg/day

Administer one cycle

m-BACOD
Methotrexate, I.V., 200 mg/m^2, days 8, 15
Leucovorin calcium, P.O., 10 mg/m^2 q6h x 8 doses beginning 24 hours after each methotrexate
   dose, days 8, 15
Bleomycin, I.V., 4 units/m^2, day 1
Doxorubicin, I.V., 45 mg/m^2, day 1
Cyclophosphamide, I.V., 600 mg/m^2, day 1
Vincristine, I.V., 1 mg/m^2, day 1
Dexamethasone, P.O., 6 mg/m^2, days 1-5

Repeat cycle every 21 days

m-BACOS
Methotrexate, I.V., 1 g/m^2, day 2
Bleomycin, I.V., 10 units/m^2, day 1
Doxorubicin, I.V., 50 mg/m^2 continuous infusion, day 1
Cyclophosphamide, I.V., 750 mg/m^2, day 1
Vincristine, I.V., 1.4 mg/m^2 (max: 2 mg), day 1
Leucovorin calcium rescue, P.O., 15 mg q6h for 8 doses, starting 24 hours after methotrexate
Methylprednisolone, I.V., 500 mg, days 1-3

Repeat cycle every 21-25 days

MINE
Mesna, I.V., 1.33 g/m^2/day concurrent with ifosfamide dose, then 500 mg P.O. 4 hours after each
   ifosfamide infusion, days 1-3
Ifosfamide, I.V., 1.33 g/m^2/day, days 1-3
Mitoxantrone, I.V., 8 mg/m^2, day 1
Etoposide, I.V., 65 mg/m^2/day, days 1-3

Repeat cycle every 28 days

Lymphoma — Non-Hodgkin's *(continued)*

MINE-ESHAP

Mesna, I.V., 1.33 g/m², administered at same time as ifosfamide, then 500 mg P.O., 4 hours after ifosfamide, days 1-3
Ifosfamide, I.V., 1.33 g/m², over 1 hour, days 1-3
Mitoxantrone, I.V., 8 mg/m², day 1
Etoposide, I.V., 65 mg/m², days 1-3

Repeat cycle every 21 days for 6 cycles, followed by 3-6 cycles of ESHAP

NOVP

Mitoxantrone, I.V., 10 mg/m², day 1
Vinblastine, I.V., 6 mg/m², day 1
Prednisone, P.O., 100 mg, days 1-5
Vincristine, I.V., 2 mg, day 8

Repeat cycle every 21 days

Pro-MACE

Prednisone, P.O., 60 mg/m², days 1-14
Methotrexate, I.V., 1.5 g/m², day 14
Leucovorin calcium, I.V., 50 mg/m² q6h x 5 doses beginning 24 hours after methotrexate dose, day 14
Doxorubicin, I.V., 25 mg/m², days 1, 8
Cyclophosphamide, I.V., 650 mg/m², days 1, 8
Etoposide, I.V., 120 mg/m², days 1, 8

Repeat cycle every 28 days

Pro-MACE-CytaBOM

Prednisone, P.O., 60 mg/m², days 1-14
Doxorubicin, I.V., 25 mg/m², day 1
Cyclophosphamide, I.V., 650 mg/m², day 1
Etoposide, I.V., 120 mg/m², day 1
Cytarabine, I.V., 300 mg/m², day 8
Bleomycin, I.V., 5 units/m², day 8
Vincristine, I.V., 1.4 mg/m² (max: 2 mg), day 8
Methotrexate, I.V., 120 mg/m², day 8
Leucovorin calcium, P.O., 25 mg/m² q6h x 4 doses, day 9
Concomitant trimethoprim/sulfamethoxazole DS, P.O., bid

Repeat cycle every 21-28 days

Single-Agent Regimens

CDA cladribine, S.C., 0.1 mg/kg/day for 5 days or 0.1 mg/kg/day I.V., for 7 days

Repeat cycle every 28 days

Rituximab, I.V., 375 mg/m², days 1, 8, 15, 22

Malignant Melanoma

CVD

Cisplatin, I.V., 20 mg/m², days 1-5
Vinblastine, I.V., 1.6 mg/m², days 1-5
Dacarbazine, I.V., 800 mg/m², day 1

Repeat cycle every 21 days

CVD + IL-21

Cisplatin, I.V., 20 mg/m²/day, days 1-4
Vinblastine, I.V., 1.6 mg/m²/day, days 1-4
Dacarbazine, I.V., 800 mg/m², day 1
IL-2, I.V., 9 million units/m² continuous infusion, days 1-4
Interferon alfa, S.C., 5 million units/m², every day, days 1-5, 7, 9, 11, 13

Repeat cycle every 21 days

Malignant Melanoma *(continued)*

Dacarbazine/Tamoxifen
Dacarbazine, I.V., 250 mg/m^2, days 1-5, every 21 days
Tamoxifen,* P.O., 20 mg/day

No Known Acronym
Dacarbazine, I.V., 220 mg/m^2, days 1-3, every 21-28 days
Carmustine, I.V., 150 mg/m^2, day 1, every 42-56 days
Cisplatin, I.V., 25 mg/m^2, days 1-3, every 21-28 days
Tamoxifen,* P.O., 20 mg/day

*Use of tamoxifen is optional.

Single-Agent Regimens

Interferon alfa-2b adjuvant therapy, I.M., 20 million units/m^2, days 1-30, **then**

10 million units/m^2 S.C., 3 times/week for 48 weeks

Interferon alfa-2a, I.M., 20 million units/m^2 3 times/week for 12 weeks

Multiple Myeloma

EDAP
Etoposide, I.V., 100-200 mg/m^2, days 1-4
Dexamethasone, P.O./I.V., 40 mg/m^2, days 1-5
Cytarabine, 1000 mg, day 5
Cisplatin, I.V., 20 mg continuous infusion, days 1-4

MP
Melphalan, P.O., 8-10 mg/m^2, days 1-4
Prednisone, P.O., 40-60 mg/m^2/day, days 1-4

Repeat cycle every 28-42 days

M-2
Vincristine, I.V., 0.03 mg/kg (max: 2 mg), day 1
Carmustine, I.V., 0.5-1 mg/kg, day 1
Cyclophosphamide, I.V., 10 mg/kg, day 1
Melphalan, P.O., 0.25 mg/kg, days 1-4 or 0.1 mg/kg, days 1-7 or 1-10
Prednisone, P.O., 1 mg/kg/day, days 1-7

Repeat cycle every 35-42 days

VAD
Vincristine, I.V., 0.4 mg/day continuous infusion, days 1-4
Doxorubicin, I.V., 9 mg/m^2/day continuous infusion, days 1-4
Dexamethasone, P.O., 40 mg, days 1-4, 9-12, 17-20

Repeat cycle every 28-35 days

VAD induction therapy followed by maintenance
Interferon alfa, S.C., 3 million units/m^2, 3 times/week
Prednisone, P.O., 50 mg, 3 times/week, after interferon

VBAP
Vincristine, I.V., 1 mg, day 1
Carmustine, I.V., 30 mg/m^2, day 1
Doxorubicin, I.V., 30 mg/m^2, day 1
Prednisone, P.O., 100 mg, days 1-4

Repeat cycle every 21 days

VBMCP
Vincristine, I.V., 1.2 mg/m^2, day 1
Carmustine, I.V., 20 mg/m^2, day 1
Melphalan, P.O., 8 mg/m^2, days 1-4
Cyclophosphamide, I.V., 400 mg/m^2, day 1
Prednisone, P.O., 40 mg/m^2, days 1-7 all cycles, and 20 mg/m^2, days 8-14 first 3 cycles only
Repeat cycle every 35 days

Multiple Myeloma *(continued)*
VCAP
Vincristine, I.V., 1 mg, day 1
Cyclophosphamide, P.O., 100 mg/m^2, days 1-4
Doxorubicin, I.V., 25 mg/m^2, day 2
Prednisone, P.O., 60 mg/m^2, days 1-4

Repeat cycle every 28 days

Single-Agent Regimens

Aldesleukin, 600,000-700,000 int. units/kg every 8 hours x 14 doses

Repeat cycle every 14 days

Dexamethasone, P.O., 20 mg/m^2 for 4 days beginning on days 1-4, 9-12, and 17-20

Repeat cycle every 35 days

Interferon alfa-2b, S.C., 2 million units/m^2, 3 times/week for maintenance therapy in selected
patients with significant response to initial chemotherapy treatment

Melphalan, I.V., 90-140 mg/m^2

Administer one cycle

Pancreatic Cancer

FAM
Fluorouracil, I.V., 600 mg/m^2, days 1, 8, 29, 36
Doxorubicin, I.V., 30 mg/m^2, days 1, 29
Mitomycin, I.V., 10 mg/m^2, day 1

Repeat cycle every 72 days

SMF
Streptozocin, I.V., 1000 mg/m^2, days 1, 8, 29, 36
Mitomycin, I.V., 10 mg/m^2, day 1
Fluorouracil, I.V., 600 mg/m^2, days 1, 8, 29, 36

Repeat cycle every 72 days

Single-Agent Regimens

Gemcitabine, I.V., 1000 mg/m^2 over 30 minutes once weekly for 7 weeks, followed by a 1-week
rest period; subsequent cycles once weekly for 3 consecutive weeks out of every 4 weeks

Sarcoma

AC
Doxorubicin, I.V., 75-90 mg/m^2 96-hour continuous infusion
Cisplatin, I.A./I.V., 90-120 mg/m^2, 6 days

Repeat cycle every 28 days

AD
Doxorubicin, I.V., 22.5 mg/m^2/day continuous infusion, days 1-4
Dacarbazine, I.V., 225 mg/m^2/day continuous infusion, days 1-4

Repeat cycle every 21 days

CYVADIC
Cyclophosphamide, I.V., 500 mg/m^2, day 1
Vincristine, I.V., 1.4 mg/m^2, days 1, 5
Doxorubicin, I.V., 50 mg/m^2, day 1
Dacarbazine, I.V., 250 mg/m^2, days 1-5

Repeat cycle every 21 days

Sarcoma *(continued)*

DI

Doxorubicin, I.V., 50 mg/m^2 bolus, day 1
Ifosfamide, I.V., 5000 mg/m^2/day continuous infusion, following doxorubicin, day 1
Mesna, I.V., 600 mg/m^2, bolus before ifosfamide, followed by 2500 mg/m^2/day, continuous infusion, for 36 hours

Repeat cycle every 21 days

HDMTX

Methotrexate, I.V., 8-12 g/m^2
Leucovorin calcium, P.O./I.V., 15-25 mg q6h for at least 10 doses beginning 24 hours after methotrexate dose; courses repeated weekly for 2-4 weeks, alternating with various cancer chemotherapy combination regimens

IE

Etoposide, I.V., 100 mg/m^2, days 1-5
Ifosfamide, I.V., 1800 mg/m^2, days 1-5
Mesna, I.V., at 20% of ifosfamide dose prior to and 4 and 8 hours after ifosfamide administration

Repeat cycle every 21-28 days

MAID

Mesna, I.V., 2500 mg/m^2/day continuous infusion, days 1-4
Doxorubicin, I.V., 15 mg/m^2/day continuous infusion, days 1-4
Ifosfamide, I.V., 2500 mg/m^2/day continuous infusion, days 1-3
Dacarbazine, I.V., 250 mg/m^2/day continuous infusion, days 1-4

Repeat cycle every 21-28 days

VAC

Vincristine, I.V., 2 mg/m^2/week (max: 2 mg), during weeks 1-12
Dactinomycin, I.V., 0.015 mg/kg (max: 0.5 mg) every 3 months for 5-6 courses, days 1-5
Cyclophosphamide, P.O., 2.5 mg/kg/day for 2 years

Single-Agent Regimens

Doxorubicin, I.V., 75 mg/m^2, day 1

Repeat cycle every 21 days

PEDIATRIC REGIMENS

Small patients have a large body surface area relative to their kg weight and could possibly be overdosed if a m^2 dosing regimen is applied. Therefore, for calculating pediatric doses of chemotherapy agents, as a general rule a child who weighs 30 kg is ~1 m^2. **For children weighing <15 kg or with surface area <0.6 m^2,** the dose per m^2 of an agent listed herein should be divided by 30 and multiplied by the weight of the child (in kg) to obtain the correct dose.

ALL, Consolidation

IDMTX/6-MP

Methotrexate, I.V. push, 200 mg/m^2, then 800 mg/m^2 as a 24-hour infusion
Mercaptopurine, I.V., 200 mg/m^2 over 20 minutes, then 800 mg/m^2 as an 8-hour infusion
Leucovorin, P.O./I.V., 15 mg/m^2 q6h x 9; begin 24 hours after end of methotrexate

ALL, Continuation

MTX/6-MP

Methotrexate, I.M., 20 mg/m^2/week, during weeks 25-130
Mercaptopurine, P.O., 50 mg/m^2/day, during weeks 25-130

ALL, Continuation *(continued)*

MTX/6-MP/VP
Methotrexate, P.O., 20 mg/m^2/week
Mercaptopurine, P.O., 75 mg/m^2/day
Vincristine, I.V., 1.5 mg/m^2 x 1 each month
Prednisone, P.O., 40 mg/m^2 x 5 days each month

ALL, Induction

PVD
Prednisone, P.O., 40 mg/m^2/day x 28 days
Vincristine, I.V., 1.5 mg/m^2/week x 4
Asparaginase, I.M., 5000 int. units/m^2 on days 2, 5, 8, 12, 15, 18

PVDA
Prednisone, P.O., 40 mg/m^2, days 1-28
Vincristine, I.V., 1.5 mg/m^2, days 2, 8, 15, 22
Daunorubicin, I.V., 25 mg/m^2, days 2, 8, 15, 22
Asparaginase, I.M., 5000 int. units/m^2 on days 2, 5, 8, 12, 15, 19

TIT (CNS Prophylaxis)
Methotrexate: 1 y: 10 mg; 2 y: 12.5 mg; ≥3 y: 15 mg
Cytarabine: 1 y: 20 mg; 2 y: 25 mg; ≥3 y: 30 mg
Hydrocortisone: 1 y: 10 mg; 2 y: 12.5 mg; ≥3 y: 15 mg

AML, Induction

CA
Cytarabine, I.V., 3 g/m^2, q12h for 4 doses
Asparaginase, I.M., 6000 int. units/m^2 3 hours after last dose of cytarabine

DA
Daunorubicin, I.V., 45 mg/m^2, days 1-3
Cytarabine, I.V., 100 mg/m^2/day, continuous infusion, days 1-7

DAT
Daunorubicin, I.V., 45 mg/m^2/day continuous infusion, days 1-3
Cytarabine, I.V., 100 mg/m^2/day continuous infusion, days 1-7
Thioguanine, P.O., 100 mg/m^2, days 1-7

DAV
Daunorubicin, I.V., 60 mg/m^2, days 3, 4, 5
Cytarabine, I.V., 100 mg/m^2 continuous infusion, days 1-2, then 30-minute infusion q12h on days
    3-8
Etoposide, I.V., 150 mg/m^2, days 6, 7, 8

HI-CDAZE
Daunorubicin, I.V., 30 mg/m^2, days 1-3
Cytarabine, I.V., 3 g/m^2, q12h, days 1-4
Etoposide, I.V., 200 mg/m^2, days 1-3, 6-8
Azacytidine, I.V., 150 mg/m^2, days 3-5, 8-10

Brain Tumors

CDDP/VP
Cisplatin, I.V., 90 mg/m^2, day 1
Etoposide, I.V., 150 mg/m^2, days 3, 4

Repeat cycle every 21 days

Brain Tumors *(continued)*

CDDP/VP-16
Cisplatin, I.V., 90 mg/m^2, day 1
Etoposide, I.V., 150 mg/m^2, days 3, 4

Repeat cycle every 21 days

COPE or "Baby Brain I"
Cycle A:
Vincristine, I.V., 0.065 mg/kg (max: 1.5 mg), days 1, 8
Cyclophosphamide, I.V., 65 mg/kg, day 1
Cycle B:
Cisplatin, I.V., 4 mg/m^2, day 1
Etoposide, I.V., 6.5 mg/kg, days 3, 4

Regimens given in alternating 28-day cycles in the sequence AABAAB

MOP
Mechlorethamine (nitrogen mustard), I.V., 6 mg/m^2, days 1, 8
Vincristine, I.V., 1.4 mg/m^2, days 1, 8
Procarbazine, P.O., 100 mg/m^2, days 1-14

MOPP
Mechlorethamine (nitrogen mustard), I.V., 3 mg/m^2, days 1, 8
Vincristine, I.V., 1.4 mg/m^2, days 1, 8
Procarbazine, P.O., 50 mg on day 1, 100 mg on day 2, then 100 mg/m^2 on days 3-10
Prednisone, P.O., 40 mg/m^2, days 1-10

Repeat cycle every 28 days

PCV
Procarbazine, P.O., 60 mg/m^2, days 8-21
Methyl-CCNU, P.O., 110 mg/m^2, day 1
Vincristine, I.V., 1.4 mg/m^2, days 8 and 29

POC
Prednisone, P.O., 40 mg/m^2, days 1-14
CCNU, P.O., 100 mg/m^2, day 1
Vincristine, I.V., 1.5 mg/m^2, days 1, 8, 15

"8 in 1"
Methylprednisolone, P.O., 300 mg/m^2 for 3 doses q6h
Vincristine, I.V., 1.5 mg/m^2
Lomustine, P.O., 100 mg/m^2
Procarbazine, P.O., 75 mg/m^2
Hydroxyurea, P.O., 3000 mg/m^2
Cisplatin, I.V., 90 mg/m^2
Cytarabine, I.V., 300 mg/m^2
Dacarbazine, I.V., 150 mg/m^2

Repeat cycle every 14 days

Single-Agent Regimen

Carboplatin, I.V., 560 mg/m^2, every 4 weeks

Lymphoma

ABVD
Doxorubicin, I.V., 25 mg/m^2, days 1, 15
Bleomycin, I.V., 10 units/m^2, days 1, 15
Vinblastine, I.V., 6 mg/m^2, days 1, 15
Dacarbazine (DTIC), I.V., 375 mg/m^2, days 1, 15

Repeat cycle every 28 days

Lymphoma *(continued)*

CHOP
Cyclophosphamide, I.V., 750 mg/m^2, days 1, 22
Doxorubicin, I.V., 40 mg/m^2, days 1, 22
Vincristine, I.V., 1.5 mg/m^2/week for 6 doses
Prednisone, P.O., 40 mg/m^2/day, for 28 days

COMP
Cyclophosphamide, I.V., 1.2 g/m^2, day 1
Vincristine, I.V., 2 mg/m^2, days 3, 10, 17, 24
Methotrexate, I.V., 300 mg/m^2, day 12
Prednisone, P.O., 60 mg/m^2, days 3-30, then taper for 7 days (max: 60 mg)

COPP
Cyclophosphamide, I.V., 500 mg/m^2, days 1, 8
Vincristine, I.V., 1.5 mg/m^2, days 1, 8
Procarbazine, P.O., 100 mg/m^2 (max: 150 mg), days 1-14
Prednisone, P.O., 40 mg/m^2, days 1-14

MOPP
Mechlorethamine (nitrogen mustard), I.V., 6 mg/m^2, days 1, 8
Vincristine, I.V., 1.4 mg/m^2, days 1, 8
Procarbazine, P.O., 50 mg, day 1, then 100 mg/m^2, days 2-14
Prednisone, P.O., 40 mg/m^2, days 1-14 in courses 1 and 4 only

OPA
Vincristine, I.V., 1.5 mg/m^2, days 1, 8, 15
Prednisone, P.O., 60 mg/m^2, days 1-15
Doxorubicin, I.V., 40 mg/m^2, days 1, 15

OPPA
Vincristine, I.V., 1.5 mg/m^2, days 1, 8, 15
Procarbazine, P.O., 100 mg/m^2, days 1-15
Prednisone, P.O., 60 mg/m^2, days 1-15
Doxorubicin, I.V., 40 mg/m^2, days 1, 15

Repeat cycle every 28 days

Burkitt's Lymphoma

Advanced Stage Burkitt's/B-cell ALL
Methotrexate, I.T., 10 mg/m^2 at hour 0
Cytarabine, I.T., 50 mg/m^2 at hour 0
Cyclophosphamide, I.V., 300 mg/m^2 q12h x 6 at hours 0-60
Vincristine, I.V., 1.5 mg/m^2 at hour 72
Doxorubicin, I.V., 50 mg/m^2 at hour 72
Followed after hematopoietic recovery by:
Methotrexate, I.T., 12 mg/m^2 at hour 0
Methotrexate, I.V. push, 200 mg/m^2, then 800 mg/m^2 as a 24-hour infusion from hours 0-24
Cytarabine, I.T., 50 mg/m^2 at hour 24
Cytarabine, I.V., 400 mg/m^2 over 48 hours from hours 24-72, with escalating doses in succeeding
    courses
Leucovorin, I.V., 30 mg/m^2 at hours 36 and 42, then 3 mg/m^2 at hours 54, 66, 78

Neuroblastoma

Cy/A
Cyclophosphamide, P.O., 150 mg/m^2/day x 7 days
Doxorubicin, I.V., 35 mg/m^2 on day 8

Pt/VM
Cisplatin, I.V., 90 mg/m^2 over 6 hours
Teniposide, I.V., 100 mg/m^2, 48 hours after completion of cisplatin

Osteosarcoma

HDMTX

Methotrexate, I.V., 12 g/m^2/week for 2-12 weeks
Leucovorin calcium rescue, P.O./I.V., 15 mg/m^2 q6h for 10 doses beginning 30 hours after the
beginning of the 4-hour methotrexate infusion (serum methotrexate levels must be monitored)

IFoVP

Ifosfamide, I.V., 1800 mg/m^2, days 1-5
Etoposide, I.V., 100 mg/m^2, days 1-5
Mesna uroprotection, I.V., 2880 mg/m^2, days 1-5

Repeat cycle every 21 days

MTX-CDDPAdr

Methotrexate, I.V., 12 g/m^2/week for 2 weeks
Leucovorin calcium rescue, I.V., 20 mg/m^2 q3h for 8 doses beginning 16 hours after completion of
methotrexate, then q6h P.O. for 8 doses
alternating with
Cisplatin, I.V., 75 mg/m^2, day 15 of cycles 1-7, then 120 mg/m^2 for cycles 8-10
Doxorubicin, I.V., 25 mg/m^2, days 15, 16, 17 of cycles 1-7

Sarcoma (Bony and Soft Tissue)

ICE

Ifosfamide, I.V., 1500 mg/m^2, days 1-3 (with mesna uroprotection)
Carboplatin, I.V., 635 mg/m^2, day 3
Etoposide, I.V., 100 mg/m^2, days 1, 2, 3

Topo/CTX

Cyclophosphamide, I.V., 250 mg/m^2 on days 1-5, followed by
Topotecan, I.V., 0.75 mg/m^2 on days 1-5

VACAdr

Vincristine, I.V., 1.5 mg/m^2/week for 6 weeks
Cyclophosphamide, I.V., 500 mg/m^2/week for 6 weeks
Doxorubicin, I.V., 60 mg/m^2, week 6
6-week rest period, then
Dactinomycin, I.V., 15 mcg/kg/day, for 5 days, followed 9 days later by
Vincristine + cyclophosphamide as above, given weekly for 5 weeks, and with
Doxorubicin given with the last treatment
or
Vincristine, I.V., 1.4 mg/m^2, day 1
Doxorubicin, I.V., 50 mg/m^2, day 1
Cyclophosphamide, I.V., 750 mg/m^2, day 1

VAC

Vincristine, I.V., 2 mg/m^2, day 1
Dactinomycin, I.V., 1 mg/m^2, day 1
Cyclophosphamide, I.V., 600 mg/m^2, day 1
or
Vincristine, I.V., 1.5 mg/m^2, day 1
Dactinomycin, I.V., 25 mcg/kg, day 1
Cyclophosphamide, I.V., 1.5 g/m^2, day 1

Repeat cycle every 21 days

VACAdr-IfoVP

Vincristine, I.V., 1.5 mg/m^2 (max: 2 mg), weekly
Dactinomycin, I.V., 1.5 mg/m^2 (max: 2 mg), every other week
Doxorubicin, I.V., 60 mg/m^2 continuous infusion over 24 hours
Cyclophosphamide, I.V., 1-1.5 g/m^2
Ifosfamide, I.V., 1.6-2 g/m^2, days 1-5
Etoposide, I.V., 150 mg/m^2, days 1-5

Sarcoma (Bony and Soft Tissue) *(continued)*

VAdrC
Vincristine, I.V., 1.5 mg/m^2 (max: 2 mg)
Doxorubicin, I.V., 35-60 mg/m^2
Cyclophosphamide, I.V., 500-1500 mg/m^2

Wilms' Tumor

VAD
Vincristine, I.V., 1.5 mg/m^2/week for 10 weeks, then every 3 weeks
Dactinomycin, I.V., 1.5 mg/m^2, every 3 weeks, alternating with
Doxorubicin, I.V., 40 mg/m^2, every 3 weeks

or

Vincristine, I.V., 1.5 mg/m^2, every 6 weeks
Dactinomycin, I.V., 15 mcg/kg x 5

or

60 mcg/kg I.V. x 1 every 6 weeks ± (add if stage III or IV)
Doxorubicin, I.V., 20 mg/m^2, every 6 weeks

HERBS AND COMMON NATURAL AGENTS

The authors have chosen to include this list of natural products and their reported uses. Due to limited scientific evidence to support these uses, the information provided here is not intended as a cure for any disease, and should not be construed as curative or healing. In addition, the reader is strongly encouraged to seek other references that discuss this information in more detail, and that discuss important issues such as contraindications, warnings, precautions, adverse reactions, and interactions.

PROPOSED MEDICINAL CLAIMS

Herb	Reported Uses
Acetyl-L-carnitine (ALC)	Alzheimer's disease; depression; diabetic peripheral neuropathy
Adrenal extract	Fatigue; stress
Aloe (*Aloe supp*)	Healing agent in wounds, minor burns, and other minor skin irritations
Alpha-Lipoic acid	Diabetes, diabetic neuropathy; glaucoma; prevention of cataracts; prevention of neurologic disorders, including stroke
Androstenedione	Increase strength and muscle mass
Aortic extract	Enhancement of the function, structure, and integrity of arteries and veins; helps to protect against various forms of vascular disease, including atherosclerosis, cerebral and peripheral arterial insufficiency, varicose veins, hemorrhoids, and vascular retinopathies such as macular degeneration
Arabinoxylane	Decreases chemotherapy-induced leukopenia; immune system enhancement (antiviral and anticancer activity); reported useful in HIV infection
Arginine	Helps lower elevated cholesterol; improvement in circulation; increases lean body mass; inflammatory bowel disease; immune enhancement; male infertility; surgery and wound healing; sexual vitality and enhancement
Artichoke (*Cynara scolymus*)	Eczema and other dermatologic problems; hepatic protection/stimulation; hypercholesterolemia; improvement in bile flow
Ashwagandha (*Withania somnifera*)	Adaptogen; chemotherapy and radiation protection; general tonic; stress, fatigue, nervous exhaustion
Astragalus (*Astragalus membranaceus*) [Milk Vetch]	Adaptogen (tonic-enhanced endurance, stamina); improvement in immune function and disease resistance; improvement in tissue oxygenation; support for chemotherapy and radiation
Bacopa (*Bacopa monniera*)	Memory enhancement and improvement of cognitive function
Beta-Carotene	Cancer prevention; cervical dysplasia; immunostimulant; photoprotection (erythropoietic protoporphyria)
Betaine hydrochloride	Digestive aid (hypochlorhydria and achlorhydria)
Bifidobacterium bifidum (*bifidus*)	Crohn's disease; diarrhea; maintenance of anaerobic microflora in the colon; ulcerative colitis
Bilberry (*Vaccinium myrtillus*)	Ophthalmologic disorders (antioxidant) including myopia, diminished acuity, dark adaptation, macular degeneration, night blindness, diabetic retinopathy, cataracts; vascular disorders including varicose veins, capillary permeability/stability, phlebitis
Biotin	Brittle nails; diabetes; diabetic neuropathy; seborrheic dermatitis; uncombable hair syndrome
Bismuth	Ulcers
Bitter melon (*Momordica charantia*)	Antiviral; hypoglycemic, impaired glucose tolerance (IGT)

(continued)

Herb	Reported Uses
Black cohosh (*Cimicifuga racemosa*)	Vasomotor symptoms of menopause; premenstrual syndrome (PMS), mild depression, arthritis
Bladderwrack (*Fucus vesiculosus*)	Rich source of iodine, potassium, magnesium, calcium, and iron; hypothyroidism; fibrocystic breast disease
Boron	Osteoarthritis; osteoporosis; rheumatoid arthritis
Boswellia (*Boswellia serrata*)	Anti-inflammatory; ulcerative colitis, arthritis
Branched-chain amino acids (BCAAs)	Muscle development and improvement in lean body mass
Bromelain (*Anas comosus*)	Digestive enzyme; proteolytic, anti-inflammatory (arthritis); sinusitis
Bupleurum (*Bupleurum falcatum*)	Chronic inflammatory disease; liver support
Calcium	Blood pressure regulation; cancer prevention; elevated cholesterol; hypertension; kidney stones; PMS; pregnancy; prevention of osteoporosis
Calendula (*Calendula officinalis*)	Antibacterial, antifungal, antiviral, antiprotozoal; vulnerary; wound-healing agent (increases wound healing by stimulating immune system)
Caprylic acid	Antifungal/antiyeast; dysbiosis
Carnitine	Congestive heart failure (CHF); enhanced athletic performance; hyperlipidemia; male infertility; weight loss
Cascara (*Rhamnus purshiana*)	Anthranquinone laxative
Cat's claw (*Uncaria tomentosa*)	Anti-inflammatory; antimicrobial (antibacterial, antifungal, antiviral); antioxidant; immunosupportive
Cayenne (*Capsicum annuum, Capsicum frutescens*)	Cardiovascular circulatory support; digestive stimulant; inflammation and pain (topical)
Chamomile, German (*Matricaria chamomilla, Matricaria recutita*)	Carminative, antispasmotic; mild sedative; anxiolytic; mouth rinse and gargle (for oral health); topical anti-inflammatory; uterine tonic
Chasteberry (*Vitex agnus-castus*)	Acne vulgaris; corpus luteum insufficiency; hyperprolactinemia and insufficient lactation; menopause; menstrual disorders, including amenorrhea, endometriosis, premenstrual syndrome
Chitosan	Weight reduction
Chlorophyll	Absorbs and suppresses odors, which makes it useful in breath fresheners, toothpastes, mouthwashes, and deodorants; anti-inflammatory, antioxidant, and wound-healing properties; exhibits bacteriostatic properties; protects against toxins
Chondroitin sulfate	Osteoarthritis
Chromium	Atherosclerosis; elevated cholesterol; elevated triglycerides; glaucoma; hypoglycemia; type 1 diabetes; type 2 diabetes; weight loss
Clove (*Syzygium aromaticum*)	Antiseptic; symptomatic relief of toothache and teething problems
Coenzyme Q_{10}	Angina; adjunct in chemotherapy; chronic fatigue syndrome; congestive heart failure (CHF); hypertension; muscular dystrophy; obesity; periodontal disease
Coleus (*Coleus forskohlii*)	Asthma, allergies; hypertension, congestive heart failure; eczema; psoriasis

(continued)

Herb	Reported Uses
Collagen (Type II)	Arthritis; first- and second-degree burns; pressure ulcers, venous stasis ulcers, diabetic ulcers (those resulting from arterial insufficiencies); surgical and traumatic wounds; topical application for wound healing
Colostrum	Antidiarrheal; antiviral; immunostimulant
Conjugated linoleic acid (CLA)	Increases metabolism, decreases body fat
Copper	Anemia; osteoporosis; rheumatoid arthritis
Cordyceps (*Cordyceps sinensis*)	Adaptogen/tonic (to promote wellness, longevity, and general health); adjunct support for chemotherapy and radiation; antioxidant; enhancement in cellular oxygenation during stress; reduction in symptoms of fatigue; immunomodulatory; enhancement of sexual vitality (males and females); hepatoprotection; improvement in endurance and stamina; support of lung, liver, and kidney function
Cranberry (*Vaccinium macrocarpon*)	Prevention of nephrolithiasis; urinary tract infection
Creatine	Enhancement of athletic performance (energy production and protein synthesis for muscle building)
Cyclo-hispro	Type 2 diabetes
Dandelion (*Taraxacum officinale*)	Leaf used as a diuretic; root used for disorders of bile secretion (cholerectic); appetite stimulation; dyspeptic complaints
Dehydroepiandrosterone (DHEA)	Antiaging; depression; diabetes; fatigue; lupus
Devil's claw (*Harpagophytum procumbens*)	Anti-inflammatory; back pain; osteoarthritis, gout, and other inflammatory conditions
Docosahexaenoic acid (DHA)	Alzheimer's disease; attention deficit disorder (ADD) and attention deficit hyperactivity disorder; Crohn's disease; diabetes; eczema, psoriasis; elevated triglycerides; hypertension; rheumatoid arthritis
Dong quai (*Angelica sinensis*)	Anemia; hypertension; improvement in energy, particularly in females; menopause, dysmenorrhea, premenstrual syndrome (PMS), and amenorrhea; phytoestrogen
Echinacea (*Echinacea purpurea, Echinacea angustifolia*)	Antiviral; arthritis (*E. augustifolia*); immunostimulant (colds and other upper respiratory infection); topical anti-infective (boils, abscesses, tonsillitis)
Elder (*Sambucus nigra, Sambucus canadensis*)	Berry used as an antiviral, antioxidant, and for influenza; flower used as an anti-inflammatory, diaphoretic, diuretic, and for colds and influenza
Ephedra (*Ephedra sinica*)	Bronchodilator in asthma; decongestant in allergies, sinusitis, hay fever; thermogenic aid in weight loss
Evening primrose (*Oenothera biennis*)	Attention deficit disorder (ADD); diabetic neuropathy; eczema, dermatitis, and psoriasis; endometriosis; hyperglycemia; irritable bowel syndrome; multiple sclerosis; omega-G6 fatty acid supplementation; PMS and menopause; rheumatoid arthritis
Eyebright (*Euphrasia officinalis*)	Eye fatigue; catarrh of the eyes
Fenugreek (*Trigonella foenum-graecum*)	Support of blood sugar regulation
Feverfew (*Tanacetum parthenium*)	Anti-inflammatory, rheumatoid arthritis; prevention of migraine headaches
Fish oils	Crohn's disease; diabetes; dysmenorrhea; eczema, psoriasis; hypertension; hypertriglyceridemia; memory enhancement; rheumatoid arthritis

(continued)

Herb	Reported Uses
Flaxseed oil	Source of omega-3 essential fatty acid; integral part of structure of cell walls and cellular membranes; necessary for the transport and oxidation of cholesterol; precursor for prostaglandins
Folic acid	Alcoholism; anemia; atherosclerosis; cancer prevention (colon and breast); cervical dysplasia; Crohn's disease; depression; gingivitis; osteoporosis; pregnancy (prevention of birth defects) and lactation
Garcinia (*Garcinia cambogia*)	Support of pancreas function and glucose regulation; weight reduction protocols
Garlic (*Allium sativum*)	Antimicrobial (bacteria and fungi); hypertension; may lower cholesterol and blood fats; mild inhibitor of platelet-activating factor; practitioners should be aware that aged garlic extracts have been reported to improve the antioxidant benefits; support of immune function
Ginger (*Zingiber officinale*)	Antiemetic; anti-inflammatory (musculoskeletal); GI distress and dyspepsia
Ginkgo (*Ginkgo biloba*)	Alzheimer's disease, dementia; asthma; increase peripheral blood flow (cerebral vascular disease, peripheral vascular insufficiency, impotence, tinnitus, and resistant depression); intermittent claudication; macular degeneration; memory enhancement; sexual dysfunction (antidepressant-induced)
Ginseng, Panax (*Panax ginseng*)	Adrenal tonic; enhancement of physical and mental performance; enhancement of energy levels; adaptation to stress; supports immune function; adjunct support for chemotherapy and radiation
Ginseng, Siberian (*Eleutherococcus senticosus*)	Adaptogen; beneficial in athletic performance; adaptation to stress (decreased fatigue); support of immune function
Glucosamine	Osteoarthritis; rheumatoid arthritis and other inflammatory conditions
Glutamine	Adjunct therapy for cancer; adjunct therapy for HIV; alcoholism; catabolic wasting processes; immunosupportive; peptic ulcers; performance enhancement; postsurgical healing; ulcerative colitis and other forms of inflammatory bowel disease
Glutathione	Hepatoprotection (alcohol-induced liver damage); immune system support; peptic ulcer disease
Golden seal (*Hydrastis canadensis*)	Mucous membrane tonifying (used in inflammation of mucosal membranes); gastritis; antimicrobial (antibacterial/antifungal); bronchitis, cystitis, and infectious diarrhea
Gotu kola (*Centella asiatica*)	Hemorrhoids (topical); memory enhancement; psoriasis; support/modulation of connective tissue synthesis; venous insufficiency; wound healing (topical)
Grapefruit seed (*Citrus paradisi*)	Antifungal, antibacterial, antiparasitic agent
Grape seed (*Vitis vinifera*)	Antioxidant; treatment of allergies, asthma; improve circulation; antiplatelet (blocks aggregation); improve capillary fragility; anti-inflammatory; arterial/venous insufficiency (intermittent claudication, varicose veins)
Green tea (*Camellia sinensis*)	Anticarcinogenic activity; antioxidant; support in cancer prevention and cardiovascular disease; chemotherapy and radiation; adjunct support for chemotherapy and radiation; may lower cholesterol; platelet-aggregation inhibitor
Ground ivy (*Hedera helix*)	Mucolytic action; upper respiratory congestion and cough
Guggul (*Commiphora mukul*)	May lower blood cholesterol levels
Gymnema (*Gymnema sylvestre*)	Diabetes, supports regulation of blood sugar levels
Hawthorn (*Crataegus oxyacantha*)	Angina, hypotension, hypertension, peripheral vascular disease, tachycardia; cardiotonic; congestive heart failure

(continued)

Herb	Reported Uses
Hops (*Humulus lupulus*)	Mild sedative and hypnotic
Horse chestnut (*Aesculus hippocastanum*)	Oral and topical used to treat varicose veins, hemorrhoids, other venous insufficiencies; deep venous thrombosis, lower extremity edema
Horsetail (*Equisetum arvense*)	Diuretic; high mineral content (including silicic acid); used to support bone and connective tissue strengthening, including osteoporosis
HuperzineA (*Huperzia serrata*)	Acetylcholinesterase inhibitor in senile dementia and Alzheimer's disease
Hydroxymethyl butyrate (HMB)	Increases muscle mass during intense exercise
5-Hydroxytryptophan (5-HTP)	Anxiety; depression; fibromyalgia; headache; migraine; obesity; sleep disorders, insomnia (stimulates the production of melatonin)
Inositol hexaphosphate (IP-6)	Anticancer agent
Iodine	Fibrocystic breast disease; goiter prevention; mucolytic agent
Ipriflavone	Prevention of and use in osteoporosis (men and women)
Iron	Anemia; menorrhagia; pregnancy; restless legs syndrome
Isoflavones (soy)	Cancer prevention; chemotherapy support; decreased bone loss; hypercholesterolemia; menopausal symptoms
Kava kava (*Piper methysticum*)	Anxiety; sedation; skeletal muscle relaxation; postischemic episodes
Lactobacillus acidophilus	Constipation; enhance immunity; hypercholesterolemia; infant diarrhea; lactose intolerance; recolonize the GI tract with beneficial bacteria during and after antibiotic use; vaginal candidiasis
Lavender (*Lavendula officinalis*)	Wound-healing agent (topical); minor burns (topical)
Lemon balm/Melissa (*Melissa officinalis*)	Antiviral agent (oral herpes virus); sedative agent (in pediatrics)
Licorice (*Glycyrrhiza glabra*)	Adrenal insufficiency (licorice); expectorant and antitussive (licorice); GI ulceration (DGL chewable products)
Liver extract	Liver tonic
Lutein	Cataracts; macular degeneration
Lycopene	Atherosclerosis; cancer prevention, especially prostate; macular degeneration
Lysine	Angina pectoris; herpes simplex; osteoporosis
Magnesium	Asthma; attention deficit hyperactivity disorder; cardiovascular disease; congestive heart failure (CHF); diabetes; epilepsy; fatigue; high blood pressure; kidney stones; migraine headaches; mitral valve prolapse (MVP); muscle cramps; nervousness; osteoporosis; premenstrual syndrome (PMS)
Malic acid	Aluminum toxicity; fibromyalgia
Manganese	Diabetes; epilepsy; osteoporosis
Marshmallow (*Althaea officinalis*)	Mucilaginous, demulcent; peptic ulceration
Mastic (*Pistacia lentiscus*)	*H. pylori* inhibitor; peptic ulcer disease
Melatonin	Insomnia; recovery from jet lag
Methionine	Liver detoxification
Methyl sulfonyl methane (MSM)	Analgesic; interstitial cystitis; lupus; osteoarthritis
Milk thistle (*Silybum marianum*)	Antidote for Poisoning by Death Cup mushroom; antioxidant, specifically for hepatic cells, liver diseases including acute/chronic hepatitis, jaundice, and stimulation of bile secretion/cholagogue; hepatoprotective, including drug toxicities (ie, phenothiazines, butyrophenones, ethanol, and acetaminophen)

(continued)

Herb	Reported Uses
Modified citrus pectin (MCP)	Anticancer activity; lowers cholesterol
Muira puama (*Ptychopetalum olacoides*)	Athletic performance enhancement; increased sexual vitality of males
N-Acetyl cysteine (NAC)	Acetaminophen toxicity; AIDS; asthma (mucolytic, antioxidant); bronchitis; cardioprotection during chemotherapy; fatigue; heavy metal detoxification; increases glutathione production
Nicotinamide adenine dinucleotide (NADH)	Chronic fatigue; Parkinson's disease; stamina and energy
Olive leaf (*Olea europaea*)	Antibiotic, antifungal, antiviral; hypoglycemic activity; antihypertensive activity
Pancreatic extract	Digestive disturbances; food allergies; celiac disease; anti-inflammatory; immune complex diseases; adjunct support for cancer therapy
Para-Aminobenzoic acid (PABA)	Peyronie's disease; scleroderma; vitiligo
Parsley (*Petroselinum crispum*)	Halitosis; antibacterial, antifungal
Passion flower (*Passiflora spp*)	Sedative
Peppermint (*Mentha piperita*)	Carminative, spasmolytic; irritable bowel syndrome
Phenylalanine	Reward deficiency syndrome in the treatment of addiction; depression; pain relief; vitiligo
Phosphatidyl choline (PC)	Alcohol-induced liver damage; Alzheimer's disease (may benefit some individuals); gallstones; hepatitis
Phosphatidyl serine (PS)	Alzheimer's disease; depression; memory enhancement
Potassium	Cardiac arrhythmias; congestive heart failure (CHF); hypertension; kidney stones
Pregnenolone	Arthritis; improved mental performance; natural precursor for the production of DHEA, cortisol, progesterone, estrogens, and testosterone in the body
Progesterone	Endometriosis; menopause symptoms; osteoporosis; PMS symptoms; prevention of breast cancer
Psyllium (*Plantago ovata, Plantago isphagula*)	Bulk-forming laxative (containing 10% to 30% mucilage)
Pygeum (*Pygeum africanum, Prunus africana*)	Symptoms associated with benign prostatic hyperplasia (BPH)
Pyruvate	Enhancement of athletic performance; obesity and weight loss
Quercetin	Allergies; atherosclerosis; cataracts; peptic ulcer
Red clover (*Trifolium pratense*)	Liquid extract used for liver detoxification and kidney detoxification; menopausal symptoms; proprietary extract contains 4 phytoestrogens
Red yeast rice (*Monascus purpureus*)	Hypercholesterolemic agent; may lower triglycerides and LDL cholesterol and raise HDL cholesterol
Rehmannia (*Rehmannia glutinosa*)	Immunosuppressive agent in rheumatoid arthritis
Reishi (*Ganoderma lucidum*)	Immunomodulation, fatigue, and hemo- and radioprotection, antihypertensive, anticonvulsive
SAMe (S-adenosyl methionine)	Cardiovascular disease; depression; fibromyalgia; insomnia; liver disease; osteoarthritis; rheumatoid arthritis

(continued)

Herb	Reported Uses
Saw palmetto (*Serenoa repens*)	Benign prostatic hyperplasia (BPH)
Schisandra (*Schizandra chinensis*)	Adaptogen/health tonic; hepatic protection and detoxification; adjunct support for chemotherapy and radiation; increased endurance, stamina, and work performance
Selenium	AIDS; atherosclerosis; bronchial asthma; cancer prevention; cardiomyopathy; cataracts; chemotherapy/radiation support; eczema
Senna (*Cassia senna*)	Anthraquinone laxative
Shark cartilage	Cancer therapy; osteoarthritis, rheumatoid arthritis
Spleen extract	Support following removal of the spleen or for individuals with weak spleen function
Stinging nettle (*Urtica dioica*)	Leaf used for allergic rhinitis; leaf increases uric acid excretion; root used for benign prostatic hyperplasia (BPH)
St John's wort (*Hypericum perforatum*)	Antiviral activity in increased doses; antibacterial, anti-inflammatory; used topically for minor wounds and infections; may be used topically for bruises, muscle soreness, and sprains; mild to moderate depression, melancholia, and anxiety
Taurine	Congestive heart failure (CHF); diabetes; epilepsy; hypertension
Tea tree (*Melaleuca alternifolia*)	**Not for ingestion**; as an antifungal, antibacterial; mouthwash for dental and oral health; burns, cuts, scrapes, insect bites
Thyme (*Thymus vulgaris*)	Antifungal; coughs and upper respiratory congestion
Thymus extract	Immunostimulant
Thyroid extract	Fatigue; immune support
Tocotrienols	Heart disease, high cholesterol; cancer prevention; protection from ultraviolet light, protection of the skin
Tribulus (*Tribulus terrestris*)	Steroidal properties (enhancement of athletic performance, increased sexual vitality)
Turmeric (*Curcuma longa*)	Antioxidant; anti-inflammatory; antirheumatic, used in arthritic problems; may lower blood lipid levels
Tylophora (*Tylophora asthmatica*)	Allergies; used in bronchial asthma
Tyrosine	Alzheimer's disease; depression; hypothyroidism; phenylketonuria (PKU); substance abuse
Uva-Ursi (*Arctostaphylos uva-ursi*)	Urinary tract infections and kidney stone prevention
Valerian (*Valeriana officinalis*)	Sedative or hypnotic; nervous tension during PMS, menopause; restless motor syndromes and muscle spasms
Vanadium	Type 1 diabetes; type 2 diabetes
Vinpocetine	Enhanced cognitive function; increased brain function (cerebral metabolic enhancing agent)
Vitamin A (Retinol)	Acne; AIDS; cancer prevention; cervical dysplasia; Crohn's disease; measles; menorrhagia; night blindness; PMS; ulcerative colitis
Vitamin B_1 (Thiamine)	Alcoholism; Alzheimer's disease; anemia (megaloblastic); congestive heart failure (CHF); diabetes; insomnia; neurological conditions (Bell's palsy, trigeminal neuralgia, sciatica, sensory neuropathies); psychiatric illness
Vitamin B_2	Cataracts; depression; migraine
Vitamin B_3	Acne vulgaris (4% niacinamide topical gel); cataracts; hyperlipidemia (hypercholesterolemia, hypertriglyceridemia); impaired glucose tolerance; intermittent claudication; osteoarthritis; prevention of myocardial infarction; Raynaud's syndrome; rheumatoid arthritis; schizophrenia; type 1 diabetes of recent onset; type 2 diabetes

APPENDIX

(continued)

Herb	Reported Uses
Vitamin B$_5$ (Pantothenic acid)	Adrenal support; allergies; arthritis; constipation; hyperlipidemia (pantethine, but not pantothenic acid, lowers cholesterol and triglycerides); rheumatoid arthritis; surgery and wound healing
Vitamin B$_6$ (Pyridoxine)	Arthritis; asthma; autism; cardiovascular disease; carpal tunnel syndrome; depression associated with oral contraceptives; diabetic neuropathy; epilepsy, B$_6$-dependant; kidney stones; MSG sensitivity; nausea and vomiting in pregnancy; peptic ulcers; PMS
Vitamin B$_{12}$ (Cobalamin)	AIDS; atherosclerosis (due to homocysteine elevation); bronchial asthma; Crohn's disease; depression; diabetic neuropathy; male infertility; memory loss; multiple sclerosis; pernicious anemia; sulfite sensitivity
Vitamin B complex-25	See individual B vitamins
Vitamin C	AIDS; allergies; asthma; atherosclerosis; cancer; cataracts; cervical dysplasia; common cold; Crohn's disease; diabetes; gingivitis; immune enhancement; Parkinson's disease; peptic ulcer; sunburn; wound healing
Vitamin D	Crohn's disease; epilepsy during anticonvulsant therapy; hearing loss; osteoporosis; psoriasis; rickets; scleroderma
Vitamin E	Alzheimer's disease; atherosclerosis; Benign prostatic hyperplasia (BPH); cancer prevention; cataracts; cervical dysplasia; diabetes; dyslipidemias; lupus; osteoarthritis; peptic ulcer; peripheral circulation; PMS; prevention of myocardial infarction; rheumatoid arthritis; sunburn
Vitamin K	Osteoporosis; synthesis of blood clotting factors
White oak (*Quercus alba*)	Soothing agent in mild inflammation of the throat and mouth
White willow (*Salix alba*)	Antipyretic; anti-inflammatory; reducing fever and in arthritic complaints
Wild yam (*Dioscorea villosa*)	Contains steroidal precursors and used in female vitality, however, conversion to progesterone in the body is poor
Yohimbe (*Pausinystalia yohimbe*)	May increase sexual vitality in men and women; male erectile dysfunction
Zinc	Acne; apthous ulcers; benign prostatic hyperplasia (BPH); common cold; Crohn's disease; diabetes; diaper rash; gastric ulcer healing; immune function; macular degeneration; male sexual vitality; osteoporosis; skin conditions, eczema; wound healing

SOUND-ALIKE COMPARISON LIST

The following list contains over 2000 pairs of sound-alike drugs accompanied by a subjective pronunciation of each drug name. Any such list can only suggest possible pronunciation or enunciation miscues and is by no means meant to be exhaustive.

New or rarely used drugs are likely to cause the most problems related to interpretation. Healthcare workers should be made aware of the existence of both drugs in a sound-alike pair in order to avoid (or minimize) the potential for error. Drug companies attempt to avoid naming different drugs with similar-sounding names; however, mix-ups do occur. Reading current drug advertisements, professional literature, and drug handbooks is a good way to avert or surely lessen such sound-alike drug errors at all levels of the healthcare industry.

Drug Name	Pronunciation	Drug Name	Pronunciation
Accolate®	(ak' cue late)	Aciphex™	(a' si fecks)
Accupril®	(ak' yu pril)	Accupril®	(ak' cue pril)
Accolate®	(ak' cue late)	Aciphex™	(a' si fecks)
Accutane®	(ak' yu tane)	Acephen®	(a' ce fen)
Accolate®	(ak' cue late)	Aciphex™	(a' si fecks)
Aclovate®	(ak' lo vate)	Aricept®	(ar' e cept)
Accubron®	(ak' cue bron)	Aclovate®	(ak' lo vate)
Accutane®	(ak' yu tane)	Accolate®	(ak' cue late)
Accupril®	(ak' cue pril)	Acthar®	(ac' thar)
Accolate®	(ak' cue late)	Acthrel®	(ak' threl)
Accupril®	(ak' cue pril)	Acthar®	(ac' thar)
Accutane®	(ak' yu tane)	Acular®	(ac' yu lar)
Accupril®	(ak' cue pril)	Acthrel®	(ak' threl)
Aciphex™	(a' si fecks)	Acthar®	(ac' thar)
Accupril®	(ak' cue pril)	Actidose®	(ac' ti dose)
Monopril®	(mon' oh pril)	Actos®	(ac' tose)
Accutane®	(ak' yu tane)	actinomycin	(ak ti noe mye' sin)
Accolate®	(ak' cue late)	Achromycin®	(ak roe mye' sin)
Accutane®	(ak' yu tane)	Actos®	(ac' tose)
Accubron®	(ak' cue bron)	Actidose®	(ac' ti dose)
Accutane®	(ak' yu tane)	Acular®	(ac' yu lar)
Accupril®	(ak' cue pril)	Acthar®	(ac' thar)
Acephen®	(a' ce fen)	adapalene	(ah dap' ah lene)
Aciphex™	(a' si fecks)	Adapin®	(ad' ah pin)
acetazolamide	(ah set ah zole' ah mide)	Adapin®	(ad' ah pin)
acetohexamide	(ah set oh heks' ah mide)	adapalene	(ah dap' ah lene)
acetohexamide	(ah set oh heks' ah mide)	Adapin®	(ad' ah pin)
acetazolamide	(ah set ah zole' ah mide)	Adipex-P®	(ad' di pex-pea)
acetylcholine	(a se teel koe' leen)	Adapin®	(ad' ah pin)
acetylcysteine	(a se teel sis' teen)	Ativan®	(at' tee van)
acetylcysteine	(a se teel sis' teen)	Adderall®	(ad' der all)
acetylcholine	(a se teel koe' leen)	Inderal®	(in' der al)
Achromycin®	(ak roe mye' sin)	Adeflor®	(a' de flor)
actinomycin	(ak ti noe mye' sin)	Aldoclor®	(al' do klor)
Achromycin®	(ak roe mye' sin)	Adipex-P®	(ad' di pex-pea)
Adriamycin™	(ade rya mye' sin)	Adapin®	(ad' ah pin)

757

APPENDIX

Drug Name	Pronunciation	Drug Name	Pronunciation
Adriamycin™ Achromycin®	(ade rya mye' sin) (ak roe mye' sin)	Aldomet® Aldoril®	(al' doe met) (al' doe ril)
Adriamycin™ Aredia®	(ade rya mye' sin) (ah red' de ah)	Aldomet® Anzemet®	(al' doe met) (an' ze met)
Adriamycin™ Idamycin®	(ade rya mye' sin) (eye da mye' sin)	Aldoril® Aldoclor®	(al' doe ril) (al' do klor)
Aerolone® Aralen®	(air' oh lone) (air' ah len)	Aldoril® Aldomet®	(al' doe ril) (al' doe met)
Afrin® aspirin	(aye' frin or af' rin) (as' pir in)	Aldoril® Elavil®	(al' doe ril) (el' ah vil)
Afrinol® Arfonad®	(af' ree nol) (arr' foe nad)	Alesse™ Aleve®	(ah less') (ah leve')
Aggrastat® Aggrenox™	(ag' gra stat) (ag' gro noks)	Aleve® Alesse™	(ah leve') (ah less')
Aggrenox™ Aggrastat®	(ag' gro noks) (ag' gra stat)	Alfenta® Sufenta®	(al fen' tah) (sue fen' tah)
Akarpine® atropine	(ay kar' peen) (a' troe peen)	alfentanil Anafranil®	(al fen' ta nil) (ah naf' ra nil)
AK-Mycin® Akne-Mycin®	(aye kay-mye' sin) (ak nee-mye' sin)	alfentanil fentanyl	(al fen' ta nil) (fen' ta nil)
Akne-Mycin® AK-Mycin®	(ak nee-mye' sin) (aye kay-mye' sin)	alfentanil remifentanil	(al fen' ta nil) (rem i fen' ta nil)
AKTob® AK-Trol®	(ak' tobe) (aye' kay-trol)	alfentanil sufentanil	(al fen' ta nil) (sue fen' ta nil)
AK-Trol® AKTob®	(aye' kay-trol) (ak' tobe)	Alferon® Alkeran®	(al' fer on) (al' ker an)
Albutein® albuterol	(al byoo' teen) (al byoo' ter ole)	Alkeran® Alferon®	(al' ker an) (al' fer on)
albuterol Albutein®	(al byoo' ter ole) (al byoo' teen)	Alkeran® Leukeran®	(al' ker an) (lu' keh ran)
albuterol atenolol	(al byoo' ter ole) (ah ten' oh lole)	Allegra® Viagra®	(al leg' ra) (vye ag' ra)
Alcaine® Alcare®	(al' kain) (al' kare)	Allerest® Sinarest®	(al' e rest) (sy' na rest)
Alcare® Alcaine®	(al' kare) (al' kain)	Allergan® Auralate®	(al' er gan) (ahl' ah late)
Aldactazide® Aldactone®	(al dak' ta zide) (al' dak tone)	allopurinol Apresoline®	(al oh pure' i nole) (aye press' sow leen)
Aldactone® Aldactazide®	(al' dak tone) (al dak' ta zide)	Alora® Aldara™	(a lor' a) (al dar' a)
Aldara™ Alora®	(al dar' a) (a lor' a)	alprazolam alprostadil	(al pray' zoe lam) (al pros' ta dil)
aldesleukin oprelvekin	(al des lu' kin) (oh prel' ve kin)	alprazolam lorazepam	(al pray' zoe lam) (lor a' ze pam)
Aldoclor® Adeflor®	(al' do klor) (a' de flor)	alprazolam triazolam	(al pray' zoe lam) (trye ay' zoe lam)
Aldoclor® Aldoril®	(al' do klor) (al' doe ril)	alprostadil alprazolam	(al pros' ta dil) (al pray' zoe lam)

Drug Name	Pronunciation	Drug Name	Pronunciation
Altace™ alteplase	(al' tase) (al' te place)	amiloride amlodipine	(ah mil' oh ride) (am lo' di pine)
Altace™ Amaryl®	(al' tase) (am' ah ril)	aminophylline amitriptyline	(am in off' i lin) (ah mee' trip ti leen)
Altace™ Amerge®	(al' tase) (ah merge')	aminophylline ampicillin	(am in off' i lin) (am pi sil' in)
Altace™ Artane®	(al' tase) (ar' tane)	amiodarone amiloride	(ah mee' oh da rone) (ah mil' oh ride)
Altenol® atenolol	(al ten' ol) (ah ten' oh lole)	amiodarone amrinone	(ah mee' oh da rone) (am' ri none)
alteplase Altace™	(al' te place) (al' tase)	amitriptyline aminophylline	(ah mee' trip ti leen) (am in off' I lin)
alteplase anistreplase	(al' te place) (ah nis' tre place)	amitriptyline imipramine	(ah mee trip' ti leen) (im ip' ra meen)
Alupent® Atrovent®	(al' yu pent) (at' troe vent)	amitriptyline nortriptyline	(ah mee trip' ti leen) (nor trip' ti leen)
amantadine ranitidine	(ah man' ta deen) (ra ni' ti deen)	amlodipine amiloride	(am lo' di pine) (ah mil' oh ride)
amantadine rimantadine	(ah man' ta deen) (ri man' ta deen)	amoxapine amoxicillin	(ah moks' ah peen) (a moks i sil' in)
Amaryl® Altace™	(am' ah ril) (al' tase)	amoxapine Amoxil®	(ah moks' ah peen) (ay moks' il)
Amaryl® Ambenyl®	(am' ah ril) (am' ba nil)	amoxicillin amoxapine	(a moks i sil' in) (ah moks' ah peen)
Amaryl® Amerge®	(am' ah ril) (ah merge')	amoxicillin Amoxil®	(a moks i sil' in) (ay moks' il)
Ambenyl® Amaryl®	(am' ba nil) (am' ah ril)	amoxicillin Atarax®	(a moks i sil' in) (at' ah raks)
Ambenyl® Aventyl®	(am' ba nil) (ah ven' til)	Amoxil® amoxapine	(ay moks' il) (ah moks' ah peen)
Ambi 10® Ambien®	(am' bee ten') (am' bee en)	Amoxil® amoxicillin	(ay moks' il) (a moks i sil' in)
Ambien® Ambi 10®	(am' bee en) (am' bee ten')	ampicillin aminophylline	(am pi sil' in) (am in off' i lin)
Amerge® Altace™	(ah merge') (al' tase)	amrinone amiodarone	(am' ri none) (ah mee' oh da rone)
Amerge® Amaryl®	(ah merge') (am' ah ril)	Anafranil® alfentanil	(ah naf' ra nil) (al fen' ta nill)
Amicar® amikacin	(am' i car) (am i kay' sin)	Anafranil® enalapril	(ah naf' ra nil) (e nal' ah pril)
Amicar® Amikin®	(am' i car) (am' i kin)	Anafranil® nafarelin	(ah naf' ra nil) (naf' ah re lin)
amikacin Amicar®	(am i kay' sin) (am' i car)	Anaprox® Anaspaz®	(an' ah prox) (an' ah spaz)
Amikin® Amicar®	(am' i kin) (am' i car)	Anaprox® Avapro®	(an' ah prox) (ah' va pro)
amiloride amiodarone	(ah mil' oh ride) (ah mee' oh da rone)	Anaspaz® Anaprox®	(an' ah spaz) (an' ah prox)

Drug Name	Pronunciation	Drug Name	Pronunciation
Anaspaz® Antispas®	(an' ah spaz) (an' te spaz)	Aplitest® Aplisol®	(ap' le test) (ap' lee sol)
Ancobon® Oncovin®	(an' coe bon) (on' coe vin)	Apresazide® Apresoline®	(ay pre' sa zide) (aye press' sow leen)
anisindione anisotropine	(ah nis in dy' one) (an iss oh troe' peen)	Apresoline® allopurinol	(aye press' sow leen) (al oh pure' i nole)
anisotropine anisindione	(an iss oh troe' peen) (ah nis in dy' one)	Apresoline® Apresazide®	(aye press' sow leen) (ay pre' sa zide)
anistreplase alteplase	(ah nis' tre place) (al' te place)	Apresoline® Priscoline®	(aye press' sow leen) (pris' coe leen)
Ansaid® Asacol®	(an' said) (as' ah col)	Aprodine® Aphrodyne®	(ap' roe dine) (af' roe dine)
Ansaid® Axid®	(an' said) (aks' id)	Aquasol® Anusol®	(ah' kwa sol) (an' yu sol)
Ansaid® Axsain®	(an' said) (aks' ane)	Aquatag® AquaTar®	(ah' kwa tag) (ah' kwa tar)
Antabuse® Anturane®	(an ta byoose') (ann' chu rane)	AquaTar® Aquatag®	(ah' kwa tar) (ah' kwa tag)
Antispas® Anaspaz®	(an' te spaz) (an' ah spaz)	ara-C Arasine®	(ah ra-cee') (ah ra seen')
Antril® enalapril	(an' trill) (e nal' ah pril)	Aralen® Aerolone®	(air' ah len) (air' oh lone)
Anturane® Antabuse®	(ann' chu rane) (an ta byoose')	Aramine® Arasine®	(air' ah meen) (ah ra seen')
Anturane® Artane®	(ann' chu rane) (ar' tane)	Aramine® Artane®	(air' ah meen) (ar' tane)
Anusol® Anusol-HC®	(an' yu sol) (an' yu sol-aych cee)	Arasine® ara-C	(ah ra seen') (ah ra-cee')
Anusol® Aplisol®	(an' yu sol) (ap' lee sol)	Arasine® Aramine®	(ah ra seen') (air' ah meen)
Anusol® Aquasol®	(an' yu sol) (ah' kwa sol)	Aredia® Adriamycin®	(ah red' de ah) (ade rya mye' sin)
Anusol-HC® Anusol®	(an' yu sol-aych cee) (an' yu sol)	Arfonad® Afrinol®	(arr' foe nad) (af' ree nol)
Anzemet® Aldomet®	(an' ze met) (al' doe met)	Aricept® Aciphex™	(ar' e cept) (a' si fecks)
Aphrodyne® Aprodine®	(af' roe dine) (ap' roe dine)	Aricept® Ascriptin®	(ar' e cept) (ah srip' tin)
A.P.L.® Aplisol®	(aye pee el') (ap' lee sol)	Artane® Altace®	(ar' tane) (al' tase)
Aplisol® Anusol®	(ap' lee sol) (an' yu sol)	Artane® Anturane®	(ar' tane) (an' chu rane)
Aplisol® A.P.L.®	(ap' lee sol) (aye pee el')	Artane® Aramine®	(ar' tane) (air' ah meen)
Aplisol® Aplitest®	(ap' lee sol) (ap' le test)	Asacol® Ansaid®	(as' ah col) (an' said)
Aplisol® Atropisol®	(ap' lee sol) (a troe' pi sol)	Asacol® Os-Cal®	(as' ah col) (os'-cal)

Drug Name	Pronunciation	Drug Name	Pronunciation
Ascriptin®	(ah srip' tin)	Augmentin®	(aug men' tin)
Aricept®	(ar' e cept)	Azulfidine®	(ay zul' fi deen)
Asendin®	(ah sen' din)	Auralate®	(ahl' ah late)
aspirin	(as' pir in)	Allergan®	(al' er gan)
asparaginase	(ah spir' ah ji nase)	Auralgan®	(ah ral' gan)
pegaspargase	(peg as' par jase)	Larylgan®	(la ril' gan)
aspirin	(as' pir in)	Auralgan®	(ah ral' gan)
Afrin®	(aye' frin or af' rin)	Ophthalgan®	(opp thal' gan)
aspirin	(as' pir in)	Avalide®	(av' ah lide)
Asendin®	(ah sen' din)	Avandia®	(ah van' de a)
Atarax®	(at' ah raks)	Avandia®	(ah van' de a)
amoxicillin	(a moks i sil' in)	Avalide®	(av' ah lide)
Atarax®	(at' ah raks)	Avandia®	(ah van' de a)
Ativan®	(at' tee van)	Coumadin®	(ku' ma din)
atenolol	(ah ten' oh lole)	Avandia®	(ah van' de a)
albuterol	(al byoo' ter ole)	Prandin™	(pran' din)
atenolol	(ah ten' oh lole)	Avapro®	(ah' va pro)
Altenol®	(al ten' ol)	Anaprox®	(an' ah prox)
atenolol	(ah ten' oh lole)	Avelox™	(av' e loks)
timolol	(tye' moe lole)	Avonex™	(av' oh neks)
atenolol	(ah ten' oh lole)	Aventyl®	(ah ven' til)
Tylenol®	(tye' le nole)	Ambenyl®	(am' ba nil)
Atgam®	(at' gam)	Aventyl®	(ah ven' til)
Ativan®	(at' tee van)	Bentyl®	(ben' till)
Atgam®	(at' gam)	Avitene®	(aye' va teen)
ratgam	(rat' gam)	Ativan®	(at' tee van)
Ativan®	(at' tee van)	Avonex™	(av' oh neks)
Adapin®	(ad' ah pin)	Avelox™	(av' e loks)
Ativan®	(at' tee van)	Axid®	(aks' id)
Atarax®	(at' ah raks)	Ansaid®	(an' said)
Ativan®	(at' tee van)	Axsain®	(aks' ane)
Atgam®	(at' gam)	Ansaid®	(an' said)
Ativan®	(at' tee van)	azatadine	(ah za' ta deen)
ATnativ®	(aye tee nay' tif)	azathioprine	(ay za thye' oh preen)
Ativan®	(at' tee van)	azathioprine	(ay za thye' oh preen)
Avitene®	(aye' va teen)	azatadine	(ah za' ta deen)
ATnativ®	(aye tee nay' tif)	azathioprine	(ay za thye' oh preen)
Ativan®	(at' tee van)	azidothymidine	(ay zi doe thy' mi dine)
atropine	(a' troe peen)	azathioprine	(ay za thye' oh preen)
Akarpine®	(ay kar' peen)	Azulfidine®	(ay zul' fi deen)
Atropisol®	(a troe' pi sol)	azidothymidine	(ay zi doe thy' mi dine)
Aplisol®	(ap' lee sol)	azathioprine	(ay za thye' oh preen)
Atrovent®	(at' troe vent)	azithromycin	(az ith roe mye' sin)
Alupent®	(al' yu pent)	erythromycin	(er ith roe mye' sin)
Atrovent®	(at' troe vent)	Azulfidine®	(ay zul' fi deen)
Natru-Vent®	(nay' tru-vent)	Augmentin®	(aug men' tin)
Attenuvax®	(at ten' yu vaks)	Azulfidine®	(ay zul' fi deen)
Meruvax®	(mur' yu vaks)	azathioprine	(ay za thye' oh preen)

Drug Name	Pronunciation	Drug Name	Pronunciation
bacitracin	(bas i tray' sin)	Bentyl®	(ben' till)
Bactrim®	(bak' trim)	Cantil®	(can' til)
bacitracin	(bas i tray' sin)	Bentyl®	(ben' til)
Bactroban®	(bak' troe ban)	Proventil®	(pro ven' till)
baclofen	(bak' loe fen)	Bentyl®	(ben' til)
Bactroban®	(bak' troe ban)	Trental®	(tren' tal)
baclofen	(bak' loe fen)	Benylin®	(ben' eh lin)
Beclovent®	(bec' lo vent)	Benadryl®	(ben' ah drill)
Bactine®	(bak' teen)	Benylin®	(ben' eh lin)
Bactrim®	(bak' trim)	Ventolin®	(ven' tow lin)
Bactrim®	(bak' trim)	Benza®	(ben' zah)
bacitracin	(bas i tray' sin)	Benzac®	(ben' zak)
Bactrim®	(bak' trim)	Benzac®	(ben' zak)
Bactine®	(bak' teen)	Benza®	(ben' zah)
Bactroban®	(bak' troe ban)	benztropine	(benz' troe peen)
bacitracin	(bas i tray' sin)	bromocriptine	(broe moe krip' teen)
Bactroban®	(bak' troe ban)	Bepridil®	(be' pri dil)
baclofen	(bak' loe fen)	Prepidil®	(pre' pi dil)
Banophen®	(ban' oh fen)	Betadine®	(bay' ta deen)
Barophen®	(bear' oh fen)	Betagan®	(bay' ta gan)
Barophen®	(bear' oh fen)	Betadine®	(bay' ta deen)
Banophen®	(ban' oh fen)	betaine	(bay' tayne)
Beclovent®	(bec' lo vent)	Betagan®	(bay' ta gan)
baclofen	(bak' loe fen)	Betadine®	(bay' ta deen)
Beminal®	(bem' eh nall)	Betagan®	(bay' ta gan)
Benemid®	(ben' ah mid)	Betagen®	(bay' ta gen)
Benadryl®	(ben' ah drill)	Betagen®	(bay' ta gen)
benazepril	(ban ay' ze pril)	Betagan®	(bay' ta gan)
Benadryl®	(ben' ah drill)	Betagen®	(bay' ta gen)
Bentyl®	(ben' till)	Betoptic®	(bay top' ik)
Benadryl®	(ben' ah drill)	betaine	(bay' tayne)
Benylin®	(ben' eh lin)	Betadine®	(bay' ta deen)
Benadryl®	(ben' ah drill)	Betapace®	(bay' ta pase)
Caladryl®	(kal' ah drill)	Betapace AF™	(bay' ta pase ay eff)
benazepril	(ban ay' ze pril)	Betapace AF™	(bay' ta pase ay eff)
Benadryl®	(ben' ah drill)	Betapace®	(bay' ta pase)
Benemid®	(ben' ah mid)	betaxolol	(be taks' oh lol)
Beminal®	(bem' eh nall)	bethanechol	(be than' e kole)
Benoxyl®	(ben ox' ill)	betaxolol	(be taks' oh lol)
Brevoxyl®	(brev ox' il)	labetalol	(la bet' ah lole)
Benoxyl®	(ben ox' ill)	bethanechol	(be than' e kole)
Peroxyl®	(per ox' ill)	betaxolol	(be taks' oh lol)
Bentyl®	(ben' till)	Betoptic®	(bay top' ik)
Aventyl®	(ah ven' til)	Betagen®	(bay' ta gen)
Bentyl®	(ben' till)	Bicillin®	(bye sil' lin)
Benadryl®	(ben' ah drill)	Wycillin®	(wye sil' lin)
Bentyl®	(ben' till)	bleomycin	(blee oh mye' sin)
Bontril®	(bon' trill)	Cleocin®	(klee' oh sin)

Drug Name	Pronunciation
Bleph®-10 Blephamide®	(blef-ten') (blef' ah mide)
Blephamide® Bleph®-10	(blef' ah mide) (blef-ten')
Bontril® Bentyl®	(bon' trill) (ben' till)
Borofax® Boropak®	(boroe' faks) (boroe' pak)
Boropak® Borofax®	(boroe' pak) (boroe' faks)
Brevibloc® Brevital®	(brev' i block) (brev' i tall)
Brevibloc® Bumex®	(brev' i block) (byoo' mex)
Brevibloc® Buprenex®	(brev' i block) (byoo' pre nex)
Brevital® Brevibloc®	(brev' i tall) (brev' i block)
Brevoxyl® Benoxyl®	(brev ox' il) (ben ox' ill)
brimonidine bromocriptine	(bri moe' ni deen) (broe moe krip' teen)
Bromfed® Bromphen®	(brom' fed) (brom' fen)
bromocriptine benztropine	(broe moe krip' teen) (benz' troe peen)
bromocriptine brimonidine	(broe moe krip' teen) (bri moe' ni deen)
Bromphen® Bromfed®	(brom' fen) (brom' fed)
bumetanide Buminate®	(byoo met' ah nide) (byoo' mi nate)
Bumex® Brevibloc®	(byoo' mex) (brev' i block)
Bumex® Buprenex®	(byoo' mex) (byoo' pre nex)
Bumex® Permax®	(byoo' mex) (per' max)
Buminate® bumetanide	(byoo' mi nate) (byoo met' ah nide)
bupivacaine mepivacaine	(byoo piv' ah kane) (me piv' ah kane)
bupivacaine ropivacaine	(byoo piv' ah kane) (roe piv' a kane)
Buprenex® Brevibloc®	(byoo' pre nex) (brev' i block)
Buprenex® Bumex®	(byoo' pre nex) (byoo' mex)

Drug Name	Pronunciation
bupropion buspirone	(byoo proe' pee on) (byoo spye' rone)
busalfan Butalan®	(byoo sul' fan) (byoo' ta lan)
buspirone bupropion	(byoo spye' rone) (byoo proe' pee on)
butabarbital butalbital	(byoo ta bar' bi tal) (byoo tal' bi tal)
Butalan® busalfan	(byoo' ta lan) (byoo sul' fan)
butalbital butabarbital	(byoo tal' bi tal) (byoo ta bar' bi tal)
Byclomine® Bydramine®	(bye' clo meen) (bye' dra meen)
Byclomine® Hycomine®	(bye' clo meen) (hye' coe meen)
Bydramine® Byclomine®	(bye' dra meen) (bye' clo meen)
Bydramine® Hydramyn®	(bye' dra meen) (hye' dra min)
Cafergot® Carafate®	(kaf' er got) (care' ah fate)
Caladryl® Benadryl®	(kal' ah drill) (ben' ah drill)
Caladryl® calamine	(kal' ah drill) (kal' ah mine)
calamine Caladryl®	(kal' ah mine) (kal' ah drill)
Calan® Colace®	(kal' an) (ko' lace)
calcifediol calcitriol	(kal si fe dye' ole) (kal si trye' ole)
Calciferol® calcitriol	(kal si' fer ole) (kal si trye' ole)
calcitonin calcitriol	(kal si toe' nin) (kal si trye' ole)
calcitriol calcifediol	(kal si trye' ole) (kal si fe dye' ole)
calcitriol Calciferol®	(kal si trye' ole) (kal si' fer ole)
calcitriol calcitonin	(kal si trye' ole) (kal si toe' nin)
calcium glubionate	(kal' see um gloo bye' oh nate)
calcium gluconate	(kal' see um gloo' koe nate)

APPENDIX

Drug Name	Pronunciation
calcium gluconate	(kal' see um gloo' koe nate)
calcium glubionate	(kal' see um gloo bye' oh nate)
Cantil®	(can' til)
Bentyl®	(ben' till)
Capastat®	(kap' ah stat)
Cepastat®	(sea' pa stat)
Capital®	(kap' i tal)
Capitrol®	(kap' i trol)
Capitrol®	(kap' i trol)
Capital®	(kap' i tal)
Capitrol®	(kap' i trol)
captopril	(kap' toe pril)
captopril	(kap' toe pril)
Capitrol®	(kap' i trol)
captopril	(kap' toe pril)
carvedilol	(kar' ve dil ole)
Carafate®	(care' ah fate)
Cafergot®	(kaf' er got)
Carbatrol®	(kar' ba trol)
Cartrol®	(kar' trol)
carboplatin	(kar' boe pla tin)
cisplatin	(sis' pla tin)
Cardene®	(kar' deen)
Cardizem®	(kar' di zem)
Cardene®	(kar' deen)
Cardura®	(kar dur' ah)
Cardene®	(kar' deen)
codeine	(koe' deen)
Cardene SR®	(kar' deen ess are)
Cardizem SR®	(kar' di zem ess are)
Cardiem	(car' dee em)
Cardizem®	(kar' di zem)
Cardizem®	(kar' di zem)
Cardene®	(kar' deen)
Cardizem®	(kar' di zem)
Cardiem	(car' dee em)
Cardizem CD®	(kar' di zem see dee)
Cardizem SR®	(kar' di zem ess are)
Cardizem SR®	(kar' di zem ess are)
Cardene SR®	(kar' deen ess are)
Cardizem SR®	(kar' di zem ess are)
Cardizem CD®	(kar' di zem see dee)
Cardura®	(kar dur' ah)
Cardene®	(kar' deen)
Cardura®	(kar dur' ah)
Cordarone®	(kor da rone')

Drug Name	Pronunciation
Cardura®	(kar dur' ah)
Cordran®	(kor' dran)
Cardura®	(kar dur' ah)
Coumadin®	(ku' ma din)
Cardura®	(kar dur' ah)
K-Dur®	(kay'-dur)
Cardura®	(kar dur' ah)
Ridaura®	(ri dur' ah)
carteolol	(kar' tee oh lole)
carvedilol	(kar' ve dil ole)
Cartia® XT	(car' te ah xt)
Procardia XL®	(pro car' dee ah xl)
Cartrol®	(kar' trol)
Carbatrol®	(kar' ba trol)
carvedilol	(kar' ve dil ole)
captopril	(kap' toe pril)
carvedilol	(kar' ve dil ole)
carteolol	(kar' tee oh lole)
Cataflam®	(kat' ah flam)
Catapres®	(kat' ah pres)
Catapres®	(kat' ah pres)
Cataflam®	(kat' ah flam)
Catapres®	(kat' ah pres)
Cetapred®	(see' ta pred)
Catapres®	(kat' ah pres)
Combipres®	(kom' bee pres)
cefaclor	(sef' ah klor)
cephalexin	(sef ah leks' in)
cefamandole	(sef ah man' dole)
cefmetazole	(sef met' ah zole)
cefazolin	(sef a' zoe lin)
cefprozil	(sef proe' zil)
cefazolin	(sef a' zoe lin)
cephalexin	(sef ah leks' in)
cefazolin	(sef a' zoe lin)
cephalothin	(sef a' loe thin)
cefmetazole	(sef met' ah zole)
cefamandole	(sef ah man' dole)
Cefobid®	(se' foh bid)
cefonicid	(se fon' i sid)
Cefol®	(cee' fol)
Cefzil®	(sef' zil)
cefonicid	(se fon' i sid)
Cefobid®	(se' foh bid)
Cefotan®	(se' foh tan)
Ceftin®	(sef' tin)
cefotaxime	(sef oh taks' eem)
cefoxitin	(se fox' i tin)

Drug Name	Pronunciation	Drug Name	Pronunciation
cefotaxime	(sef oh taks' eem)	Celebrex®	(sel' ah brex)
ceftizoxime	(sef ti zoks' eem)	Celexa®	(se lex' a)
cefotaxime	(sef oh taks' eem)	Celebrex®	(sel' ah brex)
cefuroxime	(se fyoor oks' eem)	cerebra	(cer' eh bra)
cefotetan	(sef' oh tee tan)	Celebrex®	(sel' ah brex)
cefoxitin	(se foks' i tin)	Cerebyx®	(ser' e bix)
cefotetan	(sef' oh tee tan)	Ceftin®	(sef' tin)	Celexa®	(se lex' a)
Ceftin®	(sef' tin)	Celebrex®	(sel' ah brex)
cefoxitin	(se fox' i tin)	Celexa®	(se lex' a)
cefotaxime	(sef oh taks' eem)	cerebra	(cer' eh bra)
cefoxitin	(se foks' i tin)	Celexa®	(se lex' a)
cefotetan	(sef' oh tee tan)	Cerebyx®	(ser' e bix)
cefoxitin	(se foks' i tin)	Celexa®	(se lex' a)
Cytoxan®	(sy toks' an)	Zyprexa®	(zye preks' a)
cefprozil	(sef proe' zil)	Cenestin®	(se nes' tin)
cefazolin	(sef a' zoe lin)	Senexon®	(sen' e son)
cefprozil	(sef proe' zil)	Centoxin®	(sen toks' in)
cefuroxime	(se fyoor oks' eem)	Cytoxan®	(sy toks' an)
ceftazidime	(sef' tay zi deem)	Cepastat®	(sea' pa stat)
ceftizoxime	(sef ti zoks' eem)	Capastat®	(kap' ah stat)
Ceftin®	(sef' tin)	cephalexin	(sef ah leks' in)
Cefotan®	(se' foh tan)	cefaclor	(sef' ah klor)
Ceftin®	(sef' tin)	cephalexin	(sef ah leks' in)
cefotetan	(sef' oh tee tan)	cefazolin	(sef a' zoe lin)
Ceftin®	(sef' tin)	cephalexin	(sef ah leks' in)
Cefzil®	(sef' zil)	cephalothin	(sef a' loe thin)
Ceftin®	(sef' tin)	cephalexin	(sef ah leks' in)
Cipro®	(ceh' pro)	ciprofloxacin	(sip ro floks' a sin)
ceftizoxime	(sef ti zoks' eem)	cephalothin	(sef a' loe thin)
cefotaxime	(sef oh taks' eem)	cefazolin	(sef a' zoe lin)
ceftizoxime	(sef ti zoks' eem)	cephalothin	(sef a' loe thin)
ceftazidime	(sef' tay zi deem)	cephalexin	(sef ah leks' in)
ceftizoxime	(sef ti zoks' eem)	cephapirin	(sef ah pye' rin)
cefuroxime	(se fyoor oks' eem)	cephradine	(sef' ra deen)
cefuroxime	(se fyoor oks' eem)	cephradine	(sef' ra deen)
cefotaxime	(sef oh taks' eem)	cephapirin	(sef ah pye' rin)
cefuroxime	(se fyoor oks' eem)	Ceptaz®	(sep' taz)
cefprozil	(sef proe' zil)	Septra®	(sep' trah)
cefuroxime	(se fyoor oks' eem)	cerebra	(cer' eh bra)
ceftizoxime	(sef ti zoks' eem)	Celebrex®	(sel' ah brex)
cefuroxime	(se fyoor oks' eem)	cerebra	(cer' eh bra)
deferoxamine	(de fer oks' ah meen)	Celexa®	(se lex' a)
Cefzil®	(sef' zil)	Cerebyx®	(ser' e bix)
Cefol®	(cee' fol)	Celebrex®	(sel' ah brex)
Cefzil®	(sef' zil)	Cerebyx®	(ser' e bix)
Ceftin®	(sef' tin)	Celexa®	(se lex' a)
Cefzil®	(sef' zil)	Cerebyx®	(ser' e bix)
Kefzol®	(kef' zol)	Cerezyme®	(ser' e zime)

APPENDIX

Drug Name	Pronunciation	Drug Name	Pronunciation
Ceredase®	(ser' e dase)	Citrucel®	(sit' tru cel)
Cerezyme®	(ser' e zime)	Citracal®	(sit' tra cal)
Cerezyme®	(ser' e zime)	clarithromycin	(kla rith' roe mye sin)
Cerebyx®	(ser' e bix)	erythromycin	(er ith roe mye' sin)
Cerezyme®	(ser' e zime)	Cleocin®	(klee' oh sin)
Ceredase®	(ser' e dase)	bleomycin	(blee oh mye' sin)
Cetaphil®	(see' ta fill)	Cleocin®	(klee' oh sin)
Cetapred®	(see' ta pred)	Clinoril®	(klin' oh rill)
Cetapred®	(see' ta pred)	Cleocin®	(klee' oh sin)
Catapres®	(kat' ah pres)	Lincocin®	(link' oh sin)
Cetapred®	(see' ta pred)	Clinoril®	(klin' oh rill)
Cetaphil®	(see' ta fill)	Cleocin®	(klee' oh sin)
chlorambucil	(klor am' byoo sil)	Clinoril®	(klin' oh rill)
Chloromycetin®	(klor oh my see' tin)	Clozaril®	(klo' zah rill)
Chloromycetin®	(klor oh my see' tin)	Clinoril®	(klin' oh rill)
chlorambucil	(klor am' byoo sil)	Oruvail®	(or' yu vale)
Chloromycetin®	(klor oh my see' tin)	Clinoxide®	(klin ox' ide)
Chlor-Trimeton®	(klor-try' me ton)	Clipoxide®	(kleh pox' ide)
chlorpromazine	(klor proe' ma zeen)	Clipoxide®	(kleh pox' ide)
chlorpropamide	(klor proe' pa mide)	Clinoxide®	(klin ox' ide)
chlorpromazine	(klor proe' ma zeen)	Clocort®	(klo' kort)
clomipramine	(kloe mi' pra meen)	Cloderm®	(klo' derm)
chlorpromazine	(klor proe' ma zeen)	Cloderm®	(klo' derm)
prochlorperazine	(proe klor per' ah zeen)	Clocort®	(klo' kort)
chlorpromazine	(klor proe' ma zeen)	clofazimine	(kloe fa' zi meen)
promethazine	(proe meth' ah zeen)	clonazepam	(kloe na' ze pam)
chlorpropamide	(klor proe' pa mide)	clofazimine	(kloe fa' zi meen)
chlorpromazine	(klor proe' ma zeen)	clozapine	(kloe' za peen)
Chlor-Trimeton®	(klor-try' me ton)	clofibrate	(kloe fye' brate)
Chloromycetin®	(klor oh my see' tin)	clorazepate	(klor az' ah pate)
Cidex®	(sy' decks)	Clomid®	(klo' mid)
Lidex®	(ly' decks)	clonidine	(kloe' ni deen)
Ciloxan®	(sy loks' an)	clomiphene	(kloe' mi feen)
cinoxacin	(sin oks' ah sin)	clomipramine	(kloe mi' pra meen)
Ciloxan®	(sy loks' an)	clomiphene	(kloe' mi feen)
Cytoxan®	(sy toks' an)	clonidine	(kloe' ni deen)
cimetidine	(sye met' i deen)	clomipramine	(kloe mi' pra meen)
simethicone	(sye meth'i kone)	chlorpromazine	(klor proe' ma zeen)
cinoxacin	(sin oks' ah sin)	clomipramine	(kloe mi' pra meen)
Ciloxan®	(sy loks' an)	clomiphene	(kloe' mi feen)
Cipro®	(ceh' pro)	clomipramine	(kloe mi' pra meen)
Ceftin®	(sef' tin)	desipramine	(des ip' ra meen)
ciprofloxacin	(sip ro floks' a sin)	clomipramine	(kloe mi' pra meen)
cephalexin	(sef ah leks' in)	Norpramin®	(nor' pra min)
cisplatin	(sis' pla tin)	clonazepam	(kloe na' ze pam)
carboplatin	(kar' boe pla tin)	clofazimine	(kloe fa' zi meen)
Citracal®	(sit' tra cal)	clonazepam	(kloe na' ze pam)
Citrucel®	(sit' tru cel)	clonidine	(kloe' ni deen)

Drug Name	Pronunciation	Drug Name	Pronunciation
clonazepam	(kloe na′ ze pam)	Cognex®	(kog′ neks)
clorazepate	(klor az′ ah pate)	Corgard®	(kor′ gard)
clonazepam	(kloe na′ ze pam)	Colace®	(ko′ lace)
Klonopin™	(klon′ oh pin)	Calan®	(kal′ an)
clonazepam	(kloe na′ ze pam)	Co-Lav®	(koe′-lav)
lorazepam	(lor a′ ze pam)	Colax®	(koe′ laks)
clonidine	(kloe′ ni deen)	Colax®	(koe′ laks)
Clomid®	(klo′ mid)	Co-Lav®	(koe′-lav)
clonidine	(kloe′ ni deen)	Colazal™	(koe′ la zal)
clomiphene	(kloe′ mi feen)	Clozaril®	(klo′ zah rill)
clonidine	(kloe′ ni deen)	Colestid®	(koe les′ tid)
clonazepam	(kloe na′ ze pam)	colistin	(koe lis′ tin)
clonidine	(kloe′ ni deen)	colistin	(koe lis′ tin)
clozapine	(kloe′ za peen)	Colestid®	(koe les′ tid)
clonidine	(kloe′ ni deen)	Combipres®	(kom′ bee pres)
Klonopin™	(klon′ oh pin)	Catapres®	(kat′ ah pres)
clonidine	(kloe′ ni deen)	Combivent®	(kom′ bi vent)
Loniten®	(lon′ eh ten)	Combivir®	(kom′ bi veer)
clonidine	(kloe′ ni deen)	Combivir®	(kom′ bi veer)
quinidine	(kwin′ i deen)	Combivent®	(kom′ bi vent)
clorazepate	(klor az′ ah pate)	Combivir®	(kom′ bi veer)
clofibrate	(kloe fye′ brate)	Epivir®	(ep′ ih vir)
clorazepate	(klor az′ ah pate)	Compazine®	(kom′ pah zeen)
clonazepam	(kloe na′ ze pam)	Copaxone®	(koe′ pa zone)
clotrimazole	(kloe trim′ ah zole)	Compazine®	(kom′ pah zeen)
co-trimoxazole	(koe-trye moks′ ah zole)	Coumadin®	(ku′ ma din)
clozapine	(kloe′ za peen)	Comvax®	(kom′ vaks)
clofazimine	(kloe fa′ zi meen)	Recombivax®	(ree kom′ bi vaks)
clozapine	(kloe′ za peen)	Copaxone®	(koe′ pa zone)
clonidine	(kloe′ ni deen)	Compazine®	(kom′ pah zeen)
Clozaril®	(klo′ zah rill)	Cophene®	(koe′ feen)
Clinoril®	(klin′ oh rill)	codeine	(koe′ deen)
Clozaril®	(klo′ zah rill)	Cordarone®	(kor da rone′)
Colazal™	(koe′ la zal)	Cardura®	(kar dur′ ah)
Codafed®	(kode′ ah fed)	Cordarone®	(kor da rone′)
CodAphen®	(kod′ ah fen)	Cordran®	(kor′ dran)
CodAphen®	(kod′ ah fen)	Cordran®	(kor′ dran)
Codafed®	(kode′ ah fed)	Cardura®	(kar dur′ ah)
codeine	(koe′ deen)	Cordran®	(kor′ dran)
Cardene®	(kar′ deen)	codeine	(koe′ deen)
codeine	(koe′ deen)	Cordran®	(kor′ dran)
Cophene®	(koe′ feen)	Cordarone®	(kor da rone′)
codeine	(koe′ deen)	Corgard®	(kor′ gard)
Cordran®	(kor′ dran)	Cognex®	(kog′ neks)
codeine	(koe′ deen)	Cortef®	(kor′ tef)
iodine	(eye′ oh dyne)	Lortab®	(lor′ tab)
codeine	(koe′ deen)	cortisone	(kor′ ti sone)
Lodine®	(low′ deen)	Cortizone®	(kor′ ti zone)

APPENDIX

Drug Name	Pronunciation	Drug Name	Pronunciation
Cortizone®	(kor' ti zone)	cytarabine	(sye tare' ah been)
cortisone	(kor' ti sone)	Cytosar®	(sye' to sar)
Cortrosyn®	(kor' tro sin)	cytarabine	(sye tare' ah been)
Cotazym®	(koe' ta zime)	Cytoxan®	(sy toks' an)
Cotazym®	(koe' ta zime)	cytarabine	(sye tare' ah been)
Cortrosyn®	(kor' tro sin)	vidarabine	(vye dare' ah been)
co-trimoxazole	(koe-trye moks' ah zole)	CytoGam®	(sy' to gam)
clotrimazole	(kloe trim' ah zole)	Cytoxan®	(sy toks' an)
Coumadin®	(ku' ma din)	CytoGam®	(sy' to gam)
Avandia®	(ah van' de a)	Gamimune® N	(gam' e mune en)
Coumadin®	(ku' ma din)	Cytosar®	(sye' to sar)
Cardura®	(kar dur' ah)	cytarabine	(sye tare' ah been)
Coumadin®	(ku' ma din)	Cytosar®	(sye' to sar)
Compazine®	(kom' pah zeen)	Cytovene®	(sye' toe veen)
Coumadin®	(ku' ma din)	Cytosar®	(sye' to sar)
Kemadrin®	(kem' ah drin)	Cytoxan®	(sy toks' an)
Covera®	(co ver' ah)	Cytosar-U®	(sye' to sar-u)
Provera®	(pro ver' ah)	Cytovene®	(sye' toe veen)
Cozaar®	(koe' zar)	Cytosar-U®	(sye' to sar-u)
Hyzaar®	(hi' zar)	Cytoxan®	(sye tox' an)
Cozaar®	(koe' zar)	Cytosar-U®	(sye' to sar-u)
Zocor®	(zoe' cor)	Neosar®	(ne' oh sar)
Cutivate™	(kyu' te vate)	Cytotec®	(sye' toe tek)
Ultravate®	(ul' trah vate)	Cytoxan®	(sye tox' an)
cyclobenzaprine	(sye kloe ben' za preen)	Cytotec®	(sye' toe tek)
cycloserine	(sye kloe ser' een)	Sytobex®	(sye' toe beks)
cyclobenzaprine	(sye kloe ben' za preen)	Cytovene®	(sye' toe veen)
cyproheptadine	(si proe hep' ta deen)	Cytosar®	(sye' to sar)
cyclophosphamide	(sye kloe fos' fa mide)	Cytovene®	(sye' toe veen)
cyclosporine	(sye' kloe spor een)	Cytosar-U®	(sye' to sar-u)
cycloserine	(sye kloe ser' een)	Cytoxan®	(sy toks' an)
cyclobenzaprine	(sye kloe ben' za preen)	cefoxitin	(se foks' i tin)
cycloserine	(sye kloe ser' een)	Cytoxan®	(sy toks' an)
cyclosporine	(sye' kloe spor een)	Centoxin®	(sen toks' in)
cyclosporine	(sye' kloe spor een)	Cytoxan®	(sy toks' an)
cyclophosphamide	(sye kloe fos' fa mide)	Ciloxan®	(sy loks' an)
cyclosporine	(sye' kloe spor een)	Cytoxan®	(sy toks' an)
cycloserine	(sye kloe ser' een)	cytarabine	(sye tare' ah been)
cyclosporine	(sye' kloe spor een)	Cytoxan®	(sy toks' an)
Cyklokapron®	(sye kloe kay' pron)	CytoGam®	(sy' to gam)
Cyklokapron®	(sye kloe kay' pron)	Cytoxan®	(sy toks' an)
cyclosporine	(sye' kloe spor een)	Cytosar®	(sye' to sar)
cyproheptadine	(si proe hep' ta deen)	Cytoxan®	(sy toks' an)
cyclobenzaprine	(sye kloe ben' za preen)	Cytosar-U®	(sye' to sar-u)
Cytadren®	(sy' ta dren)	Cytoxan®	(sye tox' an)
cytarabine	(sye tare' ah been)	Cytotec®	(sye' toe tek)
cytarabine	(sye tare' ah been)	dacarbazine	(da kar' ba zeen)
Cytadren®	(sy' ta dren)	Dicarbosil®	(dye kar' bow sil)

Drug Name	Pronunciation	Drug Name	Pronunciation
dacarbazine	(da kar' ba zeen)	Delacort®	(del' ah kort)
procarbazine	(proe kar' ba zeen)	Delcort®	(del' kort)
Dacriose®	(dak' ree ose)	Delcort®	(del' kort)
Danocrine®	(dan' oh crin)	Delacort®	(del' ah kort)
dactinomycin	(dak ti noe mye' sin)	Delfen®	(del' fen)
daunorubicin	(daw noe roo' bi sin)	Delsym®	(del' sim)
Dalmane®	(dal' mane)	Delsym®	(del' sim)
Demulen®	(dem' yu len)	Delfen®	(del' fen)
Dalmane®	(dal' mane)	Delsym®	(del' sim)
Dialume®	(dy' ah lume)	Desyrel®	(des' e rell)
danazol	(da' na zole)	Demadex®	(dem' ah deks)
Dantrium®	(dan' tree um)	Denorex®	(den' oh reks)
Danocrine®	(dan' oh crin)	Demerol®	(dem' eh rol)
Dacriose®	(dak' ree ose)	Demulen®	(dem' yu len)
Dantrium®	(dan' tree um)	Demerol®	(dem' eh rol)
danazol	(da' na zole)	Desyrel®	(des' e rell)
Dantrium®	(dan' tree um)	Demerol®	(dem' eh rol)
Daraprim®	(dare' ah prim)	dicumarol	(dye koo' ma role)
dapsone	(dap' sone)	Demerol®	(dem' eh rol)
Diprosone®	(dip' ro sone)	Dilaudid®	(dye law' did)
Daranide®	(dare' ah nide)	Demerol®	(dem' eh rol)
Daraprim®	(dare' ah prim)	Dymelor®	(dye' meh lor)
Daraprim®	(dare' ah prim)	Demerol®	(dem' eh rol)
Dantrium®	(dan' tree um)	Pamelor®	(pam' meh lor)
Daraprim®	(dare' ah prim)	Demulen®	(dem' yu len)
Daranide®	(dare' ah nide)	Dalmane®	(dal' mane)
Darvocet-N®	(dar' voh set-en)	Demulen®	(dem' yu len)
Darvon-N®	(dar' von-en)	Demerol®	(dem' eh rol)
Darvon-N®	(dar' von-en)	Denavir™	(den' ah vir)
Darvocet-N®	(dar' voh set-en)	indinavir	(in din' a veer)
Darvon®	(dar' von)	Denorex®	(den' oh reks)
Devrom®	(dev' rom)	Demadex®	(dem' ah deks)
Darvon®	(dar' von)	Depakene®	(dep' ah keen)
Diovan®	(dye oh' van)	Depakote®	(dep' ah kote)
daunorubicin	(daw noe roo' bi sin)	Depakote®	(dep' ah kote)
dactinomycin	(dak ti noe mye' sin)	Depakene®	(dep' ah keen)
daunorubicin	(daw noe roo' bi sin)	Depakote®	(dep' ah kote)
doxorubicin	(dox oh roo' bi sin)	Senokot®	(sen' oh kot)
Daypro®	(day' pro)	Depen®	(dee' pen)
Diupres®	(dye' yu press)	Endal®	(en' dal)
Decadron®	(dek' ah dron)	DepoCyt®	(de' po set)
Percodan®	(per' koe dan)	Depoject®	(de' po ject)
Deconal®	(dek' oh nal)	Depo-Estradiol®	(dep' oh-es tra dye' ole)
Deconsal®	(dek' on sal)	Depo-Testadiol®	(dep' oh-tes ta dye' ole)
Deconsal®	(dek' on sal)	Depogen®	(dep' oh jen)
Deconal®	(dek' oh nal)	Depoject®	(dep' oh ject)
deferoxamine	(de fer oks' ah meen)	Depoject®	(de' po ject)
cefuroxime	(se fyoor oks' eem)	DepoCyt®	(de' po set)

Drug Name	Pronunciation	Drug Name	Pronunciation
Depoject®	(dep' oh ject)	Desyrel®	(des' e rell)
Depogen®	(dep' oh jen)	Delsym®	(del' sim)
Depo-Medrol®	(dep' oh-med' role)	Desyrel®	(des' e rell)
Solu-Medrol®	(sol' yu-med' role)	Demerol®	(dem' eh rol)
Depo-Testadiol®	(dep' oh-tes ta dye' ole)	Desyrel®	(des' e rell)
Depo-Estradiol®	(dep'oh-es tra dye' ole)	Zestril®	(zes' trill)
Depo-Testadiol®	(dep' oh-tes ta dye' ole)	Devrom®	(dev' rom)
Depotestogen®	(dep oh tes' tow gen)	Darvon®	(dar' von)
Depotestogen®	(dep oh tes' tow gen)	dexamethasone	(deks ah meth' ah sone)
Depo-Testadiol®	(dep' oh-tes ta dye' ole)	desoximetasone	(des ox i met' ah sone)
Dermacort®	(der' ma kort)	Dexatrim®	(deks' ah trim)
DermiCort®	(der' meh kort)	Dextran®	(deks' tran)
Dermatop®	(der' ma top)	Dexatrim®	(deks' ah trim)
DermiCort®	(der' meh kort)	Excedrin®	(eks sed' drin)
Dermatop®	(der' ma top)	Dexedrine®	(deks' e drine)
Dimetapp®	(di meh' tap)	Dextran®	(deks' tran)
DermiCort®	(der' meh kort)	Dexedrine®	(deks' e drine)
Dermacort®	(der' ma kort)	Excedrin®	(eks sed' drin)
DermiCort®	(der' meh kort)	DexFerrum®	(deks' fer rum)
Dermatop®	(der' ma top)	Desferal®	(des' fer al)
DES®	(dee ee ess)	Dextran®	(deks' tran)
E.E.S.®	(ee ee ess)	Dexatrim®	(deks' ah trim)
deserpidine	(de ser' pi deen)	Dextran®	(deks' tran)
desipramine	(des ip' ra meen)	Dexedrine®	(deks' e drine)
Desferal®	(des' fer al)	Diaβeta®	(dye ah bay' tah)
desflurane	(des flu' rane)	Diabinese®	(dye ab' beh neese)
Desferal®	(des' fer al)	Diaβeta®	(dye ah bay' tah)
DexFerrum®	(deks' fer rum)	Zebeta®	(ze' bay tah)
Desferal®	(des' fer al)	Diabinese®	(dye ab' beh neese)
Disophrol®	(dye' so frol)	Diaβeta®	(dye ah bay' tah)
desflurane	(des flu' rane)	Diabinese®	(dye ab' beh neese)
Desferal®	(des' fer al)	Dialume®	(dy' ah lume)
desipramine	(des ip' ra meen)	Dialume®	(dy' ah lume)
clomipramine	(kloe mi' pra meen)	Dalmane®	(dal' mane)
desipramine	(des ip' ra meen)	Dialume®	(dy' ah lume)
deserpidine	(de ser' pi deen)	Diabinese®	(dye ab' beh neese)
desipramine	(des ip' ra meen)	Diamox®	(dye' ah moks)
diphenhydramine	(dye fen hye' dra meen)	Dobutrex®	(doe byoo' treks)
desipramine	(des ip' ra meen)	Diamox®	(dye' ah moks)
disopyramide	(dye soe peer' ah mide)	Trimox®	(trye' moks)
desipramine	(des ip' ra meen)	diazepam	(dye az' ah pam)
imipramine	(im ip' ra meen)	diazoxide	(dye az oks' ide)
desipramine	(des ip' ra meen)	diazepam	(dye az' ah pam)
nortriptyline	(nor trip' ti leen)	Ditropan®	(di troe' pan)
desoximetasone	(des ox i met' ah sone)	diazepam	(dye az' ah pam)
dexamethasone	(deks ah meth' ah sone)	lorazepam	(lor a' ze pam)
Desoxyn®	(de soks' in)	diazoxide	(dye az oks' ide)
digoxin	(di joks' in)	diazepam	(dye az' ah pam)

Drug Name	Pronunciation	Drug Name	Pronunciation
diazoxide	(dye az oks' ide)	Dimetane®	(dye' meh tane)
Dyazide®	(dye' ah zide)	Dimetapp®	(di meh' tap)
Dicarbosil®	(dye kar' bow sil)	Dimetapp®	(di meh' tap)
dacarbazine	(da kar' ba zeen)	Dermatop®	(der' ma top)
diclofenac	(dye kloe' fen ak)	Dimetapp®	(di meh' tap)
Diflucan®	(dye flu' can)	Dimetabs®	(di meh' tabs)
diclofenac	(dye kloe' fen ak)	Dimetapp®	(di meh' tap)
Duphalac®	(du' fa lak)	Dimetane®	(dye' meh tane)
dicumarol	(dye koo' ma role)	Dioval®	(dy' oh val)
Demerol®	(dem' eh rol)	Diovan®	(dye oh' van)
dicyclomine	(dye sye' kloe meen)	Diovan®	(dye oh' van)
diphenhydramine	(dye fen hye' dra meen)	Darvon®	(dar' von)
dicyclomine	(dye sye' kloe meen)	Diovan®	(dye oh' van)
doxycycline	(doks i sye' kleen)	Dioval®	(dy' oh val)
dicyclomine	(dye sye' kloe meen)	Diovan®	(dye oh' van)
dyclonine	(dye' kloe neen)	Zyban™	(zy' ban)
Diflucan®	(dye flu' can)	Dipentum®	(dye pen' tum)
diclofenac	(dye kloe' fen ak)	Dilantin®	(dye lan' tin)
Diflucan®	(dye flu' can)	Diphenatol®	(dye fen' ah tol)
Diprivan®	(dye' pri van)	diphenidiol	(dye fen' i dole)
Diflucan®	(dye flu' can)	diphenhydramine	(dye fen hye' dra meen)
disulfiram	(dye sul' fi ram)	desipramine	(des ip' ra meen)
digitoxin	(di ji tox' in)	diphenhydramine	(dye fen hye' dra meen)
digoxin	(di jox' in)	dicyclomine	(dye sye' kloe meen)
digoxin	(di joks' in)	diphenhydramine	(dye fen hye' dra meen)
Desoxyn®	(de soks' in)	dimenhydrinate	(dye men hye' dri nate)
digoxin	(di jox' in)	diphenidiol	(dye fen' i dole)
digitoxin	(di ji tox' in)	Diphenatol®	(dye fen' ah tol)
digoxin	(di jox' in)	Diprivan®	(dye' pri van)
doxepin	(doks' e pin)	Diflucan®	(dye flu' can)
Dilantin®	(dye lan' tin)	Diprivan®	(dip' riv an)
Dilaudid®	(dye law' did)	Ditropan®	(di troe' pan)
Dilantin®	(dye lan' tin)	Diprosone®	(dip' ro sone)
diltiazem	(dil tye' ah zem)	dapsone	(dap' sone)
Dilantin®	(dye lan' tin)	dipyridamole	(dye peer id' ah mole)
Dipentum®	(dye pen' tum)	disopyramide	(dye soe peer' ah mide)
Dilaudid®	(dye law' did)	Disophrol®	(dye' so frol)
Demerol®	(dem' eh rol)	Desferal®	(des' fer al)
Dilaudid®	(dye law' did)	Disophrol®	(dye' so frol)
Dilantin®	(dye lan' tin)	Isuprel®	(eye' sue prel)
Dilomine®	(dy' lo meen)	Disophrol®	(dye' so frol)
Dyclone®	(dye' klone)	Stilphostrol®	(stil phos' trol)
diltiazem	(dil tye' ah zem)	disopyramide	(dye soe peer' ah mide)
Dilantin®	(dye lan' tin)	desipramine	(des ip' ra meen)
dimenhydrinate	(dye men hye' dri nate)	disopyramide	(dye soe peer' ah mide)
diphenhydramine	(dye fen hye' dra meen)	dipyridamole	(dye peer id' ah mole)
Dimetabs®	(di meh' tabs)	disulfiram	(dye sul' fi ram)
Dimetapp®	(di meh' tap)	Diflucan®	(dye flu' can)

APPENDIX

Drug Name	Pronunciation	Drug Name	Pronunciation
dithranol	(di thra′ nol)	doxazosin	(doks aye′ zoe sin)
Ditropan®	(di troe′ pan)	doxepin	(doks′ e pin)
Ditropan®	(di troe′ pan)	doxazosin	(doks aye′ zoe sin)
diazepam	(dye az′ ah pam)	doxorubicin	(doks oh roo′ bi sin)
Ditropan®	(di troe′ pan)	doxepin	(doks′ e pin)
Diprivan®	(dip′ riv an)	digoxin	(di joks′ in)
Ditropan®	(di troe′ pan)	doxepin	(doks′ e pin)
dithranol	(di′ thra nol)	doxapram	(doks′ ah pram)
Diupres®	(dye′ yu press)	doxepin	(doks′ e pin)
Daypro®	(day′ pro)	doxazosin	(doks aye′ zoe sin)
dobutamine	(doe byoo′ ta meen)	doxepin	(doks′ e pin)
dopamine	(doe′ pa meen)	Doxidan®	(dox′ e dan)
Dobutrex®	(doe byoo′ treks)	doxepin	(doks′ e pin)
Diamox®	(dye′ ah moks)	doxycycline	(doks i sye′ kleen)
docusate	(dok′ yoo sate)	Doxidan®	(dox′ e dan)
Doxinate®	(dox′ eh nate)	doxepin	(doks′ e pin)
Dolobid®	(dol′ ah bid)	Doxil®	(doks′ il)
Slo-Bid®	(slo′ bid)	Doxy®	(doks′ ee)
Donnagel®	(don′ ah jel)	Doxil®	(doks′ il)
Donnatal®	(don′ ah tall)	Paxil®	(paks′ il)
Donnapine®	(don′ ah peen)	Doxinate®	(dox′ eh nate)
Donnazyme®	(don′ ah zime)	docusate	(dok′ yoo sate)
Donnatal®	(don′ ah tall)	Doxinate®	(dox′ eh nate)
Donnagel®	(don′ ah jel)	doxapram	(doks′ ah pram)
Donnazyme®	(don′ ah zime)	doxorubicin	(doks oh roo′ bi sin)
Donnapine®	(don′ ah peen)	dactinomycin	(dak ti noe mye′ sin)
dopamine	(doe′ pa meen)	doxorubicin	(doks oh roo′ bi sin)
dobutamine	(doe byoo′ ta meen)	daunorubicin	(daw noe roo′ bi sin)
dopamine	(doe′ pa meen)	doxorubicin	(doks oh roo′ bi sin)
Dopram®	(doe′ pram)	doxacurium	(doks ah kyoo′ ri um)
Dopram®	(doe′ pram)	doxorubicin	(doks oh roo′ bi sin)
dopamine	(doe′ pa meen)	doxapram	(doks′ ah pram)
doxacurium	(doks ah kyoo′ ri um)	doxorubicin	(doks oh roo′ bi sin)
doxapram	(doks′ ah pram)	doxazosin	(doks aye′ zoe sin)
doxacurium	(doks ah kyoo′ ri um)	doxorubicin	(doks oh roo′ bi sin)
doxorubicin	(doks oh roo′ bi sin)	idarubicin	(eye da roo′ bi sin)
doxapram	(doks′ ah pram)	Doxy®	(doks′ ee)
doxacurium	(doks ah kyoo′ ri um)	Doxil®	(doks′ il)
doxapram	(doks′ ah pram)	doxycycline	(doks i sye′ kleen)
doxazosin	(doks aye′ zoe sin)	dicyclomine	(dye sye′ kloe meen)
doxapram	(doks′ ah pram)	doxycycline	(doks i sye′ kleen)
doxepin	(doks′ e pin)	doxepin	(doks′ e pin)
doxapram	(doks′ ah pram)	doxycycline	(doks i sye′ kleen)
Doxinate®	(dox′ eh nate)	doxylamine	(dox il′ a meen)
doxapram	(doks′ ah pram)	doxylamine	(dox il′ a meen)
doxorubicin	(doks oh roo′ bi sin)	doxycycline	(doks i sye′ kleen)
doxazosin	(doks aye′ zoe sin)	Drisdol®	(dris′ doll)
doxapram	(doks′ ah pram)	Drysol®	(dry′ sol)

Drug Name	Pronunciation	Drug Name	Pronunciation
dronabinol	(droe nab' i nol)	Echogen®	(ek' oh jen)
droperidol	(droe per' i dole)	Epogen®	(ee' poe jen)
droperidol	(droe per' i dole)	Ecotrin®	(eh' ko trin)
dronabinol	(droe nab' i nol)	Akineton®	(ah kin' eh ton)
Drysol®	(dry' sol)	Ecotrin®	(eh' ko trin)
Drisdol®	(dris' doll)	Edecrin®	(ed' eh crin)
DuoCet™	(du' oh set)	Ecotrin®	(eh' ko trin)
Duo-Cyp®	(du' oh-sip)	Epogen®	(ee' poe jen)
Duo-Cyp®	(du' oh-sip)	Edecrin®	(ed' eh crin)
DuoCet™	(du' oh set)	Ecotrin®	(eh' ko trin)
Duphalac®	(du' fa lak)	Edecrin®	(ed' eh crin)
diclofenac	(dye kloe' fen ak)	Eulexin®	(yu leks' in)
Dyazide®	(dye' ah zide)	E.E.S.®	(ee ee ess)
diazoxide	(dye az oks' ide)	DES®	(dee ee ess)
Dyazide®	(dye' ah zide)	Efidac®	(eff' i dak)
Dynacin®	(dye' na sin)	Efudex®	(ef' yu deks)
Dyazide®	(dye' ah zide)	Efudex®	(ef' yu deks)
Thiazide®	(thye' ah zide)	Efidac®	(eff' i dak)
dyclonine	(dye' kloe neen)	Efudex®	(ef' yu deks)
dicyclomine	(dye sye' kloe meen)	Eurax®	(yoor' aks)
Dymelor®	(dye' meh lor)	Elase®	(e' lase)
Demerol®	(dem' eh rol)	Ellence®	(el' lens)
Dymelor®	(dye' meh lor)	Elavil®	(el' ah vil)
Pamelor®	(pam' meh lor)	Aldoril®	(al' doe ril)
Dynabac®	(dye' na bac)	Elavil®	(el' ah vil)
Dynacin®	(dye' na sin)	Eldepryl®	(el' de pril)
Dynabac®	(dye' na bac)	Elavil®	(el' ah vil)
DynaCirc®	(dye' na sirk)	Equanil®	(eh' kwa nil)
Dynabac®	(dye' na bac)	Elavil®	(el' ah vil)
Dynapen®	(dye' na pen)	Mellaril®	(mel' la ril)
Dynacin®	(dye' na sin)	Elavil®	(el' ah vil)
Dyazide®	(dye' ah zide)	Oruvail®	(or' yu vale)
Dynacin®	(dye' na sin)	Elavil®	(el' ah vil)
Dynabac®	(dye' na bac)	Plavix®	(plah' viks)
Dynacin®	(dye' na sin)	Eldepryl®	(el' de pril)
DynaCirc®	(dye' na sirk)	Elavil®	(el' ah vil)
Dynacin®	(dye' na sin)	Eldepryl®	(el' de pril)
Dynapen®	(dye' na pen)	enalapril	(e nal' ah pril)
DynaCirc®	(dye' na sirk)	Eldopaque Forte®	(el' do pak for' tay)
Dynabac®	(dye' na bac)	Eloquin® Forte®	(el' o kwin for' tay)
DynaCirc®	(dye' na sirk)	Eloquin® Forte®	(el' o kwin for' tay)
Dynacin®	(dye' na sin)	Eldopaque Forte®	(el' do pak for' tay)
Dynapen®	(dye' na pen)	Elixicon®	(eh lix' i con)
Dynabac®	(dye' na bac)	Elocon®	(ee' lo con)
Dynapen®	(dye' na pen)	Ellence®	(el' lens)
Dynacin®	(dye' na sin)	Elase®	(e' lase)
Dyrenium®	(dye ren' e um)	Elmiron®	(el' mi ron)
Pyridium®	(pye rid' dee um)	Imuran®	(im' yu ran)

Drug Name	Pronunciation	Drug Name	Pronunciation
Elocon®	(ee' lo con)	Epinal®	(ep' eh nal)
Elixicon®	(eh lix' i con)	Epitol®	(ep' eh tol)
Emcyt®	(em' sit)	epinephrine	(ep i nef' rin)
Eryc®	(err' ik)	ephedrine	(e fed' rin)
emetine	(em' eh teen)	EpiPen®	(ep' eh pen)
Emetrol®	(em' eh trol)	Epifrin®	(ep' eh frin)
Emetrol®	(em' eh trol)	Epitol®	(ep' eh tol)
emetine	(em' eh teen)	Epinal®	(ep' eh nal)
Empirin®	(em' pir in)	Epivir®	(ep' ih vir)
Enduron®	(en' du ron)	Combivir®	(kom' bi veer)
enalapril	(e nal' ah pril)	Epogen®	(ee' poe jen)
Anafranil®	(ah naf' ra nil)	Echogen®	(ek' oh jen)
enalapril	(e nal' ah pril)	Epogen®	(ee' poe jen)
Antril®	(an' trill)	Neupogen®	(nu' po gen)
enalapril	(e nal' ah pril)	Equanil®	(eh' kwa nil)
Eldepryl®	(el' de pril)	Elavil®	(el' ah vil)
enalapril	(e nal' ah pril)	Erex®	(err' eks)
nafarelin	(naf' ah re lin)	Urex®	(yur' eks)
enalapril	(e nal' ah pril)	Eryc®	(err' ik)
ramipril	(ra mi' pril)	Emcyt®	(em' sit)
encainide	(en' kay nide)	Eryc®	(err' ik)
flecainide	(fle kay' nide)	Ery-Tab®	(air' ee-tab)
Endal®	(en' dal)	Ery-Tab®	(air' ee-tab)
Depen®	(dee' pen)	Eryc®	(err' ik)
Endal®	(en' dal)	Erythrocin®	(ee rith' roe sin)
Intal®	(in' tal)	Ethmozine®	(eth' mo zeen)
Enduron®	(en' du ron)	erythromycin	(er ith roe mye' sin)
Empirin®	(em' pir in)	azithromycin	(az ith roe mye' sin)
Enduron®	(en' du ron)	erythromycin	(er ith roe mye' sin)
Imuran®	(im' yu ran)	clarithromycin	(kla rith' roe mye sin)
Enduron®	(en' du ron)	erythromycin	(er ith roe mye' sin)
Inderal®	(in' der al)	Ethmozine®	(eth' mo zeen)
Enduronyl®	(en dur' oh nil)	Esidrix®	(es' eh driks)
Inderal®	(in' der al)	Lasix®	(lay' siks)
Enduronyl® Forte	(en dur' oh nil for' tay)	Esimil®	(es' eh mil)
Inderal® 40	(in' der al for' tee)	Estinyl®	(es' teh nil)
enflurane	(en' floo rane)	Esimil®	(es' eh mil)
isoflurane	(eye soe flure' ane)	F.M.L.®	(ef em el)
Entex®	(en' teks)	Esimil®	(es' eh mil)
Tenex®	(ten' eks)	Ismelin®	(is' meh lin)
ephedrine	(e fed' rin)	Eskalith®	(es' ka lith)
Epifrin®	(ep' eh frin)	Estratest®	(es' tra test)
ephedrine	(e fed' rin)	esmolol	(es' moe lol)
epinephrine	(ep i nef' rin)	Osmitrol®	(os' mi trol)
Epifrin®	(ep' eh frin)	Estinyl®	(es' teh nil)
ephedrine	(e fed' rin)	Esimil®	(es' eh mil)
Epifrin®	(ep' eh frin)	Estraderm®	(es' tra derm)
EpiPen®	(ep' eh pen)	Testoderm®	(tes' toh derm)

Drug Name	Pronunciation	Drug Name	Pronunciation
Estratab®	(es' tra tab)	Eurax®	(yoor' aks)
Estratest®	(es' tra test)	Evoxac™	(ef' oh zak)
Estratab®	(es' tra tab)	Eurax®	(yoor' aks)
Estratest HS®	(es' tra test aych ess)	Serax®	(sear' aks)
Estratest®	(es' tra test)	Eurax®	(yoor' aks)
Eskalith®	(es' ka lith)	Urex®	(yur' eks)
Estratest®	(es' tra test)	Evoxac™	(ef' oh zak)
Estratab®	(es' tra tab)	Eurax®	(yoor' aks)
Estratest®	(es' tra test)	Excedrin®	(eks sed' drin)
Estratest HS®	(es' tra test aych ess)	Dexatrim®	(deks' ah trim)
Estratest HS®	(es' tra test aych ess)	Excedrin®	(eks sed' drin)
Estratab®	(es' tra tab)	Dexedrine®	(deks' e drine)
Estratest HS®	(es' tra test aych ess)	Factrel®	(fak' trel)
Estratest®	(es' tra test)	Sectral®	(sek' tral)
Ethamolin®	(ath am' oh lin)	fenoprofen	(fen oh proe' fen)
ethanol	(eth' e nol)	flurbiprofen	(flure bi' proe fen)
ethanol	(eth' e nol)	fentanyl	(fen' ta nil)
Ethamolin®	(ath am' oh lin)	alfentanil	(al fen' ta nil)
ethanol	(eth' e nol)	fentanyl citrate	(fen' ta nil sit' rate)
Ethyol®	(eth' e ole)	sufentanil citrate	(sue fen' ta nil sit' rate)
Ethmozine®	(eth' mo zeen)	Feosol®	(fee' oh sol)
Erythrocin®	(ee rith' roe sin)	Feostat®	(fee' oh stat)
Ethmozine®	(eth' mo zeen)	Feosol®	(fee' oh sol)
erythromycin	(er ith roe mye' sin)	Fer-In-Sol®	(fehr'-in-sol)
ethosuximide	(eth oh sux' i mide)	Feosol®	(fee' oh sol)
methsuximide	(meth sux' i mide)	Festal®	(fes' tal)
Ethyol®	(eth' e ole)	Feosol®	(fee' oh sol)
ethanol	(eth' e nol)	Fluosol®	(flu' oh sol)
etidocaine	(e ti' doe kane)	Feostat®	(fee' oh stat)
etidronate	(e ti droe' nate)	Feosol®	(fee' oh sol)
etidronate	(e ti droe' nate)	Feridex®	(fer' i deks)
etidocaine	(e ti' doe kane)	Fertinex®	(fer' ti neks)
etidronate	(e ti droe' nate)	Fer-In-Sol®	(fehr'-in-sol)
etomidate	(e tom' i date)	Feosol®	(fee' oh sol)
etidronate	(e ti droe' nate)	Ferralet®	(fer' ah let)
etretinate	(e tret' i nate)	Ferrlecit®	(fer' le set)
etomidate	(e tom' i date)	Ferrlecit®	(fer' le set)
etidronate	(e ti droe' nate)	Ferralet®	(fer' ah let)
etretinate	(e tret' i nate)	Fertinex®	(fer' ti neks)
etidronate	(e ti droe' nate)	Feridex®	(fer' i deks)
Eulexin®	(yu leks' in)	Festal®	(fes' tal)
Edecrin®	(ed' eh crin)	Feosol®	(fee' oh sol)
Eulexin®	(yu leks' in)	Feverall™	(fee' ver all)
Eurax®	(yoor' aks)	Fiberall®	(fye' ber all)
Eurax®	(yoor' aks)	Fiberall®	(fye' ber all)
Efudex®	(ef' yu deks)	Feverall™	(fee' ver all)
Eurax®	(yoor' aks)	Fioricet®	(fee oh' reh set)
Eulexin®	(yu leks' in)	Fiorinal®	(fee or' reh nal)

Drug Name	Pronunciation	Drug Name	Pronunciation
Fioricet®	(fee oh' reh set)	fluocinolone	(floo oh sin' oh lone)
Lorcet®	(lor' set)	fluocinonide	(floo oh sin' oh nide)
Fiorinal®	(fee or' reh nal)	fluocinonide	(floo oh sin' oh nide)
Fioricet®	(fee oh' reh set)	flunisolide	(floo nis' oh lide)
Fiorinal®	(fee or' reh nal)	fluocinonide	(floo oh sin' oh nide)
Florical®	(flor' eh kal)	fluocinolone	(floo oh sin' oh lone)
Fiorinal®	(fee or' reh nal)	fluorouracil	(flure oh yoor' ah sil)
Florinef®	(flor' eh nef)	flucytosine	(floo sye' toe seen)
flecainide	(fle kay' nide)	Fluosol®	(flu' oh sol)
encainide	(en' kay nide)	Feosol®	(fee' oh sol)
flecainide	(fle kay' nide)	fluoxetine	(floo oks' e teen)
fluconazole	(floo koe' na zole)	fluvastatin	(floo' va sta tin)
Flexeril®	(fleks' eh ril)	flurazepam	(flure az' e pam)
Floxin®	(floks' in)	temazepam	(te maz' e pam)
Flexeril®	(fleks' eh ril)	flurbiprofen	(flure bi' proe fen)
Hectoral™	(hek' to ral)	fenoprofen	(fen oh proe' fen)
Flexon®	(fleks' on)	flutamide	(floo' ta mide)
Floxin®	(floks' in)	Flumadine®	(floo' ma deen)
Flomax®	(flo' maks)	fluvastatin	(floo' va sta tin)
Fosamax®	(fos' ah maks)	fluoxetine	(floo oks' e teen)
Flomax®	(flo' maks)	F.M.L.®	(ef em el)
Volmax®	(vol' maks)	Esimil®	(es' eh mil)
Florical®	(flor' eh kal)	folic acid	(foe' lik as' id)
Fiorinal®	(fee or' reh nal)	folinic acid	(foe lin' ik as' id)
Florinef®	(flor' eh nef)	folinic acid	(foe lin' ik as' id)
Fiorinal®	(fee or' reh nal)	folic acid	(foe' lik as' id)
Floxin®	(floks' in)	Fortovase®	(for' to vase)
Flexeril®	(fleks' eh ril)	Invirase®	(in' vir ase)
Floxin®	(floks' in)	Fosamax®	(fos' ah maks)
Flexon®	(fleks' on)	Flomax™	(flo' maks)
fluconazole	(floo koe' na zole)	fosinopril	(foe sin' oh pril)
flecainide	(fle kay' nide)	lisinopril	(lyse in' oh pril)
flucytosine	(floo sye' toe seen)	Fostex®	(fos' teks)
fluorouracil	(flure oh yoor' ah sil)	pHisoHex®	(fye' so heks)
Fludara®	(floo dare' ah)	FUDR®	(ef yu dee are)
FUDR®	(ef yu dee are)	Fludara®	(floo dare' ah)
fludarabine	(floo dare' ah been)	Fulvicin®	(ful' vi sin)
Flumadine®	(floo' ma deen)	Furacin®	(fur' ah sin)
Flumadine®	(floo' ma deen)	Furacin®	(fur' ah sin)
fludarabine	(floo dare' ah been)	Fulvicin®	(ful' vi sin)
Flumadine®	(floo' ma deen)	furosemide	(fyoor oh' se mide)
flunisolide	(floo nis' oh lide)	torsemide	(tor' se mide)
Flumadine®	(floo' ma deen)	Gamimune® N	(gam' e mune en)
flutamide	(floo' ta mide)	CytoGam®	(sy' to gam)
flunisolide	(floo nis' oh lide)	Gantrisin®	(gan' tri sin)
Flumadine®	(floo' ma deen)	Gastrosed™	(gas' troe sed)
flunisolide	(floo nis' oh lide)	Garamycin®	(gar ah mye' sin)
fluocinonide	(floo oh sin' oh nide)	kanamycin	(kan ah mye' sin)

Drug Name	Pronunciation	Drug Name	Pronunciation
Garamycin®	(gar ah mye' sin)	Glycotuss®	(glye' co tuss)
Terramycin®	(tehr ah mye' sin)	Glytuss®	(glye' tuss)
Gastrosed™	(gas' troe sed)	Glytuss®	(glye' tuss)
Gantrisin®	(gan' tri sin)	Glycotuss®	(glye' co tuss)
Gemzar®	(gem' zar)	GoLYTELY®	(go lite' lee)
Zinecard®	(zin' e card)	NuLytely®	(nu lite' lee)
Genapap®	(gen' ah pap)	gonadorelin	(goe nad oh rel' in)
Genapax®	(gen' ah paks)	gonadotropin	(goe nad' oh troe pin)
Genapax®	(gen' ah paks)	gonadorelin	(goe nad oh rel' in)
Genapap®	(gen' ah pap)	guanadrel	(gwahn' ah drel)
Gengraf™	(gen' graf)	gonadotropin	(goe nad' oh troe pin)
Prograf®	(pro' graf)	gonadorelin	(goe nad oh rel' in)
Genpril®	(gen' pril)	Granulex®	(gran' u lecks)
Genprin	(gen' prin)	Regranex®	(re gra' neks)
Genprin	(gen' prin)	guaifenesin	(gwye fen' e sin)
Genpril®	(gen' pril)	guanfacine	(gwahn' fa seen)
gentamicin	(jen ta mye' sin)	guanabenz	(gwahn' ah benz)
kanamycin	(kan ah mye' sin)	guanadrel	(gwahn' ah drel)
Glaucon®	(glow' kon)	guanabenz	(gwahn' ah benz)
glucagon	(gloo' ka gon)	guanfacine	(gwahn' fa seen)
glimepiride	(glye' me pye ride)	guanadrel	(gwahn' ah drel)
glipizide	(glip' i zide)	gonadorelin	(goe nad oh rel' in)
glipizide	(glip' i zide)	guanadrel	(gwahn' ah drel)
glimepiride	(glye' me pye ride)	guanabenz	(gwahn' ah benz)
glipizide	(glip' i zide)	guanethidine	(gwahn eth' i deen)
glyburide	(glye' byoor ide)	glutethimide	(gloo teth' i mide)
glucagon	(gloo' ka gon)	guanethidine	(gwahn eth' i deen)
Glaucon®	(glow' kon)	guanidine	(gwahn' i deen)
Glucophage®	(glue' co faagsch)	guanfacine	(gwahn' fa seen)
Glucotrol®	(glue' co trol)	guaifenesin	(gwye fen' e sin)
Glucophage®	(glue' co faagsch)	guanfacine	(gwahn' fa seen)
Glutofac®	(glue' toe fak)	guanabenz	(gwahn' ah benz)
Glucotrol®	(glue' co trol)	guanfacine	(gwahn' fa seen)
Glucophage®	(glue' co faagsch)	guanidine	(gwahn' i deen)
Glucotrol®	(glue' co trol)	guanidine	(gwahn' i deen)
glyburide	(glye' byoor ide)	guanethidine	(gwahn eth' i deen)
glutethimide	(gloo teth' i mide)	guanidine	(gwahn' i deen)
guanethidine	(gwahn eth' i deen)	guanfacine	(gwahn' fa seen)
Glutofac®	(glue' toe fak)	halcinonide	(hal sin' oh nide)
Glucophage®	(glue' co faagsch)	Halcion®	(hal' cee on)
Glutofac®	(glue' toe fak)	Halcion®	(hal' cee on)
Glutose®	(glue' tose)	halcinonide	(hal sin' oh nide)
Glutose®	(glue' tose)	Halcion®	(hal' cee on)
Glutofac®	(glue' toe fak)	Haldol®	(hal' dol)
glyburide	(glye' byoor ide)	Haldol®	(hal' dol)
glipizide	(glip' i zide)	Halcion®	(hal' cee on)
glyburide	(glye' byoor ide)	Haldol®	(hal' dol)
Glucotrol®	(glue' co trol)	Halenol®	(hal' e nol)

Drug Name	Pronunciation	Drug Name	Pronunciation
Haldol®	(hal′ dol)	Hexadrol®	(heks′ ah drol)
Halog®	(hay′ log)	hexatol	(heks′ ah tol)
Haldol®	(hal′ dol)	Hexadrol®	(heks′ ah drol)
Halotestin®	(hay lo tes′ tin)	labetalol	(la bet′ ah lole)
Haldol®	(hal′ dol)	Hexalol®	(heks′ ah lole)
Stadol®	(stay′ dol)	Hexadrol®	(heks′ ah drol)
Halenol®	(hal′ e nol)	hexatol	(heks′ ah tol)
Haldol®	(hal′ dol)	Hexadrol®	(heks′ ah drol)
Halfan®	(hal′ fan)	hexatol	(heks′ ah tol)
Halfprin®	(haf′ prin)	labetalol	(la bet′ ah lole)
Halfprin®	(haf′ prin)	Histaspan®	(his′ ta span)
Halfan®	(hal′ fan)	Hespan®	(hes′ pan)
Halfprin®	(haf′ prin)	Humalog®	(hu′ ma log)
Haltran®	(hal′ tran)	Humulin®	(hu′ mu lin)
Halog®	(hay′ log)	Humulin®	(hu′ mu lin)
Haldol®	(hal′ dol)	Humalog®	(hu′ ma log)
Halog®	(hay′ log)	Hycamtin®	(hye cam′ tin)
Mycolog®	(mye′ co log)	Hycomine®	(hye′ co meen)
haloperidol	(ha loe per′ i dole)	Hycodan®	(hye′ co dan)
Halotestin®	(hay lo tes′ tin)	Hycomine®	(hye′ co meen)
Halotestin®	(hay lo tes′ tin)	Hycodan®	(hye′ co dan)
Haldol®	(hal′ dol)	Vicodin®	(vye′ co din)
Halotestin®	(hay lo tes′ tin)	Hycomine®	(hye′ coe meen)
haloperidol	(ha loe per′ i dole)	Byclomine®	(bye′ clo meen)
Halotestin®	(hay lo tes′ tin)	Hycomine®	(hye′ co meen)
halothane	(ha′ loe thane)	Hycamtin®	(hye cam′ tin)
Halotestin®	(hay lo tes′ tin)	Hycomine®	(hye′ co meen)
Halotussin®	(hay lo tus′ sin)	Hycodan®	(hye′ co dan)
halothane	(ha′ loe thane)	Hycomine®	(hye′ co meen)
Halotestin®	(hay lo tes′ tin)	Vicodin®	(vye′ co din)
Halotussin®	(hay lo tus′ sin)	Hydergine®	(hye′ der geen)
Halotestin®	(hay lo tes′ tin)	Hydramyn®	(hye′ dra min)
Haltran®	(hal′ tran)	hydralazine	(hye dral′ ah zeen)
Halfprin®	(haf′ prin)	hydroxyzine	(hye drox′ i zeen)
Hectoral™	(hek′ to ral)	Hydramyn®	(hye′ dra min)
Flexeril®	(fleks′ eh ril)	Bydramine®	(bye′ dra meen)
Hemoccult®	(he′ mo cult)	Hydramyn®	(hye′ dra min)
Seracult®	(ser′ a cult)	Hydergine®	(hye′ der geen)
heparin	(hep′ a rin)	Hydrocet®	(hye′ dro set)
Hespan®	(hes′ pan)	Hydrocil®	(hye′ dro sil)
Herceptin®	(her cep′ tin)	hydrochlorothiazide	(hye droe klor oh thye′ ah zide)
Perceptin™	(per cep′ tin)	hydroflumethiazide	(hye droe floo meth eye′ ah zide)
Hespan®	(hes′ pan)	Hydrocil®	(hye′ dro sil)
heparin	(hep′ a rin)	Hydrocet®	(hye′ dro set)
Hespan®	(hes′ pan)	hydrocodone	(hye droe koe′ done)
Histaspan®	(his′ ta span)	hydrocortisone	(hye droe kor′ ti sone)
Hexadrol®	(heks′ ah drol)		
Hexalol®	(heks′ ah lole)		

Drug Name	Pronunciation	Drug Name	Pronunciation
hydrocortisone	(hye droe kor′ ti sone)	imipramine	(im ip′ ra meen)
hydrocodone	(hye droe koe′ done)	desipramine	(des ip′ ra meen)
hydrocortisone	(hye droe kor′ ti sone)	imipramine	(im ip′ ra meen)
hydroxychloroquine	(hye droks ee klor′ oh kwin)	Norpramin®	(nor′ pra min)
hydroflumethiazide	(hye droe floo meth eye′ ah zide)	Imodium®	(i moe′ de um)
		Indocin®	(in′ doe sin)
hydrochlorothiazide	(hye droe klor oh thye′ ah zide)	Imodium®	(i moe′ de um)
		Ionamin®	(eye oh′ na min)
hydromorphone	(hye droe mor′ fone)	Imuran®	(im′ yu ran)
morphine	(mor′ feen)	Elmiron®	(el′ mi ron)
hydroxychloroquine	(hye droks ee klor′ oh kwin)	Imuran®	(im′ yu ran)
		Enduron®	(en′ du ron)
hydrocortisone	(hye droe kor′ ti sone)	Imuran®	(im′ yu ran)
hydroxyprogesterone	(hye droks ee proe jes′ te rone)	Inderal®	(in′ der al)
medroxyprogesterone	(me droks′ ee proe jes′ te rone)	Imuran®	(im′ yu ran)
		Imdur®	(im′ dure)
hydroxyurea	(hye drox ee yoor ee′ a)	Imuran®	(im′ yu ran)
hydroxyzine	(hye drox′ i zeen)	Tenormin®	(ten or′ min)
hydroxyzine	(hye drox′ i zeen)	Inapsine®	(i nap′ seen)
hydralazine	(hye dral′ ah zeen)	Nebcin®	(neb′ sin)
hydroxyzine	(hye drox′ i zeen)	indapamide	(in dap′ a mide)
hydroxyurea	(hye drox ee yoor ee′ a)	iodamide	(eye oh′ da mide)
HyperHep®	(hye′ per hep)	indapamide	(in dap′ a mide)
Hyperstat®	(hye′ per stat)	iopamidol	(eye oh pam′ i dol)
Hyperstat®	(hye′ per stat)	indapamide	(in dap′ a mide)
Nitrostat®	(nye′ troe stat)	Iopidine®	(eye oh′ pe deen)
Hytone®	(hye′ tone)	Inderal®	(in′ der al)
Vytone®	(vye′ tone)	Adderall®	(ad′ der all)
Hyzaar®	(hi′ zar)	Inderal®	(in′ der al)
Cozaar®	(koe′ zar)	Enduron®	(en′ du ron)
Idamycin®	(eye da mye′ sin)	Inderal®	(in′ der al)
Adriamycin™	(ade rya mye′ sin)	Enduronyl®	(en dur′ oh nil)
idarubicin	(eye byoo proe′ fen)	Inderal®	(in′ der al)
doxorubicin	(doks oh roo′ bi sin)	Imuran®	(im′ yu ran)
Iletin®	(il′ e tin)	Inderal®	(in′ der al)
Lente®	(len′ tay)	Inderide®	(in′ der ide)
Imdur®	(im′ dure)	Inderal®	(in′ der al)
Imuran®	(im′ yu ran)	Isordil®	(eye′ sor dil)
Imdur®	(im′ dure)	Inderal®	(in′ der al)
Inderal LA®	(in′ der al el ay)	Toradol®	(tor′ ah doll)
Imdur®	(im′ dure)	Inderal® 40	(in′ der al for′ tee)
K-Dur®	(kay′-dur)	Enduronyl® Forte	(en dur′ oh nil for′ tay)
Imferon®	(im′ fer on)	Inderal LA®	(in′ der al el ay)
interferon	(in ter fer′ on)	Imdur®	(im′ dure)
Imferon®	(im′ fer on)	Inderide®	(in′ der ide)
Roferon-A®	(roe fer′ on-ay)	Inderal®	(in′ der al)
imipramine	(im ip′ ra meen)	indinavir	(in din′ a veer)
amitriptyline	(ah mee trip′ ti leen)	Denavir™	(den′ ah vir)

Drug Name	Pronunciation	Drug Name	Pronunciation
Indocin® Imodium®	(in' doe sin) (i moe' de um)	Ismelin® Isuprel®	(is' meh lin) (eye' sue prel)
Indocin® Lincocin®	(in' doe sin) (link' oh sin)	Ismelin® Ritalin®	(is' meh lin) (ri' ta lin)
Indocin® Minocin®	(in' doe sin) (min' oh sin)	isoflurane enflurane	(eye soe flure' ane) (en' floo rane)
Indocin® Vicodin®	(in' doe sin) (vye' co din)	isoflurane isoflurophate	(eye soe flure' ane) (eye soe flure' oh fate)
Intal® Endal®	(in' tal) (en' dal)	isoflurophate isoflurane	(eye soe flure' oh fate) (eye soe flure' ane)
interferon Imferon®	(in ter fer' on) (im' fer on)	Isoptin® Isopto® Tears	(eye sop' tin) (eye sop' tow tears)
interferon 2 interleukin 2	(in ter feer' on too) (in ter lu' kin too)	Isopto® Carbachol Isopto® Carpine	(eye sop' to car' ba kol) (eye sop' to kar' peen)
interferon alfa-2a interferon alfa-2b	(in ter feer' on al' fa-too aye) (in ter feer' on al' fa-too bee)	Isopto® Carpine Isopto® Carbachol	(eye sop' to kar' peen) (eye sop' to car' ba kol)
interferon alfa-2b interferon alfa-2a	(in ter feer' on al' fa-too bee) (in ter feer' on al' fa-too aye)	Isopto® Tears Isoptin®	(eye sop' tow tears) (eye sop' tin)
interleukin 2 interferon 2	(in ter lu' kin too) (in ter feer' on too)	Isordil® Inderal®	(eye' sor dil) (in' der al)
Invirase® Fortovase®	(in' vir ase) (for' to vase)	Isordil® Isuprel®	(eye' sor dil) (eye' sue prel)
iodamide indapamide	(eye oh' da mide) (in dap' a mide)	Isuprel® Disophrol®	(eye' sue prel) (dye' so frol)
iodine codeine	(eye' oh dyne) (koe' deen)	Isuprel® Ismelin®	(eye' sue prel) (is' meh lin)
iodine Iopidine®	(eye' oh dyne) (eye oh' pe deen)	Isuprel® Isordil®	(eye' sue prel) (eye' sor dil)
iodine Lodine®	(eye' oh dyne) (low' deen)	kanamycin Garamycin®	(kan ah mye' sin) (gar ah mye' sin)
iodine Iopidine	(eye' oh dyne) (low' pi deen)	kanamycin gentamicin	(kan ah mye' sin) (jen ta mye' sin)
Ionamin® Imodium®	(eye oh' na min) (i moe' de um)	Kaochlor® K-Lor®	(kay' oh klor) (kay'-lor)
iopamidol indapamide	(eye oh pam' i dol) (in dap' a mide)	kaolin Kaon®	(kay' oh lin) (kay' on)
Iopidine® indapamide	(eye oh' pe deen) (in dap' a mide)	Kaon® kaolin	(kay' on) (kay' oh lin)
Iopidine® iodine	(eye oh' pe deen) (eye' oh dyne)	Kaopectate® Kayexelate®	(kay oh pek' tate) (kay eks' e late)
Iopidine® Lodine®	(eye oh' pe deen) (low' deen)	Kayexelate® Kaopectate®	(kay eks' e late) (kay oh pek' tate)
Ismelin® Esimil®	(is' meh lin) (es' eh mil)	K-Dur® Cardura®	(kay'-dur) (kar dur' ah)
		K-Dur® Imdur®	(kay'-dur) (im' dure)
		Kefzol® Cefzil®	(kef' zol) (sef' zil)

Drug Name	Pronunciation	Drug Name	Pronunciation
Kemadrin®	(kem' ah drin)	Lamictal®	(la mic' tal)
Coumadin®	(ku' ma din)	Ludiomil®	(lu' de oh mil)
Kenalog®	(ken' ah log)	Lamisil®	(lam' eh sil)
Ketalar®	(key' tah lar)	Lamicel®	(lam' i cel)
Ketalar®	(key' tah lar)	Lamisil®	(lam' eh sil)
Kenalog®	(ken' ah log)	Lamictal®	(la mic' tal)
Klaron®	(kla' ron)	Lamisil®	(lam' eh sil)
Klor-Con®	(klor' kon)	Lomotil®	(lo' mo til)
Klonopin®	(klon' oh pin)	lamivudine	(la mi' vyoo deen)
clonazepam	(kloe na' ze pam)	lamotrigine	(la moe' tri jeen)
Klonopin®	(klon' oh pin)	lamotrigine	(la moe' tri jeen)
clonidine	(kloe' ni deen)	labetalol	(la bet' ah lole)
K-Lor®	(kay'-lor)	lamotrigine	(la moe' tri jeen)
Kaochlor®	(kay' oh klor)	Lamisil®	(lam' eh sil)
K-Lor®	(kay'-lor)	lamotrigine	(la moe' tri jeen)
Klor-Con®	(klor'-kon)	lamivudine	(la mi' vyoo deen)
Klor-Con®	(klor'-kon)	lamotrigine	(la moe' tri jeen)
Klaron®	(kla' ron)	Lomotil®	(lo' mo til)
Klor-Con®	(klor'-kon)	lamotrigine	(la moe' tri jeen)
K-Lor®	(kay'-lor)	Ludiomil®	(lu' de oh mil)
Klotrix®	(klo' triks)	Lanoxin®	(lan oks' in)
liotrix	(lye' oh triks)	Lasix®	(lay' siks)
Komex®	(koe' meks)	Lanoxin®	(lan oks' in)
Koromex®	(kor' oh meks)	Levoxine®	(lev oks' een)
Koromex®	(kor' oh meks)	Lanoxin®	(lan oks' in)
Komex®	(koe' meks)	Levoxyl®	(le voks' ill)
K-Phos Neutral®	(kay'-fos new' tral)	Lanoxin®	(lan oks' in)
Neutra-Phos-K®	(new' tra-fos-kay)	Levsinex®	(lev' si neks)
labetalol	(la bet' ah lole)	Lanoxin®	(lan oks' in)
betaxolol	(be taks' oh lol)	Lomotil®	(lo' mo til)
labetalol	(la bet' ah lole)	Lanoxin®	(lan oks' in)
Hexadrol®	(heks' ah drol)	Lonox®	(lo' noks)
labetalol	(la bet' ah lole)	Lanoxin®	(lan oks' in)
hexatol	(heks' ah tol)	Mefoxin®	(me fox' in)
labetalol	(la bet' ah lole)	Lanoxin®	(lan oks' in)
lamotrigine	(la moe' tri jeen)	Xanax®	(zan' aks)
Lacrilube®	(lac' ri lube)	Lantus®	(lan' tus)
Surgilube®	(sur' gi lube)	Lente®	(len' tay)
lactose	(lak' tose)	Larylgan®	(la ril' gan)
lactulose	(lak' tu lose)	Auralgan®	(ah ral' gan)
lactulose	(lak' tu lose)	Lasix®	(lay' siks)
lactose	(lak' tose)	Esidrix®	(es' eh driks)
Lamicel®	(lam' i cel)	Lasix®	(lay' siks)
Lamisil®	(lam' eh sil)	Lanoxin®	(lan oks' in)
Lamictal®	(la mic' tal)	Lasix®	(lay' siks)
Lamisil®	(lam' eh sil)	Lidex®	(lye' deks)
Lamictal®	(la mic' tal)	Lasix®	(lay' siks)
Lomotil®	(lo' mo til)	Lomotil®	(lo' mo til)

781

Drug Name	Pronunciation	Drug Name	Pronunciation
Lasix®	(lay′ siks)	Levophed®	(lee′ voe fed)
Luvox®	(lu′ voks)	Levoprome®	(lee′ voe prome)
Lasix®	(lay′ siks)	Levoprome®	(lee′ voe prome)
Luxiq™	(luks′ ik)	Levophed®	(lee′ voe fed)
l-dopa	(l-doe′ pa)	levothyroxine	(lee voe thye rox′ een)
levodopa	(lee voe doe′ pa)	liothyronine	(lye oh thye′ roe neen)
l-dopa	(l-doe′ pa)	Levoxine®	(lev oks′ een)
methyldopa	(meth ill doe′ pa)	Lanoxin®	(lan oks′ in)
Lente®	(len′ tay)	Levoxine®	(lev oks′ een)
Iletin®	(il′ e tin)	Levoxyl®	(le voks′ ill)
Lente®	(len′ tay)	Levoxine®	(lev oks′ een)
Lantus®	(lan′ tus)	Levsin®	(lev′ sin)
leucovorin	(loo koe vor′ in)	Levoxyl®	(le voks′ ill)
Leukeran®	(lu′ keh ran)	Lanoxin®	(lan oks′ in)
leucovorin	(loo koe vor′ in)	Levoxyl®	(le voks′ ill)
Leukine®	(lu′ keen)	Levoxine®	(lev oks′ een)
Leukeran®	(lu′ keh ran)	Levoxyl®	(le voks′ ill)
Alkeran®	(al′ ker an)	Luvox®	(lu′ voks)
Leukeran®	(lu′ keh ran)	Levsin®	(lev′ sin)
leucovorin	(loo koe vor′ in)	Levoxine®	(lev oks′ een)
Leukeran®	(lu′ keh ran)	Levsinex®	(lev′ si neks)
Leukine®	(lu′ keen)	Lanoxin®	(lan oks′ in)
Leukine®	(lu′ keen)	Librax®	(li′ braks)
leucovorin	(loo koe vor′ in)	Librium®	(li′ bre um)
Leukine®	(lu′ keen)	Librium®	(li′ bre um)
Leukeran®	(lu′ keh ran)	Librax®	(li′ braks)
Leustatin™	(lu sta′ tin)	Lidex®	(ly′ decks)
lovastatin	(loe′ va sta tin)	Cidex®	(sy′ decks)
Levatol®	(lee′ va tol)	Lidex®	(lye′ deks)
Lipitor®	(li′ pi tor)	Lasix®	(lay′ siks)
Levbid®	(lev′ bid)	Lidex®	(lye′ deks)
Lithobid®	(lith′ oh bid)	Lidox®	(lye′ dox)
Levbid®	(lev′ bid)	Lidex®	(lye′ deks)
Lopid®	(lo′ pid)	Videx®	(vye′ deks)
Levbid®	(lev′ bid)	Lidex®	(lye′ deks)
Lorabid®	(lor′ ah bid)	Wydase®	(wye′ dase)
levobunolol	(lee voe byoo′ noe lole)	Lidox®	(lye′ dox)
levocabastine	(lee′ voe kab as teen)	Lidex®	(lye′ deks)
levocabastine	(lee′ voe kab as teen)	Lincocin®	(link′ oh sin)
levobunolol	(lee voe byoo′ noe lole)	Cleocin®	(klee′ oh sin)
levocabastine	(lee′ voe kab as teen)	Lincocin®	(link′ oh sin)
levocarnitine	(lee voe kar′ ni teen)	Indocin®	(in′ doe sin)
levocarnitine	(lee voe kar′ ni teen)	Lincocin®	(link′ oh sin)
levocabastine	(lee voe byoo′ noe lole)	Minocin®	(min′ oh sin)
levodopa	(lee voe doe′ pa)	Lioresal®	(lye or′ reh sal)
l-dopa	(l-doe′ pa)	lisinopril	(lyse in′ oh pril)
levodopa	(lee voe doe′ pa)	Lioresal®	(lye or′ reh sal)
methyldopa	(meth ill doe′ pa)	Lotensin®	(lo ten′ sin)

Drug Name	Pronunciation	Drug Name	Pronunciation
liothyronine	(lye oh thye' roe neen)	Lopid®	(lo' pid)
levothyroxine	(lee voe thye rox' een)	Levbid®	(lev' bid)
liotrix	(lye' oh triks)	Lopid®	(lo' pid)
Klotrix®	(klo' triks)	Lodine®	(low' deen)
Lipitor®	(li' pi tor)	Lopid®	(lo' pid)
Levatol®	(lee' va tol)	Lorabid®	(lor' ah bid)
lisinopril	(lyse in' oh pril)	Lopid®	(lo' pid)
fosinopril	(foe sin' oh pril)	Slo-bid™	(slo' bid)
lisinopril	(lyse in' oh pril)	Lopressor®	(lo pres' sor)
Lioresal®	(lye or' reh sal)	Lopurin®	(lo pure' in)
lisinopril	(lyse in' oh pril)	Loprox®	(loe' procks)
Risperdal®	(ris' per dal)	Lonox®	(lo' noks)
Lithobid®	(lith' oh bid)	Lopurin®	(lo pure' in)
Levbid®	(lev' bid)	Lopressor®	(lo pres' sor)
Lithobid®	(lith' oh bid)	Lopurin®	(lo pure' in)
Lithostat®	(lith' oh stat)	Lupron®	(lu' pron)
Lithostat®	(lith' oh stat)	Lorabid®	(lor' ah bid)
Lithobid®	(lith' oh bid)	Levbid®	(lev' bid)
Livostin®	(lye' voe stin)	Lorabid®	(lor' ah bid)
lovastatin	(loe' va sta tin)	Lopid®	(lo' pid)
Lodine®	(low' deen)	Lorabid®	(lor' ah bid)
codeine	(koe' deen)	Lortab®	(lor' tab)
Lodine®	(low' deen)	Lorabid®	(lor' ah bid)
iodine	(eye' oh dyne)	Slo-bid™	(slo' bid)
Lodine®	(low' deen)	lorazepam	(lor a' ze pam)
Iopidine®	(eye oh' pe deen)	alprazolam	(al pray' zoe lam)
Lodine®	(low' deen)	lorazepam	(lor a' ze pam)
Lopid®	(lo' pid)	clonazepam	(kloe na' ze pam)
Lomodix®	(lo' mo dix)	lorazepam	(lor a' ze pam)
Lovenox®	(lo' ve nox)	diazepam	(dye az' ah pam)
Lomotil®	(lo' mo til)	lorazepam	(lor a' ze pam)
Lamictal®	(la mic' tal)	temazepam	(te maz' e pam)
Lomotil®	(lo' mo til)	Lorcet®	(lor' set)
Lamisil®	(lam' eh sil)	Fioricet®	(fee oh' reh set)
Lomotil®	(lo' mo til)	Lortab®	(lor' tab)
lamotrigine	(la moe' tri jeen)	Cortef®	(kor' tef)
Lomotil®	(lo' mo til)	Lortab®	(lor' tab)
Lanoxin®	(lan oks' in)	Lorabid®	(lor' ah bid)
Lomotil®	(lo' mo til)	Lortab®	(lor' tab)
Lasix®	(lay' siks)	Luride®	(lure' ide)
Loniten®	(lon' eh ten)	losartan	(loe sar' tan)
clonidine	(kloe' ni deen)	valsartan	(val sar' tan)
Loniten®	(lon' eh ten)	Lotensin®	(lo ten' sin)
Lotensin®	(lo ten' sin)	Lioresal®	(lye or' reh sal)
Lonox®	(lo' noks)	Lotensin®	(lo ten' sin)
Lanoxin®	(lan oks' in)	Loniten®	(lon' eh ten)
Lonox®	(lo' noks)	Lotensin®	(lo ten' sin)
Loprox®	(loe' procks)	lovastatin	(loe' va sta tin)

Drug Name	Pronunciation
Lotrimin®	(low' tri min)
Lotrisone®	(low' tri sone)
Lotrimin®	(low' tri min)
Otrivin®	(oh' tri vin)
Lotrisone®	(low' tri sone)
Lotrimin®	(low' tri min)
Lotronex®	(lo' tro neks)
Lovenox®	(lo' ve nox)
Lotronex®	(lo' tro neks)
Protonix®	(pro' to niks)
lovastatin	(loe' va sta tin)
Leustatin™	(lu sta' tin)
lovastatin	(loe' va sta tin)
Livostin®	(lye' voe stin)
lovastatin	(loe' va sta tin)
Lotensin®	(lo ten' sin)
Lovenox®	(lo' ve nox)
Lomodix®	(lo' mo dix)
Lovenox®	(lo' ve nox)
Lotronex®	(lo' tro neks)
Loxitane®	(loks' e tane)
Soriatane®	(sor' e ah tane)
Ludiomil®	(lu' de oh mil)
Lamictal®	(la mic' tal)
Ludiomil®	(lu' de oh mil)
lamotrigine	(la moe' tri jeen)
Luminal®	(lu' mi nal)
Tuinal®	(tu' i nal)
Lupron®	(lu' pron)
Lopurin®	(lo pure' in)
Lupron®	(lu' pron)
Nuprin®	(nu' prin)
Luride®	(lure' ide)
Lortab®	(lor' tab)
Luvox®	(lu' voks)
Lasix®	(lay' siks)
Luvox®	(lu' voks)
Levoxyl®	(le voks' ill)
Luxiq™	(luks' ik)
Lasix®	(lay' siks)
Maalox®	(may' loks)
Maox®	(may' oks)
Maalox®	(may' loks)
Monodox®	(mon' oh doks)
magnesium sulfate	(mag nee' zhum sul' fate)
manganese sulfate	(man' gan neese sul' fate)
Maltsupex®	(malt' su peks)
Manoplax®	(man' oh plaks)

Drug Name	Pronunciation
Mandol®	(man' dole)
nadolol	(nay doe' lole)
manganese sulfate	(man' gan neese sul' fate)
magnesium sulfate	(mag nee' zhum sul' fate)
Manoplax®	(man' oh plaks)
Maltsupex®	(malt' su peks)
Maox®	(may' oks)
Maalox®	(may' loks)
Marcaine®	(mar' kane)
Narcan®	(nar' kan)
Marinol®	(mare' i nole)
Marnal®	(mar' nal)
Marnal®	(mar' nal)
Marinol®	(mare' i nole)
Matulane®	(mat' chu lane)
Modane®	(moe' dane)
Maxidex®	(maks' i deks)
Maxzide®	(maks' zide)
Maxzide®	(maks' zide)
Maxidex®	(maks' i deks)
Mazicon®	(maz' ih con)
mazindol	(may' zin dole)
Mazicon®	(maz' ih con)
Mivacron®	(mi' va cron)
mazindol	(may' zin dole)
Mazicon®	(maz' ih con)
mazindol	(may' zin dole)
mebendazole	(me ben' da zole)
Mebaral®	(meb' ah ral)
Medrol®	(med' role)
Mebaral®	(meb' ah ral)
Mellaril®	(mel' ah ril)
Mebaral®	(meb' ah ral)
Tegretol®	(teg' ree tol)
mebendazole	(me ben' da zole)
mazindol	(may' zin dole)
mecamylamine	(mek ah mill' ah meen)
mesalamine	(me sal' ah meen)
Medrol®	(med' role)
Mebaral®	(meb' ah ral)
medroxyprogesterone	(me droks' ee proe jes' te rone)
hydroxyprogesterone	(hye droks ee proe jes' te rone)
medroxyprogesterone	(me droks' ee proe jes' te rone)
methylprednisolone	(meth il pred nis' oh lone)

Drug Name	Pronunciation
medroxyprogesterone	(me droks' ee proe jes' te rone)
methyltestosterone	(meth il tes tos' te rone)
Mefoxin®	(me fox' in)
Lanoxin®	(lan oks' in)
Megace®	(me' gase)
Reglan®	(reg' lan)
Mellaril®	(mel' la ril)
Elavil®	(el' ah vil)
Mellaril®	(mel' ah ril)
Mebaral®	(meb' ah ral)
melphalan	(mel' fa lan)
Mephyton®	(meh fye' ton)
melphalan	(mel' fa lan)
Myleran®	(my' ler an)
Mepergan®	(me' per gan)
meprobamate	(me proe ba' mate)
meperidine	(me per' i deen)
meprobamate	(me proe ba' mate)
mephenytoin	(me fen' i toyn)
Mephyton®	(meh fye' ton)
mephenytoin	(me fen' i toyn)
phenytoin	(fen' i toyn)
mephobarbital	(me foe bar' bi tal)
methocarbamol	(meth oh kar' ba mole)
Mephyton®	(meh fye' ton)
melphalan	(mel' fa lan)
Mephyton®	(meh fye' ton)
mephenytoin	(me fen' i toyn)
Mephyton®	(meh fye' ton)
methadone	(meth' ah done)
mepivacaine	(me piv' ah kane)
bupivacaine	(byoo piv' ah kane)
meprobamate	(me proe ba' mate)
Mepergan®	(me' per gan)
meprobamate	(me proe ba' mate)
meperidine	(me per' i deen)
Meruvax®	(mur' yu vaks)
Attenuvax®	(at ten' yu vaks)
mesalamine	(me sal' ah meen)
mecamylamine	(mek ah mill' ah meen)
Mestinon®	(meh' sti non)
Metatensin®	(me ta ten' sin)
metaproterenol	(met ah proe ter' e nol)
metipranolol	(met i pran' oh lol)
metaproterenol	(met ah proe ter' e nol)
metoprolol	(me toe' proe lole)
Metatensin®	(me ta ten' sin)
Mestinon®	(meh' sti non)

Drug Name	Pronunciation
metaxalone	(me taks' ah lone)
metolazone	(me tole' ah zone)
methadone	(meth' ah done)
Mephyton®	(meh fye' ton)
methadone	(meth' ah done)
methylphenidate	(meth il fen' i date)
methazolamide	(meth ah zoe' la mide)
methenamine	(meth en' ah meen)
methazolamide	(meth ah zoe' la mide)
metolazone	(me tole' ah zone)
methenamine	(meth en' ah meen)
methazolamide	(meth ah zoe' la mide)
methenamine	(meth en' ah meen)
methionine	(me thye' oh neen)
methicillin	(meth i sill' in)
mezlocillin	(mez loe sill' in)
methionine	(me thye' oh neen)
methenamine	(meth en' ah meen)
methocarbamol	(meth oh kar' ba mole)
mephobarbital	(me foe bar' bi tal)
methotrexate	(meth oh treks' ate)
metolazone	(me tole' ah zone)
methsuximide	(meth sux' i mide)
ethosuximide	(eth oh sux' i mide)
methyldopa	(meth ill doe' pa)
l-dopa	(l-doe' pa)
methyldopa	(meth ill doe' pa)
levodopa	(lee voe doe' pa)
methylphenidate	(meth il fen' i date)
methadone	(meth' ah done)
methylprednisolone	(meth il pred nis' oh lone)
medroxyprogesterone	(me droks' ee proe jes' te rone)
methylprednisolone	(meth il pred nis' oh lone)
prednisone	(pred' ni sone)
methyltestosterone	(meth il tes tos' te rone)
medroxyprogesterone	(me droks' ee proe jes' te rone)
metipranolol	(met i pran' oh lol)
metaproterenol	(met ah proe ter' e nol)
metoclopramide	(met oh kloe pra' mide)
metolazone	(me tole' ah zone)
metolazone	(me tole' ah zone)
metaxalone	(me taks' ah lone)
metolazone	(me tole' ah zone)
methazolamide	(meth ah zoe' la mide)
metolazone	(me tole' ah zone)
methotrexate	(meth oh treks' ate)

Drug Name	Pronunciation	Drug Name	Pronunciation
metolazone	(me tole′ ah zone)	Midrin®	(mid′ rin)
metoclopramide	(met oh kloe pra′ mide)	Mydfrin®	(mid′ frin)
metolazone	(me tole′ ah zone)	Mifeprex®	(mye′ fe preks)
metoprolol	(me toe proe′ lole)	Mirapex®	(mir′ ah peks)
metolazone	(me tole′ ah zone)	Minizide®	(min′ i zide)
minoxidil	(mi nox′ i dill)	Minocin®	(min′ oh sin)
metoprolol	(me toe′ proe lole)	Minocin®	(min′ oh sin)
metaproterenol	(met ah proe ter′ e nol)	Indocin®	(in′ doe sin)
metoprolol	(me toe′ proe lole)	Minocin®	(min′ oh sin)
metolazone	(me tole′ ah zone)	Lincocin®	(link′ oh sin)
metoprolol	(me toe proe′ lole)	Minocin®	(min′ oh sin)
misoprostol	(mye soe prost′ ole)	Minizide®	(min′ i zide)
metyrapone	(me teer′ ah pone)	Minocin®	(min′ oh sin)
metyrosine	(me tye′ roe seen)	Mithracin®	(mith′ ra sin)
metyrosine	(me tye′ roe seen)	Minocin®	(min′ oh sin)
metyrapone	(me teer′ ah pone)	niacin	(nye′ ah sin)
Mevacor®	(me′ va cor)	minoxidil	(mi nox′ i dill)
Mivacron®	(mi′ va cron)	metolazone	(me tole′ ah zone)
Mexitil®	(meks′ i til)	minoxidil	(mi noks′ i dil)
Mezlin®	(mes′ lin)	Monopril®	(mon′ oh pril)
Mezlin®	(mes′ lin)	MiraLax™	(mir′ ah laks)
Mexitil®	(meks′ i til)	Mirapex®	(mir′ ah peks)
mezlocillin	(mez loe sill′ in)	Mirapex®	(mir′ ah peks)
methicillin	(meth i sill′ in)	Mifeprex®	(mye′ fe preks)
Miacalcin®	(my ah cal′ sin)	Mirapex®	(mir′ ah peks)
Micatin®	(my′ ca tin)	MiraLax™	(mir′ ah laks)
Micatin®	(my′ ca tin)	misoprostol	(mye soe prost′ ole)
Miacalcin®	(my ah cal′ sin)	metoprolol	(me toe proe′ lole)
miconazole	(mi kon′ ah zole)	Mithracin®	(mith′ ra sin)
Micronase®	(mye′ croe nase)	Minocin®	(min′ oh sin)
miconazole	(mi kon′ ah zole)	mithramycin	(mi thra mye′ sin)
Micronor®	(mye′ croe nor)	mitomycin	(mye toe mye′ sin)
Micro-K®	(mye′ cro-kay)	mitomycin	(mye toe mye′ sin)
Micronase®	(mye′ croe nase)	mithramycin	(mi thra mye′ sin)
Micronase®	(mye′ croe nase)	mitomycin	(mye toe mye′ sin)
miconazole	(mi kon′ ah zole)	mitotane	(mye′ toe tane)
Micronase®	(mye′ croe nase)	mitomycin	(mye toe mye′ sin)
Micro-K®	(mye′ cro-kay)	mitoxantrone	(mye toe zan′ trone)
Micronase®	(mye′ croe nase)	mitomycin	(mye toe mye′ sin)
Micronor®	(mye′ croe nor)	Mutamycin®	(mute ah mye′ sin)
Micronor®	(mye′ croe nor)	mitotane	(mye′ toe tane)
miconazole	(mi kon′ ah zole)	mitomycin	(mye toe mye′ sin)
Micronor®	(mye′ croe nor)	mitoxantrone	(mye toe zan′ trone)
Micronase®	(mye′ croe nase)	mitomycin	(mye toe mye′ sin)
Mictrin®	(mik′ trin)	Mivacron®	(mi′ va cron)
Midrin®	(mid′ rin)	Mazicon®	(maz′ ih con)
Midrin®	(mid′ rin)	Mivacron®	(mi′ va cron)
Mictrin®	(mik′ trin)	Mevacor®	(me′ va cor)

Drug Name	Pronunciation	Drug Name	Pronunciation
Moban®	(moe′ ban)	Myambutol®	(mya am′ byoo tol)
Mobidin®	(moe by′ din)	Nembutal®	(nem′ byoo tal)
Moban®	(moe′ ban)	Mycelex®	(mye′ si leks)
Modane®	(moe′ dane)	Myoflex®	(mye′ oh fleks)
Mobidin®	(moe by′ din)	Mycifradin®	(mye ce fray′ din)
Moban®	(moe′ ban)	Mycitracin®	(mye ce tray′ sin)
Mobidin®	(moe by′ din)	Myciguent®	(mye′ ci kwent)
molindone	(moe lin′ done)	Mycitracin®	(mye ce tray′ sin)
Modane®	(moe′ dane)	Mycitracin®	(mye ce tray′ sin)
Matulane®	(mat′ chu lane)	Mycifradin®	(mye ce fray′ din)
Modane®	(moe′ dane)	Mycitracin®	(mye ce tray′ sin)
Moban®	(moe′ ban)	Myciguent®	(mye′ ci kwent)
Modane®	(moe′ dane)	Mycolog®	(mye′ co log)
Mudrane®	(mud′ rane)	Halog®	(hay′ log)
Modicon®	(mod′ i kon)	Mydfrin®	(mid′ frin)
Mylicon®	(mye′ li kon)	Midrin®	(mid′ rin)
moexipril	(mo ex′ i pril)	Mylanta®	(mye lan′ ta)
Monopril®	(mon′ oh pril)	Mynatal®	(mye′ na tal)
molindone	(moe lin′ done)	Myleran®	(mye′ leh ran)
Mobidin®	(moe by′ din)	melphalan	(mel′ fa lan)
Monodox®	(mon′ oh doks)	Myleran®	(mye′ leh ran)
Maalox®	(may′ loks)	Mylicon®	(mye′ li kon)
Monoket®	(mon′ oh ket)	Mylicon®	(mye′ li kon)
Monopril®	(mon′ oh pril)	Modicon®	(mod′ i kon)
Monopril®	(mon′ oh pril)	Mylicon®	(mye′ li kon)
Accupril®	(ak′ cue pril)	Myleran®	(mye′ leh ran)
Monopril®	(mon′ oh pril)	Mynatal®	(mye′ na tal)
minoxidil	(mi noks′ i dil)	Mylanta®	(mye lan′ ta)
Monopril®	(mon′ oh pril)	Myoflex®	(mye′ oh fleks)
moexipril	(mo ex′ i pril)	Mycelex®	(mye′ si leks)
Monopril®	(mon′ oh pril)	nadolol	(nay doe′ lole)
Monoket®	(mon′ oh ket)	Mandol®	(man′ dole)
Monopril®	(mon′ oh pril)	nafarelin	(naf′ ah re lin)
Monurol™	(mon′ you rol)	Anafranil®	(ah naf′ ra nil)
Monopril®	(mon′ oh pril)	nafarelin	(naf′ ah re lin)
ramipril	(ra mi′ pril)	enalapril	(e nal′ ah pril)
Monurol™	(mon′ you rol)	Naldecon®	(nal′ dee kon)
Monopril®	(mon′ oh pril)	Nalfon®	(nal′ fon)
morphine	(mor′ feen)	Nalfon®	(nal′ fon)
hydromorphone	(hye droe mor′ fone)	Naldecon®	(nal′ dee kon)
Mudrane®	(mud′ rane)	naloxone	(nal ox′ one)
Modane®	(moe′ dane)	naltrexone	(nal treks′ one)
Murocel®	(myur′ oh cel)	naltrexone	(nal treks′ one)
Murocoll-2®	(myur′ oh coll-2)	naloxone	(nal ox′ one)
Murocoll-2®	(myur′ oh coll-2)	Naprelan®	(nap′ re lan)
Murocel®	(myur′ oh cel)	Naprosyn®	(na′ pro sin)
Mutamycin®	(mute ah mye′ sin)	Naprosyn®	(na′ pro sin)
mitomycin	(mye toe mye′ sin)	Naprelan®	(nap′ re lan)

APPENDIX

Drug Name	Pronunciation	Drug Name	Pronunciation
Naprosyn®	(na' pro sin)	Neoral®	(ne' oh ral)
naproxen	(na prox' en)	Nizoral®	(nye' zoh ral)
Naprosyn®	(na' pro sin)	Neosar®	(ne' oh sar)
Natacyn®	(na' ta sin)	Cytosar-U®	(sye' to sar-u)
Naprosyn®	(na' pro sin)	Nephro-Calci®	(nef' roe-cal' see)
Nebcin®	(neb' sin)	Nephrocaps®	(nef' ro kaps)
naproxen	(na prox' en)	Nephrocaps®	(nef' ro kaps)
Naprosyn®	(na' pro sin)	Nephro-Calci®	(nef' roe-cal' see)
Narcan®	(nar' kan)	Nephrox®	(nef' roks)
Marcaine®	(mar' kane)	Niferex®	(ny' fen eks)
Narcan®	(nar' kan)	Neptazane®	(nep' ta zane)
Norcuron®	(nor' ku ron)	Nesacaine®	(nes' ah kane)
Nardil®	(nar' dil)	Nesacaine®	(nes' ah kane)
Norinyl®	(nor' eh nil)	Neptazane®	(nep' ta zane)
Nasacort®	(nay' sa cort)	Neumega®	(new meg' ah)
Nasalcrom®	(nay' sal crome)	Neupogen®	(nu' po gen)
Nasalcrom®	(nay' sal crome)	Neupogen®	(nu' po gen)
Nasacort®	(nay' sa cort)	Epogen®	(ee' poe jen)
Nasalcrom®	(nay' sal crome)	Neupogen®	(nu' po gen)
Nasalide®	(nay' sa lide)	Neumega®	(new meg' ah)
Nasalide®	(nay' sa lide)	Neupogen®	(nu' po gen)
Nasalcrom®	(nay' sal crome)	Nutramigen®	(nu tram' eh gen)
Nasarel®	(nay' sa rel)	Neurontin®	(new ron' tin)
Nizoral®	(nye' zoh ral)	Neoral®	(ne' oh ral)
Natacyn®	(na' ta sin)	Neurontin®	(new ron' tin)
Naprosyn®	(na' pro sin)	Noroxin®	(nor oks' in)
Natru-Vent®	(nay' tru-vent)	Neutra-Phos-K®	(new' tra-fos-kay)
Atrovent®	(at' troe vent)	K-Phos Neutral®	(kay'-fos new' tral)
Navane®	(nav' ane)	nevirapine	(ne vir' ah peen)
Norvasc®	(nor' vask)	nelfinavir	(nel fin' ah vir)
Navane®	(nav' ane)	niacin	(nye' ah sin)
Nubain®	(nu' bane)	Minocin®	(min' oh sin)
Nebcin®	(neb' sin)	niacin	(nye' ah sin)
Inapsine®	(i nap' seen)	Niaspan®	(nye' ah span)
Nebcin®	(neb' sin)	niacinamide	(nye ah sin' ah mide)
Naprosyn®	(na' pro sin)	nicardipine	(nye kar' de peen)
Nebcin®	(neb' sin)	Niaspan®	(nye' ah span)
Nubain®	(nu' bain)	niacin	(nye' ah sin)
nelfinavir	(nel fin' ah vir)	nicardipine	(nye kar' de peen)
nevirapine	(ne vir' ah peen)	niacinamide	(nye ah sin' ah mide)
Nembutal®	(nem' byoo tal)	nicardipine	(nye kar' de peen)
Myambutol®	(mya am' byoo tol)	nifedipine	(nye fed' i peen)
Neocare®	(ne' oh care)	nicardipine	(nye kar' de peen)
Neocate®	(ne' oh cate)	nimodipine	(nye moe' di peen)
Neocate®	(ne' oh cate)	Nicobid®	(nye' ko bid)
Neocare®	(ne' oh care)	Nitro-Bid®	(nye' troe-bid)
Neoral®	(ne' oh ral)	NicoDerm®	(nye' co derm)
Neurontin®	(new ron' tin)	Nitroderm®	(nye' tro derm)

Drug Name	Pronunciation	Drug Name	Pronunciation
Nicorette®	(nik' oh ret)	Norcuron®	(nor' ku ron)
Nordette®	(nor det')	Narcan®	(nar' can)
nifedipine	(nye fed' i peen)	Nordette®	(nor det')
nicardipine	(nye kar' de peen)	Nicorette®	(nik' oh ret)
nifedipine	(nye fed' i peen)	Norflex®	(nor' fleks)
nimodipine	(nye moe' di peen)	norfloxacin	(nor floks' a sin)
nifedipine	(nye fed' i peen)	Norflex®	(nor' fleks)
nisoldipine	(nye' sole di peen)	Noroxin®	(nor oks' in)
Niferex®	(ny' fen eks)	norfloxacin	(nor floks' a sin)
Nephrox®	(nef' roks)	Norflex®	(nor' fleks)
Nilstat®	(nil' stat)	norfloxacin	(nor floks' a sin)
Nitrostat®	(nye' troe stat)	Noroxin®	(nor oks' in)
Nilstat®	(nil' stat)	Norgesic 40®	(nor gee' sik for' tee)
nystatin	(nye stat' in)	Norgesic Forte®	(nor gee' sik for' tay)
Nimbex®	(nim' beks)	Norgesic Forte®	(nor gee' sik for' tay)
Revex®	(rev' ex)	Norgesic 40®	(nor gee' sik for' tee)
nimodipine	(nye moe' di peen)	Norinyl®	(nor' eh nil)
nicardipine	(nye kar' de peen)	Nardil®	(nar' dil)
nimodipine	(nye moe' di peen)	Noroxin®	(nor oks' in)
nifedipine	(nye fed' i peen)	Neurontin®	(new ron' tin)
nisoldipine	(nye' sole di peen)	Noroxin®	(nor oks' in)
nifedipine	(nye fed' i peen)	Norflex®	(nor' fleks)
Nitro-Bid®	(nye' troe-bid)	Noroxin®	(nor oks' in)
Nicobid®	(nye' ko bid)	norfloxacin	(nor floks' a sin)
Nitroderm®	(nye' tro derm)	Norpace®	(nor' pace)
NicoDerm®	(nye' co derm)	Norpramin®	(nor' pra min)
nitroglycerin	(nye troe gli' ser in)	Norpramin®	(nor' pra min)
Nitroglyn®	(nye' troe glin)	clomipramine	(kloe mi' pra meen)
nitroglycerin	(nye troe gli' ser in)	Norpramin®	(nor' pra min)
nitroprusside	(nye troe prus' ide)	imipramine	(im ip' ra meen)
Nitroglyn®	(nye' troe glin)	Norpramin®	(nor' pra min)
nitroglycerin	(nye troe gli' ser in)	Norpace®	(nor' pace)
Nitrol®	(nye' trol)	Norpramin®	(nor' pra min)
Nizoral®	(nye' zoh ral)	nortriptyline	(nor trip' ti leen)
nitroprusside	(nye troe prus' ide)	Norpramin®	(nor' pra min)
nitroglycerin	(nye troe gli' ser in)	Tenormin®	(ten or' min)
Nitrostat®	(nye' troe stat)	nortriptyline	(nor trip' ti leen)
Hyperstat®	(hye' per stat)	amitriptyline	(ah mee trip' ti leen)
Nitrostat®	(nye' troe stat)	nortriptyline	(nor trip' ti leen)
Nilstat®	(nil' stat)	desipramine	(des ip' ra meen)
Nitrostat®	(nye' troe stat)	nortriptyline	(nor trip' ti leen)
nystatin	(nye stat' in)	Norpramin®	(nor' pra min)
Nizoral®	(nye' zoh ral)	Norvasc®	(nor' vask)
Nasarel®	(nay' sa rel)	Navane®	(nav' ane)
Nizoral®	(nye' zoh ral)	Norvasc®	(nor' vask)
Neoral®	(ne' oh ral)	Norvir®	(nor' vir)
Nizoral®	(nye' zoh ral)	Norvasc®	(nor' vask)
Nitrol®	(nye' trol)	Vascor®	(vas' cor)

Drug Name	Pronunciation	Drug Name	Pronunciation
Norvir®	(nor' vir)	Optiray®	(op' ti ray)
Norvasc®	(nor' vask)	Optivar™	(op' ti var)
Novacet®	(no' va set)	Optivar™	(op' ti var)
NovaSeven®	(no' va se ven)	Optiray®	(op' ti ray)
NovaSeven®	(no' va se ven)	Orabase®	(or' ah base)
Novacet®	(no' va set)	Orinase®	(or' in ase)
Nubain®	(nu' bane)	Orexin®	(or eks' in)
Navane®	(nav' ane)	Ornex®	(or' neks)
Nubain®	(nu' bane)	Orinase®	(or' in ase)
Nebcin®	(neb' sin)	Orabase®	(or' ah base)
NuLytely®	(nu lite' lee)	Orinase®	(or' in ase)
GoLYTELY®	(go lite' lee)	Ornex®	(or' neks)
Nuprin®	(nu' prin)	Orinase®	(or' in ase)
Lupron®	(lu' pron)	Tolinase®	(tole' i nase)
Nutramigen®	(nu tram' eh gen)	Ornex®	(or' neks)
Neupogen®	(nu' po gen)	Orexin®	(or eks' in)
nystatin	(nye stat' in)	Ornex®	(or' neks)
Nilstat®	(nil' stat)	Orinase®	(or' in ase)
nystatin	(nye stat' in)	Ortho-Cept®	(or' tho-sept)
Nitrostat®	(nye' troe stat)	Ortho-Cyclen®	(or' tho-sy' clen)
Ocufen®	(ok' yu fen)	Ortho-Cyclen®	(or' tho-sy' clen)
Ocuflox®	(ok' yu floks)	Ortho-Cept®	(or' tho-sept)
Ocufen®	(ok' yu fen)	Oruvail®	(or' yu vale)
Ocupress®	(ok' yu press)	Clinoril®	(klin' oh rill)
Ocuflox®	(ok' yu floks)	Oruvail®	(or' yu vale)
Ocufen®	(ok' yu fen)	Elavil®	(el' ah vil)
Ocupress®	(ok' yu press)	Os-Cal®	(os'-cal)
Ocufen®	(ok' yu fen)	Asacol®	(as' ah col)
olanzapine	(oh lan' za peen)	Osmitrol®	(os' mi trol)
olsalazine	(ole sal' ah zeen)	esmolol	(es' moe lol)
olsalazine	(ole sal' ah zeen)	Otrivin®	(oh' tri vin)
olanzapine	(oh lan' za peen)	Lotrimin®	(low' tri min)
Oncovin®	(on' coe vin)	oxaprozin	(oks a proe' zin)
Ancobon®	(an' coe bon)	oxazepam	(oks a' ze pam)
Ophthalgan®	(op thal' gan)	oxazepam	(oks a' ze pam)
Auralgan®	(ah ral' gan)	oxaprozin	(oks a proe' zin)
Ophthalgan®	(op thal' gan)	oxazepam	(oks a' ze pam)
Opthetic®	(op thet' ik)	quazepam	(kway' ze pam)
Ophthetic®	(op thet' ik)	oxybutynin	(ok i byoo' ti nin)
Ophthalgan®	(op thal' gan)	OxyContin®	(oks i kon' tin)
oprelvekin	(oh prel' ve kin)	oxycodone	(oks i koe' done)
aldesleukin	(al des loo' kin)	OxyContin®	(oks i kon' tin)
oprelvekin	(op rel' ve kin)	OxyContin®	(oks i kon' tin)
Proleukin®	(pro lu' kin)	oxybutynin	(ok i byoo' ti nin)
Optimine®	(op' ti meen)	OxyContin®	(oks i kon' tin)
Optimmune®	(op' ti mune)	oxycodone	(oks i koe' done)
Optimmune®	(op' ti mune)	oxymetazoline	(ox i met az' oh leen)
Optimine®	(op' ti meen)	oxymetholone	(ox i meth' oh lone)

Drug Name	Pronunciation	Drug Name	Pronunciation
oxymetholone oxymetazoline	(ox i meth' oh lone) (ox i met az' oh leen)	Paxil® Taxol®	(paks' ol) (tacks' ol)
oxymetholone oxymorphone	(ox i meth' oh lone) (ox i mor' fone)	Pediapred® Pedia Profen®	(pe' de ah pred) (pe' de ah pro' fen)
oxymorphone oxymetholone	(ox i mor' fone) (ox i meth' oh lone)	Pediapred® Pediazole®	(pe' de ah pred) (pe' de ah zole)
paclitaxel paroxetine	(pak le taks' el) (pa roks' e teen)	Pedia Profen® Pediapred®	(pe' de ah pro' fen) (pe' de ah pred)
paclitaxel Paxil®	(pak le taks' el) (paks' ol)	Pedia Profen® Pediazole®	(pe' de ah pro' fen) (pe' de ah zole)
Pamelor® Demerol®	(pam' meh lor) (dem' eh rol)	Pedia Profen® Prelone®	(pe' de ah pro' fen) (pree' lone)
Pamelor® Dymelor®	(pam' meh lor) (dye' meh lor)	Pediazole® Pediapred®	(pe' de ah zole) (pe' de ah pred)
Pamine® Pelamine®	(pa' meen) (pel' ah meen)	Pediazole® Pedia Profen®	(pe' de ah zole) (pe' de ah pro' fen)
Panadol® Panafil®	(pa' nah dol) (pan' ah fill)	pegaspargase asparaginase	(peg as' par jase) (ah spir' ah ji nase)
Panadol® pindolol	(pa' nah dol) (pin' doe lole)	Pelamine® Pamine®	(pel' ah meen) (pa' meen)
Panafil® Panadol®	(pan' ah fill) (pa' nah dol)	Pelamine® pemoline	(pel' ah meen) (pem' oh leen)
pancreatin Panretin®	(pan kre' ah tine) (pan ree' tin)	pemoline Pelamine®	(pem' oh leen) (pel' ah meen)
pancuronium pipercuronium	(pan kyoo roe' nee um) (pi pe kur oh' nee um)	Penetrex™ Pentrax®	(pen' e treks) (pen' traks)
Panretin® pancreatin	(pan ree' tin) (pan kre' ah tine)	penicillamine penicillin	(pen i sil' ah meen) (pen i sil' in)
Paraplatin® Platinol®	(pare ah pla' tin) (pla' ti nol)	penicillin penicillamine	(pen i sil' in) (pen i sil' ah meen)
Paregoric® Percogesic®	(pare eh gor' ik) (per coe gese' ik)	penicillin G potassium	(pen i sil' in jee poe tass' ee um)
Parlodel® pindolol	(par' loe dell) (pin' doe lole)	penicillin G procaine	(pen i sil' in jee proe' kane)
Parlodel® Provera®	(par' loe dell) (pro ver' ah)	penicillin G procaine	(pen i sil' in jee proe' kane)
paroxetine paclitaxel	(pa roks' e teen) (pak le taks' el)	penicillin G potassium	(pen i sil' in jee poe tass' ee um)
paroxetine pyridoxine	(pa roks' e teen) (peer i dox' een)	pentobarbital phenobarbital	(pen toe bar' bi tal) (fee noe bar' bi tal)
Patanol® Platinol®	(pa' ta nol) (pla' ti nol)	pentosan pentostatin	(pen' to san) (pen toe sta' tin)
Paxil® Doxil®	(paks' ol) (doks' il)	pentostatin pentosan	(pen toe sta' tin) (pen' to san)
Paxil® paclitaxel	(paks' ol) (pak le taks' el)	pentoxifylline tamoxifen	(pen toks i' fi leen) (ta moks' i fen)
Paxil® Plavix®	(paks' ol) (plah' viks)	Pentrax® Penetrex™	(pen' traks) (pen' e treks)

791

Drug Name	Pronunciation	Drug Name	Pronunciation
Pentrax®	(pen' traks)	Pertofrane®	(per' toe frane)
Permax®	(per' max)	Persantine®	(per san' teen)
Perative®	(per ah' tive)	Phazyme®	(fay' zeem)
Periactin®	(pear ee ak' tine)	Pherazine®	(fer' ah zeen)
Perceptin™	(per cep' tin)	Phenaphen®	(fen' ah fen)
Herceptin®	(her cep' tin)	Phenergan®	(fen' er gan)
Percocet®	(per' koe set)	phenelzine	(fen' el zeen)
Percodan®	(per' koe dan)	phenytoin	(fen' i toyn)
Percodan®	(per' koe dan)	Phenergan®	(fen' er gan)
Decadron®	(dek' ah dron)	Phenaphen®	(fen' ah fen)
Percodan®	(per' koe dan)	Phenergan®	(fen' er gan)
Percocet®	(per' koe set)	Phrenilin®	(fren' ni lin)
Percodan®	(per' koe dan)	Phenergan®	(fen' er gan)
Percogesic®	(per coe gese' ik)	Theragran®	(ther' ah gran)
Percodan®	(per' koe dan)	phenobarbital	(fee noe bar' bi tal)
Periactin®	(pear ee ak' tine)	pentobarbital	(pen toe bar' bi tal)
Percogesic®	(per coe gese' ik)	phentermine	(fen' ter meen)
Paregoric®	(pare eh gor' ik)	phentolamine	(fen tole' ah meen)
Percogesic®	(per coe gese' ik)	Phentermine®	(fen' ter meen)
Percodan®	(per' koe dan)	phenytoin	(fen' i toyn)
Perdiem®	(per dee' em)	phentolamine	(fen tole' ah meen)
Pyridium®	(pye rid' dee um)	phentermine	(fen' ter meen)
Periactin®	(pear ee ak' tine)	phentolamine	(fen tole' ah meen)
Perative®	(per ah' tive)	Ventolin®	(ven' to lin)
Periactin®	(pear ee ak' tine)	phenytoin	(fen' i toyn)
Percodan®	(per' koe dan)	mephenytoin	(me fen' i toyn)
Periactin®	(pear ee ak' tine)	phenytoin	(fen' i toyn)
Persantine®	(per san' teen)	phenelzine	(fen' el zeen)
Peridex®	(per' e deks)	phenytoin	(fen' i toyn)
Precedex™	(pre' se deks)	phentermine	(fen' ter meen)
Permax®	(per' max)	Pherazine®	(fer' ah zeen)
Bumex®	(byoo' mex)	Phazyme®	(fay' zeem)
Permax®	(per' max)	pHisoDerm®	(fi' so derm)
Pentrax®	(pen' traks)	pHisoHex®	(fye' so heks)
Permax®	(per' max)	pHisoHex®	(fye' so heks)
Pernox®	(per' noks)	Fostex®	(fos' teks)
Permitil®	(per' mi till)	pHisoHex®	(fye' so heks)
Persantine®	(per san' teen)	pHisoDerm®	(fi' so derm)
Pernox®	(per' noks)	PhosChol®	(fos' kol)
Permax®	(per' max)	PhosLo®	(fos' lo)
Peroxyl®	(per ox' ill)	PhosChol®	(fos' kol)
Benoxyl®	(ben ox' ill)	Phosphocol®	(fos' fo kol)
Persantine®	(per san' teen)	PhosChol®	(fos' kol)
Periactin®	(pear ee ak' tine)	Phosphocol® P32	(fos' fo kol pee thurtee tu)
Persantine®	(per san' teen)	Phos-Flur®	(fos'-flur)
Permitil®	(per' mi till)	PhosLo®	(fos' lo)
Persantine®	(per san' teen)	PhosLo®	(fos' lo)
Pertofrane®	(per' toe frane)	PhosChol®	(fos' kol)

792

Drug Name	Pronunciation	Drug Name	Pronunciation
PhosLo® Phos-Flur®	(fos' lo) (fos'-flur)	Plendil® Prinivil®	(plen' dill) (pri' ni vill)
PhosLo® ProSom™	(fos' lo) (pro' som)	Pletal® Plendil®	(ple' tal) (plen' dil)
Phosphocol® PhosChol®	(fos' fo kol) (fos' kol)	Polocaine® prilocaine	(po' loe kane) (pril' oh kane)
Phosphocol® P32 PhosChol®	(fos' fo kol pee thurtee tu) (fos' kol)	Ponstel® Pronestyl®	(pon' stel) (pro nes' til)
Phrenilin® Phenergan®	(fren' ni lin) (fen' er gan)	pralidoxime pramoxine	(pra li dox' eem) (pra moks' een)
Phrenilin® Trinalin®	(fren' ni lin) (tri' na lin)	pralidoxime pyridoxine	(pra li dox' eem) (peer i dox' een)
physostigmine Prostigmin®	(fye zoe stig' meen) (pro stig' min)	Pramosone® prednisone	(pra' mo sone) (pred' ni sone)
physostigmine pyridostigmine	(fye zoe stig' meen) (peer id oh stig' meen)	pramoxine pralidoxime	(pra moks' een) (pra li dox' eem)
pindolol Panadol®	(pin' doe lole) (pa' nah dol)	Prandin™ Avandia®	(pran' din) (ah van' de a)
pindolol Parlodel®	(pin' doe lole) (par' loe dell)	Pravachol® Prevacid®	(prav' ah kol) (prev' ah sid)
pindolol Plendil®	(pin' doe lole) (plen' dill)	Pravachol® propranolol	(prav' ah kol) (proe pran' oh lole)
pipercuronium pancuronium	(pi pe kur oh' nee um) (pan kyoo roe' nee um)	prazepam prazosin	(pra' ze pam) (pra' zoe sin)
Pitocin® Pitressin®	(pi toe' sin) (pi tres' sin)	prazosin prazepam	(pra' zoe sin) (pra' ze pam)
Pitressin® Pitocin®	(pi tres' sin) (pi toe' sin)	prazosin prednisone	(pra' zoe sin) (pred' ni sone)
Plaquenil® Platinol®	(pla' kwe nil) (pla' ti nol)	Precare® Precose®	(pre' kare) (pre' kose)
Platinol® Paraplatin®	(pla' ti nol) (pare ah pla' tin)	Precedex™ Peridex®	(pre' se deks) (per' e deks)
Platinol® Patanol®	(pla' ti nol) (pa' ta nol)	Precose® Precare®	(pre' kose) (pre' kare)
Platinol® Plaquenil®	(pla' ti nol) (pla' kwe nil)	prednisolone prednisone	(pred nis' oh lone) (pred' ni sone)
Plavix® Elavil®	(plah' viks) (el' ah vil)	prednisone methylprednisolone	(pred' ni sone) (meth il pred nis' oh lone)
Plavix® Paxil®	(plah' viks) (paks' ol)	prednisone Pramosone®	(pred' ni sone) (pra' mo sone)
Plendil® Isordil®	(plen' dill) (eye' sor dil)	prednisone prazosin	(pred' ni sone) (pra' zoe sin)
Plendil® pindolol	(plen' dill) (pin' doe lole)	prednisone prednisolone	(pred' ni sone) (pred nis' oh lone)
Plendil® Pletal®	(plen' dil) (ple' tal)	prednisone Prilosec®	(pred' ni sone) (pry' lo sek)
Plendil® Prilosec®	(plen' dil) (pry' lo sek)	prednisone primidone	(pred' ni sone) (pri' mi done)

Drug Name	Pronunciation	Drug Name	Pronunciation
prednisone	(pred' ni sone)	Prilosec®	(pry' lo sek)
promethazine	(proe meth' ah zeen)	Proventil®	(pro ven' till)
Prelone®	(pree' lone)	Prilosec®	(pry' lo sek)
Pedia Profen®	(pe' de ah pro' fen)	Prozac®	(proe' zak)
Premarin®	(prem' ah rin)	Primaxin®	(pri maks' in)
Primaxin®	(pri maks' in)	Premarin®	(prem' ah rin)
Premarin®	(prem' ah rin)	primidone	(pri' mi done)
Provera®	(pro ver' ah)	prednisone	(pred' ni sone)
Premarin®	(prem' ah rin)	Prinivil®	(pri' ni vill)
Remeron®	(reh' me ron)	Plendil®	(plen' dill)
Premphase®	(prem' fase)	Prinivil®	(pri' ni vill)
Prempro™	(prem' pro)	Prevacid®	(prev' ah sid)
Prempro™	(prem' pro)	Prinivil®	(pri' ni vill)
Premphase®	(prem' fase)	Prilosec®	(pry' lo sek)
Prepidil®	(pre' pi dil)	Prinivil®	(pri' ni vill)
Bepridil®	(be' pri dil)	Proventil®	(pro ven' till)
Prevacid®	(prev' ah sid)	Priscoline®	(pris' coe leen)
Pravachol®	(prav' ah kol)	Apresoline®	(aye press' sow leen)
Prevacid®	(prev' ah sid)	ProAmatine®	(pro am' a teen)
Prevpac™	(prev' pak)	protamine	(proe' ta meen)
Prevacid®	(prev' ah sid)	probenecid	(proe ben' e sid)
Prilosec®	(pry' lo sek)	Procanbid®	(proe can' bid)
Prevacid®	(prev' ah sid)	Procanbid®	(proe can' bid)
Prinivil®	(pri' ni vill)	probenecid	(proe ben' e sid)
PREVEN™	(pre' ven)	procarbazine	(proe kar' ba zeen)
Preveon™	(pre' vee on)	dacarbazine	(da kar' ba zeen)
PREVEN™	(pre' ven)	Procardia XL®	(pro car' dee ah eks el)
Prevnar™	(prev' nar)	Cartia® XT	(car' te ah eks tee)
Preveon™	(pre' vee on)	prochlorperazine	(proe klor per' ah zeen)
PREVEN™	(pre' ven)	chlorpromazine	(klor proe' ma zeen)
Prevnar™	(prev' nar)	Proctocort®	(prok' toe kort)
PREVEN™	(pre' ven)	ProctoCream HC®	(prok' toe cream aych see)
Prevpac™	(prev' pak)	ProctoCream HC®	(prok' toe cream aych see)
Prevacid®	(prev' ah sid)	Proctocort®	(prok' toe kort)
prilocaine	(pril' oh kane)	Prograf®	(pro' graf)
Polocaine®	(po' loe kane)	Gengraf™	(gen' graf)
prilocaine	(pril' oh kane)	Proleukin®	(pro lu' kin)
Prilosec®	(pry' lo sek)	oprelvekin	(op rel' ve kin)
Prilosec®	(pry' lo sek)	Prolixin®	(pro liks' in)
Plendil®	(plen' dill)	Proloprim®	(pro low prim)
Prilosec®	(pry' lo sek)	Proloprim®	(pro low prim)
prednisone	(pred' ni sone)	Prolixin®	(pro liks' in)
Prilosec®	(pry' lo sek)	Proloprim®	(pro low prim)
Prevacid®	(prev' ah sid)	Protropin®	(proe tro' pin)
Prilosec®	(pry' lo sek)	promazine	(proe' ma zeen)
prilocaine	(pril' oh kane)	promethazine	(proe meth' ah zeen)
Prilosec®	(pry' lo sek)		
Prinivil®	(pri' ni vill)		

Drug Name	Pronunciation	Drug Name	Pronunciation
promethazine chlorpromazine	(proe meth' ah zeen) (klor proe' ma zeen)	Protopam® Proloprim®	(proe' toe pam) (pro' low prim)
promethazine prednisone	(proe meth' ah zeen) (pred' ni sone)	Protopam® protamine	(proe' toe pam) (proe' ta meen)
promethazine promazine	(proe meth' ah zeen) (proe' ma zeen)	Protopam® Protropin®	(proe' toe pam) (proe tro' pin)
Pronestyl® Ponstel®	(pro nes' til) (pon' stel)	Protropin® Proloprim®	(proe tro' pin) (pro' low prim)
proparacaine propoxyphene	(proe par' ah kane) (proe poks' i feen)	Protropin® protamine	(proe tro' pin) (proe' ta meen)
propoxyphene proparacaine	(proe poks' i feen) (proe par' ah kane)	Protropin® Protopam®	(proe tro' pin) (proe' toe pam)
propranolol Pravachol®	(proe pran' oh lole) (prav' ah kol)	Proventil® Bentyl®	(pro ven' till) (ben' til)
propranolol Propulsid®	(proe pran' oh lole) (pro pul' sid)	Proventil® Prilosec®	(pro ven' till) (pry' lo sek)
Propulsid® propranolol	(pro pul' sid) (proe pran' oh lole)	Proventil® Prinivil®	(pro ven' till) (pri' ni vill)
Proscar® ProSom®	(pros' car) (pro' som)	Provera® Covera®	(pro ver' ah) (co ver' ah)
Proscar® Prozac®	(pros' car) (proe' zak)	Provera® Parlodel®	(pro ver' ah) (par' loe dell)
Proscar® Psorcon™	(pros' car) (sore' kon)	Provera® Premarin®	(pro ver' ah) (prem' ah rin)
Pro-Sof® Plus ProSom®	(proe'-sof plus) (pro' som)	Provera® Provir®	(pro ver' ah) (pro' vir)
ProSom® PhosLo®	(pro' som) (fos' lo)	Provir® Provera®	(pro' vir) (pro ver' ah)
ProSom® Proscar®	(pro' som) (pros' car)	Prozac® Prilosec®	(proe' zak) (pry' lo sek)
ProSom® Pro-Sof® Plus	(pro' som) (proe'-sof plus)	Prozac® Proscar®	(proe' zak) (pros' car)
ProSom® Prozac®	(pro' som) (proe' zak)	Prozac® ProSom®	(proe' zak) (pro' som)
ProSom® Psorcon™	(pro' som) (sore' kon)	Prozac® ProStep®	(proe' zak) (proe' step)
ProStep® Prozac®	(proe' step) (proe' zak)	Psorcon™ Proscar®	(sore' kon) (pros' car)
Prostigmin® physostigmine	(pro stig' min) (fye zoe stig' meen)	Psorcon™ ProSom®	(sore' kon) (pro' som)
protamine ProAmatine®	(proe' ta meen) (pro am' a teen)	Psorcon™ Psorion®	(sore' kon) (sore' ee on)
protamine Protopam®	(proe' ta meen) (proe' toe pam)	Psorion® Psorcon™	(sore' ee on) (sore' kon)
protamine Protropin®	(proe' ta meen) (proe tro' pin)	Pyridium® Dyrenium®	(pye rid' dee um) (dye ren' e um)
Protonix® Lotronex®	(pro' to niks) (lo' tro neks)	Pyridium® Perdiem®	(pye rid' dee um) (per dee' em)

795

Drug Name	Pronunciation	Drug Name	Pronunciation
Pyridium®	(pye rid' dee um)	Reglan®	(reg' lan)
pyridoxine	(peer i dox' een)	Megace®	(me' gase)
Pyridium®	(pye rid' dee um)	Reglan®	(reg' lan)
pyrithione	(peer i thye' one)	Regonol®	(reg' oh nol)
pyridostigmine	(peer id oh stig' meen)	Reglan®	(reg' lan)
physostigmine	(fye zoe stig' meen)	Renagel®	(reh' na gel)
pyridoxine	(peer i dox' een)	Regonol®	(reg' oh nol)
paroxetine	(pa roks' e teen)	Reglan®	(reg' lan)
pyridoxine	(peer i dox' een)	Regonol®	(reg' oh nol)
pralidoxime	(pra li dox' eem)	Regroton®	(re gro' ton)
pyridoxine	(peer i dox' een)	Regonol®	(reg' oh nol)
Pyridium®	(pye rid' dee um)	Renagel®	(reh' na gel)
pyrithione	(peer i thye' one)	Regranex®	(re gra' neks)
Pyridium®	(pye rid' dee um)	Granulex®	(gran' u lecks)
Quarzan®	(kwar' zan)	Regranex®	(re gra' neks)
quazepam	(kway' ze pam)	Repronex®	(re' pro neks)
Quarzan®	(kwar' zan)	Regroton®	(re gro' ton)
Questran®	(kwes' tran)	Regonol®	(reg' oh nol)
quazepam	(kway' ze pam)	Remegel®	(reh' me gel)
oxazepam	(oks a' ze pam)	Renagel®	(reh' na gel)
quazepam	(kway' ze pam)	Remeron®	(reh' me ron)
Quarzan®	(kwar' zan)	Premarin®	(prem' ah rin)
Questran®	(kwes' tran)	Remeron®	(reh' me ron)
Quarzan®	(kwar' zan)	Zemuron®	(zeh' mu ron)
quinidine	(kwin' i deen)	Remicade®	(rem' e kade)
clonidine	(kloe' ni deen)	Renacidin®	(ren ah see' din)
quinidine	(kwin' i deen)	remifentanil	(rem i fen' ta nil)
quinine	(kwye' nine)	alfentanil	(al fen' ta nil)
quinidine	(kwin' i deen)	Renacidin®	(ren ah see' din)
Quinora®	(kwi nor' ah)	Remicade®	(rem' e kade)
quinine	(kwye' nine)	Renagel®	(reh' na gel)
quinidine	(kwin' i deen)	Reglan®	(reg' lan)
Quinora®	(kwi nor' ah)	Renagel®	(reh' na gel)
quinidine	(kwin' i deen)	Regonol®	(reg' oh nol)
ramipril	(ra mi' pril)	Renagel®	(reh' na gel)
enalapril	(e nal' ah pril)	Remegel	(reh' me gel)
ramipril	(ra mi' pril)	Repan®	(ree' pan)
Monopril®	(mon' oh pril)	Riopan®	(rye' oh pan)
ranitidine	(ra ni' ti deen)	Repronex®	(re' pro neks)
amantadine	(ah man' ta deen)	Regranex®	(re gra' neks)
ranitidine	(ra ni' ti deen)	reserpine	(re ser' peen)
rimantadine	(ri man' ta deen)	Risperdal®	(ris per' dal)
ranitidine	(ra ni' ti deen)	reserpine	(re ser' peen)
ritodrine	(ri' toe dreen)	risperidone	(ris per' i done)
ratgam	(rat' gam)	Restore®	(res tore')
Atgam®	(at' gam)	Restoril®	(res' tor ril)
Recombivax®	(ree kom' bi vaks)	Restoril®	(res' tor ril)
Comvax®	(kom' vaks)	Restore®	(res tore')

Drug Name	Pronunciation	Drug Name	Pronunciation
Restoril®	(res' tor ril)	Risperdal®	(ris per' dal)
Vistaril®	(vis' tar ril)	risperidone	(ris per' i done)
Restoril®	(res' tor ril)	risperidone	(ris per' i done)
Zestril®	(zes' trill)	reserpine	(re ser' peen)
Retrovir®	(re' tro vir)	risperidone	(ris per' i done)
ritonavir	(ri ton' oh vir)	Risperdal®	(ris per' dal)
Revex®	(rev' ex)	Ritalin®	(ri' ta lin)
Nimbex®	(nim' beks)	Ismelin®	(is' meh lin)
Revex®	(rev' ex)	Ritalin®	(ri' ta lin)
ReVia®	(rev' ve ah)	Rifadin®	(rif' ah din)
ReVia®	(rev' ve ah)	Ritalin®	(ri' ta lin)
Revex®	(rev' ex)	ritodrine	(ri' toe dreen)
Rhythmin®	(rith' min)	ritodrine	(ri' toe dreen)
Rythmol®	(rith' mol)	ranitidine	(ra ni' ti deen)
ribavirin	(rye ba vye' rin)	ritodrine	(ri' toe dreen)
riboflavin	(rye' boe flay vin)	Ritalin®	(ri' ta lin)
riboflavin	(rye' boe flay vin)	ritonavir	(ri ton' oh vir)
ribavirin	(rye ba vye' rin)	Retrovir®	(re' tro vir)
Ridaura®	(ri dur' ah)	Robaxin®	(roe baks' in)
Cardura®	(kar dur' ah)	Rubex®	(rue' beks)
rifabutin	(rif ah byoo' tin)	Rocephin®	(roe sef' fen)
rifampin	(rif' am pin)	Roferon®	(roe fer' on)
Rifadin®	(rif' ah din)	Roferon®	(roe fer' on)
Ritalin®	(ri' ta lin)	Rocephin®	(roe sef' fen)
Rifamate®	(ri fam' ate)	Roferon-A®	(roe fer' on-ay)
rifampin	(rif' am pin)	Imferon®	(im' fer on)
rifampin	(rif' am pin)	ropivacaine	(roe piv' a kane)
rifabutin	(rif ah byoo' tin)	bupivacaine	(byoo piv' ah kane)
rifampin	(rif' am pin)	Roxanol®	(roks' ah noll)
Rifamate®	(ri fam' ate)	Roxicet®	(roks' ih set)
rifampin	(rif' am pin)	Roxicet®	(roks' ih set)
rifapentine	(rif' a pen teen)	Roxanol®	(roks' ah noll)
rifapentine	(rif' a pen teen)	Rubex®	(rue' beks)
rifampin	(rif' am pin)	Robaxin®	(roe baks' in)
Rimactane®	(ri mak' tane)	Rynatan®	(rye' na tan)
rimantadine	(ri man' ta deen)	Rynatuss®	(rye' na tuss)
rimantadine	(ri man' ta deen)	Rynatuss®	(rye' na tuss)
amantadine	(ah man' ta deen)	Rynatan®	(rye' na tan)
rimantadine	(ri man' ta deen)	Rythmol®	(rith' mol)
ranitidine	(ra ni' ti deen)	Rhythmin®	(rith' min)
rimantadine	(ri man' ta deen)	Salacid®	(sal as' sid)
Rimactane®	(ri mak' tane)	Salagen®	(sal' ah gen)
Riopan®	(rye' oh pan)	Salagen®	(sal' ah gen)
Repan®	(ree' pan)	Salacid®	(sal as' sid)
Risperdal®	(ris per' dal)	salbutamol	(sal byu' tu mol)
lisinopril	(lyse in' oh pril)	salmeterol	(sal me' te role)
Risperdal®	(ris per' dal)	salmeterol	(sal me' te role)
reserpine	(re ser' peen)	salbutamol	(sal byu' tu mol)

Drug Name	Pronunciation	Drug Name	Pronunciation
salsalate	(sal′ sa late)	Septra®	(sep′ trah)
sucralfate	(soo kral′ fate)	Ceptaz®	(sep′ taz)
salsalate	(sal′ sa late)	Septra®	(sep′ trah)
sulfasalazine	(sul fa sal′ ah zeen)	Sectral®	(sek′ tral)
Sandimmune®	(san′ di mune)	Septra®	(sep′ trah)
Sandoglobulin®	(san doe glo′ byu line)	Septa®	(sep′ tah)
Sandimmune®	(san′ di mune)	Seracult®	(ser′ a cult)
Sandostatin®	(san doe sta′ tin)	Hemoccult®	(he′ mo cult)
Sandoglobulin®	(san doe glo′ byu line)	Serax®	(sear′ aks)
Sandimmune®	(san′ di mune)	Eurax®	(yoor′ aks)
Sandoglobulin®	(san doe glo′ byu line)	Serax®	(sear′ aks)
Sandostatin®	(san doe sta′ tin)	Urex®	(yur′ eks)
Sandostatin®	(san doe sta′ tin)	Serax®	(sear′ aks)
Sandimmune®	(san′ di mune)	Xerac®	(zear′ ak)
Sandostatin®	(san doe sta′ tin)	Serax®	(sear′ aks)
Sandoglobulin®	(san doe glo′ byu line)	Zyrtec®	(zir′ tec)
saquinavir	(sa kwin′ ah veer)	Serentil®	(se ren′ till)
Sinequan®	(si′ ne kwan)	selegiline	(seh ledge′ ah leen)
Sarafem™	(sar′ ah fem)	Serentil®	(se ren′ till)
Serophene®	(ser′ oh feen)	Serevent®	(ser′ a vent)
Sebex®	(see′ beks)	Serentil®	(se ren′ till)
Sebutone®	(se′ byu tone)	Seroquel®	(seer′ oh kwel)
Sebex®	(see′ beks)	Serentil®	(se ren′ till)
Surbex®	(sir′ beks)	sertraline	(ser′ tra leen)
Sebutone®	(se′ byu tone)	Serentil®	(se ren′ till)
Sebex®	(see′ beks)	Serzone®	(ser zone′)
Seconal™	(sek′ oh nal)	Serentil®	(se ren′ till)
Sectral®	(sek′ tral)	Sinequan®	(si′ ne kwan)
Sectral®	(sek′ tral)	Serentil®	(se ren′ till)
Factrel®	(fak′ trel)	Surgicel®	(sir′ gee cell)
Sectral®	(sek′ tral)	Serevent®	(ser′ a vent)
Seconal™	(sek′ oh nal)	Serentil®	(se ren′ till)
Sectral®	(sek′ tral)	Serophene®	(ser′ oh feen)
Septra®	(sep′ trah)	Sarafem™	(sar′ ah fem)
selegiline	(seh ledge′ ah leen)	Seroquel®	(seer′ oh kwel)
Serentil®	(se ren′ till)	Serentil®	(se ren′ till)
selegiline	(seh ledge′ ah leen)	Seroquel®	(seer′ oh kwel)
sertraline	(ser′ tra leen)	Serzone®	(ser zone′)
selegiline	(seh ledge′ ah leen)	Seroquel®	(seer′ oh kwel)
Serzone®	(ser zone′)	Sinequan®	(si′ ne kwan)
selegiline	(seh ledge′ ah leen)	sertraline	(ser′ tra leen)
Stelazine®	(stel′ ah zene)	Serentil®	(se ren′ till)
Senexon®	(sen′ e son)	Serzone®	(ser zone′)
Cenestin®	(se nes′ tin)	selegiline	(seh ledge′ ah leen)
Senokot®	(sen′ oh kot)	Serzone®	(ser zone′)
Depakote®	(dep′ ah kote)	Serentil®	(se ren′ till)
Septa®	(sep′ tah)	Serzone®	(ser zone′)
Septra®	(sep′ trah)	Seroquel®	(seer′ oh kwel)

Drug Name	Pronunciation	Drug Name	Pronunciation
Serzone®	(ser zone')	streptomycin	(strep toe mye' sin)
sertraline	(ser' tra leen)	streptozocin	(strep toe zoe' sin)
simethicone	(sye meth' i kone)	streptozocin	(strep toe zoe' sin)
cimetidine	(sye met' i deen)	streptomycin	(strep toe mye' sin)
Sinarest®	(sy' na rest)	sucralfate	(soo kral' fate)
Allerest®	(al' e rest)	salsalate	(sal' sa late)
Sinequan®	(si' ne kwan)	Sudafed®	(sue' da fed)
saquinavir	(sa kwin' ah veer)	Sufenta®	(sue fen' tah)
Sinequan®	(si' ne kwan)	Sufenta®	(sue fen' tah)
Serentil®	(se ren' till)	Alfenta®	(al fen' tah)
Sinequan®	(si' ne kwan)	Sufenta®	(sue fen' tah)
Seroquel®	(seer' oh kwel)	Sudafed®	(sue' da fed)
Sinequan®	(si' ne kwan)	Sufenta®	(sue fen' tah)
Singulair®	(sin' gu lare)	Survanta®	(sir van' ta)
Singulair®	(sin' gu lare)	sufentanil	(sue fen' ta nil)
Sinequan®	(si' ne kwan)	alfentanil	(al fen' ta nil)
Slo-bid™	(slo'-bid)	sufentanil citrate	(sue fen' ta nil sit' rate)
Dolobid®	(dol' ah bid)	fentanyl citrate	(fen' ta nil sit' rate)
Slo-bid™	(slo'-bid)	sulfadiazine	(sul fa dye' ah zeen)
Lopid®	(lo' pid)	sulfasalazine	(sul fa sal' ah zeen)
Slo-bid™	(slo'-bid)	sulfadiazine	(sul fa dye' ah zeen)
Lorabid®	(lor' ah bid)	sulfisoxazole	(sul fi soks' ah zole)
Slow FE®	(slo' fee)	sulfamethizole	(sul fa meth' i zole)
Slow-K®	(slo'-kay)	sulfamethoxazole	(sul fa meth oks' ah zole)
Slow-K®	(slo'-kay)	sulfamethoxazole	(sul fa meth oks' ah zole)
Slow FE®	(slo' fee)	sulfamethizole	(sul fa meth' i zole)
Solu-Medrol®	(sol' yu-med' role)	sulfamethoxazole	(sul fa meth oks' ah zole)
Depo-Medrol®	(dep' oh-med' role)	sulfisoxazole	(sul fi soks' ah zole)
Somatrem®	(sow' mah trem)	sulfasalazine	(sul fa sal' ah zeen)
somatropin	(sow mah troh' pin)	salsalate	(sal' sa late)
somatropin	(sow mah troh' pin)	sulfasalazine	(sul fa sal' ah zeen)
Somatrem®	(sow' mah trem)	sulfadiazine	(sul fa dye' ah zeen)
somatropin	(sow mah troh' pin)	sulfasalazine	(sul fa sal' ah zeen)
sumatriptan	(soo ma trip' tan)	sulfisoxazole	(sul fi sox' ah zole)
Soriatane®	(sor' e ah tane)	sulfisoxazole	(sul fi soks' ah zole)
Loxitane®	(loks' e tane)	sulfadiazine	(sul fa dye' ah zeen)
sotalol	(soe' ta lole)	sulfisoxazole	(sul fi soks' ah zole)
Stadol®	(stay' dol)	sulfamethoxazole	(sul fa meth oks' ah zole)
Sporanox®	(spor' ah noks)	sulfisoxazole	(sul fi sox' ah zole)
Suprax®	(su' prax)	sulfasalazine	(sul fa sal' ah zeen)
Stadol®	(stay' dol)	sumatriptan	(soo ma trip' tan)
Haldol®	(hal' dol)	somatropin	(sow mah troh' pin)
Stadol®	(stay' dol)	sumatriptan	(soo ma trip' tan)
sotalol	(soe' ta lole)	zolmitriptan	(zohl mi trip' tan)
Stelazine®	(stel' ah zene)	Suprax®	(su' prax)
selegiline	(seh ledge' ah leen)	Sporanox®	(spor' ah noks)
Stilphostrol®	(stil phos' trol)	Suprax®	(su' prax)
Disophrol®	(dye' so frol)	Surbex®	(sir' beks)

Drug Name	Pronunciation	Drug Name	Pronunciation
Surbex®	(sir′ beks)	Tazicef®	(taz′ e sef)
Sebex®	(see′ beks)	Tazidime®	(taz′ e deem)
Surbex®	(sir′ beks)	Tazidime®	(taz′ e deem)
Suprax®	(su′ prax)	Tazicef®	(taz′ e sef)
Surbex®	(sir′ beks)	Tegison®	(teg′ i son)
Surfak®	(sur′ fak)	Talacen®	(tal′ ah sen)
Surfak®	(sur′ fak)	Tegretol®	(teg′ ree tol)
Surbex®	(sir′ beks)	Mebaral®	(meb′ ah ral)
Surgicel®	(sir′ gee cell)	Tegretol®	(teg′ ree tol)
Serentil®	(se ren′ till)	Tegrin®	(teg′ rin)
Surgilube®	(sur′ gi lube)	Tegretol®	(teg′ ree tol)
Lacrilube®	(lac′ ri lube)	Toradol®	(tor′ ah doll)
Survanta®	(sir van′ ta)	Tegretol®	(teg′ ree tol)
Sufenta®	(sue fen′ tah)	Trental®	(tren′ tal)
Symmetrel®	(sim′ et trell)	Tegrin®	(teg′ rin)
Synthroid®	(sin′ throid)	Tegretol®	(teg′ ree tol)
Synagis®	(si na′ gis)	temazepam	(te maz′ e pam)
Synalogos DC	(si nal′ gos dee′ cee)	flurazepam	(flure az′ e pam)
Synagis®	(si na′ gis)	temazepam	(te maz′ e pam)
Synvisc®	(sin′ visc)	lorazepam	(lor a′ ze pam)
Synalgos DC	(si nal′ gos dee′ cee)	Tenex®	(ten′ eks)
Synagis®	(si na′ gis)	Entex®	(en′ teks)
Synthroid®	(sin′ throid)	Tenex®	(ten′ eks)
Symmetrel®	(sim′ et trell)	Ten-K®	(ten′-kay)
Synvisc®	(sin′ visc)	Tenex®	(ten′ eks)
Synagis®	(si na′ gis)	Xanax®	(zan′ aks)
Sytobex®	(sye′ toe beks)	Ten-K®	(ten′-kay)
Cytotec®	(sye′ toe tek)	Tenex®	(ten′ eks)
Talacen®	(tal′ ah sen)	Tenormin®	(ten or′ min)
Tegison®	(teg′ i son)	Imuran®	(im′ yu ran)
Talacen®	(tal′ ah sen)	Tenormin®	(ten or′ min)
Timoptic®	(tim op′ tik)	Norpramin®	(nor′ pra min)
Talacen®	(tal′ ah sen)	Tenormin®	(ten or′ min)
Tinactin®	(tin ak′ tin)	thiamine	(thye′ ah min)
Tambocor®	(tam′ bo kor)	Tenormin®	(ten or′ min)
tamoxifen	(ta moks′ i fen)	Trovan®	(tro′ van)
Tamiflu™	(tam′ eh flu)	terbinafine	(ter′ bin ah feen)
Theraflu®	(ther′ ah flu)	terbutaline	(ter byoo′ ta leen)
tamoxifen	(ta moks′ i fen)	terbinafine	(ter′ bin ah feen)
pentoxifylline	(pen toks i′ fi leen)	terfenadine	(ter fen′ na deen)
tamoxifen	(ta moks′ i fen)	terbutaline	(ter byoo′ ta leen)
Tambocor®	(tam′ bo kor)	terbinafine	(ter′ bin ah feen)
Taxol®	(tacks′ ol)	terbutaline	(ter byoo′ ta leen)
Paxil®	(paks′ ol)	tolbutamide	(tole byoo′ ta mide)
Taxol®	(tacks′ ol)	terconazole	(ter kone′ ah zole)
Taxotere®	(taks′ oh tere)	tioconazole	(tye oh kone′ ah zole)
Taxotere®	(taks′ oh tere)	terfenadine	(ter fen′ na deen)
Taxol®	(tacks′ ol)	terbinafine	(ter′ bin ah feen)

Drug Name	Pronunciation	Drug Name	Pronunciation
Terramycin®	(tehr ah mye' sin)	Thyrolar®	(thye' roe lar)
Garamycin®	(gar ah mye' sin)	Thytropar®	(thye' troe par)
Testoderm®	(tes' toh derm)	Thytropar®	(thye' troe par)
Estraderm®	(es' tra derm)	Thyrolar®	(thye' roe lar)
testolactone	(tess toe lak' tone)	tiagabine	(tye ag' a bene)
testosterone	(tess toss' ter one)	tizanidine	(tye zan' i deen)
testosterone	(tess toss' ter one)	Tiazac®	(tye' ah zak)
testolactone	(tess toe lak' tone)	Tigan®	(tye' gan)
tetracycline	(tet ra sye' kleen)	Tiazac®	(tye' ah zak)
tetradecyl sulfate	(tetra dek' il sul' fate)	Ziac®	(zye' ak)
tetradecyl sulfate	(tetra dek' il sul' fate)	Ticar®	(tye' kar)
tetracycline	(tet ra sye' kleen)	Tigan®	(tye' gan)
Theolair™	(thee' oh lare)	Tigan®	(tye' gan)
Thiola™	(thye oh' la)	Tiazac®	(tye' ah zak)
Theolair®	(thee' oh lare)	Tigan®	(tye' gan)
Thyrolar®	(thye' roe lar)	Ticar®	(tye' kar)
Theraflu®	(ther' ah flu)	timolol	(tye' moe lole)
Tamiflu™	(tam' eh flu)	atenolol	(ah ten' oh lole)
Theraflu®	(ther' ah flu)	timolol	(tye' moe lole)
Thera-Flur	(thera'-flur)	Tylenol®	(tye' le nole)
Thera-Flur	(thera'-flur)	Timoptic®	(tim op' tik)
Theraflu®	(ther' ah flu)	Talacen®	(tal' ah sen)
Theragran®	(ther' ah gran)	Timoptic®	(tim op' tik)
Phenergan®	(fen' er gan)	Viroptic®	(vir op' tik)
thiamine	(thye' ah min)	Tinactin®	(tin ak' tin)
Tenormin®	(ten or' min)	Talacen®	(tal' ah sen)
thiamine	(thye' ah min)	tioconazole	(tye oh kone' ah zole)
Thorazine®	(thor' ah zene)	terconazole	(ter kone' ah zole)
Thiazide®	(thye' ah zide)	tizanidine	(tye zan' i deen)
Dyazide®	(dye' ah zide)	tiagabine	(tye ag' a bene)
Thiola™	(thye oh' la)	TNKase™	(tee en case')
Theolair™	(thee' oh lare)	t-PA	(tee'-pee ay)
thioridazine	(thye oh rid' ah zeen)	TobraDex®	(toe' bra deks)
thiothixene	(thye oh thix' een)	Tobrex®	(toe' breks)
thioridazine	(thye oh rid' ah zeen)	tobramycin	(toe bra mye' sin)
Thorazine®	(thor' ah zene)	Trobicin®	(troe' bi sin)
thiothixene	(thye oh thix' een)	Tobrex®	(toe' breks)
thioridazine	(thye oh rid' ah zeen)	TobraDex®	(toe' bra deks)
Thorazine®	(thor' ah zene)	tolazamide	(tole az' ah mide)
thiamine	(thye' ah min)	tolazoline	(tole az' oh leen)
Thorazine®	(thor' ah zene)	tolazamide	(tole az' ah mide)
thioridazine	(thye oh rid' ah zeen)	tolbutamide	(tole byoo' ta mide)
Thyrogen®	(thy' roe gen)	tolazoline	(tole az' oh leen)
Thyrolar®	(thye' roe lar)	tolazamide	(tole az' ah mide)
Thyrolar®	(thye' roe lar)	tolbutamide	(tole byoo' ta mide)
Theolair™	(thee' oh lare)	terbutaline	(ter byoo' ta leen)
Thyrolar®	(thye' roe lar)	tolbutamide	(tole byoo' ta mide)
Thyrogen®	(thy' roe gen)	tolazamide	(tole az' ah mide)

Drug Name	Pronunciation	Drug Name	Pronunciation
Tolinase®	(tole′ i nase)	Trental®	(tren′ tal)
Orinase®	(or′ in ase)	Tegretol®	(teg′ ree tol)
tolnaftate	(tole naf′ tate)	Trental®	(tren′ tal)
Tornalate®	(tor′ na late)	Trandate®	(tran′ date)
Tonocard®	(ton′ oh kard)	tretinoin	(tret′ i noyn)
Torecan®	(tor′ e kan)	trientine	(trye′ en teen)
Topic®	(top′ ik)	triacetin	(trye ah see′ tin)
Topicort®	(top′ ih kort)	Triacin®	(trye′ ah sin)
Topicort®	(top′ ih kort)	Triacin®	(trye′ ah sin)
Topic®	(top′ ik)	triacetin	(trye ah see′ tin)
Toradol®	(tor′ ah doll)	Tri-Levlen®	(trye′-lev len)
Inderal®	(in′ der al)	Trilafon®	(tri′ la fon)
Toradol®	(tor′ ah doll)	triamcinolone	(trye am sin′ oh lone)
Tegretol®	(teg′ ree tol)	Triaminicin®	(trye ah min′ ih sin)
Toradol®	(tor′ ah doll)	triamcinolone	(trye am sin′ oh lone)
Torecan®	(tor′ eh kan)	Triamoline®	(trye am′ oh lene)
Toradol®	(tor′ ah doll)	Triaminic®	(trye ah min′ ik)
tramadol	(tra′ ma dole)	Triaminicin®	(trye ah min′ ih sin)
Torecan®	(tor′ e kan)	Triaminic®	(trye ah min′ ik)
Tonocard®	(ton′ oh kard)	TriHemic®	(trye hee′ mik)
Torecan®	(tor′ eh kan)	Triaminicin®	(trye ah min′ ih sin)
Toradol®	(tor′ ah doll)	triamcinolone	(trye am sin′ oh lone)
Tornalate®	(tor′ na late)	Triaminicin®	(trye ah min′ ih sin)
tolnaftate	(tole naf′ tate)	Triaminic®	(trye ah min′ ik)
torsemide	(tor′ se mide)	Triamoline®	(trye am′ oh lene)
furosemide	(fyoor oh′ se mide)	triamcinolone	(trye am sin′ oh lone)
t-PA	(tee′-pee ay)	triamterene	(trye am′ ter een)
TNKase™	(tee en case′)	trimipramine	(trye mi′ pra meen)
tramadol	(tra′ ma dole)	Triapin®	(trye′ ah pin)
Toradol®	(tor′ ah doll)	Triban®	(trye′ ban)
tramadol	(tra′ ma dole)	triazolam	(trye ay′ zoe lam)
Trandate®	(tran′ date)	alprazolam	(al pray′ zoe lam)
tramadol	(tra′ ma dole)	Triban®	(trye′ ban)
Voltaren®	(vol tare′ en)	Triapin®	(trye′ ah pin)
Trandate®	(tran′ date)	Tridrate®	(trye′ date)
tramadol	(tra′ ma dole)	Trandate®	(tran′ date)
Trandate®	(tran′ date)	trientine	(trye′ en teen)
Trendar®	(tren′ dar)	Trental®	(tren′ tal)
Trandate®	(tran′ date)	trientine	(trye′ en teen)
Trental®	(tren′ tal)	tretinoin	(tret′ i noyn)
Trandate®	(tran′ date)	trifluoperazine	(trye floo oh per′ ah zeen)
Tridrate®	(trye′ date)	triflupromazine	(trye floo proe′ ma zeen)
Travatan™	(tra′ va tan)	trifluoperazine	(trye floo oh per′ ah zeen)
Xalatan®	(za la′ tan)	trihexyphenidyl	(trye heks ee fen′ i dil)
Trendar®	(tren′ dar)	triflupromazine	(trye floo proe′ ma zeen)
Trandate®	(tran′ date)	trifluoperazine	(trye floo oh per′ ah zeen)
Trental®	(tren′ tal)		
Bentyl®	(ben′ til)		

Drug Name	Pronunciation	Drug Name	Pronunciation
TriHemic®	(trye hee′ mik)	Tylenol®	(tye′ le nole)
Triaminic®	(trye ah min′ ik)	Tuinal®	(tu′ i nal)
trihexyphenidyl	(trye heks ee fen′ i dil)	Tylenol®	(tye′ le nole)
trifluoperazine	(trye floo oh per′ ah zeen)	Tylox®	(tye′ loks)
Trilafon®	(tri′ la fon)	Tylox®	(tye′ loks)
Tri-Levlen®	(trye′-lev len)	Trimox®	(trye′ moks)
Tri-Levlen®	(trye′-lev len)	Tylox®	(tye′ loks)
Trilafon®	(tri′ la fon)	Tylenol®	(tye′ le nole)
trimeprazine	(trye mep′ ra zeen)	Tylox®	(tye′ loks)
trimipramine	(trye mi′ pra meen)	Wymox®	(wye′ moks)
trimethaphan	(trye meth′ ah fan)	Tylox®	(tye′ loks)
trimethoprim	(trye meth′ oh prim)	Xanax®	(zan′ aks)
trimethoprim	(trye meth′ oh prim)	Ultane®	(uhl′ tane)
trimethaphan	(trye meth′ ah fan)	Ultram®	(uhl′ tram)
trimipramine	(trye mi′ pra meen)	Ultram®	(uhl′ tram)
triamterene	(trye am′ ter een)	Ultane®	(uhl′ tane)
trimipramine	(trye mi′ pra meen)	Ultram®	(uhl′ tram)
trimeprazine	(trye mep′ ra zeen)	Voltaren®	(vol tare′ en)
Trimox®	(trye′ moks)	Ultravate®	(ul′ trah vate)
Diamox®	(dye′ ah moks)	Cutivate™	(kyu′ te vate)
Trimox®	(trye′ moks)	Urex®	(yur′ eks)
Tylox®	(tye′ loks)	Erex®	(err′ eks)
Trinalin®	(tri′ na lin)	Urex®	(yur′ eks)
Phrenilin®	(fren′ ni lin)	Eurax®	(yoor′ aks)
Tri-Norinyl®	(tri-nor′ ih nil)	Urex®	(yur′ eks)
Triphasil®	(tri fay′ sil)	Serax®	(sear′ aks)
Triphasil®	(tri fay′ sil)	Uricit-K®	(yur′ ah sit-kay′)
Tri-Norinyl®	(tri-nor′ ih nil)	Urised®	(yur′ ih sed)
Trobicin®	(troe′ bi sin)	Uridon®	(yur′ ih don)
tobramycin	(toe bra mye′ sin)	Vicodin®	(vye′ co din)
Tronolane®	(tron′ oh lane)	Urised®	(yur′ ih sed)
Tronothane®	(tron′ oh thane)	Uricit-K®	(yur′ ah sit-kay′)
Tronothane®	(tron′ oh thane)	Urised®	(yur′ ih sed)
Tronolane®	(tron′ oh lane)	Urispas®	(yur′ ih spas)
Trovan®	(tro′ van)	Urispas®	(yur′ ih spas)
Tenormin®	(ten or′ min)	Urised®	(yur′ ih sed)
Tuinal®	(tu′ i nal)	Valcyte™	(val′ cite)
Luminal®	(lu′ mi nal)	Valium®	(val′ ee um)
Tuinal®	(tu′ i nal)	Valium®	(val′ ee um)
Tylenol®	(tye′ le nole)	Valcyte™	(val′ cite)
Tussafed®	(tus′ ah fed)	valsartan	(val sar′ tan)
Tussafin®	(tus′ ah fin)	losartan	(loe sar′ tan)
Tussafin®	(tus′ ah fin)	valsartan	(val sar′ tan)
Tussafed®	(tus′ ah fed)	Valstar™	(val′ star)
Tylenol®	(tye′ le nole)	Valstar™	(val′ star)
atenolol	(ah ten′ oh lole)	valsartan	(val sar′ tan)
Tylenol®	(tye′ le nole)	Vancenase®	(van′ sen ase)
timolol	(tye′ moe lole)	Vanceril®	(van′ ser il)

APPENDIX

Drug Name	Pronunciation	Drug Name	Pronunciation
Vanceril®	(van′ ser il)	Vicodin®	(vye′ co din)
Vancenase®	(van′ sen ase)	Hycodan®	(hye′ co dan)
vancomycin	(van koe mye′ sin)	Vicodin®	(vye′ co din)
vecuronium	(ve kyoo′ roe nee um)	Hycomine®	(hye′ co meen)
Vaniqa™	(va nee′ kwa)	Vicodin®	(vye′ co din)
Viagra®	(vye ag′ ra)	Indocin®	(in′ doe sin)
Vantin®	(van′ tin)	Vicodin®	(vye′ co din)
Ventolin®	(ven′ tow lin)	Uridon®	(yur′ ih don)
Vascor®	(vas′ cor)	vidarabine	(vye dare′ ah been)
Norvasc®	(nor′ vask)	cytarabine	(sye tare′ ah been)
Vasocidin®	(vay so sye′ din)	Videx®	(vye′ deks)
Vasodilan®	(vay so di′ lan)	Lidex®	(lye′ deks)
Vasodilan®	(vay so di′ lan)	vinblastine	(vin blas′ teen)
Vasocidin®	(vay so sye′ din)	vincristine	(vin kris′ teen)
Vasosulf®	(vay′ so sulf)	vinblastine	(vin blas′ teen)
Velosef®	(vel′ oh sef)	vinorelbine	(vi nor′ el been)
vecuronium	(ve kyoo′ roe nee um)	vincristine	(vin kris′ teen)
vancomycin	(van koe mye′ sin)	vinblastine	(vin blas′ teen)
Velosef®	(vel′ oh sef)	vinorelbine	(vi nor′ el been)
Vasosulf®	(vay′ so sulf)	vinblastine	(vin blas′ teen)
Ventolin®	(ven′ tow lin)	Vioxx®	(vye′ oks)
Benylin®	(ben′ eh lin)	Zyvox™	(zye′ voks)
Ventolin®	(ven′ to lin)	Viracept®	(vir′ uh sept)
phentolamine	(fen tole′ ah meen)	Viramune®	(vir′ ah myune)
Ventolin®	(ven′ tow lin)	Viramune®	(vir′ ah myune)
Vantin®	(van′ tin)	Viracept®	(vir′ uh sept)
VePesid®	(veh′ pe sid)	Virilon®	(vir′ ih lon)
Versed®	(ver′ sed)	Verelan®	(ver′ e lan)
verapamil	(ver ap′ a mil)	Viroptic®	(vir op′ tik)
Verelan®	(ver′ e lan)	Timoptic®	(tim op′ tik)
Verelan®	(ver′ e lan)	Visine®	(vye′ seen)
verapamil	(ver ap′ a mil)	Visken®	(vis′ ken)
Verelan®	(ver′ e lan)	Visken®	(vis′ ken)
Virilon®	(vir′ ih lon)	Visine®	(vye′ seen)
Verelan®	(ver′ e lan)	Vistaril®	(vis′ tar ril)
Vivarin®	(vye′ va rin)	Restoril®	(res′ tor ril)
Verelan®	(ver′ e lan)	Vistaril®	(vis′ tar ril)
Voltaren®	(vol tare′ en)	Versed®	(ver′ sed)
Versed®	(ver′ sed)	Vistaril®	(vis′ tar ril)
VePesid®	(veh′ pe sid)	Zestril®	(zes′ tril)
Versed®	(ver′ sed)	Vivarin®	(vye′ va rin)
Vistaril®	(vis′ tar ril)	Verelan®	(ver′ e lan)
Vexol®	(veks′ ole)	Volmax®	(vol′ maks)
VoSol®	(voe′ sol)	Flomax®	(flo′ maks)
Viagra®	(vye ag′ ra)	Voltaren®	(vol tare′ en)
Allegra®	(al leg′ ra)	tramadol	(tra′ ma dole)
Viagra®	(vye ag′ ra)	Voltaren®	(vol tare′ en)
Vaniqa™	(va nee′ kwa)	Ultram®	(uhl′ tram)

Drug Name	Pronunciation	Drug Name	Pronunciation
Voltaren®	(vol tare′ en)	Xopenex™	(zo′ pe neks)
Verelan®	(ver′ e lan)	Xanax®	(zan′ aks)
VoSol®	(voe′ sol)	Xylo-Pfan®	(zye′ lo-fan)
Vexol®	(veks′ ole)	Zyloprim®	(zye′ lo prim)
Vytone®	(vye′ tone)	Yocon®	(yo′ con)
Hytone®	(hye′ tone)	Zocor®	(zoe′ cor)
Vytone®	(vye′ tone)	Zagam®	(za′ gam)
Zydone®	(zye′ doan)	Zyban™	(zye′ ban)
Wellbutrin®	(well byu′ trin)	Zantac®	(zan′ tak)
Wellcovorin®	(well coe vor′ in)	Xanax®	(zan′ aks)
Wellbutrin®	(well byu′ trin)	Zantac®	(zan′ tak)
Wellferon®	(well′ fer on)	Zarontin®	(za ron′ tin)
Wellcovorin®	(well coe vor′ in)	Zantac®	(zan′ tak)
Wellbutrin®	(well byu′ trin)	Zofran®	(zoe′ fran)
Wellcovorin®	(well coe vor′ in)	Zantac®	(zan′ tak)
Wellferon®	(well′ fer on)	Zyrtec®	(zir′ tec)
Wellferon®	(well′ fer on)	Zarontin®	(za ron′ tin)
Wellbutrin®	(well byu′ trin)	Xalatan®	(za la′ tan)
Wellferon®	(well′ fer on)	Zarontin®	(za ron′ tin)
Wellcovorin®	(well coe vor′ in)	Zantac®	(zan′ tak)
Wyamine®	(wye′ ah meen)	Zarontin®	(za ron′ tin)
Wydase®	(wye′ dase)	Zaroxolyn®	(za roks′ oh lin)
Wycillin®	(wye sil′ lin)	Zaroxolyn®	(za roks′ oh lin)
Bicillin®	(bye sil′ lin)	Zarontin®	(za ron′ tin)
Wydase®	(wye′ dase)	Zebeta®	(ze′ bay tah)
Lidex®	(lye′ deks)	Diaβeta®	(dye ah bay′ tah)
Wydase®	(wye′ dase)	Zemuron®	(zeh′ mu ron)
Wyamine®	(wye′ ah meen)	Remeron®	(reh′ me ron)
Wymox®	(wye′ moks)	Zerit®	(zer′ it)
Tylox®	(tye′ loks)	Ziac®	(zye′ ak)
Xalatan®	(za la′ tan)	Zestril®	(zes′ trill)
Travatan™	(tra′ va tan)	Desyrel®	(des′ e rell)
Xalatan®	(za la′ tan)	Zestril®	(zes′ trill)
Zarontin®	(za ron′ tin)	Restoril®	(res′ tor ril)
Xanax®	(zan′ aks)	Zestril®	(zes′ trill)
Lanoxin®	(lan oks′ in)	Vistaril®	(vis′ tar ril)
Xanax®	(zan′ aks)	Zestril®	(zes′ trill)
Tenex®	(ten′ eks)	Zostrix®	(zos′ triks)
Xanax®	(zan′ aks)	Ziac®	(zye′ ak)
Tylox®	(tye′ loks)	Tiazac®	(tye′ ah zak)
Xanax®	(zan′ aks)	Ziac®	(zye′ ak)
Xopenex™	(zo′ pe neks)	Zerit®	(zer′ it)
Xanax®	(zan′ aks)	Zinacef®	(zin′ ah sef)
Zantac®	(zan′ tak)	Zithromax®	(zith′ roe maks)
Xanax®	(zan′ aks)	Zinecard®	(zin′ e card)
Zyrtec®	(zir′ tec)	Gemzar®	(gem′ zar)
Xerac®	(zear′ ak)	Zithromax®	(zith′ roe maks)
Serax®	(sear′ aks)	Zinacef®	(zin′ ah sef)

Drug Name	Pronunciation	Drug Name	Pronunciation
Zocor®	(zoe' cor)	Zovirax®	(zo vye' raks)
Cozaar®	(koe' zar)	Zostrix®	(zos' triks)
Zocor®	(zoe' cor)	Zyban™	(zye' ban)
Yocon®	(yo' con)	Zagam®	(za' gam)
Zocor®	(zoe' cor)	Zydone®	(zye' doan)
Zoloft®	(zoe' loft)	Vytone®	(vye' tone)
Zofran®	(zoe' fran)	Zyloprim®	(zye' lo prim)
Zantac®	(zan' tak)	Xylo-Pfan®	(zye' lo-fan)
Zofran®	(zoe' fran)	Zyloprim®	(zye' lo prim)
Zosyn®	(zoe' sin)	ZORprin®	(zor' prin)
zolmitriptan	(zohl mi trip' tan)	Zyprexa®	(zye preks' a)
sumatriptan	(soo ma trip' tan)	Celexa®	(se lex' a)
Zoloft®	(zoe' loft)	Zyprexa®	(zye preks' ah)
Zocor®	(zoe' cor)	Zyrtec®	(zir' tec)
Zonalon®	(zon' ah lon)	Zyrtec®	(zir' tec)
Zone-A Forte®	(zone'-ah for' tay)	Serax®	(sear' aks)
Zone-A Forte®	(zone'-ah for' tay)	Zyrtec®	(zir' tec)
Zonalon®	(zon' ah lon)	Xanax®	(zan' aks)
ZORprin®	(zor' prin)	Zyrtec®	(zir' tec)
Zyloprim®	(zye' lo prim)	Zantac®	(zan' tak)
Zostrix®	(zos' triks)	Zyrtec®	(zir' tec)
Zestril®	(zes' trill)	Zyprexa®	(zye preks' ah)
Zostrix®	(zos' triks)	Zyvox™	(zye' voks)
Zovirax®	(zo vye' raks)	Vioxx®	(vye' oks)
Zosyn®	(zoe' sin)	Zyvox™	(zye' voks)
Zofran®	(zoe' fran)	Zosyn®	(zoe' sin)
Zosyn®	(zoe' sin)		
Zyvox™	(zye' voks)		

TOP 200 DRUGS OF 2001*

Generic Name	Brand Name (if appropriate)	Rank
acetaminophen and codeine	----	31
acyclovir	----	149
albuterol (aerosol)	----	11
albuterol (sulfate)	----	54
alendronate	Fosamax®	44
allopurinol	----	82
alprazolam	----	10
amitriptyline	----	43
amlodipine	Norvasc®	9
amlodipine and benazepril	Lotrel®	86
amoxicillin	----	8
amoxicillin	Amoxil®	69
amoxicillin	Trimox®	35
amoxicillin and clavulanate potassium	Augmentin®	26
amphetamine mixture	Adderall®	99
aspirin	----	169
atenolol	----	4
atorvastatin	Lipitor®	2
azithromycin	Zithromax®	6
benazepril	Lotensin®	78
benzonatate	----	192
bisoprolol and hydrochlorothiazide	----	135
bupropion	Wellbutrin® SR	55
calcitonin salmon	Miacalcin®	179
captopril	----	147
carisoprodol	----	74
cefprozil	Cefzil®	139
cefuroxime	Ceftin®	145
celecoxib	Celebrex®	20
cephalexin	----	22
cerivastatin	Baycol®**	157
cetirizine	Zyrtec®	32
cimetidine	----	175
ciprofloxacin	Cipro®	51
citalopram	Celexa™	42
clarithromycin	Biaxin®	124
clarithromycin	Biaxin® XL	170
clindamycin	----	171
clonazepam	----	57
clonidine	----	91
clopidogrel	Plavix®	84
cyclobenzaprine	----	59
diazepam	----	63
diclofenac	----	188
digoxin	Digitek®	136

---

*NDC Health, "The Top 200 Prescriptions for 2001 by Number of US Prescriptions Dispensed," Available at: http://www.rxlist.com//top200.htm

(continued)

Generic Name	Brand Name (if appropriate)	Rank
digoxin	Lanoxin®	53
diltiazem	----	92
diltiazem	Cartia® XT	107
diltiazem	Tiazac®	164
doxazosin	----	100
doxycycline	----	80
enalapril	----	72
esomeprazole	Nexium™	172
estradiol	----	81
estrogens and medroxyprogesterone	Prempro™	28
estrogens (conjugated)	Premarin®	3
ethinyl estradiol and desogestrel	Mircette®	165
ethinyl estradiol and levonorgestrel	Alesse™ 28	144
ethinyl estradiol and levonorgestrel	Triphasil®	167
ethinyl estradiol and levonorgestrel	Trivora®-28	181
ethinyl estradiol and norethindrone	Loestrin® Fe	117
ethinyl estradiol and norethindrone	Necon®	143
ethinyl estradiol and norethindrone	Ortho-Novum®	102
ethinyl estradiol and norgestimate	Ortho-Cyclen®	150
ethinyl estradiol and norgestimate	Ortho Tri-Cyclen®	30
felodipine	Plendil®	180
fenofibrate	TriCor®	176
fexofenadine	Allegra®	33
fexofenadine and pseudoephedrine	Allegra-D®	98
fluconazole	Diflucan®	70
fluoxetine	----	158
fluoxetine	Prozac®	39
fluticasone	Flonase®	61
fluticasone	Flovent®	77
fluticasone and salmeterol	Advair™ Diskus®	182
fluvastatin	Lescol®	168
folic acid	----	103
fosinopril	Monopril®	109
furosemide	----	7
gabapentin	Neurontin®	49
gatifloxacin	Tequin®	186
gemfibrozil	----	115
glimepiride	Amaryl®	125
glipizide	----	141
glipizide	Glucotrol® XL	197
glyburide	----	65
glyburide and metformin	Glucovance™	162
hydrochlorothiazide	----	13
hydrochlorothiazide and triamterene	----	17
hydrocodone and acetaminophen	----	1
hydrocodone and ibuprofen	Vicoprofen®	196
hydroxyzine	----	119
ibuprofen	----	19
insulin preparations	Humulin® 70/30	142

(continued)

Generic Name	Brand Name (If appropriate)	Rank
insulin preparations	Humulin® N	90
ipratropium	Atrovent®	177
ipratropium and albuterol	Combivent®	129
irbesartan	Avapro®	152
isosorbide mononitrate	----	64
lansoprazole	Prevacid®	18
latanoprost	Xalatan®	94
levofloxacin	Levaquin™	67
levothyroxine	Levothroid®	116
levothyroxine	Levoxyl®	34
levothyroxine	Synthroid®	5
lisinopril	Prinivil®	56
lisinopril	Zestril®	25
lisinopril and hydrochlorothiazide	Zestoretic®	132
loratadine	Claritin®	12
loratadine	Claritin® RediTabs®	161
loratadine and pseudoephedrine	Claritin-D® 12 Hour	96
loratadine and pseudoephedrine	Claritin-D® 24 Hour	93
lorazepam	----	37
losartan	Cozaar®	89
losartan and hydrochlorothiazide	Hyzaar®	121
meclizine	----	120
medroxyprogesterone	----	68
metaxalone	Skelaxin®	173
metformin	Glucophage®	23
metformin	Glucophage® XR	163
methylphenidate	----	156
methylphenidate	Concerta™	160
methylprednisolone	----	87
metoclopramide	----	133
metoprolol	----	36
metoprolol	Toprol-XL®	38
metronidazole	----	138
minocycline	----	134
mirtazapine	Remeron®	154
mometasone	Elocon®	195
mometasone	Nasonex®	79
montelukast	Singulair®	62
mupirocin	Bactroban®	166
naproxen	----	48
naproxen sodium	----	194
nefazodone	Serzone®	153
nifedipine (extended release)	----	187
nitrofurantoin	Macrobid®	159
nitroglycerin	----	199
nortriptyline	----	174
nystatin	----	146
olanzapine	Zyprexa®	114
omeprazole	Prilosec®	14

(continued)

Generic Name	Brand Name (if appropriate)	Rank
omethacin	----	191
oxycodone	OxyContin®	105
oxycodone and acetaminophen	----	110
oxycodone and acetaminophen	Roxicet®	151
pantoprazole	Protonix®	126
paroxetine	Paxil™	16
penicillin V potassium	----	104
penicillin V potassium	Veetids®	131
phenazopyridine	----	200
phenobarbital	----	193
phenytoin	Dilantin®	123
pioglitazone	Actos®	95
potassium chloride	K-Dur®	75
potassium chloride	----	71
potassium chloride	Klor-Con®	127
pravastatin	Pravachol®	47
prednisone	----	29
promethazine	----	112
promethazine	Phenergan®	190
promethazine and codeine	----	148
propoxyphene and acetaminophen	----	27
propranolol	----	85
quinapril	Accupril®	45
rabeprazole	Aciphex™	122
raloxifene	Evista®	101
ramipril	Altace™	111
ranitidine hydrochloride	----	40
risperidone	Risperdal®	97
rofecoxib	Vioxx®	24
rosiglitazone	Avandia®	83
salmeterol	Serevent®	108
sertraline	Zoloft®	15
sildenafil	Viagra®	46
simvastatin	Zocor®	21
spironolactone	----	128
sulfamethoxazole and trimethoprim	Cotrim®**	76
sumatriptan	Imitrex®	118
tamoxifen	----	178
tamsulosin	Flomax®	130
temazepam	----	106
terazosin	----	113
tetracycline	----	184
theophylline	----	183
tolterodine	Detrol®	185
tramadol	Ultram®	58
trazodone	----	60
triamcinolone	----	140
triamcinolone	Nasacort® AQ	189
valacyclovir	Valtrex®	155

(continued)

Generic Name	Brand Name (if appropriate)	Rank
valproic acid and derivatives	Depakote®	198
valsartan	Diovan™	88
valsartan and hydrochlorothiazide	Diovan HCT™	137
venlafaxine	Effexor® XR	66
verapamil	----	52
warfarin	----	73
warfarin	Coumadin®	50
zolpidem	Ambien®	41

**Discontinued

NEW DRUGS INTRODUCED OR APPROVED BY THE FDA IN 2002

Brand Name	Generic Name	Use
Advicor™	niacin and lovastatin	Hypercholesterolemia and dyslipidemia
Aranesp™	darbepoetin alfa	Anemia associated with chronic renal failure
Arixtra®	fondaparinux	Deep vein thrombosis (DVT)
Avodart™	dutasteride	Benign prostatic hyperplasia (BPH)
Benicar™	olmesartan	Hypertension
Bextra™	valdecoxib	Osteoarthritis and adult rheumatoid arthritis; primary dysmenorrhea
Clarinex®	desloratadine	Seasonal allergic rhinitis
Elidel®	pimecrolimus	Atopic dermatitis
Elitek™	rasburicase	Initial management of uric acid levels
Emadine®	emedastine	Allergic conjunctivitis
Faslodex®	fulvestrant	Metastatic breast cancer
Focalin™	dexmethylphenidate	Attention-deficit/hyperactivity disorder (ADHD)
Foltx™	folic acid, cyanocobalamin, and pyridoxine	Nutritional supplement
Frova™	frovatriptan	Migraine
Geodon®	ziprasidone	Schizophrenia
Hepsera™	adefovir dipivoxil	Chronic hepatitis B
Invanz™	ertapenem	Antibacterial
Kineret™	anakinra	Rheumatoid arthritis
Lexapro™	escitalopram	Depression
Neulasta™	pegfilgrastim	Febrile neutropenia
NuvaRing®	ethinyl estradiol and etonogestrel	Prevention of pregnancy
Orfadin®	nitisinone	Hereditary tyrosinemia
Ortho Evra™	ethinyl estradiol and norelgestromin	Prevention of pregnancy
Ortho-Prefest®	estradiol and norgestimate	Menopause
Remodulin™	treprostinil	Pulmonary arterial hypertension (PAH)
Spectracef™	cefditoren	Antibacterial
Synvisc®	sodium hyaluronate/hylan G-F 20	Osteoarthritis of the knee
Tracleer™	bosentan	Pulmonary arterial hypertension
Travatan™	travoprost	Glaucoma
Tri-Luma™	fluocinolone, hydroquinone, and tretinoin	Melasma of the face
Ultracet™	acetaminophen and tramadol	Short-term (≤5 days) management of acute pain
Valcyte™	valganciclovir	Cytomegalovirus retinitis (CMV)
VFEND®	voriconazole	Antifungal
Viread™	tenofovir	HIV infections
Xigris™	drotrecogin alfa	Severe sepsis
Zelnorm™	tegaserod	Irritable bowel syndrome (IBS) in women
Zevalin™	ibritumomab	Non-Hodgkin's lymphoma

PENDING DRUGS OR DRUGS IN CLINICAL TRIALS

Proposed Brand Name or Synonym	Generic Name	Use
Amevive™	alefacept	Psoriasis
Arcoxia™	etoricoxib	Analgesic
BMS-232632	atazanavir	HIV infections
CGP-30083	eplerenone	Hypertension
Cialis™	tadalafil	Erectile dysfunction
Coiracil™	emtricitabine	HIV infections
Crestor™	rosuvastatin calcium	Hyperlipidemia
CPV	capravirine	HIV infections
Cymbalta™	duloxetine	Depression
DAPD	amdoxovir	HIV infections
D2E7	adalimumab	Arthritis
Ebritux™	cetuximab	Colon cancer
Foznol™	lanthanum carbonate	Hyperphosphatemia
Fuzeon™	enfuvirtide	HIV infections
Ketek™	telithromycin	Community-acquired pneumonia
Lumenax™	rifaximin	Traveler's diarrhea
Niviva™	vardenafil	Erectile dysfunction
PNU-140690	tipranavir	HIV infections
Qinghaosu	artesunate	Malaria
SNX-111	ziconotide	Chronic pain
Soltara™	tecastemizole	Allergic rhinitis
Spiriva™	tiotropium	Chronic obstructive pulmonary disease
Strattera™	atomoxetine	ADHD
Symlin™	pramlintide acetate	Diabetes mellitus
UroXatral™	alfuzosin	Benign prostatic hyperplasia
VX-175	fosamprenavir	HIV infections
Xyvoin™	tibolone	Osteoporosis
Zanidip™	lercanidipine	Hypertension
Zetia™	ezetimibe	Hyperlipidemia

DRUG PRODUCTS NO LONGER AVAILABLE (U.S.)

Brand Name	Generic Name
Absorbine® Antifungal	tolnaftate
Absorbine® Jock Itch	tolnaftate
Aches-N-Pain®	ibuprofen
Achromycin® Parenteral	tetracycline
Achromycin® V Capsule	tetracycline
Achromycin® V Oral Suspension	tetracycline
ACT®	fluoride
Actagen-C®	triprolidine, pseudoephedrine, and codeine
Actagen® Syrup	triprolidine and pseudoephedrine
Actagen® Tablet	triprolidine and pseudoephedrine
Act-A-Med®	triprolidine and pseudoephedrine
ACTH-40®	corticotropin
Actidil®	triprolidine
Actifed® Allergy Tablet (Night)	diphenhydramine and pseudoephedrine
Actifed® Syrup	triprolidine and pseudoephedrine
Actifed® With Codeine	triprolidine, pseudoephedrine, and codeine
Actinex®	masoprocol
Acutrim® 16 Hours	phenylpropanolamine
Acutrim® Late Day	phenylpropanolamine
Acutrim® II, Maximum Strength	phenylpropanolamine
Adalat®	nifedipine
Adipost®	phendimetrazine tartrate
Adlone® Injection	methylprednisolone
Adphen®	phendimetrazine tartrate
Adrin®	nylidrin hydrochloride
Adsorbocarpine® Ophthalmic	pilocarpine
Adsorbonac®	sodium chloride
Adsorbotear® Ophthalmic Solution	artificial tears
Advanced Formula Oxy® Sensitive Gel	benzoyl peroxide
Aeroaid®	thimerosal
Aerodine®	povidone-iodine
Aerolate® Oral Solution	theophylline
Aerosporin® Injection	polymyxin B
Afrin® Children's Nose Drops	oxymetazoline
Afrinol®	pseudoephedrine
Afrin® Saline Mist	sodium chloride
Agoral® Plain	mineral oil
AKBeta®	levobunolol
Ak-Chlor® Ophthalmic	chloramphenicol
Ak-Homatropine® Ophthalmic	homatropine
AK-Mycin®	erythromycin (systemic)
Akoline® C.B. Tablet	vitamin
AK-Spore® H.C. Otic	neomycin, polymyxin B, and hydrocortisone
AK-Spore® Ophthalmic Ointment	bacitracin, neomycin, and polymyxin B
AK-Taine®	proparacaine
AK-Zol®	acetazolamide
Ala-Tet®	tetracycline
Alazide®	hydrochlorothiazide and spironolactone
Albalon-A® Ophthalmic	naphazoline and antazoline
Albumisol®	albumin
Albunex®	albumin
Alconefrin® Nasal Solution	phenylephrine

(continued)

Brand Name	Generic Name
Aldoclor®	chlorothiazide and methyldopa
Allercon® Tablet	triprolidine and pseudoephedrine
Allerest® 12 Hour Capsule	chlorpheniramine and phenylpropanolamine
Allerest® 12 Hour Nasal Solution	oxymetazoline
Allerest® Eye Drops	naphazoline
Allerfrin® Syrup	triprolidine and pseudoephedrine
Allerfrin® Tablet	triprolidine and pseudoephedrine
Allerfrin® with Codeine	triprolidine, pseudoephedrine, and codeine
Alor® 5/500	hydrocodone and aspirin
Alphagan®	brimonidine
Alphamul®	castor oil
AL-Rr® Oral	chlorpheniramine
Aludrox®	aluminum hydroxide and magnesium hydroxide
Alu-Tab®	aluminum hydroxide
Amaphen®	butalbital compound and acetaminophen
Ambi 10®	benzoyl peroxide
Ambi® Skin Tone	hydroquinone
Amcort® Injection	triamcinolone (systemic)
Amen®	medroxyprogesterone acetate
Amin-Aid®	amino acid
Ami-Tex LA®	guaifenesin and phenylpropanolamine
Amonidrin® Tablet	guaifenesin
AMO Vitrax®	sodium hyaluronate
Amphojel®	aluminum hydroxide
Amvisc®	sodium hyaluronate
Amvisc® Plus	sodium hyaluronate
Anabolin®	nandrolone
Anacin-3® (all products)	acetaminophen
Anaids® Tablet	alginic acid and sodium bicarbonate
Anamine® Syrup	chlorpheniramine and pseudoephedrine
Anaplex® Liquid	chlorpheniramine and pseudoephedrine
Anatuss®	guaifenesin, phenylpropanolamine, and dextromethorphan
Andro/Fem®	estradiol and testosterone
Andro-L.A.® Injection	testosterone
Androlone®	nandrolone
Androlone®-D	nandrolone
Andropository® Injection	testosterone
Anergan® 25 Injection	promethazine hydrochloride
Anodynos-DHC®	hydrocodone and acetaminophen
Anoquan®	butalbital compound and acetaminophen
Antagon®	ganirelix
Antazoline-V® Ophthalmic	naphazoline and antazoline
Anthra-Derm®	anthralin
Antiben®	antipyrine and benzocaine
Antihist-1®	clemastine
Antihist-D®	clemastine and phenylpropanolamine
Antilirium®	physostigmine
Antiminth®	pyrantel pamoate
Antinea® Cream	benzoic acid and salicylic acid
Antispas® Injection	dicyclomine
Anti-Tuss® Expectorant	guaifenesin
Antivert® Chewable Tablet	meclizine hydrochloride
Antrizine®	meclizine
Antrocol® Capsule & Tablet	atropine and belladonna
Anxanil® Oral	hydroxyzine
Apacet®	acetaminophen

APPENDIX

(continued)

Brand Name	Generic Name
Apaphen®	acetaminophen and phenyltoloxamine
A.P.L.®	chorionic gonadotropin (human)
Aplitest®	tuberculin tests
----	apomorphine (now available as an orphan drug only)
Apresazide®	hydralazine and hydrochlorothiazide
Aquaphyllin®	theophylline
AquaTar®	coal tar
Aquest®	estrone
Aralen® Phosphate With Primaquine Phosphate	chloroquine phosphate and primaquine phosphate
Arcotinic® Tablet	iron and liver combination
Argyrol® S.S.	silver protein, mild
Arlidin®	nylidrin (all products)
Arm-a-Med® Isoetharine	isoetharine
Arm-a-Med® Isoproterenol	isoproterenol
Arm-a-Med® Metaproterenol	metaproterenol sulfate
A.R.M® Caplet	chlorpheniramine and phenylpropanolamine
Arrestin®	trimethobenzamide
Artha-G®	salsalate
Arthritis Foundation® Ibuprofen	ibuprofen
Arthritis Foundation® Nighttime	acetaminophen and diphenhydramine
Arthritis Foundation® Pain Reliever, Aspirin Free	acetaminophen
Articulose-50® Injection	prednisolone
A.S.A.®	aspirin
Asbron-G® Elixir	theophylline and guaifenesin
Asbron-G® Tablet	theophylline and guaifenesin
Ascorbicap®	ascorbic acid
Asendin®	amoxapine
Asmalix®	theophylline
Asproject®	sodium thiosalicylate
AsthmaHaler® Mist	epinephrine
AsthmaNefrin®	epinephrine
Atabrine® Tablet	quinacrine hydrochloride
Atolone® Oral	triamcinolone (systemic)
Atozine® Oral	hydroxyzine
Atrohist® Plus	chlorpheniramine, phenylephrine, phenylpropanolamine, and belladonna alkaloids
Atromid-S®	clofibrate
Atropair®	atropine
----	atropine soluble tablet
Aureomycin®	chlortetracycline
Avlosulfon®	dapsone
Axotal®	butalbital compound and aspirin
Azdone®	hydrocodone and aspirin
Azlin® Injection	azlocillin
Azo Gantanol®	sulfamethoxazole and phenazopyridine
Azo Gantrisin®	sulfisoxazole and phenazopyridine
Azulfidine® Suspension	sulfasalazine
B-A-C®	butalbital compound with aspirin
Bactocill®	oxacillin
BactoShield®	chlorhexidine gluconate
Bancap®	butalbital compound with acetaminophen
Banesin®	acetaminophen
Banophen® Decongestant Capsule	diphenhydramine and pseudoephedrine
Banthine®	methantheline
Bantron®	lobeline (all products)

(continued)

Brand Name	Generic Name
Barbidonna®	hyoscyamine, atropine, scopolamine, and phenobarbital
Barbita®	phenobarbital
Barc™ Liquid	pyrethrins
Basaljel®	aluminum carbonate
Baycol®	cerivastatin
Baypress®	nitrendipine
Becomject-100®	vitamin B complex
Becotin® Pulvules®	vitamins (multiple)
Beepen-VK®	penicillin V potassium
Beesix®	pyridoxine hydrochloride
Belix® Oral	diphenhydramine
Bellafoline®	levorotatory alkaloids of belladonna (all products)
Bellatal®	hyoscyamine, atropine, scopolamine, and phenobarbital
Bellergal-S®	belladonna, phenobarbital, and ergotamine tartrate
Bemote®	dicyclomine
Bena-D®	diphenhydramine
Benadryl® 50 mg Capsule	diphenhydramine hydrochloride
Benadryl® Cold/Flu	acetaminophen, diphenhydramine, and pseudoephedrine
Benahist® Injection	diphenhydramine hydrochloride
Ben-Allergin-50® Injection	diphenhydramine
Ben-Aqua®	benzoyl peroxide
Benemid®	probenecid
Benoject®	diphenhydramine hydrochloride
Benylin® Cough Syrup	diphenhydramine
Benylin DM®	dextromethorphan
Benzocol®	benzocaine
Berubigen®	cyanocobalamin
Beta-2®	isoetharine
Betachron®	propranolol
Betadine® First Aid Antibiotics + Moisturizer	bacitracin and polymyxin B
Betalene® Topical	betamethasone (topical)
Betalin® S	thiamine
Betapen®-VK	penicillin V potassium
Beta-Val® Ointment (only)	betamethasone
Betoptic®	betaxolol
Bexophene®	propoxyphene and aspirin
Biamine® Injection	thiamine hydrochloride
Bilezyme® Tablet	pancrelipase
BioCox®	coccidioidin skin test
Biodine®	povidone-iodine
Biomox®	amoxicillin
Biozyme-C®	collagenase
Biphetamine®	amphetamine and dextroamphetamine
Bisacodyl Uniserts®	bisacodyl
Blanex® Capsule	chlorzoxazone and acetaminophen
BlemErase® Lotion	benzoyl peroxide
Breezee® Mist Antifungal	miconazole
Breonesin®	guaifenesin
Brethaire®	terbutaline
Bretylol®	bretylium
Bricanyl®	terbutaline
Bromaline® Elixir	brompheniramine and phenylpropanolamine
Bromanate® DC	brompheniramine, phenylpropanolamine, and codeine
Bromarest®	brompheniramine
Bromatapp®	brompheniramine and phenylpropanolamine
Brombay®	brompheniramine

(continued)

Brand Name	Generic Name
Bromphen®	brompheniramine
Bromphen® DC With Codeine	brompheniramine, phenylpropanolamine, and codeine
Bronchial®	theophylline and guaifenesin
Bronitin® Mist	epinephrine
Bronkephrine®	ethylnorepinephrine hydrochloride
Bronkometer®	isoetharine
Bronkosol®	isoetharine
Brotane®	brompheniramine
Bucladin®-S Softab®	buclizine
Buffered®, Tri-buffered	aspirin
Buf-Puf® Acne Cleansing Bar	salicylic acid
Butace®	butalbital compound
Butalan®	butabarbital sodium
Buticaps®	butabarbital sodium
Byclomine® Injection	dicyclomine
Bydramine® Cough Syrup	diphenhydramine
Cafatine-PB®	ergotamine
Cafetrate®	ergotamine
Caladryl® Spray	diphenhydramine and calamine
Calciday-667®	calcium carbonate
Calcimar®	calcitonin
Calciparine® Injection	heparin calcium
Calphron®	calcium acetate
Cal-Plus®	calcium carbonate
Caltrate Jr.®	calcium carbonate
Camalox® Suspension & Tablet	aluminum hydroxide, calcium carbonate, and magnesium hydroxide
Cantharone®	cantharidin
Cantharone Plus®	cantharidin
Capzasin-P®	capsaicin
Carbiset® Tablet	carbinoxamine and pseudoephedrine
Carbiset-TR® Tablet	carbinoxamine and pseudoephedrine
Carbodec® Syrup	carbinoxamine and pseudoephedrine
Carbodec® Tablet	carbinoxamine and pseudoephedrine
Carbodec® TR Tablet	carbinoxamine and pseudoephedrine
Cardem®	celiprolol
Cardilate®	erythrityl tetranitrate
Cardio-Green®	indocyanine green
Cardioquin®	quinidine
Caroid®	cascara sagrada and phenolphthalein
Carter's Little Pills®	bisacodyl
Catarase® 1:5000	chymotrypsin (all products)
C-Crystals®	ascorbic acid
Cebid®	ascorbic acid
Cedilanid-D® Injection	deslanoside
Ceepryn®	cetylpyridinium
Cefanex®	cephalexin
Celectol®	celiprolol
Cenocort® A-40	triamcinolone
Cenocort® Forte	triamcinolone
Centrax® Capsule & Tablet	prazepam
Cephulac®	lactulose
Cerespan®	papaverine hydrochloride
Cesamet®	nabilone
Cetane®	ascorbic acid
Cetapred® Ophthalmic	sulfacetamide and prednisolone
Cevalin®	ascorbic acid
Charcoaid®	charcoal

(continued)

Brand Name	Generic Name
Charcocaps®	charcoal
Chenix® Tablet	chenodiol
Children's Hold®	dextromethorphan
Chlo-Amine® Oral	chlorpheniramine
Chlorafed® Liquid	chlorpheniramine and pseudoephedrine
Chlorate® Oral	chlorpheniramine
Chlorgest-HD® Elixir	chlorpheniramine, phenylephrine, and hydrocodone
Chlorofon-A® Tablet	chlorzoxazone
Chloromycetin® Cream	chloramphenicol
Chloromycetin® Kapseals®	chloramphenicol
Chloromycetin® Ophthalmic	chloramphenicol
Chloromycetin® Otic	chloramphenicol
Chloromycetin® Palmitate Oral Suspension	chloramphenicol
Chloroptic-P® Ophthalmic	chloramphenicol and prednisolone
Chloroserpine®	reserpine and hydrochlorothiazide
Chlorphed®	brompheniramine
Chlorphed®-LA Nasal Solution	oxymetazoline
Chlor-Pro® Injection	chlorpheniramine
Chlor-Rest® Tablet	chlorpheniramine and phenylpropanolamine
Chlortab®	chlorpheniramine maleate
Choledyl®	oxtriphylline
Choloxin®	dextrothyroxine
Choron®	chorionic gonadotropin (human)
Chronulac®	lactulose
Chymex®	bentiromide (all products)
Cibacalcin®	calcitonin
Cipralan®	cifenline
Cithalith-S® Syrup	lithium citrate
Citro-Nesia™ Solution	magnesium citrate
Clear Away® Disc	salicylic acid
Clear By Design® Gel	benzoyl peroxide
Clearsil® Maximum Strength	benzoyl peroxide
Clear Tussin® 30	guaifenesin and dextromethorphan
Clindex®	clidinium and chlordiazepoxide
Clistin® Tablet	carbinoxamine maleate
Clopra®	metoclopramide
Clorpactin® XCB Powder	oxychlorosene sodium
Cloxapen®	cloxacillin
Clysodrast®	bisacodyl
Cobalasine® Injection	adenosine phosphate
Cobex®	cyanocobalamin
Codamine®	hydrocodone and phenylpropanolamine
Codamine® Pediatric	hydrocodone and phenylpropanolamine
Codehist® DH	chlorpheniramine, pseudoephedrine, and codeine
Codimal-A® Injection	brompheniramine maleate
Codimal® Expectorant	guaifenesin and phenylpropanolamine
Cold & Allergy® Elixir	brompheniramine and phenylpropanolamine
ColBenemid®	colchicine and probenecid
Coldlac-LA®	guaifenesin and phenylpropanolamine
Coldloc®	guaifenesin, phenylpropanolamine, and phenylephrine
Coly-Mycin® S Oral	colistin sulfate
Comfort® Ophthalmic	naphazoline
Comfort® Tears Solution	artificial tears
Conex®	guaifenesin and phenylpropanolamine
Congess® Jr	guaifenesin and pseudoephedrine
Congess® Sr	guaifenesin and pseudoephedrine

APPENDIX

Brand Name	Generic Name
Congestant D®	chlorpheniramine, phenylpropanolamine, and acetaminophen
Constant-T® Tablet	theophylline
Contac® Cough Formula Liquid	guaifenesin and dextromethorphan
Control®	phenylpropanolamine
Control-L®	pyrethrins
Contuss®	guaifenesin, phenylpropanolamine, and phenylephrine
Contuss® XT	guaifenesin and phenylpropanolamine
Cophene-B®	brompheniramine
Cophene XP®	hydrocodone, pseudoephedrine, and guaifenesin
Co-Pyronil® 2 Pulvules®	chlorpheniramine and pseudoephedrine
Corgonject®	chorionic gonadotropin
Corliprol®	celiprolol
Cortaid® Ointment	hydrocortisone
Cortatrigen® Otic	neomycin, polymyxin B, and hydrocortisone
Cortisporin® Topical Cream	neomycin, polymyxin B, and hydrocortisone
Cortone® Acetate	cortisone acetate
Cortrophin-Zinc®	corticotropin
Cotrim®	co-trimoxazole
Cotrim® DS	co-trimoxazole
Creon®	pancreatin
Crystamine®	cyanocobalamin
Crysticillin® A.S.	penicillin G procaine
Crystodigin®	digitoxin
Cyanoject®	cyanocobalamin
Cyclospasmol®	cyclandelate (all products)
Cycofed® Pediatric	guaifenesin, pseudoephedrine, and codeine
Cycrin® 10 mg Tablet	medroxyprogesterone acetate
Cyomin®	cyanocobalamin
Dacodyl®	bisacodyl
Dakrina® Ophthalmic Solution	artificial tears
Dalgan®	dezocine
Dallergy-D® Syrup	chlorpheniramine and phenylephrine
D-Amp®	ampicillin
Danex® Shampoo	pyrithione zinc
Dapacin® Cold Capsule	chlorpheniramine, phenylpropanolamine, and acetaminophen
Darbid® Tablet	isopropamide iodide (all products)
Daricon®	oxyphencyclimine (all products)
Darvon® 32 mg Capsule	propoxyphene hydrochloride
Darvon-N® Oral Suspension	propoxyphene napsylate
Datril® Extra Strength	acetaminophen
Dayto Himbin®	yohimbine
DC 240® Softgel®	docusate
Decadron® 0.25 mg & 6 mg Tablets	dexamethasone
Decadron® Phosphate Ophthalmic Ointment	dexamethasone
Decaspray®	dexamethasone
Decholin®	dehydrocholic acid
Deficol®	bisacodyl
Degest® 2 Ophthalmic	naphazoline
Dehist®	brompheniramine maleate
Deladumone®	estradiol and testosterone
Delatest® Injection	testosterone
Del-Mycin® Topical	erythromycin (ophthalmic/topical)
Deltalin® Capsule	ergocalciferol
Delta-Tritex® Topical	triamcinolone (topical)
Del-Vi-A®	vitamin A
Demazin® Syrup	chlorpheniramine and phenylpropanolamine

(continued)

Brand Name	Generic Name
depAndrogyn®	estradiol and testosterone
depAndro® Injection	testosterone
depGynogen® Injection	estradiol
depMedalone® Injection	methylprednisolone
Depoject® Injection	methylprednisolone
Deponit® Patch	nitroglycerin
Depo-Provera® 100 mg/mL	medroxyprogesterone
Depotest® Injection	testosterone
Depotestogen®	estradiol and testosterone
Deprol®	meprobamate and benactyzine hydrochloride
Dermoxyl® Gel	benzoyl peroxide
Despec® Liquid	guaifenesin, phenylpropanolamine, and phenylephrine
Desquam-X® Wash	benzoyl peroxide
Detussin® Expectorant	hydrocodone, pseudoephedrine, and guaifenesin
Dexacen-4®	dexamethasone
Dexacen® LA-8	dexamethasone
Dexatrim® Pre-Meal	phenylpropanolamine
Dexchlor®	dexchlorpheniramine
Dexedrine® Elixir	dextroamphetamine sulfate
Dey-Dose® Isoproterenol	isoproterenol
Dey-Dose® Metaproterenol	metaproterenol sulfate
Dey-Lute® Isoetharine	isoetharine
Dialose® Capsule	docusate sodium
Dialose® Plus Capsule	docusate and casanthranol
Dialose® Tablet	docusate
Dialume®	aluminum hydroxide
Diamine T.D.®	brompheniramine
Diaparene® Cradol®	methylbenzethonium
Diapid® Nasal Spray	lypressin
Diar-aid®	loperamide
Diazemuls® Injection	diazepam
Dibent® Injection	dicyclomine
Dicarbosil®	calcium carbonate
Digepepsin®	pancreatin
Dihyrex® Injection	diphenhydramine
Dilantin-30® Pediatric Suspension	phenytoin
Dilantin® With Phenobarbital	phenytoin with phenobarbital
Dilaudid® 1 mg & 3 mg Tablet	hydromorphone hydrochloride
Dilaudid® Cough Syrup	hydromorphone
Dilocaine® Injection	lidocaine
Dilomine® Injection	dicyclomine
Dimaphen® Elixir	brompheniramine and phenylpropanolamine
Dimaphen® Tablets	brompheniramine and phenylpropanolamine
Dimetabs® Oral	dimenhydrinate
Dimetane®	brompheniramine maleate
Dimetane®-DC	brompheniramine, phenylpropanolamine, and codeine
Dimetane® Decongestant Elixir	brompheniramine and phenylephrine
Dimetapp® 4-Hour Liqui-Gel Capsule	brompheniramine and phenylpropanolamine
Dimetapp® Elixir	brompheniramine and phenylpropanolamine
Dimetapp® Extentabs®	brompheniramine and phenylpropanolamine
Dimetapp® Sinus Caplets	pseudoephedrine and ibuprofen
Dimetapp® Tablet	brompheniramine and phenylpropanolamine
Dinate® Injection	dimenhydrinate
Diocto-K®	docusate
Diocto-K Plus®	docusate
Dioctolose Plus®	docusate and casanthranol

(continued)

Brand Name	Generic Name
Dioval® Injection	estradiol
Diphenacen 50® Injection	diphenhydramine
Diphenylan Sodium®	phenytoin
Disanthrol®	docusate and casanthranol
Disonate®	docusate
Di-Spaz® Injection	dicyclomine
Di-Spaz® Oral	dicyclomine
Dispos-a-Med® Isoproterenol	isoproterenol
Dital®	phendimetrazine
Diucardin®	hydroflumethiazide
Diupress®	chlorothiazide and reserpine
Diurigen®	chlorothiazide
Dizac® Injectable Emulsion	diazepam
Dizmiss®	meclizine
Dizymes® Tablet	pancreatin
D-Med® Injection	methylprednisolone
Doktors® Nasal Solution	phenylephrine
Dolacet® Forte	hydrocodone and acetaminophen
Dolene®	propoxyphene
Dolorac™	capsaicin
Dolorex®	capsaicin
Dommanate® Injection	dimenhydrinate
Donnamar®	hyoscyamine
Donnazyme®	pancreatin
Donphen® Tablet	hyoscyamine, atropine, scopolamine, and phenobarbital
Dopar®	levodopa
Dopastat® Injection	dopamine hydrochloride
Doriden® Tablet	glutethimide
Dormarex® 2 Oral	diphenhydramine
Doxinate® Capsule	docusate sodium
Dramamine® Injection	dimenhydrinate
Dramilin® Injection	dimenhydrinate
Dramocen®	dimenhydrinate
Dramoject®	dimenhydramine
Drinex®	acetaminophen, chlorpheniramine, and pseudoephedrine
Dristan® Long Lasting Nasal Solution	oxymetazoline
Dristan® Saline Spray	sodium chloride
Dritho-Scalp®	anthralin
Drixoral® Cough & Congestion Liquid Caps	pseudoephedrine and dextromethorphan
Drixoral® Cough Liquid Caps	dextromethorphan
Drixoral® Non-Drowsy	pseudoephedrine
Dry Eye® Therapy Solution	artificial tears
Dryox® Gel	benzoyl peroxide
Dryox® Wash	benzoyl peroxide
DSMC Plus®	docusate and casanthranol
D-S-S Plus®	docusate and casanthranol
Duadacin® Capsule	chlorpheniramine, phenylpropanolamine, and acetaminophen
DuoCet™	hydrocodone and acetaminophen
Duo-Cyp®	estradiol and testosterone
Duo-Medihaler®	isoproterenol and phenylephrine
Duo-Trach® Injection	lidocaine
Duotrate®	pentaerythritol tetranitrate
Duphalac®	lactulose
Duracid®	aluminum hydroxide, magnesium carbonate, and calcium carbonate
Duract®	bromfenac (all products)
Duradyne DHC®	hydrocodone and acetaminophen

(continued)

Brand Name	Generic Name
Dura-Gest®	guaifenesin, phenylpropanolamine, and phenylephrine
Duralone® Injection	methylprednisolone
Duratest® Injection	testosterone
Duratestrin®	estradiol and testosterone
Durathate® Injection	testosterone
Dura-Vent®	guaifenesin and phenylpropanolamine
Durrax® Oral	hydroxyzine
Duvoid®	bethanechol
DV® Vaginal Cream	dienestrol
Dwelle® Ophthalmic Solution	artificial tears
Dycill®	dicloxacillin
Dyflex-400® Tablet	dyphylline
Dymelor®	acetohexamide
Dymenate® Injection	dimenhydrinate
Dyrexan-OD®	phendimetrazine
ED-SPAZ®	hyoscyamine
Effer-Syllium®	psyllium
Efodine®	povidone-iodine
Elase®-Chloromycetin® Ointment	fibrinolysin and desoxyribonuclease
Eldepryl® Tablet (only)	selegiline
Eldoquin® Lotion	hydroquinone
Elixomin®	theophylline
Elixophyllin SR®	theophylline
E-Lor® Tablet	propoxyphene and acetaminophen
Emecheck®	phosphorated carbohydrate solution
Emete-Con® Injection	benzquinamide
----	emetine hydrochloride
Emitrip®	amitriptyline
E-Mycin®	erythromycin (systemic)
E-Mycin-E®	erythromycin (systemic)
Endep® 25 mg, 50 mg, 100 mg	amitriptyline hydrochloride
Endolor®	butalbital compound and acetaminophen
Enduron® 2.5 mg Tablet	methyclothiazide
Ener-B®	cyanocobalamin
Enisyl®	l-lysine
Enkaid®	encainide
Enomine®	guaifenesin, phenylpropanolamine, and phenylephrine
Enovid®	mestranol and norethynodrel
Enovil®	amitriptyline
E.N.T.®	brompheniramine and phenylpropanolamine
Entex®	guaifenesin, phenylpropanolamine, and phenylephrine
Entozyme®	pancreatin
Entuss-D® Liquid	hydrocodone and pseudoephedrine
E-Pilo-x® Ophthalmic	pilocarpine and epinephrine
E.P. Mycin® Capsule	oxytetracycline
Equanil®	meprobamate
Equilet®	calcium carbonate
Ercaf®	ergotamine
Ergomar®	ergotamine
Ergostat®	ergotamine
Ergotamine Tartrate and Caffeine Cafatine®	ergotamine
Eridium®	phenazopyridine hydrochloride
Ery-Sol® Topical Solution	erythromycin, topical
Esidrix®	hydrochlorothiazide
E-Solve-2® Topical	erythromycin (ophthalmic/topical)
Estivin® II Ophthalmic	naphazoline

(continued)

Brand Name	Generic Name
Estradurin® Injection	polyestradiol phosphate
Estra-L® Injection	estradiol
Estro-Cyp® Injection	estradiol
Estroject-2® Injection	estradiol
Estroject-L.A.® Injection	estradiol
Estronol® Injection	estrone
Estrostep® 21	ethinyl estradiol and norethindrone
Estrovis®	quinestrol
Ethaquin®	ethaverine hydrochloride
Ethatab®	ethaverine hydrochloride
ETS-2% Topical	erythromycin (ophthalmic/topical)
Euthroid® Tablet	liotrix
Eutron®	methyclothiazide and pargyline
Evac-Q-Mag®	magnesium citrate
Evalose®	lactulose
Everone® Injection	testosterone
Excedrin® IB	ibuprofen
Exidine® Scrub	chlorhexidine gluconate
Exna®	benzthiazide
Extra Action Cough Syrup	guaifenesin and dextromethorphan
Eye-Lube-A® Solution	artificial tears
Eye-Sed® Ophthalmic	zinc sulfate
Fastin®	phentermine
Fedahist® Expectorant	guaifenesin and pseudoephedrine
Fedahist® Expectorant Pediatric	guaifenesin and pseudoephedrine
Fedahist® Tablet	chlorpheniramine and pseudoephedrine
FemCare®	clotrimazole
Femcet®	butalbital compound and acetaminophen
Femguard®	sulfabenzamide, sulfacetamide, and sulfathiazole
Femstat®	butoconazole nitrate
Fentanyl Oralet®	fentanyl
Ferancee®	ferrous sulfate and ascorbic acid
Fergon Plus®	iron with vitamin B
Fer-In-Sol® Capsule (only)	ferrous sulfate
Fermalox®	ferrous sulfate, magnesium hydroxide, and docusate
Ferndex®	dextroamphetamine sulfate
Fero-Gradumet®	ferrous sulfate
Ferospace®	ferrous sulfate
Ferralet®	ferrous gluconate
Ferralyn® Lanacaps®	ferrous sulfate
Ferra-TD®	ferrous sulfate
Fiorgen PF®	butalbital compound and aspirin
Fiorital®	butalbital compound and aspirin
Flavorcee®	ascorbic acid
Flaxedil®	gallamine triethiodide
Fleet® Flavored Castor Oil	castor oil
Fleet® Laxative	bisacodyl
Flexaphen®	chlorzoxazone
Flonase® 9 g	fluticasone
Florone®	diflorasone
Florone E®	diflorasone
Floropryl® Ophthalmic	isoflurophate
Fluonid® Topical	fluocinolone
FluorCare® Neutral	fluoride
Fluoritab®	fluoride
Fluothane®	halothane

(continued)

Brand Name	Generic Name
Flura®	fluoride
Flurate® Ophthalmic Solution	fluorescein sodium
Flurosyn® Topical	fluocinolone
Flutex® Topical	triamcinolone (topical)
Folex® Injection	methotrexate
Folex® PFS™	methotrexate
Follutein®	chorionic gonadotropin
Formula Q®	quinine
FS Shampoo® Topical	fluocinolone
Fumasorb®	ferrous fumarate
Fumerin®	ferrous fumarate
Funduscein® Injection	fluorescein sodium
Furacin® Topical	nitrofurazone
Furalan®	nitrofurantoin
Furamide®	diloxanide furoate
Furan®	nitrofurantoin
Furanite®	nitrofurantoin
G-1®	butalbital compound and acetaminophen
Gamastan®	immune globulin, intramuscular
Gammagard® Injection	immune globulin, intravenous
Gammar®	immune globulin, intramuscular
Gamulin® Rh	$Rh_o(D)$ immune globulin (intramuscular)
Gantanol®	sulfamethoxazole
Gantrisin® Ophthalmic	sulfisoxazole
Gantrisin® Tablet	sulfisoxazole
Gas-Ban DS®	aluminum hydroxide, magnesium hydroxide, and simethicone
Gastrosed™	hyoscyamine
Gee Gee®	guaifenesin
Gel-Tin®	fluoride
Gelusil® Liquid	aluminum hydroxide, magnesium hydroxide, and simethicone
Genabid®	papaverine hydrochloride
Genagesic®	guaifenesin and phenylpropanolamine
Genamin® Cold Syrup	chlorpheniramine and phenylpropanolamine
Genamin® Expectorant	guaifenesin and phenylpropanolamine
Genatap® Elixir	brompheniramine and phenylpropanolamine
Genatuss®	guaifenesin
Gencalc® 600	calcium carbonate
Gen-D-phen®	diphenhydramine hydrochloride
Gen-K®	potassium chloride
Genora® 0.5/35	ethinyl estradiol and norethindrone
Genora® 1/35	ethinyl estradiol and norethindrone
Genora® 1/50	mestranol and norethindrone
Gentrasul®	gentamicin
Geridium®	phenazopyridine
GG-Cen®	guaifenesin
Glaucon®	epinephrine
Glukor®	chorionic gonadotropin
Glyate®	guaifenesin
Glycerol-T®	theophylline and guaifenesin
Glycofed®	guaifenesin and pseudoephedrine
Glycotuss®	guaifenesin
Glycotuss-dM®	guaifenesin and dextromethorphan
G-myticin®	gentamicin
Gonic®	chorionic gonadotropin
Grisactin®	griseofulvin
Grisactin® Ultra	griseofulvin
Guaifenex®	guaifenesin, phenylpropanolamine, and phenylephrine

(continued)

Brand Name	Generic Name
Guaifenex® PPA 75	guaifenesin and phenylpropanolamine
Guaipax®	guaifenesin and phenylpropanolamine
Guaitab®	guaifenesin and pseudoephedrine
Guaivent®	guaifenesin and pseudoephedrine
GuiaCough®	guaifenesin and dextromethorphan
GuiaCough® Expectorant	guaifenesin
Guiatex®	guaifenesin, phenylpropanolamine, and phenylephrine
Guaituss CF®	guaifenesin, phenylpropanolamine, and dextromethorphan
G-well®	lindane
Gyne-Sulf®	sulfabenzamide, sulfacetamide, and sulfathiazole
Gynogen® Injection	estradiol
Gynogen L.A.® Injection	estradiol
----	halazone tablet
Haldrone®	paramethasone acetate
Halenol® Tablet	acetaminophen
Halotex®	haloprogin
Halotussin®	guaifenesin
Halotussin® DM	guaifenesin and dextromethorphan
Halotussin® PE	guaifenesin and pseudoephedrine
Harmonyl®	deserpidine
H-BIG®	hepatitis B immune globulin
Healon®	sodium hyaluronate
Healon® GV	sodium hyaluronate
HemFe®	iron with vitamins
Hep-B-Gammagee®	hepatitis B immune globulin
Heptalac®	lactulose
Herplex®	idoxuridine
Hetrazan®	diethylcarbamazine citrate
Hismanal®	astemizole
Histaject®	brompheniramine maleate
Histalet Forte® Tablet	chlorpheniramine, pyrilamine, phenylephrine, and phenylpropanolamine
Histalet® X	guaifenesin and pseudoephedrine
Hista-Vadrin® Tablet	chlorpheniramine, phenylephrine, and phenylpropanolamine
Histerone® Injection	testosterone
Histinex® D Liquid	hydrocodone and pseudoephedrine
Histor-D® Syrup	chlorpheniramine and phenylephrine
Histor-D® Timecelles®	chlorpheniramine, phenylephrine, and methscopolamine
Humibid® Sprinkle	guaifenesin
Humorsol® Ophthalmic	demecarium
HycoClear Tuss®	hydrocodone and guaifenesin
Hycomine®	hydrocodone and phenylpropanolamine
Hycomine® Pediatric	hydrocodone and phenylpropanolamine
Hydeltra-T.B.A.®	prednisolone
Hydramyn® Syrup	diphenhydramine hydrochloride
Hydrobexan® Injection	hydroxocobalamin
Hydro Cobex®	hydroxocobalamin
Hydrocodone PA® Syrup	hydrocodone and phenylpropanolamine
Hydro-Crysti-12®	hydroxocobalamin
Hydromox®	quinethazone
Hydro-Par®	hydrochlorothiazide
Hydrophed®	theophylline, ephedrine, and hydroxyzine
Hydropres®	hydrochlorothiazide and reserpine
Hydroxacen®	hydroxyzine
Hygroton®	chlorthalidone
Hy-Pam® Oral	hydroxyzine
Hyperab®	rabies immune globulin (human)
Hyper-Tet®	tetanus immune globulin (human)

(continued)

Brand Name	Generic Name
Hy-Phen®	hydrocodone and acetaminophen
HypRho®-D	Rh$_o$(D) immune globulin (intramuscular)
HypRho®-D Mini-Dose	Rh$_o$(D) immune globulin (intramuscular)
Hyprogest® 250	hydroxyprogesterone caproate
Ibuprin®	ibuprofen
Idamycin®	idarubicin
Ilopan-Choline® Oral	dexpanthenol
Ilopan® Injection	dexpanthenol
Ilosone® Pulvules®	erythromycin (systemic)
Ilozyme®	pancrelipase
I-Naphline® Ophthalmic	naphazoline
Inocor®	inamrinone (amrinone)
Intal® Inhalation Capsule	cromolyn sodium
Intercept™	nonoxynol 9
Intropin®	dopamine
Iodex-p®	povidone-iodine
Iodo-Niacin® Tablet	potassium iodide and niacinamide hydroiodide
Iophen®	iodinated glycerol
Iophen-C®	iodinated glycerol and codeine
Iophen-DM®	iodinated glycerol and dextromethorphan (all products)
Iophylline®	iodinated glycerol and theophylline
Iotuss®	iodinated glycerol and codeine
Iotuss-DM®	iodinated glycerol and dextromethorphan (all products)
I-Pentolate®	cyclopentolate
I-Phrine® Ophthalmic Solution	phenylephrine
I-Picamide®	tropicamide
Ismotic®	isosorbide
Iso-Bid®	isosorbide dinitrate
Isollyl® Improved	butalbital compound and aspirin
Isopto® Cetapred®	sulfacetamide sodium and prednisolone
Isopto® Eserine	physostigmine
Isopto® Frin Ophthalmic Solution	phenylephrine
Isopto® P-ES	pilocarpine and physostigmine
Isopto® Plain Solution	artificial tears
Isovex®	ethaverine hydrochloride
Isuprel® Glossets®	isoproterenol
I-Tropine®	atropine
Janimine®	imipramine
Jenamicin®	gentamicin
Just Tears® Solution	artificial tears
Kabikinase®	streptokinase
Kalcinate®	calcium gluconate
Kaochlor-Eff®	potassium bicarbonate, potassium chloride, and potassium citrate
Kaochlor® SF	potassium chloride
Kaodene®	kaolin and pectin
Kaopectate® Children's Tablet	attapulgite
Kaopectate® II	loperamide
Karidium®	fluoride
Karigel®	fluoride
Karigel®-N	fluoride
Kasof®	docusate
Kato® Powder	potassium chloride
Kaybovite-1000®	cyanocobalamin
Keflin®	cephalothin sodium
K-Electrolyte® Effervescent	potassium bicarbonate
Kenacort® Oral	triamcinolone (systemic)

(continued)

Brand Name	Generic Name
Kenaject® Injection	triamcinolone (systemic)
Kenonel® Topical	triamcinolone (topical)
Kestrin® Injection	estrone
K-G®	potassium gluconate
K-Gen® Effervescent	potassium bicarbonate
K-Ide®	potassium bicarbonate and potassium citrate, effervescent
K-Lease®	potassium chloride
Klerist-D® Tablet	chlorpheniramine and pseudoephedrine
Klorominr® Oral	chlorpheniramine
Klorvess® Effervescent	potassium bicarbonate and potassium chloride, effervescent
K-Lyte® Effervescent	potassium bicarbonate
K-Norm®	potassium chloride
Koate®-HS Injection	antihemophilic factor (human)
Koate®-HT Injection	antihemophilic factor (human)
Kolyum® Powder	potassium chloride and potassium gluconate
Konakion® Injection	phytonadione
Kondon's Nasal®	ephedrine
Konyne-HT® Injection	factor IX complex (human)
Kwell®	lindane
Lacril® Ophthalmic Solution	artificial tears
Lactulose PSE®	lactulose
Lamprene® 100 mg	clofazimine
Lanacane®	benzocaine
Laniazid® Tablet	isoniazid
Lanorinal®	butalbital compound and aspirin
Largon®	propiomazine
Larodopa®	levodopa
Lasan™ HP-1 Topical	anthralin
Lasan™ Topical	anthralin
Ledercillin VK®	penicillin V potassium
Lente® Insulin	insulin preparations
Lente® L	insulin preparations
Libritabs® (all products)	chlordiazepoxide
Lice-Enz® Shampoo	pyrethrins
LidoPen® I.M. Injection Auto-Injector	lidocaine
Liquaemin®	heparin
Liquid Pred®	prednisone
Liquifilm® Forte Solution	artificial tears
Liquifilm® Tears Solution	artificial tears
Listerex® Scrub	salicylic acid
Listermint® With Fluoride	fluoride
Lithane®	lithium
Lithonate®	lithium
Lithotabs®	lithium
Logen®	diphenoxylate and atropine
Lomanate®	diphenoxylate and atropine
Lorcet®	hydrocodone and acetaminophen
Lorelco®	probucol
Lorsin®	acetaminophen, chlorpheniramine, and pseudoephedrine
Losopan®	magaldrate and simethicone
Lotrimin® AF Cream	clotrimazole
Lotrimin® AF Lotion	clotrimazole
Lotrimin® AF Solution	clotrimazole
Lozi-Tab®	fluoride
LubriTears® Solution	artificial tears
Luride®-SF	fluoride

(continued)

Brand Name	Generic Name
Luvox®	fluvoxamine
Lycolan® Elixir	l-lysine
LYMErix™	lyme disease
Lyphocin® Injection	vancomycin
Maalox® Plus	aluminum hydroxide, magnesium hydroxide, and simethicone
Magalox Plus®	aluminum hydroxide, magnesium hydroxide, and simethicone
Magan®	magnesium salicylate
Magsal®	magnesium salicylate
Malatal®	hyoscyamine, atropine, scopolamine, and phenobarbital
Mallisol®	povidone-iodine
Malotuss® Syrup	guaifenesin
Mantadil® Cream	chlorcyclizine
Maolate®	chlorphenesin
Maox®	magnesium oxide
Marax®	theophylline, ephedrine, and hydroxyzine
Marezine® Injection	cyclizine hydrochloride
Marmine® Injection	dimenhydrinate
Marmine® Oral	dimenhydrinate
Marthritic®	salsalate
Max-Caro®	beta-carotene
Maximum Strength Desenex® Antifungal Cream	miconazole
Maximum Strength Dex-A-Diet®	phenylpropanolamine
Maximum Strength Dexatrim®	phenylpropanolamine
Maxolon®	metoclopramide
Maxzide®-25	hydrochlorothiazide and triamterene
Mazanor®	mazindol
Measurin®	aspirin
Meclan® Topical	meclocycline
Meclomen®	meclofenamate sodium
Medidin® Liquid	hydrocodone and guaifenesin
Medihaler-Epi®	epinephrine
Medihaler Ergotamine®	ergotamine
Medihaler-Iso®	isoproterenol
Medipain 5®	hydrocodone and acetaminophen
Medipren®	ibuprofen
Medi-Quick® Topical Ointment	bacitracin, neomycin, and polymyxin B
Medi-Tuss®	guaifenesin
Medralone® Injection	methylprednisolone
Medrapred®	prednisolone and atropine
Medrol® Acetate Topical	methylprednisolone
Mellaril-S®	thioridazine
Meprospan®	meprobamate
Mesantoin®	mephenytoin
Metahydrin®	trichlormethiazide
Metaprel® Aerosol	metaproterenol sulfate
Metaprel® Inhalation Solution	metaproterenol sulfate
Metaprel® Syrup	metaproterenol sulfate
Metaprel® Tablet	metaproterenol sulfate
Metizol® Tablet	metronidazole
Metra®	phendimetrazine tartrate
Metro I.V.® Injection	metronidazole
Metubine® Iodide	metocurine iodide
Micro-K® LS	potassium chloride
microNefrin®	epinephrine
Miflex® Tablet	chlorzoxazone and acetaminophen
Migrapap®	acetaminophen, isometheptene, and dichloralphenazone

(continued)

Brand Name	Generic Name
Milkinol®	mineral oil
Milontin®	phensuximide
Milophene®	clomiphene
Milprem®	meprobamate and conjugated estrogens
Mini-Gamulin® Rh	Rh$_o$(D) immune globulin (intramuscular)
Minocin® Tablet	minocycline
Minute-Gel®	fluoride
Miochol®	acetylcholine
Mitran® Oral	chlordiazepoxide
Modane® Soft	docusate
Moisturel® Lotion	dimethicone
Monafed®	guaifenesin
Monafed® DM	guaifenesin and dextromethorphan
Monistat i.v.™ Injection	miconazole
Monocete® Topical Liquid	monochloroacetic acid
Monocid®	cefonicid
Motrin® IB Sinus	pseudoephedrine and ibuprofen
Moxam® Injection	moxalactam
M-Prednisol® Injection	methylprednisolone
Muroptic-5®	sodium chloride
Mus-Lax®	chlorzoxazone
Mycelex®-G	clotrimazole
Mycifradin® Sulfate	neomycin
Myconel® Topical	nystatin and triamcinolone
Mylanta AR®	famotidine
Mylanta®-II	aluminum hydroxide, magnesium hydroxide, and simethicone
Mylaxen® Injection	hexafluorenium bromide
Myminic® Expectorant	guaifenesin and phenylpropanolamine
Myochrysine®	gold sodium thiomalate
Myotonachol™	bethanechol
Myphetane DC®	brompheniramine, phenylpropanolamine, and codeine
Nafazair® Ophthalmic	naphazoline
Nafcil™	nafcillin
Naldecon®	chlorpheniramine, phenyltoloxamine, phenylpropanolamine, and phenylephrine
Naldecon® DX Adult Liquid	guaifenesin, phenylpropanolamine, and dextromethorphan
Naldecon-EX® Children's Syrup	guaifenesin and phenylpropanolamine
Naldelate®	chlorpheniramine, phenyltoloxamine, phenylpropanolamine, and phenylephrine
Nalgest®	chlorpheniramine, phenyltoloxamine, phenylpropanolamine, and phenylephrine
Nallpen®	nafcillin
Nalspan®	chlorpheniramine, phenyltoloxamine, phenylpropanolamine, and phenylephrine
Nandrobolic® Injection	nandrolone phenpropionate
Naphcon Forte® Ophthalmic	naphazoline
Nasahist B®	brompheniramine
Natabec®	vitamin (multiple/prenatal)
Natabec® FA	vitamin (multiple/prenatal)
Natabec® Rx	vitamin (multiple/prenatal)
Natalins® Rx	vitamin (multiple/prenatal)
Naus-A-Way®	phosphorated carbohydrate solution
N-B-P® Ointment	bacitracin, neomycin, and polymyxin B
Nelova™ 0.5/35E	ethinyl estradiol and norethindrone
Nelova™ 1/35E	ethinyl estradiol and norethindrone
Nelova™ 1/50M	mestranol and norethindrone
Nelova™ 10/11	ethinyl estradiol and norethindrone
Neo-Calglucon®	calcium glubionate

(continued)

Brand Name	Generic Name
Neo-Castaderm®	resorcinol, boric acid, acetone
Neo-Cortef®	neomycin and hydrocortisone
NeoDecadron® Topical	neomycin and dexamethasone
Neo-Dexameth® Ophthalmic	neomycin and dexamethasone
Neo-Durabolic®	nandrolone
Neofed®	pseudoephedrine
Neo-Medrol® Acetate Topical	methylprednisolone and neomycin
Neomixin® Topical	bacitracin, neomycin, and polymyxin B
Neoquess® Injection	dicyclomine hydrochloride
Neoquess® Tablet	hyoscyamine sulfate
Neo-Synalar® Topical	neomycin and fluocinolone
Neo-Tabs®	neomycin
NeoVadrin®	vitamins (multiple)
Nephrox Suspension	aluminum hydroxide
Nervocaine® Injection	lidocaine
Nestrex®	pyridoxine
Netromycin®	netilmicin
Neucalm-50® Injection	hydroxyzine
Neuramate®	meprobamate
Neutra-Phos® Capsule	potassium phosphate and sodium phosphate
New Decongestant®	chlorpheniramine, phenyltoloxamine, phenylpropanolamine, and phenylephrine
N.G.A.® Topical	nystatin and triamcinolone
Niac®	niacin
Niacels™	niacin
N'ice®	ascorbic acid
Niclocide®	niclosamide
Nicobid®	niacin
Nicolar®	niacin
Nico-Vert®	meclizine
Nidryl®	diphenhydramine hydrochloride
Niferex Forte®	iron with vitamins
Niloric®	ergoloid mesylates
Nilstat®	nystatin
Nipride® Injection	nitroprusside sodium
Nisaval®	pyrilamine maleate
Nitro-Bid® I.V. Injection	nitroglycerin
Nitro-Bid® Oral	nitroglycerin
Nitrocine® Oral	nitroglycerin
Nitrodisc® Patch	nitroglycerin
Nitrong® Oral Tablet	nitroglycerin
Nitrostat® 0.15 mg Tablet	nitroglycerin
Noctec®	chloral hydrate
Nolamine®	chlorpheniramine, phenindamine, and phenylpropanolamine
Nolex® LA	guaifenesin and phenylpropanolamine
Noludar®	methyprylon
No Pain-HP®	capsaicin
Norcet®	hydrocodone and acetaminophen
Nordryl® Injection	diphenhydramine
Nordryl® Oral	diphenhydramine
Norethin™ 1/35E	ethinyl estradiol and norethindrone
Norlutate®	norethindrone
Norlutin®	norethindrone
Normiflo®	ardeparin
Norplant® Implant	levonorgestrel
Norzine®	thiethylperazine
Novafed®	pseudoephedrine

(continued)

Brand Name	Generic Name
Novahistine DMX® Liquid	guaifenesin, pseudoephedrine, and dextromethorphan
Novahistine® Elixir	chlorpheniramine and phenylephrine
Novahistine® Expectorant	guaifenesin, pseudoephedrine, and codeine
NP-27®	tolnaftate
NTZ® Long Acting Nasal Solution	oxymetazoline
Numzident®	benzocaine
Nursoy®	enteral nutritional therapy
Nystex®	nystatin
Octamide®	metoclopramide
Octicair® Otic	neomycin, polymyxin B, and hydrocortisone
Octocaine®	lidocaine and epinephrine
Ocusert Pilo-20®	pilocarpine
Ocusert Pilo-40®	pilocarpine
Ocutricin® Topical Ointment	bacitracin, neomycin, and polymyxin B
OmniHIB™	*Haemophilus* B conjugate vaccine
Omnipen®	ampicillin
Omnipen®-N	ampicillin
Oncet®	hydrocodone and homatropine
Opcon® Ophthalmic	naphazoline
Ophthaine®	proparacaine
Ophthalgan® Ophthalmic	glycerin
Ophthochlor® Ophthalmic	chloramphenicol
Ophthocort®	chloramphenicol, polymyxin B, and hydrocortisone
Optimoist® Solution	saliva substitute
Orabase®-O	benzocaine
Oradex-C®	dyclonine
Orajel® Brace-Aid Oral Anesthetic	benzocaine
Orasone®	prednisone
Oratect®	benzocaine
Ordrine AT® Extended Release Capsule	caramiphen and phenylpropanolamine
Oreticyl®	deserpidine and hydrochlorothiazide
Oreton® Methyl	methyltestosterone
Organidin®	iodinated glycerol
Orinase® Oral	tolbutamide
Ormazine®	chlorpromazine
Ornade® Spansule® Capsules	chlorpheniramine and phenylpropanolamine
Ornidyl® Injection	eflornithine
Or-Tyl® Injection	dicyclomine
Orudis®	ketoprofen
Osteocalcin®	calcitonin
Otic-Care® Otic	neomycin, polymyxin B, and hydrocortisone
Otic Tridesilon®	desonide and acetic acid
Otocort® Otic	neomycin, polymyxin B, and hydrocortisone
Otosporin® Otic	neomycin, polymyxin B, and hydrocortisone
Otrivin®	xylometazoline
Otrivin® Pediatric	xylometazoline
O-V Staticin®	nystatin
Oxsoralen® Oral	methoxsalen
Oxy-5®	benzoyl peroxide
----	oxyphenbutazone
Pamprin IB®	ibuprofen
Panasal® 5/500	hydrocodone and aspirin
Panscol® Lotion	salicylic acid
Panscol® Ointment	salicylic acid
Pantopon®	opium alkaloids

(continued)

Brand Name	Generic Name
Panwarfarin®	warfarin sodium
Paplex®	salicylic acid
Paradione®	paramethadione
Paraflex®	chlorzoxazone
Para-Hist AT®	promethazine, phenylephrine, and codeine
Par Decon®	chlorpheniramine, phenyltoloxamine, phenylpropanolamine, and phenylephrine
Paredrine®	hydroxyamphetamine
Paremyd® Ophthalmic	hydroxyamphetamine and tropicamide
Parepectolin®	kaolin and pectin with opium
Pargen Fortified®	chlorzoxazone
Par Glycerol®	iodinated glycerol
Parsidol®	ethopropazine (all products)
Partuss® LA	guaifenesin and phenylpropanolamine
Pathilon®	tridihexethyl
Pathocil®	dicloxacillin
Pavabid® (all products)	papaverine hydrochloride
Pavasule®	papaverine hydrochloride
Pavatine®	papaverine hydrochloride
Pavatym®	papaverine hydrochloride
Pavesed®	papaverine hydrochloride
Pavulon®	pancuronium
Paxene®	paclitaxel
PBZ® (all products)	tripelennamine
PediaPatch Transdermal Patch	salicylic acid
Pedia-Profen™	ibuprofen
Pediatric Triban®	trimethobanzamide
Pentacarinat® Injection	pentamidine
Pentids®	penicillin G potassium, oral (all products)
Pen.Vee® K	penicillin V potassium
Pepcid RPD®	famotidine
Peptavlon®	pentagastrin
Pepto® Diarrhea Control	loperamide
Percodan®-Demi	oxycodone and aspirin
Percolone®	oxycodone
Perfectoderm® Gel	benzoyl peroxide
Peritrate®	pentaerythritol tetranitrate
Peritrate® SA	pentaerythritol tetranitrate
Permitil® Oral	fluphenazine
Peroxin A5®	benzoyl peroxide
Peroxin A10®	benzoyl peroxide
Persa-Gel®	benzoyl peroxide
Pfizerpen-AS®	penicillin G procaine
Phazyme®	simethicone
Phenadex® Senior	guaifenesin and dextromethorphan
Phenahist-TR®	chlorpheniramine, phenylephrine, phenylpropanolamine, and belladonna alkaloids
Phenameth® DM	promethazine and dextromethorphan
Phenaphen®	acetaminophen
Phenaphen®/Codeine #4	acetaminophen and codeine
Phenaseptic®	phenol
Phenazine® Injection	promethazine
Phencen-50®	promethazine
Phenchlor® S.H.A.	chlorpheniramine, phenylephrine, phenylpropanolamine, and belladonna alkaloids
Phendry® Oral	diphenhydramine
Phenerbel-S®	belladonna, phenobarbital, and ergotamine tartrate
Phenergan® VC With Codeine	promethazine, phenylephrine, and codeine

APPENDIX

(continued)

Brand Name	Generic Name
Phenergan® With Dextromethorphan	promethazine and dextromethorphan
Phenetron®	chlorpheniramine
----	phenolsulfonphthalein
Phenoxine®	phenylpropanolamine
Phenurone®	phenacemide
Phenyldrine®	phenylpropanolamine
Phenylfenesin® L.A.	guaifenesin and phenylpropanolamine
Pherazine® VC With Codeine	promethazine, phenylephrine, and codeine
Pherazine® With Codeine	promethazine and codeine
Pherazine® With DM	promethazine and dextromethorphan
Phos-Ex® 62.5	calcium acetate
Phos-Ex® 125	calcium acetate
Phos-Ex® 167	calcium acetate
Phos-Ex® 250	calcium acetate
pHos-pHaid®	ammonium biphosphate, sodium biphosphate, and sodium acid pyrophosphate
Phosphaljel®	aluminum phosphate
Pilagan® Ophthalmic	pilocarpine
Pilostat® Ophthalmic	pilocarpine
Pindac®	pinacidil
Pin-Rid®	pyrantel pamoate
Plasmatein®	plasma protein fraction
Plegine®	phendimetrazine
Pneumomist®	guaifenesin
Pod-Ben-25®	podophyllum resin
Podofin®	podophyllum resin
Point-Two®	fluoride
Poladex®	dexchlorpheniramine
Polargen®	dexchlorpheniramine maleate
Poliovax® Injection	poliovirus vaccine, inactivated
Polycillin-N® Injection	ampicillin
Polycillin® Oral	ampicillin
Polycillin-PRB®	ampicillin and probenecid (all products)
Polyflex® Tablet	chlorzoxazone
Polygam® Injection	immune globulin, intravenous
Poly-Histine CS®	brompheniramine, phenylpropanolamine, and codeine
Poly-Histine-D® Capsule	phenyltoloxamine, phenylpropanolamine, pyrilamine, and pheniramine
Polymox®	amoxicillin
Pondimin®	fenfluramine
Porcelana® Sunscreen	hydroquinone
Posicor®	mibefradil (all products)
Potasalan®	potassium chloride
Pramet® FA	vitamin (multiple/prenatal)
Pramilet® FA	vitamin (multiple/prenatal)
Predair®	prednisolone
Predaject-50®	prednisolone
Predalone®	prednisolone
Predcor®	prednisolone
Predcor-TBA®	prednisolone
Predicort-50®	prednisolone
Prednicen-M®	prednisone
Preludin®	phenmetrazine hydrochloride
Premarin® With Methyltestosterone	estrogens and methyltestosterone
Prescription Strength Desenex®	miconazole
Proampacin®	ampicillin and probenecid (all products)

(continued)

Brand Name	Generic Name
Pro-Banthine®	propantheline
Pro-Cal-Sof®	docusate
Procan™ SR	procainamide
Profenal®	suprofen
Profen II DM®	guaifenesin, phenylpropanolamine, and dextromethorphan
Profen LA®	guaifenesin and phenylpropanolamine
Profilate-HP®	antihemophilic factor (human)
Progestaject® Injection	progesterone
ProHIBiT®	*Haemophilus* B conjugate vaccine
Prokine™ Injection	sargramostim
Prolamine®	phenylpropanolamine
Proloid®	thyroglobulin
Prometa®	metaproterenol sulfate
Prometh®	promethazine
Promethist® With Codeine	promethazine, phenylephrine, and codeine
Prometh® VC Plain Liquid	promethazine and phenylephrine
Prometh® VC With Codeine	promethazine, phenylephrine, and codeine
Propacet®	propoxyphene and acetaminophen
Propagest®	phenylpropanolamine
Proplex® SX-T Injection	factor IX complex (human)
Propoxacet-N®	propoxyphene and acetaminophen
Pro-Sof®	docusate sodium
Pro-Sof® Plus	docusate and casanthranol
Prostaphlin®	oxacillin
ProStep® Patch	nicotine
Prostin F₂ Alpha®	dinoprost tromethamine
Protenate®	plasma protein fraction
Prothazine-DC®	promethazine and codeine
Protilase®	pancrelipase
Protopam® Tablet	pralidoxime chloride
Protostat® Oral	metronidazole
Provatene®	beta-carotene
Pseudo-Gest Plus® Tablet	chlorpheniramine and pseudoephedrine
Psorion® Topical	betamethasone (topical)
Pyridium Plus®	phenazopyridine, hyoscyamine, and butabarbital
Queltuss®	guaifenesin and dextromethorphan
Questran® Tablet	cholestyramine resin
Quiess® Injection	hydroxyzine
Quinalan®	quinidine
Quinamm®	quinine sulfate
Quinora®	quinidine
Quiphile®	quinine sulfate
Q-vel®	quinine sulfate
Raudixin®	*Rauwolfia serpentina*
Rauverid®	*Rauwolfia serpentina*
Raxar®	grepafloxacin
Rectacort® Suppository	hydrocortisone
Redisol®	cyanocobalamin
Redux®	dexfenfluramine
Regitine®	phentolamine
Regulace®	docusate and casanthranol
Regulax SS®	docusate
Regutol®	docusate
Relefact® TRH	protirelin
Relief® Ophthalmic Solution	phenylephrine
Renoquid®	sulfacytine
Reposans-10® Oral	chlordiazepoxide

(continued)

Brand Name	Generic Name
Rep-Pred®	methylprednisolone
Resa®	reserpine
Resaid®	chlorpheniramine and phenylpropanolamine
Rescaps-D® S.R. Capsule	caramiphen and phenylpropanolamine
Rescon® Liquid	chlorpheniramine and phenylpropanolamine
Respbid®	theophylline
Rexigen Forte®	phendimetrazine
Rezulin®	troglitazone
R-Gel®	capsaicin
R-Gen®	iodinated glycerol
Rheaban®	attapulgite
Rhesonativ® Injection	$Rh_o(D)$ immune globulin
Rhinatate® Tablet	chlorpheniramine, pyrilamine, and phenylephrine
Rhindecon®	phenylpropanolamine
Rhinolar®	chlorpheniramine, phenylpropanolamine, and methscopolamine
Rhulicaine®	benzocaine
Rhuli® Cream	benzocaine, calamine, and camphor
Riobin®	riboflavin
Robafen® CF	guaifenesin, phenylpropanolamine, and dextromethorphan
Robicillin® Tablet	penicillin V potassium
Robitet®	tetracycline
Robitussin® A-C	guaifenesin and codeine
Robitussin-CF®	guaifenesin, phenylpropanolamine, and dextromethorphan
Robitussin®-DAC	guaifenesin, pseudoephedrine, and codeine
Rolatuss® Plain Liquid	chlorpheniramine and phenylephrine
Rondomycin® Capsule	methacycline hydrochloride (all products)
RotaShield®	rotavirus vaccine
Roxanol SR™ Oral	morphine sulfate
Roxiprin®	oxycodone and aspirin
Rubramin-PC®	cyanocobalamin
Rufen®	ibuprofen
Ru-Tuss® Liquid	chlorpheniramine and phenylephrine
Ru-Tuss® Tablet	chlorpheniramine, phenylephrine, phenylpropanolamine, and belladonna alkaloids
Ru-Vert-M®	meclizine
Rymed®	guaifenesin and pseudoephedrine
Rymed-TR®	guaifenesin and phenylpropanolamine
Salacid® Ointment	salicylic acid
Saleto-200®	ibuprofen
Saleto-400®	ibuprofen
Salgesic®	salsalate
Salmonine®	calcitonin
Salsitab®	salsalate
Saluron®	hydroflumethiazide
Salutensin®	hydroflumethiazide and reserpine
Salutensin-Demi®	hydroflumethiazide and reserpine
SangCya™	cyclosporine
Sanorex®	mazindol
Scabene®	lindane
Sclavo Test - PPD®	tuberculin purified protein derivative
Secran®	vitamins (multiple)
Seldane®	terfenadine
Seldane-D®	terfenadine and pseudoephedrine
Selecor®	celiprolol
Selectol®	celiprolol
Selestoject®	betamethasone
Senolax®	senna

(continued)

Brand Name	Generic Name
Septa® Topical Ointment	bacitracin, neomycin, and polymyxin B
Septisol®	hexachlorophene
Ser-A-Gen®	hydralazine, hydrochlorothiazide, and reserpine
Ser-Ap-Es®	hydralazine, hydrochlorothiazide, and reserpine
Serpalan®	reserpine
Serpasil®	reserpine
Serpatabs®	reserpine
Siblin®	psyllium
Silain®	simethicone
Silaminic® Cold Syrup	chlorpheniramine and phenylpropanolamine
Silaminic® Expectorant	guaifenesin and phenylpropanolamine
Sildicon-E®	guaifenesin and phenylpropanolamine
Siltussin-CF®	guaifenesin, phenylpropanolamine, and dextromethorphan
Sine-Aid® IB	pseudoephedrine and ibuprofen
Sinubid®	phenyltoloxamine, phenylpropanolamine, and acetaminophen
Sinufed® Timecelles®	guaifenesin and pseudoephedrine
Sinumed®	acetaminophen, chlorpheniramine, and pseudoephedrine
Sinumist®-SR Capsulets®	guaifenesin
Skelex®	chlorzoxazone
Sleep-eze 3® Oral	diphenhydramine
Sleepwell 2-nite®	diphenhydramine
Slim-Mint®	benzocaine
Slo-bid™	theophylline
Slo-Phyllin® GG	theophylline and guaifenesin
Slo-Salt®	salt substitute
Slow-K®	potassium chloride
Snaplets-EX®	guaifenesin and phenylpropanolamine
Sodium P.A.S.®	aminosalicylate sodium
Sofarin®	warfarin sodium
Solatene®	beta-carotene
Solfoton®	phenobarbital
Span-FF®	ferrous fumarate
Sparine®	promazine
Spasmoject®	dicyclomine
Spasmolin®	hyoscyamine, atropine, scopolamine, and phenobarbital
Spec-T®	benzocaine
Spectrobid® Tablet	bacampicillin
Spherulin®	coccidioidin skin test
Spironazide®	hydrochlorothiazide and spironolactone
Spirozide®	hydrochlorothiazide and spironolactone
SRC® Expectorant	hydrocodone, pseudoephedrine, and guaifenesin
Stahist®	chlorpheniramine, phenylephrine, phenylpropanolamine, and belladonna alkaloids
Staphcillin®	methicillin (all products)
Statobex®	phendimetrazine tartrate
Stemex®	paramethasone acetate
St. Joseph® Measured Dose Nasal Solution	phenylephrine
Sucostrin®	succinylcholine chloride
Sucrets® Cough Calmers	dextromethorphan
Sudafed® Cough	guaifenesin, pseudoephedrine, and dextromethorphan
Sudafed Plus® Liquid	chlorpheniramine and pseudoephedrine
Sudex®	guaifenesin and pseudoephedrine
Sufedrin®	pseudoephedrine
Sulfa-Gyn®	sulfabenzamide, sulfacetamide, and sulfathiazole
Sulfamethoprim®	co-trimoxazole
Sulfa-Trip®	sulfabenzamide, sulfacetamide, and sulfathiazole
Sultrin™	sulfabenzamide, sulfacetamide, and sulfathiazole

(continued)

Brand Name	Generic Name
Superchar®	charcoal
Superchar® With Sorbitol	charcoal
Suppress®	dextromethorphan
Surital®	thiamylal sodium
Sus-Phrine®	epinephrine
Sustaire®	theophylline
Symadine®	amantadine hydrochloride
Symmetrel® Capsule	amantadine hydrochloride
Synalar-HP® Topical	fluocinolone
Synemol® Topical	fluocinolone
Synkayvite®	menadiol sodium
Syntocinon® Nasal	oxytocin
Sytobex®	cyanocobalamin
Tabron®	vitamins, multiple
Tac™-40 Injection	triamcinolone (systemic)
Tacaryl®	methdilazine hydrochloride (all products)
TACE®	chlorotrianisene
Tamine®	brompheniramine and phenylpropanolamine
Tanac®	benzocaine
Tanoral® Tablet	chlorpheniramine, pyrilamine, and phenylephrine
Tarabine® PFS	cytarabine
Taractan®	chlorprothixene
Tavist-D®	clemastine and phenylpropanolamine
T-Caine® Lozenge	benzocaine
Tear Drop® Solution	artificial tears
TearGard® Ophthalmic Solution	artificial tears
Tebamide®	trimethobenzamide
Tedral®	theophylline, ephedrine, and phenobarbital
Tega-Vert® Oral	dimenhydrinate
Tegopen®	cloxacillin
Telachlor® Oral	chlorpheniramine
Teladar® Topical	betamethasone (topical)
Teldrin® Oral	chlorpheniramine
Teline®	tetracycline
Temaril®	trimeprazine tartrate
Temazin® Cold Syrup	chlorpheniramine and phenylpropanolamine
Ten-K®	potassium chloride
Tepanil®	diethylpropion hydrochloride
Tepanil® TenTabs®	diethylpropion hydrochloride
----	terpin hydrate
----	terpin hydrate and codeine
Terra-Cortril® Ophthalmic Suspension	oxytetracycline and hydrocortisone
Terramycin® Oral	oxytetracycline
Tesamone® Injection	testosterone
Tes-Tape®	diagnostic aids (*in vitro*), urine
Testomar®	yohimbine
Testopel® Pellet	testosterone
Tetracap®	tetracycline
Tetralan®	tetracycline
Tetram®	tetracycline
Tetramune®	diphtheria, tetanus toxoids, whole-cell pertussis, and Haemophilus B conjugate
Tetrasine® Extra Ophthalmic	tetrahydrozoline
Tetrasine® Ophthalmic	tetrahydrozoline
T-Gen®	trimethobenzamide
Theelin® Aqueous Injection	estrone
Theobid®	theophylline

(continued)

Brand Name	Generic Name
Theobid® Jr Duracaps®	theophylline
Theoclear-80®	theophylline
Theoclear®-L.A.	theophylline
Theo-Dur® Sprinkle®	theophylline
Theolair™-SR	theophylline
Theo-Organidin®	iodinated glycerol and theophylline
Theo-Sav®	theophylline
Theospan®-SR	theophylline
Theostat-80®	theophylline
Theovent®	theophylline
Theo-X®	theophylline
Therabid®	vitamins (multiple)
Thera-Flur®	fluoride
Thera-Hist® Syrup	chlorpheniramine and phenylpropanolamine
Theramine® Expectorant	guaifenesin and phenylpropanolamine
Thiacide®	methenamine and potassium acid phosphate
Thrombinar®	thrombin (topical)
Thrombostat®	thrombin (topical)
Thypinone®	protirelin
Thyrar®	thyroid
Thyro-Block®	potassium iodide
Thyroid Strong®	thyroid
Tiamate®	diltiazem
Ticon®	trimethobenzamide
Tiject-20®	trimethobenzamide
Timecelles®	ascorbic acid
Tindal®	acetophenazine maleate
Tinver®	sodium thiosulfate
Topicycline® Topical	tetracycline
Torecan® Suppository	thiethylperazine
Totacillin®	ampicillin
Totacillin-N®	ampicillin
Tral®	hexocyclium methylsulfate
Transdermal-NTG® Patch	nitroglycerin
Trans-Plantar® Transdermal Patch	salicylic acid
Travase®	sutilains
Trendar®	ibuprofen
Triafed®	triprolidine and pseudoephedrine
Triaminic® Allergy Tablet	chlorpheniramine and phenylpropanolamine
Triaminic® Cold Tablet	chlorpheniramine and phenylpropanolamine
Triaminic® Expectorant	guaifenesin and phenylpropanolamine
Triaminicol® Multi-Symptom Cold Syrup	chlorpheniramine, phenylpropanolamine, and dextromethorphan
Triaminic® Oral Infant, Drops	pheniramine, phenylpropanolamine, and pyrilamine
Triaminic® Syrup	chlorpheniramine and phenylpropanolamine
Triamonide® Injection	triamcinolone (systemic)
Triapin®	butalbital compound and acetaminophen
Triavil® 4-50	amitriptyline and perphenazine
Tri-Clear® Expectorant	guaifenesin phenylpropanolamine
Tridil® Injection	nitroglycerin
Tridione®	trimethadione
Tridione® Suppository	trimethadione
Trifed-C®	triprolidine, pseudoephedrine, and codeine
Tri-Immunol®	diphtheria, tetanus toxoids, and whole-cell pertussis vaccine
TRIKOF-D®	guaifenesin, phenylpropanolamine, and dextromethorphan
Tri-Kort® Injection	triamcinolone (systemic)
Trilog® Injection	triamcinolone (systemic)

(continued)

Brand Name	Generic Name
Trilone® Injection	triamcinolone (systemic)
Trimazide®	trimethobenzamide
Trimox® 500 mg	amoxicillin
Tri-Nefrin® Extra Strength Tablet	chlorpheniramine and phenylpropanolamine
Triofed® Syrup	triprolidine and pseudoephedrine
Tri-Phen-Chlor®	chlorpheniramine, phenyltoloxamine, phenylpropanolamine, and phenylephrine
Triphenyl® Expectorant	guaifenesin and phenylpropanolamine
Triphenyl® Syrup	chlorpheniramine and phenylpropanolamine
Tri-P® Oral Infant Drops	pheniramine, phenylpropanolamine, and pyrilamine
Triposed® Syrup	triprolidine and pseudoephedrine
Tri-Pseudo®	triprolidine and pseudoephedrine
Tristoject® Injection	triamcinolone (systemic)
Tri-Statin® II Topical	nystatin and triamcinolone
Trisudex®	triprolidine and pseudoephedrine
Tri-Tannate Plus®	chlorpheniramine, ephedrine, phenylephrine, and carbetapentane
Trivagizole 3™	clotrimazole
Trofan®	L-tryptophan
Trofan DS®	L-tryptophan
Truphylline®	aminophylline
Tryptacin®	L-tryptophan
Trysul®	sulfabenzamide, sulfacetamide, and sulfathiazole
Tucks® Cream	witch hazel
Tusal®	sodium thiosalicylate
Tusibron®	guaifenesin
Tusibron-DM®	guaifenesin and dextromethorphan
Tussafin® Expectorant	hydrocodone, pseudoephedrine, and guaifenesin
Tuss-Allergine® Modified T.D. Capsule	caramiphen and phenylpropanolamine
Tussi-Organidin®	iodinated glycerol and codeine
Tussi-Organidin® DM	iodinated glycerol and dextromethorphan (all products)
Tuss-LA®	guaifenesin and pseudoephedrine
Tusso-DM®	iodinated glycerol and dextromethorphan (all products)
Tussogest® Extended Release Capsule	caramiphen and phenylpropanolamine
Tuss-Ornade®	caramiphen and phenylpropanolamine
Two-Dyne®	butalbital compound and acetaminophen
Tylenol® Cold Effervescent Medication Tablet	chlorpheniramine, phenylpropanolamine, and acetaminophen
Tyrodone® Liquid	hydrocodone and pseudoephedrine
UAD Otic®	neomycin, polymyxin B, and hydrocortisone
ULR-LA®	guaifenesin and phenylpropanolamine
Ultralente® U	insulin zinc suspension, extended
Ultrase® MT24	pancrelipase
Unguentine®	benzocaine
Uni-Bent® Cough Syrup	diphenhydramine
Uni-Decon®	chlorpheniramine, phenyltoloxamine, phenylpropanolamine, and phenylephrine
Uni-Dur®	theophylline
Unipen®	nafcillin
Unipres®	hydralazine, hydrochlorothiazide, and reserpine
Uni-Pro®	ibuprofen
Unitrol®	phenylpropanolamine
Uni-tussin®	guaifenesin
Uni-tussin® DM	guaifenesin and dextromethorphan
Urabeth®	bethanechol
Uracel®	sodium salicylate

(continued)

Brand Name	Generic Name
Ureacin®-40 Topical	urea
Uri-Tet®	oxytetracycline
Urobak®	sulfamethoxazole
Urobiotic-25®	oxytetracycline and sulfamethizole
Urodine®	phenazopyridine
Uroplus® DS	co-trimoxazole
Uroplus® SS	co-trimoxazole
Uticort®	betamethasone (all products)
Vagitrol®	sulfanilamide
Valadol®	acetaminophen
Valergen® Injection	estradiol
Valisone® Topical	betamethasone (topical)
Valmid® Capsule	ethinamate
Valpin® 50	anisotropine methylbromide
Valrelease®	diazepam
Vamate® Oral	hydroxyzine
Vanex-LA®	guaifenesin and phenylpropanolamine
Vanoxide®	benzoyl peroxide
Vanseb-T® Shampoo	coal tar, sulfur, and salicylic acid
Vansil™	oxamniquine
Vaponefrin®	epinephrine
Vasocon Regular® Ophthalmic	naphazoline
Vasosulf® Ophthalmic	sulfacetamide and phenylephrine
Vasoxyl®	methoxamine
V-Cillin K®	penicillin V potassium
Vectrin®	minocycline
Velsar® Injection	vinblastine sulfate
Venoglobulin®-I	immune globulin (intravenous)
Verazinc® Oral	zinc sulfate
Vercyte®	pipobroman
Vergogel® Gel	salicylic acid
Vergon®	meclizine
Vermizine®	piperazine
Verr-Canth™	cantharidin
Verrex-C&M®	podophyllin and salicylic acid
Verrusol®	salicylic acid, podophyllin, and cantharidin
Versed®	midazolam
Versiclear™	sodium thiosulfate
Verukan® Solution	salicylic acid
V-Gan® Injection	promethazine hydrochloride
Vibazine®	buclizine
Vicks® 44 Non-Drowsy Cold & Cough Liqui-Caps	pseudoephedrine and dextromethorphan
Vicks® Children's Chloraseptic®	benzocaine
Vicks® Chloraseptic® Sore Throat	benzocaine
Vicks® DayQuil® Allergy Relief 4 Hour Tablet	brompheniramine and phenylpropanolamine
Vicks® DayQuil® Sinus Pressure & Congestion Relief	guaifenesin and phenylpropanolamine
Vicks® Vatronol®	ephedrine
Vioform®	clioquinol
Vioform®-Hydrocortisone Topical	clioquinol and hydrocortisone
Vistacon-50® Injection	hydroxyzine
Vistaject-25®	hydroxyzine
Vistaject-50®	hydroxyzine

(continued)

Brand Name	Generic Name
Vistaquel® Injection	hydroxyzine
Vistazine® Injection	hydroxyzine
VitaCarn® Oral	levocarnitine
Vontrol®	diphenidol
Wehamine® Injection	dimenhydrinate
Wehdryl®	diphenhydramine
Wesprin® Buffered	aspirin
40 Winks®	diphenhydramine
WinRho SD®	Rh_o (D) immune globulin (intravenous-human)
Wolfina®	*Rauwolfia serpentina*
Wyamycin S®	erythromycin
Wydase®	hyaluronidase
Wygesic®	propoxyphene and acetaminophen
Wytensin®	guanabenz
Yohimex™	yohimbine
Yutopar®	ritodrine
Zantryl®	phentermine
Zartan®	cephalexin
Zebrax®	clidinium and chlordiazepoxide
Zefazone®	cefmetazole
Zetran®	diazepam
Zolicef®	cefazolin
Zolyse®	chymotrypsin alpha (all products)
Zyban™ 100 mg	bupropion
Zymase®	pancrelipase

PHARMACEUTICAL MANUFACTURERS AND DISTRIBUTORS

AAI International
2320 Scientific Park Drive
Wilmington, NC 28405
(800) 575-4224

**Abbott Laboratories
(Pharmaceutical Products Division)**
100 Abbott Park Road
Abbott Park, IL 60064-3500
(847) 937-6100
www.abbott.com

Adams Laboratories, Inc
14801 Sovereign Road
Ft Worth, TX 76155-2645
(817) 354-3858
www.adamslaboratories.com

A P Pharma
123 Saginaw Drive
Redwood City, CA 94063
(650) 366-2626
www.advancedpolymer.com

Advanced Tissue Sciences, Inc
10933 North Torrey Pines Road
La Jolla, CA 92037-1005
(858) 713-7300
www.advancedtissue.com

Advanced Vision Research
12 Alfred Street
Suite 200
Woburn, MA 01801
(800) 579-8327
www.theratears.com

Agouron Pharmaceuticals, Inc
10350 North Torrey Pines Road
La Jolla, CA 92037-1020
(858) 622-3000
www.biospace.com

Akorn, Inc
2500 Millbrook Drive
Buffalo Grove, IL 60089-4694
(800) 535-7155
www.akorn.com

AkPharma, Inc
6840 Old Egg Harbor Road
Pleasantville, NJ 08232
(800) 994-4711
www.akpharma.com

Alcon Laboratories, Inc
6201 South Freeway
Fort Worth, TX 76134
www.alconlabs.com

Allerderm Laboratories
PO Box 2070
Petaluma, CA 94954
www.allerderm.com

Allergan Herbert Skin Care
(see Allergan, Inc)

Allergan, Inc
PO Box 19534
Irvine, CA 92623-9534
(800) 347-4500
www.allergan.com

Alliance Pharmaceutical Corp
3040 Science Park Road
San Diego, CA 92121
(858) 410-5275
www.allp.com

Allscripts Healthcare Solutions
2401 Commerce Avenue
Libertyville, IL 60048-4464
(800) 654-0889
www.allscripts.com

Almay, Inc
1501 Williamsboro Street
Oxford, NC 27565
(800) 473-8566

Alpharma, Inc
One Executive Drive
Fort Lee, NJ 07024
(201) 947-7774
www.alpharma.com

Alpharma USPD, Inc
7205 Windsor Boulevard
Baltimore, MD 21244
(800) 638-9096
www.alpharma.com

Alpha Therapeutic Corp
5555 Valley Boulevard
Los Angeles, CA 90032
(800) 421-0008
www.alphather.com

AltaRex Corp
610 Lincoln Street
Waltham, MA 02451
(888) 801-6665
www.altarex.com

Alto Pharmaceuticals, Inc
PO Box 1910
Land O'Lakes, FL 34639-1910
(800) 330-2891

Alza Corp
1900 Charleston Road
PO Box 7210
Mt View, CA 94039-7210
(800) 634-8977
www.alza.com

Amarin Pharmaceuticals, Inc
25 Independence Boulevard
Warren, NJ 07059
(908) 580-5535
www.amarinpharma.com

Ambix Laboratories
210 Orchard Street
East Rutherford, NJ 07073
(201) 939-2200
www.ambixlabs.com

Amcon Laboratories
40 North Rock Hill Road
St Louis, MO 63119
(800) 255-6161
www.amcon-labs.com

Americal Pharmaceutical, Inc
(see Akorn, Inc)

American Home Products
(see Wyeth Pharmaceuticals)

American Lecithin Company
115 Hurley Road
Unit 2B
Oxford, CT 06478
(800) 364-4416
www.americanlecithin.com

American Medical Industries
Healthcare Products
330 1/2 East Third Street
Dell Rapids, SD 57022
(605) 428-5501
www.ezhealthcare.com

American Pharmaceutical Partners (APP)
Woodfield Executive Center
1101 Perimeter Drive
Suite 300
Schaumburg, IL 60173-5837
(800) 551-7176
www.appdrugs.com

American Red Cross
1616 North Fort Myers Drive
Arlington, VA 22209
(800) 446-8883
www.redcross.org/plasma

American Regent Laboratories
One Luitpold Drive
Shirley, NY 11967
(800) 645-1706

Amgen, Inc
One Amgen Center Drive
Thousand Oaks, CA 91320-1799
(800) 282-6436
www.amgen.com

AMSCO Scientific (see Steris Labs)

Andrew Jergens Company
2535 Spring Grove Avenue
Cincinnati, OH 45214-1773
(800) 742-8798
www.jergens.com

Andrx Corp
4955 Orange Drive
Davie, FL 33314
(954) 584-0300
www.andrx.com

Angelini Pharmaceuticals
70 Grand Avenue
River Edge, NJ 07661
(201) 489-4100
www.angelini.it

Anthra Pharmaceuticals, Inc
103 Carnegie Center
Suite 102
Princeton, NJ 08540
(609) 924-2680
www.anthra.com

Antibodies, Inc
PO Box 1560
Davis, CA 95617
(800) 824-8540
www.antibodiesinc.com

Apotex Corp
2400 North Commerce Parkway
Suite 400
Weston, FL 33326
(800) 706-5575
www.apotexcorp.com

Apothecary Products, Inc
11750 12th Avenue South
Burnsville, MN 55337-1295
(800) 328-2742
www.apothecaryproducts.com

Apothecon
PO Box 4500
Princeton, NJ 08543-4500
(800) 321-1335

Apothecus Pharmaceutical Corp
220 Townsend Square
Oyster Bay, NY 11771-1532
(800) 227-2393
www.apothecus.com

Applied Genetics
205 Buffalo Avenue
Freeport, NY 11520
(516) 868-9026
www.agiderm.com

Arcola Laboratories
500 Arcola Road
Collegeville, PA 19426
(800) 472-4467

AstraZeneca Pharmaceuticals, LP
1800 Concord Pike
PO Box 15437
Wilmington, DE 19850-5437
(800) 456-3669
www.astrazeneca-us.com

Atley Pharmaceuticals, Inc
14433 North Washington Highway
Ashland, VA 23005
(804) 752-8400
www.atley.com

Aventis Behring
1020 First Avenue
PO Box 61501
King of Prussia, PA 19406-0901
(800) 504-5434
www.aventisbehring.com

Aventis Pasteur
Discovery Drive
Box 187
Swiftwater, PA 18370-0187
(800) 822-2463
www.aventispasteur.com

Axcan Scandipharm
22 Inverness Center Parkway
Suite 310
Birmingham, AL 35242
(205) 991-8085
www.axcanscandipharm.com

Bajamar Chemical Company, Inc
9609 Dielman Rock Island
St Louis, MO 63132
(888) 242-3414
www.vesselvite.com

Baker Cummins, Inc
(see Baker Norton Pharmaceuticals, Inc)

Baker Norton Pharmaceuticals, Inc
4400 Biscayne Boulevard
Miami, FL 33137-3227
(800) 735-2315
www.ivax.com

Ballard Medical Products
12050 Lone Peak Parkway
Draper, UT 84020
(800) 528-5591
www.bmed.com

Banner Pharmacaps
4125 Premier Drive
High Point, NC 27265
(800) 447-1140
www.banpharm.com

Barr Laboratories, Inc
2 Quaker Road
Pomona, NY 01970
(800) 222-0190
www.barrlabs.com

Bausch & Lomb Pharmaceuticals (BD)
8500 Hidden River Parkway
Tampa, FL 33637
(800) 323-0000
www.bausch.com

Bausch & Lomb Surgical, Inc
180 Via Verde
San Dimas, CA 91773
(800) 338-2020
www.bausch.com

Baxa Corp
13760 East Arapahoe Road
Englewood, CO 80112-3903
(800) 567-2292
www.baxa.com

Baxter Healthcare Corp
Corp Headquarters
One Baxter Parkway DF4-1W
Deerfield, IL 60015-4633
(800) 422-9837
www.baxter.com

Baxter Hyland Immuno
550 North Brand Boulevard
Glendale, CA 91203
(800) 423-2862
www.hemophiliagalaxy.com

Baxter Pharmaceutical Products, Inc
(Baxter PPI)
110 Allen Road
Liberty Corner, NJ 07938-0804
(800) 782-9375

Bayer Corp
(Biological & Pharmaceutical Division)
400 Morgan Lane
West Haven, CT 06516-4175
(203) 812-2000
www.bayer.com

Bayer Corp
(Consumer Division)
36 Columbia Road
PO Box 1910
Morristown, NJ 07962-1910
(800) 331-4536
www.bayercare.com

Bayer Corp
(Diagnostic Division)
511 Benedict Avenue
Tarrytown, NY 10591-5097
(914) 631-8000
www.bayerdiag.com

Bayer, Inc
77 Belfield Road
Etobicoke, Ontario, Canada M9W 1G6
(800) 268-1331
www.bayerdiag.com

BD Medical Systems Pharma Systems
One Becton Drive
Franklin Lakes, NJ 07417
(201) 847-4017
www.bd.com

BD Biosciences
2350 Qume Drive
San Jose, CA 95131-1807
(800) 223-8226
www.bdbiosciences.com

Beckman Coulter, Inc
4300 North Harbor Boulevard
PO Box 3100
Fullerton, CA 92834-3100
(800) 742-2345
www.beckman.com

Bedford Laboratories
300 Northfield Road
Bedford, OH 44146
(440) 232-3320
www.bedfordlabs.com

Beiersdorf, Inc
Wilton Corporate Center
187 Danbury Road
Wilton, CT 06897
(203) 563-5800
www.beiersdorf.com

Bergen Brunswig Drug Company
4000 Metropolitan Drive
Orange, CA 92868
(714) 385-4000

Berlex Laboratories, Inc
340 Change Bridge Road
PO Box 1000
Montville, NJ 07045-1000
(888) 237-5394
www.berlex.com

Berna Products
4216 Ponce de Leon Boulevard
Coral Gables, FL 33146
(800) 533-5899
www.bernaproducts.com

**Bertek
Pharmaceuticals, Inc
(Dow Hickam)**
3711 Collins Ferry Road
Morgantown, WV 26505
(304) 285-6420
www.bertek.com

Beta Dermaceuticals, Inc
PO Box 691106
San Antonio, TX 78269-1106
(210) 349-9326
www.beta-derm.com

Beutlich Pharmaceuticals
1541 Shields Drive
Waukegan, IL 60085
(800) 238-8542
www.beutlich.com

B. F. Ascher & Company, Inc
15501 West 109th Street
Lenexa, KS 66219-1308
(913) 888-1880
www.bfascher.com

Biocraft Laboratories, Inc
(see Teva Pharmaceuticals USA)

BioCryst Pharmaceuticals, Inc
2190 Parkway Lake Drive
Birmingham, AL 35244
(205) 444-4600
www.biocryst.com

Biogen
14 Cambridge Center
Cambridge, MA 02142
(800) 456-2255
www.biogen.com

BioGenex
4600 Norris Canyon Road
San Ramon, CA 94583
(800) 421-4149
www.biogenex.com

Bioglan Pharma, Inc
7 Great Valley Parkway
Suite 301
Malvern, PA 19355
(888) 246-4526
www.bioglan.com

Biomerica, Inc
1533 Monrovia Avenue
Newport Beach, CA 92663
(949) 645-2111
www.biomerica.com

Biomira USA, Inc
1002 Eastpark Boulevard
Cranbury, NJ 08512
(877) 234-0444
www.biomira.com

Biopure Corp
11 Hurley Street
Cambridge, MA 02141
(617) 234-6500
www.biopure.com

Biospecifics Technologies Corp
35 Wilbur Street
Lynbrook, NY 11563
(516) 593-7000
www.biospecifics.com

Bio-Technology General Corp
70 Wood Avenue South
Iselin, NJ 08830
(732) 632-8800
www.btgc.com

BIO-TECH Pharmacal, Inc
PO Box 1992
Fayetteville, AR 72702
(800) 345-1199
www.bio-tech-pharm.com

Birchwood Laboratories, Inc
7900 Fuller Road
Eden Prairie, MN 55344-2195
(800) 328-6156

Bird Products Corp
1100 Bird Center Drive
Palm Springs, CA 92262
(800) 328-4139
www.thermoresp.com

Blaine Pharmaceuticals
1515 Production Drive
Burlington, KY 41005
(800) 633-9353
www.blainepharma.com

Blairex Laboratories, Inc
1600 Brian Drive
PO Box 2127
Columbus, IN 47202-2127
(800) 252-4739
www.blairex.com

Blansett Pharmacal Company, Inc
PO Box 638
North Little Rock, AR 72115
(501) 758-8635

Blistex, Inc
1800 Swift Drive
Oak Brook, IL 60523-1574
(800) 837-1800
www.blistex.com

Block Drug Company, Inc
(see GlaxoSmithKline)

Bluco, Inc
28350 Schoolcraft
Livonia, MI 48150
(800) 832-4464

Bock Pharmacal Company
(see Sanofi-Synthelabo, Inc)

Boehringer Ingelheim Pharmaceuticals, Inc
900 Ridgebury Road
PO Box 368
Ridgefield, CT 06877-0368
(800) 542-6257
www.boehringer-ingelheim.com

Boehringer Mannheim (see Roche)

Bone Care International
Bone Care Center
1600 Aspen Commons
Middleton, WI 53562
(888) 389-3300
www.bonecare.com

Boots Pharmaceuticals, Inc
(see Knoll Laboratories)

Bracco Diagnostics, Inc
107 College Road East
Princeton, NJ 08540
(800) 631-5245
www.bracco.com

Braintree Laboratories, Inc
PO Box 850929
Braintree, MA 02185-0929
(800) 874-6756
www.braintreeLabs.com

Bristol-Myers Squibb Company
(Pharmaceutical Division)
PO Box 4500
Princeton, NJ 08543-4500
(800) 321-1335
www.bms.com

Bryan Corp
4 Plympton Street
Woburn, MA 01801
(800) 343-7711
www.bryancorporation.com

BTG, Inc
3877 Fairfax Ridge Road
Fairfax, VA 22030
(800) 432-4284
www.btg.com

Burroughs Wellcome Company
(see GlaxoWellcome)

Calmoseptine, Inc
16602 Burke Lane
Huntington Beach, CA 92647
(800) 800-3405
www.calmoseptineointment.com

Capellon Pharmaceuticals, Inc
7462 Dogwood Drive
Fort Worth, TX 76118
(817) 595-5820
www.capellon.com

Caraco Pharmaceutical Laboratories, LTD
1150 Elijah McCoy Drive
Detroit, MI 48202
(800) 818-4555
www.caraco.com

Cardinal Health, Inc
7000 Cardinal Place
Dublin, OH 43017
(800) 234-8701

Care Technologies, Inc
10 Corbin Drive
Darien, CT 06820
(800) 783-1919
www.clearcare.com

Carma Laboratories, Inc
5801 West Airways Avenue
Franklin, WI 53132
(414) 421-7707

Carolina Medical Products Company
PO Box 147
Farmville, NC 27828
(800) 227-6637
www.carolinamedical.com

Carrington Laboratories
2001 Walnut Hill Lane
Irving, TX 73038
(800) 527-5216
www.carringtonlabs.com

C. B. Fleet Company, Inc
4615 Murray Place
Lynchburg, VA 24506
(434) 528-4000
www.cbfleet.com

CCA Industries, Inc
200 Murray Hill Parkway
East Rutherford, NJ 07073
(800) 524-2720

Celgene Corp
7 Powder Horn Drive
Warren, NJ 07059
(732) 271-1001
www.celgene.com

Cellegy Pharmaceuticals, Inc
349 Oyster Point Boulevard
Suite 200
South San Francisco, CA 94080
(650) 616-2200

Celltech
755 Jefferson Road
Rochester, NY 14623-0000
(800) 234-5535
www.celltech.com

Centeon (see Aventis Behring)

Centers for Disease Control and Prevention
1600 Clifton Road Northeast
Atlanta, GA 30333
(800) 311-3435
www.cdc.gov

Centocor, Inc
200 Great Valley Parkway
Malvern, PA 19355
(888) 457-6399
www.centocor.com

Central Pharmaceuticals, Inc
(see Schwarz Pharma)

Cephalon, Inc
145 Brandywine Parkway
West Chester, PA 19380
(800) 782-3656
www.cephalon.com

Cetylite Industries, Inc
9051 River Road
Pennsauken, NJ 08110
(800) 257-7740
www.cetylite.com

Chattem Consumer Products
1715 West 38th Street
Chattanooga, TN 37409
(800) 366-6833
www.chattem.com

Chesapeake Biological Laboratory
PO Box 38
One Williams Street
Solomons, MD 20688
(410) 326-4281

Children's Hospital of Columbus
700 Children's Drive
Columbus, OH 43205
(614) 722-2000
www.childrenshospital.columbus.oh.us

Chiron Corp
4560 Horton Street
Emeryville, CA 94608
(510) 655-8730
www.chiron.com

Chiron Vision
(see Bausch & Lomb Surgical)

Chronimed, Inc
10900 Red Circle Drive
Minnetonka, MN 55343
(800) 444-5951
www.chronimed.com

Ciba-Geigy Pharmaceuticals
(see Novartis Pharmaceuticals Corp)

CIBA Vision
11460 Johns Creek Parkway
Duluth, GA 30097
(800) 845-6585
www.cibavision.com

Circa Pharmaceuticals, Inc
(see Watson Laboratories, Inc)

Cirrus Healthcare Products, LLC
60 Main Street
PO Box 220
Cold Spring Harbor, NY 11724
(800) 327-6151
www.earplanes.com

CIS-US, Inc
10 DeAngelo Drive
Bedford, MA 01730
(800) 221-7554

Claragen, Inc
387 Technology Drive
College Park, MD 20742
(301) 405-8593
www.claragen.com

Clay-Park Labs, Inc
1700 Bathgate Avenue
Bronx, NY 10457
(800) 933-5550
www.claypark.com

C & M Pharmacal, Inc
(see Genesis Pharmaceutical, Inc)

CNS, Inc
PO Box 1985
South Hackensack, NJ 07606-9867
(877) 553-4237
www.cns.com

Colgate Oral Pharmaceuticals
One Colgate Way
Canton, MA 02021
(800) 962-2345
www.colgate.com

Colgate-Palmolive Company
300 Park Avenue
New York, NY 10022
(800) 221-4607
www.colgate.com

CollaGenex Pharmaceuticals, Inc
41 University Drive
Suite 200
Newtown, PA 18940
(888) 339-5678
www.collegenex.com

Columbia Laboratories, Inc
2875 Northeast 191st Street
Suite 400
Aventura, FL 33180
(800) 749-1919
www.columbialabs.com

Combe, Inc
1101 Westchester Avenue
White Plains, NY 10604
(800) 431-2610
www.combe.com

Complimed Medical Research Group
1441 West Smith Road
Ferndale, WA 98248
(888) 977-8008
www.complimed.com

Conair Interplak Division
One Cummings Point Road
Stamford, CT 06904
(800) 726-6247
www.conair.com

Connaught Labs (see Aventis Pasteur)

Connetics Corp
3290 West Bayshore Road
Palo Alto, CA 94303
(888) 969-2628
www.connetics.com

Contract Pharmacal Corp
135 Adams Avenue
Hauppauge, NY 11788
(631) 231-4610
www.contractpharmacal.com

ConvaTec
(Bristol-Myers Squibb Company)
PO Box 5254
Princeton, NJ 08543-5254
(800) 422-8811
www.convatec.com

CooperVision
200 Willowbrook Office Park
Fairport, NY 14450
(800) 538-7850
www.coopervision.com

Copley Pharmaceutical
(Teva USA)
25 John Road
Canton, MA 02021
(800) 325-6111
www.copleypharm.com

Corixa
1124 Columbia Street
Suite 200
Seattle, WA 98104
(206) 754-5711
www.corixa.com

C. R. Bard, Inc
8195 Industrial Boulevard
Covington, GA 30014
(800) 526-4455
www.bardmedical.com

CVS Procare Direct
3651 Ridge Mill Drive
Columbia, OH 43026
(800) 252-6245

Cyanotech Corp
73-4460 Queen Kaahamanu Highway
Suite 102
Kailua-Kona, HI 96740
(800) 395-1353
www.cyanotech.com

Cygnus, Inc
400 Penobscot Drive
Redwood City, CA 94063-4719
(650) 369-4300
www.cygn.com

CYNACON/OCuSOFT
5311 Avenue North
Rosenburg, TX 77471
(800) 233-5469
www.ocusoft.com

Cypress Pharmaceutical, Inc
135 Industrial Boulevard
Madison, MS 39110
(800) 856-4393
www.cypressrx.com

Cytogen Corp
600 College Road East
Princeton, NJ 08540
(800) 833-3533
www.cytogen.com

CytRx Corp
154 Technology Parkway
Suite 200
Norcross, GA 30092
(770) 368-9500
www.cytrx.com

Daiichi Pharmaceutical Corp
11 Philips Parkway
Montvale, NJ 07648
(877) 324-4244
www.daiichipharm.co.jp

Dakryon Pharmaceuticals
(see Medco Lab, Inc)

Danbury Pharmacal, Inc
(Schein Pharmaceutical, Inc)
131 West Street
Danbury, CT 06810
(203) 744-7200
www.schein-rx.com

Danco Labs, LLC
PO Box 4816
New York, NY 10185
(877) 432-7596
www.earlyoptionpill.com

Daniels Pharmaceuticals, Inc
(see Jones Pharma)

Dartmouth Pharmaceuticals
38 Church Avenue
Wareham, MA 02571
(800) 414-3566
www.ilovemynails.com

Davol, Inc
100 Sockanossett Crossroad
PO Box 8500
Cranston, RI 02920
(401) 463-7000
www.davol.com

Dayton Laboratories
3337 Northwest 74th Avenue
Miami, FL 33122
(800) 446-0255
www.daytonlab.com

Del Laboratories, Inc
178 EAB Plaza
Uniondale, NY 11556
(800) 952-5080
www.dellabs.com

Delmont Laboratories, Inc
715 Harvard Avenue
PO Box 269
Swarthmore, PA 19081
(800) 562-5541
www.delmont.com

Den-Mat Corp
2727 Skyway Drive
Santa Maria, CA 93455
(800) 445-0345
www.den-mat.com

Derma Science
214 Carnegie Center
Suite 100
Princeton, NJ 08540
(800) 825-4325
www.dermasciences.com

Dermik Laboratories
500 Arcola Road
PO Box 1200
Collegeville, PA 19426
(800) 340-7502
www.dermik.com

DeRoyal Industries, Inc
200 DeBusk Lane
Powell, TN 37849
(800) 337-6925
www.deroyal.com

DexGen Pharmaceuticals, Inc
PO Box 675
Manasquan, NJ 08736
(877) DEXGEN1
www.dexgen.com

Dey LP
2751 Napa Valley Corporate Drive
Napa, CA 94558
(707) 224-3200
www.deyinc.com

Diacrin
Building 96 13th Street
Charlestown, MA 02129
(617) 242-9100
www.diacrin.com

DiaPharma Group, Inc
8948 Beckett Road
West Chester, OH 45069-2939
(800) 526-5224
www.diapharma.com

Diatide, Inc
9 Delta Drive
Londonderry, NH 03053
(603) 437-8970
www.diatide.com

Dickinson Brands, Inc
31 East High Street
East Hampton, CT 06424
(888) 860-2279

Digestive Care, Inc
1120 Win Drive
Bethlehem, PA 18017-7059
(610) 882-5950
www.pancrecarb.com

Discovery Laboratories, Inc
350 South Main Street
Suite 307
Doylestown, PA 18901
(215) 340-4699
www.discoverylabs.com

Discus Dental, Inc
8550 Higuera Street
Culver City, CA 90232
(800) 422-9448
www.discusdental.com

Dista Products Company
(see Eli Lilly & Company)

Doak Dermatologics
383 Route 46 West
Fairfield, NJ 07004-2402
(800) 405-3625
www.bradpharm.com

Dow Hickam, Inc
(see Bertek Pharmaceuticals, Inc)

Dreir Pharmaceuticals, Inc
9602 North 122nd Place
Scottsdale, AZ 85259
(800) 541-4044
www.dreirpharmaceuticals.com

DuPont Pharmaceuticals
Chestnut Run Plaza
974 Centre Road
Wilmington, DE 19805
(800) 474-2762
www.dupontpharma.com

Duramed Pharmaceuticals
5040 Duramed Drive
Cincinnati, OH 45213
(513) 731-9900
www.duramed.com

Dura Pharmaceuticals
(see Elan Pharmaceuticals)

Durex Consumer Products
3585 Engineering Drive
Suite 200
Norcross, GA 30092
(888) 566-3468
www.durex.com

Durham Pharmacal Corp
Route 145
Oak Hill, NY 12460
(888) 438-7426
www.durhampharm.com

DUSA Pharmaceuticals, Inc
25 Upton Drive
Wilmington, MA 01887
(978) 657-7500
www.dusapharma.com

Eagle Vison, Inc
8500 Wolf Lake Drive
Suite 110
PO Box 34877
Memphis, TN 38184
(800) 222-7584
www.eaglevis.com

Eckerd Drug Corp
PO Box 4689
Clearwater, FL 33758
(800) 325-3737
www.eckerd.com

Econolab
PO Box 85543
Westland, MI 48185-0543
(561) 391-5245

ECR Pharmaceuticals
PO Box 71600
Richmond, VA 23255
(804) 527-1950
www.ecrpharma.com

Effcon Laboratories, Inc
PO Box 7499
Marietta, GA 30065-1499
(800) 722-2428
www.effcon.com

E. Fougera & Company
60 Baylis Road
Melville, NY 11747
(800) 645-9833
www.fougera.com

Eisai, Inc
500 Frank W. Burr Boulevard
Teaneck, NJ 07666
(888) 793-4724

Elan Pharmaceuticals, Inc
45 Horse Hill Road
Cedar Knolls, NJ 07927
(973) 267-2670
www.elan.ie

Elan Pharmaceuticals
800 Gateway Boulevard
South San Francisco, CA 94080
(650) 877-0900
www.elan.com

Eli Lilly & Company
Lilly Corporate Center
Indianapolis, IN 46285
(800) 545-5979
www.lilly.com

EM Industries, Inc
7 Skyline Drive
Hawthorne, NY 10532
(914) 592-4660
www.emindustries.com

Enamelon, Inc
7 Cedar Brook Drive
Cranbury, NJ 08512
(888) 432-3535

Endo Pharmaceuticals, Inc
223 Wilmington Westchester Pike
Chadds Ford, PA 19317
(800) 462-3636
www.endo.com

EnviroDerm Pharmaceuticals, Inc
PO Box 32370
Louisville, KY 40232-2370
(800) 991-3376
www.ivyblock.com

Enzon, Inc
685 Route 202/206
Bridgewater, NJ 08807
(908) 575-9457
www.enzon.com

Eon Labs Manufacturing, Inc
227-15 North Conduit Avenue
Laurelton, NY 11413
(800) 526-0225
www.eonlabs.com

Epitope, Inc
8505 Southwest Creekside Place
Beaverton, OR 97008-7108
(800) 234-3786
www.epitope.com

E. R. Squibb & Sons, Inc
(see Bristol-Myers Squibb Company)

Ethex Corp
10888 Metro Court
St Louis, MO 63043-2413
(800) 321-1705
www.ethex.com

**Ethicon, Inc
(Johnson & Johnson)**
US Route 22 West
PO Box 151
Somerville, NJ 08876-0151
(800) 255-2500
www.ethiconinc.com

Everett Laboratories, Inc
29 Spring Street
West Orange, NJ 07052
(973) 324-0200
www.everettlabs.com

E-Z-EM
717 Main Street
Westbury, NY 11590
(800) 544-4624

Faulding Pharmaceuticals
650 From Road
(Mack-Cali Centre II)
5th Floor South
Paramus, NJ 07652
(201) 225-5500
www.faulding.com

Female Health Company
875 North Michigan Avenue
Suite 3660
Chicago, IL 60611-9267
(800) 635-0844
www.femalehealth.com

Ferndale Laboratories, Inc
780 West Eight Mile Road
Ferndale, MI 48220
(800) 621-6003

Ferring Pharmaceuticals, Inc
120 White Plains Road
Suite 400
Tarrytown, NY 10591
(888) 337-7464
www.ferringusa.com

Fidia Pharmaceutical Corp
2000 K Street Northwest
Suite 700
Washington, DC 20006
(202) 371-9898
www.fidiapharma.com

Fielding Pharmaceutical Company
11551 Adie Road
Maryland Heights, MO 63043
(800) 776-3435
www.fieldingcompany.com

First Horizon Pharmaceutical Corp
6195 Shiloh Road
Alpharetta, GA 30005
(800) 849-9707
www.horizonpharm.com

First Scientific, Inc
Lake Forest Plaza
2222 Francisco Drive 510-174
El Dorado Hills, CA 95762
(800) 767-2208

Fischer Pharmaceuticals, Inc
3707 Williams Road
San Jose, CA 95117
(800) 782-0222
www.dr-fischer.com

Fisons Corp (see Aventis)

Fleming & Company
1733 Gilsinn Lane
Fenton, MO 63026
(636) 343-8200
www.flemingcompany.com

Forest Pharmaceuticals, Inc
13600 Shoreline Drive
St Louis, MO 63045
(800) 678-1605
www.forestpharm.com

Freeda Vitamins, Inc
36 East 41st Street
New York, NY 10017
(800) 777-3737
www.freedavitamins.com

Fuisz Technologies, Ltd
14555 Avion Parkway
Chantilly, VA 20151
(703) 803-3260

Fujisawa Healthcare, Inc
Three Parkway North
Deerfield, IL 60015-2548
(800) 727-7003
www.fujisawa.com

Galderma Laboratories, Inc
14501 North Freeway
Fort Worth, TX 76177
(817) 961-5000
www.galderma.com

Gallipot, Inc
2020 Silver Bell Road
St Paul, MN 55122
(800) 423-6967
www.gallipot.com

Gambro, Inc
810 Collins Avenue
Lakewood, CO 80215
(800) 525-2623
www.gambro.com

Gate Pharmaceuticals
PO Box 1090
North Wales, PA 19454-1090
(800) 292-4283
www.gatepharma.com

Gebauer Company
9410 St Catherine Avenue
Cleveland, OH 44104-5526
(800) 321-9348
www.gebauerco.com

Geigy Pharmaceuticals
(see Novartis Pharmaceuticals Corp)

GenDerm Corp (see Medicis
Pharmaceutical Corp)

Gen-King (see Kinray)

Genentech, Inc
One DNA Way
South San Francisco, CA 94080-4990
(650) 225-1000
www.gene.com

General Injectables & Vaccines
US Highway 52 South
PO Box 9
Bastian, VA 24314-0009
(540) 688-4121
www.giv.com

General Nutrition, Inc
300 6th Avenue
Pittsburgh, PA 15222
(888) 462-2548
www.gnc.com

Genesis Nutrition
1816 Wall Street
Florence, SC 29501
(800) 451-7933
www.genesisnutrition.com

Genesis Pharmaceutical, Inc
1721 Maplelane Avenue
Hazel Park, MI 48030
(800) 459-8663
www.genesispharm.com

Geneva Pharmaceuticals, Inc
2655 West Midway Boulevard
PO Box 446
Broomfield, CO 80038-0446
(800) 525-8747
www.genevapharmaceuticals.com

**GenPharm International, Inc
(Medarex)**
2350 Qume Drive
San Jose, CA 95131-1807
(408) 526-1290
www.genpharm.com

Gensia Sicor Pharmaceuticals, Inc
19 Hughes
Irvine, CA 92618
(800) 729-9991
www.gensiasicor.com

GenVec, Inc
65 West Watkins Mill Road
Gaithersburg. MD 20878
(240) 632-0740
www.genvec.com

Genzyme Pharmaceuticals
One Kendall Square
Cambridge, MA 02139
(800) 868-8208
www.genzyme.com

Geodesic MediTech, Inc
2921 Sandy Pointe No. 3
Del Mar, CA 92014
(888) 357-9399
www.geodesicmeditech.com

Gerber Products Company
445 State Street
Fremont, MI 49413-0001
(800) 443-7237
www.gerber.com

Gilead
333 Lakeside Drive
Foster City, CA 94404
(800) 445-3235
www.gilead.com

Glades Pharmaceuticals, LLC
500 Satellite Boulevard
Suwanee, GA 30024
(888) 445-2337
www.glades.com

GlaxoSmithKline
One Franklin Plaza
Philadelphia, PA 19102
(888) 825-5249
www.gsk.com

**GlaxoSmithKline
Consumer Healthcare**
PO Box 1467
Pittsburgh, PA 15230
(412) 928-1000
www.gsk.com

GlaxoWellcome, Inc (see GlaxoSmithKline)

Glenwood, LLC
19 Empire Boulevard
South Hackensack, NJ 07606
(201) 221-0050
www.glenwood-llc.com

Global Pharmaceuticals, Inc
3735 Castor Avenue
Philadelphia, PA 19124
(215) 289-2220
www.globalphar.com

Global Source
3001 North 29th Street
Hollywood, FL 33020
(800) 662-7556
www.globalvitamin.com

GML Industries, LLC
PO Box 1973
Denison, TX 75020
(877) 828-4633
www.gml-industries.com

Goldline Laboratories, Inc
(see Zenith Goldline Pharmaceuticals)

Goody's Manufacturing Corp
(see Block Drug Company, Inc)

Gordon Laboratories
6801 Ludlow Street
Upper Darby, PA 19082-2408
(800) 356-7870
www.gordonlabs.com

Graham-Field Health Products, Inc
2935 Northeast Parkway
Atlanta, GA 30360
(800) 645-1023
www.grahamfield.com

Grandpa Brands Company
1820 Airport Exchange Boulevard
Erlanger, KY 41018
(800) 684-1468
www.grandpabrands.com

Gray Pharmaceutical Company (see The
Purdue Frederick Company)

Green Turtle Bay Vitamin Company
56 High Street
Summit, NJ 07901
(800) 887-8535
www.energywave.com

Greer Laboratories, Inc
639 Nuway Circle
PO Box 800
Lenoir, NC 28645-0800
(800) 438-0088
www.greerlabs.com

Guardian Laboratories
230 Marcus Boulevard
Hauppauge, NY 11788
(800) 645-5566
www.u-g.com

Guilford Pharmaceuticals, Inc
6611 Tributary Street
Baltimore, MD 21224
(410) 631-6300
www.guilfordpharm.com

Gum-Tech Industries, Inc
246 East Watkins
Phoenix, AZ 85004
(800) 676-4769

G & W Laboratories
111 Coolidge Street
South Plainfield, NJ 07080-3895
(800) 922-1038
www.gwlabs.com

Gynetics
PO Box 8509
Somerville, NJ 08876
(800) 311-7378
www.gynetics.com

Gynex (see BTG, Inc)

Halocarbon Products Corp
887 Kinderkamack Road
River Edge, NJ 07661
(201) 262-8899
www.halocarbon.com

Halsey Drug Company
(see Watson Laboratories, Inc)

Hart Health & Safety
PO Box 94044
Seattle, WA 98124
(800) 234-4278

Harvard Drug Group, LCC
31778 Enterprise Drive
Livonia, MI 48150
(800) 875-0123
www.harvarddrugs.com

Hauser Pharmaceutical, Inc
4401 East US Highway 30
Valparaiso, IN 46383
(800) 441-2309
www.hauserpharmaceutical.com

Hawthorn Pharmaceuticals, Inc
(see Cypress Pharmaceutical, Inc)

HDC Corp
628 Gibraltar Court
Milpitas, CA 95035
(800) 227-8162
www.hdccorp.com

HealthAsure, Inc
31280 Oak Crest Drive
Suite 1
Westlake Village, CA 91361-5679
(818) 706-6100
www.breathasure.com

Healthfirst Corp
22316 70th Avenue West
Unit A
Mountlake Terrace, WA 98043-2184
(800) 331-1984

Health & Medical Techniques
(see Graham-Field Health Products, Inc)

Hemacare Corp
21101 Oxnard Street
Woodland Hills, CA 91367
(877) 310-0717
www.hemacare.com

Hemagen Diagnostics, Inc
9033 Red Branch Road
Columbia, MD 21045
(800) 495-2180
www.hemagen.com

Hemispherx
One Penn Center
1617 John F. Kennedy Boulevard
6th Floor
Philadelphia, PA 19103
(215) 988-0080
www.hemispherx.com

Henry Schein, Inc
135 Duryea Road
Melville, NY 11747
(631) 843-2000
www.henryschein.com

Herald Pharmacal, Inc (see Allergan, Inc)

Hill Dermaceuticals, Inc
2650 South Mellonville Avenue
Sanford, FL 32773-9311
(800) 344-5707
www.hillderm.com

Hi-Tech Pharmaceutical, Inc
369 Bayview Avenue
Amityville, NY 11701
(631) 789-8228
www.hitechpharm.com

Hoechst-Marion Roussel, Inc (see Aventis)

Hoffmann-LaRoche
(see Roche Pharmaceuticals)

Hogil Pharmaceutical Corp
Two Manhattanville Road
Purchase, NY 10577-2118
(914) 696-7600
www.hogil.com

Hollister-Stier Laboratories, LLC
3525 North Regal Street
Spokane, WA 99207-5788
(800) 992-1120
www.hollister-stier.com

Home Access Health Corp
2401 West Hassell Road
Suite 1510
Hoffman Estates, IL 60195
(847) 781-2500
www.homeaccess.com

Hope Pharmaceuticals
8260 East Gelding Drive
Suite 104
Scottsdale, AZ 85260
(800) 755-9595
www.hopepharm.com

Horizon Pharmaceutical Corp
(see First Horizon Pharmaceutical Corp)

Huckaby Pharmacal, Inc
6316 Old LaGrange Road
Crestwood, KY 40014
(888) 206-5525
www.huckabypharmacal.com

Hyland Immuno
(Baxter)
550 North Brand Boulevard
Glendale, CA 91203
(800) 423-2090
http://baxdb1.baxter.com

Hyland Laboratories, Inc
(Standard Homeopathic Company)
210 West 131st Street
Los Angeles, CA 90061
(800) 624-9659
www.hylands.com

Hyland Therapeutics
(see Baxter Hyland Immuno)

ICI Pharmaceuticals
(see Zeneca Pharmaceuticals)

ICN Canada Ltd
Montreal, Quebec Canada

ICN Pharmaceuticals, Inc
ICN Plaza
3300 Hyland Drive
Costa Mesa, CA 92626
(800) 548-5100
www.icnpharm.com

IDEC Pharmaceuticals
3030 Callan Road
San Diego, CA 92121
(858) 431-8500

Ilex Oncology, Inc
4545 Horizon Hill Boulevard
San Antonio, TX 78229-2263
(210) 949-8200
www.ilexonc.com

Immunex Corp
51 University Street
Seattle, WA 98101
(800) 466-8639
www.immunex.com

ImmunoGen, Inc
128 Sidney Street
Cambridge, MA 02139
(617) 995-2500
www.immunogen.com

Immunomedics, Inc
300 American Road
Morris Plains, NJ 07950
(973) 605-8200
www.immunomedics.com

Immuno-US, Inc
(see Baxter Healthcare Corp)

Impax Laboratories, Inc
30831 Huntwood Avenue
Hayward, CA 94544
(510) 476-2000

InKine Pharmaceutical Company, Inc
1787 Sentry Parkway
West Building 18
Suite 440
Blue Bell, PA 19422
(215) 283-6850
www.inkine.com

INO Therapeutics, Inc
54 Old Highway 22
Clinton, NJ 08809
(908) 238-6600
www.inotherapeutics.com

Inspire Pharmaceuticals, Inc
4222 Emperor Boulevard
Suite 470
Durham, NC 27703
(919) 941-9777
www.inspirepharm.com

Interchem Corp
PO Box 1579
Paramus, NJ 07653
(201) 261-7333
www.interchem.com

Interferon Sciences, Inc
783 Jersey Avenue
New Brunswick, NJ 08901-3660
(888) 728-4372
www.interferonsciences.com

InterMune Pharmaceuticals, Inc
3280 Bayshore Boulevard
Brisbane, CA 94005
(415) 466-2200
www.intermune.com

International Medication Systems, Limited (IMS)
1886 Santa Anita Avenue
South El Monte, CA 91733
(800) 423-4136
www.ims-limited.com

Indevus Pharmaceuticals, Inc
99 Hayden Avenue
Suite 200
Lexington, MA 02421
(781) 861-8444
www.interneuron.com

Inveresk Research Group, Inc
11000 Westen Parkway
Suite 100
Cary, NC 27513
(800) 988-9845
www.inveresk-research.com

Inverness Medical Innovations
51 Sawyer Road
Suite 200
Waltham, MA 02453-3448
(781) 647-3900

Inwood Laboratories (Forest)
321 Prospect Street
Inwood, NY 11096
(800) 876-5227

Iomed, Inc
2441 South 3850 West
Suite A
Salt Lake City, UT 84120
(800) 621-3347
www.iomed.com

IOP, Inc
3151 Airway Avenue
Suite I-1
Costa Mesa, CA 92626
(800) 535-3545
www.iopinc.com

Isis Pharmaceuticals
2292 Faraday Avenue
Carlsbad, CA 92008
(760) 931-9200
www.isip.com

Ivax Pharmaceuticals, Inc
4400 Biscayne Boulevard
Miami, FL 33137
(800) 327-4114
www.ivaxpharmaceuticals.com

Jacobus Pharmaceutical Company
37 Cleveland Lane
Princeton, NJ 08540
(609) 921-7447

Janssen Pharmaceutica
1125 Trenton-Harbourton Road
Titusville, NJ 08560-0200
(800) 526-7736
www.us.janssen.com

J. B. Williams Company, Inc
65 Harristown Road
Glen Rock, NJ 07452
(201) 251-8100
www.jbwilliams.com

Jerome Stevens Pharmaceuticals, Inc
60 DaVinci Drive
Bohemia, NY 11716-2613
(631) 567-1113

J. J. Balan, Inc
5725 Foster Avenue
Brooklyn, NY 11234
(800) 552-2526
www.jjbalan.com

J & J Merck Consumer Pharmaceutical Company
Camp Hill Road
Fort Washington, PA 19034
(800) 523-3484
www.jnj-merck.com

Johnson & Johnson
One Johnson & Johnson Plaza
New Brunswick, NJ 08933
(732) 524-0400
www.jnj.com

Jones Pharma
(see King Pharmaceuticals, Inc)

J. R. Carlson Laboratories, Inc
15 College Drive
Arlington Heights, IL 60004-1985
(888) 234-5656
www.carlsonlabs.com

J. T. Baker, Inc (see Mallinckrodt Baker, Inc)

KabiVitrum, Inc (see Pharmacia Corp)

Kendall Healthcare Products
15 Hampshire Street
Mansfield, MA 02048
(800) 962-9888
www.kendallhq.com

Key Pharmaceuticals (see Schering-Plough)

King Pharmaceuticals, Inc
501 Fifth Street
Bristol, TN 37620
(800) 776-3637
www.kingpharm.com

Kingswood Laboratories, Inc
10375 Hague Road
Indianapolis, IN 46256
(800) 968-7772
www.kingswood-labs.com

Kinray
152-35 10th Avenue
Whitestone, NY 11357
(800) 854-6729
www.kinray.com

Kirkman Laboratories, Inc
6400 Southwest Rosewood Street
Lake Oswego, OR 97035
(800) 245-8282
www.kirkmanlabs.com

KLI Corp
1119 Third Avenue Southwest
Carmel, IN 46032
(800) 308-7452
www.entertainers-secret.com

Knoll Pharmaceuticals
3000 Continental Drive North
Mt Olive, NJ 07828
(800) 526-0221
www.hhplus.com

Konsyl Pharmaceuticals, Inc
4200 South Hulen
Suite 513
Fort Worth, TX 76109
(800) 356-6795
www.konsyl.com

Kos Pharmaceuticals, Inc
1001 Brickell Bay Drive
25th Floor
Miami, FL 33131
(305) 577-3464
www.kospharm.com

Kramer Laboratories, Inc
8778 Southwest 8th Street
Miami, FL 33174
(800) 824-4894
www.kramerlabs.com

K. V. Pharmaceutical Company
2503 South Hanley Road
St Louis, MO 63144
(314) 645-6600

Lacrimedics, Inc
PO Box 1209
Eastsound, WA 98245
(800) 367-8327
www.lacrimedics.com

Lactaid, Inc
7050 Camp Hill Road
Fort Washington, PA 19034
(800) 522-8243
www.lactaid.com

La Haye Laboratories, Inc
2205 152nd Avenue Northeast
Redmond, WA 98052
(800) 344-2020
www.lahaye.com

Lannett Company, Inc
9000 State Road
Philadelphia, PA 19136
(800) 325-9994
www.lannett.com

LecTec Corp
10701 Red Circle Drive
Minnetonka, MN 55343
(877) 587-2824
www.lectec.com

Lee Pharmaceuticals
1434 Santa Anita Avenue
South El Monte, CA 91733
(800) 950-5337
www.leepharmaceuticals.com

Leiner Health Products
901 East 233rd Street
Carson, CA 90745
(310) 835-8400
www.leiner.com

Lemmon Company
(see Teva Pharmaceuticals USA)

**LifeScan, Inc
(Johnson & Johnson Company)**
1000 Gibraltar Drive
Milpitas, CA 95035
(800) 227-8862
www.lifescan.com

LifeSign LLC
71 Veronica Avenue
PO Box 218
Somerset, NJ 08875-0218
(800) 526-2125
www.lifesignmed.com

Ligand Pharmaceuticals
10275 Science Center Drive
San Diego, CA 92121
(888) 550-7500
www.ligand.com

Lilly & Company (see Eli Lilly & Company)

Lincoln Diagnostics
PO Box 1128
Decatur, IL 62525
(217) 877-2531
www.lincolndiagnostics.com

Liposome Company
One Research Way
Princeton, NJ 08540
(800) 335-5476
www.liposome.com

Lotus Biochemical Corp
7335 Lee Highway
Radford, VA 24141
(423) 989-9192

LSI America Corp
4732 Twin Valley Drive
Austin, TX 78731-3537
(800) 720-5936
www.ondrox.com

Lyne Laboratories
10 Burke Drive
Brockton, MA 02301
(800) 525-0450
www.lyne.com

Lyphomed (see Fujisawa Healthcare, Inc)

3M Pharmaceuticals
3M Center
Building 275-3W-01
St Paul, MN 55133
(800) 328-0255
3m.com/pharma

Magno-Humphries Laboratories
8800 Southwest Commercial Street
Tigard, OR 97223
(503) 684-5464
www.magno-humphries.com

Mallinckrodt Baker, Inc
222 Red School Lane
Phillipsburg, NJ 08865
(314) 654-2000
www.mallbaker.com

**Mallinckrodt, Inc
(Corp Headquarters)**
675 McDonnell Boulevard
Hazelwood, MO 63042
(888) 744-1414
www.mallinckrodt.com

Marlyn Nutraceuticals, Inc
14851 North Scottsdale Road
Scottsdale, AZ 85254
(800) 462-7596

**Marsam Pharmaceuticals, Inc
(Schein Pharmaceutical, Inc)**
24 Olney Avenue
Cherry Hill, NJ 08034
(609) 424-5600
www.schein-rx.com

Martec Pharmaceutical, Inc
1800 North Topping
Kansas City, MO 64120
(800) 822-6782
www.martec-kc.com

Mason Vitamins, Inc
5105 Northwest 159th Street
Miami Lakes, FL 33014-6370
(800) 327-6005
www.masonvitamins.com

McGuff Company, Inc
3524 West Lake Center Drive
Santa Ana, CA 92704
(800) 854-7220
www.mcguffmedical.com

McNeil Consumer Healthcare
Camp Hill Road
Mail Stop 278
Fort Washington, PA 19034-2292
(800) 962-5357
www.ortho-mcneil.com

Mead Johnson Laboratories
(see Bristol-Myers Squibb Company)

Medarex
707 State Road
Princeton, NJ 08540-1437
(609) 430-2880
www.medarex.com

Medco Lab, Inc
716 West 7th Street
Sioux City, IA 51103
(712) 255-8770
www.medcolab.com

Medea Research Laboratories
200 Wilson Street
Port Jefferson, NY 11776
(516) 474-8014

Medeva Pharmaceuticals
(see Celltech)

Medicis Pharmaceutical Corp
8125 North Hayden Road
Scottsdale, AZ 85258-2463
(602) 808-8800
www.medicis.com

MedImmune, Inc
35 West Watkins Mill Road
Gaithersburg, MD 20878
(877) 633-4411
www.medimmune.com

Medisca, Inc
661 Route 3, Unit C
Plattsburgh, NY 12901
(800) 932-1039
www.medisca.com

**MediSense, Inc
(Abbott Laboratories)**
4A Crosby Drive
Bedford, MA 01730
(800) 323-9100

Medix Pharmaceuticals Americas, Inc (MPA)
12505 Starkey Road
Suite M
Largo, FL 33773
www.biafine.com

MedPointe, Inc
265 Davidson Avenue
Suite 300
PO Box 6833
Somerset, NJ 08875-6833
(732) 564-2200
www.medpointeinc.com

Medtronic, Inc
710 Medtronic Parkway
Minneapolis, MN 55432-5604
(763) 514-4000
www.medtronic.com

Menicon America, Inc
1840 Gateway Drive
Second Floor
San Mateo, CA 94404
(650) 378-1424
www.menicon.com

**Mentholatum Company, Inc
(Rohto Pharmaceutical Company)**
707 Sterling Drive
Orchard Park, NY 14127
(716) 677-2500
www.mentholatum.com

**Merck & Company
(Human Health Division)**
PO Box 4
West Point, PA 19486
(800) 672-6372
www.merck.com

Mericon Industries, Inc
8819 North Pioneer Road
Peoria, IL 61615-1561
(800) 242-6464
www.mericonindustries.com

Meridian Medical Technologies
10240 Old Columbia Road
Columbia, MD 21046
(800) 638-8093
www.meridianmeds.com

Merit Pharmaceuticals
2611 San Fernando Road
Los Angeles, CA 90065
(800) 421-9657
www.meritpharm.com

Merrell Dow (see Hoechst-Marion Roussel)

Merz Pharmaceuticals
4215 Tudor Lane
Greensboro, NC 27410
(800) 334-0514
www.merzusa.com

Methapharm, Inc
2825 University Drive
Suite 240
Coral Springs, FL 33065
(800) 287-7686
www.methapharm.com

MGI Pharma, Inc
5775 West Old Shakopee Road
Suite 100
Bloomington, MN 55437-3174
(800) 562-0679
www.mgipharma.com

Mikart, Inc
1750 Chattahoochee Avenue
Atlanta, GA 30318
(404) 351-4510
www.mikart.com

Miles Allergy (see Bayer Corp)

Miles, Inc (see Bayer Corp)

Milex Products, Inc
4311 North Normandy
Chicago, IL 60634-1403
(800) 621-1278

Miller Pharmacal Group, Inc
350 Randy Road
Unit #2
Carol Stream, IL 60188-1831
(800) 323-2935
www.millerpharmacal.com

Mission Pharmacal Company
10999 IH-10 West
Suite 1000
San Antonio, TX 78230
(800) 531-3333
www.missionpharmacal.com

Miza Pharmaceuticals, Inc
(Corp Office)
4950 Yonge Street
Suite 2001
PO Box 118
Toronto, Ontario
Canada M2N 6K1
(416) 927-0600
www.miza.com

Miza Pharmaceuticals USA, Inc
40 Main Street
Fairton, NJ 08320-0210
(856) 451-9350
www.miza.com

Monaghan Medical Corp
5 Latour Avenue
Suite 1600
PO Box 2805
Plattsburgh, NY 12901
(800) 833-9653
www.monaghanmed.com

Monarch Pharmaceuticals
(King Pharmaceuticals, Inc)
355 Beecham Street
Bristol, TN 37620
(800) 776-3637
www.monarchpharm.com

Monticello Drug Company
1604 Stockton Street
Jacksonville, FL 32204
(800) 735-0666
www.monticellocompanies.com

Moore Medical Corp
PO Box 1500
New Britain, CT 06050-1500
(800) 234-1464
www.mooremedical.com

Morton Grove Pharmaceuticals
6451 West Main Street
Morton Grove, IL 60053
(800) 346-6854
www.visitmgp.com

Muro Pharmaceuticals, Inc
890 East Street
Tewksbury, MA 01876-1496
(800) 225-0974
www.muropharm.com

Mutual Pharmaceutical Company,
Inc/United Research Laboratories
1100 Orthodox Street
Philadelphia, PA 19124
(800) 523-3684
www.urlmutual.com

Mylan Pharmaceuticals, Inc
P0 Box 4310
Morgantown, WV 26504
(800) 826-9526
www.mylanpharm.com

Nabi
(Corp Headquarters)
5800 Park of Commerce Boulevard Northwest
Boca Raton, FL 33487
(561) 989-5800
www.nabi.com

Nastech Pharmaceutical Company, Inc
45 Adams Avenue
Hauppauge, NY 11788
(631) 273-0101
www.nastech.com

NATREN, Inc
3105 Willow Lane
Westlake Village, CA 91361
(800) 992-3323
www.natren.com

Natrol, Inc
21411 Prairie Street
Chatsworth, CA 91311
(800) 326-1520
www.natrol.com

Natures Bounty, Inc
(NBTY, Inc)
90 Orville Drive
Bohemia, NY 11716
(631) 244-2055
www.naturesbounty.com

Nature's Sunshine Products, Inc
75 East 1700 South
Provo, UT 84606
(800) 223-8225
www.nsponline.com

NeoPharm, Inc
150 Field Drive
Suite 195
Lake Forest, IL 60045
(847) 295-8678
www.neopharm.com

NeoRx Corp
410 West Harrison Street
Seattle, WA 98119-4007
(206) 281-7001
www.neorx.com

Nephron Pharmaceuticals Corp
4121 34th Street
Orlando, FL 32811
(800) 443-4313
www.nephronpharm.com

Nestle Clinical Nutrition
3 Parkway North
Suite 500
Deerfield, IL 60015
(800) 422-2752

NeuroGenesis/Matrix Tech, Inc
100 Louisiana
Suite 600
Houston, TX 77002
(800) 345-8912
www.neurogenesis.com

Neutrogena Corp
5760 West 96th Street
Los Angeles, CA 90045-5595
(800) 582-4048
www.neutrogena.com

Niche Pharmaceuticals, Inc
200 North Oak Street
Roanoke, TX 76262
(800) 677-0355
www.niche-inc.com

Nnodum Corp
(Ziks)
886 Clinton Springs Avenue
Cincinnati, OH 45229
(513) 861-2329
www.zikspain.com

Nomax, Inc
40 North Rock Hill Road
St Louis, MO 63119
(314) 961-2500
www.nomax.com

Noramco, Inc
(Johnson & Johnson)
1440 Olympic Drive
Athens, GA 30608
(706) 353-4400
www.noramco.com

Norstar Consumer Products Company, Inc
5517 95th Avenue
Kenosha, WI 53144
(262) 652-8505
www.norstarcpc.com

Northern Research Laboratories, Inc
4225 White Bear Parkway
Suite 600
St Paul, MN 55110-3389
(888) 884-4675
www.northernresearch.com

Norwich Eaton (see Procter & Gamble
Pharmaceuticals)

Novartis Pharmaceuticals Corp
One Health Plaza
Building 161
East Hanover, NJ 07936-1080
(973) 781-8300
www.novartis.com

Noven Pharmaceuticals
11960 Southwest 144th Street
Miami, FL 33186
(888) 253-5099
www.noven.com

Novocol
(Septodont, Inc)
PO Box 11926
Wilmington, DE 19850
(800) 872-8305
www.septodontinc.com

Novo Nordisk Pharmaceuticals, Inc
100 College Road West
Princeton, NJ 08540
(800) 727-6500
www.novonordisk-us.com

Novopharm USA, Inc
165 East Commerce Drive
Suite 100
Schaumburg, IL 60173-5326
(800) 635-5067

Numark Laboratories, Inc
164 Northfield Avenue
Edison, NJ 08837
(800) 338-8079
www.numarklabs.com

NutraMax Laboratories, Inc
2208 Lakeside Boulevard
Edgewood, MD 21040
(800) 925-5187
www.nutramaxlabs.com

Nutricutical Solutions
6704 Ranger Avenue
Corpus Christi, TX 78415
(800) 856-7040

NutriSoy International, Inc
424 South Kentucky Avenue
Evansville, IN 47714
(888) 769-0769
www.nutrisoy.com

7 Oaks Pharmaceutical Corp
161 Harry Stanley Drive
Easley, SC 29640
(864) 850-1700

Odyssey Pharmaceuticals, Inc
72 DeForest Avenue
East Hanover, NJ 07936
(877) 427-9068
www.odysseypharm.com

Ohmeda Pharmaceuticals (see Baxter
Pharmaceutical Products, Inc)

Omnii Products
1500 North Florida Mango Road
Suite 1
West Palm Beach, FL 33409
(800) 445-3386
www.omniiproducts.com

Optics Laboratory, Inc
9480 Telstar Avenue #3
El Monte, CA 91731
(626) 350-1926
www.opticslab.com

Optimox Corp
PO Box 3378
Torrance, CA 90510-3378
(800) 223-1601
www.optimox.com

Organogenesis, Inc
150 Dan Road
Canton, MA 02021
(781) 575-0775
www.organogenesis.com

Organon, Inc
375 Mt Pleasant Avenue
West Orange, NJ 07052
(973) 325-4500
www.organon.com

Orphan Medical, Inc
13911 Ridgedale Drive
Suite 250
Minnetonka, MN 55305
(888) 867-7426
www.orphan.com

Orphan Pharmaceuticals USA
1101 Kermit Drive
Suite 608
Nashville, TN 37217
(615) 399-0700
www.orphanusa.com

Ortho Biotech, LP
700 US Highway 202
Box 670
Raritan, NJ 08869-0670
(800) 325-7504
www.orthobiotech.com

Ortho-Clinical Diagnostics
100 Indigo Creek Drive
Rochester, NY 14626
(800) 828-6316
www.orthoclinical.com

Ortho-McNeil Pharmaceutical, Inc
Route 202
Raritan, NJ 08869
(800) 631-5273
www.ortho-mcneil.com

Otsuka America Pharmaceutical, Inc
2440 Research Boulevard
Rockville, MD 20850
(800) 562-3974
www.otsuka.com

Oxford Pharmaceutical Services, Inc
One US Highway 46 West
Totowa, NJ 07512
(877) 284-9120
www.oxfordpharm.com

OXIS International, Inc
6040 North Cutter Circle
Suite 317
Portland, OR 97212
(503) 283-3911
www.oxis.com

Oxypure, Inc
3550 Morris Street North
St Petersburg, FL 33713
(888) 216-8930

Paddock Laboratories, Inc
3940 Quebec Avenue North
Minneapolis, MN 55427
(800) 328-5113
www.paddocklabs.com

Pan American Laboratories, Inc
PO Box 8950
Mandeville, LA 70470-8950
(985) 893-4097
www.panamericanlabs.com

Parkedale Pharmaceuticals
870 Parkedale Road
Rochester, MI 84307
(800) 336-7783

Parke-Davis
Pfizer Pharmaceuticals
201 Tabor Road
Morris Plains, NJ 07950
(800) 223-0432

Parnell Pharmaceuticals
PO Box 5130
Larkspur, CA 94977
(800) 457-4276
www.parnellpharm.com

Par Pharmaceutical, Inc
One Ram Ridge Road
Spring Valley, NY 10977
(800) 727-0923
www.parpharm.com

PBH Wesley Jessen
810 Kifer Road
Sunnyvale, CA 94086
(800) 538-1680

PDRx Pharmaceuticals, Inc
727 North Ann Arbor
Oklahoma City, OK 73127
(800) 299-7379
www.pdrx.com

Pecos Pharmaceutical
25301 Cabot Road
Suites 212-213
Laguna Hills, CA 92653

Pediatric Pharmaceuticals, Inc
120 Wood Avenue South
Suite 300
Iselin, NJ 08830
(732) 603-7708
www.pediatricpharm.com

Pedinol Pharmacal, Inc
30 Banfi Plaza North
Farmingdale, NY 11735
(800) 733-4665
www.pedinol.com

Permeable Technologies, Inc
712 Ginesi Drive
Morganville, NJ 07751
(800) 622-7376
www.lifestylecompany.com

Perrigo Company
515 Eastern Avenue
Allegan, MI 49010
(800) 719-9260
www.perrigo.com

Person & Covey, Inc
616 Allen Avenue
PO Box 25018
Glendale, CA 91221-5018
(818) 240-1030
www.personandcovey.com

Pfeiffer Company
71 University Avenue
Atlanta, GA 30315
(800) 342-6450

Pfizer Pharmaceuticals Group (PPG)
235 East 42nd Street
New York, NY 10017-5755
(800) 438-1985
www.pfizer.com

Pharma 21
1363 Shinly
Suite 100
Escondido, CA 92026
(760) 743-7441
www.pharma21.net

Pharmaceutical Formulations, Inc
PO Box 1904
Edison, NJ 08818-1904
(732) 985-7100
www.pfiotc.com

Pharmaceutical Specialties, Inc
PO Box 6298
Rochester, MN 55903-6298
(800) 325-8232
www.psico.com

**Pharmacia & Upjohn Company
(Ophthalmics Division)**
701 East Milham Road
Kalamazoo, MI 49001
(800) 423-4866

Pharmacia Corp
100 Route 206 North
Peapack, NJ 07977
(888) 768-5501
www.pharmacia.com

Pharmadigm, Inc
2401 Foothill Drive
Salt Lake City, UT 84109
(801) 464-6100
www.pharmadigm.com

Pharmakon Labs
6050 Jet Port Industrial Boulevard
Tampa, FL 33634
(800) 888-4045
www.pharmakonlabs.com

Pharmanex
75 West Center
Provo, UT 84601
(801) 345-9800
www.pharmanex.com

Pharma-Tek, Inc
PO Box 1148
Elmira, NY 14902
(800) 645-6655
www.pharma-tek.com

Pharmatek Laboratories, Inc
11545 Sorrento Valley Road
Suite 315
San Diego, CA 92121
(858) 350-8789
www.pharmatek.com

Pharmics, Inc
PO Box 27554
Salt Lake City, UT 84119
(800) 456-4138
www.pharmics.com

PhytoPharmica, Inc
825 Challenger Drive
Green Bay, WI 54311
(800) 553-2370
www.phytopharmica.com

Plantex USA, Inc
482 Hudson Terrace
Englewood Cliffs, NJ 07632
(201) 567-1010
www.plantexusa.com

Playtex Company
74 Commerce Drive
Allendale, NJ 07401-1600
(800) 816-5742
www.playtex.com

Plough, Inc
(see Schering-Plough Corp)

PolyMedica Corp
11 State Street
Woburn, MA 01801
(781) 933-2020
www.polymedica.com

Polymer Technology Corp
100 Research Drive
Wilmington, MA 01887
(800) 885-1241

Porton Product Limited
(see Speywood Pharmaceuticals, Inc)

Pratt Pharmaceuticals
235 East 42nd Street
New York, NY 10017-5755
(800) 438-1985

Procter & Gamble Pharmaceuticals
PO Box 231
Norwich, NY 13815
(800) 448-4878
www.pgpharma.com

ProCyte Corp
PO Box 808
Redmond, WA 98073-0808
(425) 869-1239
www.procyte.com

Protein Design Labs, Inc
34801 Campus Drive
Fremont, CA 94555
(510) 574-1400
www.pdl.com

Protein Sciences Corp
1000 Research Parkway
Meriden, CT 06450
(800) 488-7099
www.proteinsciences.com

Protherics, Inc
5214 Maryland Way
Suite 405
Brentwood, TN 37027
(615) 327-1027
www.protherics.com

**Psychemedics Corp
(Laboratory Operations)**
5832 Uplander Way
Culver City, CA 90230
(800) 522-7424
www.psychemedics.com

**Purdue Pharma, LP
(The Purdue Frederick Company)**
One Stamford Forum
201 Tresser Boulevard
Stamford, CT 06901-3431
(888) 726-7535
www.purduepharma.com

Purepac Pharmaceuticals
(see Faulding Pharmaceuticals)

Puritan's Pride
1233 Montauk Highway
PO Box 9001
Oakdale, NY 11769-9001
(800) 645-9584
www.puritanspride.com

QLT, Inc
887 Great Northern Way
Vancouver, BC
Canada V5T 4T5
(800) 663-5486
www.qlt-pdt.com

Questcor Pharmaceuticals, Inc
3260 Whipple Road
Union City, CA 94587
(510) 400-0700
www.questcor.com

Quidel Corp
10165 McKellar Court
San Diego, CA 92121
(800) 874-1517
www.quidel.com

Ranbaxy Pharmaceuticals, Inc USA
600 College Road East
Princeton, NJ 08540
(609) 720-5614
www.ranbaxy.com

Reed & Carnrick (see Schwarz Pharma, Inc)

Reese Pharmaceutical Company, Inc
10617 Frank Avenue
Cleveland, OH 44106
(800) 321-7178
www.reesechemical.com

Regeneron Pharmaceuticals, Inc
777 Old Saw Mill River Road
Tarrytown, NY 10591
(914) 345-7400
www.regeneron.com

Reid Rowell (see Solvay Pharmaceuticals)

Remel, Inc
12076 Santa Fe Drive
PO Box 14428
Lenexa, KS 66215
(800) 255-6730
www.remelinc.com

Requa, Inc
One Seneca Place
Greenwich, CT 06830
(800) 321-1085
www.requa.com

Research Triangle Institute
PO Box 12194
Research Triangle Park, NC 27709-2194
(919) 485-2666
www.rti.org

**Rexall Sundown, Inc
(Royal Numico, N.V.)**
6111 Broken Sound Parkway Northwest
Boca Raton, FL 33487
(800) 327-0908
www.rexallsundown.com

Rhone-Poulenc Rorer Pharmaceuticals, Inc
500 Arcola Road
PO Box 1200
Collegeville, PA 19426-0998
(800) 340-7502

Ribi Immunochem Research, Inc
553 Old Corvallis Road
Hamilton, MT 59840-3131
(406) 363-6214
www.ribi.com

Richardson-Vicks, Inc
(see Procter & Gamble Pharmaceuticals)

Ricola, Inc
51 Gibraltar Drive
Morris Plains, NJ 07950
(973) 984-6811
www.ricolausa.com

R.I.D., Inc
609 North Mednik Avenue
Los Angeles, CA 90022-1320
(323) 268-0635

Rite Aid Corp
30 Hunter Lane
Camp Hill, PA 17011
(717) 761-2633
www.riteaid.com

Roberts Pharmaceuticals Corp
4 Industrial Way West
Eatontown, NJ 07724
(800) 828-2088

Roche Pharmaceuticals
340 Kingsland Street
Nutley, NJ 07110
(973) 235-5000
www.rocheusa.com

Roerig
235 East 42nd Street
New York, NY 10017
(800) 438-1985

Rorer (see Rhone-Poulenc Rorer
Pharmaceuticals, Inc)

Rosemont Pharmaceutical Corp
301 South Cherokee Street
Denver, CO 80223
(800) 445-8091

Ross Products Division, Abbott Labs
625 Cleveland Avenue
Columbus, OH 43215
(800) 230-7677
www.ross.com

Roxane Laboratories, Inc
PO Box 16532
Columbus, OH 43216
(800) 962-8364
www.roxane.com

Royce Laboratories, Inc
16600 Northwest 54th Avenue
Miami, FL 33014
(800) 677-6923

R. P. Scherer, Inc
645 Martinsville Road
Suite 200
Basking Ridge, NJ 07920
(888) 636-1919
www.rpscherer.com

Russ Pharmaceuticals
(see UCB Pharmaceuticals)

Salix Pharmaceuticals, Inc
8540 Colonnade Center Drive
Raleigh, NC 27615
(919) 862-1000
www.salixltd.com

Sandoz Pharmaceuticals (see Novartis
Pharmaceuticals Corp)

SangStat, Inc
6300 Dunbarton Circle
Fremont, CA 94555
(510) 789-4300
www.sangstat.com

Sanofi-Synthelabo, Inc
90 Park Avenue
New York, NY 10016
(212) 551-4000
www.sanofi-synthelabous.com

Santen, Inc
555 Gateway Drive
Napa, CA 94558
(707) 254-1750
www.santen-inc.com

**Savage Laboratories
(Altana Inc)**
60 Baylis Road
Melville, NY 11747-2006
(800) 231-0206
www.savagelabs.com

Scandinavian Naturals
13 North 7th Street
Perkasie, PA 18944
(800) 288-2844
www.scandinaviannaturals.com

Scandipharm
(see Axcan Scandipharm)

Schaffer Laboratories
1058 North Allen Avenue
Pasadena, CA 91104
(800) 231-6725
www.schafferlabs.com

Schein Pharmaceutical, Inc
(see Watson Laboratories, Inc)

**Schering-Plough Corp
(World Headquarters)**
2000 Galloping Hill Road
Kenilworth, NJ 07033-0530
(908) 298-4000
www.schering-plough.com

Schmid Products Company
(see Durex Consumer Products)

Scholl, Inc
(see Schering-Plough Corp)

Schwarz Pharma, Inc
PO Box 2038
Milwaukee, WI 53201
(800) 558-5114
www.schwarzusa.com

SciClone Pharmaceuticals, Inc
901 Mariner's Island Boulevard
Suite 205
San Mateo, CA 94404
(650) 358-3456
www.sciclone.com

Scios
(Corp Headquarters)
820 West Maude Avenue
Sunnyvale, CA 94085
(408) 616-8200
www.sciosinc.com

Searle (see Pharmacia Corp)

Seatrace Pharmaceuticals, Inc
PO Box 7200
503 Hickman Street
Rainbow City, AL 35906
(256) 442-5023

Sepracor
(Corp Headquarters)
84 Waterford Drive
Marlborough, MA 01752
(877) SEPRACOR
www.sepracor.com

Septodont, Inc
PO Box 11926
Wilmington, DE 19850
(800) 872-8305
www.septodontinc.com

Seres Laboratories, Inc
3331-B Industrial Drive
Santa Rosa, CA 95403
(707) 526-4526
www.sereslabs.com

Serono, Inc
One Technology Place
Rockland, MA 02370
(800) 283-8088
www.seronousa.com

Shaklee Corporation
(Corp Headquarters)
4747 Willow Road
Pleasanton, CA 94588
(925) 924-2000
www.shaklee.com

Sheffield Laboratories
(Faria Ltd LLC)
170 Broad Street
New London, CT 06320
(800) 222-1087
www.sheffield-labs.com

Sherwood Davis & Geck
(see Kendall Healthcare Products)

Sherwood Medical
(see Kendall Healthcare Products)

Shionogi USA, Inc
100 Campus Drive
Florham Park, NJ 07932
(973) 966-6900

Shire US, Inc
7900 Tanners Gate Drive
Florence, KY 41042
(859) 282-2100
www.shiregroup.com

SHS North America
PO Box 117
Gaithersburg, MD 20884-0117
(800) 636-2283
www.SHSNA.com

Sidmak Laboratories, Inc
17 West Street
East Hanover, NJ 07936
(800) 922-0547
www.sidmaklab.com

Sigma-Tau Pharmaceuticals, Inc
800 South Frederick Avenue
Suite 300
Gaithersburg, MD 20877
(800) 447-0169
www.sigma-tau.com

Silarx Pharmaceuticals, Inc
19 West Street
Spring Valley, NY 10977
(914) 352-4020

SkyePharma, Inc
10 East 63rd Street
New York, NY 10021
(212) 753-5780
www.skyepharma.com

Slim Fast Foods Company
PO Box 3625
West Palm Beach, FL 33402
(877) 375-4632
www.slim-fast.com

Smith & Nephew, Inc
150 Minuteman Road
Andover, MA 01810
(978) 749-1000
www.smithnephew.com

SmithKline Beecham Pharmaceuticals
PO Box 7929
One Franklin Plaza
Philadelphia, PA 19101-7920
(800) 366-8900
www.sb.com

Solvay Pharmaceuticals
901 Sawyer Road
Marietta, GA 30062
(800) 241-1643
www.solvaypharmaceuticals-us.com

Somerset Pharmaceuticals, Inc
2202 Northwest Shore Boulevard
Suite 450
Tampa, FL 33607
(800) 892-8889
www.somersetpharm.com

Sparta Pharmaceuticals, Inc
111 Rock Road
Horsham, PA 19044
(215) 442-1700

Spectrum Chemical
Manufacturing Corp
14422 South San Pedro Street
Gardena, CA 90248-9985
(800) 772-8786
www.spectrumchemical.com

Speywood Pharmaceuticals, Inc
27 Maple Street
Milford, MA 01757-3650
(508) 478-8900

St Jude Medical, Inc
One Lillehei Plaza
St Paul, MN 55117-9913
(800) 328-9634
www.sjm.com

Star Pharmaceuticals, Inc
1990 Northwest 44th Street
Pompano Beach, FL 33064-8712
(800) 845-7827
www.starpharm.com

Squibb (see Bristol-Myers Squibb Company)

Steris Laboratories, Inc
(Schein)
620 North 51st Avenue
Phoenix, AZ 85043
(800) 692-9995

Sterling Health
(see Bayer Consumer Division)

Sterling Winthrop
(see Sanofi-Synthelabo, Inc)

Stiefel Laboratories, Inc
255 Alhambra Circle
Coral Gables, FL 33134
(888) 784-3335
www.stiefel.com

Stratus Pharmaceuticals, Inc
14377 Southwest 142nd Street
Miami, FL 33186
(800) 442-7882
www.stratuspharmaceuticals.com

SummaRx Laboratories
2525 Ridgmar Boulevard
Suite 404
Ft Worth, TX 76116
(800) 406-6900
www.summalabs.com

Summers Laboratories, Inc
103 G.P. Clement Drive
Collegeville, PA 19426-2044
(800) 533-7546
www.sumlab.com

Summit Pharmaceuticals
(see Novartis Pharmaceuticals Corp)

SuperGen, Inc
4140 Dublin Boulevard
Suite 200
Dublin, CA 94568
(800) 905-5474
www.supergen.com

Superior Pharmaceutical Company
1385 Kemper Meadow Drive
Cincinnati, OH 45240-1635
(800) 826-5035
www.superiorpharm.com

Survival Technical, Inc
(see Meridian Medical Technologies)

Swiss-American Products, Inc
4641 Nall Road
Dallas, TX 75244
(800) 633-8872
www.elta.net

Syncor
6464 Canoga Avenue
Woodland Hills, CA 91367
(800) 678-6779
www.syncor.com

Syntex Laboratories (see Roche
Pharmaceuticals)

Takeda Pharmaceuticals North America, Inc
475 Half Day Road
Suite 500
Lincolnshire, IL 60069
(847) 383-3000
www.takedapharm.com

Tanox, Inc
10301 Stella Link
Houston, TX 77025-5497
(713) 664-2288

TAP Pharmaceutical Products, Inc
675 North Field Drive
Lake Forest, FL 60045
(800) 622-2011
www.tap.com

Targeted Genetics Corp
1100 Olive Way
Suite 100
Seattle, WA 98101
(206) 623-7612
www.targen.com

Taro Pharmaceuticals USA, Inc
5 Skyline Drive
Hawthorne, NY 10532-9998
(800) 544-1449
www.taropharma.com

Taylor Pharmacal
1222 West Grand
Decatur, IL 62525

Tec Laboratories, Inc
PO Box 1958
Albany, OR 97321
(800) 482-4464
www.teclabsinc.com

Telluride Pharmaceuticals Corp
300 Valley Road
Hillsborough, NJ 08844-4656
(908) 369-1800
www.tellpharm.com

Teva Pharmaceuticals USA
1090 Horsham Road
PO Box 1090
North Wales, PA 19454-1090
(215) 591-3000
www.tevapharmusa.com

Textilease Medique Products Company
900 Lively Boulevard
Wood Dale, IL 60191
(800) 634-7680
www.textileasemedique.com

The Medicines Company
One Cambridge Center
Cambridge, MA 02142
(617) 225-9099
www.angiomax.com

Therasense
1370 South Loop Road
Alameda, CA 95402
(510) 748-5400

Thermo BioStar, Inc
6655 Lookout Road
Boulder, CO 80301
(800) 637-3717
www.thermo.com

Tishcon Corp
30 New York Avenue
Westbury, NY 11590-5910
(516) 338-0829
www.tishcon.com

Tom's of Maine, Inc
302 LaFayette Center
PO Box 710
Kennebunk, ME 04043
(800) 367-8667
www.tomsofmaine.com

Trask Industries, Inc
163 Farrell Street
Somerset, NJ 08873
(800) 579-3131

Triton Consumer Products, Inc
561 West Golf Road
Arlington Heights, IL 60005-3904
(800) 942-2009

Tweezerman
55 Sea Cliff Avenue
Glen Cove, NY 11542-3695
(800) 645-3340
www.tweezerman.com

TwinLab Laboratories, Inc
150 Motor Parkway
Hauppauge, NY 11788
(631) 467-3140
www.twinlab.com

UAD Laboratories, Inc
(see Forest Pharmaceuticals, Inc)

UCB Pharmaceuticals, Inc
1950 Lake Park Drive
Smyrna, GA 30080
(800) 477-7877
www.ucb-pharma.com

UDL Laboratories, Inc
1718 Northrock Court
Rockford, IL 61103
(800) 848-0462
www.udllabs.com

Unico Holdings, Inc
1830 2nd Avenue North
Lake Worth, FL 33461
(800) 367-4477

Unimed Pharmaceuticals
901 Sawyer Road
Marietta, GA 30062
(770) 578-9000
www.unimed.com

Unipath Diagnostics Company
47 Hulfish Street
Suite 400
Princeton, NJ 08542
(800) 321-3279
www.unipath.com

United Guardian Laboratories
230 Marcus Boulevard
Hauppauge, NY 11788
(800) 645-5566
www.u-g.com

Upjohn (see Pharmacia Corp)

Upsher-Smith Laboratories
13700 1st Avenue North
Minneapolis, MN 55441
(800) 654-2299
www.upsher-smith.com

UroCor, Inc
800 Research Parkway
Oklahoma City, OK 73104
(800) 634-9330
www.urocor.com

Urologix
14405 21st Avenue North
Minneapolis, MN 55447
(888) 229-0772
www.urologix.com

USA Nutritionals, Inc
513 Commack Road
Deerpark, NY 11729
(631) 643-0600
www.USANutritionals.com

US DenTek
1460 Cedar Lane
Suite A
Petaluma, CA 94954
(800) 433-6835

US Surgical Corp
150 Glover Avenue
Norwalk, CT 06856
(800) 722-8772
www.ussurg.com

Value in Pharmaceuticals
3000 Alt Boulevard
Grand Island, NY 14072
(800) 724-3784
www.vippharm.com

Vertex Pharmaceuticals, Inc
130 Waverly Street
Cambridge, MA 02139
(617) 444-6100
www.vpharm.com

VHA, Inc
220 East Las Colinas Boulevard
Irving, TX 75039
(800) 842-7587

Vicks Health Care Products
(see Procter & Gamble Pharmaceuticals)

Vicks Pharmacy Products
(see Procter & Gamble Pharmaceuticals)

Vision Pharmaceuticals, Inc
PO Box 400
Mitchell, SD 57301
(800) 325-6789
www.visionpharm.com

VistaPharm
1200 Corporate Drive
Birmingham, AL 35242
(205) 981-1387
www.vistapharm.com

Vitaline Corp
385 Williamson Way
Ashland, OR 97520
(800) 648-4755
www.vitaline.com

Vitamin Research Product, Inc
3579 Highway 50 East
Carson City, NV 89701
(800) 877-2447
www.vrp.com

Vivus, Inc
545 Middlefield Road
Suite 200
Menlo Park, CA 94025
(888) 345-6873
www.vivus.com

Walgreen Company
200 Wilmont Road
Dearfield, IL 60015
(847) 940-2500
www.walgreens.com

Wallace Pharmaceuticals
265 Davidson Avenue
Suite 300
PO Box 6833
Somerset, NJ 08875-6833
(732) 564-2200

Wal-Mart Stores, Inc
702 Southwest 8th Street
Bentonville, AR 72716
(501) 273-4000
www.wal-mart.com

Wampole Laboratories
2 Research Way
Princeton, NJ 08540
(800) 257-9525
www.wampolelabs.com

Warner Chilcott Laboratories
100 Enterprise Drive
Suite 280
Rockaway, NJ 07866
(973) 442-3200
www.wclabs.com

Warner Lambert Consumer Healthcare
201 Tabor Road
Morris Plains, NJ 07950
(973) 442-3200
www.warner-lambert.com

**Warrick Pharmaceuticals
(Schering Plough Corp)**
1095 Morris Avenue
Union, NJ 07083-7137
(800) 547-3869

Watson Laboratories, Inc
311 Bonnie Circle
Corona, CA 92880
(800) 272-5525
www.watsonpharm.com

West-Ward Pharmaceutical Corp
465 Industrial Way West
Eatontown, NJ 07724
(800) 631-2174

**Westwood-Squibb Pharmaceuticals
(Bristol-Myers Squibb)**
100 Forest Avenue
Buffalo, NY 14213
(800) 333-0950
www.westwood-squibb.com

W. F. Young, Inc
PO Box 1990
East Longmeadow, MA 01028-5990
(800) 628-9653
www.absorbine.com

Whitby Pharmaceuticals, Inc
(see UCB Pharmaceuticals, Inc)

**Whitehall-Robins Healthcare
(American Home Products)**
5 Giralda Farms
Madison, NJ 07940-0871
(800) 322-3129
www.whitehallrobins.com

Winthrop Pharmaceuticals
(see Sanofi-Synthelabo, Inc)

**Wisconsin Pharmacal Company
(WPC Brands)**
One Repel Road
Jackson, WI 53037
(800) 558-6614

Wm. Wrigley Jr Company
410 North Michigan Avenue
Chicago, IL 60611
(866) 787-7277
www.wrigley.com

Women First Healthcare, Inc
12220 El Camino Real
Suite 400
San Diego, CA 92130
(858) 509-1171
www.womenfirst.com

Women's Capital Corp
1990 M Street Northwest
Suite 250
Washington, DC 20036
(800) 330-1271
www.go2planb.com

Woodside Biomedical, Inc
1925 Palomar Oaks Way
Suite 105
Carlsbad, CA 92008-6526
(760) 804-6900
www.woodsidebiomedical.com

Woodward Laboratories, Inc
11132 Winners Circle
Los Alamitos, CA 90720
(800) 780-6999
www.woodwardlabs.com

Wyeth Pharmaceuticals
500 Arcola Road
Collegeville, PA 19426
(610) 902-1200
www.ahp.com/wyeth

Xoma
2910 7th Street
Berkeley, CA 94710
(800) 246-9662
www.xoma.com

Xttrium Laboratories, Inc
415 West Pershing Road
Chicago, IL 60609
(800) 587-3721
www.adultrashcreme.com

Young Dental Manufacturing
13705 Shoreline Court East
Earth City, MO 63045
(800) 325-1881
www.youngdental.com

Zanfel Laboratories, Inc
Morton, IL 61550
(800) 401-4002
www.zanfel.com

Zeneca Pharmaceuticals
(see AstraZeneca Pharmaceuticals, LP)

Zenith Goldline Pharmaceuticals
4400 Biscayne Boulevard
Miami, FL 33137-3227
(305) 575-6000
www.zenithgoldline.com

Zila Pharmaceuticals, Inc
5227 North 7th Street
Phoenix, AZ 85014-2800
(800) 922-7887
www.zila.com

Zonagen, Inc
2408 Timberloch Place, B-4
The Woodlands, TX 77380
(281) 719-3400
www.zonagen.com

ZymeTx, Inc
800 Research Parkway
Suite 100
Oklahoma City, OK 73104
(888) 817-1314
www.zymetx.com

ZymoGenetics, Inc
1201 Eastlake Avenue East
Seattle, WA 98102-3702
(206) 442-6600
www.zymogenetics.com

INDICATION/THERAPEUTIC CATEGORY INDEX

(Continued)

ALOPECIA

Antiandrogen
finasteride 272
Propecia® [US/Can] 272

Progestin
hydroxyprogesterone caproate 337
Hylutin® [US] 337
Prodrox® [US] 337

Topical Skin Product
Apo®-Gain [Can] 432
Minox [Can] 432
minoxidil........................ 432
Rogaine® [Can] 432
Rogaine® Extra Strength for Men [US-OTC] 432
Rogaine® for Men [US-OTC] 432
Rogaine® for Women [US-OTC]
.... 432

ALPHA₁-ANTITRYPSIN DEFICIENCY (CONGENITAL)

Antitrypsin Deficiency Agent
alpha₁-proteinase inhibitor 24
Prolastin® [US/Can] 24

ALTITUDE SICKNESS

Carbonic Anhydrase Inhibitor
acetazolamide 9
Apo®-Acetazolamide [Can]........... 9
Diamox Sequels® [US] 9
Diamox® [US/Can] 9

ALVEOLAR PROTEINOSIS

Expectorant
potassium iodide 531
SSKI® [US] 531

ALZHEIMER'S DISEASE

Acetylcholinesterase Inhibitor
Aricept® [US/Can] 211
Cognex® [US] 617
donepezil 211
Exelon® [US/Can]................. 575
rivastigmine 575
tacrine 617

Acetylcholinesterase Inhibitor (Central)
galantamine 292
Reminyl® [US] 292

Cholinergic Agent
Exelon® [US/Can]................. 575
rivastigmine 575

Ergot Alkaloid and Derivative
ergoloid mesylates 233
Germinal® [US] 233
Hydergine® LC [US] 233
Hydergine® [US/Can] 233

AMEBIASIS

Amebicide
Apo®-Metronidazole [Can] 426
Diodoquin® [Can] 357
Diquinol® [US] 357
Flagyl ER® [US] 426
Flagyl® [US/Can] 426
Humatin® [US/Can] 493
iodoquinol 357
MetroLotion® [US] 426
metronidazole 426
Nidagel™ [Can] 426
Noritate™ [Can] 426
Novo-Nidazol [Can] 426
paromomycin 493
Yodoxin® [US] 357

Aminoquinoline (Antimalarial)
Aralen® Phosphate [US/Can] 136
chloroquine phosphate 136

AMENORRHEA

Ergot Alkaloid and Derivative
Apo® Bromocriptine [Can] 93
bromocriptine 93
Parlodel® [US/Can] 93
PMS-Bromocriptine [Can].......... 93

Gonadotropin
Factrel® [US] 304
gonadorelin 304
Lutrepulse™ [Can] 304

Progestin
Alti-MPA [Can] 404
Aygestin® [US] 465
Crinone® [US/Can] 543
Depo-Provera® [US/Can] 404
Gen-Medroxy [Can] 404
hydroxyprogesterone caproate 337
Hylutin® [US] 337
medroxyprogesterone acetate 404
Micronor® [US/Can] 465
norethindrone 465
Norlutate® [Can] 465
Nor-QD® [US] 465
Novo-Medrone [Can] 404
Prodrox® [US] 337
Progestasert® [US] 543
progesterone 543
Prometrium® [US/Can] 543
Provera® [US/Can] 404

AMMONIACAL URINE

Urinary Acidifying Agent
K-Phos® Original [US] 528
potassium acid phosphate 528

AMMONIA INTOXICATION

Ammonium Detoxicant
Acilac [Can] 372
Cholac® [US] 372
Constilac® [US] 372
Constulose® [US] 372
Enulose® [US] 372
Generlac® [US] 372
Kristalose™ [US] 372
lactulose 372
Laxilose [Can] 372
PMS-Lactulose [Can] 372

AMYLOIDOSIS

Mucolytic Agent
acetylcysteine 11
Acys-5® [US] 11
Mucomyst® [US/Can] 11
Parvolex® [Can] 11

AMYOTROPHIC LATERAL SCLEROSIS (ALS)

Anticholinergic Agent
atropine 62
Atropine-Care® [US]............... 62
Atropisol® [US/Can] 62
Isopto® Atropine [US/Can] 62
Sal-Tropine™ [US] 62

Cholinergic Agent
Mestinon®-SR [Can].............. 556
Mestinon® Timespan® [US] 556
Mestinon® [US/Can] 556
pyridostigmine 556
Regonol® [US] 556

ANESTHESIA (LOCAL)

Local Anesthetic

Local Anesthetic, Amide Derivative

Local Anesthetic, Injectable

ANESTHESIA (OPHTHALMIC)

Local Anesthetic

ANGINA PECTORIS

Beta-Adrenergic Blocker

(Continued)

ARSENIC POISONING

ARTHRITIS

(Continued)

Nonsteroidal Anti-inflammatory Drug (NSAID), COX-2 Selective

ASCARIASIS

Anthelmintic

ASCITES

Diuretic, Loop

Diuretic, Miscellaneous

Diuretic, Potassium Sparing

ASTHMA (CORTICOSTEROID-DEPENDENT)

Macrolide (Antibiotic)

ASTHMA (DIAGNOSTIC)

Diagnostic Agent

ATELECTASIS

Expectorant

Mucolytic Agent

ATOPIC DERMATITIS

Immunosuppressant Agent

Topical Skin Product

ATTENTION-DEFICIT/HYPERACTIVITY DISORDER (ADHD)

Amphetamine

Central Nervous System Stimulant, Nonamphetamine

AUTISM

Antidepressant, Selective Serotonin Reuptake Inhibitor

Antipsychotic Agent, Butyrophenone

BACK PAIN (LOW)

Analgesic, Narcotic

Analgesic, Non-narcotic

(Continued)

BEHÇET'S SYNDROME

Immunosuppressant Agent

BENIGN PROSTATIC HYPERPLASIA (BPH)

Alpha-Adrenergic Blocking Agent

Antiandrogen

Antineoplastic Agent, Anthracenedione

BENZODIAZEPINE OVERDOSE

Antidote

BERIBERI

Vitamin, Water Soluble

BIPOLAR DEPRESSION DISORDER

Anticonvulsant

Antimanic Agent

Antipsychotic Agent

BIRTH CONTROL

Contraceptive

Contraceptive, Implant (Progestin)

Contraceptive, Oral
(Continued)

Local Anesthetic

BITES (SNAKE)

Antivenin

BITES (SPIDER)

Antivenin

Electrolyte Supplement, Oral

Skeletal Muscle Relaxant

BLADDER IRRIGATION

Antibacterial, Topical

BLASTOMYCOSIS

Antifungal Agent

BLEPHARITIS

Antifungal Agent

BLEPHAROSPASM

Ophthalmic Agent, Toxin
(Continued)

Ophthalmic Agent, Toxin *(Continued)*

BOWEL CLEANSING

Laxative

BOWEL STERILIZATION

Aminoglycoside (Antibiotic)

BREAST ENGORGEMENT (POSTPARTUM)

Androgen

Estrogen and Androgen Combination

Estrogen Derivative

BROAD BETA DISEASE

Antihyperlipidemic Agent, Miscellaneous

BROMIDE INTOXICATION

Diuretic, Loop

BRONCHIECTASIS

Adrenergic Agonist Agent

Mucolytic Agent

BRONCHIOLITIS

Antiviral Agent

BRONCHITIS

Adrenergic Agonist Agent

Antibiotic, Cephalosporin

Antibiotic, Quinolone

(Continued)

CHOLINESTERASE INHIBITOR POISONING

Antidote
pralidoxime 534
Protopam® Injection [US/Can] 534

CHORIORETINITIS

Adrenal Corticosteroid
A-HydroCort® [US/Can] 333
Alti-Dexamethasone [Can] 184
A-methaPred® [US] 423
Apo®-Prednisone [Can] 538
Aristocort® Forte Injection [US] 651
Aristocort® Intralesional Injection [US]
.... 651
Aristocort® Tablet [US/Can] 651
Aristospan® Intra-articular Injection
[US/Can] 651
Aristospan® Intralesional Injection [US/Can] 651
Betaject™ [Can] 83
betamethasone (systemic) 83
Betnesol® [Can] 83
Celestone® Phosphate [US] 83
Celestone® Soluspan® [US/Can]
.... 83
Celestone® [US] 83
Cel-U-Jec® [US] 83
Cortef® [US/Can] 333
cortisone acetate 164
Cortone® [Can] 164
Decadron®-LA [US] 184
Decadron® [US/Can] 184
Decaject-LA® [US] 184
Decaject® [US] 184
Delta-Cortef® [US] 537
Deltasone® [US] 538
Depo-Medrol® [US/Can] 423
Depopred® [US] 423
dexamethasone (systemic) 184
Dexasone® L.A. [US] 184
Dexasone® [US/Can] 184
Dexone® LA [US] 184
Dexone® [US] 184
Hexadrol® [US/Can] 184
hydrocortisone (systemic) 333
Hydrocortone® Acetate [US] 333
Kenalog® Injection [US/Can] 651
Key-Pred-SP® [US] 537
Key-Pred® [US] 537
Medrol® Tablet [US/Can] 423
methylprednisolone 423
Meticorten® [US] 538
Orapred™ [US] 537
Pediapred® [US/Can] 537
PMS-Dexamethasone [Can] 184
Prednicot® [US] 538
prednisolone (systemic) 537
Prednisol® TBA [US] 537
prednisone 538
Prelone® [US] 537
Solu-Cortef® [US/Can] 333
Solu-Medrol® [US/Can] 423
Solurex L.A.® [US] 184
Sterapred® DS [US] 538
Sterapred® [US] 538
Tac™-3 Injection [US] 651
Triam-A® Injection [US] 651
triamcinolone (systemic) 651
Triam Forte® Injection [US] 651
Winpred™ [Can] 538

CHROMOBLASTOMYCOSIS

Antifungal Agent
Apo®-Ketoconazole [Can] 367
ketoconazole 367

Nizoral® [US/Can] 367
Novo-Ketoconazole [Can] 367

CHRONIC OBSTRUCTIVE PULMONARY DISEASE (COPD)

Adrenergic Agonist Agent
AccuNeb™ [US] 18
albuterol 18
Alti-Salbutamol [Can] 18
Alupent® [US] 413
Apo®-Salvent [Can] 18
isoproterenol 362
Isuprel® [US] 362
metaproterenol 413
Novo-Salmol [Can] 18
Proventil® HFA [US] 18
Proventil® Repetabs® [US] 18
Proventil® [US] 18
Ventolin® HFA [US] 18
Ventolin® [US] 18
Volmax® [US] 18

Anticholinergic Agent
Alti-Ipratropium [Can] 358
Apo®-Ipravent [Can] 358
Atrovent® [US/Can] 358
Gen-Ipratropium [Can] 358
ipratropium 358
Novo-Ipramide [Can] 358
Nu-Ipratropium [Can] 358
PMS-Ipratropium [Can] 358

Bronchodilator
Combivent® [US/Can] 359
DuoNeb™ [US] 359
ipratropium and albuterol 359

Expectorant
potassium iodide 531
SSKI® [US] 531

Theophylline Derivative
Aerolate III® [US] 630
Aerolate JR® [US] 630
Aerolate SR® [US] 630
aminophylline 33
Apo®-Theo LA [Can] 630
Dilor® [US/Can] 221
dyphylline 221
Elixophyllin® GG [US] 631
Elixophyllin® [US] 630
Lufyllin® [US/Can] 221
Neoasma® [US] 631
Novo-Theophyl SR [Can] 630
Phyllocontin®-350 [Can] 33
Phyllocontin® [Can] 33
Quibron®-T/SR [US/Can] 630
Quibron®-T [US] 630
Quibron® [US] 631
Slo-Phyllin® [US] 630
Theo-24® [US] 630
Theochron® [US] 630
Theocon® [US] 631
Theo-Dur® [US/Can] 630
Theolair™ [US/Can] 630
Theolate® [US] 631
Theomar® GG [US] 631
theophylline 630
theophylline and guaifenesin 631
T-Phyl® [US] 630
Uniphyl® [US/Can] 630

CIRRHOSIS

Bile Acid Sequestrant
cholestyramine resin 143
LoCHOLEST® Light [US] 143
LoCHOLEST® [US] 143
Novo-Cholamine [Can] 143
(Continued)

Antitussive/Decongestant

Antitussive/Decongestant/Expectorant

Cold Preparation

(Continued)

Cold Preparation *(Continued)*

Decongestant/Analgesic

Phenothiazine Derivative

CONGESTIVE HEART FAILURE

Adrenergic Agonist Agent

Alpha-Adrenergic Blocking Agent

Angiotensin-Converting Enzyme (ACE) Inhibitor

Beta-Adrenergic Blocker

Calcium Channel Blocker

Cardiac Glycoside

Cardiovascular Agent, Other

Diuretic, Loop

Cold Preparation

Cough and Cold Combination

Expectorant

CROHN'S DISEASE

5-Aminosalicylic Acid Derivative

DEBRIDEMENT OF CALLOUS TISSUE

Keratolytic Agent

DEBRIDEMENT OF ESCHAR

Protectant, Topical

DECUBITUS ULCERS

Enzyme

Enzyme, Topical Debridement

Protectant, Topical

Topical Skin Product

DEEP VEIN THROMBOSIS (DVT)

Anticoagulant (Other)

Factor Xa Inhibitor

Low Molecular Weight Heparin

DEMENTIA

Acetylcholinesterase Inhibitor

Antidepressant, Tricyclic (Tertiary Amine)

Benzodiazepine

Ergot Alkaloid and Derivative

Phenothiazine Derivative

DENTAL CARIES (PREVENTION)

Mineral, Oral

DEPRESSION

Antidepressant

Antidepressant, Alpha-2 Antagonist

Antidepressant, Aminoketone
(Continued)

DERMATOLOGIC DISORDERS

DERMATOMYCOSIS

DERMATOSIS

(Continued)

Corticosteroid, Topical *(Continued)*

DIABETES INSIPIDUS

Hormone, Posterior Pituitary

Vasopressin Analog, Synthetic

DIVERTICULITIS

Aminoglycoside (Antibiotic)

(Continued)

ECLAMPSIA

Barbiturate

Benzodiazepine

ECZEMA

Antibiotic/Corticosteroid, Topical

Antifungal/Corticosteroid

Corticosteroid, Topical

(Continued)

EYELID INFECTION

Antibiotic, Ophthalmic

Pharmaceutical Aid

FACTOR IX DEFICIENCY

Antihemophilic Agent

FACTOR VIII DEFICIENCY

Blood Product Derivative

Hemophilic Agent

FAMILIAL ADENOMATOUS POLYPOSIS

Nonsteroidal Anti-inflammatory Drug (NSAID), COX-2 Selective

FATTY ACID DEFICIENCY

Intravenous Nutritional Therapy

Nutritional Supplement

FEBRILE NEUTROPENIA

Quinolone

FEVER

Antipyretic

FIBROCYSTIC BREAST DISEASE

Androgen

FIBROCYSTIC DISEASE

Vitamin, Fat Soluble

FIBROMYOSITIS

Antidepressant, Tricyclic (Tertiary Amine)

FOLLICLE STIMULATION

Ovulation Stimulator

FUNGUS (DIAGNOSTIC)

Diagnostic Agent

GAG REFLEX SUPPRESSION

Analgesic, Topical

Local Anesthetic

GALACTORRHEA

Ergot Alkaloid and Derivative

GALL BLADDER DISEASE (DIAGNOSTIC)

Diagnostic Agent

GAS PAINS

Antiflatulent

GASTRIC ULCER

Antacid
(Continued)

(Continued)

(Continued)

HEADACHE (SPINAL PUNCTURE)

Diuretic, Miscellaneous

HEADACHE (TENSION)

Analgesic, Narcotic

Analgesic, Non-narcotic

Barbiturate/Analgesic

Benzodiazepine

Skeletal Muscle Relaxant

HEADACHE (VASCULAR)

Analgesic, Non-narcotic

(Continued)

(Continued)

Hemostatic Agent *(Continued)*

Progestin

Sclerosing Agent

Vitamin, Fat Soluble

HEMORRHAGE (POSTPARTUM)

Ergot Alkaloid and Derivative

Oxytocic Agent

Prostaglandin

HEMORRHAGE (PREVENTION)

Antihemophilic Agent

HEMORRHAGE (SUBARACHNOID)

Calcium Channel Blocker

HEMORRHOIDS

Adrenal Corticosteroid

Anesthetic/Corticosteroid

Astringent

Local Anesthetic

HEMOSIDEROSIS

Antidote

HEMOSTASIS

Hemostatic Agent

HEPARIN POISONING

Antidote

HEPATIC CIRRHOSIS

Diuretic, Potassium Sparing

HEPATIC COMA (ENCEPHALOPATHY)

Amebicide

Aminoglycoside (Antibiotic)

Ammonium Detoxicant

INDICATION/THERAPEUTIC CATEGORY INDEX

942

(Continued)

(Continued)

Beta-Adrenergic Blocker *(Continued)*

Calcium Channel Blocker

Diuretic, Combination
amiloride and hydrochlorothiazide

Diuretic, Loop

Diuretic, Miscellaneous

Diuretic, Potassium Sparing

Diuretic, Thiazide

HYPOALDOSTERONISM

Diuretic, Potassium Sparing

HYPOCALCEMIA

Electrolyte Supplement, Oral

Vitamin D Analog

HYPOCHLOREMIA

Electrolyte Supplement, Oral

HYPOCHLORHYDRIA

Gastrointestinal Agent, Miscellaneous

HYPOGLYCEMIA

Antihypoglycemic Agent

HYPOGONADISM

Androgen

Diagnostic Agent

Estrogen Derivative

HYPOKALEMIA

Diuretic, Potassium Sparing

(Continued)

Lactrase® [US-OTC] 371

LEAD POISONING

Chelating Agent
BAL in Oil® [US] 200
Calcium Disodium Versenate® [US]
. . . . 222
Chemet® [US/Can] 608
Cuprimine® [US/Can] 497
Depen® [US/Can] 497
dimercaprol 200
edetate calcium disodium 222
penicillamine 497
succimer 608

LEG CRAMPS

Blood Viscosity Reducer Agent
Albert® Pentoxifylline [Can] 502
Apo®-Pentoxifylline SR [Can] 502
Nu-Pentoxifylline SR [Can] 502
pentoxifylline 502
Trental® [US/Can] 502

LEPROSY

Immunosuppressant Agent
thalidomide 629
Thalomid® [US/Can] 629

Leprostatic Agent
clofazimine 153
Lamprene® [US/Can] 153

Sulfone
dapsone 175

LEUKAPHERESIS

Blood Modifiers
Pentaspan® [US/Can] 501
pentastarch 501

LEUKEMIA

Antineoplastic Agent
Adriamycin® [Can] 214
Adriamycin PFS® [US] 214
Adriamycin RDF® [US] 214
asparaginase 58
busulfan 99
Busulfex® [US/Can] 99
Caelyx® [Can] 214
Cerubidine® [US/Can] 176
chlorambucil 133
cladribine 149
cyclophosphamide 169
cytarabine 171
Cytosar® [Can] 171
Cytosar-U® [US] 171
Cytoxan® [US/Can] 169
daunorubicin hydrochloride 176
doxorubicin 214
Droxia™ [US] 338
Elspar® [US/Can] 58
etoposide 259
fludarabine 275
Fludara® [US/Can] 275
Hydrea® [US/Can] 338
hydroxyurea 338
Ifex® [US/Can] 344
ifosfamide 344
Kidrolase® [Can] 58
Lanvis® [Can] 633
Leukeran® [US/Can] 133
Leustatin™ [US/Can] 149
mechlorethamine 403
mercaptopurine 410
methotrexate 417
Mithracin® [US/Can] 519
mitoxantrone 433
Mustargen® [US/Can] 403

Myleran® [US/Can] 99
Mylocel™ [US] 338
Neosar® [US] 169
Nipent™ [US/Can] 502
Novantrone® [US/Can] 433
Oncaspar® [US/Can] 495
Oncovin® [US/Can] 678
pegaspargase 495
pentostatin 502
plicamycin 519
Procytox® [Can] 169
Purinethol® [US/Can] 410
Rheumatrex® [US] 417
Rubex® [US] 214
teniposide 622
thioguanine 633
Toposar® [US] 259
tretinoin (oral) 649
Trexall™ [US] 417
VePesid® [US/Can] 259
Vesanoid® [US/Can] 649
Vincasar® PFS [US/Can] 678
vincristine 678
Vumon® [US/Can] 622

Antineoplastic Agent, Miscellaneous
arsenic trioxide 56
Trisenox™ [US] 56

Antineoplastic Agent, Monoclonal Antibody
alemtuzumab 21
Campath® [US] 21

Antineoplastic Agent, Natural Source (Plant) Derivative
gemtuzumab ozogamicin 295
Mylotarg™ [US/Can] 295

Antineoplastic, Tyrosine Kinase Inhibitor
Gleevec™ [US] 345
imatinib 345

Antiviral Agent
interferon alfa-2b and ribavirin
combination pack 355
Rebetron™ [US/Can] 355

Biological Response Modulator
interferon alfa-2a 353
interferon alfa-2b 354
interferon alfa-2b and ribavirin
combination pack 355
Intron® A [US/Can] 354
Rebetron™ [US/Can] 355
Roferon-A® [US/Can] 353

Immune Globulin
Carimune™ [US] 347
Gamimune® N [US/Can] 347
Gammagard® S/D [US/Can] 347
Gammar®-P I.V. [US] 347
immune globulin (intravenous) 347
Iveegam EN [US] 347
Iveegam Immuno® [Can] 347
Panglobulin® [US] 347
Polygam® S/D [US] 347
Venoglobulin®-S [US] 347

Immune Modulator
Ergamisol® [US/Can] 378
levamisole 378

LICE

Scabicides/Pediculicides
A-200™ Lice [US-OTC] 505
A-200™ [US-OTC] 555
Acticin® [US] 505
(Continued)

(Continued)

MOUTH INFECTION

Antibacterial, Topical

MOUTH PAIN

Pharmaceutical Aid

MULTIPLE SCLEROSIS

Antigout Agent

Biological, Miscellaneous

Biological Response Modulator

Skeletal Muscle Relaxant

MUMPS

Vaccine, Live Virus

MUMPS (DIAGNOSTIC)

Diagnostic Agent

MUSCARINE POISONING

Anticholinergic Agent

MUSCLE SPASM

Skeletal Muscle Relaxant

MYASTHENIA GRAVIS

Cholinergic Agent

Skeletal Muscle Relaxant

Adrenal Corticosteroid *(Continued)*

NEUROBLASTOMA

Antineoplastic Agent

NEUROGENIC BLADDER

Antispasmodic Agent, Urinary

NEUROLOGIC DISEASE

Adrenal Corticosteroid

NEUTROPENIA

Colony-Stimulating Factor

NIPPLE CARE

Topical Skin Product

NOCTURIA

Antispasmodic Agent, Urinary

OBESITY

Amphetamine

Miscellaneous Product

Nonsteroidal Anti-inflammatory Drug (NSAID)

(Continued)

(Continued)

Analgesic, Non-narcotic

(Continued)

Analgesic, Non-narcotic *(Continued)*

Decongestant/Analgesic

Local Anesthetic

Neuroleptic Agent

(Continued)

(Continued)

PINWORMS

Anthelmintic

PITUITARY FUNCTION TEST (GROWTH HORMONE)

Diagnostic Agent

PITYRIASIS (ROSEA)

Corticosteroid, Topical

(Continued)

(Continued)

(Continued)

Corticosteroid, Topical *(Continued)*

Keratolytic Agent

Psoralen

RESPIRATORY DISTRESS SYNDROME (RDS)

Lung Surfactant

RESPIRATORY SYNCYTIAL VIRUS (RSV)

Antiviral Agent

Immune Globulin

Monoclonal Antibody

RESPIRATORY TRACT INFECTION

Aminoglycoside (Antibiotic)

Antibiotic, Carbacephem

Antibiotic, Macrolide

Antibiotic, Miscellaneous

Antibiotic, Penicillin

Antibiotic, Quinolone

Cephalosporin (First Generation)

Cephalosporin (Second Generation)

Cephalosporin (Third Generation)

(Continued)

Corticosteroid, Topical *(Continued)*

SARCOMA

Antineoplastic Agent

SCABIES

Scabicides/Pediculicides

SCHISTOSOMIASIS

Anthelmintic

SCHIZOPHRENIA

Antipsychotic Agent

Antipsychotic Agent, Benzisoxazole

Antipsychotic Agent, Dibenzodiazepine

Neuroleptic Agent

Thioxanthene Derivative

SCLERODERMA

Aminoquinoline (Antimalarial)

Chelating Agent

SCURVY

Vitamin, Water Soluble

SEBORRHEIC DERMATITIS

Antiseborrheic Agent, Topical

Keratolytic Agent
(Continued)

Keratolytic Agent *(Continued)*

SEPSIS

Protein C (Activated)

SERUM THYROGLOBULIN (TG) TESTING

Diagnostic Agent

SHOCK

Adrenal Corticosteroid

Adrenergic Agonist Agent

Blood Product Derivative

Plasma Volume Expander

SINUSITIS

Adrenergic Agonist Agent

Aminoglycoside (Antibiotic)

Antibiotic, Miscellaneous

Antibiotic, Penicillin

Antibiotic, Quinolone

Antihistamine/Decongestant Combination

Cephalosporin (First Generation)

Cephalosporin (Second Generation)

Cephalosporin (Third Generation)

Cold Preparation

Decongestant/Analgesic

Expectorant/Decongestant

(Continued)

SJÖGREN'S SYNDROME

SKELETAL MUSCLE RELAXANT (SURGICAL)

Antifungal/Corticosteroid

Antiseborrheic Agent, Topical

Disinfectant

TISSUE GRAFT

Immunosuppressant Agent

TOOTHACHE

Local Anesthetic

TOPICAL ANESTHESIA

Local Anesthetic

(Continued)

Phenothiazine Derivative

TRANSIENT ISCHEMIC ATTACK (TIA)

Anticoagulant (Other)

Antiplatelet Agent

TRANSURETHRAL SURGERY

Genitourinary Irrigant

TUBERCULOSIS

Antibiotic, Aminoglycoside

Antibiotic, Miscellaneous

Antimycobacterial Agent

Antitubercular Agent

Biological Response Modulator

Nonsteroidal Anti-inflammatory Drug (NSAID)

TUBERCULOSIS (DIAGNOSTIC)

Diagnostic Agent

TULAREMIA

Antibiotic, Aminoglycoside

TUMOR (BRAIN)

Antineoplastic Agent

Biological Response Modulator

TURNER'S SYNDROME

Androgen

TYPHOID

Vaccine, Inactivated Bacteria

TYPHOID FEVER

Vaccine

ULCER, DIABETIC FOOT OR LEG

Topical Skin Product

(Continued)